MW01528235

Bioelectromagnetic Medicine

Bioelectromagnetic Medicine

edited by

Paul J. Rosch, M.D.

The American Institute of Stress
Yonkers
and New York Medical College
Valhalla, New York, U.S.A.

Marko S. Markov, Ph.D.

Research International
Buffalo, New York, U.S.A.

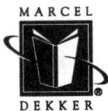

MARCEL DEKKER, INC.   NEW YORK · BASEL

Although great care has been taken to provide accurate and current information, neither the author(s) nor the publisher, nor anyone else associated with this publication, shall be liable for any loss, damage, or liability directly or indirectly caused or alleged to be caused by this book. The material contained herein is not intended to provide specific advice or recommendations for any specific situation.

Trademark notice: Product or corporate names may be trademarks or registered trademarks and are used only for identification and explanation without intent to infringe.

Library of Congress Cataloging-in-Publication Data
A catalog record for this book is available from the Library of Congress.

ISBN: 0-8247-4700-3

This book is printed on acid-free paper.

Headquarters
Marcel Dekker, Inc., 270 Madison Avenue, New York, NY 10016, U.S.A.
tel: 212-696-9000; fax: 212-685-4540

Distribution and Customer Service
Marcel Dekker, Inc., Cimarron Road, Monticello, New York 12701, U.S.A.
tel: 800-228-1160; fax: 845-796-1772

Eastern Hemisphere Distribution
Marcel Dekker AG, Hutgasse 4, Postfach 812, CH-4001 Basel, Switzerland
tel: 41-61-260-6300; fax: 41-61-260-6333

World Wide Web
http://www.dekker.com

The publisher offers discounts on this book when ordered in bulk quantities. For more information, write to Special Sales/Professional Marketing at the headquarters address above.

Copyright © 2004 by Marcel Dekker, Inc. All Rights Reserved.

Neither this book nor any part may be reproduced or transmitted in any form or by any means, electronic or mechanical, including photocopying, microfilming, and recording, or by any information storage and retrieval system, without permission in writing from the publisher.

Current printing (last digit):
10 9 8 7 6 5 4 3 2 1

PRINTED IN THE UNITED STATES OF AMERICA

Preface

A BRIEF HISTORICAL PERSPECTIVE

According to *The Yellow Emperor's Canon of Internal Medicine*, our oldest extant medical text, magnetic stones (lodestones) applied to acupuncture points were used to relieve pain and other complaints 40 centuries ago. The *Vedas*, religious scriptures of the Hindus also believed to be several thousand years old, similarly allude to the therapeutic powers of *ashmana* and *siktavati* (instruments of stone). The Greeks referred to these as *lapus-vivas* (live-stones) and Hippocrates purportedly used them to cure sterility. Egyptian physicians ascribed a variety of benefits to magnetic stones, as did early Buddhists. Tibetan monks still place bar magnets on the skull to improve the concentration and learning ability of novitiates in accordance with an age-old protocol.

In the early 1500s, the Swiss physician and alchemist Paracelsus became convinced that magnetism could restore the body's vitality and used magnets to promote healing and treat epilepsy, diarrhea, and certain types of hemorrhage. Lodestones were ground up to make powders that could be applied as magnetic salves or ingested to provide energy and stop bleeding. Such practices became very popular but were debunked in 1600 by William Gilbert in *De Magnete*. By the middle 1700s, more powerful, carbon-steel magnets had become available in Europe and there was heightened interest in their curative powers. Franz Anton Mesmer quickly became famous for his miraculous cures of everything from deafness to paralysis. In his 1775 report *On the Medicinal Uses of the Magnet*, he vividly described how he had restored health to a patient with uncontrollable seizures and numerous other nervous system complaints by feeding her iron filings and applying specially shaped magnets over affected organs. He later claimed that the healing force actually resided in his own "animal magnetism" (*magnetisomum animalem*). This was hailed as a new force analogous to Newton's gravity, and people from all over Europe waited in long lines to be treated in his Paris salon. French physicians considered him a fraud and convinced Louis XVI to establish an unbiased commission consisting of Benjamin Franklin, Antoine Lavoisier, and

Dr. J. I. Guillotin to investigate Mesmer's claims. They observed blindfolded patients who were exposed to very strong magnets and asked to describe their responses when fake objects were unknowingly substituted. The commission concluded in 1784 that magnetic healing was entirely due to the belief of the patient (placebo effect) and the power of suggestion (hypnosis). We still refer to hypnotism as "mesmerism."

Although Mesmer was thoroughly discredited, magnet therapy flourished in the United States and permanent magnet sales soared after the Civil War, particularly in the newly industrialized Western farm belts. Magnets, magnetic salves, and liniments were dispensed by traveling magnetic healers and were readily available at food and grain stores. By the turn of the century, mail-order catalogs offered magnetic soles for boots (profitable at 18 cents a pair) as well as magnetic rings, belts, caps, girdles, and other apparel that purportedly could cure anything from menstrual cramps to baldness and impotence. The king of magnetic healers was Dr. C. J. Thacher, whose Chicago's Magnetic Company in the 1920s promised "health without the use of medicine." His mail-order pamphlet explained that the energy responsible for life comes from the magnetic force of the sun, which is conducted through the rich iron content of the blood. Disease resulted when stressful lifestyles and environmental factors interfered with these healing forces. However, "magnetism properly applied will cure every curable disease no matter what the cause." The most efficient way to expedite this alleged ability of iron in the blood to transmit healing magnetic energy was to wear magnetic clothing, and almost every conceivable garment was available. A complete costume, which promised "full and complete protection of all the vital organs of the body," contained 700 magnets!

It is not clear when electricity was first used to treat illness but electric catfish native to the Nile are portrayed in Egyptian murals several thousand years old that suggest medical applications. The Roman physician Scribonius Largus used a live torpedo fish to treat a patient with gout and wrote in 46 A.D. that headaches and other pains could be cured by standing in shallow water near these electric fish. The powerful South American electric eel was introduced to Europe in 1750, and people flocked to be treated with its "natural electricity." Around the same time, the invention of the Leyden jar had dramatically demonstrated the ability of a stored electrical charge to produce muscle contractions and shocks. The publication of Mary Shelley's *Frankenstein* in 1818 stimulated interest in electricity as the source of life. Since Galvani had shown that limbs or other body parts would jump when electrical shocks were administered to animal and human cadavers, it was believed that electricity could bring the dead to life. Various "reanimation" chairs and devices were constructed, some of which may possibly have acted as pacemakers or defibrillators in the rare cases that responded. An induction coil with sponge-tipped electrodes was used in 1853 to successfully treat abnormal heart rhythms and angina. Over the next few decades, as batteries were progressively improved and electricity from generating stations became available, all sorts of "medical coils" were developed with diverse curative claims.

By the early 1900s, electrotherapeutics was viewed as a legitimate medical specialty much like the growing fields of radiology and radium therapy, and medical textbooks devoted chapters to the use of magnetism and electricity. Devices were devised to diagnose and treat anemia, hysteria, convulsions, insomnia, migraine, neuralgia, arthritis, fatigue, and all types of pain. Some were based on the proposition that each organ or individual was "tuned" to a specific electromagnetic wavelength whose application could energize or rejuvenate them. The most popular were the dynamiser and oscilloclast devised by Albert Abrams, a physician who was described by the American Medical Association in 1925 as the "dean of twentieth century charlatans." The dyanimizer was said to be so sensitive it could not only diagnose a disease from a drop of blood, photograph, or handwriting sample but also pinpoint its location in the body. The oscilloclast was then simply set to the vibratory rate of the disease to be treated and the treatment was likened to shattering a wineglass with sound vibrations. A decade later, Wilhelm Reich claimed he had discovered a universal cosmic and biological energy called orgone that permeated the universe. He constructed an orgone accumulator box he claimed could collect and accumulate orgone obtained from the atmosphere. Sitting in the accumulator would not only restore and promote health and vitality but was an effective treatment for cancer. The FDA sued and convicted him for fraud, and the court ordered his books and research burned and his equipment destroyed. Although Abrams died in prison in 1957, he still has fervent followers who believe in his theories and devices, judging from various Web sites. Other contraptions made similar extravagant but worthless claims, so it is not surprising that all bioelectromagnetic approaches came to be regarded as fraudulent. A more detailed discussion of the above is available elsewhere (1).

Unfortunately, this dismissed included legitimate research, and it is not unlikely that in some instances the baby was thrown out with the bathwater. One example may be the work of Harold Saxton Burr, whose theory of "L fields" of life showed great potential for the diagnosis of cancer and the treatment of various disorders. His research results using the comparatively crude devices available over a half century ago are now being intensively reinvestigated and confirmed with more sophisticated technology. In recent years, magnetic resonance imaging (MRI) and positive emission tomography (PET scanning) have emerged as superior diagnostic aids. Cardiac pacemakers, defibrillators, and other implantable electromedical devices have saved countless lives and eased the suffering of patients with Parkinson's disease and other debilitating disorders. The FDA has also approved specific electromagnetic devices to promote the healing of bone fractures that have failed to unite despite other interventions; this procedure has proven successful and safe in hundreds of thousands of patients over the past few decades. More recently, electromagnetic therapies for the treatment of urinary incontinence, sports injuries, and liver and kidney tumors have also been approved. Other approaches, for the treatment of osteoarthritis, pain, tinnitus, and other indications, have satisfied criteria for efficacy and safety that have led to their approval in European and other countries and that may allow them to be available in the United States under the "globalization" and "harmonization" provisions of the 1997 FDA Modernization Act.

WHY AND HOW THIS BOOK WAS WRITTEN

Permanent magnet and electromagnetic therapies are now riding the crest of a tidal wave of interest in "alternative" and "complementary" medicine. Unfortunately, charlatans, entrepreneurs, and misguided zealots with worthless devices and unfounded claims still abound. It is essential to distinguish these from authentic approaches and products. As a result, in this book we have tried to separate the wheat from the chaff by restricting contributions to evidence-based medicine supported by references in peer-reviewed publications and to provide the reader with tools and skills for evaluating the legitimacy of devices and claims. In addition to a lengthy history of quackery and fraud, another criticism that has hampered wider acceptance of bioelectromagnetic approaches is the inability to identify the mechanisms of action responsible for any benefits. We have therefore attempted to identify concepts and theories that attempt to explain the mechanisms responsible for mediating the diverse benefits of bioelectromagnetic therapies and, in some instances, how they may relate to ancient concepts of subtle energies in the body that are also found in nature. How weak environmental electromagnetic energies as well as those generated internally can produce nonthermal biological effects is not clear since the absence of detectable heat exchange would appear to violate the laws of thermodynamics.

In addition, our current concept of how communication takes place in the body is at a chemical/molecular level as we visualize small peptide and other messengers fitting into specific receptor sites on cell walls much like keys opening certain locks. Such physical structural matching that could occur only on a random-collision basis cannot explain the myriad instantaneous and automatic reactions such as those that occur in "fight or flight" responses to severe stress. As will be seen, there is an emerging paradigm of cellular communication at a physical/atomic level that may provide some answers and also provide insights into widely acknowledged but poorly understood phenomena such as the placebo effect, the power of prayer and a firm faith, telepathic communication, the benefits of acupuncture, homeopathy, therapeutic touch, various bodywork and massage therapies, and Kirlian and other low-level imaging procedures.

Another issue that has caused wariness about bioelectromagnetic therapies are safety concerns about possible increased risk of certain malignancies and birth defects resulting from proximity to high power lines, cell phones, microwave ovens, and electric blankets. It is not surprising that electromagnetic fields, like many other therapies, can be two-edged swords. For example, all the modalities we use to treat cancer, including radiation, chemotherapy, and hormonal interventions, can also cause cancer. Such effects may depend on dosage, duration of exposure, and genetic and other influences. It is not likely that any clear conclusion about adverse electromagnetic effects can be reached until more information has been obtained from long-term studies that focus on these factors. For this reason, we have refrained from participating in this debate other than to devote a chapter on the importance of dosimetry and to emphasize that no such adverse effects have been observed or seem likely in the therapies presented in this book. Indeed, those that have been proposed and implemented by Demetrio Sodi Pallares and Björn Nordenström and confirmed by others have shown stunning success in treating various malignancies. Many of the chapters in this book are based on presentations at the annual International Congress on Stress over the past decade or so, and additional information on these events can be obtained at www.stress.org.

We have also attempted in this book to trace the origin and development of various therapies, such as TENS and vagal nerve stimulation by pioneers in the field such as Norman Shealy, Donlin Long, and Jacob Zabara. Kirk Jeffrey has contributed a similar chapter on the evolution of cardiac pacemakers. We have made a concerted effort to include prominent scientists whose research may not be well known in the United States. When initially approached to serve as editor of this book, I explained that this was not my field of expertise and asked Marko Markov, a distinguished physicist, to serve as coeditor. He is also much more familiar with relevant advances in Eastern Europe and Russia, and I am grateful for his careful review of all chapters and for those he has attracted from these countries as well as his own contributions. I am also indebted to Russell Dekker for expediting this work so that the material would be current and important late-breaking advances could be included, such as radiofrequency coblation nuceloplasty for disc disease. I would also like to thank all the authors for their cooperation in responding so promptly to urgent requests for revisions necessary to adhere to this very accelerated publication schedule.

The above is a brief summary of why this book is needed and how it was assembled. I believe it is particularly appropriate to conclude with the following quotation.

> In the decade to come, it is safe to predict, bioelectromagnetics will assume a therapeutic importance equal to, or greater than, that of pharmacology and surgery

today. With proper interdisciplinary effort, significant inroads can be made in controlling the ravages of cancer, some forms of heart disease, arthritis, hormonal disorders, and neurological scourges such as Alzheimer's disease, spinal cord injury, and multiple sclerosis. This prediction is not pie-in-the-sky. Pilot studies and biological mechanisms already described in primordial terms, form a rational basis for such a statement. — *J. Andrew L. Bassett, 1992*

Andy Bassett was one of the early advocates of the use of electromagnetic fields for uniting fractures that refused to heal. Unfortunately, he died before he could see that his prophecy would come true well ahead of schedule. In many respects, this book is a tribute to him and other pioneers such as Bob Becker, Abe Liboff, Björn Nordenström, and Ross Adey who recognized the vast potential of bioelectromagnetic medicine and have helped to put it on a solid scientific footing. I am particularly delighted that we were able to obtain contributions from most of these trailblazers.

Paul J. Rosch, M.D., F.A.C.P.

REFERENCES

1. Lawrence R, Rosch PJ, Plowden J. Magnet Therapy. Rocklin, CA: Prima Press, 1998.

Contents

III. MECHANISMS OF ACTION AND THEORETICAL CONSIDERATIONS

IV. NEUROLOGIC, MUSCULOSKELETAL AND SOFT TISSUE APPLICATIONS

V. CARDIOVASCULAR DISORDERS AND CANCER

VIII. CONCLUSION

Contributors

W. Ross Adey   Loma Linda University School of Medicine, Loma Linda, California, U.S.A. RAdey43450@aol.com

Monique Azais   Unité de Recherche sur les Mouvements Anormaux de l'Enfant URMAE, Service de Neurochirurgie B, Centre Gui de Chauliac, CHU Montpellier, Montpellier, France

Tadej Badj   University of Ljubljana, Ljubljana, Slovenia. tadej.badj@robo.fe.uni-lj.si

Walter X. Balcavage   Cellular and Integrative Physiology, Indiana University School of Medicine, Terre Haute Center for Medical Education, Terre Haute, Indiana, U.S.A. wbalcava@medicine.indstate.edu

Alexandre Barbault   Symtonic S.A., Renens, Switzerland

Alim-Louis Benabid   Department of Clinical and Biological Neurosciences, INSERM, Joseph Fourier University, Grenoble, France. alimlouis.benabid@ujf-grenoble.fr

J. Benveniste   Digital Biology Laboratory, Clamart, France. jbenveniste@digibio.com

O. V. Betskii   Institute for Radio Engineering and Electronics of the Russian Academy of Sciences, Moscow, Russia

Abraham M. Blechman   Columbia University, New York, New York, U.S.A. ifnyk@aol.com

Daryl E. Bohning   The Brain Stimulation Laboratory (BSL), Psychiatry Department, and the Center for Advanced Imaging Research (CAIR), Medical University of South Carolina (MUSC), Charleston, South Carolina, U.S.A.

Martin Burian   University of Vienna Medical School, Vienna, Austria. martin.burian@akh-wien.ac.at

Ruggero Cadossi   Research and Development, Igea, Capri, Italy. cadossi@igea.it

Ivan L. Cameron   University of Texas Health Science Center, San Antonio, Texas, U.S.A.

Laura Cif   Unité de Recherche sur les Mouvements Anormaux de l'Enfant URMAE, Service de Neurochirurgie B, Centre Gui de Chauliac, CHU Montpellier, Montpellier, France. urmae@chu-montpellier.fr

Agatha P. Colbert   Oregon Center for Complementary and Alternative Medicine, Portland, Oregon, U.S.A. apcolbert@attbi.com

Phillippe Coubes   Unité de Recherche sur les Mouvements Anormaux de l'Enfant URMAE, Service de Neurochirurgie B, Centre Gui de Chauliac, CHU Montpellier, Montpellier, France. p-coubes@chu-montpellier.fr

David Cukjati   Laboratory of Biocybernetics, Faculty of Electrical Engineering, University of Ljubljana, Ljubljana, Slovenia. david@svarnun.fe.uni-lj.si

Kent Davey   American Maglev Technology, Edgewater, Florida, U.S.A. k.davey@mail.utexas.edu

Imants Detlavs   Medical-Scientific Center "ELMA-LA", Riga, Latvia. imants.detlavs@apollo.lv

Stefan Engström   Department of Neurology, Vanderbilt University Medical Center, Nashville, Tennessee, U.S.A. stefan.engstrom@vanderbilt.edu

Amandine Gannau   Unité de Recherche sur les Mouvements Anormaux de l'Enfant URMAE, Service de Neurochirurgie B, Centre Gui de Chauliac, CHU Montpellier, Montpellier, France

Mark S. George   The Brain Stimulation Laboratory (BSL), Psychiatry Department, and the Center for Advanced Imaging Research (CAIR), Medical University of South Carolina (MUSC), Charleston, South Carolina, U.S.A. georgem@musc.edu

Norman Hagfors   St. Paul, Minnesota, U.S.A. hagfors@norsen.com

W. Elaine Hardman   Pennington Biomedical Research Center, Louisiana State University, Baton Rouge, Louisiana, U.S.A.

Eric Hardouin   Unité de Recherche sur les Mouvements Anormaux de l'Enfant URMAE, Service de Neurochirurgie B, Centre Gui de Chauliac, CHU Montpellier, Montpellier, France

Simone Hemm   Unité de Recherche sur les Mouvements Anormaux de l'Enfant URMAE, Service de Neurochirurgie B, Centre Gui de Chauliac, CHU Montpellier, Montpellier, France

Sarah Hill   The Brain Stimulation Laboratory (BSL), Psychiatry Department, and the Center for Advanced Imaging Research (CAIR), Medical University of South Carolina (MUSC), Charleston, South Carolina, U.S.A. hill@musc.edu

Joshua S. Hirsch   Harvard Medical School, Beth Israel Deaconess Medical Center, Boston, Massachusetts, U.S.A.

John B. Jarding   Black Hills Regional Eye Institute, Rapid City, South Dakota, U.S.A. lowvision@bhrei.com

K. A. Jenrow Department of Neurosurgery, Henry Ford Hospital, Detroit, Michigan, U.S.A.

Kirk Jeffrey Carleton College, Northfield, Minnesota, U.S.A. kirkjeffrey@yahoo.com

Mary T. Johnson Cellular and Integrative Physiology, Indiana University School of Medicine, Terre Haute Center for Medical Education, Terre Haute, Indiana, U.S.A. mjohnson@medicine.indstate.edu

Daniel L. Kirsch Electromedical Products International, Inc., Mineral Wells, Texas, U.S.A. dan@epii.com

Tadej Kotnik Faculty of Electrical Engineering, University of Ljubljana, Ljubljana, Slovenia. tadej@svarun.fe.uni-lj.si

F. Andrew Kozel The Brain Stimulation Laboratory (BSL), Psychiatry Department, and the Center for Advanced Imaging Research (CAIR), Medical University of South Carolina (MUSC), Charleston, South Carolina, U.S.A. kozelfa@musc.edu

Marina Kurian Lenox Hill Hospital, New York, New York, U.S.A.

Martha S. Lappin Energy Medicine Developments, Burke, Virginia, U.S.A. Marlappin@aol.com

N. N. Lebedeva Institute for Higher Nerve Activity and Neurophysiology of the Russian Academy of Sciences, Moscow, Russia. N.Leb@relcom.ru

Xingbao Li The Brain Stimulation Laboratory (BSL), Psychiatry Department, and the Center for Advanced Imaging Research (CAIR), Medical University of South Carolina (MUSC), Charleston, South Carolina, U.S.A. lixi@musc.edu

Chaoyang Liang Department of Thoracic Surgery, Electrochemical Therapy Center for Tumors, China-Japan Friendship Hospital, Beijing, P. R. China.

A. R. Liboff Department of Physics, Oakland University, Rochester, Michigan, U.S.A. ARLiboff@aol.com

Bernard S. Liss MEDI Consultants, Inc., Paterson, New Jersey, U.S.A.

Saul Liss MEDI Consultants, Inc., Paterson, New Jersey, U.S.A. lissmedi@aol.com

Ganzhong Liu Department of Thoracic Surgery, Electrochemical Therapy Center for Tumors, China-Japan Friendship Hospital, Beijing, P. R. China

Donlin M. Long Johns Hopkins Hospital, Baltimore, Maryland, U.S.A. dmlong@jhmi.edu

Andres M. Lozano Department of Surgery, University of Toronto, Toronto Western Hospital Research Institute, Toronto, Ontario, Canada. lozano@uhnres.utoronto.ca

Marko S. Markov Research International, Buffalo, New York, U.S.A. msmarkov@aol.com

Harvey N. Mayrovitz College of Medical Sciences, Nova Southeastern University, Ft. Lauderdale, Florida, U.S.A. mayrovit@ix.netcom.com

Rollin McCraty HeartMath Research Center, Institute of HeartMath, Boulder Creek, California, U.S.A. rollin@heartmath.org

Alexander Mishory   The Brain Stimulation Laboratory (BSL), Psychiatry Department, and the Center for Advanced Imaging Research (CAIR), Medical University of South Carolina (MUSC), Charleston, South Carolina, U.S.A. mishory@musc.edu

Edgar Mitchell   Lake Worth, Florida, U.S.A. edgarmitchell@msn.com

Damijan Miklavčič   Faculty of Electrical Engineering, University of Ljubljana, Ljubljana, Slovenia. damijan@svarun.fe.uni-lj.si

Alon Y. Mogilner   Department of Neurosurgery, New York Medical College, Valhalla, New York, U.S.A. alon_mogilner@nymc.edu

Cédric Monnier   Unité de Recherche sur les Mouvements Anormaux de l'Enfant URMAE, Service de Neurochirurgie B, Centre Gui de Chauliac, CHU Montpellier, Montpellier, France

Ziad Nahas   The Brain Stimulation Laboratory (BSL), Psychiatry Department, and the Center for Advanced Imaging Research (CAIR), Medical University of South Carolina (MUSC), Charleston, South Carolina, U.S.A. nahasz@musc.edu

Gabi Nindl   Cellular and Integrative Physiology, Indiana University School of Medicine, Terre Haute Center for Medical Education, Terre Haute, Indiana, U.S.A. gnindl@medicine.indstate.edu

Björn E. W. Nordenström   Professor Emeritus, Karolinska Institute and Hospital, Stockholm, Sweden

Jorgen Nordenström   Huddinge University Hospital, Stockholm, Sweden. jorgen.nordenstrom@karo.ki.se

George D. O'Clock   Electrical & Computer Engineering & Technology Department, Minnesota State University, Mankato, Minnesota, U.S.A. george.oclock@mankato.msus.edu

Chiyoji Ohkubo   National Institute of Health, Tokyo, Japan. ohkubo@iph.go.jp

Hideyuki Okano*   National Institute of Health, Tokyo, Japan

James L. Oschman   Nature's Own Research Association, Dover, New Hampshire, U.S.A. joschman@aol.com

Boris Pasche   Symtonic S.A., Renens, Switzerland. b-pasche@northwestern.edu

Frank S. Prato   Lawson Health Research Institute and University of Western Ontario, London, Ontario, Canada. prato@lri.sjhc.london.on.ca

Dietmar Rabussay   Research & Development, Genetronics, Inc., San Diego, California, U.S.A. dietmarr@genetronics.com

Arra S. Reddy   Harvard Medical School, Beth Israel Deaconess Medical Center, Boston, Massachusetts, U.S.A.

Ali R. Rezai   Department of Neurosurgery, Cleveland Clinic Foundation, Cleveland, Ohio, U.S.A. rezaia@ccf.org

---

* *Current affiliation*: Pip Tokyo Co., Ltd., Tokyo, Japan.

E. Oscar Richter Department of Neurosurgery, University of Florida, Gainesville, Florida, U.S.A. richter372002@yahoo.com

Paul J. Rosch The American Institute of Stress, Yonkers, and New York Medical College, Valhalla, New York, U.S.A. stress124@optonline.net

Mitchell Roslin Lenox Hill Hospital, New York, New York, U.S.A.

James T. Ryaby OrthoLogic Corp., and Arizona State University, Tempe, Arizona, U.S.A. jryaby@olgc.com

Joseph R. Salvatore Carl T. Hayden VA Medical Center, Phoenix, Arizona, U.S.A. Joseph.Salvatore@med.va.gov

Rajmond Šavrin Institute of the Republic of Slovenia for Rehabilitation, Ljubljana, Slovenia

Steven C. Schachter Harvard Medical School, Boston, Massachusetts, U.S.A. sschacht@caregroup.harvard.edu

C. Norman Shealy Holos Institutes of Health, Inc., Fair Grove, Missouri, U.S.A. norm@shealyhealthnet.com

Ray B. Smith Electromedical Products International, Inc., Mineral Wells, Texas, U.S.A. ray@epii.com

Demetrio Sodi Pallares[*] Mexico City, Mexico

Dennis Stillings Archaeus Project, Kamuela, Hawaii, U.S.A. dstillings@kohalacenter.org

William A. Tiller Professor Emeritus, Department of Materials Science & Engineering, Stanford University, Stanford, California, U.S.A.

Gian Carlo Traina Department of Biomedical Sciences, Orthopaedic Clinic, University of Ferrara, Ferrara, Italy. tng@unife.it

Nathalie Vaysserie Unité de Recherche sur les Mouvements Anormaux de l'Enfant URMAE, Service de Neurochirurgie B, Centre Gui de Chauliac, CHU Montpellier, Montpellier, France

Georg Widera Research & Development, Genetronics, Inc., San Diego, California, U.S.A. georg.widera@alza.com

Calvin D. Williams EMF Therapeutics, Inc., Chattanooga, Tennessee, U.S.A.

Zaiyong Wang Department of Thoracic Surgery, Electrochemical Therapy Center for Tumors, China-Japan Friendship Hospital, Beijing, P. R. China

Yuling Xin Department of Thoracic Surgery, Electrochemical Therapy Center for Tumors, China-Japan Friendship Hospital, Beijing, P. R. China. suime@public3.bta.net.cn

Kaori Yamanaka Stimulation Laboratory (BSL), Psychiatry Department, and the Center for Advanced Imaging Research (CAIR), Medical University of South Carolina (MUSC), Charleston, South Carolina, U.S.A. yamanakk@musc.edu

---

[*] Deceased.

Jacob Zabara   Cyberonics, Inc., Houston, Texas, U.S.A.

Michel Zanca   Service de Médecine Nucléaire, Centre Gui de Chauliac, CHU Montpellier, Montpellier, France. m-zanca@chu-montpellier.fr

Wei Zhang   Department of Thoracic Surgery, Electrochemical Therapy Center for Tumors, China-Japan Friendship Hospital, Beijing, P. R. China

Hongchang Zhao   Department of Thoracic Surgery, Electrochemical Therapy Center for Tumors, China-Japan Friendship Hospital, Beijing, P. R. China

Bioelectromagnetic Medicine

1

Potential Therapeutic Applications of Nonthermal Electromagnetic Fields: Ensemble Organization of Cells in Tissue as a Factor in Biological Field Sensing*

W. Ross Adey

Loma Linda University School of Medicine, Loma Linda, California, U.S.A.

There are major unanswered questions about possible health risks that may arise from human exposures to various man-made electromagnetic fields where these exposures are intermittent, recurrent, and may extend over a significant portion of the lifetime of the individual. Current equilibrium thermodynamic models fail to explain an impressive spectrum of observed electromagnetic bioeffects at non-thermal exposure levels. Much of this signaling within and between cells may be mediated by free radicals of the oxygen and nitrogen species.

I. INTRODUCTION

In our solar system, the natural electromagnetic environment varies greatly from planet to planet. In the case of the planet Earth, a semiliquid ferromagnetic core generates a major and slowly migrating *static* geomagnetic field. Concurrently, there are much weaker natural *oscillating* low-frequency electromagnetic fields that arise from two major sources: in thunderstorm activity in equatorial zones of Central Africa and the Amazon basin and in lesser degree from solar magnetic storms in years of high activity in the 11-year solar sunspot cycle.

A. Comparison of Natural and Man-Made Electromagnetic Environments

All life on earth has evolved in these fields. Defining them in physical terms permits direct comparison with far stronger man-made fields that have come to dominate all civilized

---

* Portions of this chapter were first published in D. Clements-Croome, ed. Electromagnetic Environments and Safety in Buildings, London: Spon Press, 2002.

environments in the past century. Energy in the *oscillating* natural fields is almost entirely in the extremely low frequency (ELF) spectrum, with peaks at frequencies between 8 and 32 Hz, the Schumann resonances (1). Their electric components are around 0.01 V/m, with magnetic fields of 1–10 nT. These natural oscillations are ducted worldwide between the earth's surface and the ionosphere at an approximate height of 250 km. With a circumference of 41,000 km, the earth may act as a cavity resonator for this ducted propagation (at the velocity of light, 300,000 km/s), behaving resonantly at a frequency around 8Hz. Neither solar nor terrestrial sources contribute significant amounts of radiofrequency or microwave energy to the earth's biosphere, and we may contrast these weak ELF fields with the earth's much larger static geomagnetic field around 50 μT (0.5 gauss).

The earth's *static* magnetic field at 50 μT is 5000 times larger than the natural oscillations but still substantially less than a wide range of daily human exposures to static and oscillating fields in domestic and occupational environments.

Generation and distribution of electric power has spawned a vast and ever growing vista of new electronic devices and systems. They overwhelm the natural electromagnetic environment with more intense fields. They include oscillations far into the microwave spectrum, many octaves higher than the Schumann resonances. This growth of radio-frequency (RF) and/or microwave fields is further complicated by the advent of digital communication techniques. In many applications, these microwave fields, oscillating billions of times per second, are systematically interrupted (pulsed) at low frequencies. This has raised important biological and biomedical questions, still incompletely answered, about possible tissue mechanisms in detection of amplitude- and pulse-modulation of RF and/or microwave fields (2).

B. Historical Evidence on Possible Health Effects of Man-Made Environmental Fields

There are major unanswered questions about possible health risks that may arise from human exposures to various man-made electromagnetic fields where these exposures are intermittent, recurrent, and may extend over a significant portion of the lifetime of the individual. Historical correlations have been reported between growth of rural electrification in the United States and the United Kingdom and an increased incidence of childhood leukemia. A peak in childhood leukemia at ages 2 through 4 emerged de novo in the 1920s. Using U.S. census data for 1930, 1940, and 1950, Milham and Osslander (3) concluded that the peak in the common childhood acute lymphoblastic leukemia (ALL) may be attributable to electrification.

Design of modern office buildings has led to their electrification through one or more large distribution transformers that may be located in basement vaults, or in some cases, located on each floor of the building. Milham (4) has examined cancer incidence in such a building over a 15-year period and found evidence for *cumulative risks*. An analysis of linear trend in cancer incidence, using average years employed as an exposure score, was positive ($P = 0.00337$), with an odds ratio of 15.1 in workers employed longer than 5 years.

In large modern offices, the electromagnetic environment has been further complicated by introduction of local area networks (LANs) for local telephonic (voice) and data transmission. Workers may be continuously exposed to fields from a plethora of sources located on each computer and on local network controllers. Their power output is typically in the low milliwatt to microwatt range—so low that significant heating of workers' tissues is improbable. Any bioeffects attributable to their operation strongly suggest *nonthermal* mechanisms of interaction, and raise further important questions about mechanisms mediating a cumulative dose from repeated, intermittent exposures, possibly over months and years. None of these studies support tissue heating as an adequate model for bioeffects seen in a wide spectrum of laboratory experiments (see below) or in reported epidemiological findings.

The American National Standards Institute (1992) first recognized a tissue dose of 4.0 W/kg as a *thermal* (heating) tissue threshold possibly associated with adverse health effects and proposed an exposure limit in controlled environments (occupational) at 0.4 W/kg, thus creating a supposed "safety margin" of 10. For uncontrolled environments (civilian), a larger safety margin was set with a permissible exposure limit (PEL) 50 times lower at 0.08 W/kg. Since actual measurement of tissue SARs under environmental conditions is not a practical technique, PELs are typically expressed as a function of *incident field power density*, the amount of energy falling on a surface per unit area, and expressed in mW/cm^2.

More recently, the U.S. government Interagency Radio Frequency Working Group (1999) has emphasized the need for revisions recognizing nonthermal tissue microwave sensitivities:

> Studies continue to be published describing biological responses to nonthermal ELF-modulated RF radiation exposures that are not produced by CW (unmodulated) radiation. These studies have resulted in concern that exposure guidelines based on thermal effects, and using information and concepts (time-averaged dosimetry, uncertainty factors) that mask any differences between intensity-modulated RF radiation exposure and CW exposure, do not directly address public exposures, and therefore may not adequately protect the public.

II. INITIAL TRANSDUCTION OF IMPOSED MICROWAVE FIELDS AT NONTHERMAL ENERGY LEVELS t

Tissue components of environmental RF and microwave fields are consistent with two basic models. Sources close to the body surface produce *near-field exposures*, as with users of mobile phones. The emitted field is magnetically coupled directly from the antenna into the tissues. At increasing distances from the source, the human body progressively takes on properties of a radio antenna, with absorption of radiated energy determined by physical dimensions of the trunk and limbs. This is a *far-field exposure*, defined as fully developed at 10 or more wavelengths from the source and based on interactions with the electric component of the radiated field. Permissible exposure limits (PELs) have rested on measurement of microwave field energy absorbed as heat, expressed as the *specific absorption rate (SAR)* in W/kg.

There is an initial dichotomy in possible modes of interaction of cells in tissue with environmental microwave fields. It is principally determined by the separation of responses attributed to tissue heating from those elicited by certain fields at levels where frank heating is not the basis of an observed interaction. Their interpretation and possible significance has required caution in both biological and biophysical perspectives. Many of these biological sensitivities run counter to accepted models of physiological thresholds based in equilibrium thermodynamics of kT thermal collision energies. In a physical perspective, the search also continues for biological systems compatible with a first transductive step in a range of functionally effective vibrational and electromagnetic stimuli that are orders of magnitude weaker than kT. Aspects of these findings are reviewed in (Sec. IV.) Their occurrence invites hypotheses on directions of future research (5).

A. Cell Membranes as the Site of Initial Field Transductive Coupling

Collective evidence points to cell membrane receptors as the probable site of first tissue interactions with both ELF and microwave fields for many neurotransmitters (6), hormones (7,8), growth-regulating enzyme expression (9–12), and cancer-promoting chemicals (13). In none of these studies does tissue heating appear involved causally in the responses (2). Physicists and engineers have continued to offer microthermal, rather than athermal, models for these phenomena (14,15) with views that exclude consideration of cooperative organization and coherent charge states, but it is difficult to reconcile experimental evidence for factors such as modulation frequency dependence and required duration of an amplitude-modulated signal to elicit a response (*coherence time*) (11) with models based on the equilibrium dynamics of tissue heating.

B. Evidence for Role of Free Radicals in Electromagnetic Field Bioeffects

Examination of vibration modes in biomolecules, or portions of these molecules (16) has suggested that resonant microwave interactions with these molecules, or with portions of their structure, is unlikely at frequencies below higher gigahertz spectral regions. This has been confirmed in studies showing collision-broadened spectra, typical of a heating stimulus, as the first discernible response of many of these molecules in aqueous solutions to microwave exposures at frequencies below 10 GHz.

However, there is an important option for biomolecular interactions with static and oscillating magnetic fields through the medium of *free radicals* (see Refs. 17 and 18 for summaries). Chemical bonds are magnetic bonds, formed between adjacent atoms through paired electrons having opposite spins and thus magnetically attracted. Breaking of chemical bonds is an essential step in virtually all chemical reactions, each atomic partner reclaiming its electron, and moving away as a free radical to seek another partner with an opposite electron spin. The brief lifetime of a free radical is about a nanosecond or less, before once again forming a *singlet pair* with a partner having an opposite spin or for electrons with similar spins, having options to unite in three ways, forming *triplet pairs* (reviewed in Ref. 2).

During this brief lifetime, imposed magnetic fields may delay the return to the singlet pair condition, thus influencing the *rate* and the *amount of product* of an ongoing chemical reaction (19). McLauchlan points out that this model predicts a potentially enormous effect on chemical reactions for static fields in the low mT range. For oscillating fields, the evidence is less clear on their possible role as direct mediators in detection of ELF frequency-dependent bioeffects. *Spin-mixing* of orbital electrons and nuclear spins in adjacent nuclei is a possible mechanism for biosensitivities at extremely low magnetic field levels, but these interactions are multiple, complex, and incompletely understood (20). The highest level of free radical sensitivity may reside in hyperfine-dependent singlet–triplet state mixing in radical pairs with a small number of hyperfine states that describe their coupling to nearby nuclei (21,22). Although sensitivities to magnetic fields in such a system might theoretically extend down to zero magnetic field levels, singlet–triplet interconversion would need to be sufficiently fast to occur before diffusion reduced the probability of radical re-encounter to negligible levels.

Lander (23) has emphasized that we are at an early stage of understanding free radical signal transduction. "Future work may place free radical signaling beside classical intra- and intercellular messengers and uncover a woven fabric of communication that has evolved to yield exquisite specificity." A broadening perspective on actions of free radicals in all living systems emphasizes a dual role: first, as messengers and mediators in many key processes that regulate cell functions throughout life and second, in the pathophysiology of *oxidative stress diseases.*

At cell membranes, free radicals may play an essential role in regulation of receptor specificity, but not necessarily through a lock-and-key mechanism. As an example, Lander cites the location of cysteine molecules on the surface of P21-*ras* proteins at cell membranes. They may act as selective targets for nitrogen and oxygen free radicals, thereby inducing covalent modifications and thus setting the *redox potential* of this target protein molecule as the critical determinant for its highly specific interactions with antibodies, hormones, etc. Magnetochemistry studies have suggested a form of cooperative behavior in populations of free radicals that remain *spin-correlated* after initial separation of a singlet pair (24). Magnetic fields at 1 and 60 Hz destabilize rhythmic oscillations in brain hippocampal slices at 56 μT (0.35 to 3.5 nV mm^{-1}) via as yet unidentified nitric oxide mechanisms involving free radicals (23,25). In a general biological context, these are some of the unanswered questions that limit free radical models as general descriptors of threshold events.

III. SENSITIVITIES TO NONTHERMAL STIMULI: TISSUE STRUCTURAL AND FUNCTIONAL IMPLICATIONS

A. Conductance Pathways in Multicellular Tissues

In its earliest forms, life on earth may have existed in the absence of cells, simply as a "soup" of unconstrained biomolecules at the surface of primitive oceans. It is a reasonable assumption that the first living organisms existed as single cells floating or swimming in these primordial seas. Concepts of a cell emphasize the role of a bounding membrane, surrounding an organized interior that participates in the chemistry of processes essential for all terrestrial life. This enclosing membrane is the organism's window on the world around it.

For unicellular organisms that swim through large fluid volumes, the cell membrane is both a sensor and an effector. As a sensor, it detects altered chemistry in the surrounding fluid and provides a pathway for inward signals generated on its surface by a wide variety of stimulating ions and molecules, including hormones, antibodies, and neurotransmitters. These most elemental inward signals are susceptible to manipulation by a wide variety of natural or imposed electromagnetic fields that may also pervade the pericellular field. As effectors, cell membranes may also transmit a variety of electrical and chemical signals across intervening intercellular fluid to neighboring cells, thus creating a domain or ensemble of cells, often able to "whisper together" in a faint and private language. Experimental evidence suggests that these outward effector signals may also be sensitive to intrinsic and imposed electromagnetic fields.

Rather than being separated in a virtually limitless ocean, cellular aggregates that form tissues of higher animals are separated by narrow fluid channels that take on special importance in signalling from cell to cell. Biomolecules travel in these tiny "gutters," typically not more than 150 Å wide, to reach binding sites on cell membrane receptors. These gutters form the *intercellular space* (ICS). It is a preferred pathway for induced currents of intrinsic and environmental electromagnetic fields. Although it occupies only ~10% of the tissue cross section, it carries at least 90% of any imposed or intrinsic current, directing it along cell membrane surfaces. Whereas the ICS may have a typical impedance of ~4–50 ohm cm^{-1}, transmembrane impedances are ~10^4–10^6 ohm cm^{-2}.

B. Structural and Functional Organization of the Extracellular Space

The organization of cell membrane surfaces and intercellular gutters in detection of these tissue components of extrinsic and intrinsic electromagnetic fields enters the realm of *nonequilibrium* thermodynamics (26,27), characterized by *cooperative processes*, mediated by *coherent states* of electric charges on cell membrane surface molecular systems.

Spaces in the ICS are not simple saline filled channels. Numerous stranded protein molecules protrude into these spaces from the cell interior and form a *glycocalyx* with specialized receptor sites that sense chemical and electrical stimuli in surrounding fluid. Their amino sugar tips are highly negatively charged (*polyanionic*) and attract a *polycationic* atmosphere, principally of calcium and hydrogen ions. This Debye layer has an extremely high virtual dielectric constant at low frequencies ($D_k > 10^6$ at frequencies $<$ 1 kHz) (28). Biological cooperative processes occur in systems where at least one energetic parameter in that system (e.g., temperature, electric charge) has been moved far from equilibrium by the addition of external energy. This added energy may induce a population of substrate elements, all at the same higher energy level—a *coherent* energetic state. In such a system, a weak external trigger may elicit a *cooperative* process, with an energy release far greater than in the initial trigger. Capping and patching on the lymphocyte cell surface (29) offers a striking example of such a cooperative response, based on intracellular metabolic energy.

The proteins of the glycocalyx offer an anatomical substrate for the first detection of weak electrochemical oscillations in pericellular fluid, including field potentials arising in activity of adjoining cells, or as tissue components of environmental fields. Research in molecular biology has increasingly emphasized essentially direct communication between cells due to their mutual proximity. Bands of *connexin* proteins form *gap junctions* directly uniting adjoining cell membranes. Experimental evidence supports their role in intercellular signaling.

C. Tissue Detection of Low Frequency Fields and RF/Microwave Fields Amplitude-Modulated at Low Frequencies: Structural and Functional Options

Differential bioeffects, to be discussed below, have been reported between certain non-thermal RF or microwave fields with low-frequency amplitude or pulse modulation when compared to exposures to unmodulated continuous wave (CW) fields at similar power levels. The findings suggest, but do not yet establish unequivocally, that this frequency dependence may be a system property in a sequence of molecular hierarchies beyond the first transductive step. If the concept of modulation frequency-dependence continues to gain support in further research, answers must be sought as to the manner of its detection.

For ELF fields, models based on joint static-oscillating magnetic fields have been hypothesized. They include ion cyclotron resonance (30), where mono- and divalent cations, such as potassium and calcium (abundant in the cellular environment), may exhibit cyclotron resonance at ELF frequencies in the presence of ambient static fields of less than 100 µT, such as the geomagnetic field. Other models describing ELF frequency dependence have considered phase transitions (31) and ion parametric resonance (32), but interpretation of this frequency dependence based on ion parametric resonance remains unclear (33).

For amplitude- or pulse-modulated RF and/or microwave fields, there is the implication that some form of *envelope demodulation* occurs in tissue recognition of ELF modulation components, but the tissue may remain essentially transparent to the same signal presented as an unmodulated carrier wave (2,-34). However, crucial questions remain unanswered. It is not known whether biological low-frequency dependence is established at the transductive step in the first tissue detection of the field, or whether it resides at some higher level in an hierarchical sequence of signal coupling to the biological detection system (35). For ELF magnetic fields, experimental evidence points to a slow time scale in inhibition of tamoxifen's antiproliferative action in human breast cancer cells (36).

It is a principle of radio physics that extraction of ELF modulation information from an amplitude-modulated signal requires a *nonlinear element* in the detection system. This required nonlinearity may involve a spatial component, such as differential conduction in certain directions along the signal path, or the path itself may exhibit nonlinearities with respect to such factors as spatial distribution of electric charges at fixed molecular sites (so-called fixed charges), or conduction itself may involve a nonlinear quantum process, as in electron tunneling across the transverse dimensions of the cell membrane.

These constraints impose a further essential condition for demodulation to occur in the multicellular tissues of living organisms. There must be a *site for demodulation* to occur. Evidence supports a role for cell membranes to act in this way, based not only on their intrinsic structure, but also on their proximity to neighboring cells in the typical organization of tissues of the body. Typical tissue organization meets the three criteria outlined above but as a cautionary note, does not allow calculation of possible detection efficiency. Direct neighbor–neighbor cellular interactions will invite our further consideration of properties of cellular ensembles or domains in determining tissue threshold sensitivities.

1. Directional Differences in Tissue Signal Paths

As already noted, the narrow gutters of the intercellular spaces offer preferred conduction pathways, with conductivity 10^2–10^4 higher through extracellular spaces than through cell membranes (37). Thus, the intercellular spaces become preferred pathways for *conduction along (parallel to) cell membrane surfaces* and will reflect the changing directions and cross sections of a myriad channels. Although predominantly an ionic (resistive) conduction pathway, it may also exhibit reactive components, due to the presence of protein molecules in solution.

2. Nonlinearities in Extracellular Spaces Related to Electric Charge Distribution

A suggested basis for envelope demodulation at cell surfaces may reside in the intensely anionic charge distribution on strands of glycoprotein that protrude from the cell interior, forming the glycocalyx (2,38). As already noted, they provide the structural basis for specific receptor sites, and they attract a surrounding cationic atmosphere composed largely of calcium and hydrogen ions. This charge separation creates a Debye layer. In models and experimental data from resin particles, Einolf and Carstensen (28) concluded that this physical separation creates a large virtual surface capacitance, with dielectric constants as high as 10^6 at frequencies below 1 kHz. Displacement currents induced in this region by ELF modulation of an RF field may then result in demodulation.

3. Electron Tunneling in Transmembrane Conduction: Nonlinearities in Space and Time

Experimental studies of transmembrane charge tunneling by DeVault and Chance (39) and their more recent theoretical development by Moser et al. (40) offer an example of extreme functional nonlinearity within the cell membrane. Chance described temperature-independent millisecond electron transfer over a temperature range from 120K to 4K. Considering a cell membrane transverse dimension of 40 Å, Moser et al. noted that a variation of 20 Å in the distance between donors and acceptors in a protein changes the electron transfer rate by

10^{12}-fold. Concurrently in the time domain, the electron transfer rate is pushed from seconds to days, or a 10-fold change in rate for a 1.7 Å change in distance.

4. Issues of Comparability Between Bioeffects of ELF Fields, ELF-Modulated RF Fields, and Unmodulated (CW) RF Fields

From the beginning of these studies in the 1970s, it was noted that there were similarities in responses of tissues and cultured cells to environmental fields that were either in the ELF spectrum or were RF and/or microwave fields modulated at ELF frequencies. Available evidence has indicated similarities between certain cell ionic and biochemical responses to ELF fields and to RF and/or microwave fields amplitude modulated at these same ELF frequencies, suggesting that tissue demodulation of RF and/or microwave fields may be a critical determinant in ensuing biological responses.

These findings have been reviewed in detail elsewhere (2,18). They are briefly summarized here in experiments at progressively more complex levels in the hierarchies of cellular organization. Early studies described calcium efflux from brain tissue in response to ELF exposures (38,41), and to ELF-modulated RF fields (38,41–43). Calcium efflux from isolated brain subcellular particles (synaptosomes) with dimensions under 1.0 μm also exhibit an ELF modulation frequency dependence in calcium efflux, responding to 16-Hz sinusoidal modulation, but not to 50 Hz modulation, nor to an unmodulated RF carrier (44). In the same and different cell culture lines, the growth regulating and stress responsive enzyme ornithine decarboxylase (ODC) responds to ELF fields (11,45) and to ELF-modulated RF fields (9,11,12).

In more recent studies also related to cellular stress responses, Goodman and Blank and their colleagues have reported rapid, transitory induction of heat shock proteins by microtesla-level 60-Hz magnetic fields (46). In human HL60 promyelocytic cells these exposures at normal growth temperatures activated heat shock factor1 and heat shock element binding, a sequence of events that mediates stress-induced transcription of the stress gene HSP70 and increased synthesis of the stress response protein hsp70kd. Thus, the events mediating the field-stimulated response appeared similar to those reported for other physiological stressors (hyperthermia, heavy metals, oxidative stress), suggesting to the authors a general mechanism of electromagnetic field interaction with cells. Their further studies have identified endogenous levels of c-*myc* protein as a contributor to the induction of HSP70 in response to magnetic field stimulation (47), with the hypothesis that magnetic fields may interact directly with moving electrons in DNA (48–50).

Immune responses of lymphocytes targeted against human lymphoma tumor cells (allogeneic cytotoxicity) are sensitive to both ELF exposures (51) and to ELF-modulated fields, but not to unmodulated fields (52).

Communication between brain cells is mediated by a spectrum of chemical substances that both excite and inhibit transaction and transmission of information between them. Cerebral amino acid neurotransmitter mechanisms (glutamate, GABA and taurine) are influenced by ELF fields (25,53), and also by ELF-modulated microwave fields, but not by unmodulated fields. Kolomytkin et al. (6) examined specific receptor binding of three neurotransmitters to rat brain synaptosomes exposed to either 880- or 915-MHz fields at maximum densities of 1.5 mW cm^{-2}. Binding to inhibitory gamma-aminobutyric acid (GABA) receptors decreased 30% at 16 pulses/s, but was not significantly altered at higher or lower pulse frequencies. Conversely, 16 pulses/s modulation significantly increased excitatory glutamate receptor binding. Binding to excitatory acetyl choline receptors increased 25% at 16 pulses/s, with similar trends at higher and lower frequencies.

Sensitivities of GABA and glutamate receptors persisted at field densities as low as 50 μW cm^{-2}.

A selective absence of responses to unmodulated (CW) RF and/or microwave fields reported in many of these earlier studies has focused attention on establishment of threshold sensitivities to CW field exposures. De Pomerai et al. (54) have reported cellular stress responses in a nematode worm as a biosensor of prolonged CW microwave exposures at athermal levels. Tattersall et al. (55) exposed slices of rat hippocampal cerebral tissue to 700-MHz CW fields for 5–15 min at extremely low SARs in the range 0.0016–0.0044 W kg^{-1}. No detectable temperature changes ($+/- 0.1\,°$C) were noted during 15-min exposures. At low field intensities, a 20% potentiation of electrically evoked population potentials occurred, but higher field intensities evoked either increased or decreased responses. The exposures reduced or abolished chemically induced spontaneous epileptiform activity. Bawin et al. (25) also tested the rat hippocampal slice, using ELF magnetic fields. At 56 μT (0.35–3.5 nV mm^{-1}), magnetic fields destabilized rhythmic electrical oscillations via as yet unidentified nitric oxide mechanisms involving free radicals.

D. The Roles of Field Intermittency and Exposure Duration in Seeking Optimal Therapeutic Responses: Possible "Time Windows" in Trans-Membrane Signaling Paths

It has been apparent from the earliest clinical applications of pulsed magnetic fields to such problems as delayed fracture healing that continuous exposure is not an optimal technique. For example, initial tests with FDA-approved 76-Hz magnetic field generators and cultured bone samples or osteoblast cell lines revealed a range of hormonal and enzymatic responses that occurred only at the onset or immediately after termination of field exposures. In turn, similar clinical testing of various exposure schedules in bone healing led to adoption of intermittent exposure regimes (56). In B-lineage lymphoid cells exposed to 60-Hz magnetic fields, Uckun et al. (57) reported an initial stimulation of tyrosine protein kinases (PTKs) Lyn and Syk. Activation of these Src proto-oncogene PTKs is a proximal and mandatory step in the later activation of protein kinase C. They play "a myriad roles" in signal cascades affecting proliferation and survival of B lymphoid cells.

How does a cell distinguish between transient and sustained signaling? Murphy et al. (58) have shown that in 3T3 fibroblasts, the immediate early gene *c-Fos* functions as a sensor for duration of activation of *extracellular-signal-regulated kinases* (ERK-1 and ERK-2). When ERK activation is transient (30–45 min), its activity declines before the *c-Fos* protein accumulates, and under these conditions *c-Fos* is unstable. However, when ERK signaling is sustained beyond 60 min, *c-Fos* is phosphorylated by still active ERK and by RSK (90K-ribosomal S6 kinase), thus exposing a docking site for ERK (the DEF domain). Together, these data identify a time-dependent general mechanism by which cells can interpret differences in ERK activation kinetics, including control of cell cycle progression towards either differentiation or proliferation.

Rudiger et al. (59) have reported an optimal timing sequence of 5 min ON, 10 min OFF in induction of DNA single and double strand breaks in human diploid fibroblasts and blood lymphocytes. The response to 50-Hz sinusoidal magnetic fields was dose dependent with a threshold at 70 μT. Also using cultured fibroblasts, Litovitz et al. (11) determined the minimal duration that a single low-frequency modulation frequency must be sustained (*coherence time*) in order to elicit activity in the enzyme ornithine decarboxylase (ODC). Using a 915-MHz field, switching modulation frequencies from 55 to 65-Hz at coherence times of 1 s or less abolished enhancement of ODC responses, while coherence times of 10 s or longer produced full enhancement.

It is abundantly clear that such a patchwork of observations fails to provide a database that would allow selection of optimal temporal stimulus patterns in specific clinical situations. Nevertheless, they may be considered the first pointers to crucial stimulus parameters, essential in the foundations of all magnetotherapy. They emphasize the importance of further research in that direction to define both the physical characteristics of an optimal stimulus pattern, and more importantly, the cell and molecular biology in underlying tissue substrates.

IV. THE ROLE OF CELLULAR ENSEMBLES IN SETTING TISSUE THRESHOLDS FOR INTRINSIC AND ENVIRONMENTAL STIMULI

Our pursuit of mechanisms mediating tissue electromagnetic sensitivities at nonthermal levels raises questions about the relevance of observed thresholds in the sensory physiology of other modalities. By extrapolation, do these data suggest the need to explore collective properties of populations of cells in setting thresholds by forms of intercellular communication? Do cooperative processes yield one or more faint and private languages that allow ensembles of cells to whisper together in one or more faint and private languages? Do observed tissue-sensory thresholds differ significantly from thresholds measured in single cells in isolation from their neighbors?

A. Evidence for Domain Functions as a General Biological Property in Tissues

Research in sensory physiology supports this concept, i.e., that some threshold properties may reside in highly cooperative properties of populations of elements rather than in a single detector (60). Seminal observations in the human auditory system point to a receptor vibrational displacement of 10^{-11} m, or approximately the diameter of a single hydrogen atom (61,62); human olfactory thresholds for musk occur at 10^{-13} M, with odorant molecules distributed over 240 mm^2 (63); and human detection of single photons of blue-green light occurs at energies of 2.5 eV (64). In another context, pathogenic bacteria, long thought to operate independently, exhibit ensemble properties by communication through a system recognizing colony numbers as an essential step preceding release of toxins. These *quorum sensing* systems may control expression of virulence factors in the lungs of patients with cystic fibrosis (65).

1. Domain Properties in Systems of Excitable Cells

Bialek addressed the problem of the auditory receptor in quantum mechanical terms. He evaluated two distinct classes of quantum effects: a *macroquantum effect*, typified by the ability of the sensory system to detect signals near the quantum limits to measurement, and a *microquantum effect*, in which "the dynamics of individual biological macromolecules depart from predictions of a semiclassical theory." Bialek concluded that quantum-limited sensitivity occurs in several biological systems, including displacements of sensory hair cells of the inner ear. Remarkably, quantum limits to detection are reached in the ear in spite of seemingly insurmountable levels of thermal noise.

To reach this quantum limit, these receptor cells must possess amplifiers with noise performance approaching limits set by the uncertainty principle. It is equally impressive that suppression of intrinsic thermal noise allows the ear to function as though close to 0K.

Again, this suggests system properties inherent in the detection sequence. These "perfect" amplifiers could not be described by any chemical kinetic model nor by any quantum mechanical theory in which the random phase approximation is valid. The molecular dynamics of amplifiers in Bialek's models would require preservation of quantum mechanical coherence for times comparable to integration times of the detector. It is not known whether comparable mechanisms may determine electromagnetic sensitivities as a more general tissue property at cellular and subcellular levels.

Behavioral electrosensitivity in sharks and rays may be as low as $0.5 \, \text{nV mm}^{-1}$ for tissue components of electrical fields in the surrounding ocean (66). These marine vertebrates sense these fields through specialized jelly-filled tubular receptors (ampullae of Lorenzini) up to 10 cm in length, located near the snout and opening on the skin surface through minute pores. Sensing nerve cells lie in the wall of this ampullary tube. In support of a cooperative model of organization of these neurons, behavioral electrosensitivity in sharks and rays is 100 times below measurable thresholds of individual electroreceptor neurons (67).

2. Domain Properties in System of Non-excitable Cells: Culture Dimensions and "Bystander" Effects

Jessup et al. (68) have pioneered studies on the role of gravitational fields in determining trends towards either apoptosis (programmed cell death) or towards cell proliferation. Concurrently, they tested the physical configuration of cell cultures in their influence on these same trends. Based on a colorectal cancer cell line, they compared cells cultured in adherent monolayers with three-dimensional (3-D) cultures.

Biochemical measures of apoptosis and cell proliferation were tested (1) in static cultures, (2) in cultures subjected to slow rotation, and (3) in cultures exposed to the microgravity of low-earth-orbital space flight. Over the course of 6 days on earth, static 3-D cultures displayed the highest rates of proliferation and lowest apoptosis. Rotation appeared to increase apoptosis and decrease proliferation, whereas static 3-D cultures in either unit gravity or microgravity had less apoptosis. Expression of the carcinoembryonic antigen (CEA) as a marker of cell differentiation was increased in microgravity.

For ionizing radiation, the U.S. National Council on Radiation Protection (NCRP) has recommended that estimates of cancer risk be extrapolated from higher doses by using a linear, no-threshold model. This recommendation is based on the dogma that the DNA of the nucleus is the main target of radiation-induced genotoxicity and, as fewer cells are directly damaged, the deleterious effects of ionizing radiation proportionally decline. Experimental evidence seriously challenges this concept (69). They used a precision microbeam of α particles to target an exact fraction (either 100% or ≤20%) of the cells in a confluent cell population and irradiated their nuclei with exactly one α particle each. The findings were consistent with non hit cells contributing significantly to the response, designated *the bystander effect*. Indeed, irradiation of 10% of a confluent mammalian cell population with a single α particle resulted in a mutant yield similar to that observed when all the cells in the population were irradiated. Importantly, this effect was eliminated in cells pretreated with 1 mM octanol, which inhibits intercellular communication mediated by gap-junction proteins. "The data imply that the relevant target for ionizing radiation mutagenesis is larger than an individual cell."

V. CONCLUSIONS

Epidemiological studies have evaluated ELF and radio-frequency fields as possible risk factors for human health, with historical evidence relating rising risks of such factors as progressive rural electrification and, more recently, methods of electric power distribution and utilization in commercial buildings. Appropriate models describing these bioeffects are based in nonequilibrium thermodynamics, with nonlinear electrodynamics as an integral feature. Heating models, based in equilibrium thermodynamics, fail to explain an impressive spectrum of observed electromagnetic bioeffects at nonthermal exposure levels. We face a new frontier of much greater significance.

In little more than a century, our biological vista has moved from organs to tissues, to cells, and most recently, to the molecules that form the exquisite fabric of living systems. We discern a biological organization based in physical processes at the atomic level, beyond the realm of chemical reactions between biomolecules. Much of this signaling within and between cells may be mediated by free radicals of the oxygen and nitrogen species. In their brief lifetimes, free radicals are sensitive to imposed magnetic fields, including microwave fields. Free radicals are involved in normal regulatory mechanisms in many tissues. Disordered free radical regulation is associated with oxidative stress diseases, including Parkinson's and Alzheimer's diseases, coronary heart disease, and cancer.

Although incompletely understood, tissue free radical interactions with magnetic fields may extend to zero field levels. Emergent concepts of tissue thresholds to imposed and intrinsic magnetic fields address ensemble or domain functions of populations of cells, cooperatively whispering together in intercellular communication and organized hierarchically at atomic and molecular levels.

REFERENCES

1. Schumann WG. Uber elektrische Eigenschwindungen des Hohlraumes Erd-Luft-Ionosphare, erregtdurch Blitzentzladungen. Zeitschrift Angewiss J Physik 1957; 9:373–378.
2. Adey WR. Cell and molecular biology associated with radiation fields of mobile telephones. In: Stone WR, Ueno S, eds. Review of Radio Science 1996–1999. London: Oxford University Press, 1999:845–872.
3. Milham S, Osslander EM. Historical evidence that residential electrification caused the emergence of the childhood leukemia peak. Medical Hypotheses 2001; 56:290–295.
4. Milham S. Increased incidence of cancer in a cohort of office workers exposed to strong magnetic fields. Am J Indust Med 1996; 30:702–704.
5. Saunders RD, Jefferys JG. Weak electric field interactions in the nervous system. Health Phys 2002; 83:366–375.
6. Kolomytkin O, Yurinska M, Zharikov S. Response of brain receptor systems to microwave energy exposure. In: Frey AH, ed. On the Nature of Electromagnetic Field Interactions with Biological Systems. Austin, Texas: R.G. Landes, 1994:195–206.
7. Liburdy RP. Cellular studies and interaction mechanisms of extremely low frequency fields. Radio Science 1995; 30:179–203.
8. Ishido M, Nitta H, Kabuto M. Magnetic fields (MF) of 50 Hz at 1.2 μT cause uncoupling of inhibitory pathways of adenylyl cyclase mediated by melatonin 1a receptor in MF-sensitive MCF-7 cells. Carcinogenesis 2001; 22:1043–1048.
9. Byus CV, Pieper SE, Adey WR. The effects of low-energy 60 Hz environmental electromagnetic fields upon the growth-related enzyme ornithine decarboxylase. Carcinogenesis 1987; 8:1385–1389.
10. Chen G, Upham BL, Sun W. Effect of electromagnetic field exposure on chemically induced differentiation of friend erythroleukemia cells. Environmental Health Perspectives 2000; 108:967–972.
11. Litovitz TA, Krause D, Penafiel M. The role of coherence time in the effect of microwaves on ornithine decarboxylase activity. Bioelectromagnetics 1993; 14:395–403.
12. Penafiel LM, Litovitz T, Krause D. Role of modulation effects on the effects of microwaves on ornithine decarboxylase activity in L929 cells. Bioelectromagnetics 1996; 18:132–141.

13. Cain CD, Thomas DL, Adey WR. 60-Hz magnetic field acts as co-promoter in focus formation of C3H10T 1/2 cells. Carcinogenesis 1993; 14:955–960.

14. Barnes FS. The effects of ELF on chemical reaction rates in biological systems. In: Ueno S, ed. Biological Effects of Magnetic and Electromagnetic Fields. New York: Plenum Press, 1996:37–44.

15. Astumian RD, Weaver JC, Adair RK. Rectification and signal averaging of weak electric fields by biological cells. Proc Nat Acad Sci USA 1995; 92:3740–3743.

16. Illinger KH, ed. Biological Effects of Nonionizing Radiation. Washington, DC: American Chemical Society Symposium Series, No. 157, 1981:342.

17. Adey WR. Electromagnetics in biology and medicine. In: Matsumoto, H ed. Modern Radio Science. London: Oxford University Press, 1993:231–249.

18. Adey WR. Bioeffects of mobile communication fields; possible mechanisms for cumulative dose. In: Kuster N, Balzano Q, Lin JC, eds. Mobile Communications Safety. New York: Chapman and Hall, 1997:103–140.

19. McLauchlan KA. Are environmental electromagnetic fields dangerous? Physics World, 1992 January, 41–45.

20. McLauchlan KA, Steiner UE. The spin-correlated radical pairs a reaction intermediate. Molecular Physics 1994; 73:241–263.

21. Till U, Timmel CR, Brocklehurst B. The influence of very small magnetic fields on radical recombination reactions in the limit of slow recombination. Chem Phys Let 1998; 298:7–14.

22. Timmel CR, Till U, Brocklehurst B. Effects of weak magnetic fields on free radical recombination reactions. Molecular Phys 1998; 95:71–89.

23. Lander HM. An essential role for free radicals and derived species in signal transduction. FASEB J 1997; 11:118–124.

24. Grundler W, Keilmann F, Putterlik V. Mechanics of electromagnetic interaction with cellular systems. Naturwissenschaften 1992; 79:551–559.

25. Bawin SM, Satmary WM, Jones RA. Extremely low frequency magnetic fields disrupt rhythmic slow activity in rat Hippocampal slices. Bioelectromagnetics 1996; 17:388–395.

26. Binhi VN. Magnetobiology. Underlying Physical Problems. New York: Academic Press, 2002:473.

27. Scott A. Nonlinear Science: Emergence and Dynamics of Coherent Structures. Series in Applied and Engineering and Mathematics. London: Oxford University Press, 1999:474.

28. Einolf CW, Carstensen EL. Low-frequency dielectric dispersion in suspensions of ion-exchange resins. J Phys Chem 1971; 75, 1091–1099.

29. Edelman GM, Yahara I, Wang JL. Receptor mobility and receptor-cytoplasmic interactions in lymphocytes. Proc Nat Acad Sci USA 1973; 70:1442–1446.

30. Liboff AR. The "cyclotron resonance" hypothesis: experimental evidence and theoretical constraints. In: Norden B, Ramel C, eds. Interaction Mechanisms of Low-Level Electromagnetic Fields and Living Systems. London: Oxford University Press, 1992:130–147.

31. Lednev VV. Possible mechanism for the influence of weak magnetic fields on biological systems. Bioelectromagnetics 1991; 12:71–75.

32. Blackman CF, Blanchard JP, Benane SG. Empirical test of an ion parametric resonance model for magnetic field interactions with PC-12 cells. Bioelectromagnetics 1994; 15:239–260.

33. Adair RK. A physical analysis of the ion parametric resonance model. Bioelectromagnetics 1998; 19:181–191.

34. Adey WR. Tissue interactions with nonionizing electromagnetic fields. Physiological Reviews 1981; 61:435–514.

35. Engstrom S. What is the time scale of magnetic field interaction in biological systems? Bioelectromagnetics 1997; 18:244–249.

36. Harland JD, Engstrom S, Liburdy R. Evidence for a slow time-scale of interaction for magnetic fields inhibiting tamoxifen's antiproliferative action in human breast cancer cells. Cellular Biochem Phys 1999; 31:295–306.

37. Adey WR, Kado RT, Didio J. Impedance changes in cerebral tissue accompanying a learned discriminative performance in the cat. Experimental Neurology 1963; 7:259–281.

38. Bawin SM, Adey WR. Sensitivity of calcium binding in cerebral tissue to weak environmental electric fields at low frequency. Proc Nat Acad Sci USA 1976; 73:1999–2003.
39. DeVault D, Chance B. Studies of photosynthesis using a pulsed laser. I. temperature dependence of cytochrome oxidation rate in chromatin. Evidence of tunneling. Biophys J 1966; 6:825–847.
40. Moser CC, Keske JM, Warncke K. Nature of biological electron transfer. Nature 1992; 355:796–802.
41. Blackman CF, Benane SG, House DE. Effects of ELF (1-120 Hz) and modulated (50 Hz) RF fields on the efflux of calcium ions from brain tissue in vitro. Bioelectromagnetics 1985; 6:327–338.
42. Blackman CF, Elder JA, Weil CM. Induction of calcium efflux from brain tissue by radio frequency radiation. Radio Science 1979; 14:93–98.
43. Dutta SK, Ghosh B, Blackman CF. Radiofrequency radiation-induced calcium ion efflux enhancement form human and other neuroblastoma cells in culture. Bioelectromagnetics 1989; 10:7–20.
44. Lin-Liu S, Adey WR. Low frequency amplitude-modulated microwave fields change calcium efflux rates from synaptosomes. Bioelectromagnetics 1982; 3:309–322.
45. Byus CV, Kartun K, Pieper S. Increased ornithine decarboxylase activity in cultured cells exposed to low energy modulated microwave fields. Cancer Res 1988; 48:4222–4226.
46. Lin H, Opler M, Head M. Electromagnetic field exposure induces rapid transitory heat shock factor activation in human cells. J Cell Biochem 1997; 66:482–488.
47. Lin H, Head M, Blank M. Myc-activated transactivation of HSP70 expression following exposure to magnetic fields. J Cell Biochem 1998; 69:181–188.
48. Blank M, Goodman R. Electromagnetic fields may act directly on DNA. J Cell Biochem 1999; 75:369–374.
49. Blank M, Goodman R. Electromagnetic initiation of transcription at specific DNA sites. J Cell Biochem 2001; 81:689–692.
50. Blank M, Soo L. Electromagnetic acceleration of electron transfer reactions. J Cell Biochem 2001; 81:278–283.
51. Lyle DB, Ayotte RD, Sheppard AR. Suppression of T lymphocyte cytotoxicity following exposure to 6o Hz sinusoidal electric fields. Bioelectromagnetics 1988; 9:303–313.
52. Lyle DB, Schechter P, Adey WR. Suppression of T lymphocyte cytotoxicity following exposure to sinusoidally amplitude-modulated fields. Bioelectromagnetics 1983; 4:281–292.
53. Kaczmarek LK, Adey WR. Some chemical and electrophysiological effects of glutamate in cerebral cortex. J Neurobiol 1974; 5:231–241.
54. Di Pomerai D, Daniells C, David H. Non-thermal heat-shock response to microwaves. Nature 2000; 405:417–418.
55. Tattersall JE, Scott IR, Wood SJ. Effects of low intensity radiofrequency electromagnetic fields on electrical activity in rat hippocampal slices. Brain Res 2001; 904:43–53.
56. Bassett CA. The development and application of pulsed electromagnetic fields (PEMFs) for ununited fractures and arthrodeses. Clin Plast Surg 1985; 12:257–277.
57. Uckun FM, Kurosaki T, Jin J. Exposure of B-lineage lymphoid cells to low energy electromagnetic fields stimulates Lyn kinase. J Biol Chem 1995; 270:27666–27670.
58. Murphy LO, Smith S, Chen R-H. Molecular interpretation of ERK signal duration by immediate early gene products. Nature Cell Biol 2002; 4:556–564.
59. Rudiger HW, Ivancsists S, Diem E. Genotoxic effects of extremely-low-frequency electromagnetic fields on human cells in vitro. Bioelectromagnetics Society, 24th Annual Meeting, Quebec City Proceedings, Abstract 2002; 14–3:94.
60. Adey WR. Horizons in science: physical regulation of living matter as an emergent concept in health and disease. In: Bersani F, ed. Electricity and Magnetism in Biology and Medicine. New York: Kluwer/Plenum, 1998:53–57.
61. Bialek W. Macroquantum effects in biology; the evidence. Ph.D. thesis, Department of Chemistry, University of California, Berkeley, 1983:250.
62. Bialek W, Wit HP. Quantum limits to oscillator stability: theory and experiments on emissions from the human ear. Physics Lett 1984; 104A:173–178.

63. Adey WR. The sense of smell. In: Field J, Magoun HW, Hall VE, eds. Handbook of Physiology. Vol. 1. Washington, DC: American Physiological Society, 1959:535–548.

64. Hagins WA. Excitaion in vertebrate photoreceptors. In: Schmitt FO, Worden FG, eds. The Neurosciences: Fourth Study Program. Cambridge: MIT Press, 1979:183–192.

65. Erickson DL, Endersby R, Kirkham A. Pseudomonas aeruginosa quorum-sensing systems may control virulence factor expression in the lungs of patients with cystic fibrosis. Infectious Immunology 2002; 70:1783–1790.

66. Kalmijn AJ. The electric sense of sharks and rays. J Experimental Biol 1971; 55:371–382.

67. Valberg PA, Kavet R, Rafferty CN. Can low level 50/60 Hz electric and magnetic fields cause biological effects? Radiation Res 1997; 148:2–21.

68. Jessup JM, Frantz M, Sonmez-Alpin E. Microgravity culture reduces apoptosis and increases the differentiation of a human colorectal carcinoma cell line. In Vitro Cell Development and Biology-Animal 2000; 36:367–373.

69. Zhou H, Suzuki M, Randers-Pehrson G. Radiation risk to low fluences of α particles may be greater than we thought. Proc Nat Acad Sci USA 2001; 98:14410–14415.

2

Signal Shapes in Electromagnetic Therapies: A Primer

A. R. Liboff

Oakland University, Rochester, Michigan, U.S.A.

The very wide variety of electric and magnetic signals in therapeutic use today are often simply described in terms of physical observables: voltage, electric field, current, current density, and magnetic field intensity. It is important to realize that such signals can also be classified as either constant or time-varying, and that the latter can include oscillatory, pulsatile, and modulated variations. Each of these carries unique characteristics that are often claimed to be beneficial for specific indications. This chapter attempts to carefully define the parameters that underlie these various electromagnetic signal shapes without passing judgement on claims of efficacy.

I. INTRODUCTION

Electromagnetic (EM) signals are increasingly being used in both systemic and local therapeutic applications. In the following, we attempt to provide the clinician with an outline of the types of signals that are currently in use. This includes a general introductory classification of EM signals, based on how each signal varies in time.

Despite the differences in wave shape, the parameters used to measure signal intensity remain the same, whether one is interested in voltage, current, or magnetic field. Although this outline is necessarily broad and lacking in some of the finer details, hopefully it can still be used to advantage when trying to comprehend the great variety of signal shapes that are presently available.

In describing any electromagnetic regimen, one must indicate not only the signal shape, but also the nature of the signal being applied. Human tissues will respond differently to magnetic fields per se or to electric potentials either induced by a magnetic field or directly applied to the tissues. The latter two therapeutic choices, by far the most commonly employed, are indicated schematically in Fig. 1 In Fig. 1a, electrodes are used to directly connect an electrical source to the tissue under treatment. These electrodes can be located on the tissue surface or subcutaneously. The net effect is the generation of current density within

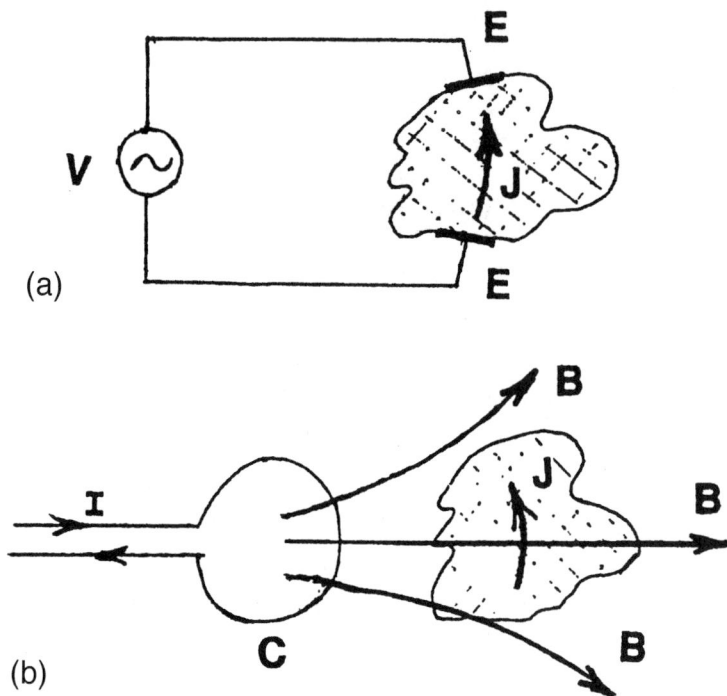

Figure 1 (a) When a potential difference V is directly attached to tissue via electrodes E, a current density J is created within the tissue. (b) A current density can also be generated in tissue when it is threaded by a magnetic field B that is changing. The field B originates in a coil C that is energized by a current I. This phenomenon of induction of electricity by a magnetic field (Faraday induction) occurs when the field changes, e.g., as an intensity change, as a relative motion between coil and tissue, or as a change in field uniformity. Note that by definition a time-varying field is one whose intensity is changing and that the higher the frequency of the field, the faster the change.

the tissue. (Current density is merely current per unit area, measured, for example, in terms of microamperes per square centimeter.) However, one can also generate meaningful current densities within tissue using Faraday's law of induction. Electrical currents will be induced within any substance that happens to be electrically conducting (such as living tissue) when this substance is located near a changing magnetic field (see Fig. 1b).

Magnetic fields can therefore provide a unique advantage in that unlike the purely electric applications pictured in Fig. 1a, they do not require electrodes and can thus be regarded as noninvasive. Two rather important examples of the equivalence pictured in Fig. 1 are found in neurology and in orthopedics. For many decades, the treatment of choice for bipolar affective disorder was electroconvulsive therapy (ECT), a procedure involving the application of large electric potentials to the brain using electrodes directly attached to the skin (1). Recently, this approach has begun to be replaced by rapid transcranial magnetic stimulation (rTMS) (2) which employs coils placed close to the head that develop large magnetic fields capable of inducing intracranial currents of the same magnitude as can be produced by ECT using electrodes. Similarly, the use of subcutaneous electrodes in the original electric treatment of choice for bony nonunions (3) was made unncessary when Bassett et al. (4) introduced pulsed magnetic fields to induce the required currents at the defect.

Whether one employs magnetic or electric fields, it is still necessary, when defining a given therapy, to specify the waveshape, i.e., how the signal develops in time. In turn the question of signal shape adds greatly to the potential complexity that accompanies electro-magnetic applications. It is critical to realize that electromagnetic therapies are intrinsically far more complicated than pharmaceutical regimens. Many clinicians fail to appreciate this complexity, applying electric or magnetic fields as they would a pharmaceutical regimen whose outcome is dependent on titer. It is important to remember that there is no such thing as a little or a lot of magnetic field.

For example, one can find high-frequency signals that have miniscule intensity, low-frequency signals with large gradients, or high-intensity magnetic fields with low duty cycles. Each of these might produce different physiological responses and have different therapeutic usefulness. It is wise for the clinician to be aware of the various factors, or metrics, the sum of which are used to define a given field.

One such factor relates to the vector nature of magnetic and electric fields. The characteristic of field uniformity has no analogue in pharmacy. Yet the interactiveness of magnetic fields is definitely a function of its uniformity. A uniform field is one that has the same intensity and direction everywhere over the region in question. As a rule this is a very difficult condition to initially provide for and also to then maintain in any given application. Figure 2 compares the lines of force for a uniform field to one which is very nonuniform.

In laboratory practice, specially designed coils (Helmholtz or Merritt coils) are often used to maintain magnetic field uniformity within the active volume of application. However, even when such specialized coil systems are employed, it is often the case that the volume within which uniform field conditions are achieved is but a small fraction of the actual volume enclosed by the coils. A good exception to this rule is found when using a properly designed (long) solenoid, where the magnetic field is highly uniform within that volume enclosed by the solenoid except near its ends. Similarly, one finds a highly uniform electric field within the volume enclosed by a parallel plate capacitor, for the case where the two parallel conducting plates are separated by a distance far less than the diameter of each plate. Unfortunately, because of the sizes that would be required to meet these criteria for uniformity, neither of these arrangements is practical when treating humans. It can be taken as a rule of thumb that none of the devices actually used in electromagnetic therapy achieve any degree of field uniformity. The situation is made even worse considering the wide range of dimensions and designs among the various devices in use, leading one to conclude that, as far as field uniformity is involved, it is highly likely that no two therapeutic devices are the same.

The most general classification of therapeutic EM signals is based not on the intensity but on how the signal varies with time (Fig. 3). This type of plot encompasses DC signals, sine wave signals, and a wide variety of pulses. For the latter two cases, sine waves and pulses, the therapeutic application usually involves the signal repeating itself periodically (Fig. 3b). The y axis in Fig. 3 is termed *signal intensity*. The signal intensity can take on many forms, depending on the parameter that is considered important to the specific therapeutic application. For example, this can refer to intensities of voltage, current, magnetic field, etc. More often than not, instead of expressing things in general terms, specific units are used to describe signal intensities: volts, millivolts, milliamperes, microamperes, microtesla, milli-gauss, etc.

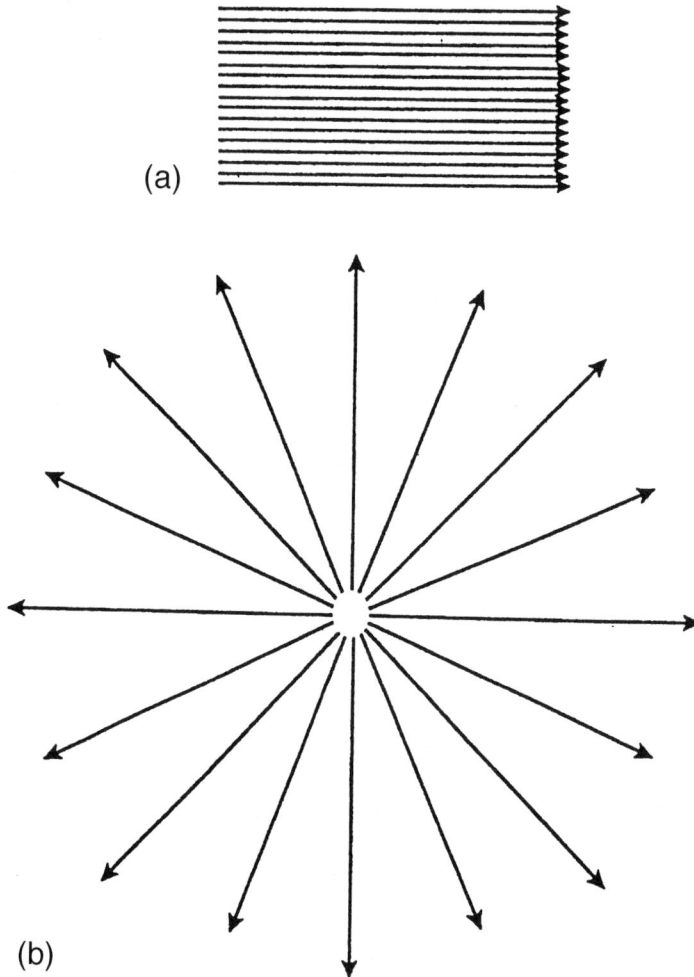

Figure 2 (a) A uniform field (either electric or magnetic) is one in which everywhere within the region of interest has the same intensity and direction. The lines of force are drawn here in two dimensions for simplicity but in reality should always be thought of as 3-dimensional. (b) Example of a very nonuniform field, namely the electric field that surrounds a single positive charge. Again, one should imagine this configuration in three dimensions, such that the radial lines of force are not only in the plane of the page but also point upward and downward. Note that the lines of force as drawn for this field have the same length as in Fig. 2a. Thus, even though this field has the same intensity as that in Fig. 2a, the fact that it is nonuniform makes it a totally different field.

II. DC SIGNALS

When an electric or magnetic field does not vary with time, it is often termed a *direct current* (DC) signal (Fig. 4). Even though the word current appears in the term DC, one often sees DC applied to voltage (DC volts) and to magnetic field (DC field). Two good examples of DC signals are the constant current supplied by an electric battery and the constant magnetic field intensity surrounding a permanent magnet. A number of other terms are used to describe the DC signal shown in Fig. 4: constant, static, electrostatic, and magnetostatic.

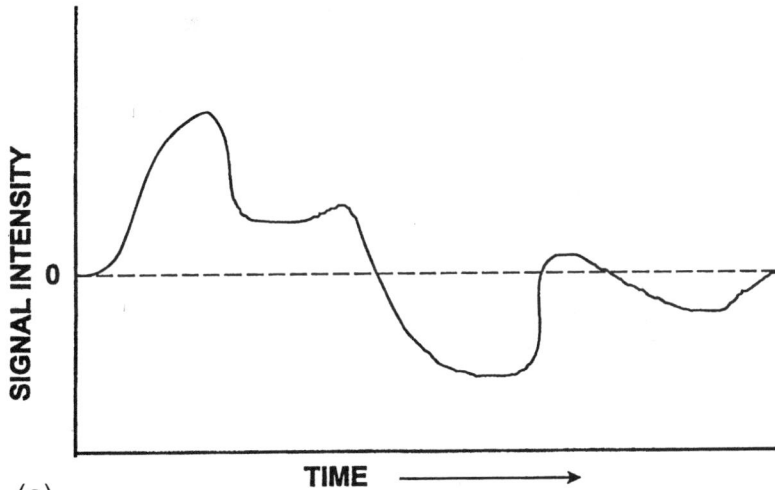

(a)

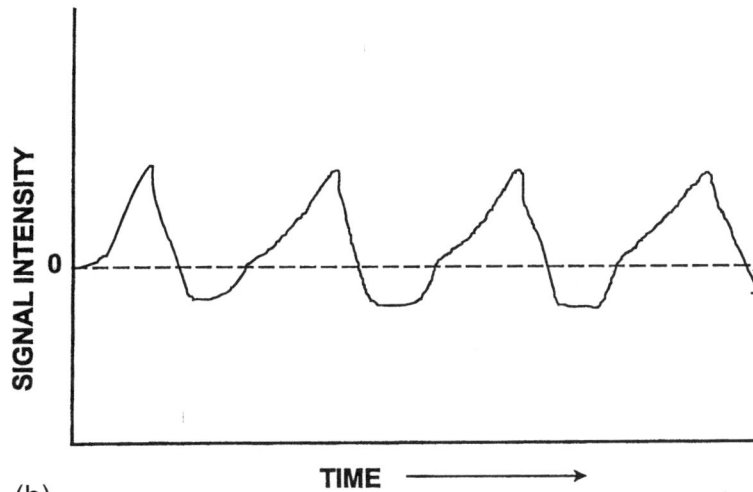

(b)

Figure 3 (a) Any type of signal variation can be plotted as a function of time. (b) When any signal, regardless of its shape, repeats itself in a regular way, the signal is termed *periodic*.

In some clinical applications, even though, say, a battery is used to supply a constant voltage to tissues, the electrical properties of these tissues may change in time so as to cause the current to vary correspondingly. For example, this happens during the healing process in both soft and hard tissues. One can adjust the current electronically to automatically compensate for such changes and thereby maintain the static nature of the application. This type of electronic compensation is achieved by means of a *constant current amplifier*.

Humans are always exposed to a very specific magnetostatic exposure, namely that due to the earth's magnetic field for geomagnetic field (GMF). This field is distributed over the surface of the earth and is maximum (approximately 65 µT) at the geomagnetic poles and minimum (approximately 25 µT) at the geomagnetic equator. It must be noted that

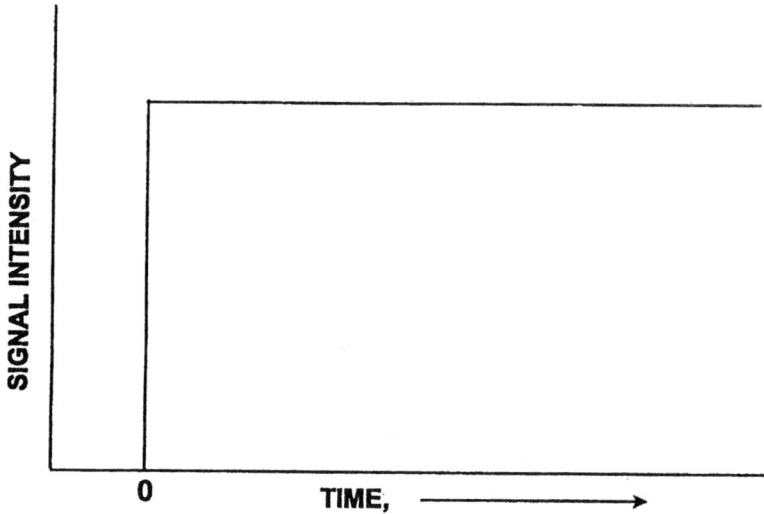

Figure 4 A DC signal plotted against time, after it is abruptly turned on at zero time.

the GMF poles and GMF equator are very different from the geographic poles and equator. At any point on the earth's surface, one can specify the GMF either in terms of the total GMF or in terms of the GMF components, i.e., the vertical component or the horizontal component.

One should be aware that the nature of magnetic fields is that these GMF components will always be directly added to magnetic signals that may be applied by the clinician. Therefore when applying therapeutic magnetic signals the GMF background field must be taken into account. The GMF can only be disregarded when its intensity is much less than the applied therapeutic signal. As a rule the GMF components can be ignored when the therapeutic intensities are more than 50–100 times larger than 50 µT. At least one therapeutic magnetic regimen is questionable since it applies magnetic fields with intensities that are approximately one millionth of the GMF. It is well to realize that in such circumstances one in effect is making the unfounded assumption that the nature of the magnetic therapeutic signal is somehow fundamentally different from that of the GMF.

There are miniscule departures from time-wise constancy in the GMF, mainly connected to the occurrence of solar storms every 11 years. Reports have surfaced (5) claiming that the GMF noise that accompanies solar storms may have physiological consequences.

Mainly because of technical improvements in permanent magnet fabrication, a number of claims have surfaced claiming that the intense (of the order of 1 T) magnetostatic fields associated with such magnets have therapeutic usefulness. The intensity of these fields may be less important than the larger magnetic gradient that is possible with high intensity permanent magnets. One such example is the MagnaBloc device (Amway Corp., Ada, MI), which produces gradients of up to 20 T/m (6).

III. SINE WAVE SIGNALS

Of all the time-varying signals utilized in EM therapeutic applications, the sine wave shape is the simplest to deal with. Some of these applications have taken advantage of the fact that electric power signals vary in a sinusoidal manner. However, there are now many devices (e.g., function generators) that are inexpensive and readily available for supplying sine wave signals that can be used as current inputs to coils for magnetic applications or voltage inputs for electric applications.

The idealized sinusoidal signal is shown in Fig. 5. Two factors are always supplied when describing any given sine wave signal: amplitude and frequency.

The amplitude is merely the maximum displacement of the signal from zero. Often one finds the term peak, or peak amplitude, used instead of amplitude. In the literature, peak amplitude can occur as volts, milliamperes, milligauss, microtesla, volts per meter, milliamperes per square centimeter (mA/cm^2), to name just a few measures of amplitude. Thus the residential magnetic field peak intensity associated with power-line fields is approximately 0.01 μT. In North America the peak voltage supplied at wall outlets is 170 V.

There is one confusing aspect to describing sine wave amplitudes. For a number of practical reasons, electrical engineers often use a slightly different terminology, referring to root-mean-square (rms) or, equally, effective (eff) values. A simple numerical factor relates the peak value of any sine wave signal to its rms value. One merely multiplies the peak value by the factor 0.7071 to obtain the corresponding rms value. Thus for the above example, the peak AC voltage in the United States and Canada of 1.70 V is the same as 120 V rms.

Another cautionary note concerning peak amplitudes is that some observers will measure the entire extent of sinusoidal signals such as shown in Fig. 4, choosing to report peak-to-peak (p–p) values. Clearly as one can see, sine waves are symmetrical about the zero axis. The positive amplitude equals the negative amplitude. Thus a peak AC voltage of 170 V is equivalent to 340 V p–p.

The frequency with which a sine wave signal repeats itself is measured in cycles per second (cps), more familiarly known as hertz (Hz) (Fig. 6). The electric power frequency in North America is 60 Hz, and in Europe it is 50 Hz. There is an enormous range of

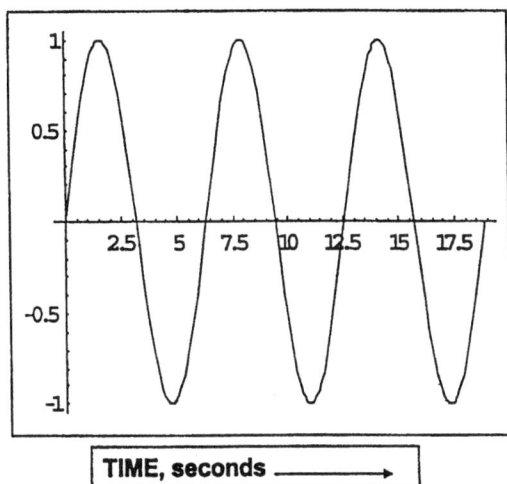

Figure 5 A sine wave, or sinusoidal, signal. Three cycles are shown. The peak amplitude is 1.0 in arbitrary units. (For example, this might be 1.0 V, 1.0 mA, or 1.0 mT). Sine wave signals have the same amplitudes above and below the horizontal zero axis. The period of the sine wave is in this case 6.3 s. The period of a sinusoidal signal is inversely equal to the frequency in Hz, when the period is measured in seconds. Therefore this sine wave signal has a frequency of 0.159 Hz.

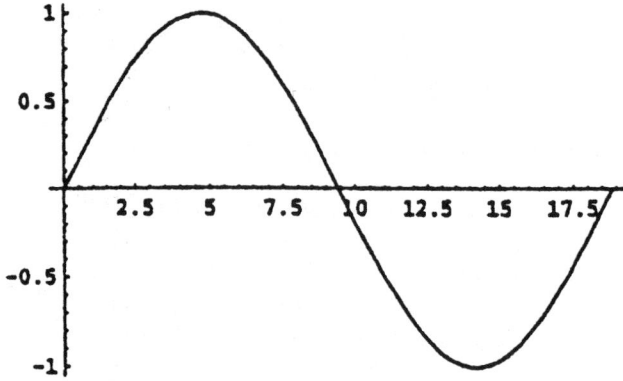

(a)

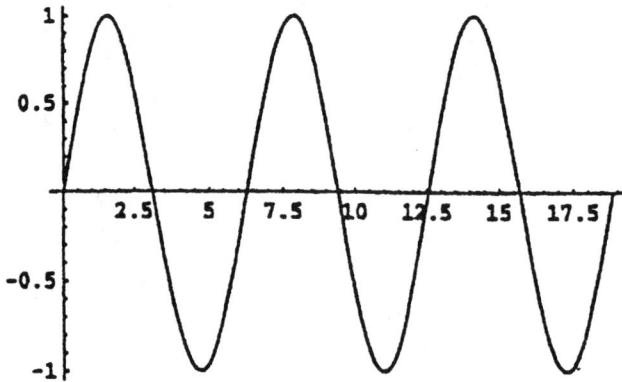

(b)

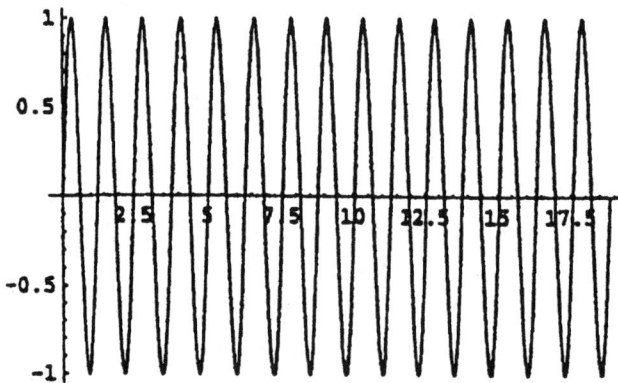

(c)

Figure 6 Three sine wave signals with different frequencies, each having an amplitude of 1.0 arbitrary units, and each plotted over the same time interval: (a) upper signal, .053 Hz; (b) middle signal, 0.159 Hz; (c) bottom signal, 0.79 Hz. The frequency of sine wave signals used in electromagnetic therapy can extend up to 50 GHz or more, where 1 GHz is equal to 1×10^9 Hz.

electromagnetic sine wave frequencies either already in use or suggested for therapeutic application. At the lower end of this range one finds extremely low frequencies (ELF), extending approximately from 3 to 300 Hz. At the upper end of this range, frequencies as high as 50 billion Hz (50 GHz) are used.

Some therapies use signals that are derived from sine waves, but slightly different. The best-known example is that of ion cyclotron resonance (ICR) (7) as shown in Fig. 7, and utilized in the repair of bony nonunions and to enhance spinal fusion (OrthoLogic Corporation, Tempe, AZ). In this case, a sinusoidal magnetic signal is applied in the same direction as a static magnetic field signal, and the amplitude of the sinusoidal signal is set equal to the intensity of the DC signal. The tissues are therefore exposed to the sum of both signals.

Another example of a nearly sine wave therapy occurs when rectification of the signal is used. Rectifying a signal means eliminating the negative part of the sine wave signal that is shown in Fig. 5, either by flipping the negative part to make it positive (full wave rectification) or merely canceling the negative part (half-wave rectification). These changes to the usual sine wave are readily achieved electronically. The idealized full rectified signal is shown in Fig. 8. For comparison, note an actual magnetic field signal (8) as measured in a therapeutic device manufactured by EMF Therapeutics (Chattanooga, TN) (Fig. 9).

One more example of a sine-wave variant occurs when employing amplitude modulation. This type of signal, illustrated in Fig. 10, involves two separate sine wave signals, with very different frequencies. The high-frequency signal is called the carrier, while the low-frequency modulated signal "rides" on the carrier. One example of this type of signal is found in the Liss Cranial Electrical Stimulator (MEDI Consultants, Inc., Paterson, NJ) (9) which uses a sinusoidal carrier signal of 15,000 Hz that is modulated either by a 15-Hz or 500-Hz signal. Yet another example of a modulated waveform is found in the use of low energy emission therapy (LEET) (10) (Symtronic S.A., Renens, Switzerland) as a treatment

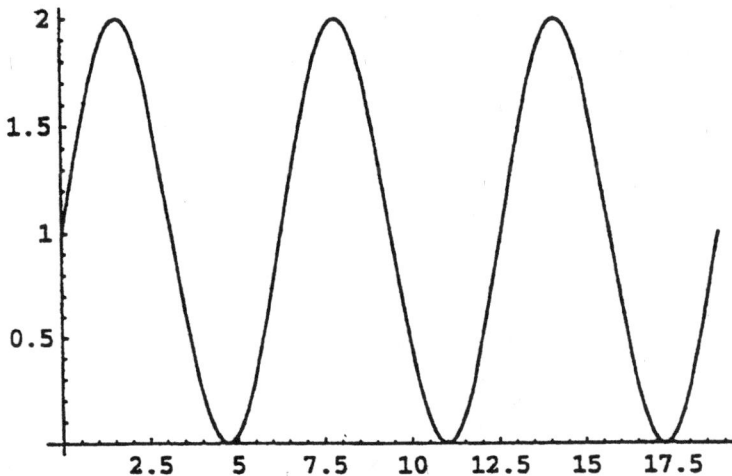

Figure 7 Adding a DC signal having an intensity of 1.0 to a sinusoidal signal having an amplitude of 1.0. Note that the midpoint of the sine wave signal intensity is now at 1.0, and is no longer at zero as was the case in Fig. 5. This illustrates the proprietary waveshapes used in ion cyclotron resonance (ICR) therapies (OrthoLogic Corporation, Tempe, AZ). For ion cyclotron resonance applications the signal intensity is given in terms of magnetic field intensity (i.e., μT or mG).

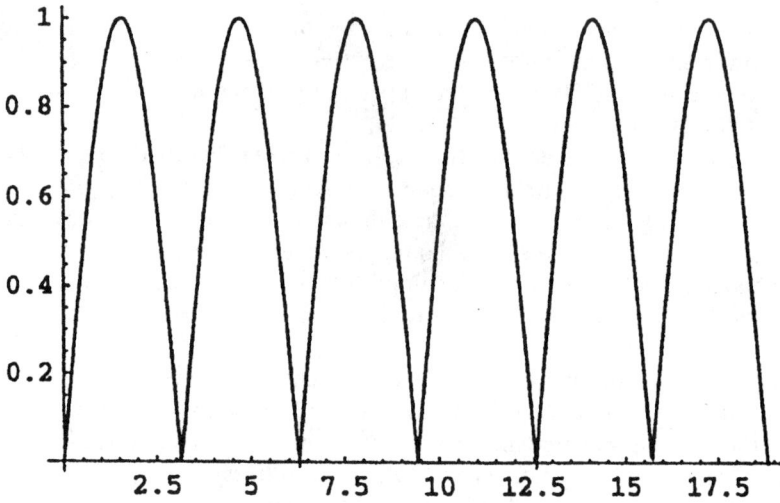

Figure 8 Rectified signal, as constructed from the sine wave signal shown in Fig. 5. The negative parts of the signal in Fig. 5 have been flipped, resulting in a signal that is everywhere positive. Note that since the rectified signal repeats itself twice as fast as the signal in Fig. 5, the new frequency is now doubled, 0.32 Hz.

for insomnia. Electrical currents modulated in this manner are supplied using electrodes attached directly to the tissues in question.

By contrast, a very special case involving two separate sine wave signals occurs when the two frequencies, instead of being very different, are close to one another (Fig. 11). Two sine waves with the same amplitude and frequencies that are slightly apart give rise to the phenomenon of beats when combined. The net frequency is in this case different from the

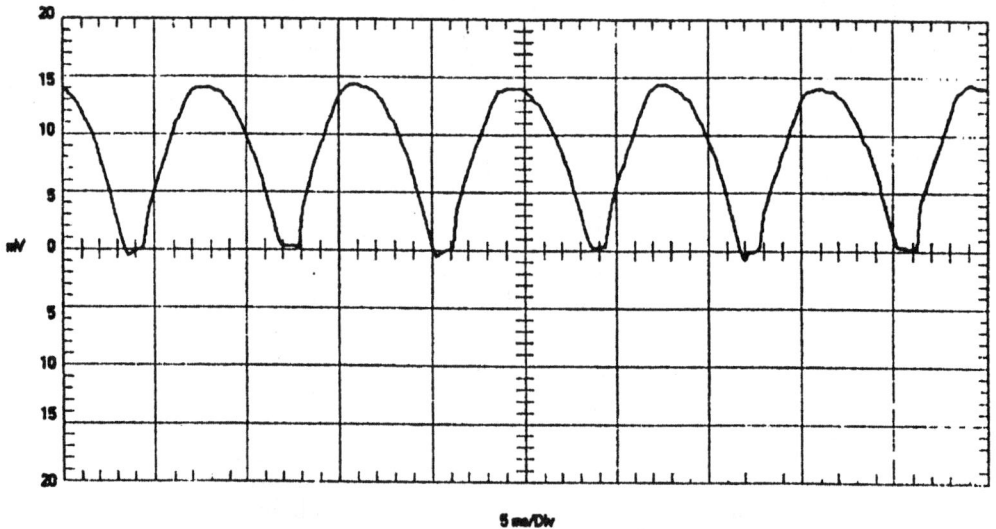

5 ms/Div

Figure 9 Rectified signal used by the EMF Therapeutics Corporation. Compare to Fig. 8. The signal intensity is measured in millivolts (mV). This signal has a frequency of 120 Hz.

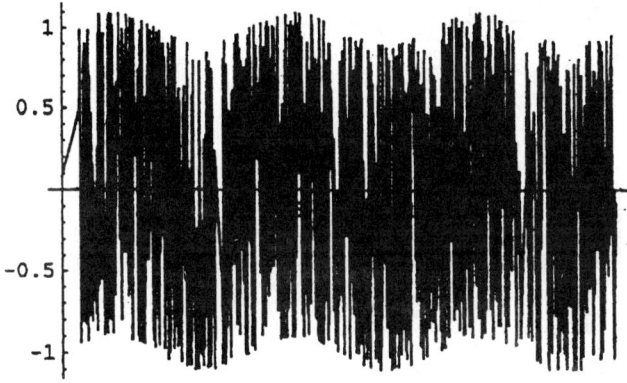

Figure 10 Example of an amplitude modulated signal. The low-frequency (0.159 Hz) signal "rides" on the carrier wave, which in this case has a frequency of 159 kHz. (One kHz equals 1000 Hz.)

two base frequencies. In AC interferential therapy (11), electrodes are used to apply two separate AC electric signals with slightly different frequencies to the tissue in question, thereby creating a means for treating the tissue with a low-frequency electric current that could not easily be applied directly.

IV. PULSED SIGNALS

A wide variety of pulsed waveshapes are used in therapeutic applications. The simplest types are either monopolar or bipolar (Fig. 12), i.e., only positive, or alternating in polarity. In

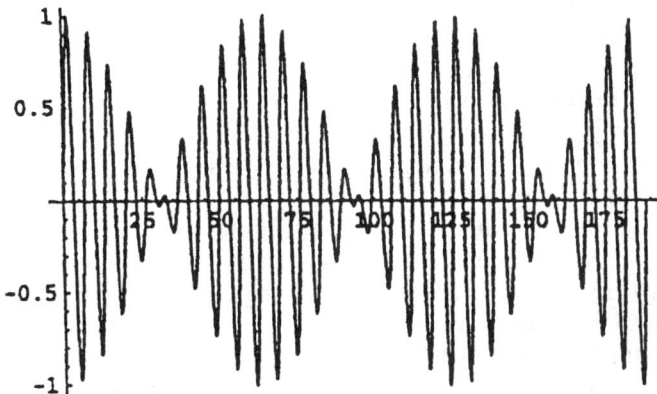

Figure 11 When two sine waves having the same amplitude and frequencies close to each other are added, one observes the phenomenon of "beats," wherein a new sine wave signal occurs whose frequency is the difference between the two original frequencies. In the example shown, the two original frequencies were 0.008 Hz apart. The beat frequency of this new signal can easily be recognized as the large variation in the amplitude of the high-frequency signal. Note that only one high-frequency signal is observed after adding the original sinusoidal signals. It has a frequency that is the average of the two original frequencies. One can also regard the new low-frequency signal is the result of an interference effect between the two high-frequency waves.

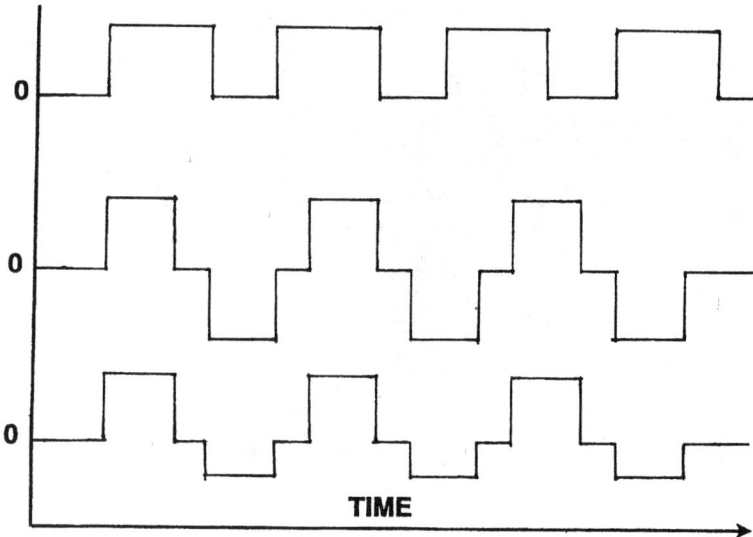

Figure 12 Three different types of pulse trains. The pulses at the top are monopolar, all positive. The lower two sets of pulses are bipolar, such that in every cycle both positive and negative values are obtained. The bottom set of bipolar pulses shows that the positive and negative amplitudes need not be the same. The positive or negative polarity in each case can refer to current direction, magnetic field direction, voltage polarity, etc.

addition, the pulse train at the bottom of Fig. 12 shows that biphasic pulses need not be symmetric about the zero axis, such that the positive amplitude is greater or smaller than the negative amplitudes. Note that the simple signals shown in Fig. 12 are periodic, that is, they repeat after a certain time. The inverse of the period is called the repetition rate, a measure of the signal that is analogous to the frequency when discussing sine wave signals. Indeed the repetition rate, in addition to being given in terms of cycles per second, is often listed in terms of hertz (Hz).

In connection with Fig. 12, the clinician should be careful not to give too much physiological meaning to the polarity of different types of signals. Tissues that are exposed, for example, to pulses that are more positive than negative, or vice versa, are not likely to respond any differently if the polarity is reversed.

The pulses as drawn in Fig. 12 are somewhat deceiving, in that the sharp leading edge of each pulse as it rises from zero to its maximum amplitude occurs over a very short time, too small to be accurately drawn (Fig. 13). It is often the case that the therapeutic value of a given pulsed signal is highly dependent on how rapidly this rise time happens. To maintain a proper control over the pulsed signals that may be used in a specific regimen, it is important for the clinician to know the rise time associated with these pulses. Note that the fall time on the back end of each pulse need not be equal to the rise time, but it is equally critical. It is usual for manufacturers of therapeutic equipment to provide, along with other measures of the device such as frequency and peak levels, the rise and fall times as well.

Thus, pulses should be regarded as expressing two types of time characteristics. The first, as mentioned above, is the period, the inverse of which is the repetition rae. The second characteristic is the rise time of the pulse. An often useful rule-of-thumb estimate of the maximum frequency of a pulse is to take the inverse of the rise time. Again as in the case of repetition rates, this maximum frequency is expressed in hertz (Hz).

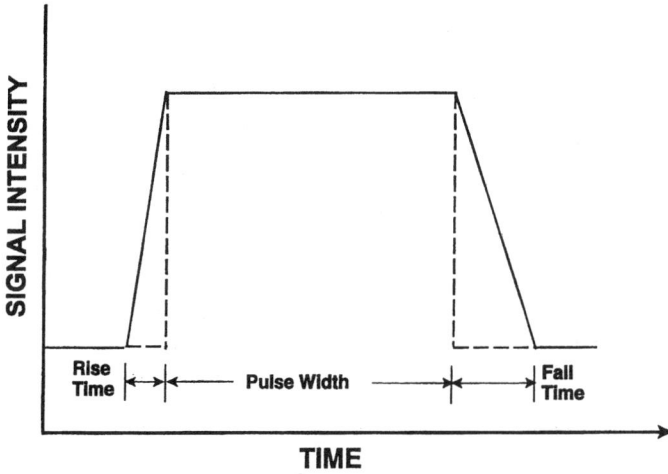

Figure 13 The ideal shape of a single pulsed waveform is never achieved in reality. Instead of the infinitely sharp edges (pictured here with dotted lines) electronic constraints invariably result in finite rise times and fall times.

It should be clear that the pulses shown in Fig. 12 can have many variations. The very simple magnetic pulsing device made by Enermed Inc (Vancouver) (12) delivers pulses with a 1-m pulse width that have signal intensities in the 5–10-μT range at a repetition rate of 4–13 Hz. A more complex signal is the pulsed signal therapy (PST) device (Bio-Magnetic Therapy Systems, Munich) (13). The PST magnetic signal, shown in Fig. 14, uses a range of many pulse widths and amplitudes in each cycle. In effect this approach finesses the problem of signal specificity, that is, the problem of not knowing precisely which waveform may result in optimum issue interaction.

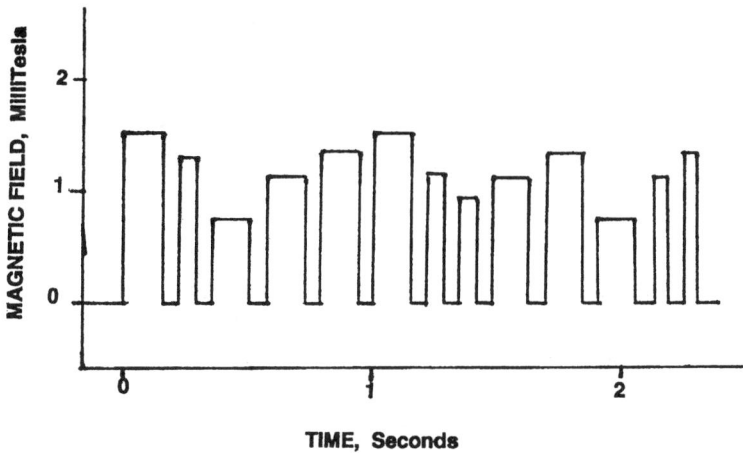

Figure 14 The pulsed signal therapy (PST) waveform is a collection of rectangular pulses, ranging in intensity from 0.5 to 1.5 mT and with various time characteristics. Although it is claimed that the overall frequency ranges from 10 to 20 Hz, it is clear that the sharp rise times occurring with each pulse must also contribute higher frequencies.

By contrast, some devices reflect less concern about the specifics of the pulse and are designed mainly to transfer energy into the tissue. For example, a much older diathermy device design (Diapulse, Inc., Great Neck, NY) (14) made use of a very narrow, very large intensity pulse, separated by long intervals of time (Fig. 15). This type of signal application, where there may be some measure of heating due to thermal effects of the electromagnetic field, is best described in terms of the signal duty cycle (Fig. 16). Higher duty cycles occur when high-intensity pulses are applied at high repetition rates, resulting in tissue heating due to transfers of energy to the tissue that are too rapid to allow for heat dissipation.

However, using electromagnetic radiation to heat tissue is now practically a thing of the past. Almost all of the electromagnetic therapy devices presently in use or planned are deliberately designed as low-duty-cycle devices in recognition of the paradigm that there may be many nonthermal medical applications for electromagnetic signals.

Perhaps the most well-known pulsed magnetic field (PMF) shape used in clinical practice was introduced by Bassett (4) as an orthopedic treatment. In this device a periodic sawtooth magnetic signal (Fig. 17) generates a rapidly changing magnetic field, shown in Fig. 18. This changing field is directly related to the induced current generated in the tissue, with the maximum current occurring when the sawtooth magnetic signal in Fig. 17 is changing most rapidly, namely when it falls from its maximum to zero.

A very similar idea, again employing a pulsatile large magnetic field is used in neurological practice to treat depression (2). A train of rather intense (of the order of tesla) magnetic pulses with repetition rates between 5 and 30 Hz are developed in coils held close to the head. In this case, as well as the similar procedure used to treat bone, the ultimate aim of the clinician is to induce electric currents within the tissue. This will always be the result when a very intense, rapidly varying magnetic field is deployed close to the body. The magnetic

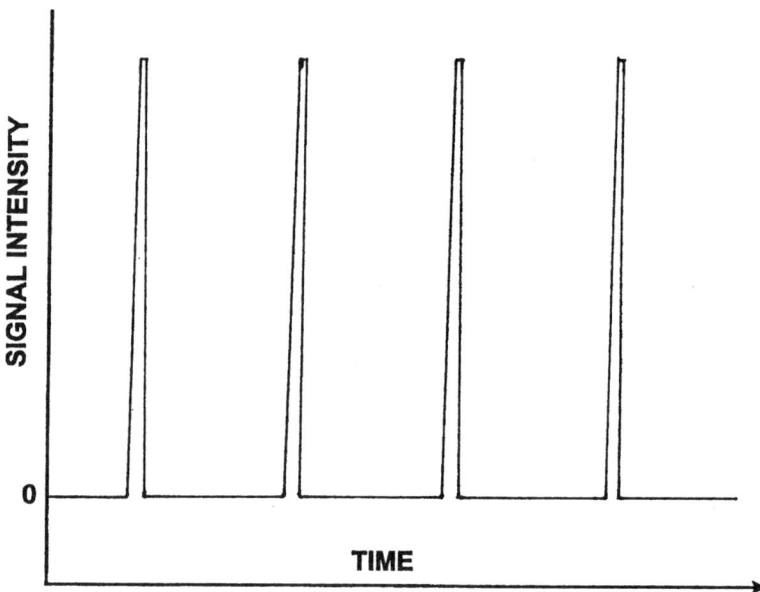

Figure 15 An example of a monophasic pulse, such as used by the Diapulse Corp in applying short microwave burst as a diathermy treatment. Even though the intensity of the pulses are large, they are extremely short (65 μs) and the time between successive pulses is rather long (1600 μs).

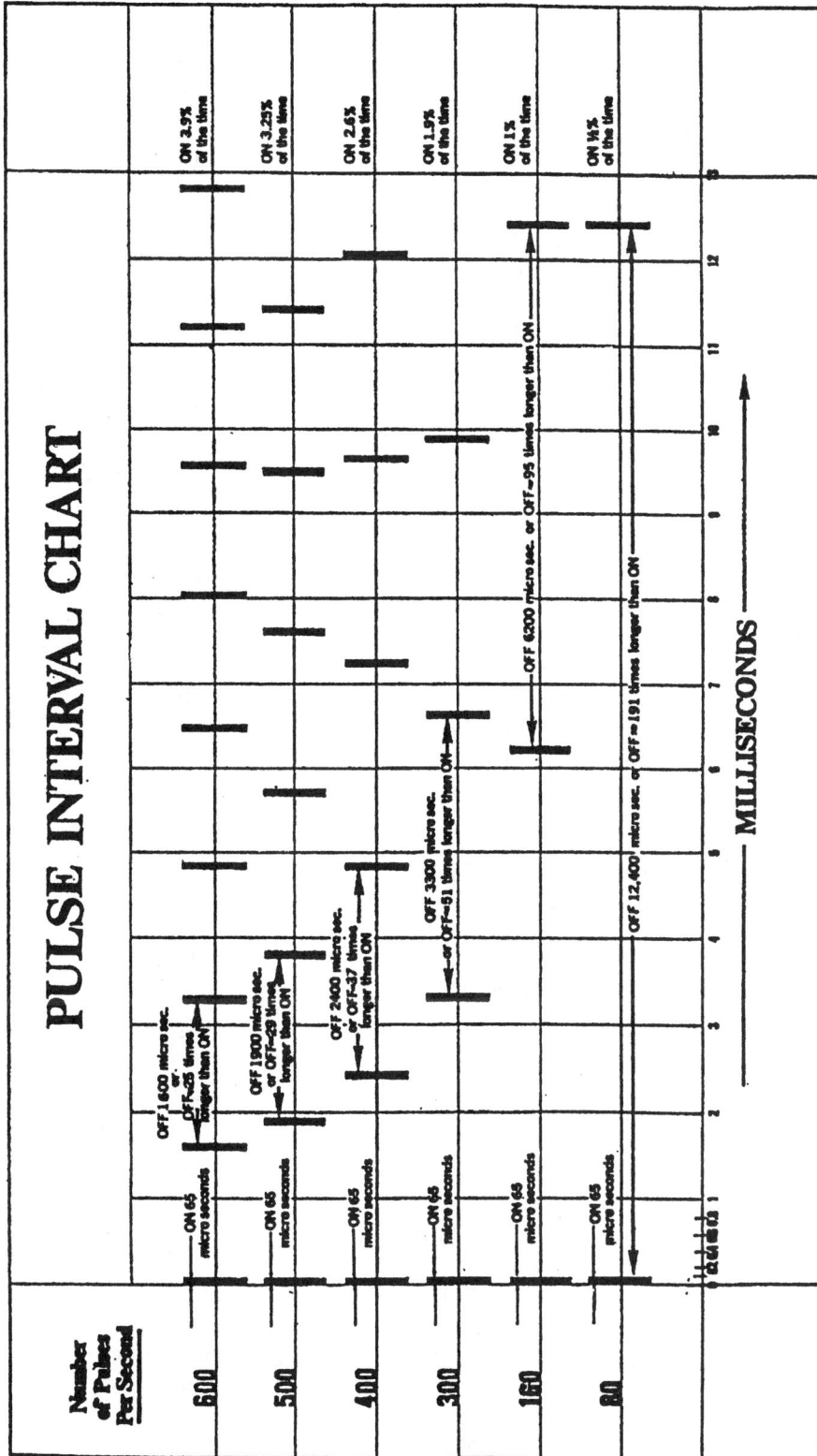

Figure 16 Illustrating the concept of duty cycle. As the number of pulses per second increases, the energy supplied to the tissue is also increased.

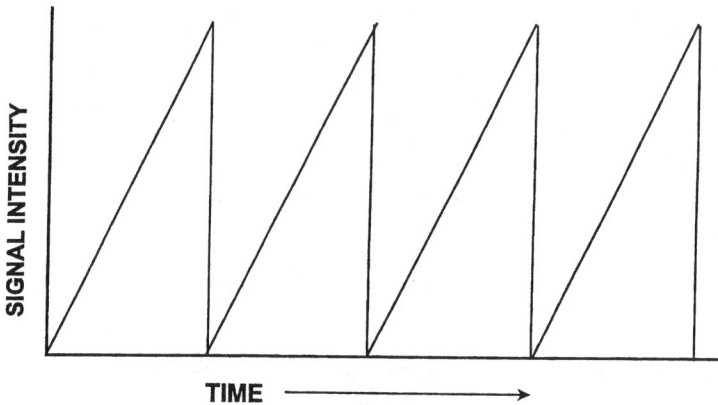

Figure 17   A sawtooth signal, characterized by a slow rise to a maximum followed by a sharp drop back to zero. When a magnetic field is generated having this shape, the rapid change in field that occurs when the current drops to zero can be used to advantage to induce large currents in tissue.

field intensity in the orthopedic case is of the order of a few millitesla, and the intensity in the neurological treatment is approximately 100–1000 times larger. (It is as yet unknown whether smaller magnetic intensities in the latter case would also be clinically effective.)

The definitions used to describe trains of magnetic pulses are very similar to those used to discuss therapeutic electrical current pulses. Instead of magnetic fields generated by coils, one has voltage sources supplying pulsatile currents to tissue by means of electrodes. One such application (15) is found in cranial electrotherapy stimulation (Electromedical Products International, Inc., Mineral wells, TX) (Fig. 19).

V. CONCLUSIONS

We have attempted to generalize for the clinician the two main types of waveforms used in electromagnetic therapy, for the most part emphasizing the newer nonthermal therapeutic applications. The most important distinction lies in the use of sinusoidal signal as opposed to pulsed signals. Within each category one finds elaborations: For sine waves one can displace the zero crossover point, one can rectify the signal, modulate the carrier frequency, or change the frequency or amplitude. Pulses can occur as bursts or trains and can enjoy different amplitudes, polarities, repetition rates, with a choice of pulse widths and rise times. All of these variations are used in therapeutic practice, both in the application of electrical currents and magnetic fields.

It is likely that the future will see combinations of such signals in therapeutic application, especially as more information filters back from the laboratory elaborating on the nature of electromagnetic interactions with living tissue.

In a number of cases, we have tried to relate the idealized specific waveform to actual devices in practice. This was done mainly to provide better understanding, and not as an endorsement for any of the devices that were mentioned. Conversely, nothing should be inferred from our failure to include other possible examples. Also, the examples that were given are made without regard to present or pending FDA approval, but solely to help the reader understand that these represent good examples of specific design features.

We hope that the outline presented in this article will help the clinician be more discerning when considering new electromagnetic therapeutic protocols. Occasionally, one

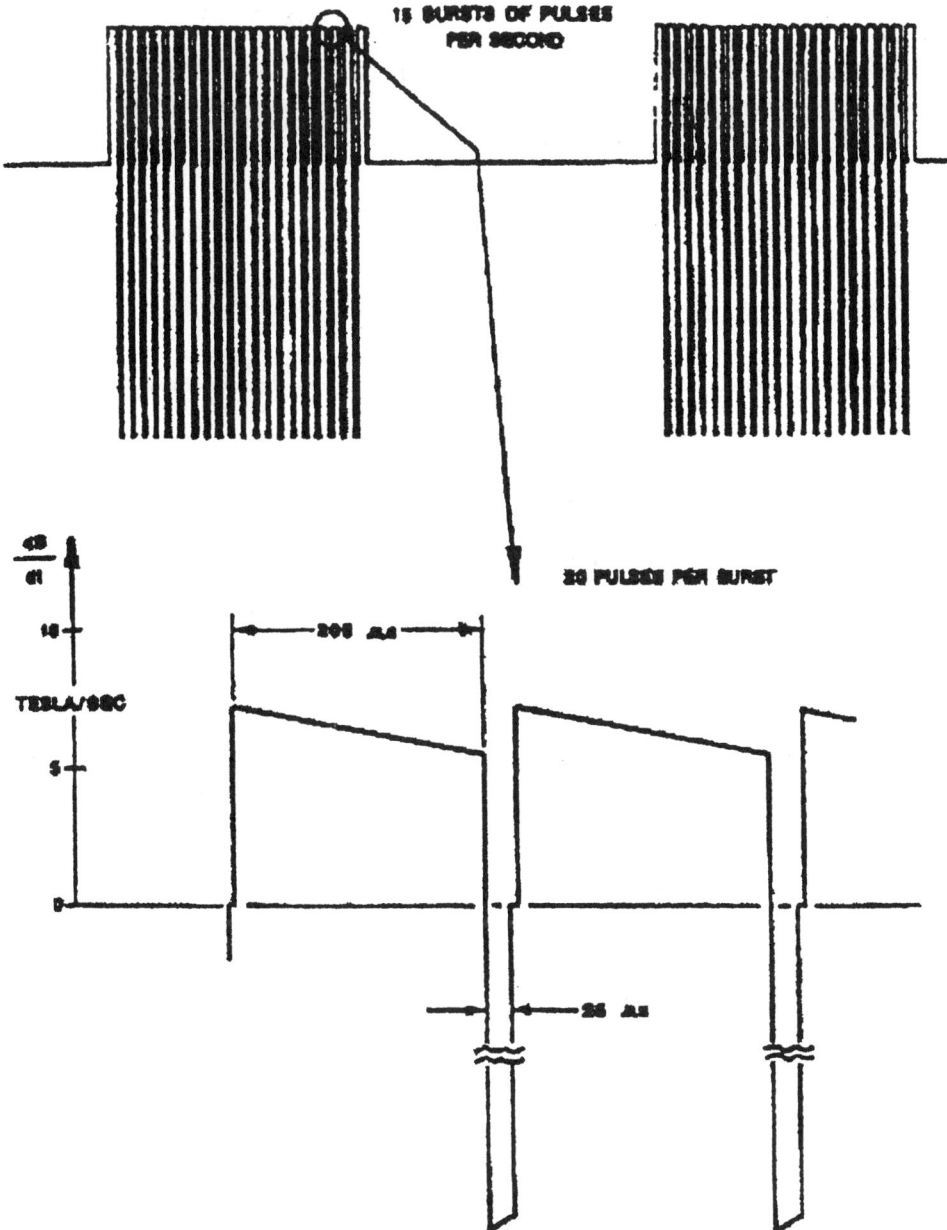

Figure 18 The EBI (ElectroBiology L. P., Parsippany, NJ) pulsed signal (PMF), originally introduced by Bassett (4). Bursts of sawtooth-shaped currents in the therapy coils produce corresponding bursts of rapidly changing magnetic field with a burst repetition rate of 15 Hz.

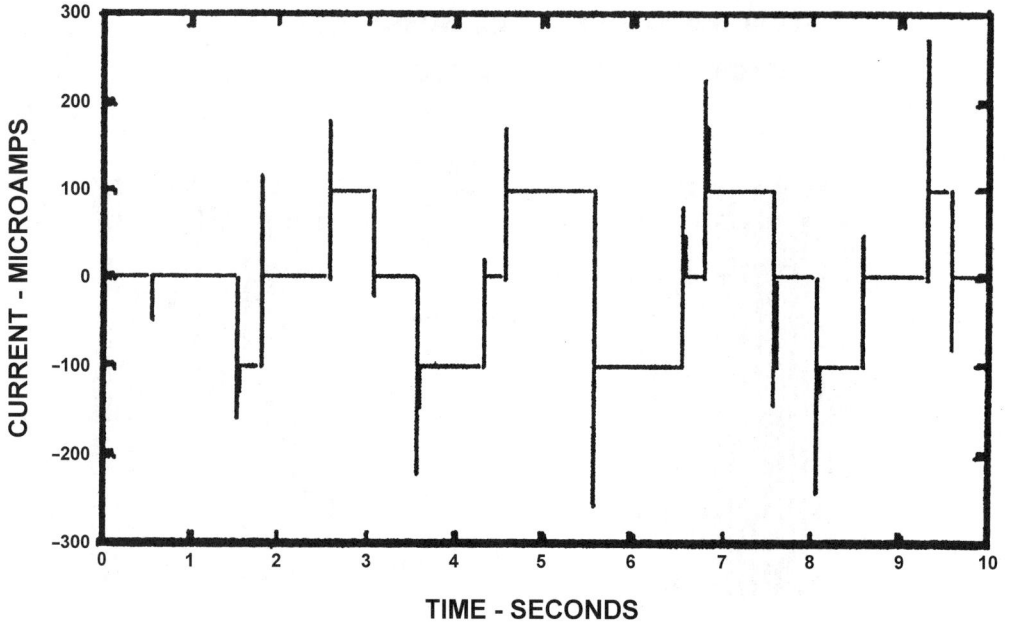

Figure 19 Electrical pulse sequence used in the α-Stim 100 device. The pulses are bipolar with repetition rates of 0.5, 1.5, and 100 Hz, and currents range from 10 to 600 μA. The high-frequency spikes at the leading and falling edges of each pulse, often seen when pulses are switched on and off rapidly, are consequences of the electronics. In this device they are part of the waveform delivered to the patient.

finds manufacturers making medical claims for a specific device without properly defining the electromagnetic characteristics of the device. Given the great variability in device design that we have shown, it is clear that the waveforms employed must be carefully delineated.

GLOSSARY

Angular frequency. Usually symbolized as Greek letter ω. Related to linear frequency f through the formula $\omega = 2\pi f$. measured in terms of rad/s (radians per second).

Athermal signal. Same as nonthermal signal.

Beat(s). The new frequency that results from adding two sine wave signals of equal amplitude but slightly different frequencies. Equal to the difference between the two original frequencies. Sometimes called the *interference frequency* or *AC interferential frequency*.

Bipolar signal. Signal composed of both positive and negative components. Sometimes called *biphasic* signal.

CES. Cranial electrical stimulation.

CMF. Combined magnetic field, formed by adding DC magnetic field to sinusoidal magnetic signal. Same as ICR when appropriate values of DC magnetic field and AC magnetic frequency are used.

Constant current amplifier. Electronic circuit that automatically adjusts the output voltage of a power supply to maintain a constant current.

Current density. Electrical current per unit cross-sectional area, measured, for example, in terms of microamperes per centimeter squared ($\mu A/cm^2$).

Duty cycle. Measure of the energy supplied by a repetitive signal over a given length of time. Dependent on the intensity of the pulsed signal and the interval between successive cycles.

ECT. Electroconvulsive therapy.

Electric field. Measure of the electric field intensity, often symbolized as *E* and specified in terms of V/cm or V/m.

Electrostatic field. A static electric field.

EMF. Two meanings: electromagnetic field, also (less correct) electromotive force, an older term for electric potential difference. Confusion follows from Faraday's law of induction, which says that a changing magnetic field (or EMF) will induce an electromotive force in an electrical conductor.

Fall time. Time interval over which pulsed signal falls to zero from its maximum value.

Faraday's law of induction. A changing magnetic field always creates an electrical potential difference. If this happens in an electrically conducting material, a current density will occur within the conducting material.

Giga. Prefix meaning one billion times, or 10^9 times larger, as in gigahertz, or GHz.

GMF. The geomagnetic field.

ICR. Ion cyclotron resonance.

Helmholtz coil. Parallel array of two circular coils where the separation between the coils is equal to the coil radius. Commonly used to provide uniformity of field at the center of the array along its axis.

Hertz (Hz). Measurement unit for frequency of sine waves. Appears often with prefix, e.g., kHz, MHz, GHz.

Kilo. Prefix indicating a factor of 1000 (10^3) larger, as in kV, kG, and kHz.

Magnetic gradient. A description of how much the magnetic field changes in any one direction, measured, for example, in terms of micro tesla per meter ($\mu T/m$).

Magnetostatic field. A static magnetic field.

Mega. Prefix meaning one million times (10^6) larger, as in MHz.

Micro. Written as Greek letter μ. Commonly used prefix in electromagnetic measurements, same as one-millionth, or 10^{-6}, e.g., μT, μA, μV. In biology, 1 μm (1 micron) is often used as a measure of distance.

Milli. Prefix in electromagnetic measurements. Equals one-thousandth (10^{-3}), e.g., mT, mV, mA.

Modulated signal. Result of adding two sinusoidal signals, usually with very different amplitudes. The lower frequency signal is the modulation signal, and the higher frequency signal is the carrier signal.

Monopolar signal. Signal which is always positive. Sometimes called *monophasic signal.*

Nano. Prefix meaning one billionth, or 10^{-9}, times smaller, as in nV, nA, and nT.

Noise. Unplanned variation in a signal that can result from random perturbations, e.g., in electronic circuitry, thermal effects.

Nonthermal signal. Signal that does not result in increase temperature within tissue.

Observable. Parameter used as a measure of a physical state, e.g., voltage, current, magnetic field.

Oscillatory. Same as periodic.

Parallel plate capacitor. Pair of parallel electrical conducting plates in which the diameter of each plate is much greater than the separation between the plates. Used to obtain highly uniform electric field between the plates.

PMF. Pulsed magnetic field. Same as PEMF.

Peak value. Maximum amplitude of sinusoidal signal.

Peak-to-peak value. Total swing in signal intensity, measured from negative minimum of sine wave to maximum positive, or simply twice the peak value.

Pico. Prefix meaning one million million times (10^{-12}) smaller, as in pV, pA, pT.

Pulsatile. Same as pulsed.

Pulse height. Maximum amplitude of pulse.

Pulse train. Sequence of pulses in one cycle. Same as pulse burst.

Pulse width. Interval of time o ver which a single pulse remains at its maximum value.

Rectified signal. Modified sine wave, always positive, either as *half-wave rectification*, lacking any negative components in wave shape, or *full-wave rectification*, with negative components of the original sine wave, flipped into the positive region.

Repetition rate. The frequency, in cycles per second, with which a periodic signal repeats itself. For a sinusoidal signal it is the same as the linear frequency. Usually applied to pulses and often given in Hz.

Rise time. Time interval over which a pulsed signal rises to its maximum value.

rms value. Root-mean-square of maximum intensity of sinusoidal signal. Numerical value equals 0.7071 times the maximum amplitude of sine wave signal. Same as effective (eff) value. With care, can also be applied to pulsed signals.

rTMS. Rapid transcranial magnetic stimulation.

Sawtooth signal. Waveform with shape similar to saw blade, either rising slowly to a maximum and falling rapidly or rising to a point slowly and than falling slowly from the point. Same as flyback waveform used in television raster return circuits.

Signature. Same as waveform.

Solenoid. Closely wound coil on long cylinder that provides excellent uniformity of field within the cylinder.

Symmetric bipolar signal. Bipolar signal that is equally positive and negative.

Static field. Electric or magnetic field that does not change in time.

TENS. Transcutaneous electrical nerve stimulation.

Thermal signal. Signal that is sufficiently energetic to measurably increase temperature within tissue.

Transient. A single pulse, usually nondescript and the result of a switching problem or unexplained perturbation such as a temporary discontinuity or nearby lightning stroke.

Uniform field. Electric or magnetic field that is everywhere within a given region constant in direction and intensity.

REFERENCES

1. Rasmussen KG, Sampson SM, Rummans TA. Electroconvulsive therapy and newer modalities for the treatment of medication-refractory mental illness. Mayo Clin Prov 2002; 77:552–556.

2. Barker AT, Freeston IL, Jalinous R, Jarrett JA. Non-invasive stimulation of motor pathways within the brain using time-varying magnetic fields. Electroencephalog Clin Neurophysiol 1985; 61:S245.
3. Lavine LS, Lustrin I, Shamos MH, Rinaldi RA, Liboff AR. Electric enhancement of bone healing. Science 1972; 175:1118–1121.
4. Bassett CAL, Pawluk RJ, Pilla AA. Acceleration of fracture repair by electromagnetic fields: a surgically non-invasive method. In: Liboff AR, Rinaldi RA, eds. Electrically Mediated Growth Mechanisms in Living Systems. Ann NY Acad Sci 1974; 238:242–262.
5. Gmitrov J, Ohkubo C. Artificial static and geomagnetic field interrelated impact on cardio-vascular regulation. Bioelectromagnetics 2002; 23:329–338.
6. Engstrom S, Markov MS, McLean MJ, Holcomb RR, Markov JM. Effects of nonuniform static magnetic fields on the rate of myosin phosphorylation. Bioelectromagnetics 2002; 23:475–479.
7. Liboff AR. Geomagnetic cyclotron resonance in living cells. J Biol Physics 1985; 13:99–102.
8. Williams CD, Markov MS. Therapeutic electromagnetic field effects on angiogenesis during tumor growth: a pilot study in mice. Electro-MagnetoBiology 2001; 20:323–329.
9. Liss S, Liss B. Physiological and therapeutic effects of high frequency pulses. Integrative Physiol Behavioral Sci 1996; 31:88–94.
10. Reite M, Higgs L, Lebet J-P, Barbault A, Rossel C, Kuster N, Amato D, Dafni U, Pasche B. Sleep inducing effect of low energy emission therapy. Bioelectromagnetics 1994; 15:67–76.
11. Schwartz RG. Electric sympathetic block: current theoretical concepts and clinical results. J Back Muscoloskeletal Rehab 1998; 10:31–46.
12. Richards TL, Lappin MS, Acosta-urquidi J, Kraft GH, Heide AC, Lawrie FW, Merrill TE, Melton GB, Cunningham CA. Double-blind study of pulsing magnetic field effects on multiple sclerosis. J Alternative Complementary Medicine 1997; 3:21–29.
13. Trock DH, Bollet AJ, Dyer RH Jr, Fielding LP, Markoll RA. A double-blind trial of the clinical effects of pulsed electromagnetic fields in osteoarthritis. J Rheum 1993; 20:456–460.
14. Hedenius P, Odeblad E, Wahlstrom L. Some preliminary investigations on the therapeutic effect of pulsed short waves in intermittent claudication. Current Therapeutic Res 1966; 8:317–321.
15. Kirsch DL, Smith RB. The use of cranial magnetic stimulation in the management of chronic pain: a review. Neurorehabilitation 2000; 14:85–94.

3

Magnetic Field Generation and Dosimetry

Stefan Engström

Vanderbilt University Medical Center, Department of Neurology, Nashville, Tennessee, U.S.A.

The physical basis of biologically significant magnetic fields is reviewed. Emphasis is placed on the importance of dosimetry issues such as how to describe, measure, and compute the three-dimensional structure of magnetic fields, particularly at their target sites.

I. INTRODUCTION

Magnetic fields are used in biological experiments and for therapeutic interventions. We need well-defined ways to generate and to characterize these exposures. This task is complicated by time-varying fields, and it becomes challenging when the fields vary in space.

This chapter will discuss various ways of producing magnetic fields. I will consider static and low-frequency time-varying magnetic field exposures. Electric fields are mentioned only inasmuch as they are induced by these magnetic fields.

Dosimetry issues will be brought up along the way—this includes appropriate ways to describe a particular field situation with complete information so that measures of action can be properly evaluated after the fact. Extra care will be paid to the generation of fields with permanent magnets where the issue of dosimetry and field penetration is a poorly defined subject when addressed at all in the current literature on magnetic field therapy.

Magnetic fields can be generated by electric currents or by permanent magnets. Neither of these sources are significantly affected by external fields and individual components are therefore directly additive (considering each vector component independently) for moderate field strengths. When ferromagnetic materials are brought into the picture the problem becomes much more difficult and numerical models usually become necessary for anything but trivial geometries.

It is safe to say that magnetic fields of relatively modest amplitudes can affect biology, but the physical mechanism by which this happens is far from clear. There is experimental evidence supporting the following:

1. Direct detection of magnetic fields is possible, with some very strong evidence in the field of animal navigation using magnetic cues (1,2).
2. Magnetically induced electric fields are involved in some examples of biological effects of time-varying magnetic fields (3,4).
3. Gradient properties of magnetic fields are relevant for the basic mechanisms at work in some experiments (5,6).

There is partial theoretical support for how each of these exposure modalities could have a biological impact, but the theoretical ideas that have scientific consensus are limited to relatively high fields and gradients (7) with a few notable exceptions (8). In a given magnetic field experiment, it is often the case that more than one of these metrics provide a possible explanation. This highlights the importance of the task of adequately describing the field so that alternative theoretical explanations may be considered after the fact.

The term *dosimetry* is sometimes used in the consideration of specific physical mechanisms, but in this paper it only carries the meaning of a physical description of the field. Similarly, *electromagnetic fields* carry different meanings. Here the term is simply used to describe magnetic fields generated with electric current. Electromagnetic fields is also used to characterize the interwoven character of electric and magnetic phenomena, but this becomes relevant only for radiation fields at distances more than a wavelength away from the field source. This is not the case for the low frequencies and static fields considered here and magnetic fields and electric fields can safely be considered in separation.

II. ELECTROMAGNETIC FIELDS

The Ampère-Laplace law (9) dictates the field from a current flowing in an arbitrarily shaped closed loop [Fig. 1, Eq. (1)]. Usually one uses circular or square coils whose symmetry allows for the generation of relatively homogenous magnetic fields and simplification of the

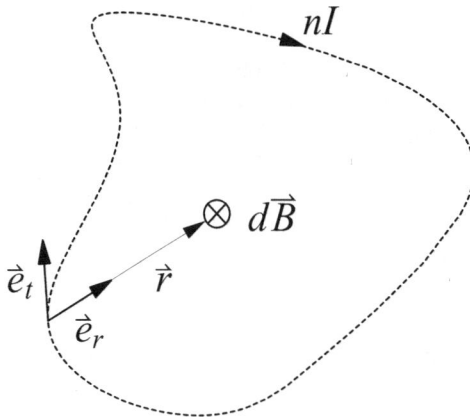

Figure 1 Geometry of the Ampère-Laplace law for calculating magnetic field induced by a current loop. $\vec{r}$ is a vector from an integration point along the loop to the field point where we are interested in the value of the resulting field at the point marked with $\otimes$ (denoting that the field vector points out of the paper). $\vec{e}_v$ and $\vec{e}_t$ are unit vectors along $\vec{r}$ and tangential to the loop, respectively.

detailed field calculation. Other than geometry, it is the amount of current flowing in a given path that determines the amplitude of the resulting field. A coil has many turns of a wire, and the determining parameter for coil arrangements becomes *ampere-turns*, the current in the coil multiplied with the number of turns of the wire [nI in Fig. 1 and Eq. (1)]:

$$\vec{B} = \frac{\mu_0 nI}{4\pi} \oint \frac{\vec{r} \times \vec{e}_r}{r^2} \, dl \tag{1}$$

Figure 1 illustrates this geometry and defines the variables of Eq. (1). Figures 2 and 3 show three current configurations which produce fields that drop off increasingly rapidly with distance from the source. μ_0 in these formulas is the permeability of vacuum ($4\pi \times 10^{-7}$ Vs/Am); this value is a useful approximation for air as well as tissue as long as there are no ferromagnetic materials involved. All formulas given here use SI units.

1. The field at a distance x from a long, straight conductor is (Fig. 2a):

   $$B_a = \frac{\mu_0}{2\pi} \frac{I}{x} \tag{2a}$$

   where is I is the current in the conductor. This is the so-called Biot-Savart formula (the loop is assumed to be closed at infinity).

2. If the wire has a parallel return path, the field is significantly reduced at some distance from the conductor (Fig. 2b). The field decreases with the inverse of the square of the distance to the wire—some distance from the wire the field is a factor δ/x of the corresponding field from a single wire, where δ is the separation of the two wires:

   $$B_b = \frac{\mu_0}{\pi} \frac{2\delta I}{4x^2 - \delta^2} \tag{2b}$$

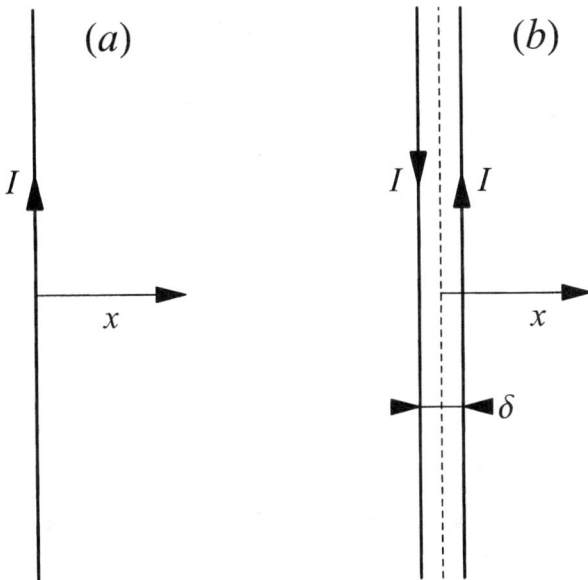

Figure 2 (a) The amplitude of the magnetic field encircling a current-carrying long wire at a distance x from the wire is inversely proportional to x. (b) If the current has a parallel return path separated a distance δ from the original wire, the field at x is reduced by a factor δ/x when x is sufficiently large compared to δ.

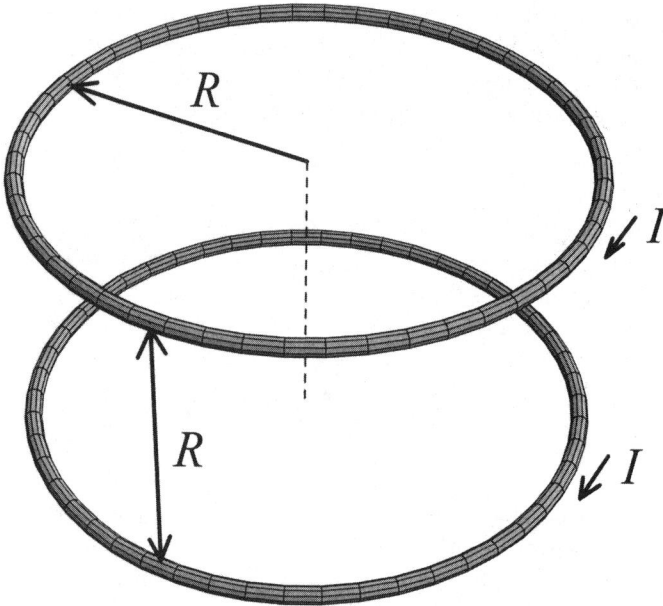

Figure 3 Helmholtz coil configuration. When two concentric circular coils are separated by a distance equal to the coil radius, we obtain a volume of homogenous magnetic field in the center of the exposure system because the gradients from the two loops tend to cancel each other in that region.

3. In laboratory exposure applications we try to maximize the field by using many turns in a localized volume. The Helmholtz coil is a tried-and-true exposure configuration for generating relatively homogenous fields in the center of the two coils (Fig. 3). At a distance from the coil pair, the field is similar to that of an isolated magnetic dipole (as is the case for all localized current sources) with the field decreasing as the inverse of the cube of the distance to the source.

While configuration (3) is used to produce homogeneous field exposures for experimentation one can increase the homogenous volume with multiple square coils with carefully selected geometry and currents (10,11). The homogeneity of the field is usually described as a volume that has field values within (say) 5% of the flux density in the center of the volume.

III. PERMANENT MAGNETS

Permanent magnets provide good options for therapeutic delivery of magnetic field exposures. No power source is needed to generate the magnetic field, and quite strong fields can be produced by magnets manufactured from neodymium-iron-boron or rare-earth–cobalt alloys. It is difficult to produce large volumes of homogeneous fields with off-the-shelf permanent magnets. However, it may be that magnetic field gradients are part of the answer to how magnetic fields are helpful in therapy and that it makes good sense to use permanent magnets in medical applications of static fields for this reason.

The dosimetry for exposures used in studies of therapeutic uses of permanent magnets in the literature is generally very rudimentary—usually the surface field strength of the magnet is reported and not much else. Ideally, the field and gradient distributions in the target tissue should be characterized. As the examples below will demonstrate, these amplitudes fall off very rapidly with distance from the magnet and great precision knowing the distance to the target volume is required if the exposures are to be at all consistent. The following discussion addresses four methods to calculate the static fields generated by permanent magnets.

A. Dipole Approximation

Isolated single magnets can be approximated with mathematical magnetic dipoles, i.e., objects with no spatial extent and defined by their location, a magnetic moment, and its orientation in space. This approximation becomes acceptable at a large enough distance away from the magnet, or in fact from any localized current source (9). For a single magnetic dipole $\vec{m}$, the absolute magnetic field at a distance r is:

$$B = \frac{\mu_0}{4\pi} \frac{m}{r^3} \sqrt{1 + 3\cos^2\theta} \tag{3}$$

where θ is the angle between the magnetic dipole and the vector $\vec{r}$. As an example (cf. Fig. 4) of this type of model, we examine the rate at which the field drops off with distance for a single magnetic dipole at the origin (Fig. 4a); a pair of antiparallel dipoles separated by a unit distance (Fig. 4b); four dipoles arranged in a square with alternating polarities (Fig. 4c).

As predicted from Eq. (3), the field decreases as the inverse third power of distance for a single dipole (Fig. 4a and 5). A popular therapeutic magnet is the configuration seen in Fig. 4b. Having more than one magnetic pole face the skin at treatment in this way is commonly called *bipolar* or *multipolar*. This is an unfortunate terminology since bipolar has connotations in psychiatry and with audiophiles, and worse, dipole and multipole have related but different meanings in physics. Far away from configuration (b) the dipole moment is zero and the next term is a quadrupole moment which decreases in field strength even more rapidly than (a) (see Fig. 5). The last considered configuration (c) is a rudimentary representation of the MagnaBloc therapeutic device. Here the quadrupole moment is also canceled and the field decline is further accelerated with distance.

B. Equivalent Magnetic Surface Charges

Permanent magnets that are uniformly magnetized can be mathematically reduced to equivalent magnetic surface charges on the pole faces (9). This reduces the problem of integrating the resulting field from the magnet from a volume magnetization to that of the two end surfaces. This is useful when there is a need to calculate the field near the magnet.

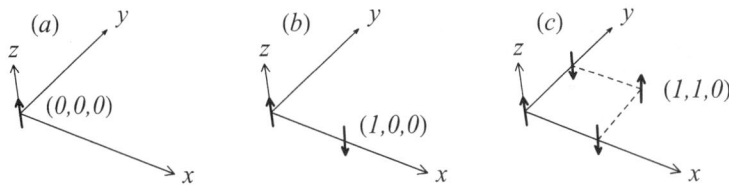

Figure 4 Magnetic dipole geometries discussed in the text. (a) A single dipole at the origin, oriented along the z axis. The field from the dipole falls off as $1/r^3$. (b) When two opposing poles are placed next to each other in the xy plane, the field amplitude drops off more rapidly at distances large compared to the separation of the dipoles. (c) A configuration corresponding to the therapeutic device MagnaBloc. The four dipoles cancel dipole and quadrupole moments at large distances from the magnets, and the field drops off even more rapidly.

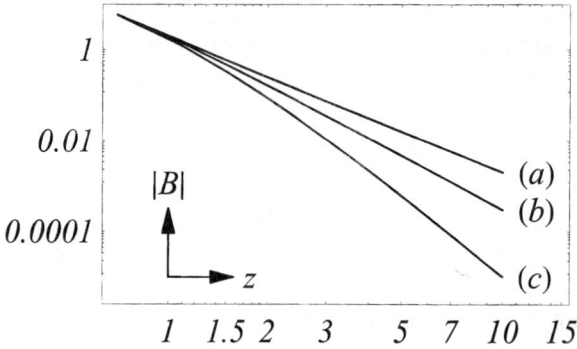

Figure 5 Rate of decline in the magnetic field amplitude ($|B|$) with distance z from the origin of the systems shown in Fig. 4. The length scale corresponds to the separation between the dipoles in Fig. 4, and the field units are arbitrary. In order to model a system of one, two, or four magnets as shown, one would scale the appropriate curve to some measurement of the field since the appropriate equivalent model dipole moment would depend on the strength and size of the constituent magnets.

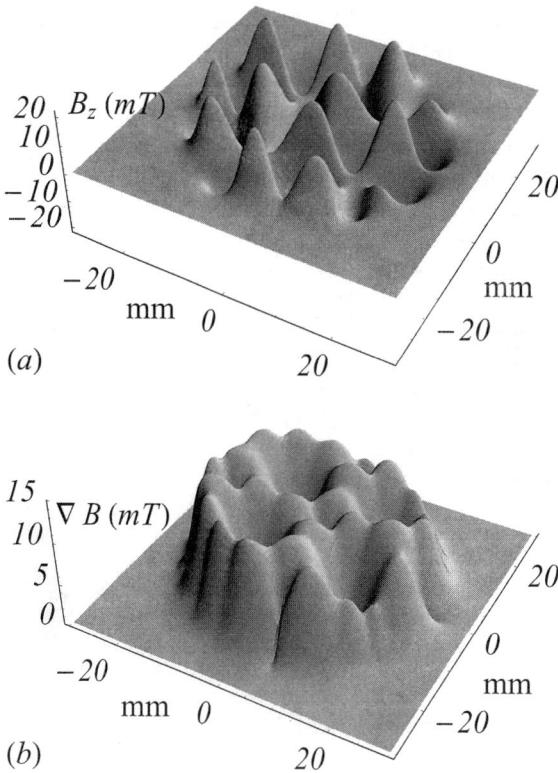

Figure 6 (a) A planar magnetic field scan of the normal component (B_z) of a therapeutic magnetic device produced by Nikken. With this information one can calculate all details of the magnetic field—field components as well as all gradient properties. (b) As an example, the absolute value of the gradient of the field magnitude near the surface of the same device calculated by the method of field continuation (12).

C. Field Measurement and Continuation

If the normal component of the field is measured with good resolution and extent in a plane, everything we need to know about the field above this plane can be calculated with relative ease, regardless of the actual sources that contribute to the field below the measured plane (12). We have utilized this extensively in calculating detailed volume dosimetry for magnetic field exposures (6). Figure 6 shows an example of a model that would be difficult to evaluate with sufficient resolution with other methods.

Another use of this method is to calculate field penetration dosimetry. One of the shortcomings of using permanent magnets for tissue treatment is that the field drops off rather rapidly as we have seen above. Figure 7 shows one way to quantify this aspect of therapeutic exposures.

D. Finite Element Methods

A finite element analysis of a particular configuration is always an option if the methods above are inadequate. This can happen when the geometry is complex or simply by the presence of ferromagnetic materials. High resolution is available with limited computational resources if there is symmetry in the problem. Figure 8 shows flux lines in an axisymmetric placebo device designed to produce an easily detectable field on one side (to protect experimental masking) and a low level field for sham exposure on the other side.

IV. INDUCED ELECTRIC FIELDS AND CURRENTS

Time-varying magnetic fields as well as motion in a magnetic field will induce electric fields and therefore currents in conductive materials. Electric fields and currents are the quantities

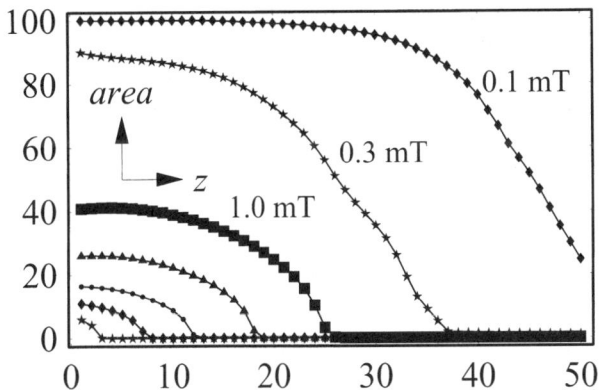

Figure 7 Contours of field penetration from the therapeutic magnetic device MagnaBloc. The contours show how large an area is covered with fields at least that large for a range of field amplitudes (0.1 mT, 0.3 mT, 1.0 mT, etc.) at a given distance from the device. As an example, we can see that in a plane 30 mm away from the device an area of approximately 35 cm^2 experiences a field larger than 0.3 mT. We can also see that 25 mm away from the device there is no exposure exceeding 1.0 mT. The contours in the lower left continue the series with (from right to left) 3.0 mT, 10 mT, 30 mT, and 100 mT.

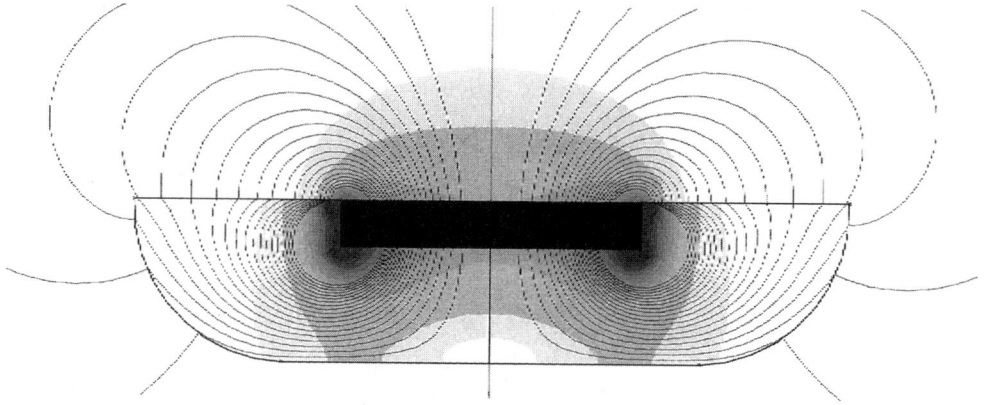

Figure 8 A cross section of a cylindrically symmetric finite element model of a magnetic placebo (sham) device. The outline is a steel casing holding a small NdFeB magnet (black), and the flux lines show how the ferromagnetic material turns the magnetic flux lines away from the bottom of the device. This allows an easily detectable field on the top side, while the bottom (treatment) side has field levels reduced by a factor 50–100. This design is one attempt to thwart inquisitive subjects in a clinical study from deducing whether they belong to the exposed or to the control group.

that describe much of our knowledge about electromagnetic signaling in biology. For this reason it is worthwhile to consider the possibility that magnetic fields act on the body through induced electric fields as opposed to through physical detectors that sense the magnetic field directly (13).

The exact field distribution in real-life situations usually requires complex solutions to Maxwell's equations, but there are two useful exact results that will provide important information about the magnitudes of the induced fields.

The force on a charge moving in a magnetic field, $\vec{F} = q\vec{v} \times \vec{B}$, can be derived from a Lorentz transformation between two frames moving at relative velocity $\vec{v}$. In this view the magnetic field $\vec{B}$ in the rest frame causes an additional electric field of magnitude $\vec{v} \times \vec{B}$ in the moving frame. This force is therefore really an electric field caused by the relative motion and generally applicable before we start considering what the system's response to this field might be.

Another exact relation is Faraday's law which states that

$$\oint_C \vec{E} \cdot \vec{dl} = -\frac{d}{dt} \int_s \vec{B} \cdot \hat{n} \, dS \tag{4}$$

The integral of the electric field ($\vec{E}$) along some closed path (C) equals the time derivative of the area integral of the magnetic field component ($\vec{B} \cdot \hat{n}$) normal to a surface S bounded by the path C. This means that we can always estimate the average field in a loop by measuring how the magnetic flux is changing inside that loop. Note that we can have a zero average even if there are fields present that exactly cancel each other over the loop, but a nonzero average indicates that a current must flow if the loop runs through a conductive medium. The time derivative in the right-hand-side of Eq. 4 considers the whole integral; so electric fields can be induced if either the field (B) or the geometry changes. The geometry changes if the loop changes size, orientation, or position in the field (14).

A. Induced Currents in a Time-Varying Field.

This is the case considered for much of the work on time-varying and especially in research on biological effects of power-frequency fields. The maximally induced average electric field is determined largely by the amplitude and frequency of the applied magnetic field and by the largest size loop that can fit inside the exposed medium. In some cases symmetry allows Eq. (4) to be used effectively, but even slight deviations from the simple cases complicate the solution (15), and in most realistic situations numerical methods are the only methods to provide detailed answers (16).

B. Motion in a Magnetic Field

Consider a person moving with velocity $\bar{v}$ perpendicular to the earth's magnetic field. According to the discussion above, an electric field is produced in the body but no current flows since there are no closure of the electric circuit. What happens is the following: Charged particles experiences the Lorentz force and become somewhat displaced as the body is accelerated, but they find a new equilibrium, and at constant velocity no currents flow.

It is a different story if the body is rotating in the field about an axis that is not collinear with the field. Faraday's law [Eq. (4)] tells us that in this case the integrated flux through some loop oscillates with the same frequency of the rotation and the average induced electric field will show the same variation as if it had seen a sinusoidal time-varying field.

Translation can induce a net electric field in our loop if we move in a gradient field since it does not matter how the change in flux density integrated over the loop surface changes.

V. GRADIENT MAGNETIC FIELDS

Magnetic fields are vector quantities meaning that we need three independent values to describe their instantaneous properties. Three Cartesian components or one amplitude and two directions provide sufficient information to describe its spatial character.

Magnetic field gradients describe how the flux density vector components vary in space implying that three spatial derivatives of three vector components ($3 \times 3 = 9$ components) are required to describe the field. If we are considering the magnetic field in a source-free region the field can be derived from a magnetic scalar potential, and we are left with six independent components. This number is further reduced by one by another constraint from Maxwell's equations: $\nabla \cdot \bar{B} = 0$.

Another gradient measure is describing how the field amplitude varies by taking the gradient of the absolute magnitude of the flux density: ∇B. It should be noted that this is not a complete description of the gradient field since different fields could conceivably produce the same gradient measure (see Fig. 6 for an example of this type of metric).

Yet another way to express gradients is one that our research group at Vanderbilt has found to have predictive power for experiments in our laboratory—we divide the gradient components into parts parallel and perpendicular to the local field vector. This description is useful if one expects a spatially isotropic distribution of the biological detectors that sense the field and/or its gradients. If they are isotropic, then the absolute field conveys all the necessary mechanistic information instead of the usual three components of the field vector. Similarly, only the two gradient components above are needed to completely describe the gradient aspect of the system if the isotropy assumption holds.

VI. FIELD SUPRESSION

Sometimes it is of interest to reduce the level of magnetic field exposure:

    1. Field nulling or shielding: In conducting a biological experiment it is often essential to compare results to a sample which is exposed to no field or to a controlled field level. For fields of similar magnitude (or smaller) to that of the earth's magnetic field, it is essential to measure and document the local field. Unless the geomagnetic field is part of the experimental hypothesis, it might even be a good idea to remove it altogether from the experiment. This can be achieved by compensatory coils that generate a field of equal magnitude but oriented in the opposite direction, or one can use μ-metal enclosures in which to perform the experiments. μ-Metal is an alloy with very high magnetic permeability so that the field lines tend to follow the μ-metal shell and not enter the enclosed volume. Interestingly, nulling the field with a μ-metal enclosure appears to have biological consequences as well (17), although the physical mechanism is unclear at this point.

    2. Somebody concerned with exposure from magnetic fields generated as a side effect of using electric power might want to find ways to reduce this exposure. Shielding the field is rarely a practical solution for this purpose. Better solutions involve using distance (magnetic fields drop off rapidly with distance to the source) and by solving improper wiring and grounding problems: if a current-carrying wire has its return current in a different path, then the examples in Fig. 2 shows us how to mitigate the situation by running the return current along the same path.

    3. If we are studying the therapeutic effects of devices constructed from permanent magnets, it is important to use a sham, or placebo, device that has a significantly different field character than the device under study. However, a subject in such a study is likely to try to divine if he is the subject of the active or the placebo treatment; so it becomes relevant to provide an ineffective device that still exhibits some detectable form of magnetism. (See Fig. 8 for an example.)

VII. CONCLUSIONS

Since the physical transduction mechanism responsible for magnetic field effects in biology remains elusive, it is essential to completely characterize the field exposures so that alternative explanations can be reviewed in the future.

    The bulk of carefully controlled work on the effects of magnetic fields has considered static or low-frequency spatially uniform fields. The dosimetry issues for these types of studies have been adequately addressed in the literature (11), and most papers in these topics report adequate dosimetry for replication: generation of the field, types of coils, field intensity, degree of spatial uniformity, frequency or waveform of the applied field, exposure duration, and how sham conditions were maintained and masked.

    This level of control has been generally lacking from studies of the effects of permanent magnets, and a different set of priorities has to be observed as characterizing the spatial variation becomes our primary concern. In a gradient field some measure of the distribution of field magnitudes become necessary and careful control of the relative positioning of the exposure device and target becomes crucial since the field varies so strongly in the vicinity of a permanent magnet. Practically, one needs to specify the magnets carefully (e.g., type or composition, size, the manufacturer's rating, surface magnetic field). An effort should be made to calculate an average field distribution in the target; a minimum would be an average and standard deviation of the absolute field distribution. As mentioned above, a tricky issue in clinical studies is how sham controls are executed—it is important that the study subjects are unable to differentiate between field and sham treatments.

REFERENCES

1. Phillips JB. Magnetic Navigation. J Theor Biol 1996; 380:309–319.
2. Lohmann KJ, Hester JT, Lohmann CMF. Long-distance navigation in sea turtles. Ethology Ecology Evolution 1999; 11(1):1–23.
3. DiCarlo AL, Mullins JM, Litovitz TA. Thresholds for electromagnetic field-induced hypoxia protection: evidence for a primary electric field effect. Bioelectrochemistry 2000; 52:9–16.
4. Liburdy RP. Calcium signaling in lymphocytes and ELF fields. Evidence for an electric field metric and a site of interaction involving the calcium ion channel. Febs Lett 1992; 301:53–59.
5. McLean MJ, Holcomb RR, Wamil AW, Pickett JD. Blockade of sensory neuron action potentials by a static magnetic-field in the 10 mT range. Bioelectromagnetics 1995; 16:20–32.
6. Engström S, Markov MS, McLean MJ, Holcomb RR, Markov JM. Effects of non-uniform static magnetic fields on the rate of myosin phosphorylation. Bioelectromagnetics 2002; 23:475–479.
7. Adair RK. Static and low-frequency magnetic field effects: health risks and therapies. Rep Prog Phys 2000; 63:415–454.
8. Timmel CR, Cintolesi F, Brocklehurst B, Hore PJ. Model calculations of magnetic field effects on the recombination reactions of radicals with anisotropic hyperfine interactions. Chem Phys Lett 2001; 334:387–395.
9. Jackson JD. Classical Electrodynamics. 3rd ed. New York: Wiley, 1999.
10. Merritt R, Purcell C, Stroink G. Uniform magnetic field produced by three, four, and five square coils. Rev Sci Instrum 1983; 54:879–882.
11. Misakian M, Sheppard AR, Krause D, Frazier ME, Miller DL. Biological, physical, and electrical parameters for in-vitro studies with ELF magnetic and electric-fields—a primer. Bioelectromagnetics Suppl 1993; 2:1–73.
12. Engström S. A Green function method for calculating properties of static magnetic fields. Bioelectromagnetics 2001; 22:511–518.
13. Engström S, Fitzsimmons R. Five hypotheses to examine the nature of magnetic field transduction in biological systems. Bioelectromagnetics 1999; 20:423–430.
14. Ptitsyna NG, Villoresi G, Dorman LI, Iucci N, Tyasto MI. Natural and man-made low-frequency magnetic fields as a potential health hazard. Physics–Uspekhi 1998; 41:687–709.
15. McLeod BR, Pilla AA, Sampsel MW. Electromagnetic-fields induced by helmholtz aiding coils inside saline-filled boundaries. Bioelectromagnetics 1983; 4:357–370.
16. Gandhi OP, Kang G, Wu D, Lazzi G. Currents induced in anatomic models of the human for uniform and nonuniform power frequency magnetic fields. Bioelectromagnetics 2001; 22:112–121.
17. Choleris E, Del Seppia C, Thomas AW, Luschi P, Ghione S, Moran GR, Prato FS. Shielding, but not zeroing of the ambient magnetic field reduces stress-induced analgesia in mice. Proc Royal Soc London Series B Biolog 2002; 269:193–201.

4

Image-Guided Electromagnetic Therapy

Frank S. Prato

*Lawson Health Research Institute and University of Western Ontario,
London, Ontario, Canada*

Medical imagery techniques facilitate the targeting of electromagnetic therapies to achieve more precise results and to evaluate their efficacy more accurately. These modalities include molecular imaging, mapping endogenous electromagnetic activity (particularly in the heart and brain), multi-modality image integration, and image-guided therapy.

I. INTRODUCTION

Today (2002) we are at a threshold for the acceptance of electromagnetic therapy as a clinically accepted form of therapy for such diverse diseases as unipolar depression, Parkinson's disease, and sleep disorders and the treatment of debilitating chronic and acute pain. This threshold is high because (1) electromagnetic field therapy is suspect because of its present relegation to the alternative medicine market, (2) electromagnetic field therapy has been practiced with questionable spcificity where there is often a claim that one exposure regime cures all, and (3) contemporary medicine only accepts new methods after extensive testing often needing extensive clinical trials. For example, in the well-established and accepted methods of drug therapy, a new pharmaceutical to reduce the incidence of stroke recently required testing in over 6600 patients who were each followed for two years (1). Such trials are very expensive and number of patients large because the incremental improvement in outcome is small compared to existing therapy.

For electromagnetic therapy to scale this threshold we need applications that have significant beneficial effects and that are targeted to specific clinical problems. This requires specific delivery of physical therapy with a pronounced and specific outcome measure. It is the thesis of this chapter that medical imaging, including present and future forms, will guide and target electromagnetic therapy so that it is very effective. Medical imaging will provide the means by which electromagnetic therapy (1) can be targeted to specific medical problems and (2) can be used to objectively evaluate the effectiveness of that therapy. Hence image-guided electromagnetic therapy will be the decisive approach to ensure that electromagnetic therapy becomes clinically accepted.

In the rest of this chapter I will summarize the present and future capability of medical imaging, summarize the future potential of electromagnetic field therapy, and provide examples of present and predicted future forms of image-guided electromagnetic field therapy.

II. MEDICAL IMAGING: PRESENT AND RESEARCH DIRECTIONS

Contemporary imaging research can be classified into four areas: molecular imaging, imaging or mapping of endogenous electromagnetic activity primarily in the heart and the brain, multimodality image integration, and image-guided therapy.

A. Molecular Imaging

Molecular imaging involves both the development of new imaging methods and the enhancement of existing methods. Much of this development has been ratified by the need of nondestructive small animal imaging to follow phenotypic manifestations of gene and cell therapies. Some of these methods, such as optical imaging (2), are limited to the small animal domain, whereas others like positron emission tomography (PET) (3) and to a lesser extent magnetic resonance imaging (MRI) (4) are scalable to the adult human. Of particular interest to the future of electromagnetic therapy are the current developments in PET. PET imaging involves the use of organic compounds labeled with a radioactive nucleus that emits positrons. Since the radioactive nuclei are isotopes of carbon, nitrogen, oxygen, and fluorine, any naturally occurring compound can be labeled (5). This allows the creation of images, which are functional, and biochemical maps of the human body. Hence, one can image parameters such as blood flow, glucose metabolism, or dopamine receptor densities in patients suffering from diseases like depressioin, dementia, or schizophrenia. In the study of pain, opioid receptor distribution activity and concentration can be imaged (6–11).

In the future it may be possile to use molecular imaging to determine exactly when a particular gene is turned on using a *reporter gene* (3). (A reporter gene is one that "reports" by changing the image when a particular biochemical event occurs.) Hence, if electro-magnetic fields were to "turn on" a particular gene, then that event could be "imaged" noninvasively in a human.

B. Endogenous Electromagnetic Activity

Of particular interest for electromagnetic therapy is the mapping of endogenous electro-magnetic activity in the brain. There are two basic approaches. One is to image the cortical activity in the brain using an array (between 16 and 128) of electrical detectors placed over the skull. The electroencephalogram (EEG) from each of the array of detectors is then used to show the electrical activity as a function of the time as it evolves on the brain surface (the brain cortex). This technology is limited to measuring the electrical activity in the cortex unless electrodes are placed directly into deeper brain regions as is clinically done to identify the epileptic focus in some patients (12). However, here we are only interested in essentially non-invasive imaging methods.

To get to deeper brain structures magnetoencephalography (MEG) must be used (12). In this method the EEG electrodes are replaced by MEG detectors known as SQUIDs, or superconducting quantum interference devices (13,14). However, to identify the actual magnetic dipoles within the brain has been a difficult mathematical problem. This in general has been solved by reducing the number of allowed dipoles to 6 or less and assuming that they correspond to activated regions of the brain previously identified by other imaging methods such as fMRI (15,12). The mapping of endogenous electromagnetic fields is of considerable interest as it may be that exposure to exogenous sources may affect, at least temporarily, endogenous electromagnetic fields. This has certainly been the case in transcranial magnetic stimulation (TMS) in which very strong fields are used (16,17) and recently reported for very weak extremely low frequency magnetic fields (18) and as well in some cases of exposure to the brain from cell phones like radiofrequency fields (19).

C. Multimodal Image Integration

Multimodality image integration involves taking images from different imaging systems (MRI, x-ray CT, PET, ultrasound, etc.) and overlapping them into the same 3-dimensional (3-D) space (20). For example, an MRI image would provide the anatomical location of an increase in brain metabolism measured using PET. Images from different modalities can be registered, i.e., superimposed into a common 3-D space using software, or they can be collected with hybrid, multimodality imaging systems so that in principal the images are already superimposed together.

In electromagnetic therapy we could use image integration to demonstrate in what part of the brain (taken with MRI) the therapy caused a biochemical change (taken with PET). Besides integrating medical imaging methods with each other, there is also the integration of electromagnetic mapping with medical imaging (15). This is particularly useful in EEG and MEG brain mapping. For example, locating the source of an activated magnetic dipole in the brain is often achieved using MRI to constrain the search to within a region of the brain (15).

D. Image-Guided Therapy

Image-guided therapy is an extremely fast developing area. Development in molecular imaging and image integration are having a profound influence on the accuracy of image-guided therapy. Today it is routine to use real-time ultrasound-guided therapy for the treatment of breast cancer (21). However, image-guided surgery is only one of many possibilities. These others include image-guided tomotherapy for the delivery of ionizing radiation so that malignant tumors are damaged by imaging radiation while the surrounding healthy tissue is spared (22). Another future example will be image-guided drug therapy.

For example, in the future, imaging of neurotransmitter concentrations in the brain will allow the determination of the effectiveness of different drugs for the treatment of brain disorders such as schizophrenia or depression or bipolar disease or dementia (23). In the future it will be possible to practice image-guided electromagnetic field therapy. Not only will imaging indicate the exact anatomical target, but it will also be needed to design the electromagnetic field characteristics that will produce the specific therapy desired while at the same time reducing unwanted side effects.

III. FUTURE POTENTIAL OF ELECTROMAGNETIC FIELD THERAPY

It has been more than a century now since the discovery of x-rays and their potential use in diagnostic medicine. Since that time it has been determined that ionizing radiation can be used to effectively diagnose disease and treat cancer. It has also been established that ionizing radiation can be detrimental to health. Can we expect a similar capability from nonionizing electromagnetic radiation? I believe so. Clearly nonionizing EM has a place in diagnostic medicine with the spectacular growth of magnetic resonance imaging over the last two decades. Also, recognizing that radio-frequency and microwave radiation can efficiently deposit significant energy into biological samples has resulted in the presence of a microwave oven in almost every home in the developed world. If nonionizing electromagnetic fields can produce nonthermal, nonstochastic deterministic effects, then I predict that there will be significant use of these fields for therapeutic and diagnostic purposes.

Of course, as with ionizing electromagnetic radiation, we will have to keep in mind the potential for detrimental effects. The establishment of such effects has been and will be very important. However, success in the application to therapy (here I will focus on therapy rather than diagnosis) is very dependent on knowledge of the initial biophysical detection mechanism and the cascade of events from this initial event to the desired therapeutic result. Imaging will be essential in the determination of such mechanisms in humans.

IV. EXAMPLES OF IMAGE-GUIDED ELECTROMAGNETIC THERAPY

A. Repetitive Transcranial Magnetic Stimulation

Repetitive transcranial magnetic stimulation (rTMS) is presently being investigated as a method for treatment of depression and many other conditions (24). A strong electrical pulse is sent through a coil, which generates a strong time-changing magnetic field of the order of 10,000 T/s (25). When placed against the human skull this time-changing magnetic field induces a strong current in the brain. To date the pulses used have been very simple with respect to possible information content; basically either single pulses (TMS) or repetitive single pulses at 1 to 20 Hz (rTMS) are used. To optimize the method of magnetic field therapy a number of questions need to be answered which include

1. For a specific disease what is the anatomical target, e.g., what part of the brain?
2. For that target what is the needed induced current?
3. For that induced current what are the possible effects on surrounding tissues?
4. What is the optimal pulse pattern?

Imaging methods can help with all of these questions. For example superposition of 3-D MRI images with the magnetic field distributions have allowed stimulation of structures within the motor cortex to 5-mm spatial resolution (26,27). Further, MRI determined 3-D brain tissue conductivity maps have allowed the calculation of the 3-D distribution of induced current densities in the brain giving the needed values for the target sites and the surrounding tissue (28–30). These MRI approaches will allow refinement of TMS and rTMS for various disease states. However, imaging can also provide the needed information on the type of pulse sequence that should be used to activate the magnetic field coils. Some investigators have shown that PET studies of brain blood flow and metabolism in patients with depression can predict the effectiveness of rTMS for different pulse sequences and the targeting of different brain structures (31). PET can then be used to follow up the effectiveness of therapy by showing how quickly brain blood flow and metabolism return to normal levels. It has been further shown by using EEG brain mapping methods how the brain's electrical activity responds within milliseconds after a single TMS pulse and the connectivity of the initial stimulated site to other sites in the brain which subsequently become activated (16,17,32–34).

I believe that this example of image-guided TMS therapy shows us the way to apply imaging and mapping of endogenous electromagnetic fields to guide all forms of electromagnetic therapy. First, we must know the nonionizing radiation dosimetry; imaging (e.g.,

MRI) indicates the magnetic field dosimetry at specific anatomical sites or targets and dosimetry in remote regions to be spared therapy (29). Second, we must know the secondary dosimetry, which is dependent on the mechanisms of detection and the cascade of events to the desired outcome. So if, as is assumed with TMS, the detection is by induced electromotive force, which has its biological effect through induction of current, then imaging (e.g., MRI, EEG) is used to determine the secondary dosimetry. Third, we must know how therapy at a specific site affects function and/or biochemistry at a remote site. This can be achieved by passive and active imaging (EEG, MEG, fMRI, PET) and can tell us, for example, how the treatment to one area of the brain is detected in another area. Fourth, imaging tells us the effectiveness of the therapy. For example, we determine if abnormal function and/or biochemistry returns to normal (PET, SPECT, fMRI, EEG, MEG). Fifth and finally, we repeat steps 1 to 4 again and again to optimize the treatment through an understanding of mechanism. Much of what follows is a hypothesis of how this could be undertaken.

B. Pain Therapy

Image-guided electromagnetic pain therapy will significantly alter the management of both acute and chronic pain. Today we know that whole animal exposure to pulsed extremely low frequency magnetic fields can both (1) augment opioid-induced analgesia and induce analgesia (35,36) and (2) attenuate opioid-induced analgesia (37,38). However, before such therapy can be effective for the masses, we must discover the mechanism and specifically the target tissue.

Recently there has been considerable interest in imaging pain centers in the brain using MRI and PET (39–45). New knowledge regarding the mechanism of action of analgesic drugs is accumulating, and we are actually starting to understand more about the placebo effect with imaging studies allowing us to differentiate between areas of the brain activated by placebo compared to those from analgesics (46,47). For electromagnetic pain therapy we need to discover (1) the mechanism with respect to detection and the cascade of events leading to the analgesic effect, (2) the anatomical targets, and (3) the optimal pulsed magnetic field waveform. It is only through sophisticated imaging methods that we can gather this information.

First, we need to establish, using imaging, how pulsed magnetic field therapy affects pain centers in the brain. For example, we can ask whether or not such therapy affects the somatosensory detection of pain or the higher brain functions associated with cognitive process including the placebo effect (39,48,49). This can be done using fMRI and PET in acute pain studies or using PET, SPECT (single photon emission computed tomography), or MRI (brain blood flow) to determine basal conditions in patients treated for chronic pain. Imaging studies can tell us how patients treated for chronic pain respond to acute pain.

Besides such uses of active imaging methods, it is postulated that, passive imaging in the form of brain mapping (EEG and MEG) could be used to determine how (1) treatment to one brain site is electrically connected to other sites and (2) how the exposing pulsed magnetic field can be optimized for the individual patient. Monitoring brain electromagnetic activity during pulsed magnetic field therap and after therapy may allow tuning of the pulse sequence for individual patients. Hence imaging will guide all aspects of electromagnetic pain therapy including the pulsed magnetic field temporal design and the preferred spatial localization. It wil even be possible to use imaging to target pulsed magnetic field therapy to areas of the brain associated with negative drug side effects with the purpose of reducing those unwanted side effects.

C. Molecular Imaging

Molecular imaging will allow the observation of when a gene is "turned on." For example, there have been a number of proposals indicating how the magnetic field controlled production of heat shock proteins (HSP) can be used therapeutically. A number of independent research laboratories (50–54) have proposed that an extremely low frequency magnetic field (ELFMF) can induce significant levels of heat shock proteins (HSP) that can be used to reduce permanent damage to the heart from ischaemic injury. Like the analgesic application of electromagnetic field therapy, this has been demonstrated in small animals uniformly exposed to ELFMF. For human application it will be necessary to ensure that the increase in HSP occurs in the heart muscle (myocardium), that the levels are high enough to anticipate a therapeutic effect, and that the heart response is favorable. All of this can be done with imaging. In fact, in the future molecular imaging will allow the determination of exactly when transcription of a particular gene has started. Hence, if magnetic fields can affect gene expression, human imaging will report exactly when and where increased transcription and/or protein expression is occurring in the human body.

V. SUMMARY

The present explosion in the development, integration, and use of medical imaging for image-guided therapies is an unprecedented event in the field of imaging. In a brief 5 years it has allowed the new magnetic field technology transcranial magnetic stimulation to be accepted as mainstream medicine in a number of jurisdictions. This was quickly achieved, however, partly because the mechanism was believed to be known and the technology was targeted to replace a more invasive physical therapy, i.e., electroconvulsive shock. For other magnetic field therapies to become mainstream requires significant effort. However, the use of imaging to guide this development will quicken acceptance through specificity of treatment and evaluation of outcome using the hard measures associated with medical imaging.

REFERENCES

1. Wong NN. Aggrenox: an aspirin and extended release dipyridamole combination. Heart Disease 2001; 3:340–346.
2. Sharpe J, Ahlgren U, Perry P, Hill B, Ross A, Hecksher-Sorensen J, Baldock R, Davidson D. Optical projection tomography as a tool for 3D microscopy and gene expression studies. Science 2002; 296:541–545.
3. Blasberg R. Imaging gene expression and endogenous molecular processes: molecular imaging. J Cereb Blood Flow Metab 2002; 22:1157–1164.
4. Bulte JW, Duncan ID, Frank JA. In vivo magnetic resonance tracking of magnetically labeled cells after transplantation. J Cereb Blood Flow Meta 2002; 22:899–907.
5. Iwata R. Reference Book for PET Radiopharmaceuticals, 2001.
6. Wagner KJ, Willoch F, Kochs EF, Siessmeier T, Tolle TR, Schwaiger M, Bartenstein P. Dose-dependent regional cerebral blood flow changes during remifentanil infusion in humans: a positron emission tomography study. Anesthesiology 2001; 94:732–739.
7. Smith JS, Zubieta JK, Price JC, Flesher JE, Madar I, Lever JR, Kinter CM, Dannals RF, Frost JJ. Quantification of delta-opioid receptors in human brain with N1′([11C]methyl) naltrindole and positron emission tomography. J Cereb Blood Flow Metab 1999; 19:956–966.
8. Koeppe MJ, Duncan JS. PET: Opiate neuroreceptor mapping. Adv Neurol 2000; 83:145–156.
9. Willoch F, Tolle TR, Wester HJ, Munz F, Petzold A, Schwaiger M, Conrad B, Bartenstein P.

Central pain after pontine infarction is associated with changes in opioid receptor binding: a PET study with 11C-diprenorphine. Am J Neuroradiol 1999; 29:686–690.

10. Jones AK, Kitchen ND, Watabe H, Cunningham VJ, Jones T, Luthra SK, Thomas DG. Measurement of changes in opioid receptor binding in vivo during trigeminal neuralgic pain using (11C) diprenorphine and positron emission tomography. J Cereb Blood Flow Metab 1999; 19:803–808.

11. Wester HJ, Willoch F, Tolle TR, Munz F, Herz M, Oye I, Schadrack J, Schwaiger M, Bartenstein P. 6-O-(2-[18F]fluoroethyl)-6-O-desmethyldiprenorphine ([18F]DPN): synthesis, biologic evaluation, and comparison with [11C]DPN in humans. J Nucl Med 2000; 41:1279–1286.

12. Ueno S. Biomagnetic approaches to studying the brain. IEEE Eng Med Biology 1999; 108–120.

13. Clarke J. SQUIDS. Scientific American, 1994; 46–53.

14. Ryhanen T, Knuutila J. SQUID magnetometers for low-frequency applications. J Low Temp Phys 1989; 76:287–288.

15. Babiloni F, Carducci F, Del Gratta C, Roberti GM, Cincotti F, Bagni O, Romani GL, Rossini PM, Babiloni C. Multimodal integration of high resolution EEG, MEG and functional magnetic resonance data. IJBEM 1999; 1:62–74.

16. Paus T, Jech R, Thompson CJ, Comeau R, Peters T, Evans AC. Transcranial magnetic stimulation during positron emission tomography: a new method of studying connectivity of the human cerebral cortex. J Neurosci 1997; 17:3178–3184.

17. Ilmoniemi RJ, Virtanen J, Ruohonen J, Karhu J, Aronen JH, Naatanen R, Katila T. Neuronal responses to magnetic stimulation reveal cortical reactivity and connectivity. Neuroreport 1997; 8:3537–3540.

18. Cook CM, Thomas AQ, Prato FS. Human resting EEG is affected by exposure to a pulsed ELF magnetic field. Neuroreport, Oct. 2002. Submitted to.

19. Cook CM, Thomas AW, Prato FS. Human electrophysiological and cognitive effects of exposure to ELF magnetic and ELF modulated RF and microwave fields: a review of recent studies. Bioelectromagnetics 2002; 23:144–157.

20. Slomka PJ, Mandel J, Downey D, Fenster A. Evaluation of a voxel-based registration of 3-D power Doppler ultrasound and 3-D magnetic resonance angiographic images of carotid arteries. Ultrasound Med Biol 2001; 27:945–955.

21. Surry K, Smith W, Campbell L, Mills G, Downey D, Fenster A. The development and evaluation of a three-dimensional ultrasound-guided breast biopsy apparatus. Med Image Anal 2002; 6:301.

22. Ling CC, Humm J, Larson S, Amols H, Fuks Z, Leibel S, Koutcher JA. Towards multi-dimensional radiotherapy (MD-CRT): biological imaging and biological conformality. Int J Radiation Oncology Biol Phys 2000; 47:551–560.

23. Theberge J, Bratha R, Drost DJ, Menon RS, Malla A, Takhar J, Neufeld RW, Rogers J, Pavlosky W, Schaefer B, Densmore M, Al-Semaan Y, Williamson PC. Glutamate and glutamine measured with 4.0 T proton MRS in never-treated patients with schizophrenia and healthy volunteers. Am J Psychiatry 2002; 159:1944–1946.

24. Wassermann EM. Risk and safety of repetitive transcranial magnetic stimulation: report and suggested guidelines. International Workshop on the Safety of Repetitive Transcranial Magnetic Stimulation Electroncephalography and Clinical Neurophysiology 1998; 108:1–16.

25. Ueno S, Tashiro T, Harada K. Localized stimulation of neural tissues in the brain by means of paired configuration of time-varying magnetic fields. J Appl Phys 1988; 64:5862–5864.

26. Ueno S, Matsuda T, Fujiki M, Hori S. Localized stimulation of the human motor cortex by means of a pair of opposing magnetic field. Digest of IEEE Intermag Conf GD-10, Washington DC, 1989.

27. Ueno S, Matsuda T, Fujiki M. Vectorial and focal magnetic stimulation of the brain for the understanding of the functional organization of the brain. IEEE Trans Magn 1990; 26:1539–1544.

28. Ueno S. Impedence magnetic resonance imaging: A method for imaging of impedance distributions based on magnetic resonance imaging. J Appl Physics 1998; 83:6450–6452.

29. Masaki, Sekino, Ueno S. Numerical calculations of current distributions in electric stimulation and magnetic stimulation of the brain. Int Union Radio Science, 27th General Assembly, August 17–24, 2002.

30. Liu R, Ueno S. Calculating the activating function of nerve excitation in inhomogeneous volume conductor during magnetic stimulation using the finite element method. IEEE Trans Magn 2000; 36:1700–1796.

31. Kimbrell TA, Dunn RT, George MS, Danielson AL, Willis MW, Repella JD, Benson BE, Herscovitch P, Post RM, Wassermann EM. Left prefrontal-repetitive transcranial magnetic stimulation (rTMS) and regional cerebral glucose metabolism in normal volunteers. Psychiatry Res 2002; 115:101–113.

32. Strafella AP, Paus T, Barrett J, Dagher A. Repetitive transcranial magnetic stimulation of the human prefrontal cortex induces dopamine release in the caudate nucleus. J Neurosci 2001; 21:1–4.

33. Bourtros NN, Berman RM, Hoffman R, Miano AP, Campbell D, Ilmoniemi R. Electroencephalogram and repetitive transcranial magnetic stimulation. Depression and Anxiety 2000; 12:166–169.

34. Nobler MS, Teneback CC, Nahas Z, Bohning DE, Shastri A, Kozel FA, George MS. Structural and functional neuroimaging of electroconvulsive therapy and transcranial magnetic stimulation. Depression and Anxiety 2000; 12:144–156.

35. Thomas AW, Kavaliers M, Prato FS, Ossenkopp K-P. Analgesic effects of a specific pulsed magnetic field in the land snail, *cepaea nemoralis*: consequences of repeated exposures, relations to tolerance and cross-tolerance with DPDPE. Peptides 1998; 19:333–342.

36. Prato FS, Kavaliers M, Thomas AW. Extremely low frequency magnetic fields can either increase or decrease analgaesia in the land snail depending on field and light conditions. Bioelectromagnetics 2000; 21:287–301.

37. Prato FS, Carson JJL, Ossenkopp K-P, Kavaliers M. Possible mechanisms by which extremely low frequency magnetic fields affect opioid function. FASEB 1995; 9:807–814.

38. Choleris E, Del Seppia C, Thomas AW, Luschi P, Ghione S, Moran GR, Prato FS. Shielding, but not zeroing of the ambient magnetic field reduces stress-induced analgesia in mice. Proc R Soc Lond 2002; 269:193–201.

39. Tolle TR, Kaufmann T, Siessmeier T, Lautenbacher S, Berthele A, Munz F, Zieglgansberger W, Willoch F, Schwaiger M, Conrad B, Bartenstein P. Region-specific encoding of sensory and affective components of pain in the human brain: a positron emission tomography correlation analysis. Am Neuro Assoc 1999, 40–47.

40. Bromm B. Brain images of pain. News Physiol Soc 2001; 16:244–249.

41. Treede R-D, Kenshalo DR, Gracely RH, Jones AKP. The cortical representation of pain. Pain 1999; 79:105–111.

42. Casey KL. Forebrain mechanisms of nociception and pain: analysis through imaging. Proc Natl Acac Sci 1999; 96:7668–7674.

43. Talbot JD, Marrett S, Evans AC, Meyer E, Bushnell MC, Duncan GH. Multiple representations of pain in human cerebral cortex. Science 1991; 1353–1355.

44. Hsieh J-C, Stone-Elander S, Ingvar M. Anticipatory coping of pain expressed in the human anterior cingulate cortex: a positron emission tomography study. Neuroscience Letters 1999; 262:61–64.

45. Derbyshire SWG, Jones AKP, Devani P, Friston KJ, Feinmann C, Harris M, Pearce S, Watson JDG, Frackowiak RSJ. Cerebral responses to pain in patients with atypical facial pain measured by positron emission tomography. J Neurol Neurosurg Psychiatry 1994; 57:1166–1172.

46. Leuchter AF, Cook IA, Witte EA, Morgan M, Abrams M. Changes in brain function of depressed subjects during treatment with placebo. Am J Psychiatry 2002; 159:122–129.

47. Petrovic P, Kalso E, Petersson KP, Ingvar M. Placebo and opioid analgesia imaging a shared neuronal network. Science 2002; 295:1737–1740.

48. Zubieta JK, Smith YR, Bueller JA, Xu Y, Kilbourn MR, Jewett DM, Meyer CR, Koeppe RA,

Stohler CS. Regional mu opioid receptor regulation of sensory and affective dimensions of pain. Science 2001; 293:311–315.

49. Jones AK, Liyi Q, Cunningham VV, Brown DW, Ha-Kawa S, Fujiwara T, Friston KF, Silva S, Luthra SK, Jones T. Endogenous opiate response to pain in rheumatoid arthritis and cortical and subcortical response to pain in normal volunteers using positron emission tomography. Int J Clin Pharamacol Res 1991; 11:261–266.

50. Goodman R, Blank M. Insights into electromagnetic interaction mechanisms. J Cellular Physiol 1992; 192:16–22.

51. DiCarlo AL, Farrell JM, Litovitz T. Myocardial protection conferred by electromagnetic fields. Circulation 1999; 99:813–816.

52. Carmody S, Wu SL, Lin H, Blank M, Skopicki H, Goodman R. Cytoprotection by electromagnetic field-induced hsp70: a model for clinical application. J Cellular Biochem 2999; 79:453–459.

53. Ventura C, Maioli M, Pintus, Gottardi G, Bersani F. Elf-pulse magnetic fields modulate opioid peptide gene expression in myocardial cells. Cardiovascular Res 2000; 45:1054–1064.

54. Albertini A, Zucchini P, Noera G, Cadossi R, Napoleone CP, Pierangeli A. Protective effect of low frequency low energy pulsing electromagnetic fields on acute experimental myocardial infarcts in rats. Bioelectromagnetics 1999; 20:372–377.

5

The Theology of Electricity

Electricity, Alchemy, and the Unconscious

Dennis Stillings
Archaeus Project, Kamuela, Hawaii, U.S.A.

My interest in the history of electrical theory and practice was stimulated by Carl Jung's *Psychology and Alchemy*, which allowed me to trace the myths, metaphors, and archetypal images of 18th-century electrical thinking back to alchemical and even early Gnostic writings. I subsequently became familiar with *The Theology of Electricity* by Ernest Benz, who claimed that "the discovery of electricity was accompanied by a most significant change in the image of God" that led to a "completely new understanding of the relation of body and soul, of spirit and matter..." This chapter will explain, explore and expand upon these aspects of what might be referred to as "the electric unconscious."

I. INTRODUCTION

In late 1968, I began work as a research librarian at Medtronic, Inc., a major manufacturer of medical devices, in particular, the implantable cardiac pacemaker. Late in that year, Earl Bakken, founder of Medtronic, approached me about a special project: collect the history of bioelectricity and electromedicine in the form of printed materials and original devices. This project eventually led to the establishment of a museum and rare book collection (1).

Before this project, I had no interest at all in electricity even though I had studied physics both in high school and at the University of Minnesota. In the late 1960s, I was immersed in German studies in graduate school, where my chief interest lay in applying the methods of C. G. Jung's analytical psychology to the interpretation of literature, and I was also happily occupied teaching eighteenth century humanities at the University of Minnesota. It was through Jung's work, especially *Psychology and Alchemy*, that I first came to develop an interest in the history of electrical theory and practice, since, through Jung, I was able to see that much of the imagery and nomenclature of alchemy had been transferred, virtually unchanged, into the language and speculations of the emerging electrical science. When I perceived this, I was able to trace the myths, metaphors, and

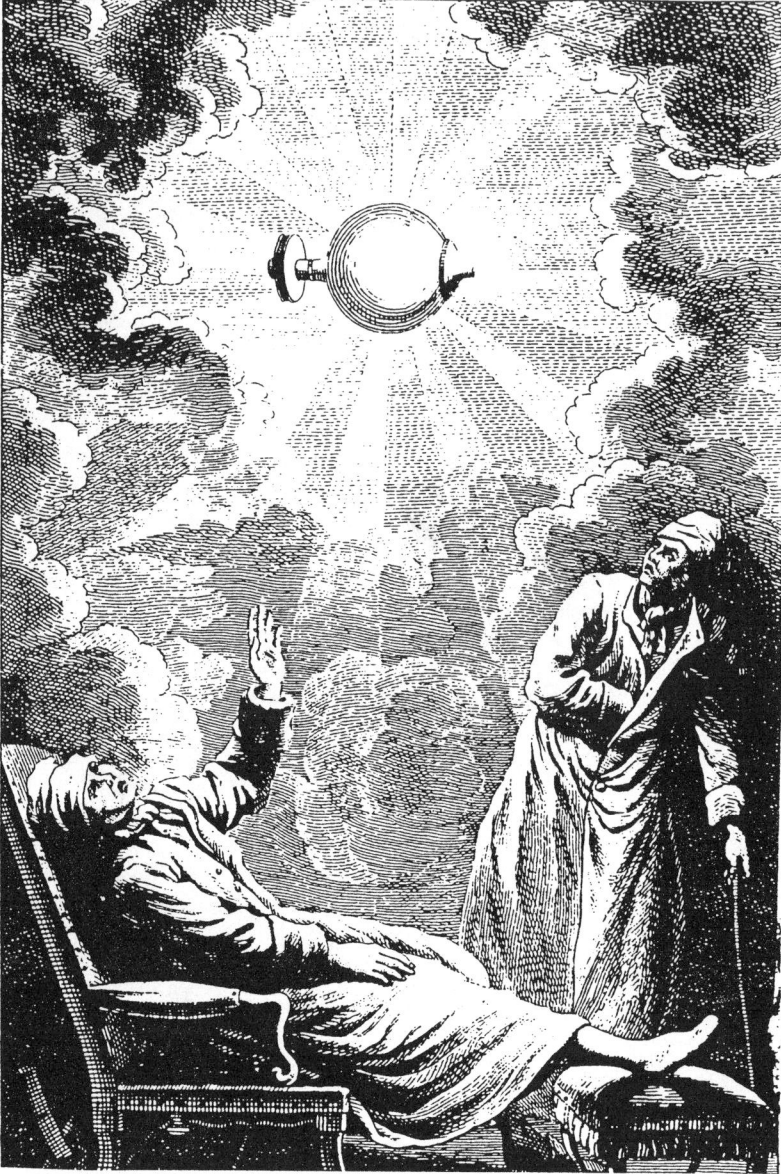

From Abbé Sans [Pierre de Saint Lazare], *De la Guérison de la Paralysie par l'Électricité* (Penpignan, 1771).

archetypal images that permeated eighteenth century electrical thinking back to alchemical and even to early Gnostic writings.

In 1972, at the 24th International Conference of the History of Medicine in Budapest, I presented a paper which emphasized some of the early images and ideas that led to the association of the cardiovascular system with electrical activity (2). In the course of the conference, I was approached and asked if I knew of the recently published work by Ernst Benz, *Theologie der Elektrizität* (Mainz, 1970). I had not heard of the book, but I resolved to obtain a copy upon my return to Minneapolis. A couple of years went by before I finally got the book through a foreign book search service. A brief glance at the contents caught my attention: it looked as though Benz had also perceived the hermetic background of early electrical philosophizing. I commissioned Wolfgang Taraba, then Chairman of the University of Minnesota German Department, to translate the work (3).

II. BENZ'S AGENDA

Benz's main concern in *The Theology of Electricity* is the "interrelationship of the religious and scientific consciousness." More specifically, Benz intends to establish the claim that the "discovery of electricity and the simultaneous discovery of magnetic and galvanic phenomena were accompanied by a most significant change in the image of God." Furthermore, Benz claims that these discoveries led to a "completely new understanding of the relation of body and soul, of spirit and matter...." (4)

Benz illustrates his interest in the traditional split between science and religion by juxtaposing the personalities and perceptions of Benjamin Franklin and Franz Anton Mesmer. In terms of Jungian typology, Franklin might be said to represent the archetypical American extraverted, sensation-thinking type—the empiricist and practical manipulator of the external world. Mesmer, on the other hand, is portrayed as operating within the realms of intuition and feeling. Ill-adapted to the practicalities of making his methods acceptable to the powers that be, he is tuned to cosmic feeling, an empathy with the workings of nature. According to his personality type, Franklin might argue that a ball is spherical, hard, and suitable for a number of uses; Mesmer might say that it is gold-colored, round, and therefore a symbol of spiritual value and cosmic wholeness. This type-determined difference in perception and thinking, expanded and generalized, lies close to the heart of the persistent opposition between religion and science: Franklin's side giving dominant value to the facts and objects of external reality; Mesmer's, to the inner subjective states evoked by the object.

The "electrical theologians" saw electricity as the "primordial light" investing matter with living evolutionary force. God is no longer merely a "clock maker" who stands apart from His created world; He enters into it in the most intimate way. This view of the role of God as interacting with the world foreshadows so-called process theology (5). Benz looks forward to the time when religion and science will resolve their apparent differences, and sees the work of the electrical theologians as demonstrating that science and religion motivate each other.

III. A BRIEF HISTORY OF EARLY ELECTROMEDICINE AND BIOELECTRICITY

Electrical and magnetic phenomena have always been associated with the soul, divine judgment, and psychic matters. Thunderbolts of Zeus were cast down upon those who offended him. Amber and other electrics were perceived as having "soul." Ancient Sumerians wore magnetic amulets engraved with images of Marduk (6)—"He-Who-Causes-Action-at-a-Distance"—to ward off evil spirits (Fig. 1). It is possible that primitive peoples used pools of electric fish [the Mediterranean torpedo (Fig. 2) and Nile catfish were available in Europe and the Middle East, the electric eel in Central and South America] for the purpose of exorcising spirits by means of subconvulsive electroshock therapy (7). Along these lines, electroexorcism was used by Joseph Priestley (1733–1804) (8), a theologian and also the first historian of electricity. This peculiar therapy has been practiced down into our own century (9).

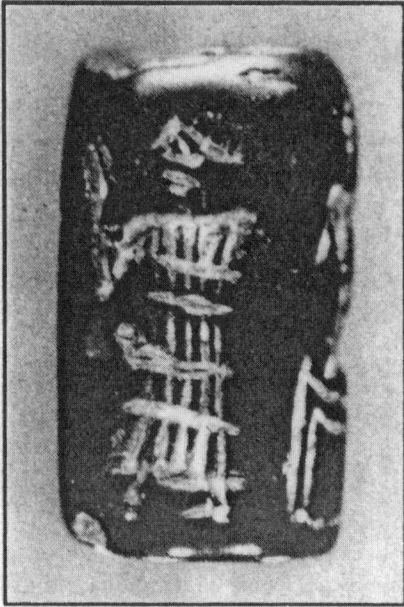

Figure 1 Sumerian cylinder seal of magnetite, c. 2500 B.C., with figure of Marduk. (Courtesy of The Bakken.)

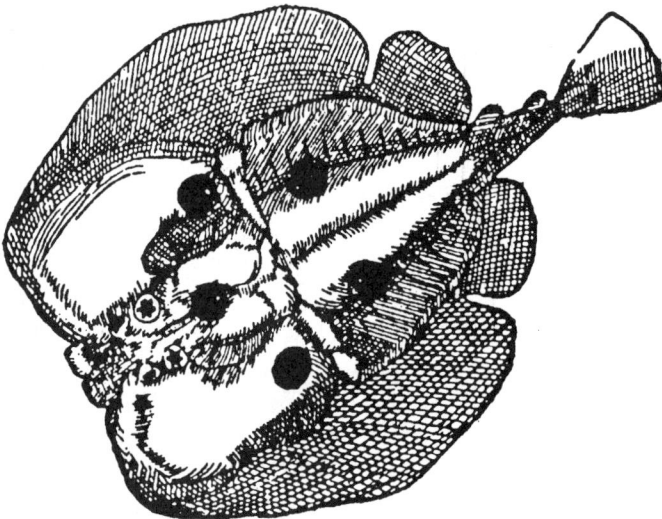

Figure 2 The Mediterranean torpedo. This fish is capable of a 100 + -V discharge. Courtesy of The Bakken.

Medical applications of the discharge of electric fish for treatment of headache, arthritis, and anal prolapse were recorded by Scribonius Largus (10) and Dioscorides (11) in the second century A.D. The electrical discharge of the live Mediterranean torpedo was used by Dawud al Antaki in the sixteenth century for the treatment of epilepsy (12).

FRANKENSTEIN;

or,

THE MODERN PROMETHEUS.

IN THREE VOLUMES.

Did I request thee, Maker, from my clay
To mould me man? Did I solicit thee
From darkness to promote me?——
PARADISE LOST.

VOL. I.

London:
PRINTED FOR
LACKINGTON, HUGHES, HARDING, MAVOR, & JONES,
FINSBURY SQUARE.

1818.

(Courtesy of the Bakken).

At the time of Harvey and Gilbert, the role of electricity and/or magnetism in the physiological functioning of the body was already a matter of serious speculation (13). By the mid-eighteenth century, it was assumed by many prominent physicians and physiologists that electricity was indeed intrinsic to the life processes of both animals and humans (14). The Galvanic-Volta controversy over the existence and nature of "animal electricity" (15) and many French experiments on the applications of electrical current to freshly decapitated corpses (Fig. 3) (16) made it appear quite plausible that electricity was the vital fluid and that its proper application could raise even the dead. The great Frankenstein myth, intuited and articulated by Mary Shelley in her book *Frankenstein; or, The Modern Prometheus* (Courtesy of the Bakken.) (17) was not, at the time, considered to be merely an imaginative flight of fancy. During the late eighteenth and early nineteenth centuries, electrical resurrection was probably considered, from the scientific point of view, not much more

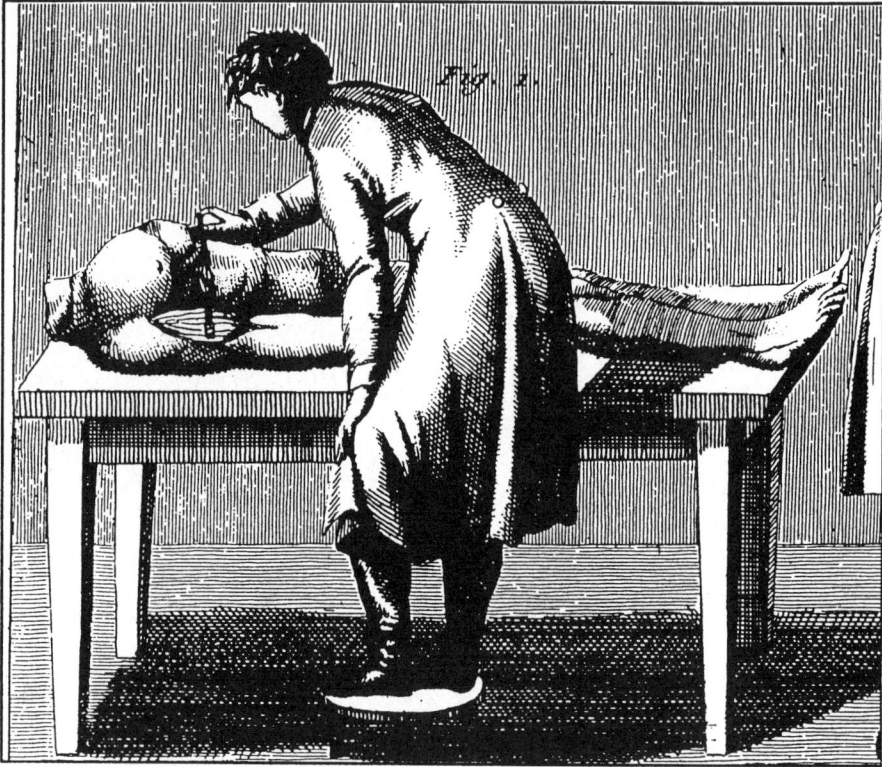

Figure 3 Galvanic experimentation on decapitated criminals. From Giovanni Aldini, *Essai Théoretique et Experimental stir le Galvanisme* (Paris, 1804). Courtesy of The Bakken.

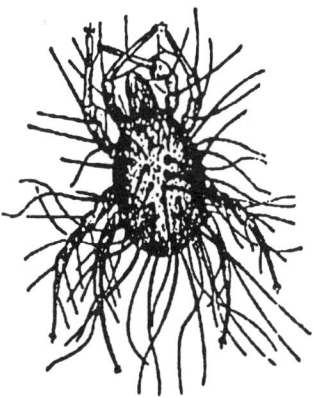

Figure 4 *Acarus electricus.* From H. M. Noad, *Lectures on Electricity* (London, 1849).

than a short-term extrapolation from what was then known about the effects of electricity on fresh corpses. In fact, about 1836, the amateur scientist Andrew Crosse created an uproar in England and earned a reputation as an "atheist, a blasphemer, a reviler of religion," and a "would-be Frankenstein" for using an electrochemical process, not merely to create life, but life in a very specific form—that of the insect *Acarus electricus* (Fig. 4) (18). Considering this history, it is small wonder that electricity continued to be under theological scrutiny. Even as late as the 1930s, Albert S. Hyman, a New York physician who developed an early version of the artificial cardiac pacemaker, was attacked by religious proponents for interfering with the divine will (19)—a judgment curiously reserved for electrical physicians, since it can be argued that a wide variety of other medical interventions do the same.

IV. ALCHEMY DIVIDES AND CONQUERS

As I collected early eighteenth century writings on electricity, it soon became clear to me that a great deal of the symbolism, and even the nomenclature, of alchemy had been carried over into the new electrical theorizing (20). Merely scanning the titles of early books on electricity confirms this. Electricity is the "ethereal fire," the "desideratum," the "quintessential fire,"

THE

DESIDERATUM:

OR,

ELECTRICITY

Made PLAIN and USEFUL.

By

A LOVER OF MANKIND AND OF COMMON SENSE,

THE REVEREND JOHN WESLEY,
1759.

Second Edition,

WITH AN APPENDIX ON THE ELECTRICITY OF
MODERN TIMES.

LONDON:
BAILLIÈRE, TINDALL, AND COX,
20 KING WILLIAM STREET, STRAND.

MDCCCLXXI.]

(Courtesy of the Bakken.)

the *medicina catholica* (courtesy of the Bakken.), the "cheap thing to be found everywhere"; it is the long-sought panacea—terms all used to characterize the nature and properties of the philosophers' stone. The transfer of the belief in the universal medical efficacy of the philosophers' stone to electricity was reflected in the utterly promiscuous use of electro-therapies in the treatment of disease from the mid-eighteenth century until well into our own. This archetypally based belief continues, down to the present day, to motivate claims by quacks—and occasionally by serious medical practitioners as well—for the extraordinary unrecognized medical value of electricity, magnetism, and electromagnetic waves (21).

Since the philosophers' stone was also identified with Jesus Christ (22) and hence the divine itself, this aspect also appears in speculations about the nature of electricity (Fig. 5). According to the electrical theologians, electricity is the very light of creation (23), a light

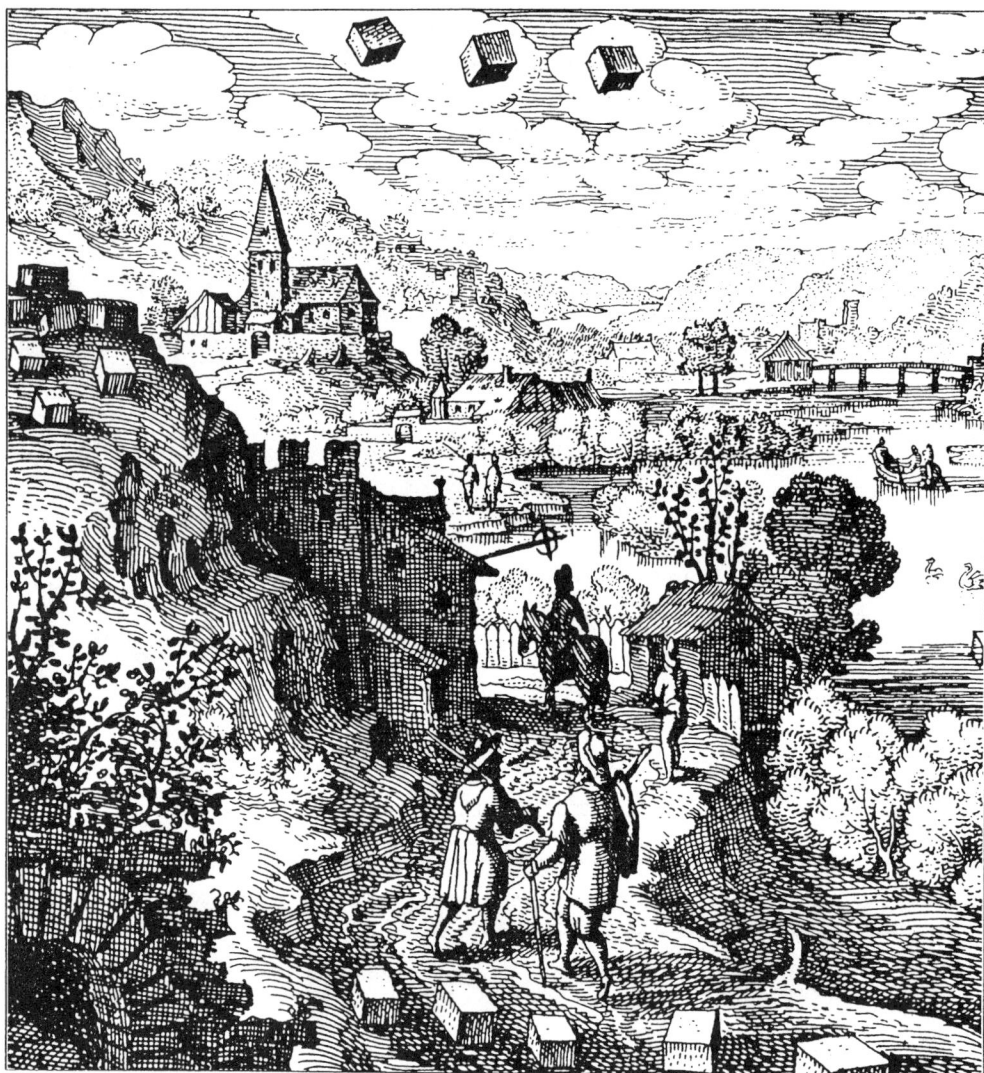

Figure 5   "Ubiquity of the Philosophers' Stone." (From Michael Maier, *Atalanta Fugiens*, 1617.)

that informs matter and is the impetus toward its evolution into higher and higher forms (24).

Alchemy has its roots in gnosticism (25). It is therefore tempting to look for images in the Gnostic writings that relate to alchemy and electrical theorizing. If one is familiar with the principles and operation of eighteenth-century glass-sphere electrostatic generators the following passage is very suggestive, especially in connection with the thoughts of electrical theologians (26):

> [The] power [of the spheres], as it became purified, was gathered back to the higher world by Melchisedec, the Great Receiver or Collector of Light, it being continually liberated by the spheres being made to turn more rapidly, that is to say by the quickening of evolution owing to the influx of light. The substance... is ... described as...the matter out of which souls are made.

In a discussion of the Manichaean Gnostic sect, Marie-Louise von Franz cites their belief that "God created the real world as a machine designed to liberate...light" (Fig. 6) (27). It is also of interest that Otto von Guericke, in his experiments on electricity and

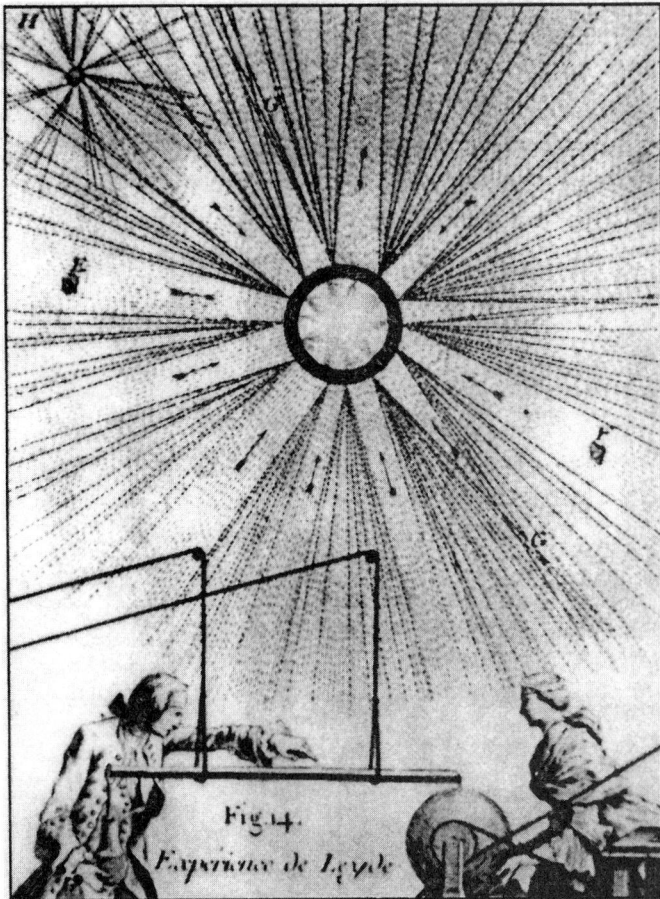

Figure 6 Electrical effluents and affluents. From Abbé Nollet, *Essai sur l'électricité des corps*, 1750. (Courtesy of The Bakken.)

gravitation (28), constructed, in 1660, a spherical "terrella" (29) made of sulfur. This little "model of the world" produced sparks (Fig. 7).

In our own day, this connection of electrical phenomena with religious ideas appears in cultish beliefs about the power of certain electromagnetic fields for good or evil. Electromagnetic waves, particularly those of extremely low frequency (ELF) are especially suited for attracting archetypal projections of properties normally ascribed to the divine: omnipresence (they penetrate almost anything), omnipotence (they are supposed to cause a wide variety of specific effects against which there is virtually no protection), and they are invisible. Michael A. Persinger, a neuroscientist with considerable experience in bioelectrical and biomagnetic effects, touches on this aspect (30):

> The persistence of an interest in the effects of magnetic fields can also be traced to psychological factors. Every researcher's personal environment is a product of language and the processes by which it is generated. Despite maturational (developmental) shifts in the cognitive schemes by which we assimilate information, there are concepts from previous stages [archetypal images–ED.] that remain. One of them is the fascination with invisible forces (animism). This idea serves as a conceptual core around which cluster ideas of infantile mysticism, paranormal experiences and sometimes a modified form of omnipotence. It is so closely tied to the concept of self that if care is not taken, magnetotherapies become a personal quest. It acquires the dynamics of a belief.

Electricity was the last of the classical sciences to be born—at a time when the rule of the materialistic, mechanistic view of nature and man was gathering full steam. The electrical science developed as a sort of subversive material-spiritual "fifth column" within the body of an otherwise mechanistic science and medicine. In physiology, even at present, chemical

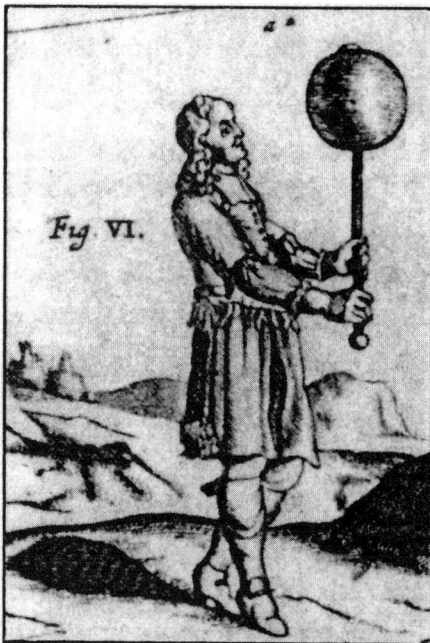

Figure 7 Otto von Guericke demonstrating electrical effects with a sulfur "terrella." From his *Experimenta nova (ut vocantur) magdeburgica de vacuo spatio* (Amsterdam, 1672).

factors are emphasized over the accompanying electrical events. This one-sided emphasis persists to a degree that makes one suspect that bioelectricity still raises the specter of vitalism among modern scientists and medical practitioners. According to Robert O. Becker and Andrew A. Marino (31):

> Practically from the time of its discovery, electromagnetic energy was identified by the vitalists as being the "life force," and consequently it has occupied a central position in the conflict between [mechanism and vitalism] for the past three centuries. While the modern view of the role of electromagnetic energy in life processes is not that of the mysterious force of the vitalists, it has nevertheless inherited the emotional and dogmatic aspects of the earlier conflict.

Electricity still evokes, on an unconscious level, images of that paradoxical figure of alchemy, Mercurius, (32) and of the elusive vital fluid that transcends the merely mechanical. Indeed, the paradoxes of modern quantum mechanis and the endless popular speculations on the role of consciousness in the material world, not to mention the actual transmutations of metals now possible using particle accelerators, are the outward manifestation of symbols that drove alchemy and now drive modern physics. (33)

But alchemy was fundamentally a *monstrum compositum*, an expression of underlying symbols hopelessly enmeshed within an essentially undiscriminated mixture of psyche and substance. After centuries of collective concern chiefly for otherwordly things, the world and the matter of which it is constituted had become, for the Western man of the fifteenth century, a great *fascinosum*—a fascination that would extend to the present day. The fifteenth- and sixteenth-century voyages of exploration and the golden age of alchemy therefore coincide. At first the world and matter were great mysteries, knowledge-vacuums that drew forth a flow of projected fantasies, fantasies that have become, for us, a gold mine of images revealing the structure and dynamics of the psyche. Mind became intimately bound up with matter, and this condition was expressed in the obscure symbolism of alchemical formulas. With the beginnings of modern chemistry and physics, the unconscious dynamics of alchemical symbolism split into two directions: one was that of mainstream science and technology; the other, a more subterranean and quieter path, lent impetus to the development of psychology and the discovery of the unconscious. Electricity, expressing what appeared to be both material and immaterial aspects, was not readily stripped of the ancient symbolic projections it had acquired; hence, by its ambiguous and pradoxical nature, it brought philosophers into yet closer contact with the unconscious, the very essence of which is ambiguity and paradox. On the other hand, material science could not pull itself entirely clear of the alchemistic residuum that adhered to electrical theorizing, thus permitting the symbols carried by electricity to drive modern science toward accomplishment that strongly echo the goals of alchemy: the transmutation and spiritualization (*sublimatio*) of matter (Fig. 8).

The lack of a concept of the unconscious, the failure actually to achieve the transmutation of metals, and the rise and success of mechanistic science all hastened the demise of alchemy. But with the splitting off of alchemy into an exoteric "alchemy of matter"—i.e., normal chemistry and physics—the psychic residuum made it possible for an intuitive perception of the existence of the unconscious psyche to arise.

V. THE ELECTRICAL UNCONSCIOUS

An examination of how the electrical theologians conceived of the role of that primordial light, electricity, reveals how close they were able to come to the beginnings of a psychology of the unconscious. For the electrical theologians, there is not only a "conscious and

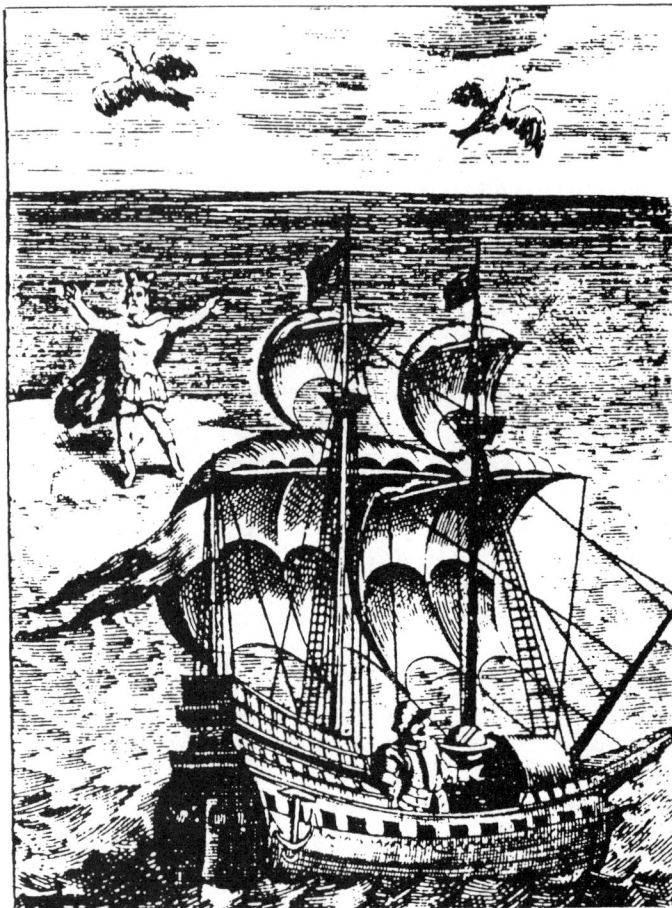

Figure 8 The "Grand Peregrination" by ship—the search for wholeness. The alchemists connected the imagery of world exploration with their own discoveries in matter and in the psyche. (From Michael Maier, *Viatorium*, 1651.)

rational" life, but a "sensory, growth-like, sensitive" life. This "sensuous soul" (the unconscious) is electric and is nourished by the "electrical fire" (read *libido* or *psychic energy*). Man is a being "involved in all levels of life—the material, vegetable, animal." His soul "has deep roots in pre-human realms." Man's spiritual life is rooted "in the organic structures and physico-chemical processes of his bodily existence." Not only is the "animalistic" soul the "nourishment of the rational soul," but the rational soul "needs this substratum in order to function" (34). The two should generate thoughts that stand in opposition to one another. And in a clear prefiguration of Jung's conception of the effects of complexes and archetypes, Oetinger (cited in Benz) says that the images that arise out of the "animistic soul" must be overcome by conscious reflection or meditation, lest "you [be] forced to act according to the needs of the body" (35). The texts Benz examines seem not only to refer to the fact of a conscious and unconscious mind but to address the more dynamic influence of the one on the other, including the compensatory function of the unconscious, and the drive toward individuation as freedom from the opposites.

It is worth noting that the beginnings of quantum theory coincide with the rise of the depth psychology of Sigmund Freud (36). Jung, in fact, saw Freud's work as an unconscious return to the fundamental psychological and spiritual problems raised by alchemy (37). Jung himself was, of course, heavily motivated by the ideas and images of alchemy—and even had a remarkable and persistent fantasy in his mid-teens in which images of alchemy and electricity were combined (38):

> I was the king of an island in a great lake like a sea, stretching from Basel Strassburg. The island consisted of a mountain with a small medieval town nestling below. At the top was my castle, and on its highest tower were things like copper antennae which collected electricity from the air and conducted it into a deep vault underneath the tower. In this vault there was a mysterious apparatus that turned the electricity into gold. I was so obsessed with this fantasy that reality was completely forgotten.

This recounting of his fantasy was in response to a letter from Aniela Jaffé in which she reported the following dream (39):

> I am in a deep cellar, together with a boy and an old man. The boy has been given an electric installation for Christmas: a large copper pot is suspended from the ceiling and electric wires from all directions make it vibrate. After some time there are no more wires; the pot now vibrate from atmospheric electric oscillations.

Clearly, the modern mind still brings forth the images that gripped the electrical theologians. What we are apparently witnessing is the playing out of the alchemical problem of the unification of the opposites of spirit and matter, soul and body. Jung believed that the ultimate nature of the psyche—which he conceived of as an intermediate state between mind and matter—would be approached by psychology from one side and by quantum physics from the other (40). Certainly this is happening. Such endeavors are the conscious reflection of a ferment below the level of collective consciousness. The social problems of our day involve questions of soul and body, spirit and matter, good and evil, male and female—precisely those issues that, a half-millennium ago, were prefigured in the flasks and fevered brains of the alchemists (Fig. 9).

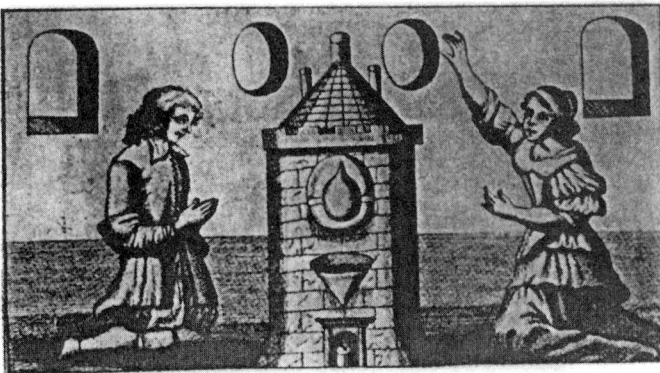

Figure 9 An alchemist and his *soror mystica* kneeling by the furnace and praying for God's blessing (*Mutus liber*, 1702).

REFERENCES

1. The Bakken: A Library and Museum of Electricity in Life. 3537 Zenith Ave. S., Minneapolis, MN.
2. Stillings D. The early history of attempts at electrical control of the heart: Harvey to Hyman. Acta Congressus internationalis XXIV Historiae Artis Medicinae. Budapest: Museum Bibliotheca et Archivum Historiae Artis Medicinae de I. Ph. Semmelweis Nominata, 1976: 73–80.
3. Published as Benz E. The theology of electricity. Allison Park, Pa: Pickwick Publications, 1989.
4. Benz E. The Theology of Electricity. Allison Park, Pa: Pickwick Publications, 1989:2.
5. "Process theology"—derived from the philosophy of Alfred North Whitehead—emphasizes evolutionary views of the cosmos ("God's body") and a dynamic, living God who participates in the world.
6. Two examples of cylinder seals made of magnetite, once in the Editor's collection, are now in The Bakken.
7. Kellaway P. The part played by electric fish in the early history of bioelectricity and electrotherapy. Bull Hist Med 1946; 20:112.
8. The Dictionary of National Biography, Vol. XVI, repr. Oxford 1967–1968:360.
9. Wickland CA. Thirty Years Among the Dead. London: Spiritualist Press, 1968. This book was first published in 1924.
10. Scribonius Largus. De compositionibus medicamentorurn. Liber unus, antehac nusquarn excusus: Joanne Ruellio. Paris, 1528.
11. Pedanius Dioscorides of Anazarbos. The Greek herbal of Dioscorides, illustrated by a Byzantine A.D. 512, Englished by John Goodyer A.D. 1655. London: Hafner, 1968. Facsimile of 1934 edition.
12. Leibowitz JO. Electroshock therapy in Ibn-Sina's canon. J Hist Med 1957; 12:71.
13. Stillings D. Early attempts at electrical control of the heart: Harvey to Hyman. Artifex 1986; 5(3):1.
14. Hoff HE. Galvani and the pre-galvanian electrophysiologists. Ann Sci 1936; 1:157.
15. Dibner B. Galvani-Volta: A Controversy that Led to the Discovery of Useful Electricity. Norwalk, Conn: Burndy Library, 1952.
16. Since most of these experiments were carried out in France during the Revolution, there was no shortage of such material.
17. Shelley M. Frankenstein; or, the modern Prometheus. London: Lackington, Hughes, Harding, Mayor, and Jones, 1818. A copy of the first edition may be seen at The Bakken.
18. Gould RT. Crosse's acari. In: Gould RT, ed. Oddities: A Book of Unexplained Facts. New Hyde Park, N.Y.: University Books, 1965:117–123.
19. Schechter DC. Background of clinical cardiac electrostimulation, pt. V: Direct electrostimulation of heart without thoracotomy. New York State Journal of Medicine March 1, 1972; 72(3):612–619.
20. It is noteworthy that one of the earliest electrical generators (c. 1734) was constructed from an alembic by Georg Matthias Bose. Both the neck and the spherical body of the vessel were used as electrical generators. See Hackmann WD. Electricity from Glass: the History of the Frictional Electrical Machine 1600–1850. Alphen aan den Rijn: Sijthoff & Noorhoff, 1978, pp. 68ff.
21. Of course, other exotic "energies" have been posited that are even more fundamental and efficacious—"odic force," "orgone energy," "eloptic energy," "scalar waves," "etheric waves," etc.
22. Jung CG. Psychology and alchemy. In: Jung CG, ed. Collected Works 1953; Vol. 12. CW 12. London: Routledge and Kegan Paul, 1953:406ff.
23. That is, the first light mentioned in Genesis I: 3–4.
24. Benz E. The Theology of Electricity. Allison Park, Pa: Pickwick Publications, 1989:46ff.
25. Jung CG. Psychology and alchemy. In: Jung CG, ed. Collected Works. Vol. 12. London: Routledge & Kegan Paul, 1953:453ff.
26. Mead GRS. Summary of the contents of the so-called Pistis Sophia treatise. In: Mead GRS, ed. Fragments of a Faith Forgotten. New Hyde Park, N.Y.: University Books, 467.

27. von Franz M-L. Dreams. Boston & London: Shambhala, 1991:85. For further discussion of this Manichaean "machine," see Legge, F. Forerunners and Rivals of Christianity. New Hyde Park, N.Y.: University Books, 1964; II:297.

28. von Guericke, O. Experiments nova magdeburgica ... Amsterdam, 1672.

29. Making "terrellas" was a favorite pastime of the alchemists. See Jung CG. Psychology and Alchemy, Collected Works, vol. 12. London: Routledge & Kegan Paul, 1953.

30. Persinger MA. The modern magnetotherapies. In: Marino AA, ed. Modern Bioelectricity. New York: Marcel Dekker, 1988:590.

31. Becker RO, Marino AA. Electromagnetism and Life. Albany: State University of New York Press, 1982:4.

32. For a discussion of the electricity/Mercurius parallels, see Stillings D. The primordial light: electricity to paraelectricity. Archaeus 1984; 2(1):81–90.

33. For a clear and concise discussion of how science and technology arise from symbols and why early protosciences sometimes prefigure modern discoveries, see Jung CG. On psychic energy. In: Jung, CG, ed. The Structure and Dynamics of the Psyche, CW 8. New York: Pantheon Books, 1960:45ff.

34. Benz E. The Theology of Electricity. Allison Park, Pa: Pickwick Publications, 1989:56ff.

35. One is reminded hereof Goethe's "Two souls, alas, do dwell within my breast." St. Paul's version of this is to be found in Romans 7:19–20: "For the good that I would I do not: but the evil which I would not, that I do. Now if I do that I would not, it is no more I that do it, but sin that dwelleth in me."

36. Max Planck formulated quantum theory in 1900, the same year that Freud's *The Interpretation of Dreams* was published.

37. Jung CG. Psychology of the transference. In: Jung CG, ed. The Practice of Psychotherapy, CW 16. New York: Pantheon Books, 1954:315.

38. Jung CG. Letters 1: 1906–1950. Princeton, N.J.: Princeton University Press, 1973:325f.

39. Jung CG. Letters 1: 1906–1950. Princeton, N.J.: Princeton University Press, 1973:325n.

40. A considerable literature exists on this subject. Perhaps the best of these works is Jahn, RC and BJ Dunne's Margins of Reality: The Role of Consciousness in the Physical World. San Diego: Harcourt Brace Jovanovich, 1987. See also Jahn and Dunne's "Collected Thoughts on the Role of Consciousness in the Physical Representation of Reality"—"Appendix B" in their laboratory publication PEAR 83005.1B, On the quantum mechanics of consciousness with application to anomalous phenomena. Princeton, N.J.: Princeton Engineering Anomalies Research Laboratory, 1984. For a superb discussion of the Gnostic and alchemical roots of modern technology, electricity included, see Davis, E., *Techgnosis: Myth, Magic + Mysticism in the Age of Information*. New York: Three Rivers Press, 1998.

6

Recent Developments in Bioelectromagnetic Medicine

James L. Oschman

Nature's Own Research Association, Dover, New Hampshire, U.S.A.

Recent advances confirm the presence of an energy field in and around the body that can provide diagnostic information and also be utilized to validate the efficacy of non-traditional therapies and determine which may be particularly effective for certain complaints and conditions. The development of our understanding of these biofields will be traced with a focus on elucidating the scientific basis of energy medicine.

I. HISTORICAL BACKGROUND

The history of bioelectromagnetic medicine has been marked by confusion, controversy, and a profusion of quack devices. A number of individuals, such as Anton Mesmer, Albert Abrams, and Wilhelm Reich, introduced energy 'therapies' that are widely considered to be fraudulent, although they continue to have many supporters.

At the turn of the twentieth century (1900) a variety of electrotherapeutic devices were in widespread use by medical doctors. All sorts of energy gimmicks were being sold to the public. Extravagant claims were made, but this was before the Food and Drug Administration (FDA) existed and before there was any requirement or tradition for scientific testing such as in clinical or experimental trials. For example, the "$18.00 Giant Power Heidelberg Electric Belt," sold in the 1902 catalog of the Sears Roebuck Company, was described as providing "the most wonderful relief and cure of all chronic and nervous diseases, disorders, and weaknesses peculiar to men, no matter from what cause or how long standing."

It was outrageous and completely unsubstantiated claims such as this and comparable problems with drugs, foods, and cosmetics that led to the Pure Food and Drug Act of 1906 and the formation of the FDA. A few years later, the Carnegie Foundation commissioned Abraham Flexner to conduct a comprehensive and independent study of the nation's medical schools. Flexner's 1910 report led to the reorganization of medical education (1).

Clinical teaching facilities were moved to closer geographical proximity to university science departments. This was the beginning of modern scientific medical education based on clinical research.

With the abolishment of electrotherapy devices came a period when academics frowned upon anyone who even brought up the subject of electromagnetic therapy. But a few scientists continued to pursue research on biological electricity and made significant progress, although their findings were, until recently, largely ignored. We shall look at some of the early work and see how it is being successfully applied in clinical medicine. Bioelectromagnetic approaches are used in both diagnosis and treatment, and we shall take a close look at some examples of each.

II. BIOELECTROMAGNETIC MEDICINE TODAY

In clinical medicine, there are many devices using different forms of energy for diagnosis and treatment. X-rays and MRIs fall into the diagnostic category. Passive measures of the fields produced by the body are also important in diagnosis: electrocardiograms, electroencephalograms, electroretinograms, electromyograms, and their biomagnetic counterparts, magnetocardiograms, magnetoencephalograms, magnetoretinograms, magnetomyograms, etc.

As recently as 10 years ago, most physicians and biomedical researchers were certain that the human body did not have any sort of energy field around it, and now medical decisions are being made on the basis of biofield measurements. It is important to appreciate that the standard methods of recording electrical fields with electrodes on the skin surface provide much less information than the corresponding biomagnetic measurements. The reason for this is that the electrical resistances of the various tissues vary by a factor of about 30. Bioelectric fields generated within the body by tissues such as the heart and brain take the paths of least electrical resistance, so the patterns measured at the body surface are intricate and difficult to interpret. In contrast, the magnetic permeabilities of the various tissues are all about the same, approximately 1, as in a vacuum. Hence the biomagnetic measures provide a picture of internal activities that has a much higher spatial resolution.

Modern researchers have developed the magnetic biopsy (2), the electrical biopsy (3), and the optical biopsy (4). Transcutaneous nerve stimulators, cardiac pacemakers and defibrillators, lasers, electrocautery, and pulsing magnetic field therapy are examples of treatment modalities that are part of conventional medicine. Controversy or not, energy medicine is alive and well in hospitals, clinics, and research centers.

From the historical perspective, transcutaneous electrical nerve stimulation (TENS) and pulsing electromagnetic field therapies (PEMFs) played a vital role in rehabilitating electromedicine.

In the meantime, various hands-on energy approaches are making their way into the hospital setting, at least in some locations. Here in New England, in Wentworth-Douglass Hospital, surgeons inform their patients that Reiki treatments are available pre- and post-operatively. It is a popular program and is spreading to other hospitals, many of which have established departments of integrative medicine to provide access to acupuncture, massage, Reiki, and other popular complementary therapies that were virtually unmentionable in hospitals a few years ago.

Acupuncture has been used by millions of Americans and is now recognized by the National Institutes of Health (NIH) and the FDA. The FDA regulates acupuncture needles as medical devices, and rates them in the category of 'safe and effective.' In collaboration with the FDA, the NIH conducted a 2 $\frac{1}{2}$-year study of acupuncture, electrical acupuncture, and microcurrent therapies and published their Consensus Statement in November 1997 (5). The Consensus Statement concludes (5)

> While it is often thought that there is substantial research evidence to support conventional medical practices, this is frequently not the case. This does not mean that these treatments are ineffective. The data in support of acupuncture are as strong as those for many accepted Western medical therapies. One of the advantages of acupuncture is that the incidence of adverse effects is substantially lower than that of many drugs or other accepted medical procedures used for the same conditions.

This information is provided to indicate that a complementary medical modality such as acupuncture can be accepted and used widely even though the underlying mechanisms involved remain a subject of ongoing research. In terms of the theme of this chapter, modern developments in meridian theory are extremely useful in exploring the basis for the various electromagnetic technologies, as the meridians are essential parts of the body's "circuitry" that both produces and responds to energy fields. Recent research is describing the nature of the interactions between the acupuncture needle and the connective tissue into which it is inserted (6,7).

Healing Touch and Therapeutic Touch are energy therapies taught in many nursing schools, are practiced widely, and are often reimbursed by health insurance. Nurse practitioners have a basic science background and have started many well-designed research projects to explore the basis and efficacy of these techniques. Valuable information is being obtained by studying the ways these methods affect living tissues.

It seems incomprehensible to some that the tiny energy fields radiating from the hands of a therapist or generated by the piezoelectric effect from the pressures used in massage or other hands-on methods could conceivably affect physiological processes within the body. However, we now know that these fields are similar in strength and frequency to those emitted by the proven therapeutic devices to be described below. This is an important point for those who design electrotherapeutic devices because we are discerning that living tissues are far more sensitive to external fields than previously realized. After a period when physicists were certain that observed sensitivities to nonionizing and nonthermal radiations were physically impossible, we now know that biological systems defy the simple logic that larger stimuli should produce larger responses. For many living systems, extremely weak fields can be more effective than strong fields (8). This is possible because of two important phenomena, cellular amplification and stochastic resonance, to be discussed below.

III. PULSING ELECTROMAGNETIC FIELD THERAPY

Given the stifling academic atmosphere of the times, and the FDA's reluctance to approve electromagnetic therapies of any kind, the acceptance of pulsing electromagnetic field therapy for bone healing was a milestone. In his last scientific paper, C. Andrew L. Bassett (1924–1994) summarized the history of this development (9). Much credit is due Bassett and his colleagues at Columbia University, College of Physicians and Surgeons, in New York for their persistence in overcoming daunting regulatory hurdles and entrenched skepticism to bring this technology into mainstream medicine. The first FDA approval was obtained in 1979.

In the mid-1800s, electric stimulation was the method of choice for slow-healing bone fractures (10). Direct currents were passed through needles inserted directly into the fracture gap. The method was successful for bone fractures but was soon abused by being applied to more and more human ailments, from cancer to colds, contributing to the backlash that led to the abolition of all electrotherapies.

In the 1950s and 1960s, there was a resurgence of interest in the United States and Japan when the validity of DC stimulation of bone healing was confirmed in animal studies (11,12). Basic research into the mechanisms involved led to a detailed understanding of the way energy fields stimulate the recruitment of bone-forming cells at a fracture site. Apparently the DC currents mimic the injury potentials generated in bone by a fracture (13). Artificial microampere currents seem to trigger a response similar to that involved in the normal repair process.

Soon it was realized that the microcurrents could be induced to flow in the fracture site noninvasively by magnetic induction: pulsing electromagnetic fields (PEMFs) provided by coils placed around the cast would induce current flows through the fracture site (Fig. 1). Extensive multicenter clinical trials have confirmed the effectiveness of both electrical (14,15) and magnetic (16) fields for bone healing. By 1982, Bassett was able to report an overall success rate at Columbia Presbyterian Medical Center in New York of 81%; internationally, 79%, and in other patients in the United States, 76%. Treatment with PEMFs was effective in 75% of 332 patients with an average 4.7 year disability duration, an average of 3.4 previous operative failures to produce union, and a 35% rate of infection (16).

Basic research on cells in culture, animals, and clinical studies led to specific information on the frequency, amplitude, orientation, and exposure characteristics required to activate specific processes in specific cells (17). As a result, we now have a sophisticated understanding of the mechanism of action of bioelectromagnetic therapies—with a detailed picture of the cascade of reactions taking place from the cell surface to the cytoplasm and on to the nucleus and genes—where selective effects on transcription and translation have been documented (18). Figure 2 summarizes the scheme as it is presently understood. A single

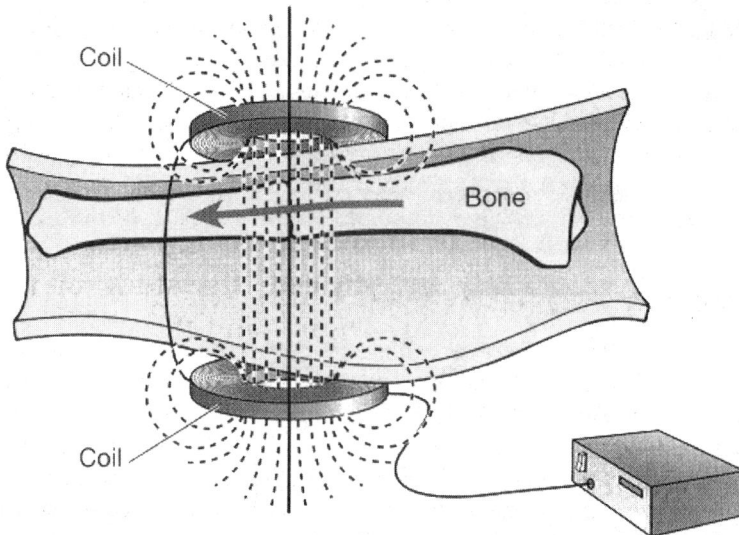

Figure 1 Pulsed electromagnetic field therapy (PEMF) involves passing currents through coils adjacent to an injury such as a bone fracture. The magnetic fields induce a current flow in the bone (arrow) that jump-starts the healing process, even in an nonunion that has failed to heal for many years. (From Ref. 55, Fig. 6.1A, p. 74; used by permission of Churchill Livingstone, Edinburgh.)

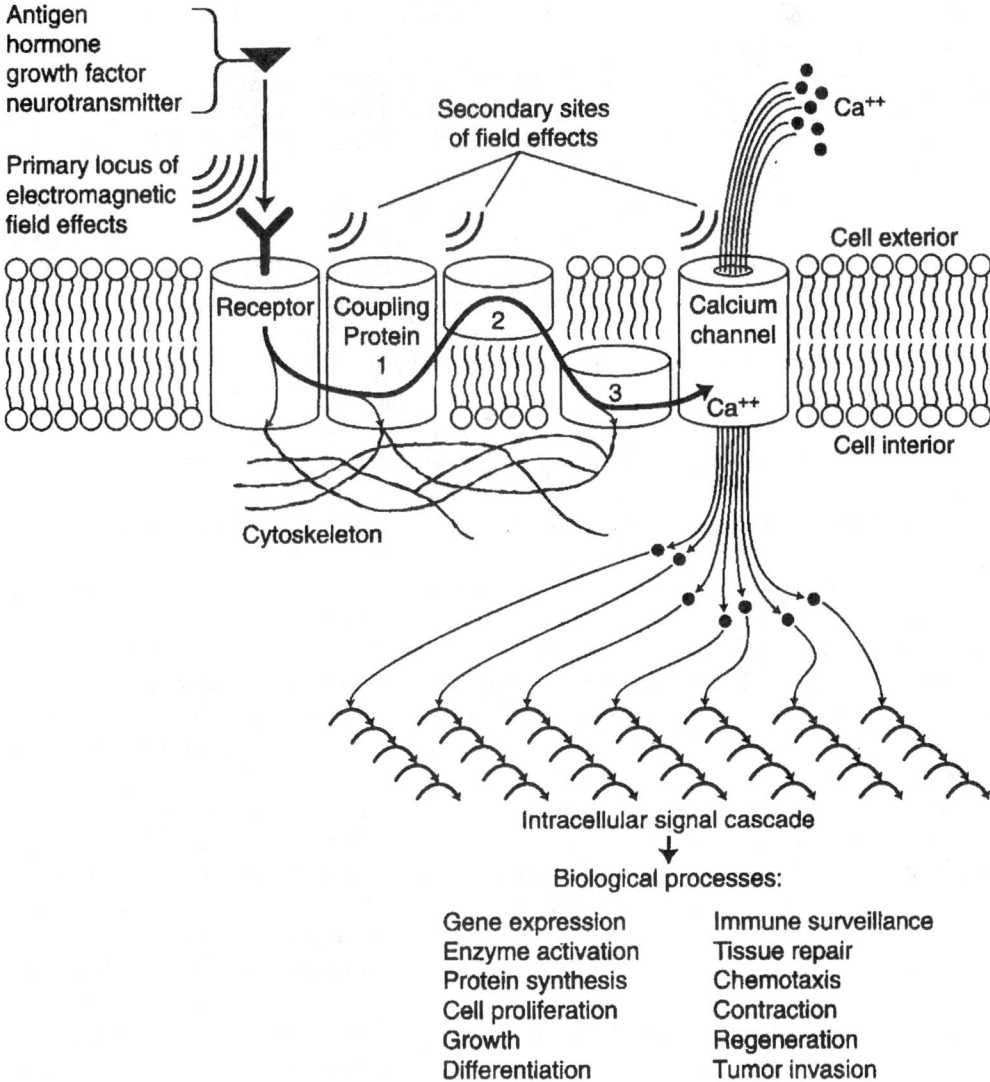

Figure 2 The cellular cascade and amplification process that provides a basis for the effects of pulsing electromagnetic field therapies as well as various complementary therapies such as Reiki, Therapeutic Touch, Healing Touch, Polarity Therapy, Cranialsacral, etc. (From Ref. 50, Fig. A-1, p. 253; used by permission of Churchill Livingstone, Edinburgh.)

antigen, hormone, pheromone, growth factor, smell or taste or neurotransmitter molecule, or a single photon of electromagnetic energy can produce a cascade of intracellular signals that initiate, accelerate, or inhibit biological processes. This is possible because of enormous amplification—a single molecular event at the cell surface can trigger a huge influx of calcium ions, each of which can activate an enzyme. The enzymes, in turn, act as catalysts, greatly accelerating biochemical processes. The enzymes are not consumed by these reactions and can therefore act repeatedly. Some of the reactions are sensitive to electromagnetic fields, some are not, and others have not yet been tested. Some frequencies enhance calcium entry, while others diminish it. Steps in the cascade involving free radical formation are likely targets of magnetic fields.

Bone healing is stimulated by minute currents, far smaller than those that could produce significant tissue heating. This is explained by the cellular amplification process described in the 1994 Nobel Prize in Physiology of Medicine (19). The subject is discussed further in the chapter by W.R. Adey in this book (Chapter 1).

An additional mechanism, unanticipated by the physicists who were convinced that the biologists were hallucinating about the extreme sensitivity of living systems, is stochastic resonance. This is a process that enables both living systems and electronic devices to detect signals that are far smaller than ambient noise. The noise in a biological or electronic system actually plays a constructive role in detecting weak rhythmic signals. The regular periodic signal entrains ambient noise to boost the signal strength to a detectable level (20,21).

Patients with fracture nonunions now have a vastly improved clinical prognosis. The PEMF method is just as successful as surgical repair, without the attendant hazards (17). The appropriate electromagnetic fields are very specific, inexpensive to apply, and devoid of risks.

Bassett estimated that there are some 2 million long-bone fractures in the United States every year, of which some 5% fail to heal normally within 3–6 months. Some never heal, leading to prolonged disability and even amputation. By 1995, Bassett could state that PEMF was used in the treatment of more than 300,000 un-united fractures, with no untoward events or hazards observed. Approximately 20% of the 100,000 tardy fracture unions are treated by this riskless method each year, the remainder being repaired by an operation that costs 2–3 times as much and that carries a significant complication rate.

Since 1979, when PEMFs were first approved by the FDA for treating nonunions, more than 17,500 members of the approximately 20,000-member American Academy of Orthopedic Surgeons have prescribed the method, most on multiple occasions.

Bassett and his colleagues also researched the use of PEMFs on other musculoskeletal problems and had considerable success. These include osteoarthritis, osteonecrosis, osteochondritis dessecans, osteogenesis imperfecta, and osteoporosis. Sadly, more widespread application of PEMF for these conditions is limited by FDA restrictions that require separate clinical trials and approvals on an indication-by-indication basis, in spite of the mechanistic, animal, and human data that have been accumulated. Industry simply cannot justify the huge expenditures needed to meet FDA requirements that would lead to wider use of this valuable technology. Fortunately, the extensive basic research and clinical data published by Bassett are available should the regulatory climate change so these methods can be made more widely available.

IV. PEMF EFFECTS ON SOFT TISSUES

After decades of clinical success with the use of PEMF for bone, attention turned naturally to injuries of soft tissues, such as nerve, skin, muscle, and tendon and the pain associated with those injuries. Unlike the situation in the late 1800s, however, these applications are being developed with appropriate mechanistic understandings (22) and clinical verification. Siskin and Walker summarize the results with various soft tissues (23). The following effects have been observed:

Enhanced capillary formation
Decreased necrosis
Reduced swelling

Diminished pain

Faster functional recovery

Reduction in depth, area, and pain in skin wounds

Reduced muscle loss after ligament surgery

Increased tensile strength in ligaments

Acceleration of nerve regeneration and functional recovery.

V. SINE WAVE DEVICES

In 1979, Blackman and colleagues (24) confirmed earlier reports of Bawin and others (25) showing that DC magnetic fields play a role in determining the biological effectiveness of weak intensity extremely low frequency (ELF) magnetic fields. On the basis of these findings, the distinguished American researcher, Abraham R. Liboff and his colleagues developed the ion cyclotron resonance (ICR) concept (26).

Robert O. Becker, in Cross Currents, provides a simplified explanation of this important phenomenon (27). An ion exposed to a steady magnetic field will begin to move in a circular or orbital motion at right angles to the applied field. Energy is transferred from the field to the charged particle. Cyclotron resonance is a mechanism that enables very low strength electromagnetic fields, acting in concert with the earth's geomagnetic field, to produce significant biological effects by enhancing movements of important ions such as sodium, potassium, and calcium across the cell membrane. Calculations using the equations for ICR indicate that the frequencies for the oscillating fields needed to produce resonance with biologically important ions are in the ELF region. Further research by Liboff and others has provided experimental and theoretical support for the concept, and other labs have confirmed cellular responses to cyclotron resonance conditions for specific ions.

Within two years after Liboff's discovery, it was applied practically to the same problem as Bassett had tackled originally, namely the repair of bony nonunions. The ICR application is fundamentally different from all pulsed electromagnetic therapies in that the magnetic signal that is applied is a sine wave. Rather than the intensity, the emphasis shifted to the frequency of the signal. Today, two ICR devices are approved for use by the FDA: the first for the treatment of nonunions, and the second for spinal fusion following back surgery.

VI. OTHER PULSING FIELD DEVICES

Naturally, clinical success with PEMF and ICR has led many creative and ingenious inventors to develop other applications for a wide range of other disorders. Although some of these have supportive scientific studies (28,29) and are approved by regulatory agencies in other countries with strict standards for proving safety and efficacy, attempts to gain FDA approval have been frustrating and disappointing. I have met a number scientists and therapists who have successfully or unsuccessfully dealt with the regulatory issues, and none have had a positive experience. Protection of the public from useless and ineffective technologies is essential, and the FDA has played a vital role in this process. But protection must be properly balanced with encouragement and openness for new and potentially useful approaches.

The overall impression is that the American public is being overly protected, particularly from the enormous potential offered by electromagnetic therapies. Many opportunities for treatments with better clinical outcomes have been abandoned or have moved to other countries. This creates the dilemma for the patient as to whether they should seek help across the border where these treatments are available but where clinical trials are generally not conducted with the same rigor as in the United States. In some sense, the babies are, sadly, being tossed out with the bath water. There is an urgent need to find better ways of distinguishing the wheat from the chaff and for encouraging the very promising biomedical research on bioelectromagnetics. One has the impression that the extravagant claims for electrotherapies a hundred years ago created an atmosphere of confusion and bias that was seized upon by the pharmaceutical industry, leading to its current virtual monopoly on medical treatments.

VII. TRANSCUTANEOUS ELECTRICAL NERVE STIMULATION

Another crucial step in the revival of electrotherapeutics was the development of transcutaneous electrical nerve stimulation (TENS). In 1965, Melzack and Wall proposed the gate control theory of pain (30). A few years later, C. Normal Shealy, M.D., a neurosurgeon who had been routinely implanting dorsal column stimulators (DCS) that he had developed to control pain, discovered that the electric signals could be introduced from the skin surface, providing pain control without the risks of surgery (31). After a lengthy and difficult interaction with the FDA, the TENS unit was recognized as safe and effective, and there are now more than 100 different FDA approved devices in this category, with some 250,000 TENS units prescribed annually in the United States alone. Like Bassett, Shealy deserves much credit for persisting with the regulatory process, for his work has had a huge impact in pain management and reduced suffering for a very large patient population.

   As this book is going to press, Dr. Shealy is announcing a new and improved model of his device, known as the She/Li Tens. The new design is based on years of continuing investigation following on the success of the earlier TENS system, and the development of a remarkable treatment protocol known as the five circuits or *sacred rings*. The device is showing excellent results not only for treatment of pain but also for depression, rheumatoid arthritis, migraine headache, and diabetic neuropathy (e.g., Ref. 32).

VIII. HAROLD SAXTON BURR AND ENERGY FIELD DIAGNOSIS

Harold Saxton Burr obtained his Doctor of Philosophy degree at Yale in 1915 and became a full professor at Yale School of Medicine in 1929. He was appointed E.K. Hunt Professor of Anatomy in 1933 and remained in the post for 40 years. He is one of several investigators who utilized their secure tenured status to research highly controversial subjects.

   In 1932, Burr began a series of studies on the role of electricity in ontogeny and disease. From his earlier work on the development of the nervous system, he realized how little was known about the control of form in animals. Molecular genetics was showing how the parts of the body are manufactured, but there was little understanding of the "blueprint" that directs their assembly into cells, tissues, organs, and the whole organism. This is a mystery that continues to this day, as we see genomics being superseded by proteonomics. Many assume that the pattern or blueprint for the body resides in the genome, but the truth is that this has never been documented and the real source of morphogenetic information must at least in part be elsewhere. Chapter 10 by Mitchell, on quantum holography, provides an important and cutting-edge perspective on this subject.

   Burr's work on energy fields from 1932 to 1956 was way out of step with the mainstream medicine and biology of the time. This was a period of explosive growth in pharmaceutical medicine and the application of x-rays for diagnosis. Antibiotics were winning the "war on disease," and the thrust of medical research and public interest was toward "a pill for every problem." Scientific and medical progress occurred at a seemingly dazzling pace. In this heady atmosphere there was little interest in Burr's essential findings, i.e., that living systems produce energy fields that can be measured and that are useful for diagnosis of disease. Moreover, Burr was convinced that application of appropriate energy fields could counteract pathological processes.

The abundance of untested and highly questionable electromagnetic devices created an atmosphere in which electromedicine was held in suspicion. This definitely created an opportunity for the rapidly growing pharmaceutical industry, which spent a large portion of its income on advertising, educating physicians, and conducting research on the benefits of various drugs. In spite of great promise, comparable funding has never been available for electromagnetic medicine.

The general academic consensus during Burr's tenure at Yale was that energy therapies and "healing energy" were nonsense concepts. Those who thought they were benefiting from energy therapies of any kind were considered by many to be victims of deception, illusion, trickery, fakery, quackery, hallucination, or the placebo effect. Scientists were certain that any energy field around an organism would be far too weak to be detected. If such a field existed, it surely had no biological significance. This perspective has changed completely with the development of modern biomagnetic measurement techniques, particularly the superconducting quantum interference device (SQUID).

IX. EARLY EXPERIMENTS ON TUMORS

In the 1920s, Fricke and Morse noted differences in electrical impedance and capacitance properties of normal and benign tissue and malignant tumors (33). This was a landmark study because it opened up the possibility of studying the electronic and dielectric properties of living systems. But many years passed before research of this kind was taken up by modern investigators.

In 1940, Burr and his colleagues induced tumors in mice by applying a carcinogen, benzpryene, and followed the electrical potentials at skin points across the axillary areas (34). There was an initial hyperelectrical inflammatory response, followed by a return to normal, and then a wave of hypoelectrical activity. The original data were graphed for the first time by Brewitt in 1996 (35) and are shown in Fig. 3. Further work by Burr, also summarized by Brewitt, substantiated that measurements of skin voltage could indicate physiological states such as cancer, wound healing, central nervous system activity, drug use, sleep, development, and reproductive cycles.

These studies laid the foundation for the electrical and electronic correlates of disease. Interestingly, it was during this same period that Nobel Laureate Albert Szent-Györgyi began his studies of electronic biology with his observation that protein molecules must be semiconductors (36). While this view was initially opposed, it was not long before it was determined that most if not all biological molecules have semiconductor properties (37). The application of electrical and electronic properties of tissues for diagnosis and treatment has, until recently, evolved slowly.

Electromagnetic cancer detection advanced in 1991, when Swarup and colleagues (38) showed that the electrical conductivity of tumors differed when measured at radio frequencies between 104 and 108 Hz. Specifically, tumor conductivities were lower than normal tissues when measured at 104–106 Hz, while they were higher than normal tissues when measured at 106–108 Hz. When measurements were made directly on the tumors, conductivities were 6.0–7.5 times higher than normal tissue (39). Further research in vitro

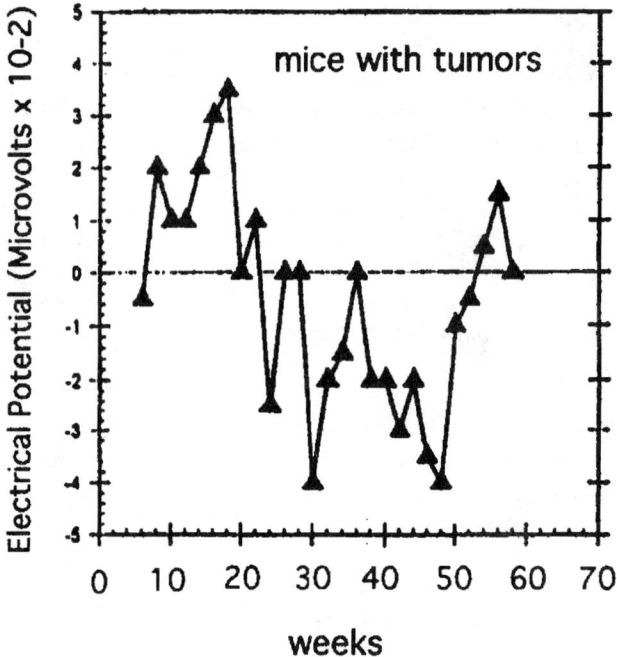

Figure 3 Tumors in mice were induced by applying a carcinogen, benzpryene, and followed the electrical potentials at skin points across the axillary areas (34). (Reproduced by permission of the Journal of Naturopathic Medicine.)

(40–42) and in vivo (43,44) confirmed that electrical and electronic properties could be used for cancer detection.

X. DEVELOPMENT OF PRACTICAL DIAGNOSTIC TOOLS FOR BREAST CANCER

It is a big step from direct measurements of electrical and dielectric properties of surgically removed tumors to a practical noninvasive diagnostic tool. In 1998, Cuzick and colleagues (45) described a noninvasive electropotential test based on Burr's original observation that cancer results in electrical disturbances that can extend to the skin surface. Rapidly proliferating and transformed cells have electrically depolarized cell membranes compared with normal cells (46–48). The diagnostic method involves placing a specially designed array of sensors in the region of a suspected lesion (Fig. 4). The test requires a 10-min equilibration period followed by less than 1 min of data acquisition that results in a depolarization index.

A multicenter study of the method was carried out at eight breast centers in five European countries. Tests were performed on 661 patients scheduled for biopsy. The electropotential tests showed 55% specificity and 90% sensitivity for palpable lesions (49). Funds were raised to seek FDA approval, but this has not happened so far.

In the meantime, another group, T-Scan has developed a promising device based on electrical impedance scanning. A low-level electric signal is transmitted into the body and the resulting electric field is measured by sensors in a noninvasive probe placed on the breast. Measurements are made over several frequencies using proprietary algorithms that create and display real-time capacitance and conductivity images of the breast. Malignant tissue

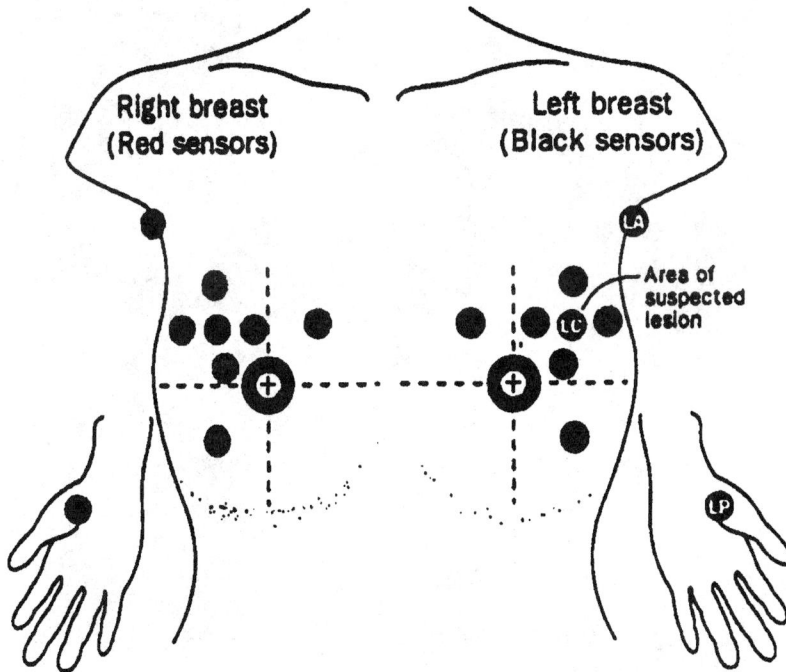

Figure 4 A non-invasive electropotential test based on Burr's original observation that cancer results in electrical disturbances that can extend to the skin surface.

differs from normal breast tissue in electrical properties because of differences in water and electrolyte content, changes in membrane permeability, and differences in orientation and packing density of cells (50). An earlier version, called TS2000, was subjected to an international, multicenter trial and received approval from the FDA in April 1999 for use as an adjunct to mammography (51). If a lesion looked suspicious on a mammogram, the TS 2000 exam could be used to determine whether a patient has cancer cells without the need for a biopsy. Clinical trials are continuing.

The current device (Figure 5) is called the T-Scan 2000ED (for early detection). The device has been improved and simplified from earlier versions, and is now suitable for use in the office of a gynecologist. It is particularly valuable for screening young women who do not get routine mammography and for whom the cancer rate is increasing at an alarming rate. Regular screening of younger women can save many lives because cancers in younger women tend to be more aggressive. Unlike any other diagnostic tool, the 2000 ED is capable of detecting tumors smaller than one centimeter in size, which is considered a biological "breaking point" affecting overall survival (52). In contrast to other technologies, the testing does no harm in terms of pain or radiation, and it is effective on women who have dense breast tissue.

These examples of electromagnetic diagnosis are presented to introduce the reader to what this author considers to be the frontier opportunity for modern medicine. There is no question that research into the solid state electronic semiconductor properties of living matter will lead to new understandings of the role of bioelectromagnetics in life and disease. To emphasize the importance of this topic, a recent issue of the IEEE Transactions on Medical Imaging is devoted to electrical impedance tomography (53).

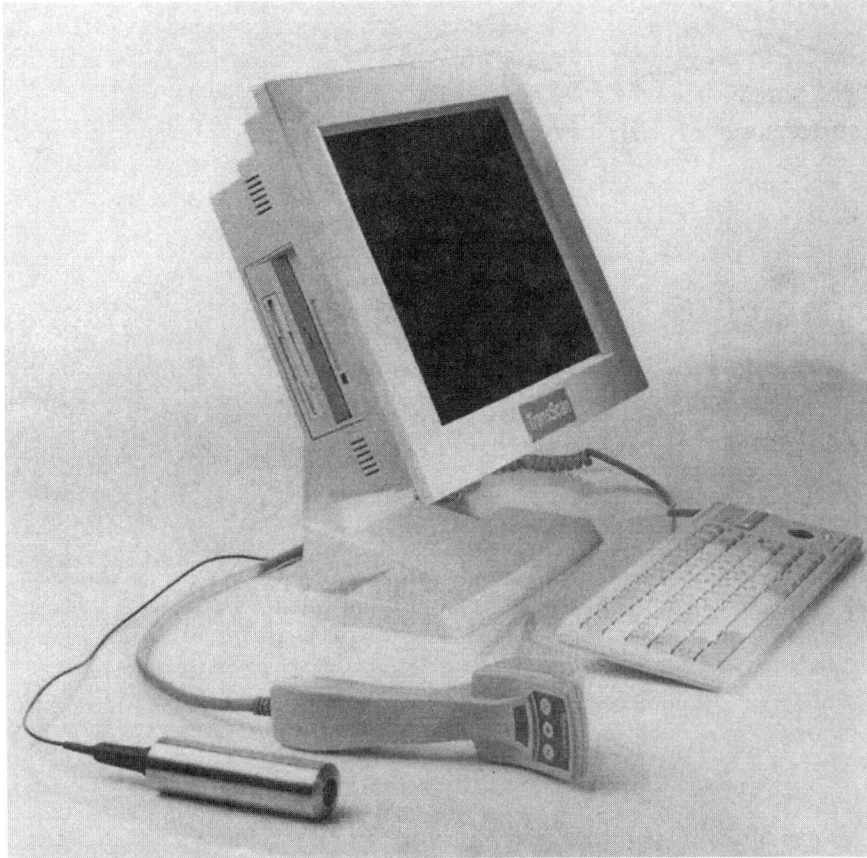

Figure 5 The T-Scan™ 2000ED (for Early Detection). (Illustration used courtesy of TransScan Medical, Inc., 70 Hilltop Road, Suite 2300, Ramsey, NJ 07446, and TransScan Medical, Ltd., Ramat Gabriel Industrial Zone, POB 786, 10550 Migdal HaEmek, Israel.)

XI. THE SUBSTRATE FOR BIOELECTROMAGNETIC INTERACTIONS

Precisely what is it within the body that interacts with electrical impedance scanners and other diagnostic tools and that responds to fields applied to the body? It is obvious that the fluid systems of the body, including the circulatory system and extracellular fluids of various kinds, will act as virtual antennas for externally applied fields. These fluids are highly conductive because they contain electrically charged ions, predominantly sodium, potassium, and chloride. More subtle but perhaps far more significant effects occur because the proteins and other molecules comprising the tissues are semiconductors.

Mention has been made of the early development of biological electronics and applications of solid-state physics to living systems. We now know that the human body is composed of an interconnected semiconductor fibrous matrix that extends into its every nook and cranny. Macroscopically, this system consists of the connective tissues that form bones, tendons, fascia, cartilage, and ligaments and that also form the matrix of all organs and glands. All of the great systems of the body, the musculature, vasculature, nervous system, digestive tract, integument, and lymphatics are composed of connective tissue that gives them their characteristic form and physical properties. Cell biologists have now

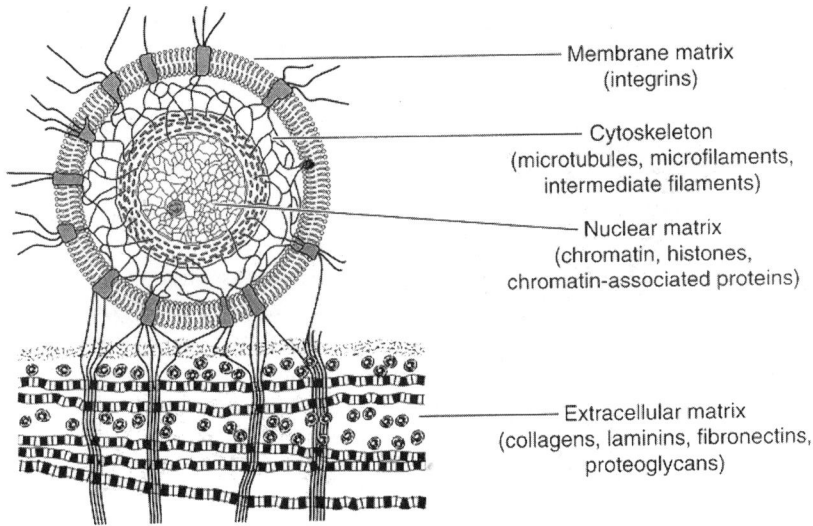

Figure 6 The living matrix consists of the classical connective tissue or extracellular matrix (shown at the bottom) plus the cellular matrix composed of the cytoskeleton and the nuclear matrix. The strands and fibers are continuous across the cell surface membrane matrix by virtue of the integrins. (The drawing is adapted from K. J. Pienta and D. S. Coffey. Cellular harmonic information transfer through a tissue tensegrity–matrix system, Medical Hypotheses 34:88–95, 1991, and is used by permission from Medical Hypotheses.)

discerned how this continuous fibrous system connects with cell surfaces and cell interiors via transmembrane proteins such as the integrins (54). Figure 6 details the extracellular matrix and its continuity with the cytoskeleton and nuclear matrix. The entire system is termed the *living matrix* (55). It is significant that all components of this continuous system are liquid crystalline semiconductors (56,57), features that confer a variety of interesting properties to the material substance of the body. Future developments in bioelectromagnetics will undoubtedly emerge from the study of the living body as an integrated electronic and protonic circuit.

XII. CONCLUSIONS

While skepticism remains, modern science has essentially resolved the issues that have surrounded bioelectromagnetics and that have led to so much bitter controversy in the past. This progress is vitally important for the future evolution of medicine. The energetic perspective has, perhaps more than any other, been blinded by confusion and debate, significantly slowing medical progress. The confusion and controversy have benefited the very profitable pharmaceutical approach, which has dominated modern medicine in spite of its enormous costs and debilitating side effects. By following the energetic thread that runs through all therapies we are opening up a discussion that is having a dramatic impact on the future of medicine.

The developments summarized in this chapter are the tip of the iceberg in terms of the bioelectromagnetic therapies that are available or are being developed. After talking with researchers around the country, it is apparent that bioelectromagnetics offers a tremendous opportunity to create a new and more effective kind of medicine with very specific effects and virtually no toxic side effects. Inordinately complex and arbitrary regulatory hurdles are hindering the emergence of this field, and another way of separating the wheat from the chaff is definitely needed if we are to survive the current crisis in health care and experience the full potential bioelectromagnetic medicine has to offer. For we are living in a time when the health care system is in severe crisis due to high costs, and we are experiencing several epidemics simultaneously, e.g., cancer and AIDS and chronic exposure to deadly toxins such as pesticides of all kinds and Aspartame and related sugar substitutes.

Energetic phenomena serve as a focal point for discussing both causes and treatments in new and productive ways. Many of the complementary therapies have energetic concepts as part of their theoretical base, and these methods not only are becoming quite popular, but also show promise for treating the chronic patient whose problems are the most costly in terms of suffering and in terms of health-care dollars, and whose lingering difficulties often frustrate the conventional physician.

ACKNOWLEDGMENTS

For valuable suggestions and comments, I am profoundly indebted to Drs. Paul Rosch, Karl Maret, Abe Liboff, and Marko Markov.

REFERENCES

1. Bassett CAL, Chokshi HR, Hernandez E, Pawluk RJ, Strop M. In: Brighton CT, Black J, Pollack SR, eds. Electrical Properties of Bone and Cartilage: Experimental Effects and Clinical Applications. New York: Grune and Stratton, 1979:427.
2. Farrell DE. Assessment of iron in human tissue: The magnetic biopsy. In: Williamson SJ, Romani GL, Kaufman L, Modena I, eds. Biomagnetism: An Interdisciplinary Approach. New York: Plenum, 1983:483–500.
3. Scholz B. Towards virtual electrical breast biopsy: Space-frequency MUSIC for trans-admittance data. IEEE Trans on Medical Imaging 2002; 21(6):588–595.
4. Tearney GJ, Brezinski ME, Bouma BE, Boppart SA, Pitris C, Southern JF, Fujimoto JG. In vivo endoscopic optical biopsy with optical coherence tomography. Science 1997; 276(5321): 2002–2003.
5. The complete document from the NIH may be found on the World Wide Web by searching for National Institutes of Health Consensus Statement on Acupuncture, 1997.
6. Langevin HM, Churchill DL, Cipolla MJ. Mechanical signaling through connective tissue: a mechanism for the therapeutic effect of acupuncture. FASEB J 2001; 15:2275–2282.
7. Langevin HM, Churchill DL, Fox JR, Badger GJ, Garra BS, Krag MH. Biomechanical response to acupuncture needling in humans. J Appl Physiol 2001; 91(6):2471–2478.
8. Ho MW, Popp FA, Warnke U. Bioelectrodynamics and Biocommunication. Singapore: World Scientific, 1994.
9. Bassett CAL. Bioelectromagnetics in the service of medicine. In: Blank M, ed. Electromagnetic fields: biological interactions and mechanisms. Advances in Chemistry Series 250. Washington DC: American Chemical Society, 1995:261–275.
10. Lente RW. Cases of un-united fracture treated by electricity. NY J Med 1859; 5:317.
11. Yasuda I. Fundamental aspects of fracture treatment. J Kyoto Med Soc 1953; 4:395–406.
12. Bassett LS, Pawluk RJ, Becker RO. Effects of electric currents on bone in vivo. Nature 1964; 204:652.
13. Borgens RB. Exogenous ionic currents traverse intact and changed bone. Science 1984; 225(4661):478–482.

14. Brighton CT, Black J, Friedenberg ZB, Esterhai JL, Day LJ, Connolly JF. A multicenter study of the treatment of non-union with constant direct current. J Bone Joint Surg Am 1981; 63(1):2–13.

15. Mammi GI, Rocchi R, Cadossi R, Massari L, Traina GC. The electrical stimulation of tibial osteotomies. Double blind study. Clin Orthop 1993; 288:246–253.

16. Bassett CAL, Mitchell SUN, Gaston SR. Pulsing electromagnetic field treatment in ununited fractures and failed arthroeses. JAMA 1982; 247(5):623–628.

17. Bassett CAL. Fundamental and practical aspects of therapeutic uses of pulsed electromagnetic fields (PEMFs). Crit Rev Biomed Eng 1989; 17(5):451–529.

18. Bassett CAL, Chokshi HR, Hernandez E, Pawluk RJ, Strop M. In: Brighton CT, Black J, Pollack SR, eds. Electrical Properties of Bone and Cartilage; Experimental Effects and Clincal Applications. New York: Grune and Stratton, 1979:427.

19. Gilman AG. G proteins and regulation of adenylyl cyclase. Nobel Lecture presented December 8 1994. In: Ringertz N, ed. Nobel Lectures Physiology or Medicine. Singapore: World Scientific, 1991–1995:182–212.

20. Wiesenfeld AK, Moss F. Stochastic resonance and the benefits of noise. In: Ice ages to crayfish and SQUID's. Nature 1995; 373:33–36.

21. Bulsara AR, Gammaitoni L. Tuning into noise. Physics Today, March 1996:39–45.

22. Goodman R, Henderson A. Exposure of salivary gland cells to low-frequency electromagnetic fields alters polypeptide synthesis. Proc Natl Acad Sci USA 1988; 85(11):3928–3932.

23. Siskin BF, Walker J. Therapeutic aspects of electromagnetic fields for soft-tissue healing. In: Blank M, ed. Electromagnetic fields: biological interactions and mechanisms. Advances in Chemistry Series 250. Washington DC: American Chemical Society, 1995:227–285.

24. Blackman CF, Elder JA, Weil CM, Bename SG, Eichinger DC, House DE. Induction of calcium-ion efflux from brain tissue by radio-frequency radiation: effects of modulation frequency and field strength. Radio Science 1979; 14(6S):93–98.

25. Bawin SM, Kaczmarek LK, Adey WR. Effects of modulated very high frequency fields on specific brain rhythms in cats. Brain Research 1975; 58:365–384.

26. Liboff A. Geomagnetic cyclotron resonance in living cells. J Biol Phys 1985; 13:99–102.

27. Becker RO. Cross Currents. Los Angeles: Jeremy P. Tarcher, 1990:236.

28. Trock DH, Bollet AJ, Markoll R. The effect of pulsed electromagnetic fields in the treatment of osteoarthritis of the knee and cervical spine. Report of randomized, double blind, placebo controlled trials. J Rheumatol 1994; 21(10):1903–1911.

29. Trock DH, Bollet AJ, Dyer RH Jr, Felding LP, Miner WK, Markoll R. A double-blind trial of the clinical effects of pulsed electromagnetic fields in osteoarthritis. J Rheumatol 1993; 20(12): 2166–2167.

30. Melzack R, Wall PD. Pain mechanisms: a new theory. Science 1965; 150:971.

31. Shealy CN, Mortimer JT, Reswich JB. Electrical stimulation of pain by stimulation of the dorsal column: preliminary clinical reports. Anesth Analg 1967; 45:489.

32. Shealy CN, Cady RK, Cox RH. Pain, stress and depression: psychoneurophysiology and therapy. Stress Medicine 1995; 1:65–77.

33. Fricke H, Morse S. The electric capacity of tumors of the breast. J Cancer Res 1926; 16:310–376.

34. Burr HS, Smith GM, Strong LC. Electrometric studies of tumors induced in mice by the external application of benzpyrene. Yale J Biol Medicine 1940; 12:711–717.

35. Brewitt B. Quantitative analysis of electrical skin conductance in diagnosis: historical and current views of bioelectric medicine. J Naturopathic Medicine 1996; 6(1):66–75.

36. Szent-Gyrögyi A. The study of energy levels in biochemistry. Nature 1941; 148:157–159.

37. Rosenberg B, Postow E. Semiconduction in proteins and lipids-its possible biological import. Annals of the New York Academy of Sciences 1969; 158(1):161–190.

38. Swarup A, Stuchly SS, Surowiec A. Dielectric properties of mouse MCA1 fibrosarcoma at different stages of development. Bioelectromagnetics 1991; 12:1–8.

39. Smith SR, Foster KR, Wolf GL. Dielectric properties of VX-2 carcinoma versus normal liver tissue. IEEE Trans Biomed Eng 1986; BME-33:522–524.

40. Singh B, Smith CW, Hughes R. In vivo dielectric spectrometer. Med Biol Eng Comput 1979; 17:45–60.

41. Jossinet J. Variability of impedivity in normal and pathological breast tissue. Med Biol Eng Comput 1996; 34:346–350.

42. Jossinet J. The impedivity of freshly excised human breast tissue. Physiol Meas 1998; 19:61–75.

43. Morimoto T, Kinouchi Y, Iritani T, Kimura S, et al. Measurement of the electrical bio-impedance of breast tumors. Eur Surg Res 1990; 22:86–92.

44. Morimoto T, et al. A study of the electrical bio-impedance of tumors. J Invest Surg 1993; 6(1):25–32.

45. Cuzick J, Holland R, Barth V, Davies R, Faupel M, Fentiman I, Frischbier HJ, LaMarque JL, Merson M, Sacchini V, Vanel D, Veronesi U. Electropotential measurements as a new diagnostic modality for breast cancer. Lancet 1998; 352(9125):359–363.

46. Binggeli R, Weinstein RC. Membrane potentials and sodium channels: hypotheses for growth regulation and cancer formation based on changes in sodium channels and gap junctions. J Theoretical Biol 1986; 123(4):340–377.

47. Goller DA, Weidema WF, Davies RJ. Transmural electrical potential difference as an early marker in colon cancer. Arch Surg 1986; 121:345–350.

48. Marino AA, Iliev IG, Schwalke MAA, Gonzales E, Marler KC, Flanagan CA. Association between cell membrane potential and breast cancer. Tumor Biology 1994; 15:82–89.

49. Cuzick J. Continuation of the International Breast Cancer Intervention Study (IBIS). European Journal of Cancer 1998; 34(11):1647–1648.

50. Scholz B, Anderson LR. On electrical impedance scanning-principles and simulations. Electromedica 2000; 68:35–44.

51. FDA Approves new breast imaging device. FDA Talk Paper 1999; T99-18, http://www.fda.gov/bbs/topics/ANSWERS/ANS00950.html.

52. Michaelson JS, Silverstein M, Wyatt J, Weber G, Moore R, Halpern E, Kopans DB, Hughes K. Predicting the survival of patients with breast carcinoma using tumor size. Cancer 2002; 95:713–723.

53. Electrical impedance tomography. IEEE Trans Medical Imaging 2002; 21(6):1–712.

54. Horwitz AF. Integrins and health. Discovered only recently, these adhesive cell surface molecules have quickly revealed themselves to be critical to proper functioning of the body and to life itself. Scientific American 1997; 276:68–75.

55. Oschman JL. Energy Medicine: the scientific basis. Edinburgh: Churchill Livingstone, 2000: 41–68.

56. Ho M-W. Coherent energy, liquid crystallinity and acupuncture. Talk presented to British Acupuncture Society, 2 October 1999. http://www.i-sis.org/acupunc.shtml.

57. Ho M-W, Knight D. The acupuncture system and the liquid crystalline collagen fibers of the connective tissues. Am J Chinese Medicine 1988; 26:251–263.

7

Evolution of Electrotherapy: From TENS to Cyberpharmacology

C. Norman Shealy

Holos Institutes of Health, Inc., Fair Grove, Missouri, U.S.A.

Saul Liss and Bernard S. Liss

MEDI Consultants, Inc., Paterson, New Jersey, U.S.A.

The use of electricity in medicine is reviewed with special emphasis on its use for the treatment of pain that culminated in dorsal column stimulation and our development of the TENS device. We later found that pain relief could be enhanced with cranioelectrical stimulation which also relieved symptoms of depression via effects on serotonin. This chapter reviews effects on a host of other neurotransmitters following cranio-electrical and electroacupuncture techniques that have led to an appreciation of five specific energetic circuits: the Ring of Fire, Ring of Air, Ring of Water, Ring of Earth, and Ring of Crystal. The acupuncture sites and cyberpharmacologic significance of each of these are explained.

I. INTRODUCTION

The use of electricity, interestingly, is almost as old as acupuncture. As early as 2750 B.C. individuals were exposed to shocks produced by electric eels (1). Static electricity was created by rubbing amber at least as early as 400 B.C. Modern medical electrotherapy, however, began in the late 1700s. A wide variety of electrotherapy devices were patented throughout the nineteenth century. Unfortunately, the Flexner Report in 1910 almost wiped out electrotherapy and except for the fortuitous discovery of a naturopathic invention, the Electreat, we might not have modern electrotherapy. In 1919, C. W. Kent of Peoria, Illinois patented the Electreat, which came to the attention of Shealy at a time when he was introducing the concept of dorsal column stimulation (DCS) and resurrected the Electreat in clinical trials in the mid-1960s (2).

II. ELECTREAT TO DCS AND TENS

In an attempt to demonstrate to patients what they might feel with dorsal column stimulation, Shealy used the Electreat and encouraged engineers to develop a modern solid-state device.

DCS had a brief enthusiastic period of usage, but its complications led Shealy to discontinue it in 1973. It was his conclusion that the risk in benign pain did not justify any risk of possible paralysis. In recent years, DCS has been somewhat resurrected and is used today more often to treat reflex sympathetic dystrophy (RSD) than to treat other forms of pain. Shealy has not recommended it for that use, however, because he has found that intravenous magnesium works quite adequately in most patients with RSD.

In 1975, Liss brought to Shealy his earliest device, the Pain Suppressor; that and its later evolution will be discussed in Sec. IV, Modulated Electric Energy Stimulator. Shealy first noted that when the Pain Suppressor was applied transcranially, it caused a visual flicker, and shortly thereafter he demonstrated that cranial electrical stimulation (CES) significantly raised levels of serotonin (3). This is the first known example of *cyberpharmacology*, the use of electrical stimulation to modify pharmacologic neurochemistry. Since that time, Shealy and his colleagues have used the original Pain Suppressor and LISS TENS devices in well over 20,000 patients.

Shealy later demonstrated that use of the Liss device transcranially relieved depression in patients within 2 weeks without the use of drugs. If patients discontinued use of the stimulator over the next several months, the depression would return. Later work by Shealy and colleagues demonstrated that the addition of photostimulation, education, and music to cranial stimulation led to a significant relief of depression in 85% of patients who had failed pharmacological agents. Long-term follow-ups have revealed that at least 70% of patients with chronic depression can be maintained long term with only the LISS Cranial Stimulator transcranially, photostimulation, education, and music. This approach to depression is at least twice as effective as any known antidepressant drugs and without complications (4–9). Even more critically, a recent landmark article by the American Psychological Association emphasizes that "the pharmacological effects of antidepressants are clinically negligible." They proceed to suggest "alternative experimental designs for the evaluation of antidepressants (10)." We suggest that the treatment of choice is cyberpharmacology.

III. ELECTROACUPUNCTURE TO GIGATENS

In 1966, Shealy began applying electrical current to acupuncture needles. Interestingly, when the first medical delegation from the People's Republic of China visited this country in 1972, they indicated that electroacupuncture had begun in China about the same time. Unquestionably, the application of standard pulsed direct current (DC) to the acupuncture needles improved its efficacy moderately. However, Liss and Shealy were invited to visit the Ukraine Council of Ministers Research Center Vidhuk in Kiev 11 years ago and learned there that nuclear physicists and physicians had been working with a much higher frequency device, which they call *microwave resonance therapy*.

It was the belief of these scientists that each organ essentially has a vector potential of current from the organ to the surface of the body along the meridians discovered in acupuncture, which they called *channels*. The heart, for instance, projects its energy from the upper anterior chest down the ulnar side of the arm to the tip of the little finger and back. These scientists state that human DNA resonates at 54 to 78 GHz, and they believe that illness results not from a loss of frequency but a loss of intensity or total energy in a given channel (11). By 1994, they had already treated some 200,000 patients with a wide variety of illnesses claiming success of 50% in narcotic addicts and 6- to 24-month remission in over 90% of rheumatoid arthritics. Some of the Ukrainian devices were obtained and modified for research done in this country by Shealy, who has confirmed that remarkably beneficial effects from this type of current can be obtained in several illnesses, which will be discussed in a later section.

IV. MODULATED ELECTRICAL ENERGY STIMULATORS

Modulated electric energy stimulators are devices that utilize the physics characteristics of the body to have a beneficial clinical effect on the human in reducing pain and symptoms of depression, anxiety, and insomnia and are authorized by the FDA for these indications. Researchers have reported that they have already used these devices to reduce spasticity, enhance alertness, and increase attention span in the normal and increase the cognitive performance of neuronally deficient children. One researcher even developed safety information for use on the heads of children from 2.5 to 7.5 years of age. The authors conceived this application of the stimulator technology by analyzing the physics character-istics of the body and attempted to match the dynamic electrical impedance of the body with a stimulation pattern that the body could then convert into an internal signal that could be used constructively to help the body help itself.

A. Principles of Operation

1. Using the Electrical Characteristics of the Body

Modulated electrical energy stimulators utilize the principles of carrier-frequency penetra-tion, which places very low electrical charge on the bulk capacitance of the body or head of an individual in such a manner that when the current from the said stimulator is turned off for 33.3 μs, the charge can leak from the bulk capacitance into the resistance of the tissue. This activity causes a current to flow inside the body, which apparently has been able to alter the level of certain neurobiochemicals, as will be described subsequently. A modulated waveform, which philosophically turns the carrier waveform off and on and has been found to have certain bioactive effects on the human physiology, is impinged on the carrier.

2. Physics of the Body

The study of physics states that all matter (including the body) has electrical characteristics: resistive, capacitive, or inductive. There are some parts of the heart system that contain inductive characteristics, but in the main, the body and head are mostly capacitive and resistive (including semiconductorlike characteristics which are a very special form of conducting or resistive circuits).

For the record, resistive characteristics are those that impede the flow of current; capacitive characteristics include the ability to store an electrical charge. This has been observed in conjunction with the bulk capacitance of the body. If a researcher connected a capacitance meter or a power factor meter to measure the capacitance of the body, they would definitely find measurable capacitance associated therewith. The electrical equivalent circuit is shown in Fig. 1. When two contacts are placed on the body from a LISS Cranial or Body Stimulator (LCS or LBS), we observe the effect of the contact impedance and the epidermis as a parallel network of both resistance and capacitance. The next series element in the body is the dermis, which looks electrically like a resistor (as the signals begin to exit from the body or head), as does the nerve (also in series with the previous elements). Finally, the

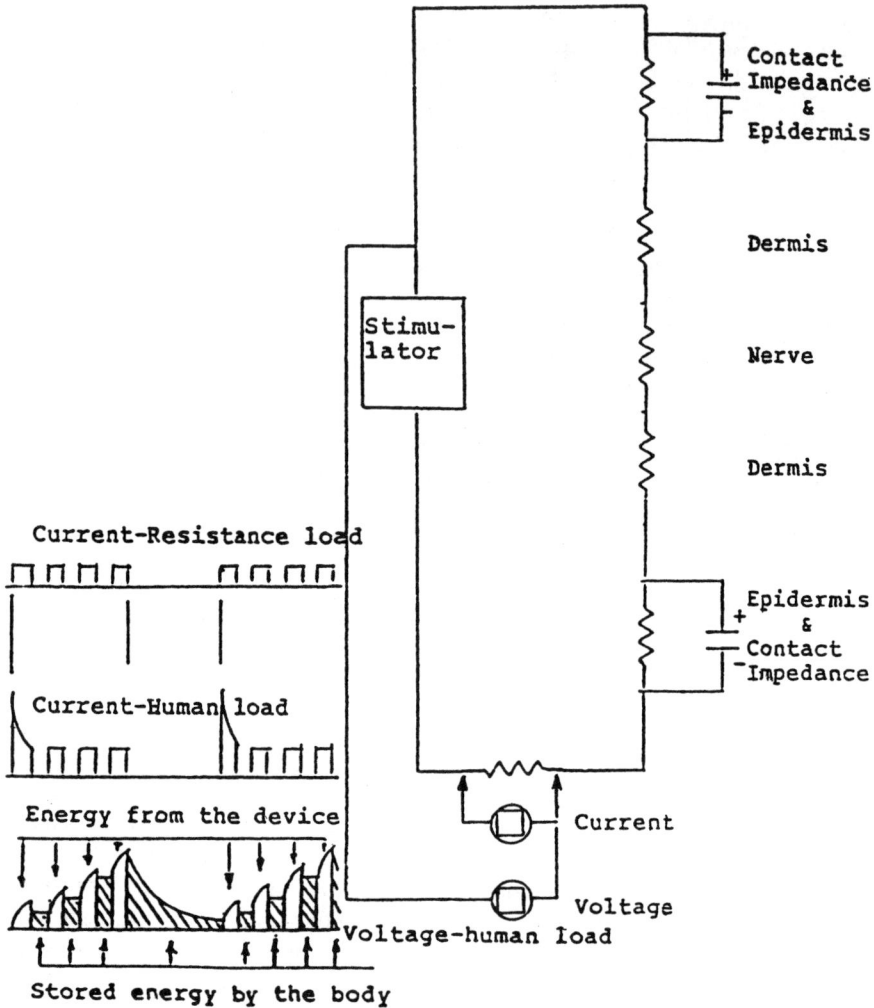

Figure 1 Equivalent circuit of the body.

exiting epidermis and contact impedance, appear as the same type of resistance and capacitance network as seen in the initial part of this analysis.

To test such a circuit, we must connect the stimulator in series both with the body or head circuit and a current-reading resistor, across which we attach an oscilloscope. This in turn can display the pattern of current that flows through the test system. Another oscilloscope, which should be connected above the stimulator and beyond the current-reading resistor, will present the pattern of the voltage, which represents the "pressure" that pushes the current through the impedance of the body (or head).

3. The Gathering Effect

Figure 2 shows the impact of the body's electrical circuit altering the wave shape of the LBS where the voltage rises from zero with the first pulse of energy in an exponential fashion, but when the pulse attempts to return to zero, it does not do so because the electrical charge from the device is stored on the bulk capacitance of the body and dissipates it when the high-speed

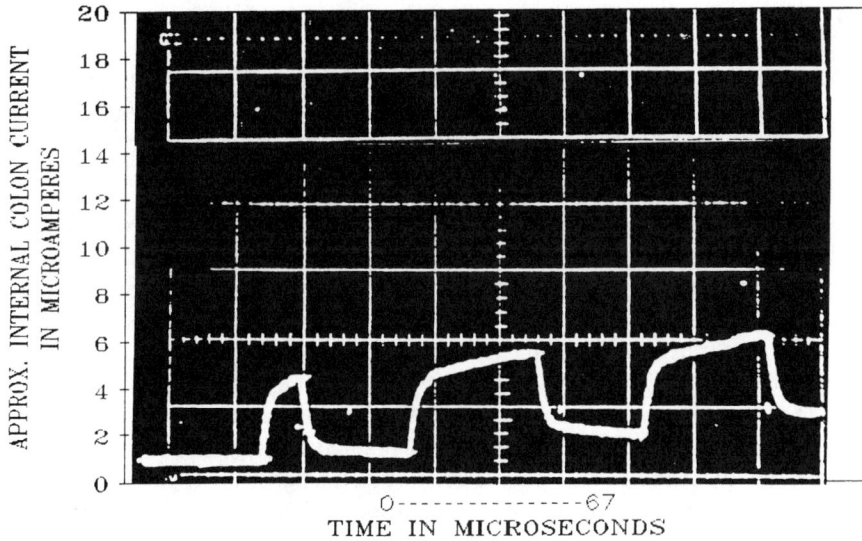

Figure 2 The gathering effect showing the energy storage of in vitro sigmoid colon stimulated by modulated electric energy stimulator.

pulse (15,000 Hz) is momentarily turned off (for 33.3 μs). During the off time of 33.3 μs, the stored energy leaks off through the body's own resistance (or equivalent), making a voltage step from which the second pulse is initiated. Continuation of this process is called the *gathering effect*, one pulse building on the level of the previous pulse—until an equilibrium is achieved.

4. The Triggering Phenomenon of the Body

The triggering concept is based on the assumption that it takes a certain amount of energy for a nerve signal to cross the synapse (12). When there is less than the required amount of energy present at the junction of the nerves under study, no signal will cross the synapse. When this occurs in a motor circuit, the affected muscle will not function. Similarly, in a sensory nerve or memory system, there will be no consequent change in perception or transference of the memory information. The disturbance can also occur in the emotional systems of the brain and mind thus bringing a cloud over the individual's whole thought processes or behavior. Sir John Eccles was the first to demonstrate signal transmission across the synapse as it related to intercellular resting potential in neurons. Sufficient energy at the synapse, therefore, appears to be essential for neurons that are involved in adaptive physiological mechanisms to function effectively and achieve homeostatic balance.

A research team at the Max Planck Institute of Biochemistry in Martinsried, Germany have built a new type of junction between a microscopic spot on a silicon chip and a corresponding spot on the neuron of a leech and have demonstrated that "an electric voltage applied to the interior of the chip produces an electric field that induces a charge inside the cell (13)." They showed, furthermore, that when this charge reaches a certain level, the cell fires, initiating the electrochemical sequence by which nerve cells communicate with their neighbors.

The apparent requirement of an increment of triggering energy to be present for an event to transpire is well known in nature. In chemistry, for example, reactants must reach a "temperature of reaction" for an effect to take place. Similarly, in mechanics, stiction (static friction) must be overcome for motion to take place.

We hypothesize that in physiology, while the factors for an action may be present, if the triggering energy is absent or insufficient, no action will occur. We suggest that in some cases, introducing the current of the LCS or the LBS facilitates the physiologic action.

5. Demodulation

Demodulation is the process of separating the audio frequency or the video signal from the carrier waveform in radio and television transmission, respectively. There is a circuit in radio and television that includes the lumped constant equivalent of resistors, capacitors, and semiconductors. Such a circuit separates the modulating frequency (or information) from the carrier frequency that transmits the signals through the atmosphere. We dial the radio to carrier frequency (500,000 to 1,600,000 Hz), but we listen to the radio-transmitted audio frequency (15 to 15,000 Hz), and we see the video results of frequencies ($\pm$100,000 Hz), while the television carrier frequencies can be 88,000,000 to 108,000,000 Hz.

Granbard reported that the electrical characteristic of a lobster stomatogastric ganglion includes the property of demodulation, normally the property of a semiconductor circuit in a communication device (14). Thus, circuit rectification, which occurs in demodulation appears to be present in certain neural systems.

The modulated energy of the present and predecessor devices can be utilized in a variety of sites on the human head and body to provide the signal for the nervous system to demodulate the stimulator energy into the information that the organism needs to help alter the neurochemical levels of certain substances. Having learned how to bring energy into the anatomy, the real challenge lies in how to utilize it to enhance the body's ability to reduce its own disease symptoms.

Hence, contact placement, the combination of contacts, and integration into a complete treatment regimen may need to take place at a particular time of day in the circadian cycle of the substance being targeted. Moreover, the sequence of treatments must be adapted to the disorder being treated.

6. Waveforms of the LCS and the LBS

The low-frequency oscillograph in Fig. 3 is that of the SBL202-B and that of the SBL502-B LBS.

Figure 4 shows the timing relationships among the various constituent waveforms. Please note that in Fig. 4a, the 15,000 Hz carrier frequency is modulated by both the first modulator of Fig. 4b, 15 Hz, and the second modulator of Fig. 4c, 500 Hz, to form the total waveform of both the SBL202-B LCS and the SBL502-B LBS.

B. Implications of Neurobiochemicals Altered by Electrical Stimulation

The modulated electric energy stimulator technology, herein described, is backed by 27 peer-reviewed published studies, 27 patents, and six authorizations to market from the federal regulatory agency. These stimulators have been shown to alter the level of serotonin and beta-endorphin in both the cerebral spinal fluid (CSF) and the blood plasma, as well as cortisol, ACTH, GABA, DHEA, neurotensin, and human growth hormone in blood plasma under certain specified conditions (9).

As a result of the alteration in the levels of these neurochemicals, the following clinical sequelae can be expected.

Pain control and management

Depression and mood management

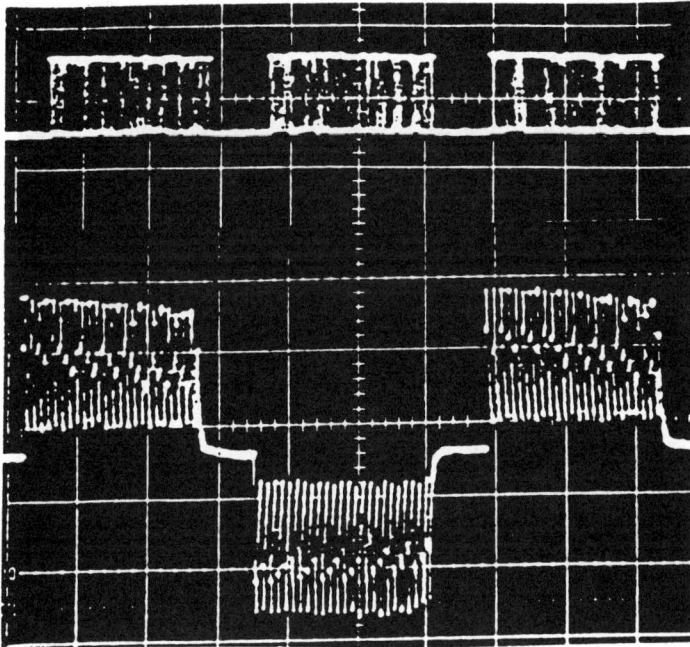

Figure 3 Output of LCS & LBS. A. Resistance load (monopolar) and (upper) B. Human load (bipolar) (lower).

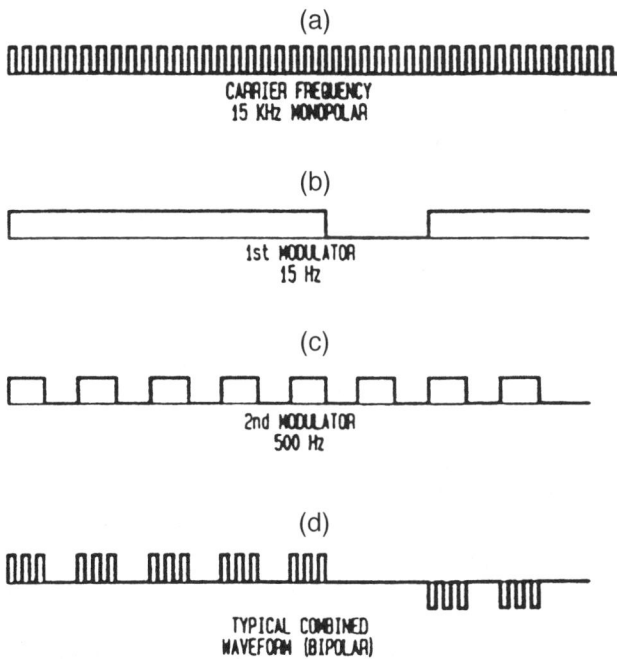

(a)

CARRIER FREQUENCY
15 KHz MONOPOLAR

(b)

1st MODULATOR
15 Hz

(c)

2nd MODULATOR
500 Hz

(d)

TYPICAL COMBINED
WAVEFORM (BIPOLAR)

Figure 4 LCS and LBS constituent waveforms.

Reduce the symptoms of anxiety and/or phobic disorder

Reduce the symptoms of Insomnia

Relaxation

Rebalane hypothalamic–pituitary–adrenal axis

Reduce spasticity in the musculature

Enhance dehydroepiandrosterone (DHEA)

Enhance the immune system

Enhance alertness and increase attention span.

Let us consider the mechanisms for drugs which affect serotonin, as compared to the action of the subject stimulator. Mood enhancing drugs and migraine headache drugs increase serotonin in a synapse by one of three mechanisms:

Reuptake inhibition

Monoamine oxidase inhibitor

Bind to the particular subreceptor site.

The modulated energy stimulators have been shown to use the capacitance of the body to store an electrical charge temporarily. This causes a gathering effect by creating an electrical storage condition on the bulk capacitance of the body. Thus, the authors have learned how to convert the energy from an external 9-V battery into an internal current, which, we believe, causes the alteration in the level of serotonin and the other neurobiochemicals noted above.

Pain control and pain management have been reported by Cassuto (15), Graziano (16), and Shealy (17) and can be understood from the biochemical work of Shealy (18), Closson (19 20), LISS (12), and Shealy (21). Experience has shown that the rise in serotonin and beta-endorphin in both the cerebral spinal fluid and the blood plasma are likely responsible for the pain control and management benefit to the patients using the modulated energy stimulators.

Depression, mood management, anxiety and/or phobic disorder, and insomnia are all classified as serotonergic-dependent symptoms. Therefore, if we can see the rise in serotonin, then it is easy to understand why these symptoms are reduced following an electrical treatment with the modulated energy stimulators.

Relaxation of the human is represented by the reduction in the plasma level of cortisol. Cortisol is recognized as the "fight or flight" neurochemical in the body. Therefore, in order to relax the body, it is understandable why the reduction in cortisol indicates systemic relaxation.

Balancing the hypothalamic–pituitary–adrenal (HPA) axis is the function of ACTH (which rises following electrical stimulation with the modulated energy stimulators). However, there is a paradox when we analyze the biochemical level changes. In hundreds of assays following the electrical stimulation with the LISS stimulators, cortisol levels go down (representing systemic relaxation) while ACTH rises in the plasma measurements made to date. These two biochemicals normally rise and fall together, but in this situation, that is not the case. We are at a loss at this time to explain this consistent paradox.

GABA is the neurobiochemical responsible for reducing spasticity in the body. It is one of two inhibiting neurobiochemicals and is, thereby, very important in balancing the action of complementary muscle actions (e.g., agonist vs. antagonist).

Dehydroepiandrosterone (DHEA) is the leading neurobiochemical in the aging process and directly involved in enhancing the immune system. Dr. Shealy found that the use of 12 acupuncture sites in a specified order, once per day for a total of 15 to 20 min/day can enhance the level of DHEA an average of 225% within a 12-week period (22). Compare this statistic to the use of progesterone cream, used for 6 months, which resulted in an average enhancement of 60%. With the use of the LISS Body Stimulator on the "ring-of-fire" points for 12 weeks, one of eight people had a reduced level, while seven of the eight volunteers averaged 225% increase in that same time period. The characteristics of the waveform are critical to make this application work. The use of this technology for the enhancement of DHEA, by itself, can help the senior to a higher quality of life, and thereby enhanced independence.

It is apparent that with the cost of nursing home care averaging $50,000 per person per year,if we are able to save an average of only one—month delay in entering a nursing home,the gross saving would be $4,000,000 for every 1000 people. If we saved each of the seniors over 65 during the 1993 census, society could be saved $132 billion for each month of delay. Society, in this context, includes the individual, family, responsible organization like a union, major industry, or the appropriate government agency.

The clinical performance of the subject modulated energy stimulators has been documented in 27 peer-reviewed published studies in various applications such as

Depression

Pain

Headache

Cerebral palsy spasticity reduction

Learning disabilities (including ADHD, dyslexia, and austism)

Enhancement of dehydroepiandrosterone (DHEA)

Alteration of serotonin and beta-endorphin in both the CSF and the blood plasma

Alteration in the blood plasma level of cortisol, ACTH, and GABA

Dental applications for

Restorative procedures without Novocaine

TMJ pain control and muscle relaxation

Increasing the alertness and attention span in normal volunteers beyond the treatment time

Safety for transcranial use on children

C. Studies and Implications in Levels: Neurobiochemicals

1. Double-Modulated Carrier-Frequency Stimulators

Electrical stimulation via double-modulated carrier-frequency stimulators (DMCFS) can alter the level of certain neurotransmitters, such as serotonin, beta-endorphin, GABA, and even DHEA without the use of drugs (3,19,20,22,23). Over the last 24 years, research has been accomplished that indicates, in hundreds of normal volunteers and patients, that these neurobiochemical levels are altered after either transcranial stimulation with the LISS Cranial Stimulator or on the body with the LISS Body Stimulator (which are electrically identical).

Significant benefits have been demonstrated in pain control (15,16), headache management (24–30), reducing the need for amputating diabetic legs (S. Weinstein, personal communication1987 and S. Wolf, personal communication 1995), depression symptom reduction (4,5), and in the research mode, cerebral palsy and other brain-injured patients spasticity reduction (31–36), and relieving symptoms of learning disabilities (37).

2. *LISS Cranial Stimulators and LISS Body Stimulators*

LISS Cranial Stimulators and LISS Body Stimulators come in two different electrical characteristics. Monopolar, where each positive burst of energy from 0 to a plus value of 4 mA is "on" for 50 ms and "off" for 16.7 ms. Each combination of on time and off time comprise 66.7 ms, which is the period of the 15-Hz signal and is followed by the same burst of positive energy. Since this pattern of energy is only varying from zero to positive value, there is a modicum of direct current. We have observed increases in blood flow and alterations in the level of certain neurobiochemicals such as (see Fig. 1):

Serotonin

Cortisol

ACTH

Beta-endorphin

Bipolar LISS Cranial and Body Stimulators are devices where each positive burst of energy, varying from 0 to a plus value of 4 mA is on for 50 ms and off for 16.7 mA and is followed b a comparable negative burst of energy equal and opposite polarity to the initial burst. This *balanced energy* method provides a net zero direct current. We have seen no blood flow increase from this waveform, but blood testing has shown almost twice the amount of neurobiochemical changes following bipolar stimulation, stimulation compared to that of the monopolar (see Fig. 5). The net frequency of this modulated device is 7.5 Hz.

Note that the monopolar device is able to increase blood flow toward the black contact and alters the level of certain neurobiochemicals, noted above. The bipolar version has not shown such increase in blood flow, but it has shown alteration of the same neurobiochemicals approximately twice that of the monopolar device. Therefore, clinically, if there is a need to reduce pain through the increase of the flow of blood in the body, as in diabetic neuropathy, Raynaud's disease, and multiple sclerosis, or out of the head, as in migraine headache, use the monopolar device. If there is a need to reduce pain by altering the level of neurobiochemicals, such as in chronic back and other musculoskeletal body pain, facial pain, or pain secondary to neural dysfunctions, such as reflex sympathetic dystrophy syndrome (RSDS), then use the bipolar device.

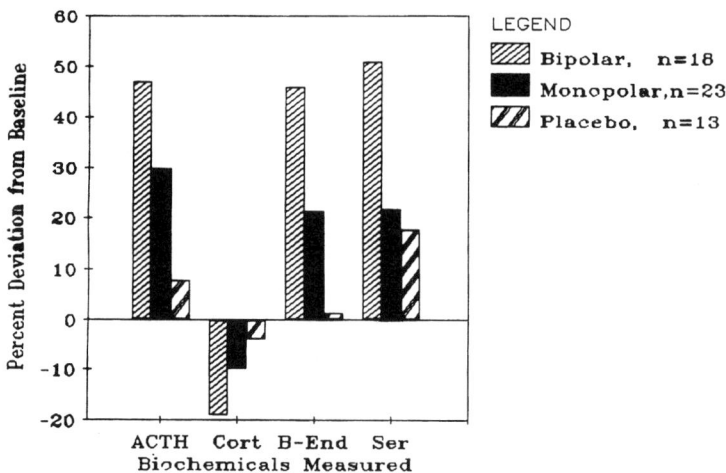

Figure 5 Baseline measurements following 20-min transcranial stimulation vs. placebo testing.

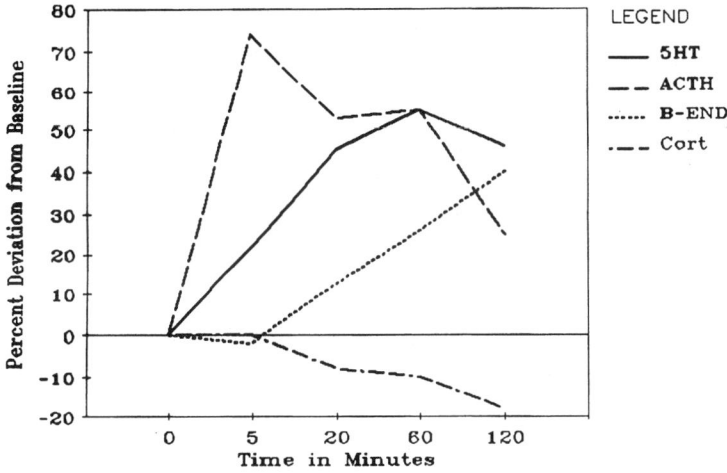

Figure 6 Kinetic neurobiochemical effects following transcranial stimulation (40). Average biochemical changes in two subjects following 20 min stimulation with LISS cranial stimulator #201 = M.

The kinetics of the post-transcranial-stimulation blood plasma measurements, shown in Fig. 6, indicate that during the first 5 mins, there is no alteration in the level of cortisol. However, during the same time there is a 75% increase in ACTH, which over the rest of 2 h reduces to 25% over baseline, while the cortisol reduces to −12.5% (in the direction indicating relaxation). It takes 20 min for the serotonin to rise to its maximum of 50% over baseline, which is maintained for the rest of the 2 h. Beta-endorphin continued to increase over the 2-h period. The only conclusion taken by the author is that this study must be replicated and extended to at least 4 h or more. However, it certainly hints that 20 min of stimulation with the LISS Cranial Stimulator likely triggers the body's long-term neurobiochemical reactions. Cerebral spinal fluid and blood plasma neurobiochemical measurements are shown in Fig. 7 (38).

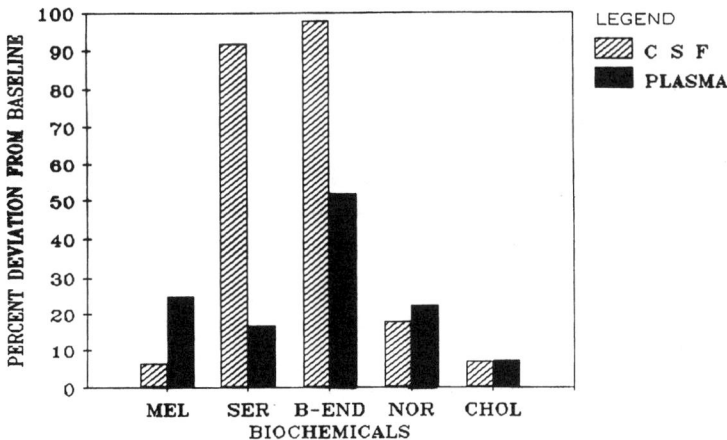

Figure 7 Cerebral spinal fluid and blood plasma tests. Biochemical changes in five subjects following 20 min transcranial stimulation with LCS (averages).

A study was done in 1985 by William J. Closson, Ph.D., which indicated that the best conventional TENS device did not cause the significant changes in blood plasma neuro-biochemical levels noted above. These differences were presented at the Fourth International Montreux Congress on Stress (39,40) (Fig. 8).

The principal neurobiochemicals measured to date include those shown in Table 1. The next consideration in understanding the mechanisms of neurotransmitters in the body relates to the precursors of some of the critical neurobiochemicals (Table 2).

D. Data Summation and Analysis: Standard Screen

The original intent of evaluating the neurobiochemical levels was Dr. Shealy's desire to explore the foundation of pain control. Therefore, the following screen was chosen:

Serotonin (pain tolerance, depression, insomnia)

Beta-endorphin (pain control, sense of well being)

Cortisol (systemic relaxation with decrease)

ACTH (anti-inflammatory, balance of HPA axis)

Over the years, 92 normals have been measured for changes in serotonin and beta-endorphin, while 73 have been assayed for cortisol and 78 for ACTH. Figure 9 shows the information noted herein.

Figures 10–12 show patients with various pathologies also screened with the same protocol but with dysfunctions of pain, depression, multiple sclerosis, and dental restorative pain. Figure 10 shows the effect of the modulated electrical stimulators on 23 pain patients, 11 depressed patients, and 14 normals, for comparison. Figure 11 shows the stimulators' effects in changing the plasma levels of ACTH for 15 multiple sclerosis patients and 10 normals (5 active and 5 placebo). Figure 12 shows the beneficial effects on 22 dental patients who had been initially treated with transcranial stimulation to enhance the basic screen of neurobiochemicals prior to the restorative process. Please note that following the preparation for the cavities, the neurobiochemical levels basically were reduced from the effect of the procedure imposing pain on the patient. It is interesting to know that the neurobiochemical

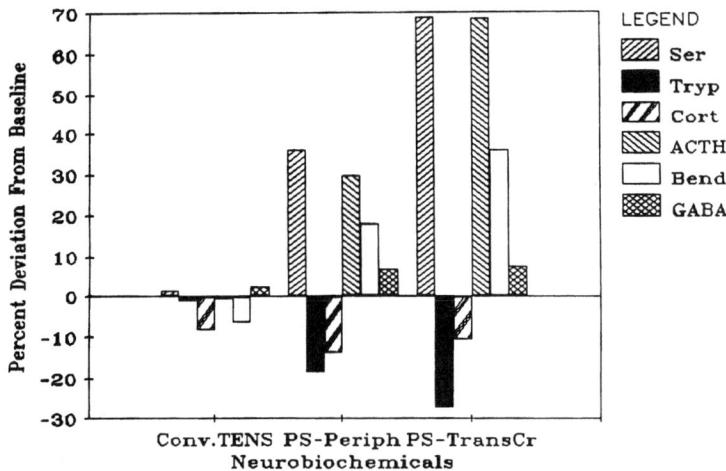

Figure 8   Neurobiochemical measurements following stimulation with devices of differing waveform.

Table 1 Neurobiochemicals Changes Following Electrical Stimulation with the LISS Stimulators and Implications Thereof

Substance	Alteration	Measured in Plasma	C S F
A. Serotonin	Increases	X	X
B. Beta-Endorphin	Increases	X	X
C. Tryptophan	Decreases	X	
D. Cortisol	Decreases	X	
E. ACTH	Increases	X	
F. GABA	Increases	X	
G. DHEA	Increases	X	

Substance	Implications
A. Serotonin	1. Mood management
	2. Pain tolerance
	3. Insomnia symptom reduction
	4. Cardiovascular control
B. Beta-Endorphin	Endogenous morphinelike biochemical
C. Tryptophan	Precursor to serotonin
D. Cortisol	Systemic relaxation (upon decrease)
E. ACTH	Hypothalmus / pituitary / adrenal axis
F. GABA	1. Neural inhibitor
	2. Involved with spasticity reduction
G. DHEA	1. Principal neurochemicals in aging
	2. Involved with immune system
	3. Involved with endocrine system

levels did not return to the original baseline but were considerably higher than the original baseline for both serotonin and beta-endorphin, the premier neurobiochemical associated with the pain management process. We opine that the postoperative benefit in pain control (approximately 4 h) was due to the fact that the pretreatment cranial application of the modulated electric stimulators created the elevated levels of both serotonin and beta-endorphin that gave rise to the prolonged benefit following the dental procedures.

Over the years 140 normals have been measured before and after active device stimulation with various neurobiochemical assays, while 18 additional tests were made on

Table 2 Neurobiochemicals and Associated Precursors

Neurobiochemical	Precursor amino acid
1. Serotonin	Tryptophan
2. Dopamine	Tyrosine
3. Norepinephrine	Tyrosine (via dopamine)
4. Epinephrine	Tyrosine (via norepinephrine)
5. Acetylcholine	Lecithin

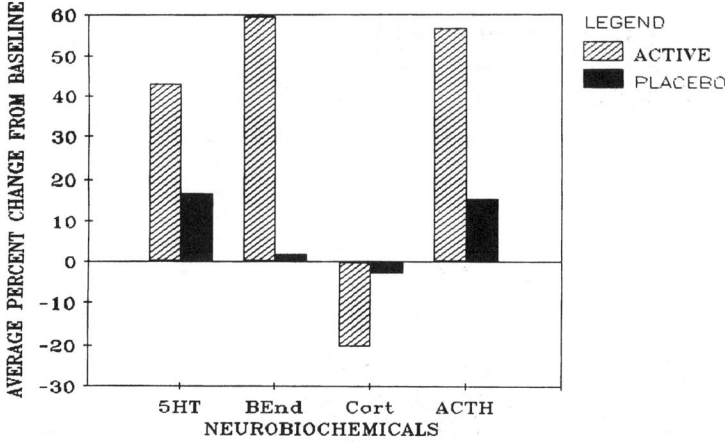

Figure 9 Analysis of normals tested with either active or placebo modulated electrical energy stimulators.

normals before and after placebo device treatment. The same type of testing was done on patients with multiple sclerosis, pain, depression, headache, diabetic neuropathy, and dental restorative procedures. Two hundred fifty-two patients were treated with an active device and 14 patients were treated with a placebo device.

E. Discussion

It has been shown that the tissue of the body contains electrical characteristics, which can be utilized to help the body help itself. Since the alteration of certain neurobiochemicals in the body and head can have a salutary impact on reducing the symptoms of depression, anxiety, insomnia, and pain, MEDI has now demonstrated the alteration of some of the same neu-

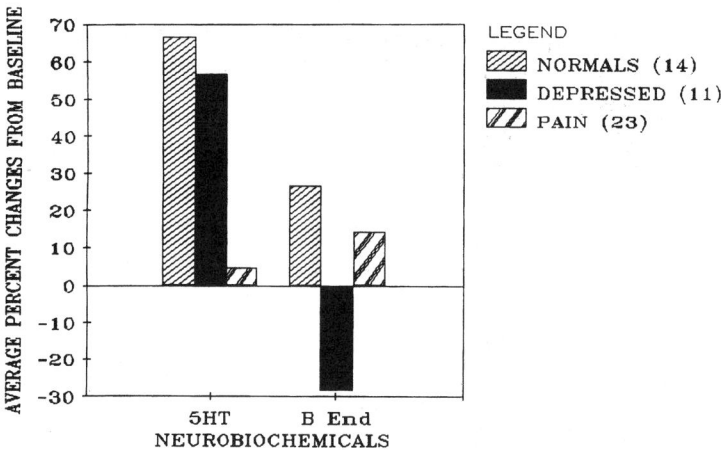

Figure 10 Neurobiochemical measurements following stimulation with modulated electric stimulators on patients with pain and depression compared to normals.

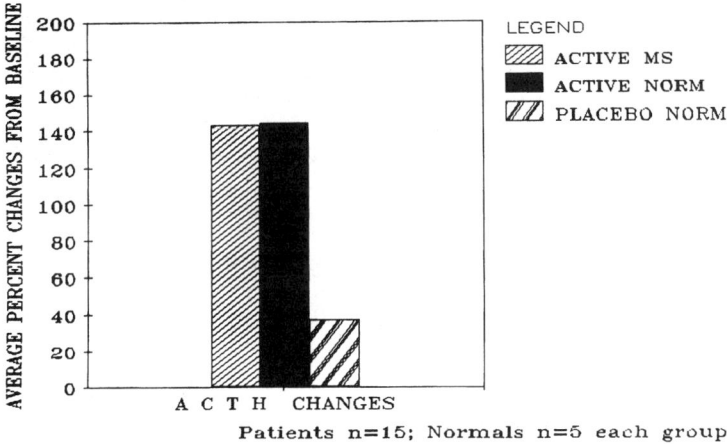

Figure 11 ACTH changes following stimulation with modulated electric stimulators on patients with multiple sclerosis compared to normals.

robiochemicals that specific drugs attempt to manage. If drugs work for the particular patient, then the physician in charge of that patient would do well to use them. However, there are a significant number of patients with pathology associated with depression, anxiety, insomnia, and pain for whom the drugs are not adequate. Their bodies and organic systems frequently are allergic or are overly sensitive to some of the side effects or drug interaction dysfunctions unique to that particular person. For those types of patients, the capability of the modulated electric energy stimulators may be a viable alternative. It is for them and their responsible, caring physician that this presentation is dedicated.

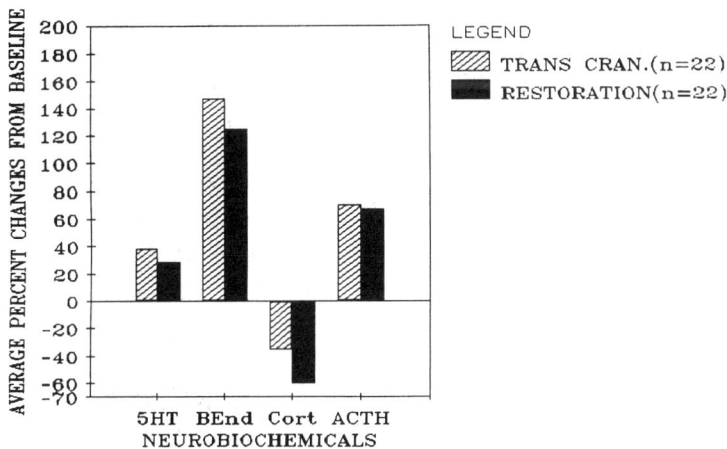

Figure 12 Comparison between the levels of neurobiochemicals resulting from transcranial pretreatment with modulated electric stimulators compared to those levels following dental restorative procedures. Note that the imposed pain reduced the levels of serotonin, beta-endorphin, and ACTH.

F. Conclusion

The use of the double-modulated cranial and/or body electrical stimulators can utilize the body's bulk capacitance to cause an internal current to flow. That internal current, flowing through its own resistance, can increase a voltage that may be able to facilitate triggering energy of a neural system. Tests have also confirmed that certain neurobiochemical levels have been altered following the use of the subject double-modulated electrical nerve stimulators. Those measured include the following:

Serotonin
Beta-endorphin
Cortisol
ACTH
GABA
DHEA
Neurotensin
Human growth hormone

V. FIVE SPECIFIC ENERGETIC CIRCUITS

Shortly after returning from the Ukraine, Shealy began development of five specific circuits in the human body. These circuits have demonstrated that specific cyber pharmacological techniques may be practical. The first of these came in response to his seeking ways of raising dehydroepiandrosterone (DHEA), the most critical hormone in the human body for maintaining health and longevity. He discovered that electrical stimulation with either the LISS TENS or the GigaTENS from the Ukraine raised DHEA an average of 60%. The effect was virtually the same whether one used the LISS TENS or the GigaTENS.

Even more critically, the increase in DHEA appears to be greater in older, more depleted individuals. Our numbers are small, but some older individuals experienced DHEA enhancement of well over 500%.

Clinical experiments later revealed that the stimulation of this particular 12-point circuit, which he called the *ring of fire*, not only raised DHEA, but was clinically beneficial in 70% of patients with rheumatoid arthritis, 75% of patients with migraine, 80% of individuals with diabetic neuropathy, and 70% of individuals with depression (22,41,42). Note that the use of the Liss on specific acupuncture points, the ring of fire, is even more effective for depression than its use transcranially. This result alone strongly suggests that 50 million Americans experiencing the "clinically negligent" effects of antidepressants, should be given the safe, effective alternative of cyberpharmacological ring-of-fire therapy! Stimulation transcranially with the LISS Stimulator does not raise DHEA but raises primarily beta-endorphin and serotonin, and when the stimulators are applied to only half of the ring-of-fire points, there is no increase in DHEA. Interestingly, in diabetic neuropathy, there was no improvement with the LISS TENS on the ring of fire, but there was with the GigaTENS.

About the time of the completion of the work with the ring of fire, Shealy discovered that the old Electreat, which he had always considered more effective than any of the modern solid-state TENS devices, included in its output, pulses in the 54- to 78-GHz range at amplitudes of 50 to 100 dB, essentially equivalent to the output of the Ukrainian devices. Based upon that, he redesigned this device and has later patented it as the She-Li TENS. It has been approved by the FDA for manufacture and sale as other TENS on prescription by a physician. Considerable additional work has now been done with the She-Li TENS and the LISS Cranial Stimulator, since the Ukrainian GigaTENS devices are not available in this country yet.

Acupuncture points for the ring of fire are

K3	Midway between the tip of medial malleolus and tendo calcaneus.
CV2	In the superior border of the pubic symphysis, on the midline of the abdomen.
CV6	One and one-half (1.5) cun below the umbilicus, on the midline of the abdomen
B22	One and one-half (1.5) cun lateral to the lower border of the spinous process of the first lumbar vertebra
MH6	On the ulnar side of the wrist, on the radial side of the tendon M. flexor carpi ulnaris, below pisiform bone
LI18	Three cun lateral to the thyroid cartilage, between the sternal head and the clavicular head of the sternocleidomastoid muscle
CV18	On the midline of the abdomen, 1.6 cun above the line of two nipples, at the level of the third intercostal rib
GV20	Seven cun above the posterior hairline, midway on a line connecting the apex of both ears

The distance between the two creases marking the joints of the distal and middle phalanges of the middle finger is 1 cm.

The second circuit that Shealy investigated is one that he has called the *ring of air*. This 13-point circuit significantly raises neurotensin. Neurotensin is a major marker for states of increased mental lucidity, the states in which holographic awareness is enhanced. Electrical stimulation of the ring of air with either the LISS or the She-Li TENS increases neurotensin up to 500% (43).

Neurotensin is an endogenous tridecapeptide found in the central nervous system and has been postulated to be a neurotransmitter found in synapses and the hypothalamus, amygdala, basal ganglia, and dorsal grey matter of the spinal cord. Neurotensin plays a role in pain perception, but its analgesic effects are not blocked by opiod antagonists. It also affects pituitary hormone release and gastrointestinal activity. Two important aspects of neurotensin's action on the central nervous system are possible involvement in the etiology of schizophrenia and its analgesic properties. It has thus been suggested that neurotensin may have neurolepticlike activity within the central nervous system.

Acupuncture points for the ring of air are

Sp1A	On the medial side of the great toe, 0.1 cun posterior to the corner of nail.
Liv3	Between the first and second toe, 2 cun proximal to the margin of the web.
S36	Three cun below lateral side of patella, one finger breadth from anterior crest of the tibia.
L1	On the lateral aspect of the chest, in the interspace of the first and second rib, 6 cun lateral to the midline of the chest.
G20	In the depression between the M. sternocleidomastoid and the upper portion of the M. trapezius. Specifically, between the depression directly inferior to the occipital protuberance and the mastoid.

GV1   Midway between the top of coccyx and the anus.

GV16   Directly below the occipital protuberance, in the midline, in a depression 1 cun above the hairline.

GV20   Seven cun above the posterior hairline, midway on a line connecting the apex of both ears.

The third circuit investigated by Shealy was the Ring of Water, another 13-point circuit that has been studied only with the She-Li TENS. Activation of the Ring of Water optimizes aldosterone in those individuals where the baseline aldosterone level is low but it has not been seen to raise aldosterone above the upper limit of normal. Shealy theorizes that stimulation of the *ring of water* with stimulation of the ring of fire will aid in weight loss, an experiment currently underway.

Acupuncture points for the ring of water are

SP4   On the medial aspect of the foot, in a depression at the anterior and inferior border of the first metatarsal bone, at the junction of the "red and white" skin

H7   On the ulnar side of the wrist, on the posterior border of the pisiform bone, in the depression at the radial side of the tendon M. flexor carpi ulnaris

B10   One and three-tenths (1.3) cun lateral to the midline of first and second cervical vertebrae, on the lateral side of M. trapezius

B13   One and one-half (1.5) cun lateral to the lower border of the spinous process of the third thoracic vertebrae

CV14   Six cun above the umbilicus, on the midline of the abdomen

TH16   Posterior and inferior to the mastoid process, in the posterior border at M. sternocleidomastoid, at the level of the angle of the mandible

GV8   Below the spinous process of the ninetieth thoracic vertebra

GV20   Seven cun above the posterior hairline, midway on a line connecting the apex of both ears

The fourth circuit is the *ring of earth*, stimulation of which with either the She-Li TENS or the LISS TENS, significantly raises calcitonin (44). Calcitonin has a wide variety of physiological effects including maintenance of bone density as well as in treatment of a wide variety of pain problems. Exogenously administered, calcitonin carries some risk of anaphylaxis and is quite expensive. In a pilot study done by Shealy, six patients who had at least a measurable level of calcitonin initially had a significant increase in calcitonin levels after a single application of electrical stimulation to 13 specific acupuncture points. It is of considerable interest that all four individuals with no measurable calcitonin had temperatures well below normal. Shealy has demonstrated that subclinical hypothyroidism may be corrected by administration of iodine. This raises the interesting possibility that thyroid function must be normal for activation of calcitonin enhancement after electrical stimulation of the ring of earth. This circuit is of particular interest since osteoporotic hip fracture is a leading cause of death in the elderly. A major study of this potential is currently beginning.

Acupuncture points for the ring of earth are

K1   In the depression at the junction of the anterior and middle third of the sole in a depression between the second and third metatarso-phalangeal joint when the toes are plantar flexed.

B54   Exact midpoint of the popliteal transverse crease.

B60   Between the posterior border of the external malleolus and the medial aspect of tendo calcaneus at the same level as the tip of the malleolus.

LI16   In the depression between the clavico-acromal extremity and the spine of the scapulae.

ST9   Posterior to the common carotid artery on the anterior border of M. sternocleidomastoid, lateral to the thyroid cartilage.

SI17   Posterior to the angle of the jaw on the anterior border of M. sterno-cleidomastoid.

GV20   Seven cun above the posterior hairline, midway on a line connecting the apex of both ears.

Finally, the fifth circuit discovered by Shealy is called the *ring of crystal*. Stimulation with either the LISS TENS or the She-Li TENS reduces free radicals about 80%. In about 10% of individuals, it appears that the She-Li TENS is more effective than the LISS TENS, but for most individuals there is no appreciable difference in the effectiveness of the She-Li TENS or the LISS TENS in activating the ring of crystal. The value of reducing free radicals in everyone is obvious, since oxidative stress is the major cause of illness and death (45).

Acupuncture points for the ring of crystal are

SP4   On the medial aspect of the foot, in a depression at the anterior and inferior border of the first metatarsal bone, at the junction of the "red and white" skin

GB30.5   Two cun lateral of the greater trochanter to major trochanter, lateral side of the upper leg

CV8.5   One-half (0.5) cun above the umbilicus

GV4.5   On the spinous process of the second lumbar vertebra

CV14.5   Six and one-half (6.5) cun above the umbilicus on the midline of the abdomen

GV7.5   On the spinous process of the ninetieth thoracic vertebra

GV14.5   On the spinous process of the third cervical vertebra

CV23   Midline of the neck, midway between the tip of the cricoid cartilage and the border of the mandible

GB11   In the depression 1 cun posterior of the horizontal line of the auricle

GV20   Seven cun above the posterior hairline, midway on a line connecting the apex of both ear

Implications of these specific neurochemical circuits are quite extraordinary. For instance, neurotensin deficiency is not particularly necessary factor for most people, but the modulating effect of the ring of air could be particularly useful in some patients with severe psychological diseases because of the neuroleptic effects of neurotensin. Similarly, the ring of water may not be of great clinical importance except in those older individuals who have difficulty with water and mineral metabolism. However, low DHEA is rampant in our society with about 98% of individuals being low or deficient by the time they reach age 80. Osteoporosis is the most common cause of death in the elderly. The recent report that Primpro is not only ineffective long-term but carries risks enhances the potential for using the ring of earth to enhance calcitonin production and potentially treat and prevent osteoporosis. Finally, free radicals are the major biochemical cause of disease and death and appear to increase their negative effects as indivuduals age. Thus, raising DHEA, calcitonin, and reducing free radicals by sequentially stimulating the rings of fire, earth, and crystal has a theoretical potential for significant benefit in enhancing health and prolonging life.

TENS has led far beyond pain relief to a new scientific principle, cyberpharmacology. It is reasonable to expect that further research will yield increasing ability to restore neuro-homeostasis. Refinements in technique, current, and specific circuits offer the potential for safer and more effective therapy than chemical agents. It is already apparent that many disorders are much more effectively treated with electrotherapy than with chemotherapy. Stimulation of the five rings suggests the potential for significant extension of a healthy life, perhaps even doubling life expectancy (46).

REFERENCES

1. Kellaway P. The part played by electric fish in the early history of bioelectricity and electrotherapy. Bull Hist Med 1946; 20:112–132.
2. Shealy CN, Mortimer JT, Becker DP. Electrical inhibition of pain by dorsal column stimulation: preliminary clinical report. Anesthesia Analgesia. Current Researches 1967; 46:489–491.
3. Shealy CN. Effects of transcranial neurostimulation upon mood and serotonin production: a preliminary report. Il dolore 1979; 1:13–16.
4. Shealy CN, Cady RK, Wilkie RG, Cox RH, Liss S, Closson W. Depression: a diagnostic neurochemical profile and therapy with cranial electrical stimulation (CES). J Neurol Orthopaedic Med Surg 1989; 10(4):319–321.
5. Shealy CN, Cady RK, Veehoff D, Houston R, Burnetti M, Cox RH, Closson W. The neurochemistry of depression. Am J Pain Management 1992; 2:13–16.
6. Shealy CN. The physical roots of depression. Vision, Association of Unity Churches 1990; 3:11–13.
7. Shealy CN. Depression: The common denominator in dis-ease. Venture Inward 1993; 9(3):16–19.
8. Shealy CN, Cady RK, Veehoff DC, Cox RH, Houston R, Atwell M. Nonpharmaceutical treatment of depression using a multimodal approach. Subtle Energies 1993; 4(2):125–134.
9. Shealy CN, Cady RK, Cox RH. Pain stress and depression: Psychoneurophysiology and therapy. Stress Medicine 1995; 11:75–77.
10. Kirsch I, Moore TJ, Scoboria A, Nicholls SS. The Emperor's new drugs: An analysis of antidepressant medication data submitted to the U.S. Food and Drug Administration. Prevention and Treatment 2002; 5(article 23).
11. Shealy CN. Microwave resonance therapy: Innovations from the Ukraine. Greene County Med Bull 1993; 47(3):15–17.
12. Liss S, Liss B. Physiological and therapeutic effects of high frequency pulses. Integrative Physiol Behavioral Sci 1996; 31(2):88–94.
13. Fromherz P. Neurons talk to chips and chips talks to nerve cells. J Phys Rev Lett, August 21, 1995.
14. Granbard K, Heartline DK. Full-wave rectification from a mixed electrical, chemical synapse. Science Rep 1987; 237:535–537.
15. Cassuto J, Liss S, Bennett A. The use of modulated energy carried on a high frequency wave for the relief of intractable pain. Int J Clin Pharmacol Res 1993; 13(4):239–241.
16. Graziano JM. Retrospective analysis of acute and chronic pain control in physical therapy and rehabilitation with the Pain Suppressor. Chicago Pain Conference, Chicago, IL, May 1997.
17. Shealy CN. Characteristics of pain reduction. Chicago Pain Conference, Chicago, IL, May 1997.
18. Shealy CN. External electrical stimulation: types, techniques and results. Neuroelectric News 1976; 6:4–9.
19. Closson W. Transcutaneous electrical nerve stimulation and adrenocorticotropic hormone production. Polypeptide Meeting, George Washington University, Washington, DC, May 1997.

20. Closson W. Changes in blood biochemical levels, following treatment with TENS devices of differing frequency composition. Fourth International Montreux Congress on Stress, Montreux, Switzerland 1992.

21. Thomlinson P, Shealy CN. Successful holistic treatment of chronic depression. Twenty-second International Conference on the Unity of the Sciences, Seoul, Korea, February 9–13, 2000.

22. Shealy CN. Electrical stimulation raises DHEA and improves diabetic neuropathy. Stress Medicine 1995; 11:215–217.

23. Rosch PJ. DHEA and the fountain of youth. Newsletter of the American Institute of Stress 1995; Number 8.

24. Solomon S, Guglielmo K. Treatment of headache by transcutaneous electrical stimulation. Headache J 1985; 25(1).

25. Solomon S, Elkind A, Freitag F, Gallagher RM, Moore K, Swerdlow B, Malkin S. Safety and effectiveness of cranial electrotherapy in the treatment of tension headaches. Headache J 1989; 29(7).

26. MacGregor EA, Bennett A, Liss S, Wilkinson MIP. Transcranial electrical stimulation in migraine prophylaxis. European Headache Conference, 1993.

27. Markovich SE. Post traumatic headaches. Nineth Annual Meeting of the Neuroelectric Society, Marco Beach, FL, December 1977.

28. Romano TJ. The usefulness of cranial electrotherapy in the treatment of headache in fibromyalgia patients. Am J Pain Management 1993; 1(1).

29. Terezhalmy GT, Ross GR, Holmes-Johnson E. Transcutaneous electrical nerve stimulation treatment of TMJ-MPDS patients. Ear, Nose, Throat J, 1982.

30. Morrison H, Liss B, Liss S. Cranial electrical stimulation for treatment of stress-related pain. Sixth International Montreux Congress on Stress, Montreux, Switzerland, February 1994.

31. Malden JW, Charash LI. Transcranial stimulation for the inhibition of primitive reflexes in children with cerebral palsy. Neurology Rep APTA 1985; 9(2).

32. Logan MP. Improved mechanical efficiency in cerebral palsy patients treated with a cranial electrotherapy stimulator (CES). American Academy of Cerebral Palsy and Developmental Medicine Conference, October 1988.

33. Sornson R, Liverance D, Armstrong G, Zelt B. Neurotransmitter modulation benefits adolescent cerebral palsy students. Am J Electromedicine, February 1989.

34. Reilly MA, Light KE. Movement efficiency: Effects of transcranial stimulation on a single subject with cerebral palsy. Presented and published by the Forum on Efficacy of Physical Therapy Treatment for Patients with Brain Injury. Combined Sections Meeting of the American Physical Therapy Association, 1990.

35. Hunt TF. Senior Thesis: Transcranial electrical stimulation as a means of treating neuropathological disorders in children, University of Utah Division of Physical Therapy, 1986.

36. Childs, A. Case Study: Fifteen-cycle cranial electrotherapy stimulation for spasticity. Brain Injury 1993; 7(2).

37. Okoye R, Malden JW. Use of neurotransmitter modulation to facilitate sensory integration. Neurol Sec Am Phys Therapy Assoc 1986; 10(4).

38. Cady R, Shealy CN. Cerebrospinal fluid and plasma neurochemicals: Response to cranial electrical stimulation. Study grant from the Charlson Foundation 1991.

39. Liss S, Liss BS, Closson WJ. Baseline analysis—normals with 20 minute transcranial treatment using LISS cranial stimulators (monopolar, bipolar and placebo). Fourth International Montreux Congress on Stress, Montreux, Switzerland 1992.

40. Liss S, Malden J. Average biochemical changes in 2 subjects following 20 minutes stimulation with LISS cranial stimulator #201-M. Fourth International Montreux Congress on Stress, Montreux, Switzerland, 1992.

41. Cox RH, Shealy CN, Cady RK, Cadle R, Richards G. Successful treatment of rheumatoid arthritis with GigaTENS™. J Neurol Orthopaedic Med Surg 1996; 17(1):31.

42. Shealy CN, Myss CM. The ring of fire and DHEA: A theory for energetic restoration of adrenal reserves. Subtle Energies 1995; 6(2):167–175.

43. Shealy CN, Borgmeyer, V, Thomlinson P. Intuition, neurotensin and the ring of air. Subtle Energies and Energy Medicine 2002; 11(2):145–150.

44. Shealy CN, Borgmeyer VM. Calcitonin enhancement with electrical activation of a specific acupuncture circuit. Am J Pain Management. In press.

45. Shealy CN, Borgmeyer VM, Thomlinson RP. Reduction of free radicals by electrical stimulation of specific acupuncture points. Submitted for publication.

46. Shealy CN. The Methuselah Potential for Health and Longevity. Fair Grove, MO:Brindabella Books, 2002.

8

Origin and Evolution of Vagal Nerve Stimulation: Implications for Understanding Brain Electrodynamics, Neuroendocrine Function, and Clinical Applications

Jacob Zabara

Cyberonics, Inc., Houston, Texas, U.S.A.

Vagal nerve stimulation had its roots in the "animal electrical fluid" vs. bioelectricity debate between Galvani and Volta. It was stimulated by Sherrington's concept of inhibition as a coordinative factor in integrating nervous system activity and the recognition that nerve stimulation effects were due to depolarization or hyperpolarization of nerve and muscle membrane potentials. As will be explained, vagal nerve stimulation also involves a negarive feedback action, a filtering action, and a switching effect. Variations in these may explain its wide clinical applications ranging from epilepsy, depression and anxiety, to obesity and insulin resistance that are discussed in other chapters in this book.

I. ANIMAL ELECTRICAL FLUID AND BIOELECTRICITY

When Galvani discovered "animal electricity" in muscle and nerve, Volta doubted its authenticity and criticized Galvani on the basis that the electricity was external to muscle or nerve tissue and subsequently invented the voltaic pile battery in an attempt to prove he was right. Actually, both Galvani and Volta were correct, but Volta could not comprehend that electricity was also present in nerve and muscle, albeit of a much different nature than that flowing through a metal conductor. As a result, electricity developed into a central and critical investigation of physics and bioelectricity existed for many years as a backwater or underground stream. It seemed a worthwhile challenge to combine the electricity of physics with the electricity of biology and apply the result to medicine.

In a series of experiments that began in Bologna around 1780, Luigi Galvani showed that an electrical stimulus from a Leyden jar or static electricity generator could cause contraction of muscles in a frog's leg by applying the charge to either the muscle or its nerve.

In an effort to demonstrate that lightning was a similar electrical spark as Benjamin Franklin had proposed, Galvani suspended frog legs with brass hooks from an iron railing during a thunderstorm and observed that the muscles contracted coincident with a lightning strike. However, contractions also occurred when there was no evidence of thunderstorm activity as well as in the laboratory if a nerve–muscle preparation was put into contact with two dissimilar metals. Since this happened indoors when no external source of electricity was present, Galvani theorized that the frog's muscles were generating what he called *animal electricity*, to distinguish it from the "natural" electricity in lightning or that produced by machines. He viewed the muscle as being similar to a small Leyden jar stored with electricity and proposed that the application of an external charge caused an attraction of opposite electrical charges on its inside and outside surfaces that made the muscle contract. He published his conclusions in a 1791 essay titled *De Viribus Electricitatis in Motu Musculari Commentarius* (Commentary on the Effect of Electricity on Muscular Motion).

Allessandro Volta repeated Galvani's experiments at the University of Pavia and confirmed that applying probes made of two different metals to nerves caused contraction of the muscles they were connected to. However, he rejected Galvani's Leyden jar model and offered the alternative hypothesis that external electricity was being generated by the contact between two different kinds of metal. His explanation was that the frog muscle functioned only as a detector of the small differences in external electrical potential. To support this theory, he built an electrical storage (voltaic) pile consisting of a series of two different metal disks separated by cardboard disks soaked with acid or salt solutions that is still the basis of modern wet-cell batteries and was the first method developed to generate a sustained electrical current.

Although Volta had refuted the notion of any "animal electric fluid," Galvani was able to prove that animal tissue was indeed a source of electricity since he could cause a muscle to contract by touching the exposed muscle of one frog with the nerve of another when there was no contact with any metal and published his results in the supplement of an anonymous 1794 book titled *Dell'uso e Dell'attività Dell'arco Conduttore Nella Contrazione dei Muscoli* (On the Use and Activity of the Conductive Arch in the Contraction of Muscles). Volta persisted in his attempts to dispute the existence of animal electricity and the controversy was resolved by Alexander von Humboldt in 1797. He explained that both were right as well as wrong by demonstrating that electrical flow mediated by moist tissue contact with dissimilar metals and that generated by animal tissue were two genuine but different phenomena.

The Galvani-vs.-Volta debate is one of the most interesting episodes in the history of science. Both were gentlemen with high scientific principles, in contrast to their supporters who often clashed violently in public and academic confrontations. Volta wrote that Galvani's work "contained one of the most beautiful and most surprising discoveries" and was actually responsible for coining the term *galvanism* Volta's name is commemorated in *volt* and *voltage* and his demonstration of the voltaic pile to the French Academy of Science prompted Napoleon to appoint him a count of Lombardy.

Edgar Adrian summarized this in *The Mechanism of Nervous Action* (1932) as follows:

> . . . and if we are really to date the present era from any one experiment, a good case could be made for an observation in medical physics in the year 1786. Galvani of Bologna was investigating the effects of static and atmospheric electricity on the muscles. He had prepared the body of a frog and had fixed a brass hook in the vertebral canal intending to hang it upon the terrace outside his house. He placed the frog on an iron plate so that the hook touched the iron, and when it did so the body moved. "*En motus in rana spontanei, vorii, haud infrequentes!*" and when the

movements ceased, they would be revived by pressing the hook more firmly against the iron. Galvani had produced an electric current and had the wit to realize that he had done so.

It was some time before the full meaning of this observation was understood, for the role of the frog's muscles was uncertain. Galvani had made other experiments which led him to believe that a muscle could generate electricity in the absence of metals, and it was known that a fish, the torpedo, could give a severe electric shock. For a few years, until 1792, it seemed that Galvani's phenomena was due to a form of electricity which was peculiar to living tissues. Enthusiasts held that this "Animal Electricity" was the true life force, that it would explain movement and sensation and lead to the cure of all kinds of nervous disease. Then Volta pricked the physiologists' bubble by showing that when the two metals were used, the frog acted merely as indicator and a source of moisture. The electric current occurred in inanimate systems, life was not an essential ingredient, and the science of electrodynamics became a branch of physics and not of medicine or biology.

Prior to Galvani, terms like *anima* and *animal spirits* had been used by Aristotle, Galen, and others to refer to some source of energy in the body. William Gilbert, physician to Queen Elizabeth I, introduced the term *electrica* (derived from the Greek *electra* for amber) to describe what would later be known as static electricity to distinguish it from magnetism. (Gilbert W., *De Magnete, Magneticisique Corporibus, et Magno Magnete Tellure*. London, 1600). *Electricity* was first used by the physician Sir Thomas Browne in 1646 as follows, "Electricity, that is, a power to attract strawes or light bodies, and convert the needle freely placed" (Browne, Sir Thomas. *Pseudodoxia Epidemica*; 1646: Bk II, Ch. 1. London, 1660). The French philosopher René Descartes, explained movement and muscular contraction in terms of a complex mechanical interaction of threads, pores, passages, and "animal spirits" in which he conceived of a type of fluid motion in nerve–muscle to explain the stimulus-response reflex. [Descartes R. *De Homine* (Treatise of Man), Leiden, 1662]. Around the same time, the English physician and anatomist Thomas Willis also viewed animal spirits as running up a sensory nerve and down a motor nerve. The theoretical existence of an energetic organic "fluid" different from water was hypothesized by many seventeenth century philosophers and scientists, including Sir Isaac Newton, who wrote of "a certain most subtle spirit which pervades and lies hid in all gross bodies," and that "all sensation is excited, and the members of animal bodies move at the command of the will, namely, by the vibrations of this spirit, mutually propagated along the solid filaments of the nerves, from the outward organs of sense to the brain, and from the brain into the muscles" (Newton, Sir Isaac, *Principia Mathematica*, London, 1687).

Galvani's remarkable experiments shifted the paradigm that nerves functioned like water pipes or channels as Descartes had proposed, but rather as conductors that carried electricity generated directly by organic tissue. Galvani established the basis for the biological investigation of nerve conduction that eventually led to the development of neurophysiology as a distinct discipline. Sherrington later acknowledged this in his 1905 Silliman lectures at Yale when describing man as (Sherrington, CS. *The Integrative Action of the Nervous System*, Yale University Press, New Haven, 1906)

> . . . a reflex creature which not only breathes and stands but rises and walks, or runs and attitudinizes, looking up at a shelf, or scanning the floor. . . . Slowly and surely the ensuing century's analysis resolved this aspect of the spirits of the animal into transient electrical potentials traveling the fibers of the nervous system. They were no longer "spirit" but were becoming a physical event describable under energy.

Kolliker and Muller placed the nerve portion of a nerve–leg preparation of one frog on the beating heart of another frog and demonstrated that the frog's leg contracted with each heart contraction (Kolliker A, Muller H: Zweiter Bericht über die im Jahr1854/55 in der physiologischen Anstalt der Universität Wurzburg angestellten Versuche. Vll. Nachweis der negativen Schwankung des Muskelstroms am naturlich sich contrahirender Muskel. *Verh Phys-Med Ges Wurzb* 1856; 6:528.). The study of animal electricity seemed to hold the clue to an understanding of life and had attracted pioneers like Emile DuBois-Reymond, Eduard Pflüger, and Hermann Helmholtz. By 1848 Du Bois Reymond had published two large volumes on the subject, and the use of electric currents for stimulation had become a general method of research. As Adrian noted, "It is difficult to conceive of any other method which has done so much to show us how the body works for it gives us a means of throwing a muscle or a nerve into activity at will by an agency, which does no damage and can be precisely controlled."

However, it was clear that bioelectricity and electricity traveling through metal conductors had quite different characteristics. Du Bois-Reymond built a *Froschwecker* (frog alarm) to show that an impulse traveling along a stimulated nerve moved too slowly to be considered a current such as that conducted by a wire. In this Rube Goldberg contraption, a frog leg contracted to move a lever and ring a bell in response to a discharge from an electric fish. In 1868 his student, Julius Bernstein, proposed that the impulse was not a current but rather a disturbance in ionic properties that traveled along the nerve fiber at a slower rate. While this hypothesis is generally accepted, the source of the energy to pump these ions is still not clear.

Lord Edgar Douglas Adrian and Sir Charles Scott Sherrington shared the 1932 Nobel Prize in Physiology or Medicine "for their discoveries regarding the functions of neurons" and their acceptance speeches summarize the state of knowledge 70 years ago. In his Nobel lecture, entitled The Activity of the Nerve Fibres, Adrian noted

> The nerves do their work economically, without visible change and with the smallest expenditure of energy. The signals which they transmit can only be detected as changes of electrical potential, and these changes are very small and of very brief duration.... The grading and coordination of muscular activity is a subject which has been so greatly illuminated by my friend Sir Charles Sherrington that I mention my own work as a very small supplement to his. It has dealt as before with the signals which are sent by the individual nerve fibres, and its results emphasize the close correspondence between the sensory and motor activities of the nervous system.... On the whole it appears that the frequency of the impulses varies over a more restricted range in the motor than in the sensory discharge, but the two are so closely alike that the mechanism of the sense organ and of the motor nerve cell must have much in common. They have, of course, the common factor of a nerve fibre which can only respond in one way, but the likeness goes beyond this. Also the particular frequencies which commonly occur are lower than they would be if determined solely by the characteristics of the nerve fibre. In quiet breathing, for instance, at each expansion of the lungs the sense organs of the vagus send up a train of impulses rising to a frequency of about 20 a second at the height of inspiration, and simultaneously the movement of expansion is being produced by trains of motor impulses rising to much the same frequency and almost indistinguishable from the discharge in the sensory fibres. In fact the motor nerve cells seem to be acting just like a collection of sense organs responding to a rhythmic stretch... Resemblances of this kind show that there is an underlying unity of response in the various parts of the neurone in spite of their differentiation into axon, dendrites or terminal arborizations.

Sherrington's lecture, Inhibition as a Coordinative Factor, is even more relevant to vagal nerve stimulation (VNS) as indicated by the following excerpts.

That a muscle on irritation of its nerve contracts had already long been familiar to physiology when the 19th century found a nerve which when irritated prevented its muscle from contracting. This observation seemed for a time too strange to be believed. Its truth did not gain acceptance for ten years; but at last in 1848 the Webers accepted the fact at its face value and proclaimed the vagus nerve to be inhibitory of the heart muscle. Two hundred years earlier Descartes, in writing the *De Homine*, had assumed that muscle was supplied with nerves which caused muscular relaxation. An analogous suggestion was put forward by Charles Bell in 1819. The inhibition suggested was in each case peripheral. The role of inhibition in the working of the central nervous system has proved to be more and more extensive and more and more fundamental as experiment has advanced in examining it. Reflex inhibition can no longer be regarded merely as a factor specially developed for dealing with the antagonism of opponent muscles acting at various hinge joints. Its role as a coordinative factor comprises that, and goes beyond that. In the working of the central nervous machinery, inhibition seems as ubiquitous and as frequent as is excitation itself. The whole quantitative grading of the operations of the spinal cord and brain appears to rest upon mutual interaction between the two central processes "excitation" and "inhibition", the one no less important than the other.

It was by this circuitous route that electrical stimulation of nerve and muscle finally emerged as an investigational tool for the pursuit of medical applications. The basis of these effects was subsequently found to reside in the depolarization or hyperpolarization of nerve and muscle membrane potentials. It is now clear that the nerve propagates a signal that is not passive like a current in a conducting metal, but active and continually generated as an action potential along the length of the axon. However, when the action potential reaches the end of the axon the signal changes from a digital all-or-none to a nonpropagated potential. At the *synapse* (a term coined by Sherrington) it gives rise to an active, interactive phase of excitation or inhibition of adjacent neurons. From my perspective, synapses resemble computer chips in that they are components of an integrative system that coordinates all the organs, tissues, and functions. However, their "memory" may be greater, since it would seem that each synapse "knows" what every other synapse is doing, perhaps by a field effect. The electroencephalogram (EEG) may represent an example of this.

II. THE NEURON AND RETICULAR THEORIES

The neuron theory can be said to have its origin with the statement of cell theory by Schlieden and Schwann about 1840. During the next 50 years, there was an enormous effort dedicated to the description of cells in the nervous system. The reason the anatomists of that time had such great difficulty picturing nervous system cells was the initial straightforward picture of what a cell looked like in general. The anatomic word *cell* was borrowed from the name of a room in a monastery where monks lived, called a *monastery cell*. The monastery cell was a simple rectangular or square room which resembled what the early workers such a sHooke saw in biologic preparations such as sponge and which were labeled by them as biologic *cells*. This early picture of a biologic cell did not conform to anything that the anatomists of the nineteenth century could see in the nervous system. Instead, the anatomists saw a bizarre collection of rounded bodies interspersed between a fabric of long fibrous processes, but there did not appear to be any consistent connection between these two entities. Because of these difficulties in observing a discrete anatomic structure that could be called a cell, the leading nineteenth century explanation of the structure of the nervous systems was "the reticular theory." The reticular theory stated that the nervous system was structured as a continuous network of nervous processes in which the proto-plasm of one nerve fiber ran continuously into the protoplasm of another nerve fiber without a break or anatomic separation between them.

The controversy between the neuronists and the reticularists continued to develop until it reached a peak at the time of the Nobel Prize presentations in 1906. At this point, the cell had been established as being the basic structure of all organs, except for the nervous system. The neuron theory and the reticular theory each had vigorous supporters with perhaps Camillo Golgi and Ramón y Cajal representing the most capable leaders of their respective camps. Golgi, an Italian physician and cytologist, also at the University of Pavia, had devised the silver nitrate method of staining nervous tissue, which allowed him to demonstrate the existence of a kind of nerve cell with many short, branching extensions or dendrites that connected to other nerve cells. This came to be known as the *Golgi cell*. Cajal, a Spanish physician and histologist at the University of Madrid, improved Golgi's silver nitrate stain, which enabled him to clearly differentiate neurons from other cells and to trace the structure and connections of nerve cells in gray matter and the spinal cord. As the date for the Nobel Prize Award for Physiology or Medicine approached, scientists hotly debated whether Golgi or Cajal would be the recipient, since this would settle the neuron vs. reticular controversy. Both were eminent scientists, but if one received the prize, it would mean automatic defeat for the other's theory, and some felt that Golgi had the advantage since he had developed the technique Cajal had used to support his neuron theory.

The Nobel Prize committee rose to the occasion by presenting the award to both Golgi and Cajal, essentially corroborating the correctness of both theories. They seemed to support the thesis, which Golgi himself stated in his acceptance speech, that in certain regions the nervous system was composed of neurons and in others it was composed of a reticulum. It would have been contradictory to propose that one region of the nervous system could consist of both neurons and a reticulum since these ideas were antagonistic, unless one postulated that the nervous system had the potential to change from a collection of neurons to a reticulum or the reverse as the situation warranted. The single individual who was the most important in the decision of this controversy was Sherrington, who was viewed by most of his contemporaries as more of a physiologic philosopher rather than a classical physiologist.

Sherrington's involvement in the controversy developed in the following way. He was sent to Spain as a physician to treat the populace when a plague had suddenly emerged. While there, he literally bumped into Cajal who informed him in detail about the evidence in support of the neuron theory. Sherrington was so impressed by Cajal that on his return to England he immediately undertook to defend the neuron theory. His support of the neuron theory also derived from his experimental research on the reflex contraction of extensor and flexor muscles. Extensor muscles when contracting tend to extend the limb, whereas flexor muscles tend to flex it. Sherrington called the relationship between flexor and extensor muscles *antagonistic* since flexion and extension of the limb cannot occur simultaneously. Contraction of extensor muscles naturally opposes flexion of the limb and vice versa. He found that in order for a smooth flexion of the limb to occur, the extensor muscles must relax before or during the contraction of flexor muscles. This relaxation is determined by special activity in the nervous system called *inhibition*.

Sherrington determined that the inhibition in the reflex extension and flexion experiments occurred in the spinal cord and wondered whether there were special structures or sites within the spinal cord that might represent the locus of inhibition. Here, the neuron theory came to his aid. If the protoplasm of one nerve cell stops before the beginning of another nerve cell, then there exists a gap or separation between nerve cells. Even though this separation is microscopic, it is still logical to inquire what material it might contain. Cajal had stated that the gap contains a basement cement, which is nonviable, but Sherrington did not agree. He believed that the membrane of one nerve cell was juxtaposed to the membrane of another nerve cell, and with his characteristic wit, referred to this anatomic arrangement as "nerve cells holding hands." He called this the *synapse*, from the Greek word for connection or junction, and this is where inhibition takes place.

Vagal nerve stimulation (VNS) includes inhibition in its actions but goes beyond this. Inhibition is defined electrodynamically as a polarization or hyperpolarization of the synaptic membranes, which means that it counteracts the depolarization of excitation, so that threshold is much more difficult to achieve. However, VNS also involves a negative feedback action, a filtering action, and a switching effect that can best be explained as follows. Our present conception is that the neuron functions on the basis of three types of electrical phenomenon:

1. A resting membrane potential
2. An action potential produced by a decrease of the resting membrane potential to a threshold level that then self-propagates
3. A synaptic potential which occurs at junctions between neurons

In contrast to the synaptic potential, the action potential is all-or-none due to a threshold for activation, so that the neuron is functioning in a nonlinear fashion, and therefore, the amount and pattern of current does not linearly correlate with the neuron's output. This can lead to confusion if it is assumed that an increase of stimulating current automatically leads to a corresponding increase in nerve output because the relationship is not a straight line response but more like a logarithmic curve.

Several early twentieth century events have largely shaped our present electrical orientation to brain and nerves. Willem Einthoven, a Dutch physician, developed the electrocardiograph, for which he received the Nobel Prize in 1924 and in 1929. Hans Berger in Germany invented the electroencephalograph to measure and record brain waves. Around the same time, Joseph Erlanger, a U.S. physiologist, in collaboration with Herbert Gasser, one of his students, found that a cathode-ray oscilloscope could demonstrate the characteristic wave pattern of an impulse generated in a stimulated nerve fiber and that amplification allowed them to study its components. In 1932, they found that the fibers of a nerve conduct impulses at different rates depending on the thickness of the fiber, and that each fiber had a different threshold of excitability. Thus, a stimulus of different intensity was required to create an impulse, and they also found that different fibers transmitted different kinds of impulses that were represented by different types of waveforms. Erlanger and Gasser shared the 1944 Nobel Prize for discovering that fiber within the same nerve cord possess different functions.

The primary problem was how the nervous system functioned with respect to whether the basis of communication was electrical or chemical, or both, which Sherrington referred to as the *integrative action* of the nervous system. He approached this with the reflex as his conceptual and experimental tool in an attempt to coordinate the balance between organs and tissues, the autonomic and somatic motor systems, as well as consciousness and behavior. Sherrington's overall goal was to describe the unifying or integrating process within the nervous system, which brought the diverse functions of the organs and tissues into a coordinated global action. However, he believed that the physical and psychological functions of the nervous system were integrated separately and interacted only at certain times, so that this opened the door to separate integrations instead of a single all-encompassing process. For instance, he went on to separate other functions of the nervous system, of which the most important was the distinction between the autonomic nervous system and voluntary somatic motor functions. The autonomic or involuntary nervous system regulated the internal environment, and somatic motor responses dealt more with influences on the external environment. But are these divisions really necessary in light of contemporary data showing that some autonomic functions are under volitional control. Is it possible to forge the autonomic and somatic motor together into a common integration? One of the misleading conclusions or assumptions arising out of Sherrington's divided integrations was that the autonomic nervous system had virtually no afferent neurons, and thus was an efferent or motor system in contrast to the somatic motor which was both somatic and motor. The main purpose of VNS is to activate afferent portions of the vagus, which, of course, would be impossible if none were present.

Sherrington was an ingenious and accomplished experimenter, and it is surprising that he did not investigate whether the vagus nerve had any afferent input. In actuality, approximately 80% of the vagus is afferent, and some indication of the relatively large predominance of afferent neurons began to emerge early on when cardiovascular, respiratory, abdominal, etc., afferents were discovered. However, at the time I began the experiments with VNS, the vagus was still considered to be primarily efferent, and I believe my experiments were perhaps the first to demonstrate the functional predominance of the afferents of the vagus nerve and their clinical importance. This is in addition to the afferent neurons with specific functional connections to the cardiovascular, respiratory, and abdominal systems. Since there are about 90,000 neurons in the vagus nerve, and about 20,000 are efferent, this leaves about 70,000 afferent neurons. Several questions stood out at the beginning of my VNS studies. Did all of these thousands of neurons have some clinical relevance or was it only some subset that might be minute? Secondly, how did these thousands of unspecified neurons interact with higher centers in the brain? It was known that most of the afferent neurons terminated in the nucleus tractus solitarius, with a relatively small group ending in the area postrema region or the trigeminal nucleus. While these synaptic sites are in the most hind portion of the brain, tracts emerge from these areas to innervate many other regions of the brain.

These myriad tracts from the vagus to many other brain locations demonstrate that vagus impulses can have far reaching effects on higher centers, but this does not mean that they have any clinical applications. My reasoning was that for this to happen, vagal stimulation would have to act to restore normalcy to some complex electrochemical cerebral system that had become unstable for some reason. To explore this underlying electrochemical system, it is necessary to begin with Sherrington and the reflex.

To explore this, it was necessary to begin with Charles Sherrington's "The Integrative Action of the Nervous System," which was the paradigm of the nervous system that formed the basis for neurological research and the diagnosis of neurologic disorders. His major question was how were the organs and tissues of the body coordinated into a functionally complete system in which each organ acted in concert with all other organs and tissues. In Sherrington's words: "This integrative action in virtue of which the nervous system unifies from separate organs an animal possessing solidarity, an individual, is the problem before us in these lectures." Sherrington methodically pursued this goal through most of his life and, in this effort, defined the synapse as the junction between nerve cells, the two main underlying processes of excitation and inhibition, the local motor circuit, etc. It was a remarkable achievement, especially considering the primitive nature of the technology available to him at the time. It consisted of levers connected at one end to muscles and at the other resting on a kymograph drum covered by a cylindrical roll of smoked paper on which was registered the muscle movements, that would later by preserved with shellac. It has always seemed amazing to me that this primitive methodology gave rise to his results that have survived the advances provided by sophisticated modern technologies.

Sherrington approached the problem of integration from both ends of the spectrum. At the lowest level of integration was the reflex and at the highest was consciousness. At the conscious level, he was unable to maintain a single coordinating unifying mechanism and had to rely on two apparently independent integrations. Sherrington enumerated the central problem in the understanding of integration as follows:

> Enough has been said to stress that in the sequence of events a step is reached where a physical situation in the brain leads to a psychical which however contains no hint of the brain or any other bodily part. . . . The suggestion has to be, it would seem, two continuous series of events, one physico-chemical, the other psychical, and at times interaction between them.

This was essentially the same as the duality framework of brain and mind that Descartes had elaborated three centuries earlier. It was at the reflex level that Sherrington presented a simple integration of stimulus and response, which can occur without the participation of mind or consciousness. However, the process at the reflex level is still complex with motor nerves going to the muscle and afferent nerves acting as feedback from the muscle. There are also neurons, whose activity originates in the reticular formation of the brain, that act to produce a set point or tone of the muscle. Sherrington considered the higher brain functions to be an integration or combination of these basic reflex patterns. He appreciated that afferent and set-point neurons were important in reflex muscle contractions, but he missed their great significance as the inherent components of a system, in the sense of what we today call *system analysis*. Without this understanding, an analysis or investigation of the integrative action of the nervous system was not possible. Sherrington kept the reflex as an almost linear input-output relationship, the most primitive analysis possible, and incapable of explaining the intricacies of brain electrodynamics.

In justice to Sherrington, system analysis and cybernetics came into being much later with the origins of complex electrical circuitry. In addition, the first application was not to the nervous system, but to the cardiovascular system in terms of neurons from the heart and blood vessels as a kind of negative feedback. Understanding system analysis and cybernetics is crucial in explaining VNS effects. What is the importance of thousands of unidentified afferent neurons of the vagus if not to produce negative feedback for brain stability? The input-output of the reflex must be superimposed upon an inherent feedback and set-point structure that corresponds to complex electrical circuits. It is their inherent structure that constitutes the mechanism of VNS. A major consideration is that when all the components of the circuit are brought together, there must be stability. I believed the same was true of the nervous system, that what we call *nervous system illness* is often a reflection of some instability, and that this instability or illness could be "cured" by negative feedback, analogous to what can occur in a complex electrical circuit. What follows is an account of the tortuous route that had to be taken to establish the basic mechanisms underlying VNS, determining the validity of these findings in the laboratory and determining their potential clinical applications.

At this point, it was important to harmonize or at least coordinate my theories with those of Sherrington. Adrian and others, and do basic experiments in autorhythmic nerve discharge, vomiting, respiration, heart, and autonomic nervous system function. It would then be necessary to combine the results of these endeavors into a single, critical experimental model demonstrating the control of brain instability by vagal nerve stimulation. The prime example of brain instability is seizure activity, which is also a serious clinical problem; so that supportive evidence would be derived not only from animal experiments but also clinical studies. I could do the basic animal experiments myself, but the clinical investigations would involve a far-flung effort requiring considerable investment capital to establish a start-up company, obtain FDA approval for clinical trials, patient ethics concerns that would be acceptable to a hospital or other Institutional Review Boards, and numerous other obstacles.

III. OBSERVATIONS

A basic observation derives from physics and engineering. As circuits became much more complicated, they might easily generate resonance in the form of an extreme oscillation that rendered the circuit inoperable. Such resonance could simply result from a strong electrical signal in the environment entering the circuit that was then amplified in its oscillation. An antidote to this is negative feedback achieved by simply feeding a very small portion of the output signal back (inverted) to the input where it is amplified simultaneously with the environmental signal, thereby neutralizing it to prevent resonance.

It occurred to me that perhaps vagal afferents could be considered as being analogous to negative feedback. For instance, certain cardiovascular afferents are assumed to be a kind of negative feedback for the cardiovascular systems, such as carotid sinus afferents to lower blood pressure. Why couldn't the brain have vagal afferents that might act as negative feedback? Stability of the brain suggests that its functions are performing optimally and in perfect balance whereas a condition such as epilepsy represented periods when the brain is unstable as reflected by an abnormal EEG and oscillatory muscular movements. It seemed feasible that stimulation of vagal afferents could supply the kind of negative feedback that would stabilize the brain and stop or prevent resonance instability. However, electrical stimulation of vagal afferents has at least one significant difference from physiological stimulation in that the nerves discharge together rather than gradually. Would the brain accept these almost synchronized volley of action potentials? For instance, after a period of time, most drugs are resisted or rejected by the brain. Would this also happen with VNS? Our results with animals and patients were quite different from those seen with drugs. Not only was there no rejection, but effectiveness with VNS actually increased over months or years so that the brain not only did not reject VNS but rather seemed to welcome it. One caveat in this regard is that the optimal parameters of VNS have still not been determined and it may not be effective in certain patients.

A personal observation relates to my wife's pregnancy when we chose the Lamaze technique for childbirth in preference to anesthesia. Ferdinand Lamaze had visited the maternity wards in Russia where he was told that certain respiratory maneuvers diminished childbirth pain by Pavlovian conditioning. Instead, Lamaze concluded that these strenuous respiratory efforts merely distracted the woman from the pain of labor. The Lamaze approach uses strenuous breathing techniques to assist contractions and relaxation methods that allow a woman to separate muscle groups and work with one part of her body while deliberately relaxing the rest of it. I observed the others in our group performing what I concluded was hyperventilation and the same maneuvers during labor and felt that the process achieved was primarily physiological. Stretch receptors were activated by this lung expansion to produce a high frequency of afferent vagal action potentials resulting in regularization of uterine and abdominal contractions and a decrease of pain. I suspected that these vagal afferents had access to some central command system subserving many functions.

In the course of performing other experiments, I made observations that I thought might be relevant to the development of VNS for clinical applications. One of the most important was to place VNS within the concept of a physiological system with input, output, negative and positive feedback, etc., which is especially critical if VNS is relevant to an electrodynamic system of the brain. All too often, there has been satisfaction in simply stating that a certain neurotransmitter or neurotransmitters was the key factor in transmitting messages, whereas it is the brain's overall electrical connectivity that is most critical and is actually responsible for neurotransmitter effects.

The cardiovascular system has perhaps been the most intensively investigated physiological system with respect to electrical connectivity. It also combines vagus neurons in both the afferent and efferent loops with an input and an output. I investigated the resonance or oscillation in the system and found that these are most likely due to a delay between the input and output and probably due to the conduction time of action potentials, and the relatively slow contraction time of the smooth muscle of the vessel walls. In complex electrical circuits, the delay can be also a basis of resonance; so first of all, the electrodynamics appeared to be critical for stable brain function. Second, vagal neurons appeared to be playing a significant role in system function and stabilization. Might not vagal afferents be playing a similar role for the brain as a whole?

Another important observation was made in relation to emesis. I had noticed the projectile vomiting of my son, and initiated an experiment where vomiting was triggered by electrical stimulation of vagal abdominal afferents. It is a somewhat common experience that an adult may attempt to control a vomiting episode by deep respiration, so I stimulated respiratory afferents in the cervical vagus nerve and was encouraged to find that this did prevent vomiting. It seemed that emesis had some of the characteristics of a seizure:

1. Rhythmic contraction of muscles and diaphragm
2. Change in the conscious state
3. Uncontrolled muscle contractions and behavior
4. Multiple etiologies that might precipitate vomiting

I decided to investigate other causative events that resulted in vomiting to determine whether vagal afferent stimulation might be equally effective.

My first experiments were with a potentially toxic substance, which can cause emesis by action on the chemoreceptor trigger zone in the brain stem that apparently has a direct neural connection with the emetic center. Here again, vagal afferent stimulation also prevented vomiting. Is it possible to view emesis as a kind of "physiological seizure"? What prevents vomiting from continuing indefinitely? Was this a consequence of negative feedback by vagal afferents? With respect to seizures, could something similar be occurring with vagal afferents to prevent seizures from continuing indefinitely? Was it conceivable that the stability of the brain in general depends upon some sort of negative feedback that involves vagal afferents? After all, vagal afferents represent feedback from virtually all the organs and systems responsible for preserving the stability of life, function, and behavior.

I decided to pursue motion sickness, another cause of emesis. Monkeys experience motion sickness with horizontal acceleration, but not vertical acceleration, and cats experience motion sickness with vertical acceleration, but not horizontal acceleration. In both animals, I was able to demonstrate that vomiting could be prevented by cervical vagus stimulation. Although the term *sickness* is used to describe motion-induced vomiting, it is not a sickness in the usual sense but rather a disturbance or imbalance produced by some combination of visual and semicircular canal interaction.

Vomiting is usually explained as an attempt to expel some toxic substance from the stomach, which obviously does not apply to motion sickness. Here, vagal afferents apparently counteract an imbalance consequent to a contradictory receptor input to the brain. The important point here is that vagal afferents can correct this imbalance. Was it possible that vagal afferents could prevent or reverse other imbalances in the brain by similar stabilizing activities? Although vagal neurons innervate virtually all the internal organs, this does not apply to striated muscle that is the basis of behavior. Striated muscle can have its own local negative and positive feedback. But in a complex electronic circuit, the negative feedback element doesn't connect with all the circuit elements, but is a function of the output. The internal organs represent a more than sufficient output of the brain for such a purpose. Autorhythmic electrical potentials and currents arise in many parts of the brain. How do they arise and are they important in the action of VNS? The function of most of these autorhythmic potentials remains elusive but that of the respiratory center is well known, as it drives the respiratory musculature. Vagal afferents can inhibit this electrical activity, and since a seizure has the characteristics of a self-generating process, it may be inhibited by VNS.

The central problem of the action potential still remains. What is the nature of the neural code that underlies the transmission of information? Historically, in the initial period of action potential observations, it was concluded that since the spike is digital, i.e., all or none, that the information is a function of the frequency of action potential generation. This was later found to be only a general approximation primarily relating to Sherrington's concept of the central excitatory state. For instance, changes in excitation or central excitatory state corresponded to a change in the frequency of excitatory fiber spikes. However, changes in interspike intervals were observed to be a more accurate indicator, even in excitability changes. There ensued a period of intensive accumulation of interspike interval histograms, and analysis of these histograms based on a statistical analysis was pursued. However, this period also appears to be drawing to a close, apparently because so much is left unanswered by even this sophisticated analysis, even in the area of excitability. The basic assumption of information transmission is still retained, i.e., that the spike is essentially a marker of time intervals. The question then emerges as to how a collection of time intervals represents the different physical energies transduced by the receptor and how the brain reinterprets these time intervals into a picture of the "real world," i.e., information in the brain–mind domain.

A new approach appears to be necessary to go beyond the very simplest level of analysis as occurred with frequency and interspike interval studies. Perhaps the first level of analysis is to determine what type of order obtains in an assemblage of spike intervals. The predominant view at present is to consider the spike intervals as approximately linear within limits and representing corresponding changes in excitation. This approach has produced the concept of excitation at a synapse as a function of spike intervals reaching the synapse and releasing a neurotransmitter whose concentration is a function of these intervals. The excitation potential is an inverse function of interval length. Thus, this view presupposes an inherent order or linearity in spike generation and reception. The other view is that spike generation is a random process and excitation changes are a function of an assemblage of random spike intervals.

A new approach should be based upon a more fundamental physical basis. Perhaps, simply counting the number of spikes or intervals between spikes is much too simplistic to yield significant results. One way of looking at this is in terms of the operations the brain must perform to be able to decode the information transmitted by spikes from the receptors. Does the brain simply reconstitute the original generator potential from the receptor? It appears to be very unlikely that this would be sufficient to determine the informational content. The other side of the problem is how are the various environmental energies reconstituted in the brain from an assemblage of spiked time intervals. Leaving aside for now the very different subjective qualities, how does the brain "know" that different energies are involved, since all the brain "sees" are these time intervals marked by spikes? I decided to bypass these important questions with a simple pragmatic approach of testing the frequency of VNS stimulation since I had found that a certain frequency range proved to be the most effective in interrupting seizures.

IV. THE CRITICAL EXPERIMENT

An experimental model was developed in canines to exhibit generalized seizures as a demonstration of brain electrodynamic instability that could be inhibited by repetitive electrical stimulation of the cervical vagus nerve. Seizures or tremors were induced by injection boluses of strychnine or pentylenetetrazol at 1 to 4-min intervals. Vagal stimulation stopped ongoing seizures in 0.5–5 s. Strychnine induces seizures by action in the brain stem, and pentylenetetrazol does so by action on the cortex. Thus, this experimental model was able to test the two major sites of clinical seizure generation, and alpha-chloralose was the anesthetic utilized to allow maximal seizure generalization. Strychnine was selected because of extensive information on its physiological actions and the forceful, rhythmic movements of alternating flexor and exterior muscles were recorded. Would stimulation of vagal afferents terminate a kind of electrical resonance in the brain responsible for producing these convulsive movements? If so, vagal afferents could be considered as providing something analogous to negative feedback to stabilize brain networks. Another possibility was that efferent neuron activation could also be having some effect on seizures. However, there was significant restriction on the intact efferent neurons for three reasons:

1. The polarization of the anode blocked the conduction of a number of these efferents.
2. In the clinical setting with the stimulator model used, the current was apparently not sufficient to activate C fibers.
3. The electrodes were to be placed beneath the branching of the superior cardiac nerve.

We were also able to demonstrate that activity in the efferent neurons had no effect on seizures by cutting the nerve distal to the electrodes.

More research is required to describe the groups of action potentials of different stimulation parameters, the most important being current frequency and pulse duration. The stimulation of the vagus nerve can result in complicated physical events depending on the characteristics of threshold, refractory periods, and conduction velocity. The three major groups of neurons, called *A*, *B*, and *C*, have different characteristics, and thus behave in a different fashion electrically. At present, it appears that A or B fibers can inhibit seizures, and although early claims suggested that C fibers could inhibit seizures, this has not been verified in recent research. And the effect of C fibers on seizures is still not clear. In addition, there are four groups of A fibers whose individual roles remain to be elucidated. It will be necessary to determine whether there are selective nerve fibers that alone are responsible for seizure inhibition or whether inhibition is a function of many thousands of vagal afferents. There is also the question as to whether there are vagal afferents that can actually be excitatory and thus oppose afferent inhibition of seizures. Thus, the simple term *VNS* belies a host of imponderables, but, nonetheless, all capable of being resolved by experimental inquiry with present technology. However, as will be explained, the term *NeuroCybernetic Prosthesis* (NCP) would appear to more properly describe the complex process involved in both the nerve and the brain.

A major intent of these experiments was to observe the ranges of stimulus parameters that produced antiseizure effects to determine whether there were optimum parameters. This could be crucial for constructing an effective clinical device and establishing the protocol for future experiments and eventually therapy. The number of combinations of stimulus parameters is astronomical when one considers the duration of the stimulus train and how often it is repeated. Of equal importance is the nonlinear relationship between stimulation and nerve responses. There is a progression of A fibers being activated at the lower currents to C fibers at the higher currents, and the progression is not linear but in discrete jumps. In addition, there may be four groups of A fibers and two groups of C fibers, each with a different threshold and other electrical properties. Is there one group that is most effective or is it simply a question of stimulating a sufficient number of neurons? Also, as previously indicated, could there be any excitatory groups that act in an opposite fashion to prevent inhibition?

The conclusion was that effectiveness is based on two mechanisms:

1. A direct process stopping the seizure
2. A long-term process of accumulation of repetitive stimulations which steadily reduces seizure magnitude or frequency.

While there was some indication of pro-seizure activity, this excitation was limited apparently to the duration of stimulation. An important observation was that the duration of seizure suppression extended beyond the period of stimulation since in these acute experiments, the period of seizure inhibition lasted four times the duration of stimulation. It was suggested that this extended inhibition would continue to increase over time in chronic experiments on conscious epileptic animals as manifested by a steady decrease in seizure frequency or magnitude over a period of weeks, months, or even years. This has now been confirmed in thousands of patients. Our hypothesis was that this effect was due to a decreasing synaptic receptor sensitivity. In any event, there appears to be present at least two components of the inhibitory process: a rapidly rising and decaying phase and a slowly rising and decaying phase.

An important question is whether this is an accidental result, i.e., a nonphysiological consequence of vagal afferent impulses interfering in some way with seizure activity in the brain, or a physiological result? The indications are that it is truly a physiological result in spite of the fact that there has been no evidence heretofore of fundamental vagal afferent involvement in seizures. The direct and indirect evidence is

1. The minute currents generated in the brain by vagal afferents
2. The stability of the background EEG during VNS
3. The thousands of vagal afferents for which no specific function has been identified
4. The long-term beneficial effect of VNS over months or years documented in animals and patients.

I therefore came to the conclusion, based on experimental and clinical results, that VNS could prevent or stop brain electrodynamic instability in an analogous manner in which negative feedback prevents electrical instability. It seemed possible that brain instability might be the basis of many illnesses that VNS could alleviate, such as depression.

V. BRAIN ELECTRODYNAMICS

One of the problems is that stimulation is not a precise term, since it can include not only electrical but pharmacological and physiological agents as well as diverse forms of energy. The term *neurocybernetic prosthesis* was specifically utilized to avoid this imprecision and also to indicate the underlying mechanism of action and clinical application. The device is called *NCP*, and, in a sense, VNS can be considered to be the first generation of NCPs. It is true that vagus nerve stimulation is part of the action of the NCP, but it is only a means to an end; the real center of action is in the brain, which results as a consequence of correctly applying VNS. In relation to electrical stimulation, the effective action occurs within 500 ms for A neurons and somewhat longer for C neurons. This is because stimulation only refers to a transient electrical change that is akin to an "activation energy," and then the neuron "takes over" with a relatively large explosion of energy represented by the action potential and its propagation along the neuron. For VNS, the goal is to use a small quantity of energy to harness this large quantity of neural energy. VNS is apparently able to do this because the nerve is electrically structured at its ends to respond to a depolarization, i.e., a decrease in its membrane potential. This property continues throughout most of the extent of the neuron, even though there seems to be no physical reason for it to do so. The basis of this property is presumed to be explained by the Hodgkin–Huxley hypothesis that the electrical stimulation "opens" the pores of the neuronal membrane so that sodium ion, which is at a higher concentration outside the neuron, can "diffuse" rapidly into the neuron and thus generate the main portion of the action potential.

The major question is that with such a transient electrical current, is it possible to initiate a change in brain electrodynamics? For instance, the seizure represents a synchronization of neuronal discharge that can involve millions of neurons. Can the activation of a few hundred or even a few thousand vagal afferents prevent this massive brain discharge of electrical potentials? On the surface, it does not appear possible because we are not putting energy into an electrical circuit but only in the transient stimulation of the membrane, so that the brain must activate its own electrical energetics to end the seizure discharge. How is it possible then that the brain's electrodynamics can be stabilized by VNS? A process akin to negative feedback appears to be a reasonable explanation. Since vagal afferents express a kind of negative feedback in circulatory, heart, and respiratory functions, why not also in a global electrodynamic way for the brain as a whole. Stability of the brain may be of utmost importance in certain brain disorders. Thus, a relatively small current acts similarly to a relatively small electric signal in negative feedback circuits, and this stimulation current is amplified by the synaptic output in the brain.

The role of the neuron in brain electrodynamics is almost as great a question today for biology and medicine as it was in the time of Galvani. Although the existence of bioelectricity is now commonly accepted, its origin or origins and potential applications remain to be determined. The main reason for this in my opinion is that most attention has emphasized neurotransmitters, receptors, and pharmacological agents and the focus initiated by du Bois-Reymond and others has largely dissipated. However, in the 1920s and 1930s with the arrival of the amplifier and oscilloscope, these efforts were revived by

Adrian, Matthews, and others in England and by Forbes, Erlanger, and Gasser in the U.S. as well as others in Europe.

The controversy began with the question of how the electrical charge transversed the synapse from one neuron to another. It was known that the action potential reaching the axonal terminal was transformed into a synaptic potential that was not self-propagating but decremented in magnitude as it spread along the terminal branch. In terms of standard electronics, the action potential might be considered a digital signal whereas the synaptic potential is analog. It is interesting that these two potentials are the two main categories of electrical change in the nervous system, whether in the brain, spinal cord, or peripherally. The resting membrane potential is the basic electrical polarization upon which these two potentials can play their game. Synaptic potentials are of two types:

1. Depolarization of the membrane, called an *excitatory synaptic potential*, because it causes discharge of the action potential
2. Hyperpolarization of the membrane, called an *inhibitory synaptic potential* since it can prevent discharge of the action potential.

This has led me to conclude that VNS prevents the excitation causing seizures because of hyperpolarization effects.

Another controversy has centered on whether the means of crossing the synaptic gap between neurons was via chemical or electrical processes. This debate had its sponsors on each side who were known in the trade as the "juice" or "sparks" boys. Support for the neurotransmitters began with the experiments of Henry Dale, who demonstrated acetylcholine release at synapses. Later, a number of leading sparks boys such as John Eccles converted to the concept of neurotransmitters, which rapidly became the leading model of brain processes. In this scheme, the action potentials and synaptic potentials were viewed primarily as a method of releasing neurotransmitters. However, neurotransmitters acted primarily to change the membrane potential, and formulating a hypothetical mechanism for brain electrodynamics requires much more than this. For example, Clerk Maxwell was confused by the problem of how capacitors worked since the capacitor interrupted electrical connectivity so that there should have been no current. Maxwell concluded that in actuality, electrical connectivity was not broken because a field existed between the capacitor plates and through the dielectric, a concept that eventually led to the discovery of generation of electromagnetic waves. It might be reasonable to investigate the possible existence of a field effect of the NTS which could act like a switch to turn synaptic clusters on or off based on a depolarization produced by vagal afferents.

The mechanism of VNS is based on a polarization field, which is a resultant of an ensemble of synaptic membrane potentials. Axon polarization is changed (depolarization) by stimulation to produce the action potential which is conducted (by a series of successive depolarizations) to the nucleus of the tractus solitarius (NTS) where synaptic polarization changes occur, as well as neurotransmitter actions. Specific functions (or programs) can be switched on or off by changes in this polarization field, similar to a digital switch. For instance, the NTS subserves the functions of respiration, cardiovascular, vomiting, etc.; respiration can be switched off temporarily so that vomiting can occur. The NTS is connected to other brain areas to produce a similar effect on the polarization field there.

As an undergraduate at Johns Hopkins, I was influenced by Detlev Bronk, who was a student of E. D. Adrian, began Biophysics at the University of Pennsylvania, and became President of Johns Hopkins the year I enrolled. A close associate of Detlev Bronk was Frank Brink who had assigned me to study the physiology of oxygen uptake by peripheral nerve. I was very impressed by the capability of technology to follow the invisible movement of oxygen through the nerve cell and believed I was being shown a powerful tool for insight into a fascinating universe, although I knew I still only slightly understood the full implications. Curtis Marshall, in Neurosurgery and Director of the EEG laboratory, introduced me to epileptic patients, the electroencephalogram and temporal lobe surgery. He was one of the few scientists who was doing what I had been taught, namely, that the goal of medical research was its clinical application, i.e., a combination of basic and applied research. However, in subsequent years, the division between basic and applied research had increased to the extent that I felt it would be impossible for me to achieve this goal since I had begun to doubt that the existing brain paradigm could lead to an explanation or therapy for epilepsy or other brain disorders.

When Detlev Bronk assumed the presidency of The Rockefeller Institute, I left the Biophysics Department and went to The Institute of Neurological Sciences at the University of Pennsylvania where Louis Flexner was the Director and where I was introduced to a wide range of research and clinical disciplines. John Dempsher, my thesis supervisor, was a dedicated researcher, and with his invaluable help, I pursued my research project on the virus-infected nervous system, with a model system that Dempsher had developed. I used electrical recording and stimulating technology to investigate the model and saw that the complex electrical changes produced by the virus in the nerve cell went far beyond what could be appreciated using standard stimulation or pharmacological techniques. The question arose that if these electrical changes could be reversed would this stop the infection? It was much later that I came to the conclusion that electrical stimulation of afferent nerves could prevent brain instability or illness based upon a number of other experimental models with which I had subsequently worked. Would electrical stimulation of afferent neurons be less effective than direct brain stimulation? Could electrical stimulation be as effective as pharmacological treatment? It seemed possible since neurotransmitters were released as a consequence and these would act at the designated local receptor, which should be safer than drugs. I pursued these questions in various experimental models, especially the one asking whether the vagus was part of the integrative system or simply an input into it.

My laboratory investigations and analysis led to the pursuit of support for a clinical trial in epilepsy and funding was obtained from three venture capital firms. This was based on the data and my patent as presented in a business plan to initiate a start-up company called Cyberonics to develop pilot studies for obtaining FDA approval for a clinical trial of VNS. Cyberonics went public in 1994 and obtained FDA approval in 1997, the year after I retired as Professor of Physiology from Temple University. Cyberonics began with about five employees and now stands at about 300, based in Houston, Texas. It was possible to expand investigation into several other serious brain illnesses including depression and Alzheimer's, and preliminary research is proceeding in a number of other brain problems. Many researchers and clinicians became involved to make this possible, but appreciation is especially due to the patients, their bravery in pursuing a new therapy, and the people at Cyberonics, in particular Reese Terry and Skip Cummins, whose guidance was invaluable.

The scrutiny of VNS as a clinical therapy or research procedure has recently began, and it is difficult to say at present whether my theoretical and experimental results will be substantiated. However, projects in depression, Alzheimer's, etc., are progressing so that within a few years, a definitive answer may be forthcoming. I have attempted to present the history of VNS in the framework of previous investigators, at least seven of whom have been Nobel Prize recipients for their contributions to our understanding of how the nervous system functions. Although the significance of VNS had been overlooked by these researchers, they nonetheless set a basis upon which a viable approach to VNS could proceed. I owe a debt to these investigators and their dedication to this subject, which hopefully, my efforts may have partly repaid.

Adrian's "The Mechanism of Nervous Action" (1932) gave two major reasons for clinical applications of electrical stimulation: safety and precision. However, safety depends on several factors, the most important being the exact site of stimulation and the magnitude of the current. Stimulation in the brain is not as safe and may not be as precise as stimulation of a peripheral nerve, which is why VNS may have advantages over deep brain stimulation in certain situations. More importantly, carefully controlled VNS appears to be safer than pharmacological agents and possibly more effective based on results in patients non-responsive to antiepileptic drugs. In view of the fact that VNS has primarily been utilized in patients refractory to pharmacological treatment, its results are fairly impressive, and some of its potential applications are discussed in the chapters by Stephen Schachter and Mitchell Roslin. VNS is still in its infancy. I have little doubt that as further experience is obtained and technologic advances are implemented therapeutic results will be significantly improved. Finally, I would like to thank Paul J. Rosch for contributing to this chapter in addition to his valuable editorial suggestions.

V. SUGGESTED READING

Manon-Espaillat R, Hoenig E, Zabara J, Rosenwasser R. Minimal changes to the vagus nerve and brainstem after two years of simulation. Epilepsia 1982; 33(3):100.

Martin WH, Pratt H, Zabara J, Rosenwasser R, Manon-Espaillat R. Electrically evoked vagal nerve potentials in humans. Epilepsia 1991; 32:53–54.

Meschersky RM, Rozenschtein GS. Instability of the central nervous system. Brain Research 1969; 13:367–375.

Terry R, Tarver WB, Zabara J. The neurocybernetic prosthesis system. PACE 1991; 14:86–93.

Terry R, Tarver WB, Zabara J. An implantable neurocybernetic prosthesis system. Epilepsia 1990; 31(suppl 2):33–37.

Wiener N. Cybernetics. Cambridge, Ma: MIT Press, 1965.

Zabara J, Dempsher J. The role of acetycholine and cholinesterase in sympathetic ganglia. J Neuropharmacol, 1962:259–264.

Zabara J. Reflex and autorhythmicity: A formal model. Mathematical Biosciences, 1969:33–38.

Zabara J. Autorhythmic structure of the brain: synaptic equivalence and connective feedback. Cybernetica 1973:77–98.

Zabara J. Inhibition of experimental seizures in canines by repetitive vagal stimulation. Epilepsia 1992; 33(6):1005–1012.

Zabara J. Neuroinhibition of Xylazine induced emesis. Pharmacol & Toxicology 1988; 63:70–74.

Zabara J. Inhibitory Neuron Control of Seizure Epeirogenesis [abstr]. Hamberg: International Congress of Neurology, 1985.

Zabara J. Peripheral Control of Hypersynchronous Discharge in Epilepsy. Electroenceph Clin Neurophys 1985; 61:162.

Zabara J. Time course of seizure control to brief, repetitive stimuli. Epilepsia 1985; 26:518.

Zabara J. Neuroinhibition in the regulation of emesis. In: Bianchi AL, Grelot L, Miller AD, King L, John Libby, eds. Mechanisms and Control of Emesis 1992; 223:285–295.

Zabara J. Controlling seizures by changing GABA receptor sensitivity. Epilepsia 1987; 28:604.

9

Chronic Therapeutic Brain Stimulation: History, Current Clinical Indications, and Future Prospects

Alon Y. Mogilner
New York Medical College, Valhalla, New York, U.S.A.

Alim-Louis Benabid
INSERM, Joseph Fourier University, Grenoble, France

Ali R. Rezai
Cleveland Clinic Foundation, Cleveland, Ohio, U.S.A.

Although electrical stimulation of the brain has been utilized for over half a century advances over the past decade have increased the avility of this modality to dramatically improve patients with Parkinson's disease, chronic pain syndromes, epilepsu, tremor, dystonia, and other movement disorders. Promising results have been also been obtained in patients suffering from brain injury, obsessive-compulsive, and eating disorders.

First performed over 50 years ago, chronic electrical stimulation of the human brain has only recently begun to achieve its clinical potential. The dramatic benefit of the technique in the treatment of severe movement disorders including Parkinson's disease and tremor has spurred its use in a number of other disease conditions, including pain, epilepsy, and psychiatric disorders, while other emerging indications await.

I. HISTORICAL OVERVIEW

The relationship between electricity and biology was known to the Romans of the first century A.D., who used the electrical discharges of the torpedo fish to treat headaches and gout. Following the observation made by Luigi Galvani (1737–1798) that twitches could be elicited by touching the leg of a frog with two metallic wires, Jean Aldini, professor of anatomy in Bologna in 1804, performed what could be considered as the first human electrical brain stimulation by applying a conductor from a Volta battery to the scalp of a subject who experienced a strong discharge. Aldini then wrote, "It seems highly probable that electrical stimulations might have in the future important therapeutic applications," and half a century later, in 1855, Duchenne de Boulogne published a monograph reporting his experience in physiology and therapeutics (1).

In 1870, Gustav Fritsch and Eduard Hitzig of Germany reported that electrical stimulation of the canine frontal lobes could elicit contralateral body movements (2). While these authors refer to stimulation of the human brain in a footnote, it is unclear whether they stimulated the brain surface directly or transcutaneously via an electrode placed on the mastoid process (3). Similar findings in the dog were reported three years later by David Ferrier of London (4). The first unequivocal report of direct stimulation of the human brain was by Roberts Bartholow of Cincinnati, Ohio in 1874 (3–6). Having read the work of these pioneers, Bartholow proceeded to perform the same on humans, writing, "Having had a case recently in which a considerable portion of the posterior lobes of the brain was exposed by disease without any interruption of its functions, I ventured to make some experiments on the plan pursued by Fritsch and Hitzig and Ferrier" (7).

Bartholow inserted insulated needle electrodes through the exposed dura and brain of a 30-year-old woman with a scalp defect secondary to an erosive basal cell carcinoma. Electrical stimulation produced a variety of effects, including contractions of the contralateral extremities, unpleasant sensory experiences, and, with increasing amounts of current, focal and then generalized seizures. Ultimately, the patient exhibited recurrent seizure activity over the next few days and expired soon thereafter. Postmortem examination performed by Bartholow revealed multiple electrode tracts, as well as extensive sagittal sinus thrombosis and a subdural empyema.

After finding considerable disapproval with his actions in the scientific community, Bartholow later wrote in a letter to the British Medical Journal (8),

> To repeat such experiments with the knowledge we now have that injury will be done by them...would be in the highest degree criminal. I can only now express my regret that the facts which I hoped would further, in some slight degree, the progress of knowledge, were obtained at the expense of some injury to the patient.

It was not until 74 years later that this technique was used for therapeutic purposes. The first neurosurgeon to do so was J. L. Pool of Columbia University's Neurological Institute (9), who considered brain stimulation as an alternative to the ablative psychosurgical procedures of his era. In 1948, via open craniotomy, Pool implanted a silver electrode in the caudate nucleus of a woman suffering from depression and anorexia, who, incidentally, suffered from advanced Parkinson's disease. Electrical stimulation via an implanted induction coil was carried out over a period of 8 weeks and improved her mood as well as her appetite. Stimulation was discontinued only after one of the wires broke. (No mention was made of the effects of stimulation on her Parkinson's disease.) That same year, Pool placed a stimulating electrode in the cingulate gyrus of a psychotic patient—the results of which were not reported. No specific rationale was provided by Pool for the target selection in these two patients. By the time Pool published these results in 1954 in the Journal of the American Geriatric Society, similar psychiatric neurosurgical procedures had been performed by others, most notably R. G. Heath (10) at Tulane University, starting in 1950.

Heath and co-workers implanted electrodes in the septal region of patients, the majority of whom were schizophrenics, but also in four patients suffering from diffuse metastatic carcinoma with intractable pain, as well as one patient with advanced rheumatoid arthritis. The electrodes were placed in a region anterior and inferior to the foramen of Monro at the base of the anterior portion of the septum pellucidum. Anatomic and physiologic studies in animals by Heath and colleagues had demonstrated that electrical activation of the septal region resulted in an electroencephalograpic activation of motor cortex. The initial patients were schizophrenics, and a deactivation of motor cortex was thought by Heath and colleagues to be a key etiologic component of the disease. Thus, a target which would activate frontal cortex was chosen (10). Stimulation was applied at a frequency of 100 Hz with a 1-ms square wave pulse, at voltages up to 20 V. All patients reported pain relief from electrical stimulation. Pool, using Heath's stereotactic technique, reported pain relief in one patient with septal stimulation. Nevertheless, Pool stated that brain stimulation should "probably be used only in desperate cases in which there is virtually nothing else to offer" (9). In 1960, Heath and Mickle reported their long-term follow-up data on patients undergoing septal stimulation for the treatment of both schizophrenia and chronic pain. Chronic stimulation of the septal region successfully relieved pain in all patients (11).

During the same time period, another technical development in neurosurgery significantly influenced the evolution of brain stimulation. Stereotactic neurosurgery, introduced by Spiegel and Wycis in 1947 (12), offered a less invasive alternative to open neurosurgical ablative procedures pioneered by Egaz Moniz in Portugal for the treatment of psychiatric disorders and movement disorders. At that time, these conditions were treated surgically with procedures including prefrontal lobotomy and pedunculotomy, performed via craniotomy with its associated morbidity. It soon became evident that this technology was well suited for the placement of stimulating electrodes into the brain (13) with decreased risk to the patient as compared with open procedures. Consequently, the histories of brain stimulation and stereotactic neurosurgery became inextricably linked.

While Heath and colleagues began using the stereotactic method to place their stimulating electrodes for the treatment of psychiatric disorders and chronic pain, intraoperative electrical stimulation became part and parcel of functional stereotactic neurosurgery for the treatment of movement disorders. Intraoperative stimulation was routinely used prior to placement of a lesion, both to verify the efficacy of the planned lesion and to detect any adverse side effects (13). By 1960, Hassler had reported his observations that electrical stimulation of the globus pallidus had opposite effects on tremor, depending on the frequency of stimulation (14,15). Stimulation at 4–8 Hz was noted to evoke tremor, while higher frequency stimulation at 25–100 Hz could reduce or even arrest it. Indeed, Spiegel and Wycis reported that low-frequency stimulation of the globus pallidus could elicit or augment tremor—no note was made of tremor arrest via stimulation (16). Throughout literature, the effects of intraoperative electrical stimulation were reported, mentioning either a worsening or an alleviation of symptoms, including tremor, incidentally providing information about the parameters that were employed, in particular low or high frequency, without a specific rationale. This did not lead to the recognition of a clear relationship between the excitatory or inhibitory observed effects and the frequency of the stimulus.

As neurosurgery for psychiatric disorders fell out of favor by the 1960s, chronic pain became the sole indication for brain stimulation, in parallel to attempts to control spasticity and epilepsy by stimulation of the cerebellum (17). Furthermore, the advent of levodopa for the treatment of Parkinson's disease in the late 1960s resulted in a significant reduction in the number of functional neurosurgical procedures performed during that era. Brain stimulation for the treatment of movement disorders, as we shall see later in this article, continued to be performed by a small number of neurosurgeons during the 1970s and 1980s for a variety of clinical indications, with a variety of different targets and stimulation parameters. The modern era of stimulation for movement disorders can be considered to start in 1987, when A. L. Benabid (Grenoble, France) first reported the use of high-frequency (130 Hz or greater) ventralis intermedius (Vim) thalamic stimulation for the treatment of tremor (18). The introduction of bilateral subthalamic nucleus stimulation by Benabid in 1993 further demonstrated the remarkable efficacy of this technique in treating the cardinal symptoms of Parkinson's disease, including not only tremor but rigidity, bradykinesia, and gait and postural instability.

II. MECHANISM OF ACTION

The exact mechanism of action of brain stimulation remains unknown. There is now sufficient evidence to suggest that brain stimulation exerts its effects via a number of differing but interrelated mechanisms which come into play depending on the site being stimulated, the disease entity being treated, and the stimulation parameters used. Undoubtedly, the clinical effects seen with brain stimulation reflect the complex combination of inhibition and activation of cell bodies and axons and depend on the orientation of the electrode, the cytoarchitecture of the structure being stimulated, as well as the frequency, pulse width, and duration of stimulation.

The similarity between the clinical effects of high-frequency stimulation and ablative procedures, particularly for the thalamic and pallidal targets, suggest that high-frequency deep-brain-stimulating (DBS) effects a functional inhibition of the target structure (19). An in vitro study in the rat demonstrated that high-frequency (100–250 Hz) stimulation of subthalamic nucleus resulted in a transient blockade of the persistent sodium current as well as L- and T-type calcium currents, results also consistent with an inhibitory effect of stimulation (20), while others report inhibition of the subthalamic nucleus (STN) following high-frequency stimulation (21).

Other studies have shown the opposite result, namely that high frequency stimulation acts via an excitatory mechanism by increasing neuronal output of the target structure (22). It has therefore been suggested that HFS, rather than simply inhibiting a hyperactive structure, acts via a resynchronization of abnormal output patterns present in disease (23,24) or via a "jamming" of these abnormal patterns by HFS providing physiologic white noise (21). Clearly, further studies are needed to improve our understanding of these complex mechanisms.

III. EQUIPMENT

The electrode used for chronic stimulation, known as a *deep-brain-stimulating* (DBS) electrode (Medtronic Inc., Minneapolis, MN), is a 1.27-mm-diameter quadripolar platinum–iridium lead (Fig. 1). Each of the four contacts is 1.5 mm long and, depending on the model of the electrode, is separated by either 0.5 or 1.5 mm of insulation. The electrode is connected via an extension lead tunneled subcutaneously to an implanted pulse generator (Fig. 2a and b). Stimulation can be unipolar, bipolar, or multipolar, as each of the electrode contacts can be used as an anode or cathode providing a variety of different electrical field patterns. Stimulation parameters include frequency in the range of 2–185 Hz, a voltage range of 0–10.5V, and square wave pulse widths ranging from 60 to 450 μs. The stimulators are programmed via portable device which communicates with the implanted generator via telemetry. Stimulation can be performed continuously or intermittently and can be programmed to cycle on and off during fixed time intervals. Patients are able to activate and deactivate the stimulator via handheld controllers and can modify a subset of the stimulation parameters within given limits set by the medical team. The degree of patient control, particularly for brain stimulation for movement disorders, is limited in the United

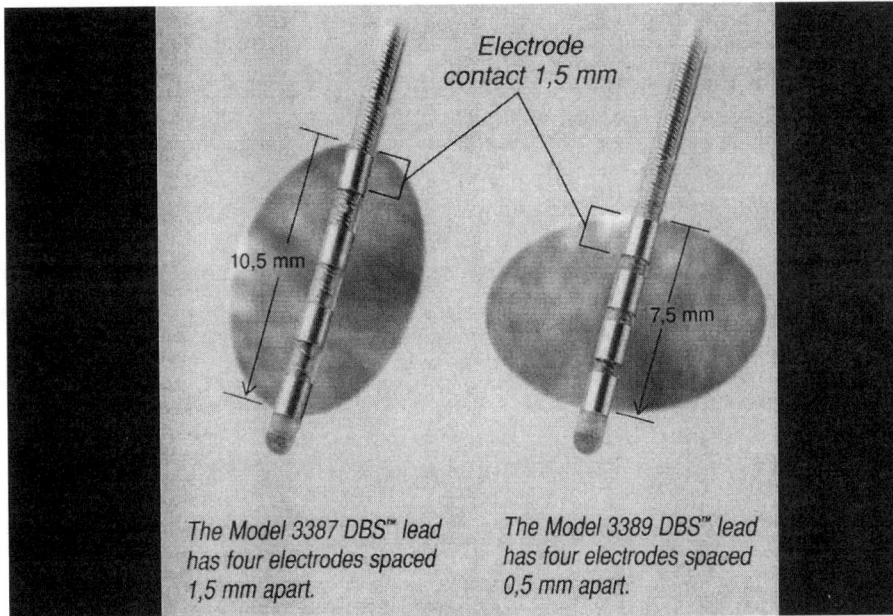

Figure 1 Quadripolar DBS electrode. Photograph of the four-pole-contact electrode. Each contact is made of platinum/iridium alloy and is 1.27 mm in diameter. The insulated interpole distance is 1.5 mm or 0.5 mm depending on the model (courtesy of Medtronic).

States by the Food and Drug Administration (FDA). For example, patients with subthalamic, thalamic, or pallidal stimulators in the United States can only activate or deactivate the device, but cannot modify stimulus parameters.

IV. SURGICAL PROCEDURE

Stereotactic neurosurgical techniques allows the localization of any brain structure with millimeter precision. Anatomic localization is achieved with stereotactic imaging via imaging modalities such as MRI, CT, and ventriculography. Dramatic advances in image processing technology allow for rapid, automated fusion of different imaging modalities (Fig. 3). For example, a high-resolution MRI scan obtained prior to stereotactic frame placement can be fused with a CT scan obtained with the frame in place, allowing for both increased patient comfort as well as removing any potential MRI image distortion induced by the frame. Stereotactic atlases, in which cadaver brains were sliced and oriented with respect to landmarks such as the anterior and posterior commissures (25–28), can be "morphed" to a particular patient's anatomic imaging data, allowing for further increased ease of target selection.

Similarly, a number of methods of physiologic verification of the anatomical target exist: microelectrode recording (MER), semimicroelectrode recording, and macrostimulation. Both microelectrode and semimicroelectrode recording attempt to define the boundaries of a given structure based on the known spontaneous and/or evoked electrical activity of that structure and surrounding structures. Macrostimulation, stimulation through a relatively large diameter electrode (on the order of 1 mm diameter), is used in all DBS cases prior to final implantation of the electrode. Macrostimulation allows the physician to assess for both the therapeutic effects of stimulation (reduction of tremor, rigidity, or pain),

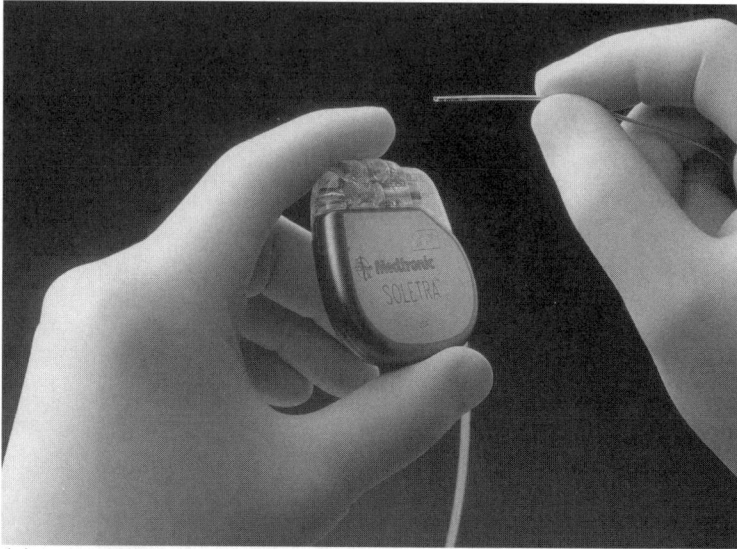

(a)

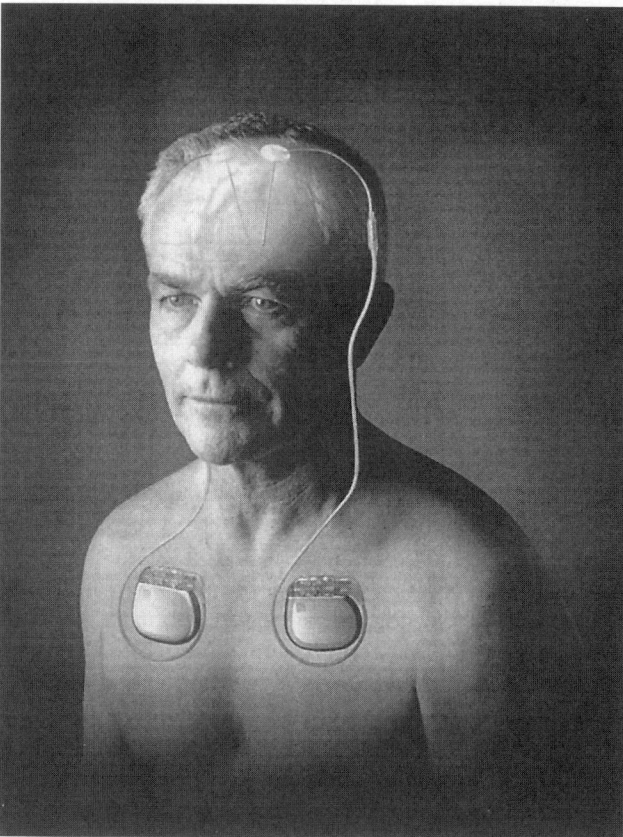

(b)

Figure 2 Pulse generator and DBS electrode. (a) Photograph of the pulse generator device that is implanted in the infraclavicular region. (b) Photograph showing the overall configuration and positioning of the implanted bilateral electrodes and pulse generators (courtesy of Medtronic).

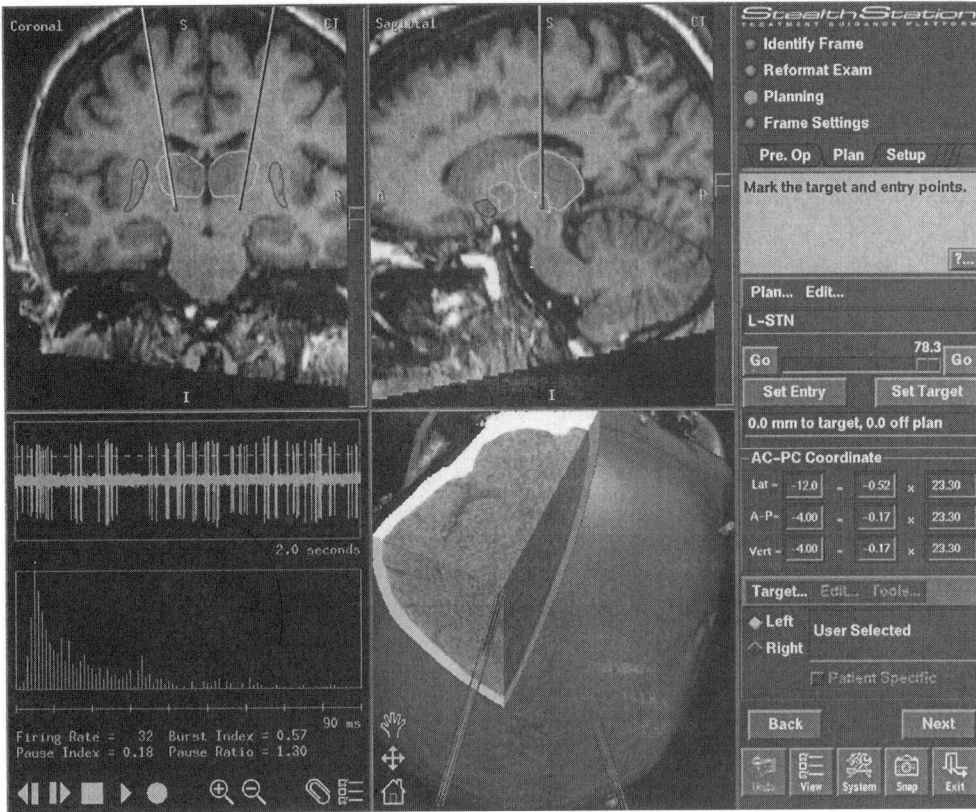

Figure 3 Computer-guided brain targeting and navigation. Operative computers combine different imaging modalities such as CT and various MRI sequences, along with brain and patient-specific atlases, to provide the target and best trajectory of approach to that target. In this case, an actual path in the brain is shown in the axial, sagittal, coronal, and three-dimensional planes, toward the target—the subthalamic nucleus (STN).

as well as for possible untoward effects (i.e., paresthesias, motor contractions, ocular deviation). As the stimulation parameters used during this testing phase are usually similar to those that will be used for chronic stimulation, macrostimulation should approximate the effects of chronic therapy.

A trial period, where the stimulating wires are externalized for durations on the order of days to weeks and various stimulation combinations are evaluated for clinical efficacy, is routinely used for pain therapy. Such trial periods were used more frequently in the past for movement disorder therapy. Currently, given the demonstrated efficacy of DBS for movement disorders, DBS electrodes are routinely permanently implanted without a prolonged trial period in movement disorder surgery. The pulse generators may be implanted at the same sitting or at a later date.

V. CLINICAL INDICATIONS

While the earliest uses of brain stimulation were for the treatment of chronic pain, the most common indication over the past 15 years remains movement disorders, specifically Parkinson's disease and essential tremor. The dramatic success of DBS therapy in movement disorders has spurred renewed interest in other applications including pain, epilepsy, and psychiatric disorders. A summary of common clinical indications and target sites is shown in Fig. 1.

A. Movement Disorders

1. Thalamic Stimulation

Benabid's initial reports (18,29) suggested that chronic Vim stimulation may be useful in those patients who have already undergone unilateral thalamotomy with persistent symptoms on the nonoperated side. He noted that the thalamotomy provided better tremor relief but that this was most likely due to the frequency limit of 130 Hz on the stimulator. He stated that the optimal frequency appeared to be about 200 Hz, close to the current standard frequency of 185 Hz. His 1991 report in *Lancet* reported up to 29-month (mean 13 months) follow-up on 26 patients with Parkinson's disease (30). Complete relief or major improvement in the tremor was noted in 88% of cases. His report of 8-year follow-up of 80 patients demonstrated the effect to be robust, with half the patients able to decrease dopaminergic medication by at least 30%. However, Vim stimulation was only effective for tremor and not other Parkinsonian symptoms (31). On the other hand, Vim stimulation was clearly seen to be the surgical treatment of choice for essential tremor, a benign condition in which tremor is the only symptom. Since that time, thalamic stimulation has been well established as a safe and effective treatment of refractory Parkinsonian and essential tremor, with results as good as traditional thalamotomy and with fewer associated significant adverse events (32–34).

a.   Other Tremor Types—Multiple Sclerosis: Head and Voice Tremors.   In 1980, Brice and McLellan (Lancet, 1980) reported their successful suppression of upper extremity tremor in three patients with multiple sclerosis (MS). Their targets included both the midbrain and the basal ganglia. The effect was durable during the reported 6-month follow-up period. There have been few reports dedicated to DBS for multiple sclerosis-related tremor, but these patients are frequently included in other series of DBS patients. The largest dedicated series is that of Montgomery et al. (35), involving 15 patients treated with chronic Vim stimulation. While tremor was generally improved, tachyphylaxis was common and frequent programming changes were required. Other small series with similar results have been reported (36,37).

Multiple small series have demonstrated the potential of thalamic DBS for treating intractable head and voice tremor. The largest series of patients with head tremor is that of Koller et al. (38) in which 38 patients were followed for 12 months. Twenty-four of these patients underwent blinded clinical evaluations. Stimulation significantly reduced head tremor in both the blinded and nonblinded groups. Other small series and the European Multicenter Trial also seem to indicate that bilateral thalamic stimulation is a valid treatment for head tremor (33,39). The European trial and Carpenter (40) found minimal improvement in voice tremor with thalamic DBS. In both cases, however, larger well-designed trials are needed before making firm conclusions about the utility of DBS for these conditions.

2. Subthalamic Nucleus Stimulation

Unlike the Vim thalamus and globus pallidus, the subthalamic nucleus (STN) was previously not considered for lesioning procedures in Parkinson's disease (PD). This was due to fear of causing hemiballism, a well-documented effect of STN lesions in previously normal individuals experiencing intracerebral hemorrhage in this area (41). The impetus for targeting the subthalamic nucleus resulted from a number of studies in the MPTP-lesioned primate model of PD, beginning in the mid to late 1980s.

After animal studies confirmed an increased glutaminergic (excitatory) STN output in Parkinson's (42), STN lesions in MPTP-treated monkeys were clearly demonstrated to alleviate the symptoms of PD (43–45), and high-frequency STN was shown to be effective as well in these animals (42). Armed with these experimental findings, Benabid, in 1993, implanted a stimulating electrode in the STN of a 51-year-old patient with severely disabling akinetic-rigid PD with severe on-off fluctuations (46). The first patient was reported in 1994 and a lengthier paper followed in 1995 describing the first three patients to have electrodes implanted chronically in the STN. The activities of daily living (ADL) score portion of the Unified Parkinson's Disease Rating Scale (UPDRS) improved over 50%, as did motor scores. Some stimulation-induced hemiballismus was noted but was controlled by adjusting the stimulation. One-year follow-up of 24 patients with bilateral STN stimulators demonstrated that UPDRS ADL and motor scores improved by 60% in the off-medication state. The UPDRS subscores for akinesia, tremor, rigidity, and gait also improved, in contrast to the results seen with Vim stimulation (47). Since that time, the STN is increasingly becoming the preferred target for chronic electrical stimulation in PD at most centers, effective in treating the cardinal manifestations of the disease, with improvements in motor function of approximately 80% using the standardized UPDRS rating scale. Furthermore, levodopa intake is reduced following surgery by approximately 50%, resulting in a significant decrease in drug-induced dyskinesias (48,49).

Side effects appear to be mild in most cases. In those patients who experience an increase in dyskinesias soon after initiating chronic stimulation, a reduction in the dose of dopaminergic medications or an adjustment in stimulation parameters usually suffices to alleviate the problem. Postoperative confusion is more common in elderly patients. In addition, a small number of patients have experienced mood alterations, apparently associated with a more ventral electrode placement closer to or in the substantia nigra pars reticulata (50). While one study reported an overall cognitive decline in 30% of patients after 1 year of bilateral STN stimulation (51), a number of other studies have shown no significant cognitive deterioration with chronic STN stimulation (52–54).

3. Globus Pallidus Internus (GPi) Stimulation

Given the known beneficial effects of lesioning of the posterior ventral globus pallidus in alleviating many of the cardinal symptoms of Parkinson's disease including rigidity, bradykinesia, gait dysfunction, tremor, as well as reducing the severity of levodopa-induced dyskinesias (55), the GPi became the next target for chronic stimulation. GPi stimulation is currently used by a number of centers for the treatment of refractory Parkinson's disease, with beneficial effects on these cardinal manifestations of PD and reduction in dyskinesias similar to that obtained by pallidotomy.

A series of 36 patients demonstrated that bilateral pallidal stimulation results in a median motor improvement of 37% and an increase from 28 to 64% of the day without disabling involuntary movements (47). A number of studies have demonstrated the beneficial effects of GPi stimulation on dyskinesias, on-off fluctuations, and tremor (47,56–58).

4. GPi Versus STN Stimulation for Parkinson's Disease

A handful of head-to-head comparisons of GPi and STN stimulation have been published. The largest multicenter study found that STN stimulation was significantly more efficacious (47). Burchiel conducted a randomized trial of pallidal versus STN stimulation. While the results off medication were similar for the two groups, pallidal, but not subthalamic, stimulation improved Parkinsonian symptoms while patients were in the medication-on state. Furthermore, while rigidity, bradykinesia, and tremor were equally affected by both targets, axial symptomatology was relieved only by GPi stimulation. However, only STN stimulation provided enough relief to allow patients to reduce their medication dosage (59). Other reports also favored the STN (60–62). Clearly, larger randomized studies are needed to settle this debate.

5. *Other Movement Disorders*

With the success of DBS for PD and tremor, investigators have attempted to expand the range of indications for the procedure. Dystonia, with a long history of neurosurgical treatment, has always been a target for DBS, and reports continue to emerge describing its use in dystonia with a variety of subcortical targets. However, dystonia is extremely heterogenous, with a widely varying clinical spectrum and multiple etiologies (generalized vs. focal, idiopathic, genetic, posttraumatic, poststroke, etc.), making the assembly of large patient populations problematic.

Recent reports have demonstrated the efficacy of deep brain stimulation of the thalamus and GPi for various forms of dystonia, with more benefical effects on primary and generalized dystonias as opposed to secondary and focal dystonias and with the suggestion that the GPi may be a more suitable target (63–70).

The procedure is complicated in these patients by their very disease in that cervical torsion complicates frame placement, imaging, and image fusion. Moreover, patient tolerance of the procedure is limited as they are restrained in a fixed frame for several hours. In addition, cervical torsion puts these patients at high risk for such complications as lead fracture and other wound-related complications. Future directions point towards expanding the use of DBS for the treatment of other movement disorders. Both Tourette's syndrome and Huntington's chorea are thought to be amenable to DBS therapy (71,72).

B. Brain Stimulation for Chronic Pain

In contrast to the field of movement disorder surgery, there are few systematic, multicenter controlled trials of brain stimulation for pain in the literature. However, the demonstrated efficacy of brain stimulation for movement disorders will assure that the technology to perform these procedures will be routinely available and may thus result in a return to favor of some of these procedures.

The initial use of brain stimulation for pain control by Pool, Heath, and others targeted the so-called affective state of the individual and thus was viewed more as a psychosurgical intervention. Targets stimulated included the septal region, cingulate gyrus, and caudate nucleus. Subsequently, other subcortical sites were targeted, and recently the precentral cortex appears to show promise in selected patients.

1. *Subcortical Targets*

Sensory thalamic (VC or VP) stimulation, first reported by Mazars and colleagues, (73–75) results in the production of paresthesias in the area of pain, associated with pain relief, similar to that obtained with stimulation of the dorsal columns of the spinal cord. The exact mechanism by which paresthesia-evoking thalamic stimulation results in pain relief is not known. One concept is that deafferentation causes an abnormal firing pattern in thalamic neurons and that thalamic stimulation inhibits this abnormal neural activity (76–78). Gerhardt et al. showed that stimulation of the VC in monkeys caused inhibition of spinothalamic neurons' evoked responses to noxious cutaneous stimulation (79). Benabid demonstrated that VC stimulation inhibited the response of parafascicular nucleus (Pf) cells to noxious stimuli (80).

Stimulation of the periacqueductal gray, first reported in 1969, provided yet another proposed pathway of analgesia, via a presumed opioid-related mechanism (81–83). PAG/PVG stimulation is indicated for pain classified as *nociceptive,* which is defined as pain caused by direct activation of the nociceptors (mechanical, chemical, and thermal) found in various tissues. Examples of nociceptive pain include cancer pain from bone or tissue invasion, or noncancer pain secondary to degenerative bone and joint disease or osteoarthritis. This type of pain stands in contrast to *neuropathic* or deafferentation pain, which results from an injury or dysfunction of the central or peripheral nervous system. Examples include thalamic pain, stroke, traumatic or iatrogenic brain or spinal cord injuries, phantom limb or stump pain, postherpetic neuralgia, and various peripheral neuropathies. The sensory thalamus is usually considered a more appropriate target for neuropathic pain conditions. The overall long-term successful pain control reported in the literature with stimulation is approximately 60% for nociceptive pain and 50% for neuropathic pain (84).

2. Motor Cortex (Precentral) Stimulation

One of the most promising recent developments in neurostimulation for pain control is that of epidural motor cortex stimulation (MCS), first reported by Tsubokawa and colleagues. Tsubokawa and colleagues found that stimulation of the precentral motor cortex resulted in effective pain relief (85,86), relief far better than observed with postcentral somatosensory stimulation. Stimulation was applied for 5–10 min at a time from 5 to 7 times during the day, with frequencies of 50–120 Hz, pulse width 0.1–0.5 ms, and current <1 mA. Stimulation parameters were adjusted to be below the threshold for a motor response. The analgesic effects had a "halo" effect, lasting at times for hours after stimulation was discontinued.

An increasing number of groups are now reporting promising results with this technique. The largest series with the longest follow-up in the literature comprises 32 patients spanning a 4-year period, reported by Nguyen and colleagues (87). Ten of the 13 patients with central pain (77%) and 10 of the 12 patients with neuropathic facial pain had experienced substantial pain relief (75%). At this time, the questions remaining to be answered include: indications for surgery, surgical technique, and optimal stimulation parameters to maximize long-term clinical benefit. Unlike paresthesia-producing (i.e., sensory thalamic) stimulation, motor cortex stimulation does not usually induce paresthesias, making this technique ideal for double-blinded controlled studies.

The mechanism of action of MCS is a subject of debate. While some have postulated that direct projections from motor cortex to sensory cortex can provide for a stimulation-induced modulation of abnormal sensory cortical activity present in pain states, others suggest that descending corticothalamic projections play an important role in the generation of analgesia (85,86,88).

C. Brain Stimulation—Other Emerging Areas

1. Epilepsy

Initial attempts at seizure control using brain stimulation utilized stimulation of the cerebellar cortex. Irving Cooper (17,89–92) was the first to employ cerebellar stimulation for epilepsy. Cooper hypothesized that the massive inhibitory Purkinje cell outflow of the cerebellum could modulate abnormal cortical epileptogenic activity "as the pedals of a mighty organ modulate the output of its chimes"(93). While Cooper reported significant seizure reduction in 56% of patients, other clinical trials failed to demonstrate any benefit (94,95).

Stimulation of the anterior nucleus of the thalamus for epilepsy was first reported by Cooper as well (96,97). The rationale for choosing the anterior nucleus involved its important role in the limbic circuitry, receiving projections from the mammilary bodies and projecting to the hippocampus, amygdala, cingulate, orbitofrontal cortex, and caudate. It was thought that anterior nucleus stimulation would modulate abnormal epileptiform activity within the limbic system. Although exact details of the stimulation were not provided, he reported that in five of six patients with intractable seizures, anterior nucleus stimulation reduced seizures by more than 60% in five of six cases, with 30% average decrease in medication requirements.

Velasco et al. were the first to employ bilateral centromedian (CM) nucleus stimulation for the treatment of epilepsy (98), and their long-term results in 13 patients were recently reported (99). Stimulation parameters were 60 Hz, 4–6V, alternating right and left sides. With a mean follow-up of 41 months, they noted a significant decrease (defined as >80% seizure reduction) in the incidence of generalized tonic-clonic seizures and atypical absence seizures, but no change, in the incidence of complex partial seizures.

Recent reports of seizure control following subthalamic nucleus stimulation (100–102), combined with confirmatory data in a rat model (103–105), suggest that the STN may be a future target for seizure control using brain stimulation.

2. Psychiatric Disorders

Since the early reports of Pool over a half a century ago, there have been few advances in the use of brain stimulation to treat psychiatric conditions. While lesioning procedures including cingulotomy, capsulotomy, subcaudate tractotomy, and limbic leukotomy have all been employed for the treatment of refractory obsessive-compulsive disorder (OCD) and, to a lesser degree, major affective disorder, chronic electrical stimulation of these lesioning targets has only recently been reported. Nuttin et al. placed quadripolar electrodes bilaterally in the anterior limbs of the internal capsules of four patients suffering from severe OCD. Beneficial effects were seen in three patients (106).

A recent report of transient depression induced by high-frequency stimulation of the substantia nigra pars reticulata (50), using the lower poles of an electrode placed for subthalamic nucleus stimulation, raise the intriguing possibility that STN and/or SNr stimulation may be a putative target for future intervention.

3. Eating Disorders

A long history of animal studies of hypothalamic function has elucidated two hypothalamic regions related to food intake: the ventromedial nucleus as a satiety center and lateral nucleus as a hunger center (107–109). Destruction of the ventromedial nucleus in animals leads to hyperphagia and obesity, while lesions of the lateral nucleus lead to weight loss. Over 25 years ago, Quaade et al. performed low-frequency stimulation of the lateral hypothalamic nucleus in morbidly obese patients as a prelude to electrocoagulation, without significant long-term benefit (110). As Benabid and colleagues have reported preliminary work with both lateral and ventromedial hypothalamic stimulation in an animal model (100), others may follow his lead in investigating this potential application of brain stimulation.

Table 1 Current Stimulation Targets for Various Disease States

Condition	Stimulation Targets
Movement Disorders	Ventral intermediate nucleus of thalamus (Vim)
	Subthalamic nucleus (STN)
	Globus pallidus internus (Gpi)
Tremor	Ventral intermediate nucleus of thalamus (Vim)
Parkinson's disease	Ventral intermediate nucleus of thalamus (Vim)
	Subthalamic nucleus (STN)
	Globus pallidus internus (Gpi)
Dystonia	Ventral intermediate nucleus of thalamus (Vim)
	Globus pallidus internus (Gpi)
Chronic pain	Ventralis caudalis nucleus of thalamus (VC)
	Periacqueductal/periventricular gray (PAG/PVG)
	Medial lemniscus (ML)
	Internal capsule (IC)
	Motor cortex (MC)
Epilepsy	Centromedian nucleus of thalamus (CM)
	Anterior nucleus of thalamus (AN)
	Subthalamic nucleus (STN)
Psychiatric disorders	Internal capsule (IC)
	Cingulate gyrus
Brain injury states	Intralaminar nucleus of the thalamus (IL)
	Midbrain reticular formation (RF)

4. Brain Injury States

In 1949, Moruzzi and Magoun (111) described the reticular activating system of the brainstem, an area which, when stimulated, evokes arousal responses and EEG desynchronization. Within the thalamus, stimulation of the midline projection nuclei (i.e., intralaminar and centromedian) was noted to be effective in eliciting these responses in animals (112). Based on these observations, a number of targets have stimulated in comatose patients in an attempt to increase their level of consciousness. The midbrain reticular formation, intralaminar thalamus, other thalamic nuclei, and the globus pallidus all have been stimulated without evidence of dramatic improvement (113–116). It is quite possible that the severe degree of brain damage in these patients may have precluded any possibility of functional recovery. A recent proposal to revisit intralaminar stimulation in a less severely disabled group of patients, described as *minimally conscious* (117) appears promising. Since these patients may not be able to provide informed consent, ethical issues will most likely limit the number of these surgeries performed until that time where a strong multidisciplinary effort is made to address the use of these techniques in these patients (118). (Table 1)

VI. CONCLUSIONS

Advances in anatomical and functional imaging and improvements in device technology, coupled with an increased understanding of the pathophysiology of various neurologic disorders, have provided us with the ability to reversibly modulate the nervous system. It is important to emphasize, however, that the technique still remains in its infancy. Future advances in this technology will undoubtedly arise as a result of safer and less invasive surgical methods as well as from the development the next generation deep-brain-stimulation devices with combined closed loop electrical and chemical sensing and output functions. Finally, continued advances in the neurosciences will provide for the extension of this technology to treat other disease conditions.

REFERENCES

1. De Boulogne D. De l'électrisation localisée et son application à la physiologie, à la pathologie et à la thérapeutique. Paris: J.B. Bailliere, 1855.
2. Fritsch G, Hitzig E. On the electrical excitability of the cerebrum (translated from the German). In: Bonin Gv, ed. Some Papers on the Cerebral Cortex. Springfield, IL: Charles C. Thomas, 1960:73–96.
3. Thomas RK, Young CD. A note on the early history of electrical stimulation of the human brain. J Gen Psychol 1993; 120:73–81.
4. Morgan JP. The first reported case of electrical stimulation of the human brain. J Hist Med Allied Sci 1982; 37:51–64.
5. Sheer DE. Electrical Stimulation of the Brain. Austin: University of Texas Press, 1961.
6. Zimmermann M. Electrical stimulation of the human brain. Hum Neurobiol 1982; 1:227–229.
7. Bartholow R. Experimental investigations into the functions of the human brain. Am J Med Sci 1874; 67:305–313.
8. Bartholow R. Letter to the editor. Brit Med J 1874; 3:727.
9. Pool JL. Psychosurgery in older people. J Am Geriat Soc 1954; 2:456–465.
10. Heath R. Studies in schizophrenia: a multidisciplinary approach to mind-brain relationships. Cambridge, MA: Harvard University Press, 1954.
11. Heath R, Mickle W. Evaluation of 7 years' experience with depth electrode studies in human patients. In: Ramey E, O'Doherty D, eds. Electrical Studies in Unanesthetized Brain. New York: Harper & Brothers, 1960:214–217.
12. Spiegel EA, Wycis HT, Marks M, Lee AJ. Stereotaxic apparatus for operations on the human brain. Science 1947; 106:349–350.
13. Spiegel EA, Wycis HT. Chronic implantation of intracerebral electrodes in humans. In: Sheer DE, ed. Electrical Stimulation of the Brain. Austin: University of Texas Press, 1961:37–44.
14. Hassler R, Riechert TFM Physiological observations in stereotaxic operations in extrapyramidal motor disturbances. Brain 1960; 83:337–350.
15. Hassler R. Thalamic regulation of muscle tone and the speed of movements. In: Purpura DP, Yahr MD, eds. The Thalamus. New York: Columbia University Press, 1966:419–438.
16. Spiegel EA, Wycis HT, Baird HW, Szekely EG. Physiopathologic observations on the basal ganglia. In: Ramey E, O'Doherty DS, eds. Electrical Studies on the Unanesthetized Brain. New York: Harper & Brothers, 1960:192–213.
17. Cooper IS. Effect of chronic stimulation of anterior cerebellum on neurological disease. Lancet 1973; 1:206.
18. Benabid AL, Pollak P, Louveau A, Henry S, de Rougemont J. Combined (thalamotomy and stimulation) stereotactic surgery of the VIM thalamic nucleus for bilateral Parkinson disease. Appl Neurophysiol 1987; 50:344–346.
19. Benabid AL, Benazzous A, Pollak P. Mechanisms of deep brain stimulation. Mov Disord 2002; 17(suppl 3):S73–S74.
20. Beurrier C, Bioulac Bernard, Audin J, Hammond C. High-frequency Stimulation produces a transient blockade of voltage-gated currents in subthalamic neurons. J Neurophysiol 2001; 85:1351–1356.
21. Dostrovsky JO, Lozano AM. Mechanisms of deep brain stimulation. Mov Disord 2002; 17(suppl 3):S63–S68.
22. Vitek JL. Mechanisms of deep brain stimulation: excitation or inhibition. Mov Disord 2002; 17(suppl 3):S69–S72.

23. Montgomery EB Jr, Baker KB. Mechanisms of deep brain stimulation and future technical developments. Neurol Res 2000; 22:259–266.

24. Vitek JL. Surgery for dystonia. Neurosurg Clin N Am 1998; 9:345–366.

25. Andrew J, Watkins ES. A Stereotaxic Atlas of the Human Thalamus. Baltimore: Williams and Wilkins, 1969.

26. Morel A, Magnin M, Jeanmonod D. Multiarchitectonic and stereotactic atlas of the human thalamus [published erratum appears in J Comp Neurol 1998 Feb 22;391(4):545]. J Comp Neurol 1997; 387:588–630.

27. Schaltenbrand G, Wahren W. Atlas for Stereotaxy of the Human Brain. Stuttgart: Thieme, 1977.

28. Talairach J, David M, Tournoux P, Corredor H, Kvasina T. Atlas d'Anatomie Stéréotaxique. Paris: Masson, 1957.

29. Benabid AL, Pollak P, Hommel M, Gaio JM, de Rougemont J, Perret J. [Treatment of Parkinson tremor by chronic stimulation of the ventral intermediate nucleus of the thalamus]. Rev Neurol 1989; 145:320–323.

30. Benabid AL, Pollak P, Gervason C. Long-term suppression of tremor by chronic stimulation of the ventral intermediate thalamic nucleus. Lancet 1991; 337:403–406.

31. Benabid AL, Pollak P, Gao D. Chronic electrical stimulation of the ventralis intermedius nucleus of the thalamus as a treatment of movement disorders. J Neurosurg 1996; 84:203–214.

32. Schuurman PR, Bosch DA, Bossuyt PM. A comparison of continuous thalamic stimulation and thalamotomy for suppression of severe tremor [see comments]. N Engl J Med 2000; 342:461–468.

33. Limousin P, Speelman JD, Gielen F, Janssens M. Multicentre European study of thalamic stimulation in parkinsonian and essential tremor. J Neurol Neurosurg Psychiatry 1999; 66:289–296.

34. Koller W, Pahwa R, Busenbark K. High-frequency unilateral thalamic stimulation in the treatment of essential and parkinsonian tremor. Ann Neurol 1997; 42:292–299.

35. Montgomery EB Jr, Baker KB, Kinkel RP, Barnett G. Chronic thalamic stimulation for the tremor of multiple sclerosis. Neurology 1999; 53:625–628.

36. Geny C, Nguyen JP, Pollin B. Improvement of severe postural cerebellar tremor in multiple sclerosis by chronic thalamic stimulation. Mov Disord 1996; 11:489–494.

37. Schulder M, Sernas T, Mahalick D, Adler R, Cook S. Thalamic stimulation in patients with multiple sclerosis. Stereotact Funct Neurosurg 1999; 72:196–201.

38. Koller WC, Lyons KE, Wilkinson SB, Pahwa R. Efficacy of unilateral deep brain stimulation of the VIM nucleus of the thalamus for essential head tremor. Mov Disord 1999; 14:847–850.

39. Berk C, Honey CR. Bilateral thalamic deep brain stimulation for the treatment of head tremor. Report of two cases. J Neurosurg 2002; 96:615–618.

40. Carpenter MA, Pahwa R, Miyawaki KL, Wilkinson SB, Searl JP, Koller WC. Reduction in voice tremor under thalamic stimulation. Neurology 1998; 50:796–798.

41. Lee MS, Marsden CD. Movement disorders following lesions of the thalamus or subthalamic region. Mov Disord 1994; 9:493–507.

42. Benazzouz A, Gross C, Feger J, Boraud T, Bioulac B. Reversal of rigidity and improvement in motor performance by subthalamic high-frequency stimulation in MPTP-treated monkeys. Eur J Neurosci 1993; 5:382–389.

43. Bergman H, Wichmann T, DeLong M. Reversal of experimental parkinsonism by lesions of the subthalamic nucleus. Science 1990; 249:1346–1348.

44. Aziz TZ, Peggs D, Agarwal E, Sambrook MA, Crossman AR. Subthalamic nucleotomy alleviates parkinsonism in the 1-methyl-4-phenyl- 1,2,3,6-tetrahydropyridine (MPTP)-exposed primate. Brit J Neurosurg 1992; 6:575–582.

45. Aziz TZ, Peggs D, Sambrook MA, Crossman AR. Lesion of the subthalamic nucleus for the alleviation of 1-methyl-4- phenyl-1,2,3,6-tetrahydropyridine (MPTP)-induced parkinsonism in the primate. Mov Disord 1991; 6:288–292.

46. Pollak P, Benabid AL, Gross C. Effects of the stimulation of the subthalamic nucleus in Parkinson disease. Rev Neurol 1993; 149:175–176.

47. Group TD-BSfPsDS. Deep-brain stimulation of the subthalamic nucleus or the pars interna of the globus pallidus in Parkinson's disease. N Engl J Med 2001; 345:956–963.

48. Limousin P, Krack P, Pollak P. Electrical stimulation of the subthalamic nucleus in advanced Parkinson's disease. N Engl J Med 1998; 339:1105–1111.

49. Krack P, Limousin P, Benabid AL, Pollak P. Chronic stimulation of subthalamic nucleus improves levodopa-induced dyskinesias in Parkinson's disease [letter]. Lancet 1997; 350:1676.

50. Bejjani BP, Damier P, Arnulf I. Transient acute depression induced by high-frequency deep-brain stimulation [see comments]. N Engl J Med 1999; 340:1476–1480.

51. Dujardin K, Krystkowiak P, Defebvre L, Blond S, Destee A. A case of severe dysexecutive syndrome consecutive to chronic bilateral pallidal stimulation. Neuropsychologia 2000; 38:305–1315.

52. Perozzo P, Rizzone M, Bergamasco B. Deep brain stimulation of the subthalamic nucleus in Parkinson's disease: comparison of pre- and postoperative neuropsychological evaluation. J Neurol Sci 2001; 192:9–15.

53. Pillon B, Ardouin C, Damier P. Neuropsychological changes between "off" and "on" STN or GPi stimulation in Parkinson's disease. Neurology 2000; 55:411–418.

54. Ardouin C, Pillon B, Peiffer E. Bilateral subthalamic or pallidal stimulation for Parkinson's disease affects neither memory nor executive functions: a consecutive series of 62 patients. Ann Neurol 1999; 46:217–223.

55. Laitinen L, ATB, Hariz M. Leksell's posteroventral pallidotomy in the treatment of Parkinson's disease. J Neurosurg 1992; 76:53–61.

56. Ghika J, Villemure JG, Fankhauser H, Favre J, Assal G, Ghika-Schmid F. Efficiency and safety of bilateral contemporaneous pallidal stimulation (deep brain stimulation) in levodopa-responsive patients with Parkinson's disease with severe motor fluctuations: a 2-year follow-up review. J Neurosurg 1998; 89:713–718.

57. Volkmann J, Sturm V, Weiss P. Bilateral high-frequency stimulation of the internal globus pallidus in advanced Parkinson's disease. Ann Neurol 1998; 44:953–961.

58. Galvez-Jimenez N, Lozano A, Tasker R, Duff J, Hutchison W, Lang AE. Pallidal stimulation in Parkinson's disease patients with a prior unilateral pallidotomy. Can J Neurol Sci 1998; 25:300–305.

59. Burchiel KJ, Anderson VC, Favre J, Hammerstad JP. Comparision of Pallidal and Subthalamic Nucleus Deep Brain Stimulation for Advanced Parkinson's Disease: Results of a Randomized, Blinded Pilot Study. Neurosurgery 1999; 45:1375–1384.

60. Allert N, Volkmann J, Dotse S, Hefter H, Sturm V, Freund HJ. Effects of bilateral pallidal or subthalamic stimulation on gait in advanced Parkinson's disease. Mov Disord 2001; 16:1076–1085.

61. Volkmann J, Allert N, Voges J, Weiss PH, Freund HJ, Sturm V. Safety and efficacy of pallidal or subthalamic nucleus stimulation in advanced PD. Neurology 2001; 56:548–551.

62. Krack P, Poepping M, Weinert D, Schrader B, Deuschl G. Thalamic, pallidal, or subthalamic surgery for Parkinson's disease? J Neurol 2000; 247(suppl 2):II122–II134.

63. Kumar R, Dagher A, Hutchison WD, Lang AE, Lozano AM. Globus pallidus deep brain stimulation for generalized dystonia: clinical and PET investigation. Neurology 1999; 53:871–874.

64. Krauss JK, Pohle T, Weber S, Ozdoba C, Burgunder JM. Bilateral stimulation of globus pallidus internus for treatment of cervical dystonia [letter]. Lancet 1999; 354:837–838.

65. Lozano AM, Kumar R, Gross RE, et al. Globus pallidus internus pallidotomy for generalized dystonia [see comments]. Mov Disord 1997; 12:865–870.

66. Islekel S, Zileli M, Zileli B. Unilateral pallidal stimulation in cervical dystonia. Stereotact Funct Neurosurg 1999; 72:248–252.

67. Thompson TP, Kondziolka D, Albright AL. Thalamic stimulation for choreiform movement disorders in children. Report of two cases. J Neurosurg 2000; 92:718–721.

68. Sellal F, Hirsch E, Barth P, Blond S, Marescaux C. A case of symptomatic hemidystonia improved by ventroposterolateral thalamic electrostimulation. Mov Disord 1993; 8:515–518.

69. Tronnier VM, Fogel W. Pallidal stimulation for generalized dystonia. Report of three cases. J Neurosurg 2000; 92:453–456.

70. Vercueil L, Krack P, Pollak P. Results of deep brain stimulation for dystonia: a critical reappraisal. Mov Disord 2002; 17(suppl 3):S89–S93.

71. Bonelli RM, Gruber A. Deep brain stimulation in Huntington's disease. Mov Disord 2002; 17:429–430. Discussion 431–432.

72. Vandewalle V, van der Linden C, Groenewegen HJ, Caemaert J. Stereotactic treatment of Gilles de la Tourette syndrome by high frequency stimulation of thalamus [letter]. Lancet 1999; 353:724.

73. Mazars GL, Merienne L, Ciolocca C. Stimulations thalamiques intermittents antalgiques. Note Préliminaire. Revue Neurol 1973; 128:273–279.

74. Mazars GL. Intermittent stimulation of nucleus ventralis posterlateralis for intractable pain. Surgical Neurology 1975; 4:93–95.

75. Mazars GL, Merienne L, Ciolocca C. Treatment of certain types of pain by implantable thalamic stimulators. Neurochirurgie 1974; 29:117–124.

76. Lenz F, Tasker R, Dostrovsky J. Abnormal single-unit activity recorded in the somatosensory thalamus of a quadriplegic patient with central pain. Paine 1987; 31:225–236.

77. Lis-Planells M, Tronnier V, Rinaldi P. Neural activity of medial and lateral thalamus in a deafferentation model. Soc Neuroscience Abstr 1992; 18:288.

78. Rinaldi P, Young R, Albe-Fessard D. Spontaneous neuronal hyperactivity in the medial and intralaminar thalamic nuclei of patients with deafferentation pain. J Neurosurgery 1991; 74: 415–421.

79. Gerhart K, Yezierski R, Fang Z, Willis W. Inhibition of primate spinothalamic tract neurons by stimulation in ipsilateral or contralateral ventral posterior lateral (VPL) thalamic nucleus: Possible Mechanisms. J Neurophysiol 1983; 59:406–423.

80. Benabid AL, Henriksen SJ, McGinty JF, Bloom FE. Thalamic nucleus ventro-postero-lateralis inhibits nucleus parafascicularis response to noxious stimuli through a non-opioid pathway. Brain Res 1983; 280:217–231.

81. Reynolds D. Surgery in the rat during electrical analgesia induced by focal brain stimulation. Science 1969; 164.

82. Richardson DE, Akil H. Pain reduction by electrical brain stimulation in man. Part 2: chronic self-administration in the periventricular gray matter. J Neurosurg 1977; 47:184–194.

83. Richardson DE, Akil H. Pain reduction by electrical brain stimulation in man. Part 1: acute administration in periaqueductal and periventricular sites. J Neurosurg 1977; 47:178–183.

84. Kumar K, Toth C, Nath RK. Deep brain stimulation for intractable pain: a 15-year experience. Neurosurgery 1997; 40:736–746. Discussion 746–747.

85. Tsubokawa T, Katayama Y, Yamamoto T, Hirayama T, Koyama S. Chronic motor cortex stimulation in patients with thalamic pain. J Neurosurg 1993; 78:393–401.

86. Tsubokawa T, Katayama Y, Yamamoto T, Hirayama T, Koyama S. Chronic motor cortex stimulation for the treatment of central pain. Acta Neurochir Suppl 1991; 52:137–139.

87. Nguyen JP, Lefaucheur JP, Decq P, et al. Chronic motor cortex stimulation in the treatment of central and neuropathic pain. Correlations between clinical, electrophysiological and anatomical data. Pain 1999; 82:245–251.

88. Peyron R, Garcia-Larrea L, Deiber MP. Electrical stimulation of precentral cortical area in the treatment of central pain: electrophysiological and PET study. Pain 1995; 62:275–286.

89. Cooper IS. Effect of stimulation of posterior cerebellum on neurological disease. Lancet 1973; 1:1321.

90. Cooper IS, Amin I, Riklan M, Waltz JM, Tung PP. Chronic cerebellar stimulation in epilepsy. Arch Neurol 1976; 33:559–570.

91. Cooper IS, Amin I, Gilman S. The effect of chronic cerebellar stimulation upon epilepsy in man. Trans Am Neurol Assoc 1978; 98:192–196.

92. Cooper IS. Cerebellar Stimulation in Man. New York: Raven Press, 1978.
93. Cooper IS, Amin I, Gilman S, Waltz JM. The effect of chronic stimulation of cerebellar cortex on epilepsy in man. In: Cooper IS, Riklan M, Snider RS, eds. The Cerebellum, Epilepsy, and Behavior. New York: Plenum, 1974:122.
94. Van Buren JM, Wood JH, Oakley J, Hambrecht F. Preliminary evaluation of cerebellar stimulation by double-blind stimulation and biological criteria in the treatment of epilepsy. J Neurosurg 1978; 48:407–416.
95. Wright G, McLellan D, Brice A. A double-blind trial of chronic cerebellar stimulation in twelve patients with epilepsy. J Neurol Neurosurg Psychiatry 1984; 47:769–774.
96. Cooper IS, Upton AR, Amin I. Reversibility of chronic neurologic deficits. Some effects of electrical stimulation of the thalamus and internal capsule in man. Appl Neurophysiol 1980; 43:244–258.
97. Cooper IS, Upton AR. Therapeutic implications of modulation of metabolism and functional activity of cerebral cortex by chronic stimulation of cerebellum and thalamus. Biol Psychiatry 1985; 20:811–813.
98. Velasco F, Velasco M, Ogarrio C, Fanghanel G. Electrical stimulation of the centromedian thalamic nucleus in the treatment of convulsive seizures: a preliminary report. Epilepsia 1987; 28:421–430.
99. Velasco F, Velasco M, Jimenez F. Predictors in the treatment of difficult-to-control seizures by electrical stimulation of the centromedian thalamic nucleus [In Process Citation]. Neurosurgery 2000; 47:295–304. Discussion 304–305.
100. Benabid AL, Koudsié A, Pollak P. Future Prospects of Brain Stimulation. Neurological Research 2000; 22:237–246.
101. Benabid AL, Minotti L, Koudsie A, de Saint Martin A, Hirsch E. Antiepileptic effect of high-frequency stimulation of the subthalamic nucleus (corpus luysi) in a case of medically intractable epilepsy caused by focal dysplasia: a 30-month follow-up: technical case report. Neurosurgery 2002; 50:1385–1391. Discussion 1391–1392.
102. Loddenkemper T, Pan A, Neme S. Deep brain stimulation in epilepsy. J Clin Neurophysiol 2001; 18:514–532.
103. Deransart C, Le BT, Marescaux C, Depaulis A. Role of the subthalamo-nigral input in the control of amygdala-kindled seizures in the rat. Brain Res 1998; 807:78–83.
104. Deransart C, Vercueil L, Marescaux C, Depaulis A. The role of basal ganglia in the control of generalized absence seizures. Epilepsy Res 1998; 32:213–223.
105. Vercueil L, Benazzouz A, Deransart C. High-frequency stimulation of the subthalamic nucleus suppresses absence seizures in the rat: comparison with neurotoxic lesions. Epilepsy Res 1998; 31:39–46.
106. Nuttin B, Cosyns P, Demeulemeester H, Gybels J, Meyerson B. Electrical stimulation in anterior limbs of internal capsules in patients with obsessive-compulsive disorder [letter]. Lancet 1999; 354:1526.
107. Anand BK, Brobeck JR. Hypothalamic control of food intake in rats and cats. Yale J Biol Med 1951; 24:123–140.
108. Anand BK, Brobeck JR. Localization of a "feeding center" in the hypothalamus of the rat. Proc Soc Exp Biol Med 1951; 77:323–324.
109. Anand BK, Dua S. Feeding Responses induced by electrical stimulation of the hypothalamus in cat. Indian J Med Res 1955; 43:113–122.
110. Quaade F, Vaernet K, Larsson S. Stereotaxic stimulation and electrocoagulation of the lateral hypothalamus in obese humans. Acta Neurochir 1974; 30:111–117.
111. Moruzzi G, Magoun HW. Brainstem reticular formation and activation of the EEG. Electroencephalogr Clin Neurophysiol 1949; 1:455–473.
112. Magoun HW. The Waking Brain. Springfield, Ill: Charles C. Thomas, 1958.
113. Hassler R, Ore GD, Bricolo A, Dieckmann G, Dolce G. EEG and clinical arousal induced by bilateral long-term stimulation of pallidal systems in traumatic vigil coma. Electroencephalogr Clin Neurophysiol 1969; 27:689–690.

114. Sturm V, Kuhner A, Schmitt HP, Assmus H, Stock G. Chronic electrical stimulation of the thalamic unspecific activating system in a patient with coma due to midbrain and upper brain stem infarction. Acta Neurochir 1979; 47:235–244.

115. Tsubokawa T, Yamamoto T, Katayama Y, Hirayama T, Maejima S, Moriya T. Deep-brain stimulation in a persistent vegetative state: follow-up results and criteria for selection of candidates. Brain Inj 1990; 4:315–327.

116. Cohadon F, Richer E. [Deep cerebral stimulation in patients with post-traumatic vegetative state. 25 cases]. Neurochirurgie 1993; 39:281–292.

117. Schiff ND, Rezai AR, Plum F. A neuromodulation strategy for rational therapy of complex brain injury states. Neurol Res 2000; 22:267–272.

118. Fins JJ. A proposed ethical framework for interventional cognitive neuroscience: a consideration of deep brain stimulation in impaired consciousness. Neurol Res 2000; 22:273–278.

10

Quantum Holography: A Basis for the Interface Between Mind and Matter

Edgar Mitchell
Lake Worth, Florida, U.S.A.

Quantum holography, a recently discovered attribute of all physical matter, provides a new conceptual tool to understand subtle complexities and processes of biological systems. Some of these cannot be explained by Newtonian physics but become comprehensible using this new approach, which may lead to exciting new advances in biology and medicine.

I. INTRODUCTION

The effects of mind, emotional support systems, stress management, the placebo effect, and other subtle factors affecting health have been long noted and documented. The missing ingredient for serious clinical study within mainstream science of such effects has been the absence of a cause-and-effect link within the accepted scientic and medical paradigm. Electromagnetic and quantum effects, operating below the scale of chemical description have now become recognized as fertile ground for understanding these subtle linkages. The experimental bioelectric evidence reported by Tiller in this publication represent a significant advance in probing the linkage to mind of this level of bioelectromagnetic activity. In this chapter a related and interacting phenomenon is reported.

Quantum holography, a recently discovered attribute of all physical matter, and initially validated by experimental work with functional magnetic resonance imaging (fMRI) tomography, provides a new conceptual tool to understand quantum level processes of biological systems, including the mind–matter interface. Quantum coherence has for decades been considered of importance, of practical usefulness, and studied only in the domain of isolated nuclear particles. However, research over the past two decades clearly demonstrates that nature exhibits quantum properties at all scales sizes (1,2). Classical descriptions of the physical, chemical, and electromagnetic properties of inanimate matter are useful but incomplete tools for the complexities of microbiology and medicine. This chapter describes quantum holography, its foundations, mathematical formalism, and implications for further research, particularly in the field of microbiology and mind–brain–consciousness studies.

II. BACKGROUND

The emergence of quantum information theory almost 60 years following the formulation of quantum mechanics, and more than 30 years following Shannon's classic information theory, opens new techniques to probe below chemical and electrical models of living systems. Although disputed and often ignored until recent years, the deep complexities of microbiology are now clearly seen to be dependent upon quantum and electromagnetic processes operating at more subtle levels of reality than have been previously described.

The initial formulations of quantum theory focused upon subatomic particles, their interactions and energy transfers. This was based on the observation that light and atomic particles exhibit both particle and wave characteristics called the *wave–particle duality*. Depending upon what experiment was conducted, one could observe wave or particle characteristics but not both simultaneously. However, particles involved in a process together will subsequently exhibit quantum entanglement that remains, whatever separate paths the entangled particles subsequently follow. The entangled (or coherence) property of the particles most often of concern is *spin* or *polarization* of the ensemble of particles. The *nonlocal* correlation of particle properties has been the subject of debate and concern for 75 years as it suggests instantaneous action at a distance. It has spawned several interpretations of the deeper meaning of quantum mechanics and was challenged by Einstein as "spooky action at a distance" and in violation of his special relativity. Only a decisive experiment by Alain Aspect and his team, in Paris, in 1982, finally established unequivocally that "nonlocal quantum correlation" is indeed a property of entangled quantum particles at a distance, but the issue of superluminal speeds still remains unresolved (3).

Hidden beneath the accepted standard formalism of the Schrödinger equation, which is still largely used today by practicing physicists, is useable information carried by entangled quantum entities. The standard formalism, its interpretations and utilization in practice, over the years has ignored or denied that the information from quantum entanglement was useful, usable, or could be recovered. Research during the last two decades of the twentieth century into the possibilities of quantum computing, however, has demonstrated that quantum entanglement not only can be employed to develop quantum computing technology but has been fundamental in natural evolution to shape both inanimate and biological systems. The brain and body, it appears, may be viewed as a naturally evolved, massively parallel, multitasking, learning, quantum computing system. The concept of the quantum hologram is a key ingredient in understanding these underlying quantum processes.

The mathematical formalism initially used in quantum mechanics and largely still used in particle research focuses on the classical variables of energy, position, momentum, velocity, and spin of individual particles. But quantum information theory uses equally valid and equally long-standing formalism of Dirc and Weyl to look at frequencies and phase relationships (Tiller's R domain in this book), which reveals the hidden information. Matrix formulation of the Weyl–Heisenberg noncommutative, nilpotent, Lie group algebra forms the basis for understanding quantum holography (4,5). In these analyses one is less concerned with energy transfer from particle to particle, or with individual particle dynamics, than in the subtle dynamics of the spin entanglement of *groups* of atoms and molecules. Biomolecules in cells are entangled in quantum processes from the moment of fertilization and can be caused to release the information of their quantum states. Frequency and phase become the new quantum measurables of this mathematical formalism. As frequency and phase entanglement are the properties of laser holographic technology as well, this natural process was labeled quantum holography.

III.   WHAT IS QUANTUM HOLOGRAPHY?

All matter absorbs and reemits quanta of energy at the molecular level from and into the underlying field of quantum fluctuations called *zero point energy* (ZPE). When studied in isolation, emission and absorption are considered random exchanges of energy between particles. However, the emissions from complex matter are now understood to exhibit quantum coherence also and thus carry information nonlocally about the event history of quantum states of the emitting matter. Walter Schempp used the mathematical formalism of the Weyl–Heisenberg nilpotent Lie group algebra to expand quantum information theory. He validated this approach by significantly improving the definition and specificity of magnetic resonance imaging tomography (6), and in this process discovered the inherent information content of the emitter–absorber model of quantum mechanics. Schempp and Peter Marcer subsequently expanded the theory of the quantum hologram to propose that prokaryote, DNA molecules, and neurons exchange information with their environment via this nonlocal quantum mechanism (7–9). This suggests that all biomatter, from simple cells to organisms on all scale sizes, are informationally interconnected internally by nonlocal quantum coherence and externally with the larger environment by their coherent quantum emissions: the quantum hologram.

The mathematical formalism requires that phase-conjugate adaptive resonance (PCAR) exists between the emitting object and its colocated quantum hologram. Likewise, PCAR must exist for any reception or recording of the holographic information. Physically this may be interpreted as a standing wave between object and receptor, or mathematically as equal waves traveling in opposite directions between object and receptor. For example, synthetic aperture radar operates on a similar principle (PCAR) using electromagnetic pulses. And sound waves in an organ pipe have an analogous mathematical description.

A laser hologram exhibits the distributive property. This means that a small part of a holographic record (for example, a hologram recorded on photographic film) contains the entire record of the recorded image, but with less visual brightness when reconstructed optically. Quantum holography appears to operate similarly in that emissions from complex matter, for example, biomatter, carry information about the entire organism. The fact that living cells in any organism evolve and grow from more simple cells, under the guidance of DNA molecules, implies quantum entanglement throughout the organism and its composite parts, with an associated instantaneous exchange of information through adaptive resonance. Thus some information about the entire organism is carried in the quantum emissions from its parts.

Two seminal papers by R. Noboli (10,11) to account for the function of glial cells show that wave conjugation occurs spontaneously such that both virtual and real images of recorded information are elicited by wave diffraction—a result consistent with and required by quantum holography and validated in fMRI research. Further, the ongoing work of Roger Penrose, Oxford (12), and Stuart Hameroff, University of Arizona (13), in their studies of microtubules and the emergence of consciousness in the brain is consistent with quantum holographic theory, such that one may view the microtubules as phase gates in managing holographic information.

IV. IMPLICATIONS OF QUANTUM HOLOGRAPHY

1. All matter, including biomatter and brains, must be regarded as quantum systems exhibiting internal quantum coherence as well as entanglement with the larger environment. Both classical and quantum properties must be understood in order to have complete information about the system.

2. The nonlocal information carried by the quantum hologram, ubiquitously in nature, elevates information to the same level of importance as energy in physical theories. Utilizing information is a basic definition of intelligence, thus even inanimate nature must be considered in some sense intelligent.

3. The numinous attribute we call *mind*, as distinguished from the physical brain, is likely associated with the quantum hologram (14,15).

4. Classical descriptions of the five normal senses are incomplete in that the brain must mix classical space–time information for the five senses, by phase gating, withthe nonlocal quantum holographic information in order for PCAR to occur. PCAR is necessary so that objects in the 3D Cartesian theatre of reality appears as they actually are rather than as just images inside the brain (15).

One may demonstrate this point simply by snapping one's fingers and noting that the sound seems to emanate from the location of the fingers, not as a point in the brain. This is modeled mathematically as phase conjugation, such that the real signal and a virtual signal created by the brain coincide. PCAR is a necessary condition for all the senses in order to perceive accurately the 3D reality, and certainly conveys evolutionary advantage over sensing modalities lacking this mechanism. For vision, close one eye. Reality continues to appear 3D, just the field of vision is reduced. That is to say, the stereoscopic binocular effect to explain 3D vision is incomplete.

5. Sensing quantum holographic information without normal sensory confirmation may be responsible for a host of phenomena related to remote viewing, telepathy, intuition, the "twin effect," the "phantom limb" effect, etc.

6. The experiments of Jacques Benveniste (16), with "memory of water," in which aqueous solutions were diluted until no molecules of the original substance remained, yet the solution retained pharmaceutical effectiveness, is easily explained with quantum holographic theory. Although Benveniste's career was severely damaged by rejection of his findings by mainstream science, his results, plus quantum holography as an explanatory mechanism correctly establish homeopathy as a valid pharmaceutical approach.

7. The measurables of quantum holography are frequency and phase, with information encoded in the phase relationships about the event history of the emitting object. Thus the encoded information from biomatter will have a signature frequency spectrum analogous to fingerprints or DNA from humans. It should, therefore, be possible to diagnose abnormal cell and organ functions at more subtle levels than chemical and electrical analysis. To do so would validate the twentieth-century approach in radionics, which, missing the quantum information, still falls short of the mark and is incomplete.

An example from modern astronomy will illustrate how this can be accomplished. Laser light (coherent photons) are beamed into the atmosphere and reflected back from the interfering air mass. The twinkling light from astronomical objects is then corrected with a computer for the air-mass interference to remove the atmospheric noise from the starlight. Even newer techniques, using quantum holographic theory, are being tested to phase gate starlight with nonlocal holographic input from the star to improve the imaging even more, as has been accomplished with fMRI (17). Similarly, quantum holographic formalism can be used to improve reception and recording of low-level emanations from cell structure to improve diagnosis

8. If the quantum wave and phase information as described in Ref. 7 for anomalies within the biomatter can be discretely captured, then in principle sending back an antiwave (wave of opposite phase) should have a therapeutic effect. Some scant evidence exists to suggest this is true. If further validated as true, then the mounting evidence for the efficacy of remote therapy through touch and mental effects would have a causal basis.

V. CONCLUSIONS

Quantum holography was been validated initially with fMRI technology. New technologies such as pattern recognition technology are picking up this subtle quantum information formalism to enhance definition, specificity, and flexibility in computer recognition of human faces (15) and, as previously stated, astronomy. Significant additional research is needed to validate and implement this nonlocal information mechanism as a fundamental factor in the organization, evolution and functioning of biomatter and for understanding complex organisms like the human. The evidence for the existence of nonlocal interconnections in animal and human sensory perceptions has been building to irrefutable statistical significance for more than five decades (18), but without a proper explanatory mechanism. Any other anomalous experimental results in classical science would have been accepted with far less statistical validity. However, the quantum hologram most likely provides the missing link for these findings and provides the basis for more intense research into the mysterious interface between mind and matter.

Study of the existing scientific and medical literature in which mathematical formalism is used reductively to study biomatter reveals the limitation of classical mathematical approaches to quantum-, electromagnetic-, and chemical-level phenomena. The complex interactions in living matter usually defy adequate understanding through simple reductionism only, as all these levels of process interact and influence each other, requiring a level of holistic thinking and analysis outside existing paradigms.

REFERENCES

1. Wilson K. The renormalization group and critical phenomena. Reviews of Modern Physics July 1983; 55(3):583–600.
2. Marcer P, Mitchell E, Schempp W. Self Reference, the dimensionality and scale of quantum mechanical effects, critical phenomena and qualia. Sixth International Conference on Computing Anticipatory Systems. In publication.
3. Chubylalo AE, Pope V, Smirnov-Reuda R, Eds. Instantaneous Action at a Distance in Modern Physics: Pro and Contra. Commack, NY: NOVA, 1999.
4. Schempp W. Harmonic Analysis on the Heisenberg group with applications in signal theory. Pitman Notes in Mathematics Series. 14. London: Longman Scientific and Technical, 1986.
5. Schempp W. Magnetic Resonance ImagingMathematical Foundations and Applications. New York: John Wiley, 1998.
6. Schempp W. Sub-Reimannian geometry and clinical magnetic resonance tomography. Math Meth Appl Sci 1999; 22:867–922.
7. Marcer P, Schempp W. The model of the prokaryote cell as an anticipatory system working by quantum holography. In: Dubois D, ed. Proceedings of the First International Conference on Computing Anticipatory Systems, Liege, Belgium, August 11–15, 1997:307–313.
8. Marcer P, Schempp W. A mathematically specified template for dna and the genetic code, in terms of the physically realizable processes of quantum holography. In: Fedorec, Marcer, eds. Proceeding of Greenwich (University) Symposium on Living Computers, 1996:45–62.
9. Marcer P, Schempp W. Model of the neuron working by quantum holography. Informatica 1997; 21:519–534.

10. Noboli R. Schrodinger wave holography in the brain cortex. Phys Rev A 1985; 32(6):3618–3626.
11. Noboli R. Ionic waves in animal tissue. Phys Rev A 1987; 35(4):1901–1922.
12. Penrose R. Quantum computation, entanglement and state reduction. Philosophical Transactions: Mathematical, Physical and Engineering Sciences, Aug 15, 1990; 356(1743):1927–1939.
13. Hameroff S. Quantum computation in brain microtubules? The Penrose-Hameroff 'Orch Or' model of consciousness. Philosophical Transactions: Mathematical, Physical and Engineering Sciences, Royal Society of London, Aug 15, 1998; 356(1743):1869–1896.
14. Mitchell E. Nature's Mind: The Quantum Hologram. ISCAS, 1999:295–312.
15. Marcer P, Mitchell E. What is consciousness? In: Van Loocke Philip, ed. The Physical Nature of Consciousness. Advances in Consciousness Research series. Amsterdam: John Benjamins B.V., 2001:45–174.
16. McTaggart L. The Field. London: HarperCollins, 2001, Chap. 4.
17. Binz E, Schempp W. Quantum Holography and Its Symbols: A Conceptual Survey, Institute of Noetic Sciences. In publication.
18. Radin D. The Conscious Universe. New York: HarperEdge, 1997.

11

Subtle Energies and Their Roles in Bioelectromagnetic Phenomena

William A. Tiller

Professor Emeritus, Stanford University, Stanford, California, U.S.A.

Various studies are presented to illustrate how human consciousness and intentionality can generate subtle energy fields that are translated into electromagnetic fields having significant biochemical and physiologic effects. Such subtle energies can also be stored in an electrical device and utilized to change the pH of a solution, increase the in vitro thermodynamic activity of enzymes and increase the in vivo ratio of ATP to ADP in developing fruit fly larvae to significantly reduce the maturation time to adult flies.

I. INTRODUCTION

The existing formalism for the quantum mechanical (QM) paradigm of physics is perhaps the greatest stumbling block that we have in trying to understand the essential differences that exist between bioelectromagnetism (bio-EM) and conventional electromagnetism (EM). Most scientists and engineers tend to think that bio-EM is just conventional electricity and magnetism applied to biological systems—it is not! In this chapter and the next, we show why it is not and how to begin revealing the differences.

To help the reader understand these differences, Sec. II deals briefly with key concepts and definitions that need to be comprehended in order to grasp the viewpoint of this chapter. In Sec. III, some general psychoenergetic experimental data will be utilized to illustrate how human bio-EM can be very different than conventional EM. In this section, one particular example will be utilized to show how human consciousness can generate subtle energy fields that, in turn, translate into experimentally measurable EM-fields. In Sec. IV, recent experimental studies by the author and his colleagues regarding some very robust effects of human intention on "conditioning" the experimental space to a higher EM gauge symmetry state will be presented. In turn, this higher symmetry level strongly influences physical reality via altered material properties manifesting in experimental measurements. In the next chapter, this work is extended to show why humans, and probably all vertebrates, contain a higher EM gauge symmetry state system functioning in their bodies and this system *strongly* influences their bio-EM. Here, we will see how subtle information–energy fields convert, in part, to measurable E and H fields and how conscious intent can act as a true thermodynamic variable to influence the magnitude of E and H, the only fields we can instrumentally quantify at the moment. There, we finally get to discussing some quantitative differences between bio-EM and standard EM. There, a multidimensional theoretical model is presented that both rationalizes the aforementioned experimental observations and provides a meaningful quantitative basis for expanding our QM paradigm. Finally, the next chapter closes by returning to day-to-day expectations for one area of near-future applications of bio-EM and subtle energies in the area of medical therapeutics.

II. SOME CONCEPTS AND DEFINITIONS (1,2)

A. De Broglie's Particle–Pilot Wave Concept

Classical mechanics dealt only with particles whereas this concept, which became one of the cornerstones of QM, is perhaps best illustrated by Fig. 1. De Broglie proposed that every particle had a pilot wave envelope enclosing it and moving at the particle's velocity. This concept required that, as this pilot wave envelope moved along, some new wave components moved into the envelope while some old wave components moved out. Calling the particle wave velocity v_p and an individual wave component velocity v_w, relativity theory requires that the following relationship hold (3)

$$v_p v_w = c^2 \tag{1}$$

where c is the velocity of light. Since $v_p < c$ always, $v_w > c$ always, and these waves were dubbed "information" waves in order to not make trouble for relativity theory.

Although in QM, de Broglie's concept (proven experimentally) became known as wave-particle *duality*, this author proposes that nature expresses itself simultaneously via its particle aspect and its information wave aspect. This means that the quantitative magnitude of *any* physical measurement is comprised of two parts: (1) the coarse particulate part and (2) the fine information wave part. Here, it is important for us to realize that all the waves of

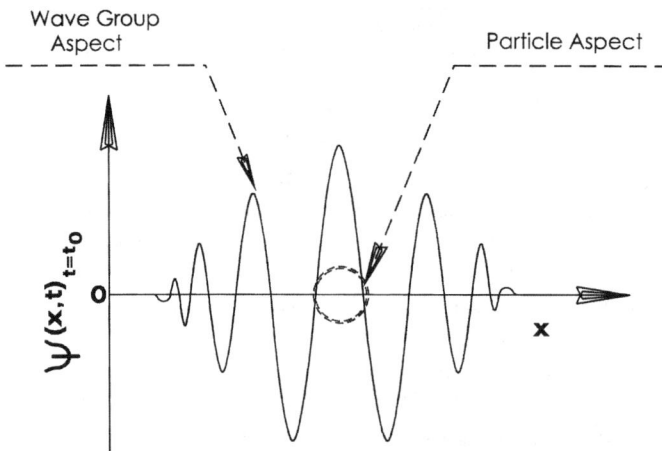

Figure 1 A group of pilot waves for a physical particle located somewhere in the group.

our cognitive experience are merely modulations of particle fluxes or particle densities in space-time. All the continuum type EM waves, drawn in electrical engineering textbooks, are actually de Broglie's information waves traveling through the vacuum level of substance.

B. The Vacuum Level of Substance

The fundamental particles making up our atoms and molecules are so tiny that they occupy only a miniscule amount of the total space. The remainder of that space (99.999 + %) is the vacuum level of substance. This particular vacuum, like that between the planets, *is not empty*. For QM and relativity theory to be internally self-consistent, others have calculated that it must contain an energy density, in mass units, of 10^{94} g/cm^3. This is a huge number. What it means in more practical terms is that provided we can assume our universe to be flat (and current day astronomers say that we can), there is a trillion times more latent energy stored in the volume of a single hydrogen atom's vacuum level than in all the mass of all the planets and all the stars in our universe out to a radius of 20 billion light-years. Thus, the vacuum level of substance is what we must look to for our scientific and technological future.

C. Gauge Symmetry

In current physics, one of the key discussions that connects the *Gauge* condition to important concepts and hypotheses is that associated with the big bang concept. Here, one encounters a description of energy and eventually matter undergoing evolutionary changes of state, from states of higher fundamental symmetry to states of lower fundamental symmetry (4). At amazingly short times in this proposed process, gauge transformations occurred from very high symmetry states and progressively drop to the lower state of the SU(2) EM gauge and then on down to the U(1) EM gauge symmetry level—our present cognitive domain.

Symmetry changes for matter still occur at the U(1) gauge level but these all involve collective interactions described as changes of state of the plasma $\rightarrow$ gas $\rightarrow$ liquid $\rightarrow$ solid kind as the temperature continues to fall. Further lowering of temperature leads to magnetic dipole ordering in some materials, electron pairing in others and phonon–photon coherence development in still others. All of this is a manifestation of the lowering of the Gibb's free energy for the system.

We are all familiar with the simple symmetry rule of rotational invariance, examples being 60° for the snowflake, 90° for the cube and 120° for the triangle. For the U(1) EM gauge symmetry state, it is a little more complex with the major requirements being (1) the coexistence of electric monopoles and magnetic dipoles, (2) Maxwellian equations for EM, (3) Abelian algebra applies ($XY - YX = 0$, where X and Y are unique fields), and (4) a completely disordered vacuum level. On the other hand, for the SU(2) EM gauge symmetry state [a higher Gibb's free energy state than the U(1) state], the situation is still more complex in some ways. Here, the major requirements for this chapter are (1) the coexistence of both electric and magnetic monopoles, (2) non-Maxwellian EM equations (5), (3) non-Abelian algebra ($XY - YX \neq 0$), and (4) the existence of domains of order in the vacuum (6).

What one notes regarding the big bang process is that, *unimpeded by consciousness inputs*, thermodynamics will drive the system towards a lower and lower Gibb's free energy state.

D. The Conditioning of Space

This involves the sustained use of human intention at a particular spatial location. This raises the EM Gauge symmetry condition, metastably at first and then, eventually, to a sufficiently high state that a symmetry phase transition can be nucleated at the vacuum level of that location. This stabilizes the higher symmetry state for an extended period of time (years). But perhaps can be destabilized by the reverse intention.

E. Our Particular Biconformal Base-Space Frame of Reference (F.R.) (1,2)

The current reference frame for QM is distance-time, (x,y,z,t), and this is fine provided no mathematical singularities are present. However, QM abounds in singularities and relativity theory has a major one at $v = c$. Based on Eq. (1), Fig. 2 illustrates this latter singularity. When mathematical singularities are present in the domain of interest, it is well known that the expansion of any mathematical function about a point in the domain requires the use of Laurent's procedure rather than Taylor's procedure, which is usually used. As an example, for the Gibb's free energy function G, we must use

$$G(z) = \underbrace{\underbrace{G(z_0) + \sum_{n=1}^{\infty} a_n(z - z_0)^n}_{\text{Taylor}} + \sum_{n=1}^{\infty} b_n(z - z_0)^{-n}}_{\text{Laurent}} \tag{2a}$$

where z_0 is the point about which we are expanding. In the thermodynamics of homogeneous systems, only the first ordered terms are considered. Typically, one either lets z represent the thermodynamic intensive variables of P, T, n_j, etc., (P = pressure, T = temperature, n = number of moles of chemical species j, etc.) or the distance-time coordinates, (x, y, z, t) (2,7). For our interest here, it is the first-order expansion terms in distance-time that are important so Eq. (2a) shows us that we have terms involving (x, y, z, t) plus terms involving $(x^{-1}, y^{-1},$

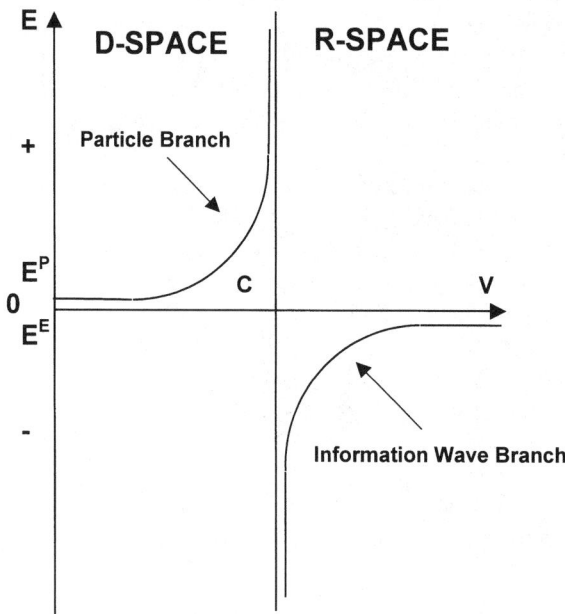

Figure 2 Energy-velocity diagram for a D-space particle ($v < c$ branch) and its R-space pilot wave conjugate ($v > c$ branch).

z^{-1}, t^{-1}). If we define $b_1' = b_1/2\pi$, $kj = 2\pi/(z_j - z_{j_0})$ and $z_j = (x, y, z, t)$, then we can begin to see our biconformal base-space reference frame developing out of Eq. (2a). It is two, four-dimensional subspaces, (x, y, z, t) and its reciprocal $(x^{-1}, y^{-1}, z^{-1}, t^{-1})$ or (k_x, k_y, k_z, k_t). The reciprocal coordinates are all frequencies, x^{-1} = number per unit distance = a spatial frequency and t^{-1} = number per unit time or a temporal frequency. Thus, Eq. (2a), in its first-order form but with all coordinates represented, becomes

$$G - G_0 \approx a_x(x - x_0) + a_y(y - y_0) + a_z(z - z_0) + a_t(t - t_0)$$

$$+ b_x' k_x + b_y' k_y + b_z' k_z + b_t' k_t \tag{2b}$$

$$= \text{D-space } (x, y, z, t) \text{ terms} + \text{R-space}(k_x, k_y, k_z, k_t) \text{ terms}$$

Here D-space refers to direct space, while R-space refers to its reciprocal space. Together, they form a unique 8 space.

One of the beautiful things about this particular biconformal base-space RF is that it naturally separates into particle space (D-space) and information wave space (R space). Another is that the D-space contribution allows only local forces while the R-space contribution allows nonlocal forces. This is because things that are far away and far apart in D space (like planets and stars) are very close together in the low-frequency domain of R space. A third important outcome of choosing this particular RF is that, for such reciprocal 4 spaces, mathematics *requires* that any substance quality in D space be quantitatively related to its conjugate equilibrium quality in R space by a *Fourier transform* type of relationship and vice versa. This latter outcome means that, for *any* physical measurement Q_M, we must have

$$Q_M = Q_D + Q_R \tag{3}$$

And we have a quantitative pathway connecting Q_R to Q_D (the Fourier transform). Thus, we must begin to look at physical reality as consisting of two layers: (1) the coarse, particulate layer which we all cognitively access and (2) the fine information wave layer, which most of us do not presently cognitively access because it functions at the vacuum level of nature.

F. Deltron Coupling

As we will see later in Sec. IV, a strong DC magnetic field polarity effect occurs on the pH of water when the water is in a conditioned space (2) but not when it is in an unconditioned space [the U(1) EM Gauge symmetry state]. The fact that such a polarity effect can arise would seem to suggest that magnetic monopoles are somehow being accessed. This implies that the information wave aspect of substance may be "written" by the magnetic mono-poles. If this is so, then the actual existence of any form of EM requires a meaningful although not direct interaction between electric monopole substance traveling at $v < c$ and magnetic monopole substance traveling at $v > c$ [see Eq. (1)]. Let us invent a higher dimensional coupling substance that is *outside* the constraints of relativity theory and can travel at both $v < c$ to interact with D-space substances *and* at $v > c$ to interact with R-space substances. I label this coupling substance "deltrons" from the next higher dimension (9 space), which I have elsewhere (1) designated as the domain of emotion.

G. Subtle Energies

We are all familiar with the four fundamental forces of gravitation, electromagnetism, the long-range nuclear force, the short-range nuclear force and the energies that they give rise to.

Subtle energies are none of these! Subtle energies need not be weak, but they are elusive because we do not presently have direct detection probes for them. At this point in time, it is thought that all subtle energies reside at *the vacuum level* of nature (see Fig. 3). At present only the information wave substance and the deltron substance have been articulated and discriminated by this author. However, acupuncture energies, homeopathy energies, remote viewing energies, etc., are all thought to fall into the R-space category.

H. Equilibrium Cluster Populations

Many scientists hold the naive view that all liquids, and particularly pure water, are completely homogeneous down to the atomic or molecular level and exhibit structural characteristics in complete accord with the random network model proposed over a half-century ago for glasses (8). However, nothing could be further from the truth and even the nano-scale heterogeneous perspective of water's structure has grown greatly in the last few decades and is available in some fine reviews (9). This topic is considered here because it is so relevant to medical therapeutics.

From a theoretical perspective (10), one naturally expects pure water to contain a wide spectrum of thermodynamically distinguishable species because the configurational entropy contribution of each unique species lowers the bulk free energy of water. The equilibrium population, N_i^*, of each unique species i, is given by $N_i^* = N_0 \exp(-\Delta G_{F_i}/kT)$, where N_0 is the monomer H_2O concentration available for forming these new species, kT is the thermal

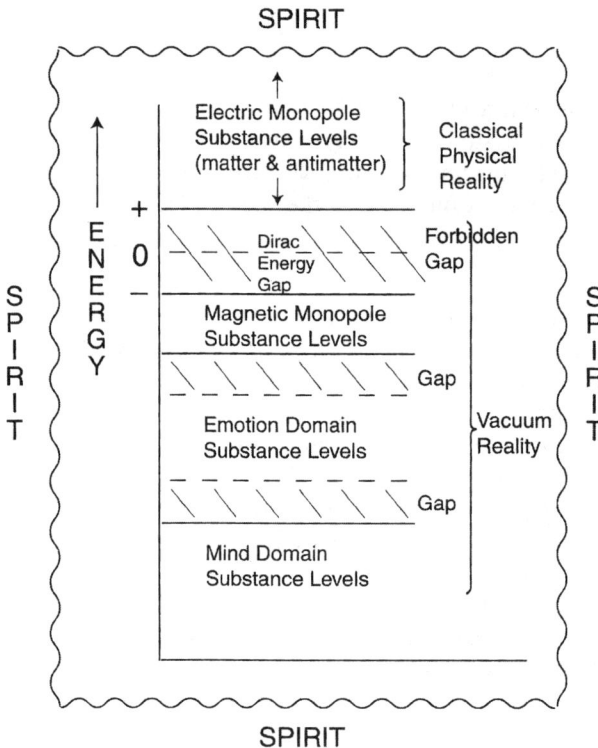

Figure 3 An energy level diagram embracing both classical physical substance and "unseen" vacuum substances.

energy and ΔG_{F_i} is the free energy of formation of the i species from this multispecies "soup." These species range from H^+, OH^- and monometric H_2O in the H-bonded network to clusters, differentiated by both polymorphic structure and size, and to microvoids of varying size and internal gas content. Although the statistical ensemble of these associated entities exhibits a stable equilibrium population distribution at any particular temperature and pressure, a particular cluster may dissociate and another re-form at a high frequency to stabilize the total ensemble on time average. Whenever N_i falls below or exceeds N_i^*, a thermodynamic driving force exists to change N_i toward N_i^* at the fastest rate allowed by the local reaction kinetics. It is also important to note that a specific solute, j, added to water also has a specific equilibrium population, N_j^*, given by the above formula with ΔG_{F_i} equal to the free energy of solution for j. However, the concentration of this species can only be changed by dilution with pure water or by the addition of more solute. Since all of these various N_i^* and N_j^* species are enfolded into the bulk water host via surrounding envelopes of H bonds that join the general H bond network of the water and, since overall free energy minimization of the total system may be constrained by the availability of such H bonds, solute agglomeration might be an anticipated result below some specific degree of dilution (11). If H bond availability can be a thermodynamic and perhaps a kinetic rate-limiting constraint in water, this suggests that a large fraction of the H_2O molecules present in bulk water are associated with unique complexes of the types delineated above. From the foregoing, one must expect great heterogeneity in the fluid aspect of human cells.

I. External Field Effects

General electric E and magnetic H field effects on the thermodynamic properties of a homogeneous liquid can be inferred from Refs. 2 and 10. However, the nano-scale heterogeneity of water discussed above introduces several new and important factors that need to be addressed here. This arises from the fact that our standard environment contains a DC magnetic field, AC electromagnetic fields of a wide range of frequencies plus atmospheric ion-generated DC electric fields. For either DC or AC fields, the clusters and microbubbles have different electric and magnetic susceptibilities relative to bulk water. Thus both electric and magnetic dipoles are induced at these interfaces (12) and, for nonuniform fields, will migrate towards the high field regions under the influence of dielectrophoresis and diamagnetophoresis (13) forces. These quasiparticles will migrate towards the high-field regions of the bulk water sample where many will annihilate ($N_i > N_i^*$) while new cluster/nanobubble creation events must occur in the low field regions ($N_i < N_i^*$) adding to the overall dynamism of change. It has been shown recently that magnetically shielded water stays for a remarkably long time in metastable states without actively moving towards equilibrium and that miniscule H fields greatly enhance the rate of pH and ORP progression towards some stationary state with the rate of progression increasing strongly with the magnitude of H (14). Abundant experimental data exists to confim many strange effects associated with electromagnetic field effects and water (15). Surprisingly, when the water is first degassed before EMF exposure, these strange effects are absent (16). Direct electron microscope evidence also exists for magnetic field alteration of the Helmholtz layer thickness at solid–water interfaces (17).

Perhaps a simple example from medical therapeutics will best illustrate the complexity of the issues here. Suppose we have a device placed around a human's knee that creates a macroscopically uniform AC electromagnetic field intensity (E^2 and H^2) outside the knee. One might quickly assume that nothing will happen inside the knee because this imposed field is macroscopically uniform. However, inside the knee, the structure is polyphase (bone, cartilage, tendons, fluid, "colloids", ions, etc.) and thus heterogeneous with respect to electric and magnetic susceptibilities. This means that, *inside* the knee, the E and H fields are macroscopically very nonuniform and it is these internal environment fields that drive "colloids" and small dipoles to drift towards the local high field regions. Further, with the passage of time, these "colloids" and small dipoles concentrate in certain regions and now create *DC fields* which, in turn, initiate local ion movements (electrophoresis) to neutralize such induced DC fields.

The main point to be communicated by this final section is that the presence of any structural heterogeneities in water leads to local heterogeneities in electric permittivity and magnetic permeability and these, in turn, respond directly or indirectly to ambient E and H fields so as to cause drift movement of such moieties in the solution. Such long-range movement upsets the homeostasis of the solution with a variety of interesting consequences.

III. SOME GENERAL, BACKGROUND PSYCHOENERGETIC DATA

In a recent book, Radin (18) has provided clear and incontrovertible evidence to support the existence of extra sensory perception (ESP) capabilities in humans. Although the effect size is small for the average population, it is clearly nonzero. This field also has its superstars, like a Michael Jordan or a Tiger Woods, where the effect size can be very large. Ingo Swann (19) and Edgar Cayce (20) are two names that come readily to mind. For today's medicine, this type of data sheds strong light on the so-called placebo effect. The prevailing medical view is that nothing real has occurred and that any improvement is delusional. In Benson's work (21) among patients receiving a variety of treatments they believed in, but for which medicine finds no physiological basis, treatments were effective 70% to 90% of the time. However, when the physicians doubted whether these treatments actually worked, their effectiveness dropped to 30–40%.

Similar belief-related success was observed in Stewart Wolf's work (22) with women who experienced persistent nausea and vomiting during pregnancy. First, sensors were positioned in their stomachs so that contractions could be recorded. Next, they were given a drug that they were told would cure their nausea. In fact, they were given Ipecac. However, because of their belief, the women reversed the laboratory-proven action of the drug and their measured stomach contractions damped down to negligible values. Further, Enserink (23) has pointed out that "when companies started testing drugs for obsessive-compulsive disorder back in the mid-1980s, the placebo response rate was almost zero. As time went on, this response rate began to creep upward, up to a point when one could reasonably conclude that some clinical trials failed because of high placebo response rates." A very recent meta-analysis of 19 antidepressant drug trials revealed that the placebo effect on average accounted for 75% of the effect of *real* drugs. Although many feel that this data represents a kind of soft underbelly that both academic and industry researchers are more comfortable leaving out of sight, others are fascinated by the power of the placebo effect viewing it not as a problem but as a source of insight into mental health. Going even further, what is it saying about the *actual* laws of nature, as distinct from our metaphysical assumptions about them, and *why* has the magnitude of the placebo effect increased so remarkably in the last 20 years?

Another major psychoenergy experiment involves the conscious cognition of objects, terrain, atmospheric conditions, and so forth located hundreds to thousands of miles away, given only the coordinates of the location. This experiment, originally conceived, conducted and developed by Ingo Swann and given the name *remote viewing*, was refined and perfected by him in association with Puthoff and Targ (24) at Stanford Research International. For government service remote viewers, successful completion of a training program required a minimum of 85% accuracy with respect to the coordinates of 20 blind targets. In some cases time coordinates, past or future, were also involved.

A more familiar mode of remote viewing involves one's ability to "tune in" to a specific individual and view a specific remote locality through that individual's eyes. This mode of remote viewing ability is more easily acquired and has been replicated in many laboratories around the world (24).

Dossey (25), Tart and Katra (26) plus many others have clearly shown that humans are not only capable of highly accurate long-range cognition of local details plus events but they are also capable of eliciting human health transitions at such distant locations. From Dossey's three eras of medicine model, Era III-Medicine is defined by *nonlocal* approaches to healing (25). It views the mind as unbounded and unconfined to points in space and time so that this category of healing events may bridge persons who are widely separated from each other. This category of medicine goes well beyond today's view of physics so that mind, not matter, is ultimately considered as being primary. Expanding on nonlocal force and influence effects, a great deal of data (27) is now available to show that both Qigong masters and adepts can significantly influence materials and processes both locally and nonlocally located. For example, Yan Xin emitted his Qi into samples of tap water both from a local

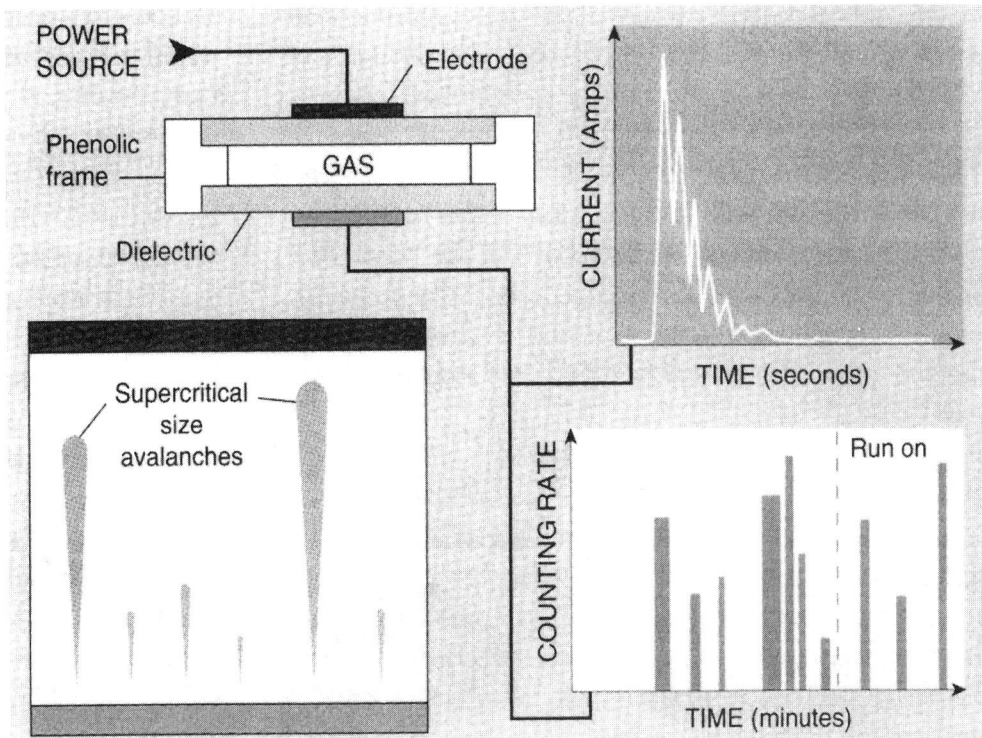

Figure 4 The gas-discharge experimental setup comprised a high-fidelity, high-voltage power source, the gas discharge device, and a monitoring system. This schematic illustration shows electron avalanches passing through the gas, a typical oscilloscope tracing of total electron avalanche current vs. time and a plot of the count rate as a function of time during an experimental run.

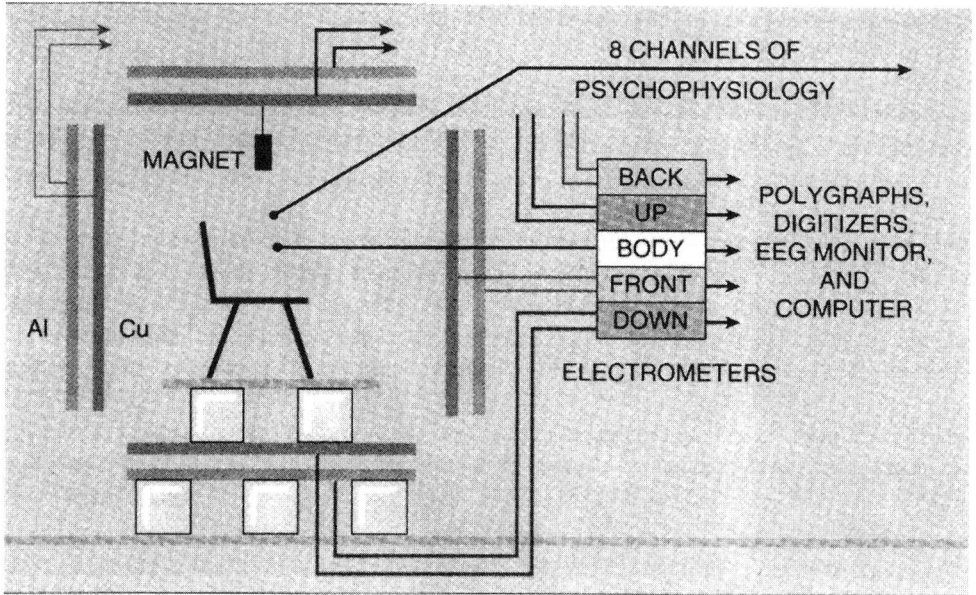

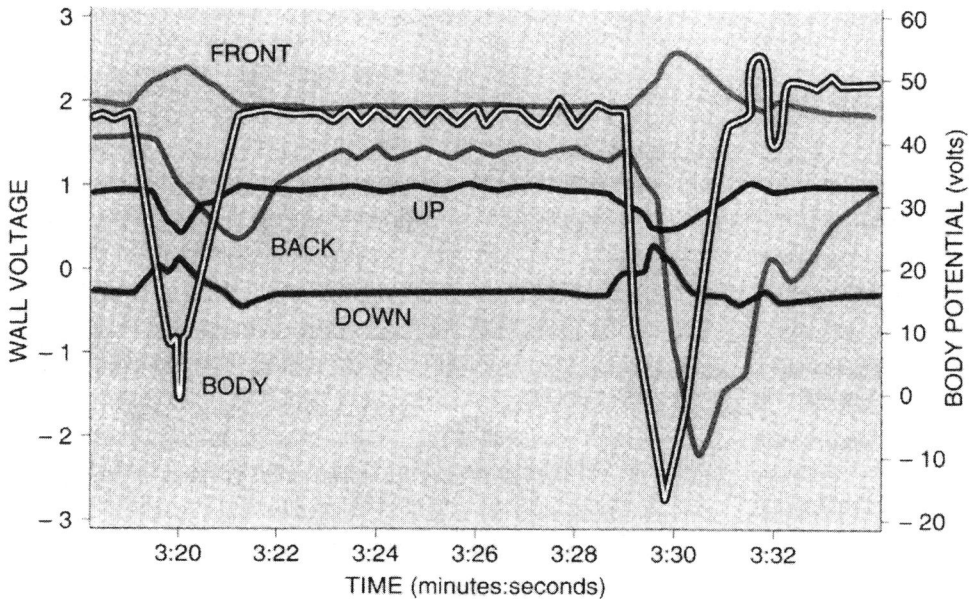

Figure 5 In the copper-walled meditation room, four pairs of insulated copper and aluminum panels float in electrical space around a research chair, which also floats electrically, insulated from the "down" panel by glass construction blocks. Signals from the subject's body and from the four copper walls are fed into electrometers, and data from all channels are forwarded to polygraphs, digitizers, and a computer. The graph shows an example of simultaneous body and wall potentials.

arrangement and via a nonlocal arrangement (~7 km away) and any change in the water's Raman spectrum was investigated (28). There are two peaks in the Raman spectrum of normal water: one very large peak is at 3430 cm^{-1}, corresponding to the stretching vibrational mode of OH, and one weak at 1635 cm^{-1}, corresponding to the bending vibration mode for HOH. Before Yan Xin's Qi emission, this is what was observed for all samples. However, after Qi emission, there was a huge peak (~18 times higher than the normal peak at 3430 cm^{-1}) ranging from 1000 cm^{-1} to 3000 cm^{-1} observed in the Raman spectrum for the water samples. This huge peak decayed by ~2/3 within the first 1.5 h and had completely disappeared after ~2 h from Qi emission, leaving a Raman spectrum that was essentially identical to that of the untreated water.

All of the aforementioned works are examples of subtle energies producing substantial effects on physical reality! Now, let me provide a few examples from this author's own work (1,29).

In the 1970s, I carried out a series of experiments with a man whose bio-EM field was such that he had a unique ability with cameras and its photographic film. Whenever he took a picture while he was experiencing a particular familiar feeling in his seventh cervical and

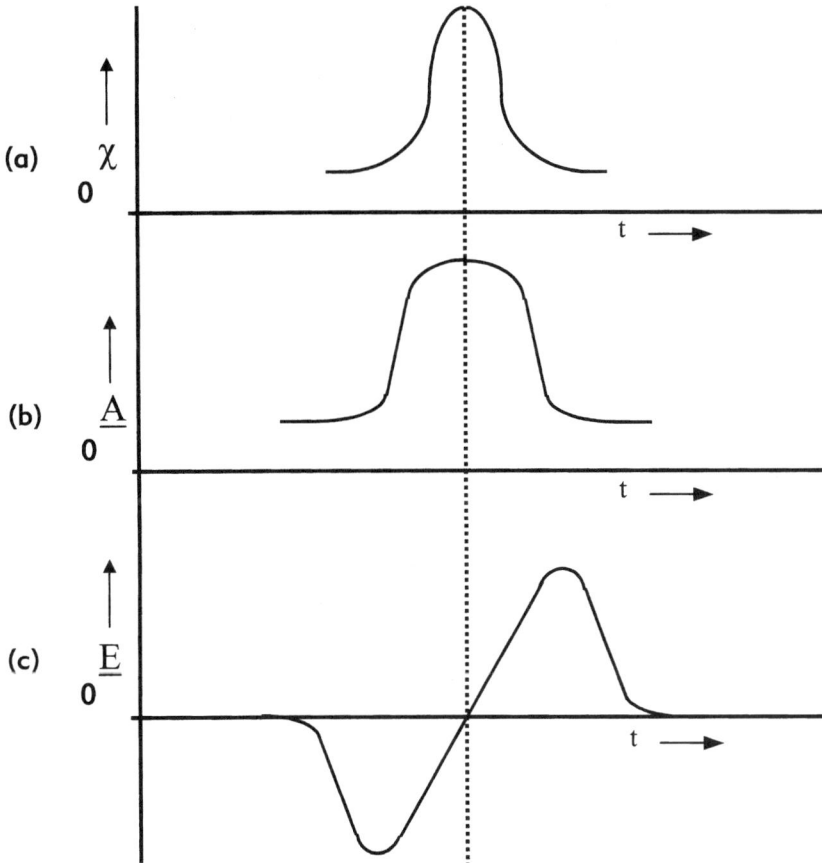

Figure 6 Schematic illustration of a subtle energy pulse χ, which generates the magnetic vector potential pulse A shown in (b), which, in turn, generates the electric field E shown in (c) at some specific origin in the healer's physical body.

fourth thoracic vertebrae, some striking anomaly would appear in the photograph. His held intention during the picture-taking process was, he said, "to reveal God's universe."

My experiments with him used two cameras, one of them sensitized by keeping it close to his body for several days and the other unsensitized. Both cameras were mounted on the same tripod and tripped with a single shutter release. Ordinary colored film was used in both cameras and was processed by its manufacturer, and the subject was never allowed to touch the film. Often, though not always, pictures taken with the sensitized camera showed one or more people as if they were partially transparent, or translucent, so that objects located behind them could be seen "through" them (29,30). The pictures from the unsensitized camera appeared normal. On other occasions, clear pictures were taken via the sensitized camera with the lens cap firmly in place on the camera (30).

My interpretation of this phenomenon is that

1. Some radiations exist in nature that can travel through materials that are opaque to visible light.
2. Because of some presently unknown quality inherent in the subject's biofield, these radiations can be detected by film in the sensitized camera.
3. Some time is required for the camera placed in this special human energy field to acquire its anomalous capacity.
4. The anomalous capacity leaks away in about an hour or so unless continuously pumped by the energy field of the subject.

In a second set of studies (29,30), an AC voltage at 450 Hz was applied to dielectric-coated electrodes that bounded at 2 mm layer of gas in a sandwichlike gas discharge device (see Fig. 4). The applied voltage peak to the device was kept 10% to 15% below the breakdown voltage for the layer of gas, and electron "microavalanches" passing through the gas were monitored by a pulse counter that could be set to count any pulse over a predetermined size.

Typically, the pulse counter was set to just miss the largest avalanches traveling across the gas. Thus, the system was poised but yielding a zero count for many hours until a human subject attempted to influence it. Almost a thousand or so experimental runs involved a

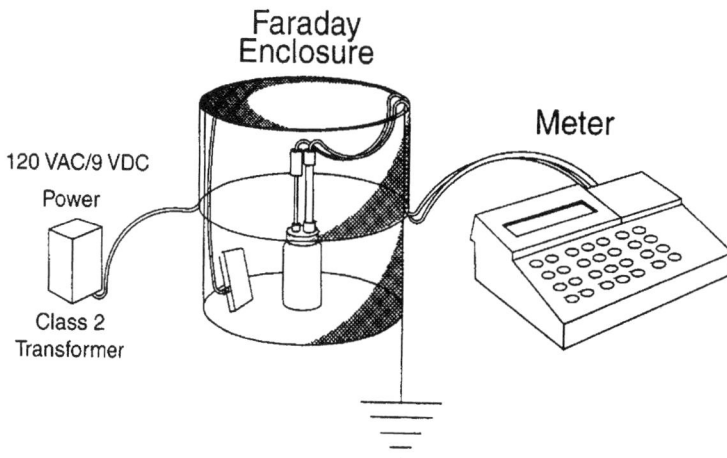

Figure 7 Schematic drawing of experimental setup used in simultaneous exposure to a device and pH plus temperature measurements.

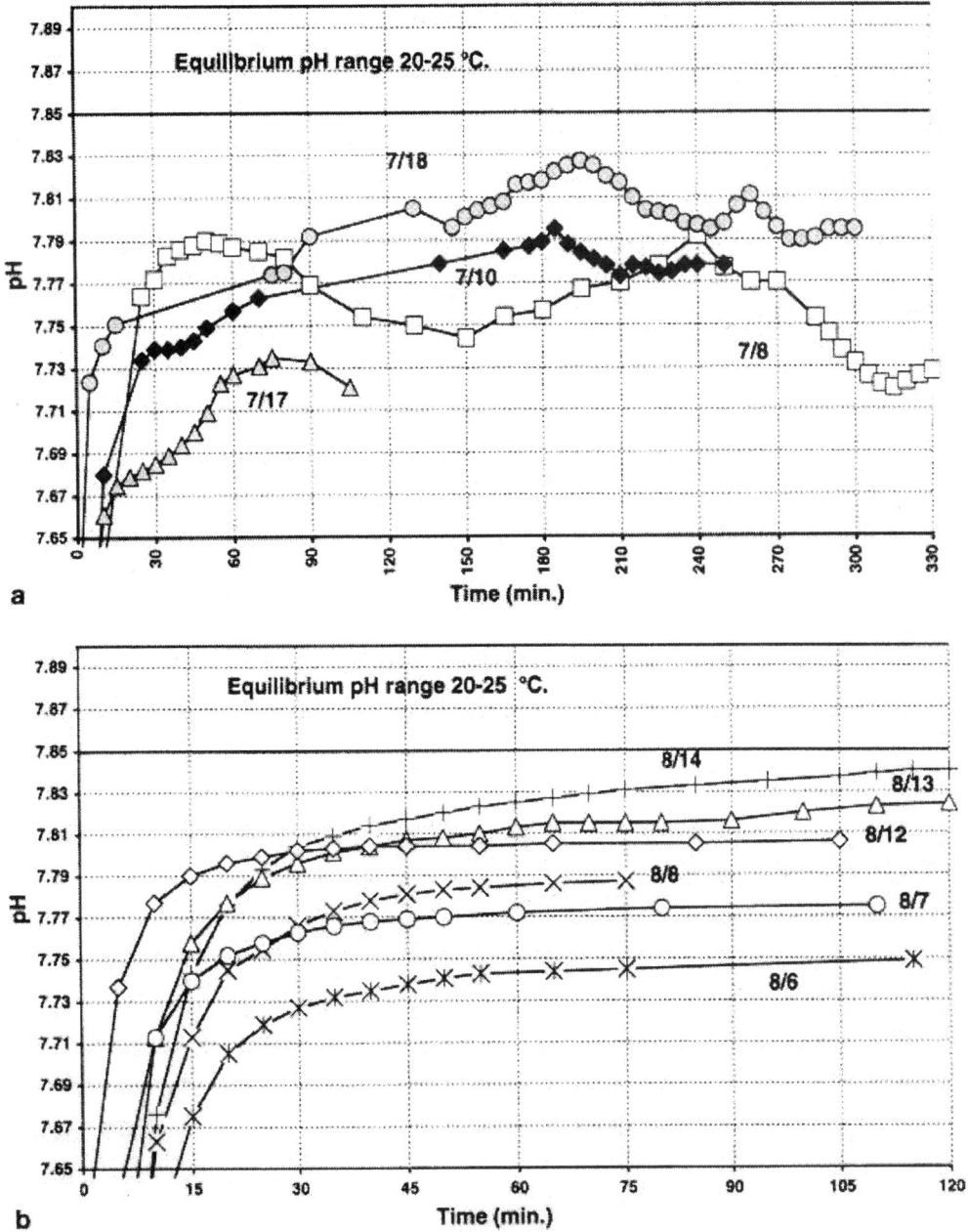

Figure 8   pH vs. time for 50/50 dilution of Castle Rock Water with purified H$_2$O. (a) Measurements were made on a solution that had been exposed to an *unimprinted* three-oscillator device on 7/7/97. Note irregular pH behavior and oscillation of pH in the days following exposure. (b) Measurements were made on a solution that had been exposed to the *imprinted* three-oscillator device on 8/5/97. Note monotonically increasing pH behavior and steady increase in pH in the days following exposure.

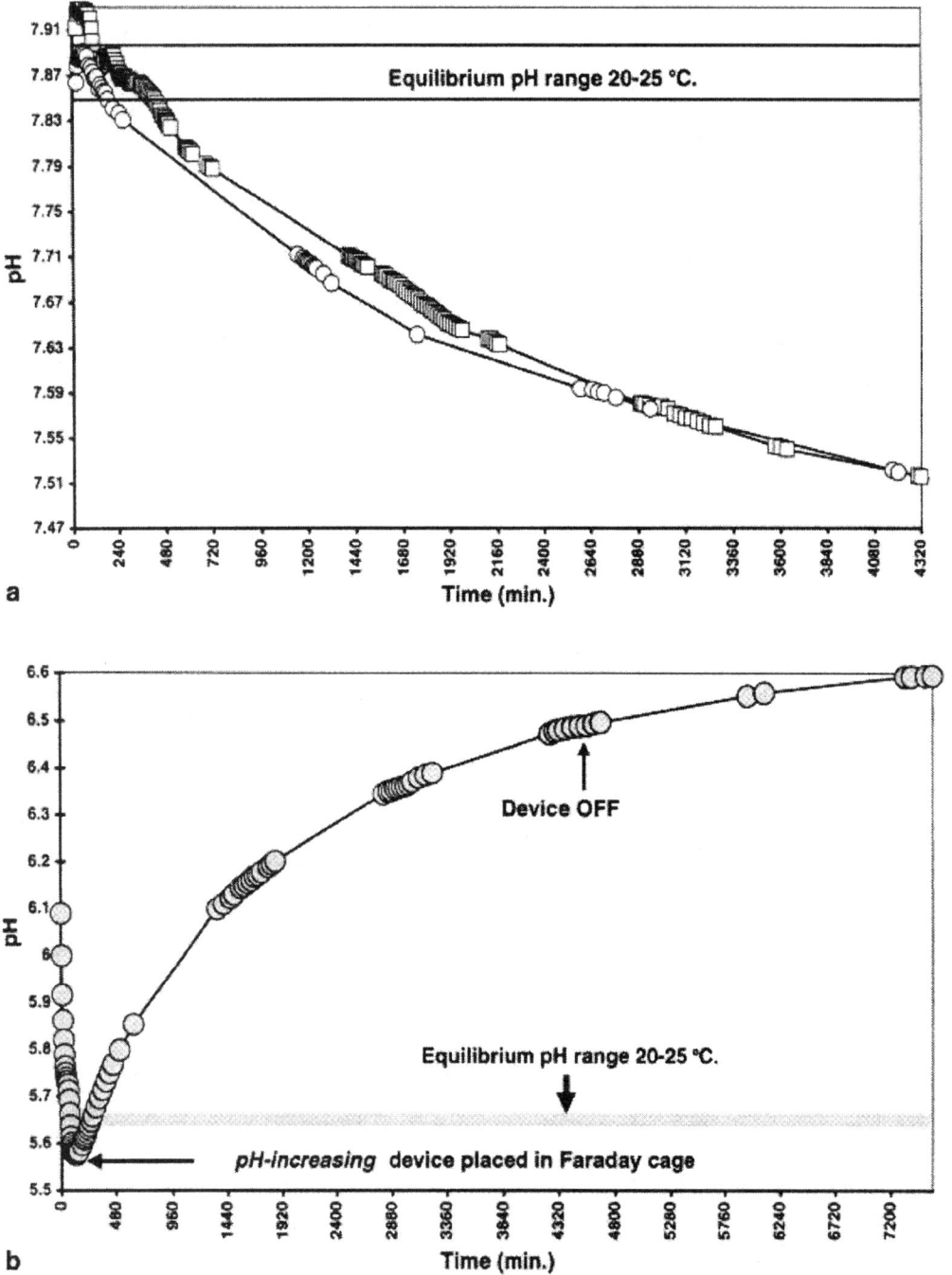

Figure 9 (a) pH vs. time for 50/50 dilution of Castle Rock Water with purified H$_2$O. Measurement of pH was done simultaneously with exposure to the imprinted *pH-lowering* device for the data points depicted by square but only after exposure for the data points depicted by circles. (b) pH vs. time of pure water in equilibrium with laboratory air during exposure to *pH-increasing* IIED.

person holding their hands about 6 in. from the device and *intending* to increase the count rate. Over a 5-min/period of such intending, the number of recorded pulses often went from zero to the 50,000 range.

If the subject's hands were not held near the device but the intention was still to increase the count rate, total counts could still be increased from zero to a range of 10,000 to 20,000 counts within 5 min. If, during the same type of experiment, the subject's intention was directed *away* from the device by being focused on a different mental task, no change in the count rate occurred, and the total counts was still zero at the end of 5 min even though the subject's hands were straddling the device.

From these results, I deduced that

1. People manifest a heretofore undetected energy that has the property of increasing both electron microavalanche size and number in a nearby gas discharge system.
2. A person can direct the flow of this energy in a chosen direction by their mind.
3. The mind–electron interaction can be effective over appreciable distances.

Elmer Green and his associates at the Menninger Clinic devised a simulated healing experiment involving an accomplished healer in a specially designed environment in a larger

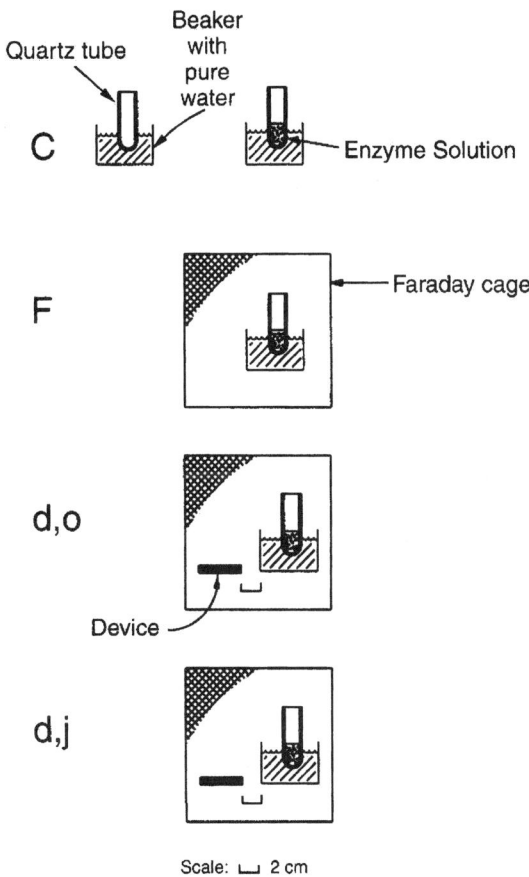

Figure 10 Schematic drawing of the side-by-side experimental configuration for the four simultaneous ALP treatments.

room (29,30) (see Fig. 5). The healer, wired to a variety of electrophysiological measurement instruments, stood or sat on an electrically insulated framework placed within four large, square copper walls (one in front, one behind, one above, and one below). Electrically insulated electrometers simultaneously recorded the voltages of these four walls plus that from an electrode placed on the healer's earlobe.

Instead of the 10- or 15-mV baseline reading with 1-mV ripples that are typical of the human body, it was observed that the healer's body voltage often plunged by 30 to 300 V and then returned to baseline within 0.5 to 10 s. This astoundingly large voltage pulse is about 100,000 times normal. Correlated pulses of 1 to 5 V appeared on each of the four copper walls. In a 30-min simulated healing session, the healer manifested 15 of these anomalously large pulses.

From this experiment, I generated a theoretical model (31) of a nondirectly observable subtle energy pulse emitted from some locations in the healer's body which was transduced through a series of stages and manifested as an electric dipole pulse at a specific location in the healer's body (see Fig. 6). With this model and the experimental data, I was able to make a quantitative analysis from the 15 pulses (31).

In 13 of the 15 pulses, the place of origin in the healer was the lower abdomen. The dipole was predicted to extend from the ear (negative charge end) to the feet (positive charge end), and it required quite small current flows for a very short time to achieve the result (~5 nA flowing for ~1 s). Such a current flow is much less than that typically observed when two different acupuncture points on the body are connected.

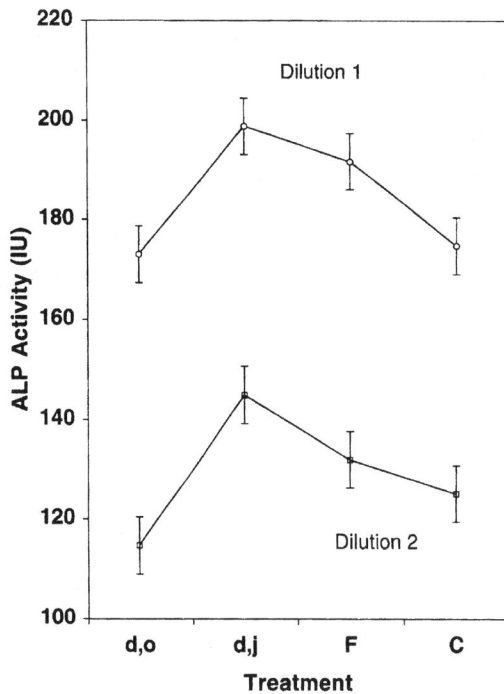

Figure 11 Statistical means data on ALP activity for the four simultaneous treatments (dilution 1 is 100 ml ALP solution plus 150 ml purified water; dilution 2 is 100 ml ALP solution plus 200 ml purified water).

For the other two anomalous pulses, it was necessary to propose the formation of two simultaneous electric dipole pulses to account for the different type of data observed. From this data, the location of the second dipole was predicted to be in the head (31).

What I deduced from this study was that (1) the healer's intention to heal can manifest, ultimately, as large, observable electric voltage pulses in physical reality, (2) some medium exists that couples the non directly observable subtle energy to an observable physical energy, and (3) a precise mathematical analysis can be generated to concretize this elusive concept.

From what is to come in Sec. VI, a hypothesized subtle energy field, χ, is pulsed in time. This is transduced to a magnetic vector potential, A, profile in time of a gaussianlike shape. From our conventional U(1) EM gauge symmetry equations, this leads to the type of E-field pulse illustrated in Fig. 6(c) which, in turn, causes ion movement in the electrolyte of the body to create a charge dipole of the type needed to rationalize the experimental data.

IV. SOME ROBUST EFFECTS OF HUMAN INTENTION ON SPACE CONDITIONING

For the past several years, my colleagues and I have been conducting specific target experiments on the use of Intention Imprinted Electrical Devices (IIEDs) to influence both

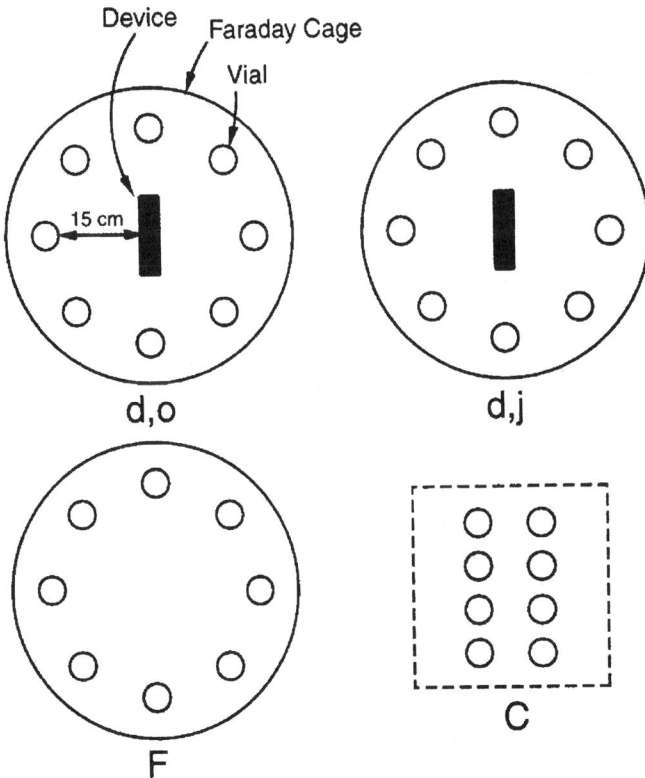

Figure 12 Experimental configuration for the simultaneous, four-treatment, side-by-side, in vivo larval development study.

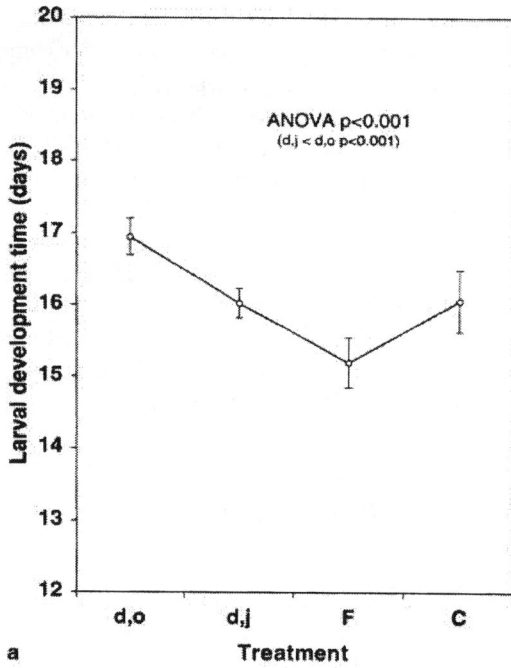

a

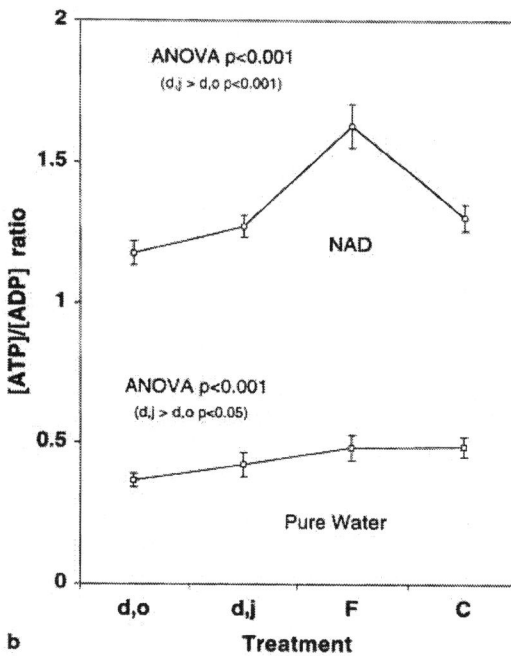

b

Figure 13   (a) Means for larval development time vs. treatment and (b) [ATP]/[ADP] ratio for the larvae vs. treatment (means).

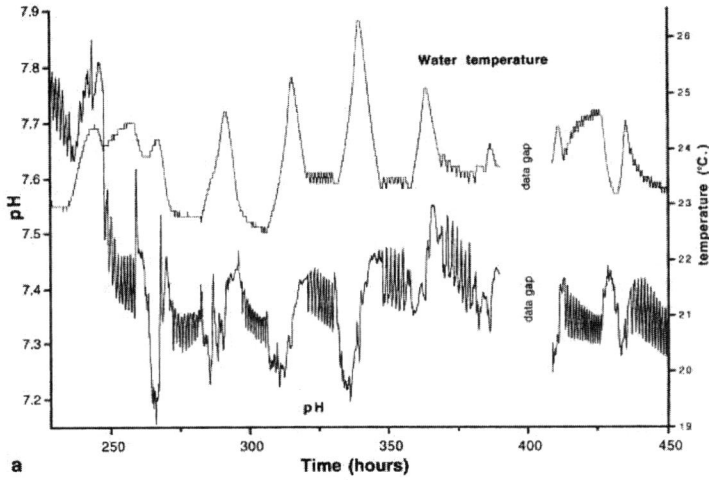

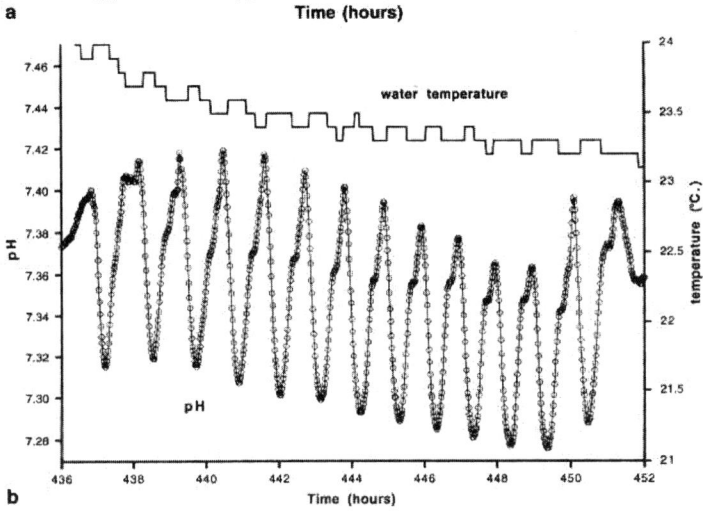

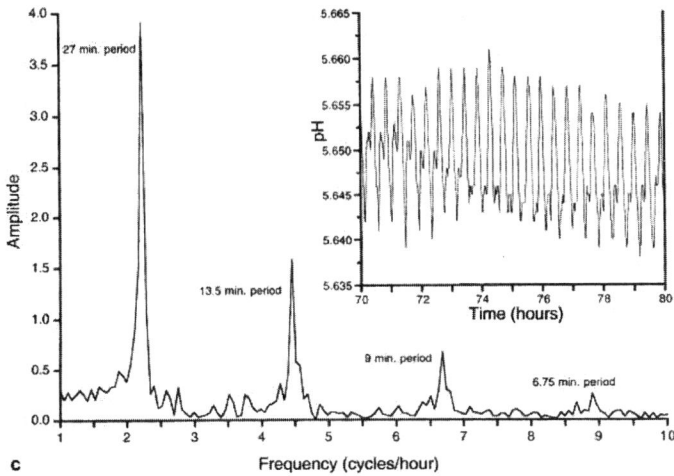

Figure 14 (a) pH and temperature changed with time for pure water containing fine-grained $ZnCO_3$ particulates. The plots reveal both long t_L and short t_s periods of undulations. (b) An expanded short interval from (a) illustrating the regularity of the t_s oscillations. Note the inverse correlation between pH oscillations and temperature fluctuations. (c) Amplitude spectra data via Fourier transform for part of the real-time data set (shown in inset) depicted in the lowest plot in Figure 15.

inanimate and animate materials with respect to some of their properties (2). For each target experiment, one starts with two identical simple electronic devices housed in 17.8 cm × 7.6 cm × 2.5 cm black plastic boxes. One isolates them from each other by first wrapping them in aluminum foil and then storing them in separate electrically grounded Faraday cages (FCs). One is left as is and is designated as the "control." The other is taken out of its FC, unwrapped, and "charged" with the specific intention or the particular target experiment under consideration. It is then rewrapped in Al foil and returned to its FC.

This charging process involved the services of four highly qualified meditators to "imprint" the device with the specific intention following a specific protocol (see the appendix of section IA in Ref. 2). Then, on separate days, the control device and the imprinted device were shipped via Federal Express about 3000 km to a laboratory where the actual target experiments were conducted by others.

When not in use, the devices were always wrapped in Al foil and stored in individual FCs. This was found to be necessary because without it, even if the devices were separated by 100 m and in the off state, the control device gradually became imprinted with that specific intention and we eventually lost our "control." Following this isolation procedure, we could maintain the imprint charge in the active device for ~4 months before reimprinting was felt to be needed.

A. Target Experiment 1

Here, the specific intention was to either increase or decrease the pH of aqueous solutions and purified water (ASTM type 1) by one full pH unit. Separate IIEDs were needed for

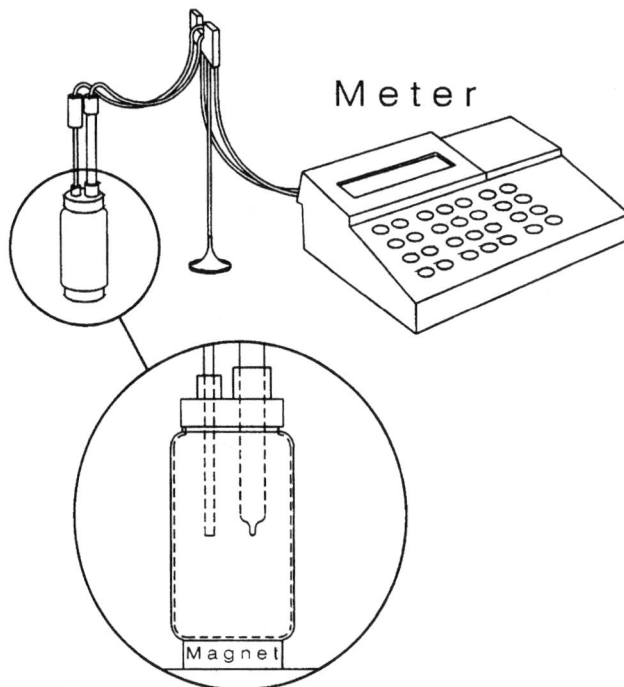

Figure 15 Conditioned locale pH changes with time for purified water with either the north pole or south pole of a DC magnetic field aligned vertically upwards (at 100 and 500 G).

$\Delta pH = +1$ and $\Delta pH = -1$. Thus, considering both, a swing of hydrogen ion concentration by a factor of 10^2 was attempted without any intentional chemical additions except those entering via contact with the local air atmosphere. The experimental setup used is shown in Fig. 7 where a modern, high-quality pH meter (accuracy of ± 0.01 pH-unit, resolution of 0.001 pH-unit) and a high-quality temperature probe (accuracy of $\pm 0.012°C$, resolution of $0.001°C$) were utilized. The device was merely placed ~ 15.25 cm (6 in.) from the water and turned on (total radiated electromagnetic energy $< 10^{-6}$ W).

Figure 8 demonstrates an obvious differnce in the coherence state for one of the aqueous solutions, exposed for 2 h to either an unimprinted device (Fig. 8a) or to an imprinted device (Fig. 8b) and then monitored for several subsequent days (2). For the unimprinted device the subsequent pH readings are erratic while, for the imprinted device, the pH readings monotonically vary over time and step in an orderly fashion from day to day. The readings were taken from $\sim 9:00$ A.M. to 11:00 A.M. every day and start each day with the buffer calibration. Later, in a separate experiment, the pH electrode was placed in the test solution which initially drives the pH downward to equilibrate with the solution (initial transient deleted).

Figure 9 demonstrates results with two different IIEDs, one with the intention to *decrease* the pH by one full unit (Fig. 9a) and the other with the intention to *increase* the pH by one full pH unit (Fig. 9b). The tests were made using different solutions so the equilibrium pH ranges were quite different. The purified water was ASTM type 1 (resistivity ≥ 18.2 MΩ cm, TOC < 5 ppb) water, while the Castle Rock water is a naturally occurring spring water with total dissolved solids (TDS) of about 95 mg/l and $[Ca^{2+}]/[Mg^{2+}] = 2.0$. In these par-

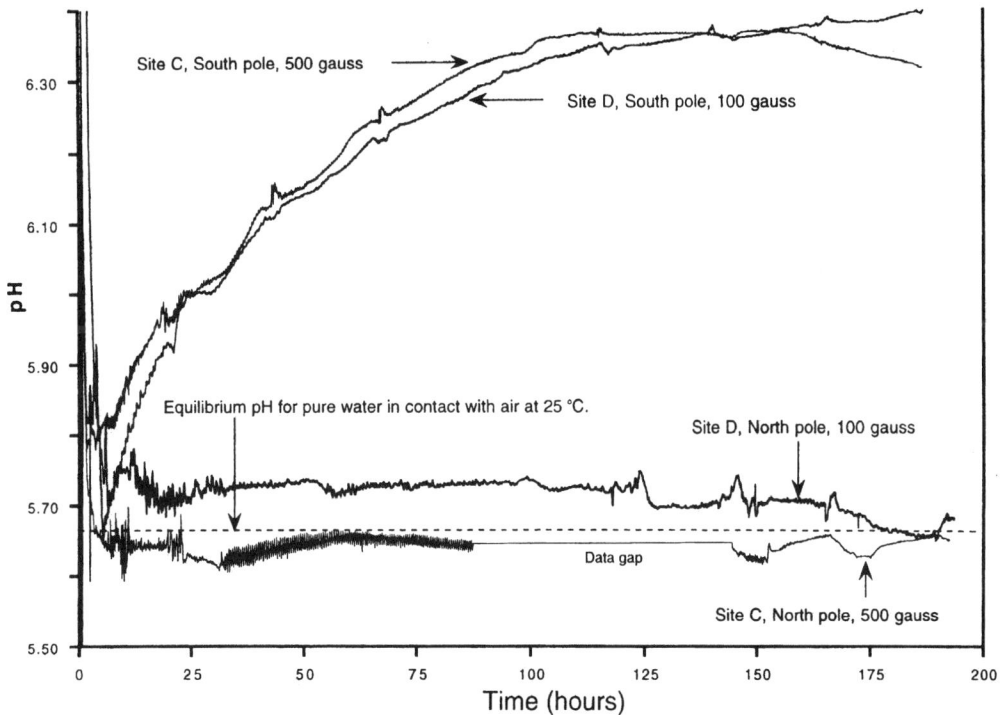

Figure 16 Experimental setup for testing changes due to a DC magnet placed under the water vessel with either the N pole or the S pole aligned upwards.

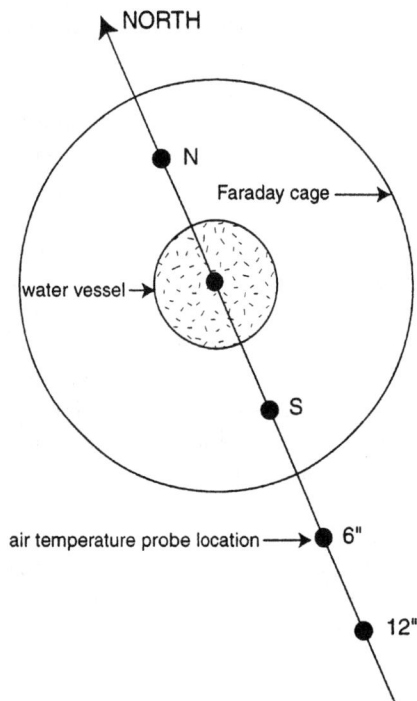

Figure 17 Schematic illustration of air and water temperature probe locations relative to a centrally located water vessel in an electrically grounded Faraday cage.

ticular experiments, the pH change over ∼5 days (7200 min) was ∼−0.5 pH units for the pH-decreasing IIED and ∼+1 pH units for the pH-increasing IIED, relative to the equilibrium pH range at 20–25°C for each experiment. When one uses a control device (unimprinted) instead of an IIED, the pH tends to stay in the equilibrium range or very close to it.

B. Target Experiments 2 and 3

To show the scope of this new potential technology, I briefly demonstrate its application in the area of biological materials (both inert and living) as well. Details, only of interest to biologists, are provided in Ref. 2.

Figure 18 (a) Pure water with zinc carbonate particulates in vessel in Faraday cage. Simultaneous measurement of air and water temperature plus pH in the Fig. 17 configuration on 5/12/99 to 5/13/99. Note the precise frequency correlation for the three variables. (b) Four real-time temperature vs. time plots for simultaneous air temperature measurements made at the N, S, and 6-in. positions of Fig. 17 plus the water temperature inside the vessel (5/11/99). (c) Fourier transformed amplitude spectra data for a 8.5-h interval of (b) (between hour 9 and 17.5). The fundamental period is 46.5 min and five harmonics can be observed. (d) Fourier transform comparison of both water T-oscillation and pH-oscillation data in the water vessel of Fig. 17 on 5/10/99. Real-time oscillation data shown in inset. The fundamental period is 36.6 min and three harmonics can be discerned.

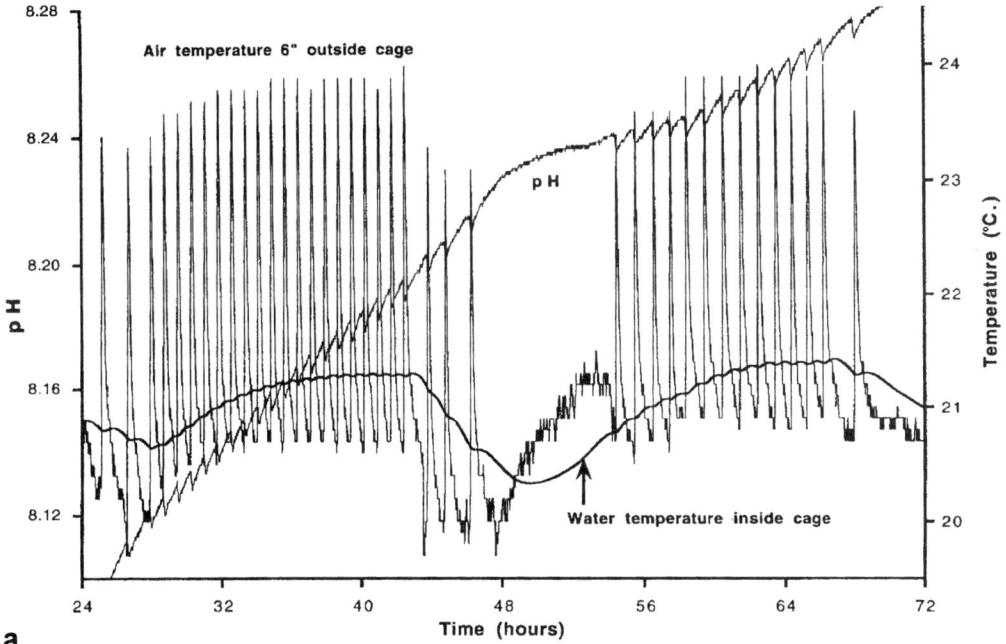

a

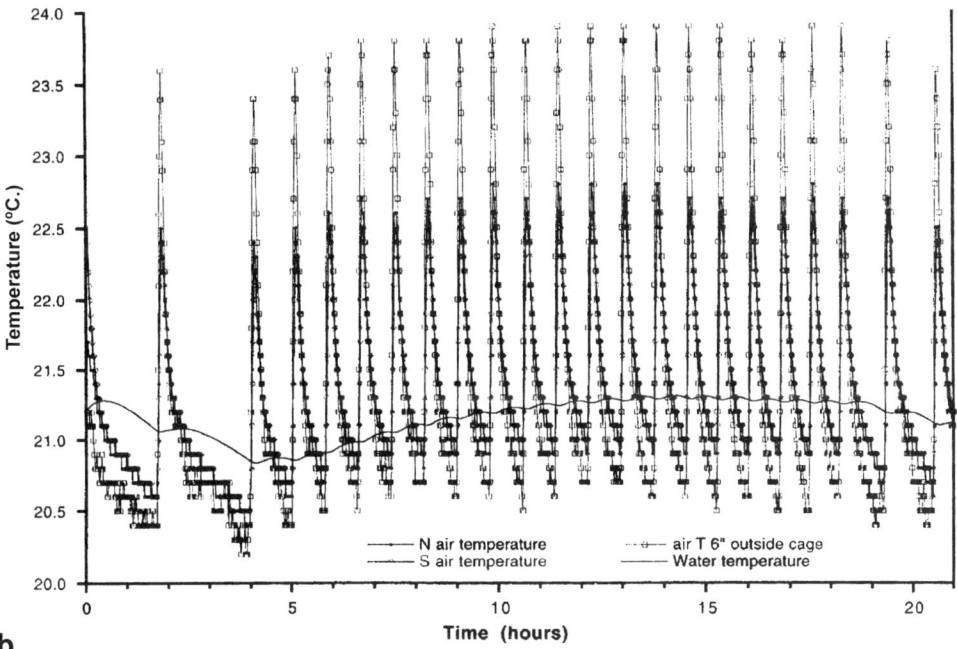

b

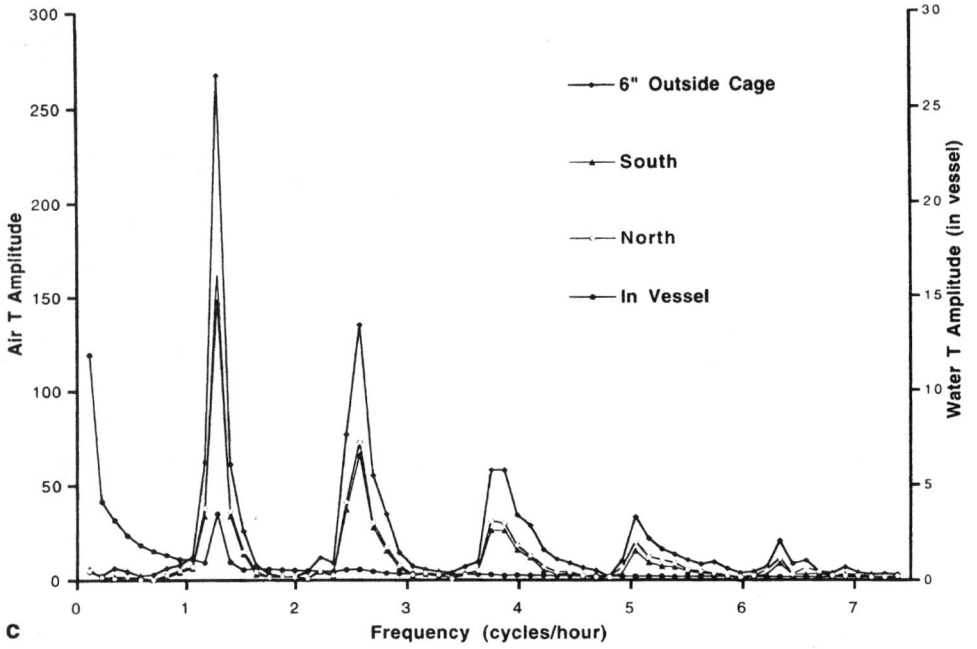

c

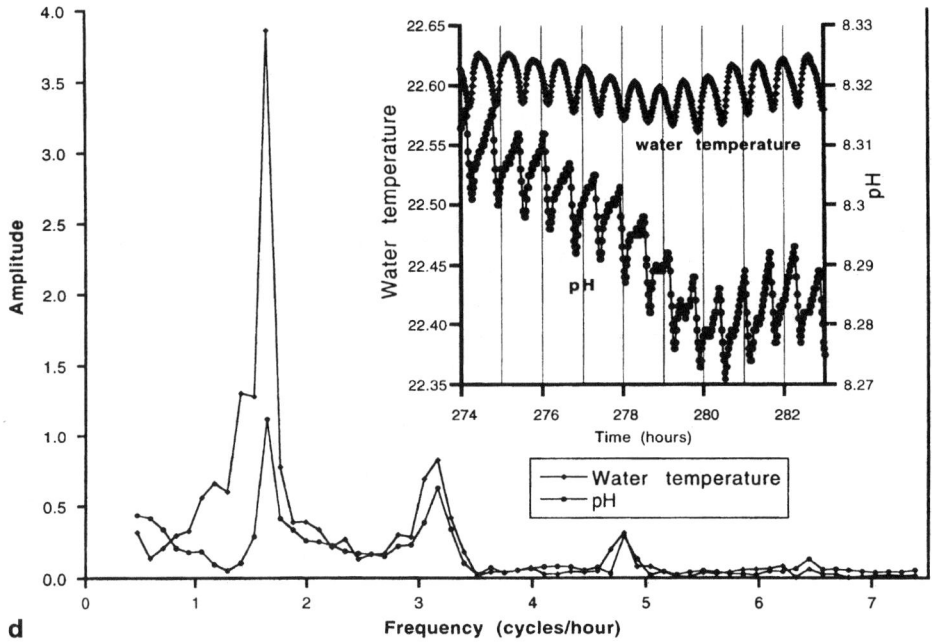

d

Figure 18 Continued.

For target experiment 2, the specific IIED intention was to increase the in vitro thermodynamic activity of a specific liver enzyme, alkaline phosphatase (ALP). Four simultaneous, side-by-side variants were conducted on the same shelf in an incubator (held at 4°C) as shown in Fig. 10. Comparisons could then be readily made between the control ALP solution (*C*) and

1. ALP solution placed in a small but otherwise empty grounded FC (*F*)
2. The same as (1) but with an activated *imprinted* device (*d, j*) present
3. The same as (1) but with an activated *unimprinted* device (*d, o*) present

The first comparison, (*C*) with (*F*), allows one to assess the effect of the broad band ambient EMFs in the incubator on the ALP activity. The second comparison, (*F*) with (*d, o*), allows one to assess the effect of low power (less than 1 μW) and specific frequency (three frequencies in the 1–10-MHz range) EMFs on ALP activity. The third comparison, (*d, j*) with (*d, o*), allows one to assess the effect of imprinted human intention, at constant EMF output, on ALP activity. In addition, simultaneous correlations between any and all of these different experimental states are available.

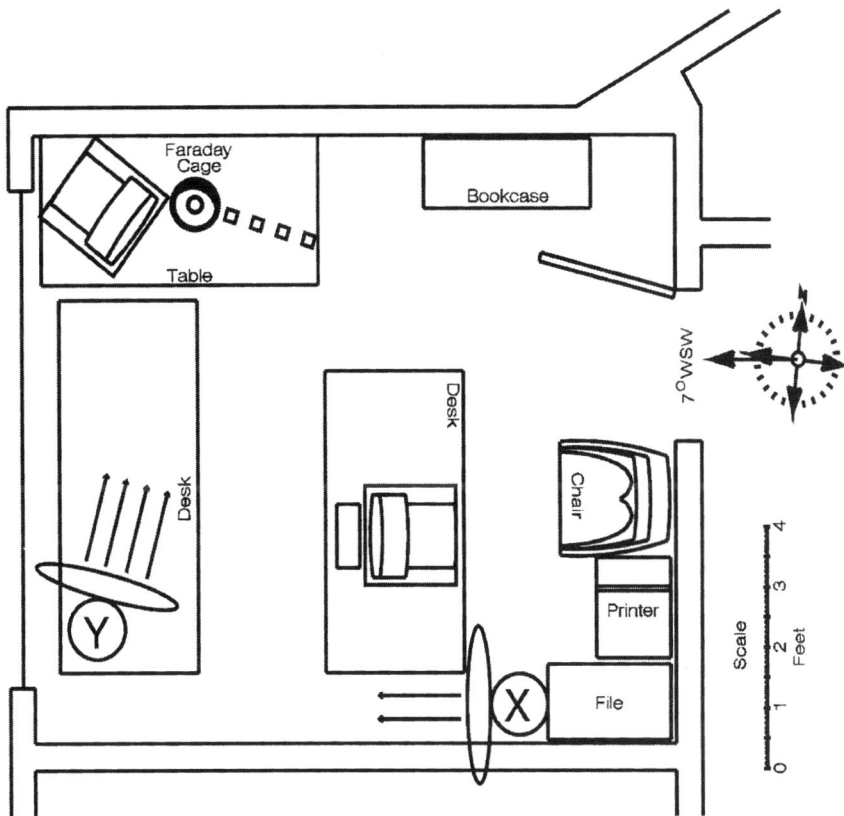

Figure 19   Forced convection experiment using a mechanical fan to perturb the air around a series of aligned temperature measurement probes. Fan location positions (X is on the floor, Y is on a desk) relative to the water vessel in a Faraday cage on upper left table top and a line of temperature probes (small boxes) 6 in. (15.24 cm) apart.

The results of this experiment, in terms of means with their standard deviations, are provided in Fig. 11. The data were assessed via the ANOVA statistical procedure, and based on this, pairwise comparison with Tukey post hoc tests were examined. Visual inspection of Fig. 11 and the ANOVA indicated that both the treatment and the dilution significantly modified ALP activity. The treatment rankings for both dilutions were $(d, j) > (F) > (C) > (d, o)$ and the Tukey post hoc comparisons between treatments indicated that

1. (d, j) was significantly ($p < 0.001$) greater than (d, o) and also significantly ($p < 0.005$) greater than (C).
2. (F) was significantly ($p < 0.011$) greater than (C).

For target experiment 3, the specific IIED intention was to increase the in vivo ratio of ATP to ADP in developing fruit fly (*Drosophila melanogaster*) larvae so as to significantly reduce their development time to the adult fly stage. Once again, we incorporated four simultaneous experimental variants in a side-by-side positioning on a laboratory bench top (at 18°C and 55% relative humidity) as indicated in Fig. 12. The four treatments investigated were as follows:

1. (C): the control culture of 30 larvae (0–4 h old) transferred to a single vial containing nonstressful food
2. (F): a similar culture inside an otherwise empty Faraday cage
3. (d, o): culture as in (2) but containing an *unimprinted* device in the "on" state
4. (d, j): culture as in (2) but containing an *imprinted* device in the "on" state

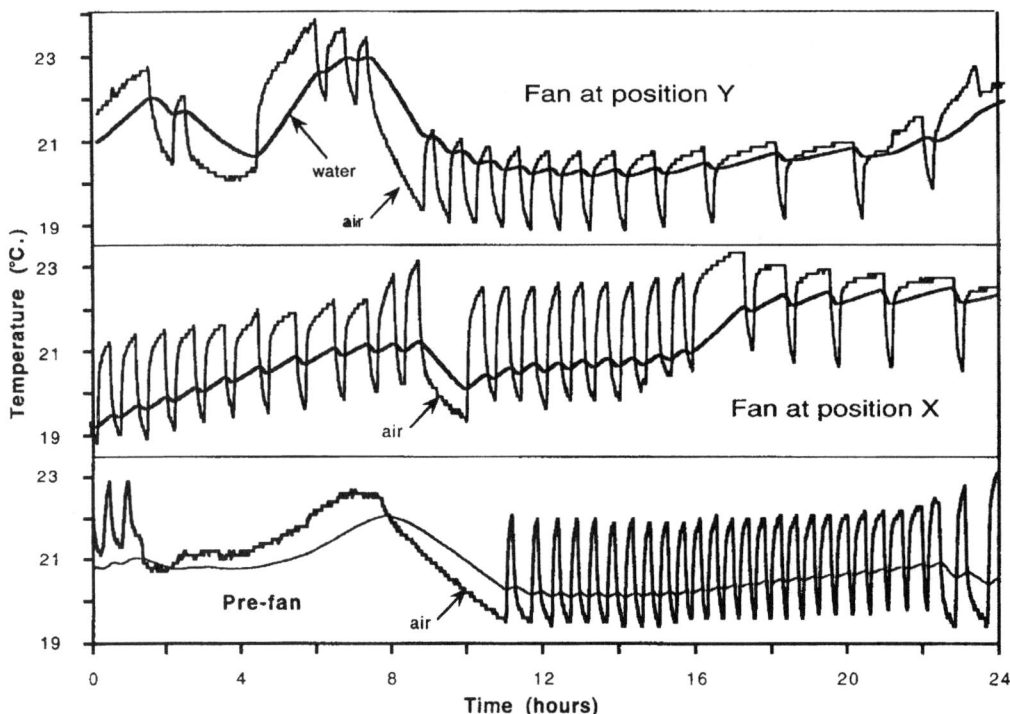

Figure 20 Temperature oscillation in air [1 ft (30.5 cm) outside FC] and water (inside FC), with and without the fan operating.

Our larval assay used high-performance liquid chromatography (HPLC) to measure changes in levels of ATP, ADP, and AMP present in larval homogenate samples. From this, the [ATP]/[ADP] ratio was readily determined. Larval development time (LDT) is defined as the time taken for half of the surviving adults to emerge. We assessed LDT and [ATP]/[ADP] ratio in a total study involving approximately 10,000 larvae and 7000 adult flies over an 8-month period (2). For the [ATP]/[ADP] ratio assessment, we utilized a specific added amount of either nicotinamide adenine dinucleotide (NAD) or purified water to the larval homogenate samples for a set time period.

The experimental data is presented in Fig. 13 as means with standard deviations arising from ANOVA statistical procedures and Tukey post hoc tests. For both results, the ANOVA gives $p < 0.001$ overall. In terms of our basic hypothesis concerning the influence of intention-augmented EMFs on larval fitness, this data provides robust support from LDT with $(d, j) < (d, o)$ at the $p < 0.001$ level of statistical significance. The unexpected findings that $(F) < (C)$ at $p < 0.001$ and that $(F) << (d, o)$ at $p < 0.0001$ illustrates that both random ambient EMFs and specific high-frequency EMFs (even at quite low power levels) are significant stressors for *D. melanogaster*. The finding that the [ATP]/[ADP] ratio practically mirrors the LDT data for the added NAD case, at a high Pearson correlation value, strongly supports the connection between energy availability to the cells and

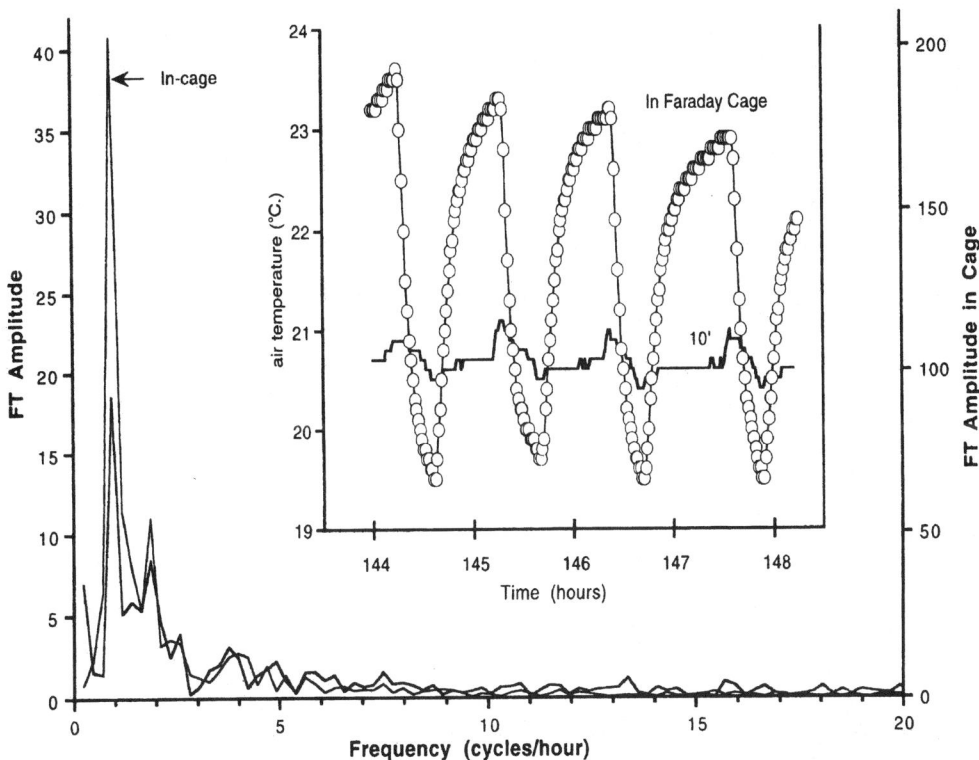

Figure 21 Amplitude spectra from Fourier analysis of air, T-oscillation real-time data (see inset) both in the FC and 10 ft (3.05 m) away outside the closed door of Fig. 19. Note the high correlation between the oscillations measured at locations separated by 10 ft (3.05 m), a closed door and a FC.

organism fitness as well as the profound importance of NAD to overall metabolic activity. Finally, it is important to note that, even for the added pure water case, the different treatments gave an overall statistically significant effect ($p < 0.001$).

C. Target Experiment 4

During the course of the preceding experiments, it began to be apparent that some type of "conditioning" process was going on in the particular locale associated with continued use of the IIEDs in that locale. In the purified water experiments locale, after some incubation period, we began to observe oscillations (2) in air temperature, water temperature, water pH, and water electrical conductivity whose amplitude often exceeded 10^2 times the sensitivity of our detection systems (see Fig. 14). In other nearby locales (~6–15 m away), where no previous IIED studies had taken place, no such oscillations were observed.

In Fig. 14a, one sees the presence of both highly periodic short-period (<2 h) and long-period (>20 h) oscillations in both pH and temperature. Figure 14b is an expanded scale view of one oscillation train from Fig. 14a (near the end) to illustrate the "lawful" nature of the pH waveform. These oscillations are among the largest amplitude pH oscillations we recorded. Figure 14c provides the amplitude spectrum for a pH-oscillation wavetrain from Fig. 14a which demonstrates how periodic even the lowest amplitude pH oscillations can be.

To probe the nature of this conditioning, we conducted a DC magnetic field polarity experiment using the experimental setup shown in Fig. 16. With this configuration, one can

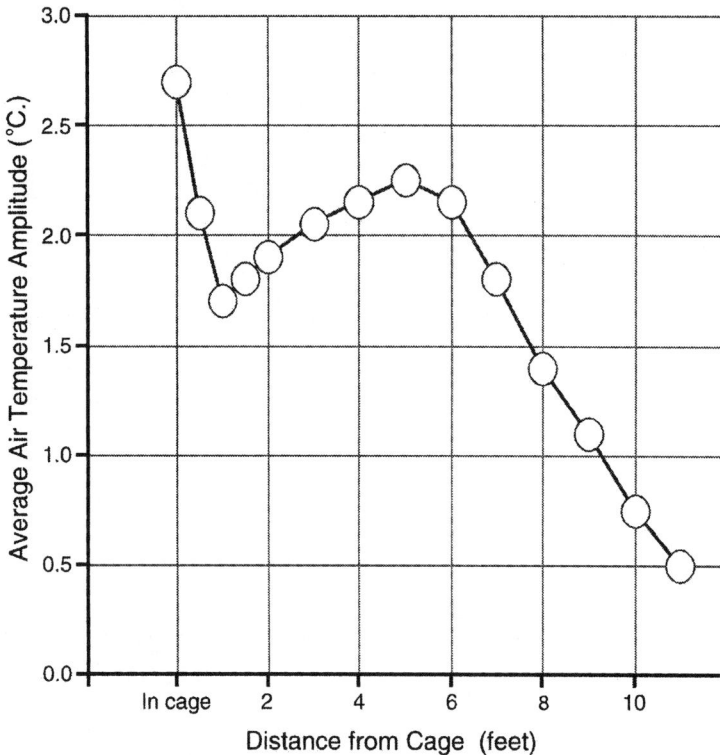

Figure 22 Composite amplitude vs. distance plot for air, T oscillations in the Fig. 17 geometry (between August and September 1999).

readily measure any water pH changes associated with the north pole vs. the south pole pointing upwards without altering the basic cylindrical symmetry of the field. When one conducts this pH measurement experiment in a typical laboratory environment were no conditioning has occurred, one observes two things:

1. There is no measurable difference between the N-pole up case and the S-pole up case.
2. There is no measurable pH change in the water for either field polarity (for field strengths ≤ 500 G).

On the other hand, when one makes such measurements in a "conditioned" locale, the results are remarkably different. There, one generally finds a marked difference for $\Delta pH = pH(S) - pH(N)$. Figure 16 demonstrates an example wherein ΔpH grows in magnitude with the passage of time to attain a maximum value of ~ 0.60 pH units.

To demonstrate both simultaneous water and air temperature (T) oscillations plus the correlation between them, a Faraday cage with a central water vessel was set up in one conditioned space (purified water plus 1 gm of fine-grained $ZnCO_3$ powder, surface area = 21.4 m2/g, was added to 250 ml of ASTM-type 1 purified water in a polypropylene bottle). High-resolution digital thermometers were located with the local geometry shown in Fig. 17. Figure 18a shows the air T oscillations at the 15.25 cm (6″) location outside the cage plus the water T and water pH in the vessel located inside the cage. Figure 18b is an expanded view of the data collected just before that shown in Figure 18a while Figure 18c shows the amplitude

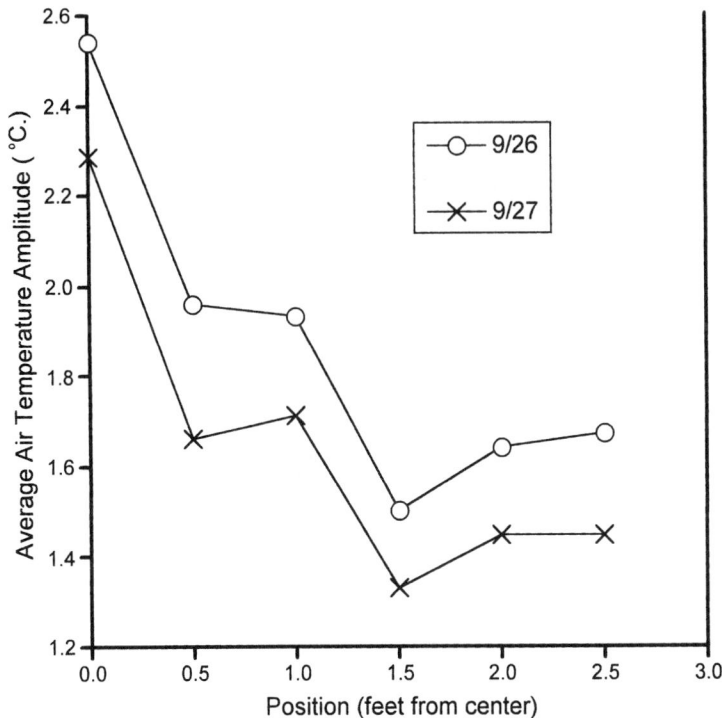

Figure 23 Average air, T-oscillation amplitude vs. distance plot for Fig. 17 geometry 1 and 2 days after removal of the FC and water vessel (the former FC edge was located at 0.5 ft).

spectrum for a portion of this data (from hour 9 to hour 17.5 in Fig. 18b). These air T oscillations are huge (~230 times our best measurement accuracy and ~3500 times the resolution), and all have the same waveform. Figure 18d illustrates the comparative amplitude spectra data for simultaneous T and pH oscillations taken in this vessel of water two days earlier (oscillation data shown in inset). Again, the same wave shape (revealed by the nesting of the amplitude spetra) is exhibited for these two very different material properties.

To illustrate that the Fig. 18 results were not generated by some type of natural convection phenomenon, a mechanical fan experiment was conducted in a strongly conditioned space. The focus of this experiment was to see if the air T oscillations would be strongly influenced by the forced convection from a mechanical fan. The furniture arrangement in the conditioned room, including both the location of the water vessel inside its Faraday cage (similar to Fig. 17 configuration) adjacent to a monitoring computer and the two fan locations, X (one on the floor) and Y (on a desktop) is shown in Fig. 19. Temperature measurements outside of the Faraday cage occurred at 15.25-cm (6-in.) intervals out to 3.35 m (11 ft). High-resolution digital thermometers (resolution = 0.001°C) were used in the water and at 30.5 cm (1 ft) outside the cage. Lower resolution, digital thermometers (resolution = 0.1°C) were used in the air inside the cage and at all other locations outside the cage. All measurements were computer monitored.

Earlier measurements had shown that the major floor–ceiling temperature gradients occurred between the floor and ~1 m (3–4 ft) above the floor; thus, we started with the fan at position X (on the floor) and operated it for 55 h. Later, the fan was moved to position Y

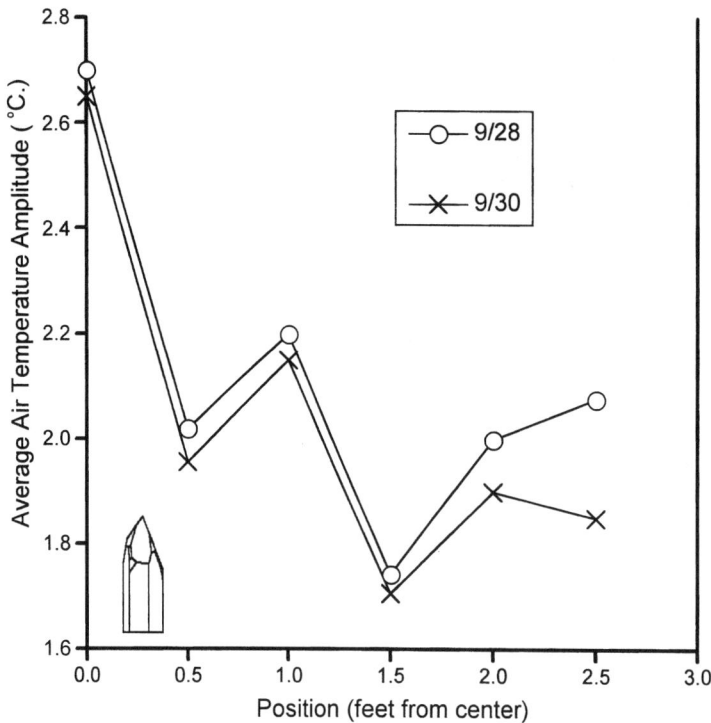

Figure 24 Average air, T-oscillation amplitude vs. distance plot on the phantom profile immediately after placing a natural quartz crystal (*c* axis up) between position 0.0 and 0.5 ft as shown.

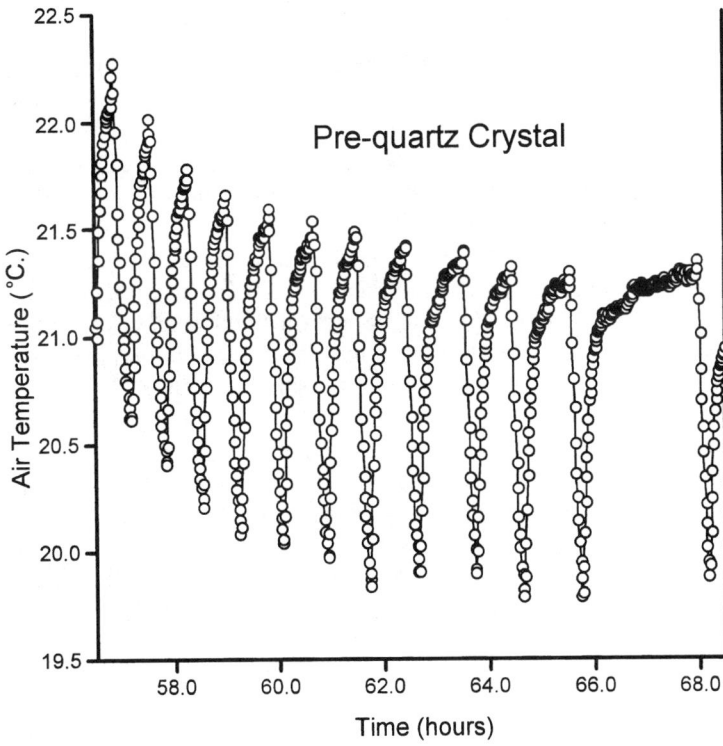

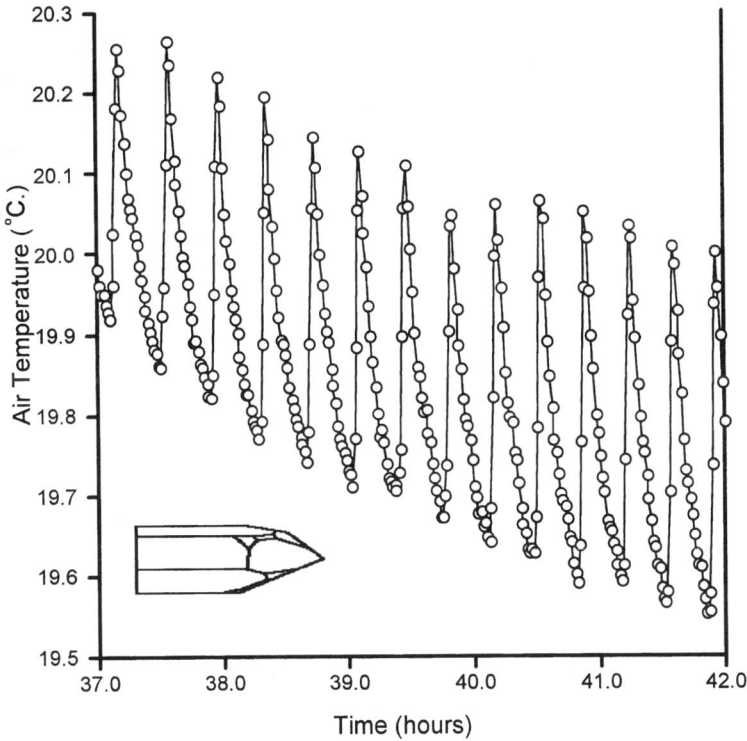

Figure 25 Comparison of air, T-oscillation amplitude, frequency, and waveform between the pre-quartz crystal condition and the condition immediately after changing the orientation of the quartz crystal to the *c*-axis horizontal position.

and operated for 42 h. For comparison purposes, a 24-h period, real-time record of the T oscillations for the three cases of (1) no fan, (2) fan at X, and (3) fan at Y are given in Fig. 20. From Fig. 20, it seems clear that these T oscillations neither cease nor change in a significant way due to the operation of the fan. It is also clear that the total oscillation ΔT excursion is a large percentage (sometimes 100%) of the total diurnal temperature variation in this room.

Since the 3-m (10-ft) measuring point was in the hallway outside the office depicted in Fig. 19, it was possible to close the office door and compare the T oscillations both inside the Faraday cage with those outside in the hallway. It was apparent that the air T-oscillation amplitudes did decline significantly with distance from the FC. However, they were still measurable more than 3 m away. The inset in Fig. 21 shows the simultaneous, real-time data at these two locations. The Fourier analysis for these two oscillation data sets reveals that they share the same basic wave harmonics, despite the fact that they were separated by a 3-m (10-ft) distance, a closed door and a Faraday cage. Clearly, it is predominantly something other than standard air that is being monitored here (perhaps the vacuum phase within the air molecules?)!

The variation of T-oscillation amplitude from inside the FC to a point out in the hall ~11 ft away is shown in Fig. 22. This is certainly a very anomalous profile with the secondary maximum being prominently present. This profile certainly establishes the water vessel and its surrounding FC as a type of "source" for the temperature oscillations. After removal of this D-space "conditioning center", the air T-oscillation amplitude profile remained and only decayed over a period of weeks to months. Figure 23 displays the "phantom" profile, a very anomalous result indeed (2). When a natural quartz crystal (6 in. long in the c-axis direction and 3 in. in diameter) was placed near the now absent "source" center with the c axis upwards, a sharpened definition and small increase of the phantom T-oscillation amplitude profile occurred (see Fig. 24), with no meaningful change in the shape of the T-oscillation waveform. However, when the crystal was rotated to lay with a prism face flat on the table and its c axis aligned with the row of thermometers and its apex pointing away from the center position, *immediately* the T-oscillation amplitude waveform changed dramatically (see Fig. 25). The oscillation amplitude decreased by about a factor of 4–5, the oscillation frequency increased by a factor of 2–3 and the oscillation wave shape became inverted.

This very anomalous behavior led us to strongly propose that we were *not* dealing with properties of D space coarse particulate substance here but rather with the R space fine information wave substance from the coarsest level of the vacuum.

ACKNOWLEDGMENTS

I wish to thank Ditron LLC and The Samueli Institute for partial support of this work.

REFERENCES

1. Tiller WA. Science and Human Transformation: Subtle Energies, Intentionality and Consciousness. Walnut Creek: Pavior Publishing, 1997.
2. Tiller WA, Dibble WE Jr, Kohane MJ. Conscious Acts of Creation: The Emergence of a New Physics. Walnut Creek: Pavior Publishing, 2001.
3. Eisenberg RM. Fundamentals of Modern Physics. New York: John Wiley & Sons, 1961:140–146.
4. 't Hooft G. Gauge theories of forces between elementary particles. Scientific American 1980; 242(6):104.
5. Barrett TW. Comments on the Harmuth Ansatz: Use of a magnetic current density in the

calculation of the propagation velocity of signals by amended Maxwell theory. IEEE Transactions on Electromagnetic Compatibility 1988; 30:419.

6. Tiller WA, Dibble WE Jr, Kohane MJ. Conscious Acts of Creation: The Emergence of a New Physics. Walnut Creek: Pavior Publishing, 2001:170.

7. Tiller WA, Dibble WE Jr, Kohane MJ. Conscious Acts of Creation: The Emergence of a New Physics. Walnut Creek: Pavior Publishing, 2001:248–249 and 302–304.

8. Bernal JD. Proc Roy Soc 1964; A 280:299.

9. Ludwig R. Water: From Clusters to the Bulk. Angew Chem Int 2001; 40:1808–1827.

10. Tiller WA. The Science of Crystallization: Microscopic Interfacial Phenomena. Cambridge: Cambridge University Press, 1991:327–347.

11. Samal S, Geckler KE. Unexplained solute aggregation in water on dilution. Chem Comm 2001, 2224–2225.

12. Jackson JD. Classical Electrodynamics. New York: John Wiley & Sons, 1962:110–116.

13. Pohl HA. Dielectrophoresis. Cambridge: Cambridge University Press, 1978:5–18.

14. Yamashita M. Effects of Magnetic Fields and Electromagnetic Fields on Water and Aqueous Solutions: Experimental Study. Ph.D. dissertation, Geophysics, Stanford University, Stanford, CA, 2001.

15. Tiller WA, Dibble WE Jr, Kohane MJ. Conscious Acts of Creation: The Emergence of a New Physics. Walnut Creek: Pavior Publishing, 2001:62–68.

16. Colic M, Morse D. Effects of amplitude of RF EM radiation on aqueous suspensions and solutions. J Coll Interf Sci 1998; 200:265, and Mechanisms of the long term effects of EM radiation on solutions and suspended colloids. Langmuire 1998; 14:783.

17. Higashitani IK; Oshitani J. Measurement of magnetic effects on electrolyte solutions by atomic force microscope. Trans I Chem Eng 1977; 75B:115, and Magnetic effects on thickness of adsorbed layer in aqueous solutions evaluated directly by atomic force microscope. J Coll Interf Sci 1998; 204:363.

18. Radin DI. The Conscious Universe. San Francisco: Harper Edge, 1997.

19. Swann I. To Kiss Earth Goodbye. New York: Hawthorn Books Inc., 1975.

20. Sugrue T. There is a River: The Story of Edgar Cayce. New York: Holt, Rinehart and Winston, 1942.

21. Benson H, Stark M. Timeless Healing: The Power and Biology of Belief. New York: Scribner, 1996.

22. Wolf S. Educating Doctors. New Brunswick: Transaction Publishers, 1997.

23. Enserink M. Can the placebo be the cure? Science 1999; 284:238.

24. Puthoff HE, Targ R. A perceptual channel for information transfer over kilometer distances: Historical perspective and recent research. Proceedings of the IEEE 1976; 64:329.

25. Dossey L. Meaning and Medicine: Lessons From a Doctor's Tales of Breakthrough and Healing. New York: Bantam Books, 1991.

26. Targ R, Katra J. Miracles of Mind: Exploring Nonlocal Consciousness and Spiritual Healing. Novato: New World Library, 1998.

27. Zuyin L. Scientific QiGong Exploration: The Wonders and Mysteries of Qi. Malvern: Amber Leaf Press, 1997.

28. Zuyin L. Scientific QiGong Exploration: The Wonders and Mysteries of Qi. Malvern: Amber Leaf Press, 1997:91–98.

29. Tiller WA. Subtle Energies. Sci Med 1999; 6(3):28–33.

30. Tiller WA. Science and Human Transformation: Subtle Energies, Intentionality and Consciousness. Walnut Creek: Pavior Publishing, 1997 (Chap. 1).

31. Tiller WA, Green EE, Parks PA, Anderson S. Towards explaining anomalously large body voltage surges on exceptional subjects: Part I, The electrostatic approximation. J Sci Expl 1995; 9:331.

12

Electromagnetism Versus Bioelectromagnetism

William A. Tiller

Professor Emeritus, Stanford University, Stanford, California, U.S.A.

Most scientists and engineers mistakenly believe that bioelectromagnetic phenomena can be comprehended in terms of conventional electrical and magnetic forces acting on biological systems. Eletromagnetic gauge symmetry physics concepts and definitions explain why this is not true by demonstrating the differences between electromagnetism and bioelectromagnetism.

I. INTRODUCTION

Because, as indicated in the previous chapter, a higher EM gauge symmetry state than the U(1) state has a higher thermodynamic free energy than the U(1) state (see Fig. 1), this means that useful work can be pumped from any of these states X, Y, SU(2), Z, etc., to the U(1) gauge symmetry world. Thus, if a single organ or system of the human body was elevated to one of these higher symmetry states at birth and the rest of the body was not, seemingly all functions of the body could be driven via this energy source to exhibit what we call life, i.e., the heart would pump blood, nerve synapses would switch on and off, electric currents would flow, the brain would be activated to direct various body processes, etc. Interestingly, experimental data shows us that there is at least one important body system that is at one of these higher EM gauge symmetry states!

It is a fairly common experience in advanced kinesiology studies that a practitioner can slide a small circular DC magnet (with a central hole) onto the tip of their finger and, bringing this finger–magnet into the biofield of a particular muscle group of a patient, can either strengthen or weaken this muscle group depending upon which pole points towards the muscle group. The S pole facing the group strengthens the muscle's response while the N pole facing the group weakens the muscle's response. Thus, it is the acupuncture meridian system (in the R-space layer of the human biobodysuit) that is at a higher EM Gauge symmetry state (probably the SU(2) Gauge symmetry state) (1). What the Asian culture has called *Qi* (or *chi*) for millennia is what flows in this meridian–chakra system driven by this

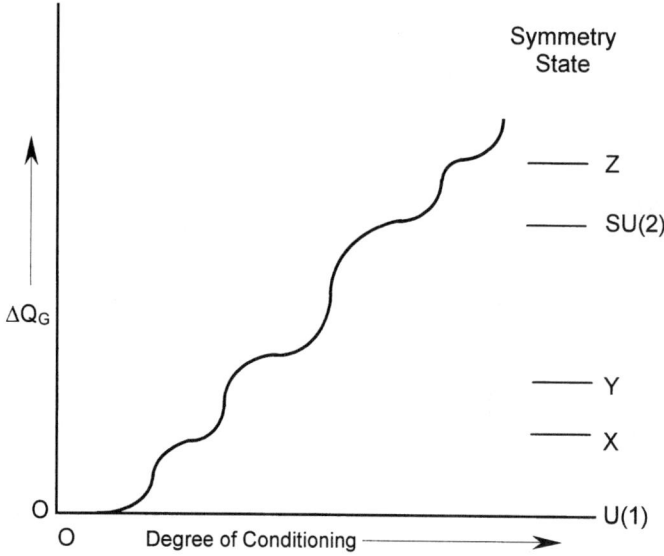

Figure 1 Schematic illustration of free-energy change ΔQ_G from the ground symmetry state, U(1), as the degree of locale conditioning increases.

EM gauge symmetry "pump." This pump drives everything else in the physical body and is what we call the *life force*.

The general picture that I would like to leave with the reader as I close this introduction relates to how we operate in life with respect to another; whether we be a minister, a healer, a medical doctor, an acupuncturist, or just a spouse and parent. This picture is illustrated via Fig. 2 for the practitioner–client interaction. Usually, all five components are intimately involved in the interaction even though the practitioner, using some device, may only

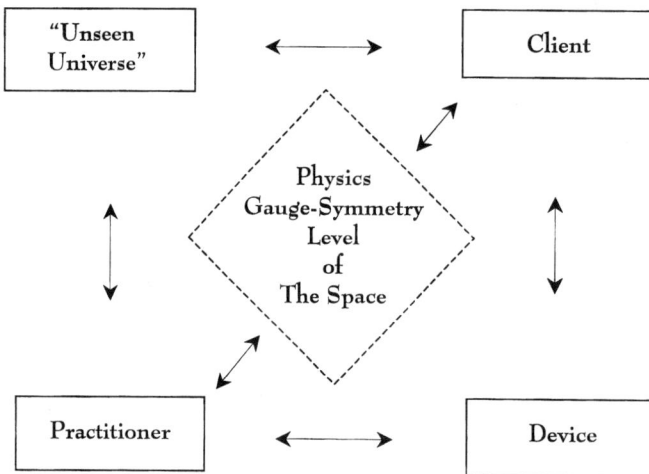

Figure 2 Illustration of the five key ingredients involved in every human action and every human interaction.

acknowledge that they and the client are involved. It is the practitioner's love, compassion, devotion to service, and intent that can elicit the unseen assistance of the universe to co-raise the EM gauge symmetry of the intervening space allowing the intention to be more empowered. Even saturating the device with activated deltrons is an important factor in the overall effectiveness of the process. It is via being fully appreciative of this entire operating system in all the processes of our lives that we can collectively lift the gauge symmetry state throughout our entire world and move us forward into the next phase of our great human adventure.

This seems remarkably like the general human experience wherein a group of well-intended individuals come into a room to meditate together, pray together, meaningfully commune from a "spiritual" perspective together, etc. Then, an elevated and tangible "field of consciousness" seems to fill the room and one doesn't want to leave this room. When the group eventually leaves, a residue of the experience remains in the room and slowly disperses. If this gathering meets daily in the same room for the same purpose then, after years to decades of such processing, the room takes on a seemingly permanent "conditioning" that can be tangibly felt by most individuals when walking singly into the room. Some of these sites become what we currently call *sacred spaces*.

On a more technical and theoretical level, our working hypothesis concerning nature's structural element involved in the laboratory conditioning process is that we are changing the degree of order in the physical vacuum state of the room. This vacuum fills the spaces between all the atoms and molecules of the room as well as most of the space within all the atoms and molecules of the room. This vacuum is thought to contain unseen substances that today's science has not explored in any detail. However, its normal state is postulated to be highly energetic, chaotic, and completely random (disordered). Our IIED work suggests that human consciousness, specifically human intention, can interact with this vacuum stuff and alter its degree of order in a seemingly permanent way. Since material properties are EM gauge symmetry specific, changing the local EM gauge symmetry state via our focused intention, the Qi-Prana pump changes the material properties of that local space to some degree.

II. ELECTROMAGNETISM VERSUS BIOELECTROMAGNETISM

From a macroscopic and U(1) EM gauge viewpoint, the interaction of matter with an electric field occurs in two ways: (1) as a conduction of mobile charge carriers through the material (called *conduction* current) and (2) as a polarization or electric dipole formation in the material (called *displacement* current). The former is always in phase with the electric field E, leading to a conductivity σ', while the latter is always out of phase with E leading to a conductivity σ''. The total electrical conductivity of the material is thus σ, given by

$$\sigma = \sigma' + i\sigma'' \tag{1}$$

where $i = \sqrt{-1}$ and means a counterclockwise rotation by $90°$. Alternatively, and equivalently, these two material response effects may be considered as the out-of-phase and in-phase electrical permittivities, ε'' and ε', respectively, of the material. Once again, these may be lumped together as a complex permittivity, ε, given by

$$\varepsilon = \varepsilon' - i\varepsilon'' \tag{2}$$

the conversion relations between Eqs. (1) and (2) are

$$\sigma = i\omega\varepsilon \qquad \sigma' = \omega\varepsilon'' \qquad \sigma'' = \omega\varepsilon' \tag{3}$$

where ω is the angular frequency of the applied voltage source to the material ($V = V_0 \exp i\omega t$).

Our sample material can be thought of as a "leaky" capacitor of capacitance C ($C = \varepsilon' A/d$, where A is the cross-sectional area and d is the length of our material). The charge built up along this capacitor is Q, and the charging current I_C is given by

$$I_C = \frac{dQ}{dt} = \frac{d(CV)}{dt} = i\omega CV \tag{4a}$$

and I_C is said to lead V by 90°. Simultaneously, the conduction current, I_σ (called a *loss* current, here) is given by

$$I_{\sigma'} = GV = \frac{A\sigma' V}{d} \tag{4b}$$

where G is the conductance of the material. The total current I is thus

$$I = I_C + I_{\sigma'} = i\omega CV + GV = (i\omega\varepsilon' + \sigma')C_0 \frac{V}{\varepsilon_0} \tag{4c}$$

where $C = C_0(\varepsilon'/\varepsilon_0)$ and C_0 is the capacitance when our material is replaced by normal vacuum having electric permittivity ε_0. Using Eqs. (1) to (3), we have

$$I = i\omega\varepsilon\, V\frac{C_0}{\varepsilon_0} = \sigma\, V\frac{C_0}{\varepsilon_0} \tag{4d}$$

in terms of either the complex permittivity or the complex conductivity description, respectively.

From an electric circuit viewpoint, the foregoing simultaneous conduction and displacement processes are seen as a resistor and capacitor in parallel as illustrated in Fig. 3a, where the resistance is $R = d/A\sigma'$. The time constant τ for charging up this circuit is $\tau = RC = \varepsilon/\sigma$ and its impedance Z is $Z = R/(1 + i\omega\tau)$ with $I = V/Z$.

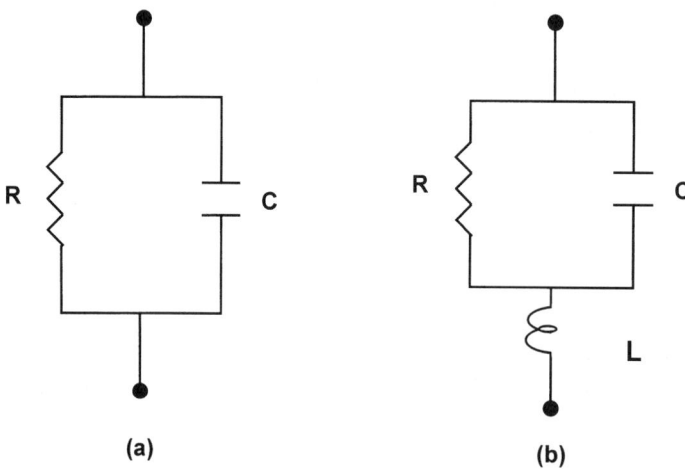

Figure 3 Electrical equivalent circuits for a material displaying both conduction current flow (due to R) and displacement current flow (due to C) for the two cases, (a) where magnetic field energy storage is neglected and (b) where it is not (L is the inductance).

The bottom line point of the foregoing discussion is that from an electrical response viewpoint, the material medium is considered to contain both electric monopoles and electric dipoles that respond to the driving electric potential.

Going a little further, from Ampere's law, we learn that current flow induces a clockwise circulating magnetic field, H, in the plane perpendicular to the direction of the current flow. The quantitative expression of this law is that the line integral of H around a closed path is equal to the current I enclosed ($\oint H \cdot d\ell = I$). The spatial distribution of this magnetic field in the medium around our material sample is given by

$$H = \frac{I}{2\pi r} \tag{5}$$

for a long straight sample, where r is the radial distance from the wire. The magnetic flux density B at any location r is just given by

$$B = \mu H \tag{6}$$

where μ is the magnetic permeability of this surrounding medium in units Henrys per meter (Hm^{-1}). Thus, since analysis shows us that energy $\tilde{E} = \frac{1}{2}\mu H^2$ per unit volume is stored in this field, our circuit diagram for this overall process must change from that of Fig. 3a to that of Fig. 3b to incorporate this effect.

From Faraday's law, one also learns that there is an EMF induced in a closed electrical circuit due to any change in the magnetic flux linking it (a kind of magnetic displacement current). Expanding this type of discussion, Maxwell's general equations for electromagnetism in materials can be simplified into four mathematical expressions: one derived from Ampere's law, one from Faraday's law, and two from Gauss' law. These are shown in Fig. 4 and indicate that the U(1) EM gauge state is "source" free with respect to magnetic charge [Eq. (1) of Fig. 4]

One last perspective addition to the foregoing discussion of conventional electromagnetism is to note that, just as the electrostatic potential (or voltage) V is given by Eq. (7a).

$$V = \frac{1}{4\pi\epsilon} \int_v \frac{\rho_e \, dv}{r} \tag{7a}$$

where ρ_e is the electric charge density and the integration is over the entire volume of electric charge, we can also define a magnetic potential, A_e, which is given by Eq. (7b) and is a vector:

$$A_e = \frac{\mu}{4\pi} \int_v \frac{J_e}{r} dv \tag{7b}$$

where J_e is the electric current density. Now, from the two potentials V and A_e, both the electric field E and the magnetic field H in the U(1) EM gauge symmetry state are readily given by

$$E = -\nabla V - \frac{\delta A_e}{\delta t} \tag{8a}$$

and

$$H = \frac{1}{\mu} \nabla X A_e \tag{8b}$$

$$\nabla \cdot \underline{B} = 0 \qquad\qquad (1)$$

$$\nabla \times \underline{E} + \frac{\partial \underline{B}}{\partial t} = 0 \qquad\qquad (2)$$

$$\nabla \cdot \underline{D} = \rho \qquad\qquad (3)$$

$$\nabla \times \underline{H} - \left(\underline{J} + \frac{\partial \underline{D}}{\partial t} \right) = 0 \qquad\qquad (4)$$

with

$$\underline{D} = \varepsilon \underline{E} = \varepsilon_0 (\underline{E} + \underline{P}); \qquad \underline{B} = \mu \underline{H} = \mu_0 (\underline{H} + \underline{M})$$

and in S. I. units, $\qquad \varepsilon_0 = 8.854 \times 10^{-12} \ (J^{-1} C^{-2} m^{-1})$,

$$\mu_0 = 4\pi \times 10^{-7} \ (J \, s^2 C^{-2} m^{-1}).$$

$\underline{B}$ is the magnetic flux density, $\underline{H}$ is the magnetic field strength,

$\underline{E}$ is the electric field strength, $\underline{D}$ is the electric displacement,

ρ is the electric charge density, $\underline{J}$ is the electric current density,

$\underline{P}$ is the electric polarization, $\underline{M}$ is the magnetization,

ε is the electric permittivity, (ε_0 is the vacuum value), and

μ is the magnetic permeability (μ_0 is the vacuum value).

Figure 4 The classical Maxwell equations.

Here, t is time, ∇ represents the gradient operation, while ∇X represents the curl operation. From Eq. (7b), one sees that A_e is collinear with the electric current so ∇X in Eq. (8b) just represents a clockwise screw operation along the locus of this electric current. To completely define A_e, standard electromagnetic practice is to set $\nabla \cdot A_e = 0$ (which is the same as saying that A_e is a constant spatially). This may be acceptable for the U(1) EM gauge symmetry state, but it is unlikely to hold true for the higher EM gauge symmetry states of Fig. 1.

As a bridge to our consideration of higher EM gauge symmetry states, we must also incorporate separate response characteristics of the vacuum level of substance (fine information wave level) into the foregoing description. A simple initial procedure for this is illustrated by the parallel circuit diagram of Fig. 5a. An important refinement of this approach is illustrated in Fig. 5b.

In Fig. 5a, Z_{cp} is the electrical impedance of the coarse particulate level with the electrical equivalent circuit of Fig. 3b and Z_v is the impedance of the vacuum level. In Fig. 5b, the subscripts R, δ, and D stand for R space, deltron, and D space, respectively. For the U(1) EM gauge state, we have

$$\frac{1}{z} = \frac{1}{z_V} + \frac{1}{z_{CP}} \approx \frac{1}{z_{CP}} \qquad\qquad (9a)$$

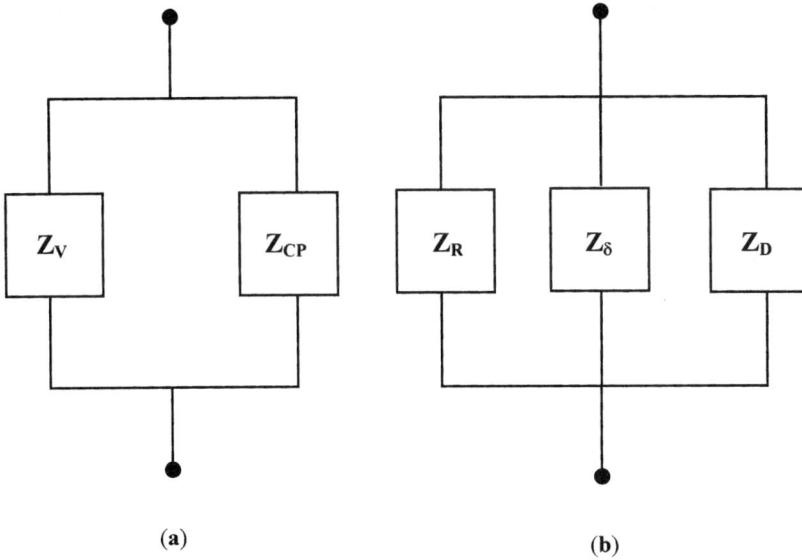

Figure 5 Two equivalent electromagnetic circuit illustrations for total physical reality; i.e., both the coarse particulate level (subscript *CP*) and the fine information wave level [subscript *V* in (a)] for the two cases, (a) neglecting separation of deltrons and (b) discriminating D-space, R-space, and deltron levels.

or

$$\frac{1}{z} = \frac{1}{z_R} + \frac{1}{z_\delta} + \frac{1}{z_D} \approx \frac{1}{z_D} \tag{9b}$$

since z_V and $(1/z_R + 1/z_\delta)^{-1} \sim 0$ for this state. Thus, the experimentally measured impedance, z is $\approx Z_{CP} = Z_D$. However, for higher EM gauge symmetry states, we must consider that magnetic charge ρ_{mj} is present and that the vacuum permeability/permittivity has changed to μ'_{0j}/ϵ'_{0j} (due to the possibility of both magnetic and electric dipoles manifesting in the vacuum), where *j* refers to the particular higher EM gauge symmetry state (*X*, *Y*, SU(2), or *Z*, in Fig. 1) under consideration.

Now, returning to our simple material example of Fig. 3b, A_e from Eq. (7b) is expected to act on the magnetic charge ρ_{mj} to produce a magnetic conduction current J_{mc_j} and a magnetic displacement current J_{md_j} along the same vector direction (the same as J_e). This new axial total magnetic current, $J_m = J_{mc} + J_{md}$, will give rise to a circulatory E field and associated electric current in the perpendicular plane. Likewise, the magnetic polarization due to J_{md} creates a B field (like a magnetic capacitor) in this axial direction. Thus, overall, a material in one of these higher gauge symmetry states will exhibit both axial and circulatory fields in the perpendicular plane for both E and B. One also sees that

$$A_j = A_{e_j} + A_{mj} = \frac{\mu}{4\pi} \int_v \frac{J_e}{r} dv + \frac{1}{4\pi\mu'_{0j}} \int_v \frac{\tilde{\rho}_{mi}}{r} dv \tag{10a}$$

and

$$V_j = V_{e_j} + V_{m_j} = \frac{1}{4\pi\epsilon} \int_v \frac{\rho_e}{r} dv - \frac{\epsilon'_{0j}}{\sigma_m 4\pi} \int_v \frac{(\delta\tilde{J}_{mj}/\delta t)}{r} dv \tag{10b}$$

The tilde over ρ_{mj} and J_{mj} indicates that we do not know the nature of these quantities; however, it is perhaps reasonable to think of them as tensors of some unknown rank. The right-hand term in Eq. (10b) comes from the application of Faraday's law to the magnetic current, and because of this tensorial nature, it is also not clear that this term has the mathematically correct formulation.

Applying this conceptualization to humans, whose body's fine information wave level of substance is most probably in the SU(2) EM gauge symmetry state, one sees that their bioelectromagnetism is significantly different that conventional electromagnetism. Following Barrett's lead (2) Fig. 6 shows us how SU(2) EM gauge symmetry equations of electromagnetism differ from those of the U(1) gauge symmetry state. The actual experimentally measured manifestation of higher gauge symmetry electromagnetism will be somewhat different than that provided by Eq. (9a) because these are based on the Fig. 5a approximation. However, in reality, one must take into account the deltron coupling between the D-space and R-space aspects of substance. Thus, the Fig. 5b approximation is required for the proper mathematical formulation. It will require careful experimentation in conditioned spaces to sort this out.

$$\nabla \cdot \underline{B} = \rho_m \tag{1}$$

$$\nabla \times \underline{E} + \frac{\partial \underline{B}}{\partial t} + g_m = 0 \tag{2}$$

$$\nabla \cdot \underline{E} = \rho_e \tag{3}$$

$$\nabla \times \underline{H} - (g_e + \frac{\partial \underline{D}}{\partial t}) = 0 \tag{4}$$

$$g_e = \sigma \underline{E} \quad ; \quad g_m = s \underline{H} \tag{5}$$

U(1) Symmetry	SU(2) Symmetry
$\rho_e = \dot{\underline{J}}_0$	$\rho_e = \dot{\underline{J}}_0 - iq(\underline{A} \cdot \underline{E} - \underline{E} \cdot \underline{A})$
$\rho_m = 0$	$\rho_m = - iq(\underline{A} \cdot \underline{B} - \underline{B} \cdot \underline{A})$
$g_e = \underline{J}$	$g_e = iq[\underline{A}_0, \underline{E}] - iq(\underline{A} \times \underline{B} - \underline{B} \times \underline{A}) + \underline{J}$
$g_m = 0$	$g_m = iq[\underline{A}_0, \underline{B}] + iq(\underline{A} \times \underline{E} - \underline{E} \times \underline{A})$
$\sigma = \underline{J} / \underline{E}$	$\sigma = (iq[\underline{A}_0, \underline{E}] - iq(\underline{A} \times \underline{B} - \underline{B} \times \underline{A}) + \underline{J}) / \underline{E}$
$s = 0$	$s = (iq[\underline{A}_0, \underline{B}] + iq(\underline{A} \times \underline{E} - \underline{E} \times \underline{A})) / \underline{H}$

Here, g_e, g_m, ρ_e, ρ_m, σ, s and $\underline{A}$ stand, respectively, for electric current density, magnetic current density, electric charge density, magnetic charge density, electric conductivity, magnetic conductivity, and magnetic vector potential, respectively.

Figure 6   Amended Maxwell's equations with symmetry parameters.

III. A MULTIDIMENSIONAL THEORETICAL MODEL (3,4)

The key elements of this model are

1. A network of nodal points that act as transponders and/or transducers for consciousness-wave–energy-wave conversion. The nodal point network functions on three size scales with the two larger grids being superlattice-like grids for the primary grid at the smallest size scale.

2. Spirit activates the driving consciousness-wave pattern for its specific intention and the nodal points in the grid convert these consciousness-wave patterns into various kinds of energy-wave patterns. These energy-wave patterns communicate with the various types of particles and agglomerations of particles within the interstices of the appropriate nodal point network.

3. Because these three nodal networks, when perfectly ordered, form reciprocal hexagonal lattices to each other, any quality of substance in the space of one network is related to the complementary quality in another network via a Fourier transform relationship.

To use the big bang concept for illustrative purposes, this model proposes that at the inception of our universe there preexisted the mind and emotion domain substructures of the vacuum (see Fig. 7). Thus, directed intention from the domain of spirit has a ready mechanism for creating the big bang process. As alluded to above, the key structural element of the mind domain is a 10-dimensional network of active nodal points in a close-packed arrangement with a lattice spacing of $\lambda_M \approx 10^{-27}$ m (so this network forms an extremely fine grid closely related to the fundamental Planck length and Planck time). These nodal points are undetectable by the tools of today's physics.

During the condensation phases of the big bang, both the substances and the nodal networks of R space and D space are formed. The latter via a type of self-induced coherence of superposed consciousness waves broadcast from the mind domain nodal points. We will label these three nodal networks (NN) as NN_M, NN_R, and NN_D, where the subscripts are used to distinguish the particular level of the model. Thus, this primary lattice of mind nodal points contains within itself two potential superlattices of nodal points that are reciprocals to each other (see Fig. 8). The first sublattice, NN_R, is also a reciprocal of the primary mind lattice, NN_M. The use of the word *potential* here is meant to imply that these particular nodal points must first form (via some process of organization) and then they must organize themselves into an array, which originally will be a relatively random array. This then proceeds through various stages of ordering to eventually become a relatively perfect 4-dimensional periodic lattice. The closest analogue to this in the world of materials science is *superlattice* formation in a host lattice of atoms. Let us now proceed with the description of the fully ordered state of these three nodal networks.

For NN_R, this first superlattice to NN_M has uniquely identifiable nodal points at $\lambda_R \sim 10^{-17}$ m and, at a 3-space level, is also of a close-packed hexagonal type but rotated counterclockwise by 90° with respect to NN_M (see Fig. 8a). In fact, the NN_R are located at certain sites in the NN_M separated by $\sim 10^{10}$ primary sites and have their own unique identifiable nature. The second superlattice, NN_D, is also formed from uniquely identifiable nodal points at a spacing of $\lambda_D \sim 10^{-7}$ m. It is a superlattice to the NN_R and, at a 3-space level, is also of the hexagonal close-packed type but rotated counterclockwise a further 90° with respect to the NN_R. Figure 8a represents an illustrative picture of these three nodal structures in perfect lattice form (but with much reduced spacing between the superlattice

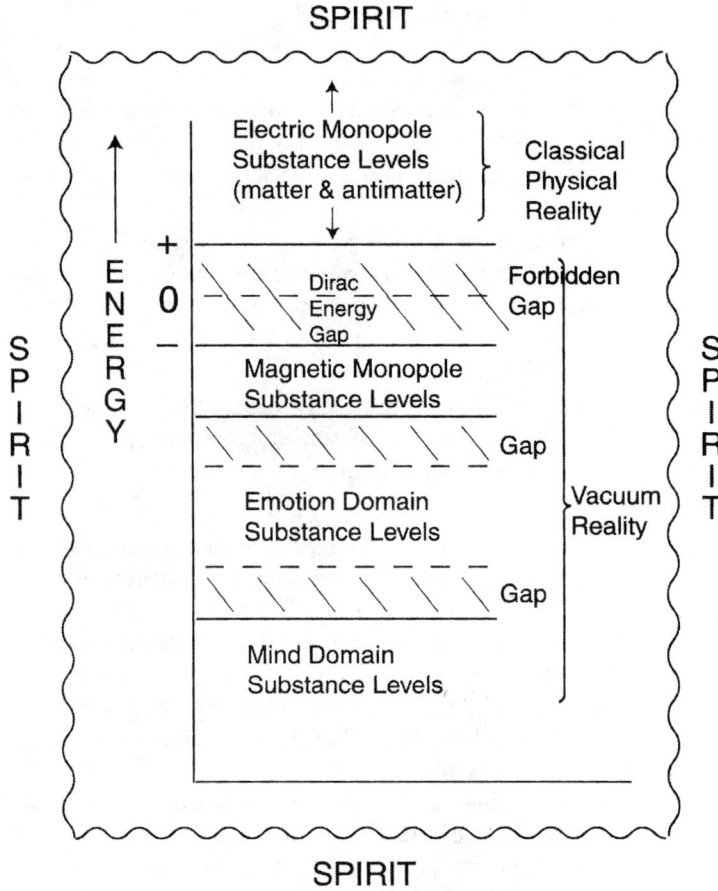

Figure 7 An energy level diagram embracing both classical physical substance and "unseen" vacuum substances.

nodal points); however, relative to the sites in the NN_M lattice, those in the NN_R lattice are thought to have a spacing $\sim 10^{10}$ times larger while those in the NN_D lattice have a spacing $\sim 10^{20}$ times larger.

Figure 8b illustrates how the situation might look when defects and disorder of the NN_R and NN_D are present. As already stated, order–disorder transformations are thought to be involved in the two coarsest networks so they can exhibit amorphous, polycrystalline, or single crystal type of character. Here, one grain is thought to differ from another by the orientation of some special nodal point property, e.g., special spin vector, tensor, torsion.

These grids of nodal points are unique in that the waves traveling through the networks exhibit qualities of consciousness as distinct from energies. The conversion from consciousness to energies occurs at the nodal points themselves. It is also thought that the major components of life energy for humans are radiated from the NN_R and NN_D. Thus, the larger is the size or number of regularly spaced radiators in the array, the greater will be the amount (and fidelity) of the information transferred from the NN_M as well as energy transferred to the human from the NN_R and NN_D making the individual more conscious and more vital.

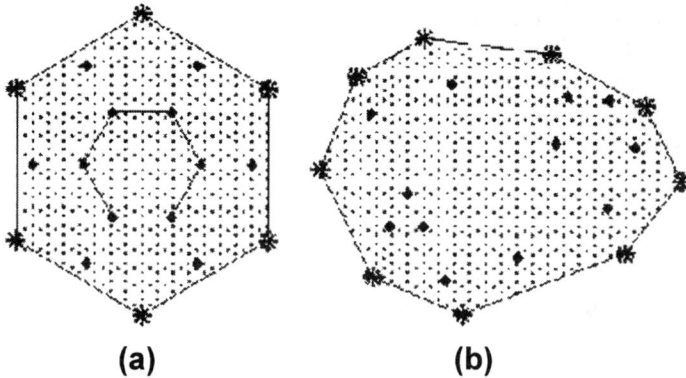

(a) **(b)**

Figure 8 Illustrative plan view of the three nodal networks: (a) in a perfectly ordered state and (b) in the normally disordered state (except for the mind domain network). The proposed size scale change from network to network is $\sim 10^{10}$.

The structural character of the nodal networks are though to be influenced by three main forces:

1. Cosmological scale forces driven from higher dimensional realms
2. Individual human internal harmony vs. disharmony
3. Collective humanity's internal harmony vs. disharmony

When all the forces are beneficial, the NN form relatively perfect lattices of very large extent (e.g., Fig. 8a) and humans manifest amazingly large consciousness and energy densities. When the reverse occurs, the NN form an almost amorphous arrangement and humans manifest only very small amounts of consciousness and life energy. In between, the NN structure is polycrystalline (e.g., Fig. 8b) and the larger the size of the average NN grain, the greater will be the amount of consciousness and life energy flowing through the individual.

Generally, from the perspective of this model, a saint has reached a high state of inner self-management at mental and emotional levels so that the body substance radiation fields are harmonized and synchronized. This supports a superlattice ordering process to occur at the NN level so that grain growth occurs and the average NN grain size increases. Such individuals manifest an abundant energy output even with negligible physical food intake. Their Qi-Prana pumps are optimally functioning.

Figure 7 has been used to express the various energy bands involved in this model. Here, one can discriminate the classical physical reality (positive energy states) from the vacuum reality (negative energy states), once one defines the zero energy state as being located in the middle of what we will label the *Dirac energy gap*. This choice of zero energy state is historical and arbitrary. In the new paradigm it would seem more reasonable to shift it to the bottom of Fig. 7. Then, all of the energies in the diagram are positive. The presently described quantum mechanical reality is thought to include this classical physical reality plus some aspects of the upper band of the vacuum reality.

The experimentally observed reality, which this chapter has largely focused on, includes the classical physical reality (D space), the mathematical modulus of the upper band (R space) of the vacuum reality, plus both the deltron activation function from the middle vacuum reality band and the intention imprint "boundary condition" imposed on the lower vacuum reality band. The details of the nodal network structures in Fig. 8 are intimately related to the details of the energy levels in the energy bands of Fig. 7. One goal of the present work is to expand our current quantum mechanical perspective via the "biconformal base-space interpretation" so as to develop a quantitative predictability of experimentally observable events that incorporates (1) the details of both the magnetic and the electric monopole substance levels, (2) the intention imprint as a boundary condition (BC) imposed on R space, and (3) a parameterized version of the deltron activation function. Sometime in the distant future we will have learned enough to expand the perspective sufficiently that the intention imprint, BC, can be moved to the NN_M level and the deltron activation function can be expressed in much more fundamental terms. Then we will have created a level of physics that truly incorporates the human qualities of emotion and mind into observable reality.

In the U(1) gauge experimental world, one doesn't detect any significant object shape effects, at least not for objects of macroscopic size. Presumably, this is because the magnitude of the effect in normal cases is so small that it is down amongst the noise for the current levels of measurement accuracy. This could be interpreted to mean that the shape's R-space modulus is small because the cosmic background level of deltron coupling is quite small. For a system in a linear regime of deltron coupling, the deltron effect would cancel out of the normalized modulus (4) and this becomes a baseline pattern effect for the particular shape (4). To empower the pattern to have a marked physical measurement contribution, through enhanced deltron activation, this additional factor must be incorporated into the theory in a mathematical fashion. At our present level of understanding, we simply define the deltron activation factor as C_δ (k, t, . . .), where the dots represent other as yet undelineated variables, and we incorporate it into Eqs. (11a) and (11b), which describe the R-space Fourier transform, $F(k)$, for the particular D-space quality distribution, ρ_s, in a material plus the inverse Fourier transform to convert from the R-space quality distribution to its equilibrium D-space counterpart.

$$T: \qquad \hat{F}(k) = \frac{1}{(2\pi)^{1/2}} \int_{D \text{ space}} \hat{\rho}_s C_\delta e^{i2\pi sk} \, ds \tag{11a}$$

$$T^{-1}: \qquad \hat{\rho}(s)C_\delta = \frac{1}{(2\pi)^{1/2}} \int_{R \text{ space}} \hat{F}(k) e^{-i2\pi sk} \, dk \tag{11b}$$

Here the superscript ˆ notifies us that enhanced deltron activation is being taken into account. Equation (11) can also be used when only the cosmic background level of deltron activation, $C_\delta = C_{\delta_0}$, is present. In such a case, C_{δ_0} can be treated as a constant and brought out from under the integral sign, so it disappears in the expression for the normalized modulus (4).

IV. APPLICATIONS IN THE ELECTROPHYSIOLOGY AREA

The main portion of this and the previous chapter has focused on three aspects of the larger reality: (1) the coarse particulate level, (2) the fine information wave level, and (3) the deltron coupling medium from the domain of emotion. These can be thought of as three unique layers of substance in the human body with particular infrastructure development and features of all three are present and convoluted together in every type of electrophysiological measurement made by today's medicine. If we could deconvolve these three aspects, bioelectromagnetic medicine would have made an enormous step forward. Well, the mathematics is now available to allow us to do just that. It will not be laid out here, but it has been demonstrated by recent publications (5,6).

Let us use EEG measurements to illustrate the principle. At present, we take time-dependent electric voltage measurements at N unique spatially separated points on the head and immediately Fourier transform this $V(r_j, t)$, $j = 1, 2,...,N$, data to obtain a frequency domain representation. We then use this result as a diagnostic tool. However, this raw data is a type of mixture from three different layers in the human so the diagnostic power is not as great as it might be. In Refs. 5 and 6, respectively, we have shown (1) how to take spatially varying data and calculate its complementary spectral amplitude profile at the R-space level and (2) how to take time-varying data and calculate its complementary spectral amplitude profile at the R-space level. Combining this same type of analysis procedure into a 4-space distance-time set of data, the full four-dimensional R-space spectral amplitude profile that generated this data set can be calculated. In addition, the general equations also allow one to calculate the deltron activation function profile yielding this particular D-space and R-space result. Now, with this addition, the same experimental data-gathering procedure provides explicit information on (1) the patient's D-space coarse particulate brain, (2) R-space fine information wave brain, and (3) one aspect of the emotion domain brain.

Such mathematical procedures can also be applied to all other electrophysiological measurements on the human body so that future medicine will be able to experimentally manifest a richer perspective on the state of health and pathology for the "whole" human.

ACKNOWLEDGMENT

I wish to thank Ditron, L.L.C., and The Samueli Institute for partial support of this work.

REFERENCES

1. Tiller WA. Subtle Energies and Their Roles in Bioelectromagnetic Phenomena, 2003. This book, previous chapter.
2. Barrett TW. Comments on the Harmuth Ansatz: Use of a magnetic current density in the calculation of the propagation velocity of signals by amended Maxwell theory. IEEE Trans Electromagnetic Compatibility 1988; 30:419.
3. Tiller WA. Science and Human Transformation: Subtle Energies, Intentionality and Consciousness. Walnut Creek, CA: Pavior Publishing, 1997.
4. Tiller WA, Dibble WE Jr, Kohane MJ. Conscious Acts of Creation: The Emergence of a New Physics. Walnut Creek, CA: Pavior Publishing, 2001.
5. Tiller WA, Dibble WE Jr. Anomalous temperature oscillation behavior near a "source" in a "conditioned" space. Part II: A biconformal base-space theoretical interpretation. www.tiller.org.
6. Tiller WA, Dibble WE Jr. Towards general experimentation and discovery in "conditioned" laboratory spaces. Part III: A theoretical interpretation of non-local information entanglement. www.tiller.org.

13

A Fundamental Basis for the Effects of EMFs in Biology and Medicine: The Interface Between Matter and Function

J. Benveniste

Digital Biology Laboratory, Clamart, France

Our current key–keyhole concept of random collision communication in the body cannot explain the myriad biochemical and physiologic reactions that can occur instantaneously and automatically. A new paradigm of electromagnetic signaling may explain these and other well-accepted but poorly understood observations.

I. INTRODUCTION

Why should any fields that are nonmaterial by essence act on biological constructions, which, as everybody knows since the beginning of modern biological research, are exclusively made of matter? I remember attending a presentation at a FASEB meeting in the United States about 10 years ago on the effect of electromagnetic fields (EMF) on living matter. At the end of the talk, the presenter was quite apologetic: "It is clear that EMF act on living matter but we don't know really why since this effect does not fit into classical molecular biology". Another interesting comment is from Tian Yow Tsong (1):

> A prominent biochemist, in a recent conversation with the author, even labeled study of this type of cell-to-cell communication as "astrology" and maintained that signals could only be carried by "the substance of chemistry," such as molecules or ions. Although any activity of a cell or an organism must ultimately be accountable or linked to reactions of molecules, these reactions can be and most likely are driven by physical forces. Here we will consider how communications through space by force fields (electrical, magnetic, pressure, etc., i.e., the substance of physics) may also accomplish similar tasks and are universally used by cells and organisms.

What is striking in these quotations is the neglect by classical biology of the existence of physical interactions between cells and molecules. T. Y. Tsong himself seems to consider that there are two ways of communication, one which is supposed to be strictly molecular and one which is physical.

II. THE MOLECULAR SIGNAL: FROM PTOLEMEUS TO NEWTON

An interesting aspect of this near blindness of current biology is the universal use of the words *molecular signal* or *signaling*. These words, along with *molecular genetics*, are certainly the most used nowadays by biologists at large. Readers of these pages may be willing to experience personally the reality of this biological black hole. It would be surprising if in any nearby university there were not one conference a month dealing directly or indirectly with molecular signaling. The experiment that I have myself practiced quite often is the following: attend the conference. At the end, ask the following question: I am not a specialist in molecular signaling, but I heard repeatedly the word *signal, signal, signal....* Would you please tell me what is the physical nature of the molecular signal?

The result is rather funny, most lecturers and participants reaching near catalepsy. In fact, they do not understand the question. Most of the time an answer will come such as "the molecule is the signal". It is clear that biologists confuse the origin of the signal with the signal itself (everybody knows that if a man waves a red flag to stop a train, the signal is the red flag, not the man) and that they are reluctant to envision the role of physical forces in the generation and transmission of the signal. It took me several years to realize with astonishment that the cornerstone of biology, i.e., the communication between molecules, relies on a Ptolemean concept, which postulates that the exchange of information takes place following a mere physical contact between coalescent molecules. The newtonian principle of action between two distant bodies without any material connection has not yet penetrated biology.

III. FROM THE "MEMORY OF WATER" TO DIGITAL (ELECTROMAGNETIC) BIOLOGY

Starting from the surprising result (surprising, to say the least, for the "normal" biologist that I was at that time) that water could convey and keep for quite for a long time the specific molecular message, I reached, through several experimental steps, the conclusion that molecular signal could be mimicked by electromagnetic signals in the sound range. The well-known emissions of frequency spectra by molecules, which is the basis of molecular spectroscopy, appear not only to be a physical characteristics but seems to be generating the specific molecular signal that is instrumental in the exchange of information between molecules, probably via the phenomenon of coresonance.

The history of my involvement with "high dilutions" is summarized in Table 1.

IV. SIX BIOLOGICAL SYSTEMS

Meanwhile, we have developed several biological systems that allow us to extend the concept of high dilutions being capable of mimicking the effect of the original molecule. Besides the basophil degranulation (1984–1986), we have done hundreds if not thousands of experiments on isolated perfused guinea-pig heart according to Langendorff (1990–1998) and in the same time period, activation of human neutrophils by electronically transmitted PMA. Then, in 1997–1998, we worked on a skin test (guinea pig or rabbit) and on an antigen–antibody precipitation system, which allows us to remotely detect any antigen or groups of

Table 1 History of High Dilution (Dubbed the "Memory of Water")

1984	Fortuitous discovery of basophil degranulation triggered by high dilution of anti-IgE antiserum
1988	Publication in Nature, followed by an "inquiry"
1991	Erasing of high dilution activities by an oscillating magnetic field (series of blind experiments in collaboration with a CNRS team)
1992	Electronic transfer (via an amplifier) of biological information to a tube of water
1995	Digitization: recording then replay of the biological signal using a computer
1998	Activation by agitation of a solution at very low concentration (down to 10^{-14}M)

antigens. The latter has been our main supporting procedure for research along with the effect of digitally recorded heparin and heparin like substances on plasma or fibrinogen clotting, developed in 1999. More recently we have constructed an automatic analyzer which performs the digital technique without any human intervention.

We do not have enough space in this short review to show experimental results on all these systems. We have presented these results at many FASEB meetings along these years and recently succeeded, in spite of open censorship from main scientific journals, to publish one full article (2). A complete bibliography can be found at http://www.digibio.com/cgi-bin/node.pl?lg = us&nd = n4_7.

V. THE FLYING MOLECULES

One of our most spectacular experiments was performed in 1996 between Northwerstern University, Chicago and our laboratory in Clamart-Paris, France. Molecular solutions of ovalbumin, acetylcholine, and, as control, dextran or water were recorded in Chicago using a purpose-designed transducer and a computer equipped with a sound card. The recordings were sent coded to us either on diskettes or by E-mail. Results on 25 files are summarized as follows: The variation in coronary flow of ovalbumin-sensitized guinea-pig isolated hearts induced by digitally recorded ovalbumin was (in percent $\pm$ 1 SD) 24.0 $\pm$ 1.4 (number of measures = 30), whereas that induced by digitally recorded water was 4.4 $\pm$ 0.3 (n = 58); p = 4.5 e − 17. The effect of naive water was 4.9 $\pm$ 0.3 ns (n = 41) compared to d water, and that of molecular ovalbumin was 0.1 μM 28.9 $\pm$ 3.7 ns (n = 19) compared to digital ovalbumin. Specificity of the system was absolute: no effect was seen when the ovalbumin signal was applied to hearts from nonsensitized animals. Similarly, atropine but not antihistamine inhibited the acetylcholine digital signal as well as the real molecule.

This experiment, I believe, unequivocally demonstrates that the specific molecular signal can be recorded, transmitted at long distance and then reapplied to the relevant biological system, where it induces the same effect as the original molecule. It is for this experiment that I was awarded a second ig-nobel prize. Problem is that no scientific criticism was voiced by the distinguished jury, composed of self-appointed guardians of the scientific purity. Here it is worth noting that our high-dilution experiments have been replicated by six independent laboratories, one doing it twice. How many replications are required for a work to be considered as replicated?

VI. TWO WORKHORSES

Our present main experimental systems are (1) the inhibition of fibrinogen coagulation by digital anticoagulant (see www.digibio/video); (2) the precipitation of antigen–antibody

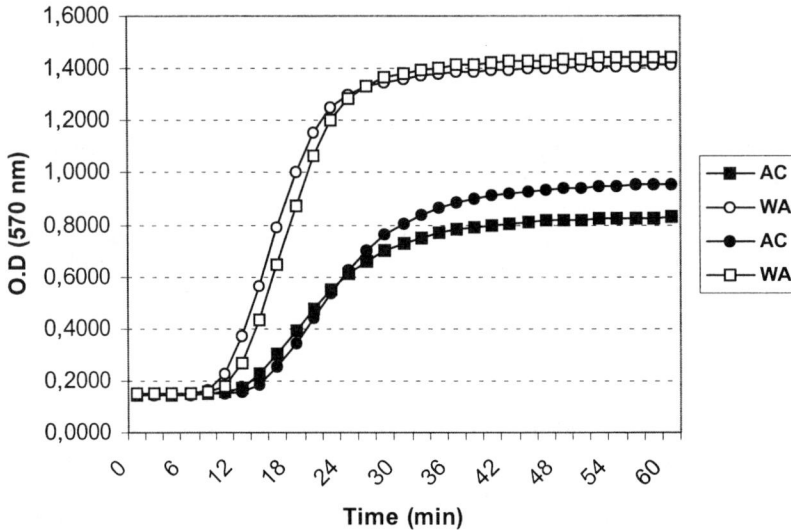

Figure 1   Thrombin-induced fibrinogen coagulation after exposure to anticoagulant (AC) or water (WA) signals. Blind experiment performed by an automatic analyzer (July 5, 2002).

complexes following exposure to the signal of the specific antigen or antibody. The latter method could allow us to remotely detect the presence of microbes (bacteria, viruses, parasites, fungi).

Figure1 is a representative example of inhibition of coagulation by the signal of an anticoagulant. We have performed hundreds of such experiments.

VII.   CONCLUSIONS

This set of results provides an answer for our initial question: EMF act on living matter because the mode of communication between molecules, which is essential to life, is electromagnetic in nature. Molecules communicate like a radio set that receives waveforms carrying specific information from the station to which it is tuned to coresonate and to none other. This communication takes place through water molecules surrounding all biological molecules. Water may have an amplifying role. Some of our data indicate that the signal is indeed emitted by the molecules but is finally conveyed by water, quite similarly to the strings of a violin, which do not create music unless affixed to the resonating wooden box. Also, we have clear evidence of an influence of some humans on our experiments. This may apply to classical biology too.

These results represent a small theoretical step forward. That molecules emit specific frequencies has been known for decades. We claim, and we believe we have shown, that they use these frequency spectra as their major means of communication. The heretofore physically undefined molecular signal appears to be composed of hertzian waves at least in the sound range. This is not a scientific revolution, as stated by conservative scientists who accused us of "negating the existence of molecules, hence two centuries of research." We simply replace the arrow which is supposed to represent the interaction of two ligands with a symbol representing the waveforms that support this interaction, Fig 2.

The Current Theory:
"structural matching"   **The Proposed Theory:**
                                    "electromagnetic signals"

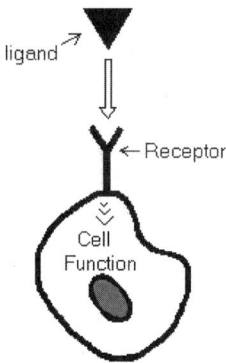

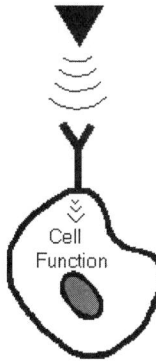

The 3D structure of the ligand
matches that of the receptor.
Physical proximity induces
receptor conformational
changes which in turn triggers
the cascade of events
prompting cell function

Proximity favors co-resonance
of ligand-receptor specific EM
signals. Resonance amplifies
molecule conformational
changes at all steps of the
cascade inducing cell function.

Figure 2   Molecular signaling.

Since a vast array of technological devices are now at our disposal to record, transmit, analyze, modify, and digitize these types of signals, this advance could profoundly change our views and our experimental approaches to biology and medicine. The now obvious failure of classical structural biology to explain the complex mechanisms supporting life and provide solutions to its disorders shows that it is about time that biology makes, at long last, its Newtonian revolution, that is, going from matter to energy.

REFERENCES

1.   Tsong TY. Deciphering the language of cells. Trend Biochem Sci 1989; 14:89–92.
2.   Thomas Y. Activation of human neutrophils by electronically transmitted phorbol-myristate acetate. Medical Hypotheses 2000; 54:33–39.

14

Electromagnetic Techniques in Neural Therapy

K.A. Jenrow

Henry Ford Hospital, Detroit, Michigan, U.S.A.

A.R. Liboff

Oakland University, Rochester, Michigan, U.S.A.

Neuroelectromagnetic therapies vary widely with respect to the nature of the signal, but they can be classified into three main categories based on distinctions in current densities and frequencies. These may achieve their biological effects via different mechanisms. Since electromagnetic stimulation of the brain for neurologic and behavioral disorders is often based on empiric observations, a clearer understanding of mechanisms of action might provide useful information to improve treatment results.

I. INTRODUCTION

The use of electromagnetism in nonthermal therapeutic procedures follows from an increasing number of laboratory observations suggesting a wide range of heretofore unsuspected physiological effects, observed both in vivo and in vitro, resulting from the application of electric or magnetic fields. Early therapeutic applications made use of surface or subcutaneous electrodes to produce appropriate current densities within selected tissues. However, it is now apparent that time-varying magnetic fields can be used to advantage to produce equivalent current densities in these tissues. This was first demonstrated by Bassett (1), who used a pulsed magnetic field (PMF) to obtain the same results in repairing bony nonunions as had been previously obtained with the use of electrodes embedded in the defect (2). Although the clinical use of electromagnetic fields may have initially surfaced in connection with bone repair, there is presently a good deal of interest in applying such fields within the central nervous system to treat both behavioral and neurological problems.

The direct application of electric signals to the brain via electrodes is now widely used in a variety of therapeutic procedures. Some of these therapies induce currents within large regions of the brain and are associated with a wide range of effects. Cranial electrical stimulation (CES) has been used to treat problems from chronic pain (3) to tension headaches (4). Electrical currents applied directly to the head have also been used as an adjunct to anesthetics (5) and for the treatment of insomnia via low energy emission therapy (LEET) (6). Analogous stimulation at higher intensity can be used to produce an electroconvulsive shock (ECS) that forms the basis of electroconvulsive therapy (ECT), which remains in use for the treatment of affective disorders (7). More focused application of electrical signals presently involves the delivery of deep brain stimulation (DBS) via permanently indwelling electrodes. DBS of the globus palladius, thalamus, or subthalamic nucleus is widely used for the treatment of tremor, rigidity, and dyskinesia associated with Parkinson's disease and other movement disorders (8). Application of DBS at other sites is presently being investigated for treating epilepsy (9) and OCD (obsessive compulsive disorder) (10).

Electric stimulation can also exert its effects on the brain indirectly via stimulation of afferent sensory pathways. Vagal nerve stimulation (VNS) is presently in wide use as an anticonvulsant therapy and is believed to exert its effects via activation of the diffuse afferent projections of the vagus nerve to the ascending reticular formation, hypothalamus, thalamus, amygdalohippocampal complex, and insular cortex (11). VNS has also been suggested as a treatment for a variety of other psychiatric and behavioral disorders (12,13). Spinal cord stimulation (SCS) involves the delivery of electrical stimulation to ascending pain pathways via chronically implanted electrodes and is used to alleviate pain associated with peripheral nerve injury and rhizopathy (14). Finally, functional electrical stimulation (FES) of descending motor pathways is used as a means of inducing muscle contraction when the integrity of these pathways is compromised (15), effectively replacing the electrical signal that has been lost due to spinal cord injury, stroke, head injury, cerebral palsy, ALS, MS, or CNS tumors (16).

Compared to electrical stimulation, the use of magnetic fields as a means of generating induced currents within the brain for therapeutic purposes is in its infancy. Most recent reports have centered around the use of TMS (transcranial magnetic stimulation) (17), which was originally applied as a single pulse but has subsequently been applied repetitively (rTMS) because of its broader therapeutic possibilities. rTMS shares many of the behavioral and biochemical actions of ECS but without requiring seizure induction (7). In fact, at lower frequencies rTMS appears to be anticonvulsant, whereas at higher frequencies rTMS can be used to induce seizures to assist in the localization of seizure foci in epileptics or as an alternative to electrical stimulation for ECT (7). rTMS is being explored as a potential treatment for depression (18), mania (19), schizophrenia (20), obsessive-compulsive disorder (21), and Parkinson's disease (22). It appears to exert its effects through regionally-specific changes in monoamine neurotransmitter levels and turnover rates within the brain (23,24).

The efficacy of both the electric and magnetic therapies mentioned above appears generally to be mediated by induced current densities within the brain; however, a number of other electromagnetic therapies are reported to affect neural function, which do not appear to be connected to any comparable change in current. Following the discovery in the Ukraine (25) that microwave signals at frequencies of 50 GHz and higher can affect behavior, so-called microwave relaxation therapy (MRT) has been used extensively in Russia. More than 250,000 patients per year receive clinical applications of MRT, although the greater fraction of these are treated for purported benefits to the immune system rather than for purposes of relaxation (26). The frequencies involved are remarkably high, ranging from 40 to 80 GHz (1 GHz = 1×10^9 Hz). There is some question as to the mode of interaction, considering the enormous reduction in intensity that occurs when very high frequencies are applied to human tissue, to say nothing about the weak intensities that are employed, of the order of 1 μW/cm^2.

Another case where one observes electromagnetic effects on the nervous system that do not appear to depend upon induced current density occurs under the condition of ion cyclotron resonance (ICR). This approach is based on the now broadly confirmed empirical observation (27) that combinations of relatively weak DC and sinusoidal magnetic fields "tuned" to the charge to mass ratios of ions such as calcium, magnesium, and potassium can significantly affect biological response in a wide variety of systems. There is an interesting parallel to the use of pulsed magnetic fields originally introduced by Bassett (1). In much the same way as PMFs were first clinically employed in treating bony nonunions, ICR has been established as an equally effective treatment for the same problem (28), even though the current densities used are much lower than those induced using pulsed magnetic fields. Futhermore, just as PMFs were subsequently found to be effective in neurotherapy, there is now excellent evidence (29) that ICR magnetic field combinations also affect rat brain, especially in connection with learning and memory.

Finally, another interesting modality involves application of static magnetic fields. Magnetostatic fields in the range of 1 to 4 mT have been reported to significantly alter cortical electrical activity in epileptic patients (30–32). These effects seem to require specific exposure timing sequences and do not manifest uniformly among individuals. Approximately half of those examined responded significantly to field exposure by either increasing or decreasing epileptiform spike activity (32).

Our present level of ignorance regarding the respective mechanisms of action of the electric and magnetic therapies considered above limits us to a strictly empirical classification. Evaluating these therapies in terms of their associated induced currents, however, affords an opportunity to frame this classification in terms of their most relevant physical parameter. Viewed in this light, there is a clear distinction between therapies that produce current densities that approximate or exceed those associated with endogenous processes within the CNS and therapies whose current densities are seemingly insignificant with respect to this standard. In the former case, the therapeutic effects appear to be a function of both the magnitude and frequency of the induced currents, whereas in the latter case the therapeutic effects appear to be primarily a function of frequency alone. This contrast is illustrated by comparing rTMS with CES. The currents produced by rTMS are approximately 1000 times larger than those produced by CES and yet the therapeutic effects of both of these therapies are frequency dependent (3–5,7,21,33). This suggests that the relative contributions of magnitude and frequency to the effects produced by their respective induced currents may differ between these therapies and that they may, therefore, be mediated by profoundly different mechanisms of action within the brain. Considering these therapeutic effects in relation to currents and frequencies associated with endogenous processes within the CNS may facilitate a better understanding of how these therapies work while simultaneously providing an improved picture of the intrinsic electromagnetic character of brain function.

II. NEOCORTICAL CURRENT DENSITIES

One of the most interesting aspects concerning the role of electromagnetism in neural function is that the measurement parameters used in electromagnetic therapies are different from those used in diagnostic procedures. The most commonly employed techniques for determining the electromagnetic properties of the human brain for diagnostic purposes are the electroencephalogram (EEG), and to a lesser extent the magnetoencephalogram (MEG). The EEG measures potential differences between various points on the scalp as a function of time (typically expressed in microvolts). There have been attempts to relate these time-varying potential differences to the corresponding current sources, but because the required calculations can be daunting, the experimental end point in EEG analyses has traditionally been limited to observed voltage measurements. The MEG yields a magnetic field measurement (typically expressed in femtoTesla (or 10^{-15} T), and since all magnetic fields are ultimately the result of electrical current, the source currents in MEG are also implicit. The analysis of MEG data to determine current localization is more direct however, because the magnetic field is not significantly attenuated or distorted as it propagates outward from its source. It is most convenient to assume that the geometry of the source is a current dipole (typically expressed in ampere meters), though it actually reflects cooperative interactions among local groups of perhaps a million pyramidal cells, conducting charge to produce a coherent current. The current dipoles obtained in this manner are commonly of the order of 10 nAm (10×10^{-9} Am).

Even though neither EEG nor MEG techniques deal with end points that one can readily relate to current density, the levels associated with endogenous processes within the brain have been estimated. One estimate by Nunez (34) sets the current density associated with the spontaneous EEG at 30 nA/mm^2, whereas another estimate (35) sets this value at 100 nA/mm^2. It may be helpful to use this value, representing the normal or intrinsic current density, as a reference or standard with which to compare electromagnetic therapeutic current densities. Such a standard may prove useful in evaluating the efficacy of different types of electromagnetic therapies. For purposes of discussion, we will arbitrarily adopt the value at the lower end of the estimated range as a baseline for the intrinsic current density, 30 nA/mm^2.

For those devices whose efficacy appears to depend primarily on current density, the largest currents are achieved for the case of transcranial magnetic stimulation. During TMS, a magnetic field of 2 T is produced within the brain in a time interval of 100 μs, resulting in a local rate of change of magnetic field of $dB/dt = 2 \times 10^4$ T/s (33). This is an extremely large rate of change of magnetic field, almost 3000 times greater than the time rate of change of magnetic field used in bone repair (1), approximately 7 T/s. It must be emphasized that the current density induced within the brain is directly proportional to how quickly the magnetic field changes. Additionally, the current density induced in any specific brain structure by a rapidly changing magnetic field is directly proportional to the effective radius of that structure and inversely proportional to the square of its distance from the coil. The *effective radius* can be defined as that distance equivalent to the radius of an imaginary circle having the same cross-sectional area as that cross-sectional portion of the structure that is parallel to the plane of the coil. Table 1 lists seven such structures, along with their cross-sectional areas and distances below the scalp (36). The current density for each of these structures is calculated using the rate of change $dB/dt = 2 \times 10^4$ T/s, along with the corresponding effective radius and the depth of the structure. Even for the smallest structure indicated, the corpus striatum, the current density resulting from TMS is approximately 10 times that of the naturally occurring EEG. This ratio becomes very large for the cortical structures, ranging from 1000 to 3000.

The maximum voltage induced in the brain by TMS is approximately 3 Volts (33), which implies* an enormous current density, on the order of 70,000 nA/mm^2. This value is 2000 times larger than the current density associated with spontaneous EEG. By contrast, Nunez (34) estimates that the current densities associated with epileptic seizures are typically 10–100 times larger than the spontaneous EEG figure of 30 nA/mm^2. It is worth noting in this regard that TMS treatments can trigger seizure activity (21) in a small number of patients.

---

* This estimate is arrived at assuming that the electric field is induced in a cross section of the brain immediately below the scalp with a circular cross-sectional area having an effective radius of 7 mm.

Table 1   Estimated Current Densities in Neural Structures Resulting from TMS Application[a]

Structure	Area (mm^2)	Effective radius (mm)	Depth (mm)	Current density (nA/mm^2)
Frontal lobe	4712	38.7	10	1×10^5
Parietal lobe	4000	35.7	10	9×10^4
Temporal lobe	3534	33.5	10	7×10^4
Occipital lobe	874	16.7	10	4×10^4
Hippocampus	507	12.7	50	1800
Thalamus	475	12.3	85	400
Corpus striatum	242	8.8	80	300

[a] Calculations assume that the rate of change of magnetic field $dB/dt = 2 \times 10^4$ T/s at 10 mm below TMS coil, that the magnetic field drops off inversely with depth below the 10-mm point, and that the conductivity of brain tissue is 0.25 S/m (37). Lateral cross-sectional areas are given for each of the cortical lobes, and dorsal for the hippocampus.

For the case of CES, time-varying electric voltages are applied to the brain through electrode entry points such as the earlobes (3), the upper palate (6), or directly to the scalp (38). The maximum current supplied by the α-Stim device (3) is well below 1 mA (1 milliampere), ranging between 10 and 600 μA. If we assume that this current is 100 μA, one can estimate a very representative value for the mean CES current density supplied by this device, namely 3 nA/mm^2. Therefore, in contrast to the large current densities associated with TMS, we find a current density that is only one tenth of that associated with spontaneous EEG. Given the large disparity between the current densities associated with TMS and CES, it is likely that the effects produced by these therapies are mediated via very different mechanisms.

III. THE IMPORTANCE OF FREQUENCY

The second key parameter in neuroelectromagnetic therapeutic applications is frequency. The possibility that a particular frequency, or even a range of frequencies, might have therapeutic significance suggests that the underlying mechanisms of action are also frequency dependent. This reflects a growing awareness among neuroscientists that endogenously generated oscillatory states within the brain and their associated frequencies have functional significance. It is generally proposed that these oscillations act to modulate or "gate" information flow into major processing centers such as the cortex via the thalamus and the hippocampus via the perforant path by affecting prolonged shifts in resting membrane potential (38,39). It has also been suggested that oscillations represent the most efficient means of affecting a change of state within, and between, neuronal networks with similar resonance characteristics. Finally, it appears that transient gamma oscillations (20–80 Hz) observed in connection with sensory input and processing may be involved in binding distributed processing spread over multiple cortical areas to produce a coherent representation of a stimulus pattern (39,40). It may be that the mechanisms of action of some electromagnetic therapies involve coupling to these endogenous oscillatory processes within the brain, which are themselves frequency dependent.

The manner in which synchrony is established and maintained within neural networks is not yet fully understood. It was originally thought that the so-called brain waves associated with the EEG were mediated by reciprocal interactions between inhibitory interneurons and feedback connections within thalamocortical networks (41), with the resultant oscillations being an emergent property of the network (40) (Fig. 1). More recently it has been established that such interactions are also mediated by local-circuit feedback and by the ion conductance properties of neuronal membranes, giving rise to intrinsic oscillatory states (39). Neurons with these conductance properties exhibit oscillatory behavior even in the absence of synaptic interaction and are therefore referred to as *pacemaker neurons*.

Other mechanisms involved in neural synchronization include gap junctions and field effects, both of which require a juxtaposition of cell membranes (42). *Gap junctions* are protein complexes that form between closely packed neurons and provide low-resistance electrical pathways. *Field effects* are electrical interactions mediated by ions and/or electric fields propagating through intra- and extracellular space. Though not prevalent within the mammalian CNS, gap junctions have been shown to play a prominent role in synchronizing adjacent pacemaker neurons within the inferior olive (IO) (43), and in the generation of high frequency (200 Hz) oscillations within the hippocampus (44). Field effects have also been demonstrated in the hippocampus, where intrinsically generated field potentials apparently participate in the generation of 3–10 Hz oscillations known as *rhythmic slow activity* (RSA) (45). Field effects are facilitated by the parallel alignment of pyramidal neurons within this structure, which promotes intracellular current flow and the emergence of synchronous subthreshold membrane potential oscillations among them (45). Similar subthreshold oscillations are generated synaptically in cortical neurons and may form the basis of the resonance-induced increase in cooperativity observed during cortical oscillations (46). Resonance interactions have been proposed to explain the reduction in amplitude of cortical oscillations that occurs with increasing frequency, which suggest that as frequency increases, the contributing neurons or neural networks are either reduced in number or dissipated (40).

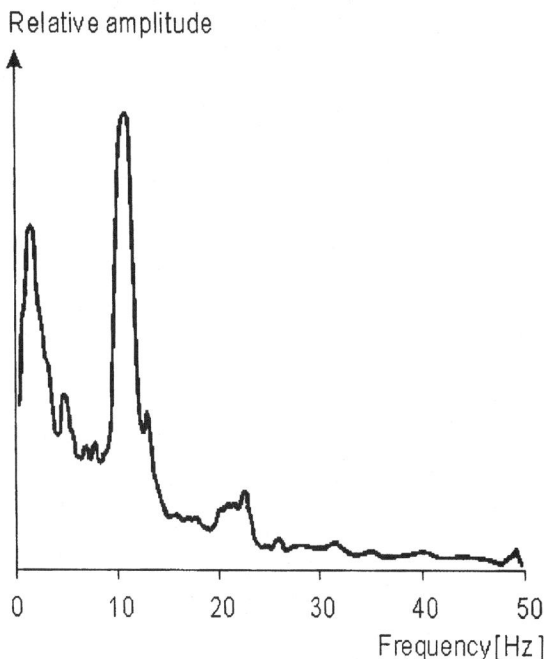

Figure 1 Typical frequency spectrum of the (awake) spontaneous EEG. With sleep, the spectrum shifts to include more low-frequency components and the 8–13-Hz α-rhythm is greatly diminished.

Although certain aspects of these oscillatory phenomena have been well characterized (39–41), much remains unknown regarding the relationship between specific oscillatory states and events at the cellular level and the means by which they exert their broader influence within the brain. Synchronous subthreshold membrane potential oscillations bear some resemblance to other subthreshold oscillations within neurons that are known to involve calcium-dependent signaling pathways (47), suggesting the possibility that neurons posses a form of cellular memory regarding their oscillatory history. It may also be possible that oscillations within one cerebral structure can influence adjacent structures in a manner that does not involve an explicit recruitment.

The uniformity with which the various oscillatory states of the brain are observed among individuals suggests strongly that the underlying mechanisms are, to some extent, hardwired. From a therapeutic standpoint, it is not clear that merely passing a frequency-specific signal through a region that ordinarily exhibits these endogenous oscillations will necessarily couple to the underlying circuitry. Nevertheless there are reports suggesting that certain intrinsic oscillations within the brain can be altered by external electromagnetic signals. Large corrective changes (48) are observed in the EEG of patients following the application of the α-Stim CES signal (3). Exposures to a 0.1 mT magnetic field oscillating in the range 5–10 Hz has also been shown to affect the frequency distribution of human EEG (49). In addition, a large body of work (45,50–52) has found that oscillatory states in rat and guinea pig hippocampus are altered by exposure to electric and magnetic fields.

Unfortunately, except for pacemakerlike devices, where reinforcement of a well-characterized signal frequency is clearly advantageous, not enough is presently known about the various brain oscillations to design devices that would provide therapeutic benefits at certain frequencies. However, this has not prevented the emergence of frequency-specific devices that are based on empirical observation. As an example, consider that although TMS was originally designed to provide possible therapeutic benefit because of its unique means of generating large current densities within the brain, it was later determined that different patient responses are observed as the pulse frequency (i.e., repetition rate) is increased to levels approaching 50 Hz (53). Responses such as mood modification can be opposite for low and high TMS frequencies. However, it must be noted that such responses may not represent a purely frequency-specific mechanism. For example, the large current densities associated with TMS may initiate an event, say, an ionic displacement current, that conceivably entails a long relaxation time before equilibrium is reestablished. If this were the case, the effect of TMS pulses following one another quickly could result in an additive process, where the event is progressively enhanced with each succeeding pulse. Nevertheless, it is clear that coupling within circuits that ordinarily exhibit endogenous oscillatory characteristics is made easier if the exogenous signal intensity is substantial. Thus the possibility that rTMS signals are capable of exhibiting frequency-specific effects cannot be ruled out.

More difficult to explain are effects where the induced currents are minuscule relative to those associated with endogenous oscillations. In some instances such effects appear to additionally depend upon the static magnetic field, which is most commonly the geomagnetic field (GMF). This is suggested by reports (29,54–56) indicating that learning, memory, and aggressive behavior are altered by magnetic field combinations corresponding to ion cyclotron resonance (ICR) conditions (27). One of the key aspects of ICR magnetic field exposures is their explicit dependence on magnetic field frequency. ICR effects on learning and memory make a circumstantial case for the involvement of the n-methyl d-aspartate (NMDA) glutamate receptor subtype in these effects. The regulatory properties of this receptor are mediated by removal of a Mg^{2+} block, which permits Ca^{2+} conduction into the cell through a highly permeable channel.

ICR magnetic exposures tuned to Mg^{2+} have been shown to enhance learning in rats, whereas exposures tuned to Ca^{2+} tend to impede it. In the most recent of these experiments (29) Mg^{2+} stimulation was achieved at 63 Hz, whereas the frequency for Ca^{2+} stimulation was 38 Hz, both in the presence of a simultaneously applied 50 µT static magnetic field, which approximates the GMF intensity. The implication of this work is that in the presence of the GMF (for those regions where its intensity is 50 µT) there will be one behavioral response when a 63-Hz field is applied and an opposite type of response when a 38-Hz magnetic field is used. The alternating field intensity used in these experiments was only 35 µT, which is lower than the field associated with TMS by a factor of 50,000. Moreover, the rate of change of a 38-Hz sine wave magnetic field is reduced by at least a millionfold from the value estimated for TMS pulses, namely 20,000 T/s. Thus, the current densities achieved in such ICR exposures are perhaps 10^{10} to 10^{11} smaller than the current densities accompanying TMS.

Still more evidence that the GMF may play a role in brain function follows from observations (57) indicating that the activation of calmodulin, a key Ca^{2+} binding protein found in all neural tissues, is sharply dependent on the GMF. It has also been reported (58) that calmodulin activation is altered by ICR combined magnetic fields.

IV. CLASSIFYING ELECTROMAGNETIC THERAPIES

We have previously suggested (59) that electromagnetic neural therapies might be considered in terms of three categories: subtle, gross, and disruptive. Following is a tentative attempt at classifying some of the better known electric and magnetic therapeutic modalities in terms of these categories.

Subtle interaction techniques exhibiting global effects:

    Cranial electric stimulation
    Ion cyclotron resonance
    Millimeter radiation therapy

Gross interaction techniques exhibiting specific effects:

    Deep brain stimulation
    Functional electrical stimulation
    Vagal nerve stimulation
    Transcutaneous electrical nerve stimulation
    Electric sympathetic nerve block
    Low-energy emission therapy
    Repetitive transcranial magnetic stimulation (?)

Disruptive interaction techniques, acting globally and specifically:

    Electroconvulsive shock therapy
    Transcranial magnetic stimulation
    Repetitive transcranial magnetic stimulation

The *disruptive* category includes both TMS and ECS procedures, where the currents that are applied or induced are well in excess of 1000 times those arising naturally in connection with the spontaneous EEG. Instead of replacing or reinforcing endogenous electrical or chemical signals, there is an apparent therapeutic advantage in applying signal strengths that are so large that the dynamics in the existing neural networks are temporarily suspended. In the words of Hallett, "TMS can transiently disrupt activity in focal brain regions ..." (60). Putting this another way, there is no known neural signal source that matches the current densities associated with either ECS or TMS. The disruptive nature of TMS and rTMS clearly has enormous potential benefit for those suffering from the types of neurological disorders that respond to abrupt and discontinuous changes in the distribution and pattern of activity within neural currents.

The second category includes nondisruptive signals with appreciable intensities that are highly specific. We term these gross because they tend to be immediately obvious in terms of function. Examples include VNS, FES, DBS, LEET, and possibly rTMS. In the latter case, even though a single pulse develops current densities that cannot be classified as specific, the clinical frequencies that one finds attached to rTMS in the literature may turn out to be highly specific. Other examples in this category include pain-controlling devices that deliver, to surface nerves in the skin, electrical currents sufficiently large to affect neuronal discharge. Transcutaneous electrical nerve stimulator (TENS) (61) typically uses 50–500 μs pulses in the milliampere range, while patients with complex regional pain are often treated with electric sympathetic nerve block (62). The latter applies much higher currents, in excess of 100 mA. Ordinarily this level of current can be problematic, but the frequencies that are employed in this procedure, up to 20 kHz, allow such currents to be used safely.

In the *subtle* category one finds signals that, although neurologically effective, have current densities that can be a factor of 10^{10} smaller than those associated with the disruptive TMS signals. This classification includes both the ICR and CES signals, both so weak that a functional relationship to the neural end point is difficult to establish. Because the power levels involved in millimeter radiation therapy (MRT) are extremely small, to the degree where they defy any known interaction mechanism, this modality must be similarly classified. Whatever efficacy is attached to the subtle therapy category, it is probably strongly determined by the signal frequency.

V. DISCUSSION

The classification system proposed above represents an initial attempt to group electromagnetic therapies according to their induced current densities and/or particular aspects of their application. Our attempt to partially characterize neuroelectromagnetic therapies in terms of current density is in line with guidelines for human exposure to time–varying magnetic fields established by the World Health Organization (63). These guidelines point out that "induced electric current densities can be used as the decisive parameter in the assessment of the biological effects at the cellular level." They suggest that the threshold current density for biological effects is 10 nA/mm^2, a value approximately consistent with what we have termed the *baseline intrinsic current density*. They further suggest that the current density threshold for potentially harmful effects is 1000 nA/mm^2, a value approximately the same as current densities associated with TMS. Note that range of current densities defined by these thresholds exclude those associated with the category we termed *subtle*. Thus, there appear to be neurological effects associated with current densities that are 10–100 times smaller than the threshold for biological effects suggested by WHO guidelines.

Evaluating these therapies in terms of their associated induced current densities avoids the potential confusion concerning whether the fields being applied are electric or magnetic. The fundamental issue at hand is the manner in which these induced currents produce their effects within the CNS. Obviously, this involves some form of coupling to constituent elements within the CNS milieu, which could conceivably encompass processes ranging from those at the molecular level to those involving broadly distributed neuronal networks. Such coupling seems more plausible where the therapeutically induced currents approximate the baseline intrinsic current density within the brain or where they dramatically exceed it as is the case for ECT and rTMS. As alluded to above, therapeutic effects in which the induced currents are dramatically less than this baseline are more difficult to account for. In either case, however, the precise mechanisms of action remain a mystery, and we are left with only the empirical evidence of a therapeutic effect, which at best is only suggestive of an underlying mechanism.

In the extreme case of very large current densities resulting from ECT or rTMS, the effects tend to be heterogeneously distributed within the brain and to involve multiple neurotransmitter systems. For rTMS, the effects vary depending upon stimulus intensity, stimulus frequency, the proximity of a given region of the brain to the coil, and whether treatments are delivered acutely or chronically. These often involve regionally specific changes in monoamine transmitter levels and turnover rates within the brain, principally norepinepherine and serotonin, which partially mirror changes in these neurotransmitter systems associated with ECT (23,64,65).

Neurophysiological effects of rTMS have also been observed. Frequency-dependent inhibition (72) or enhancement (66) of motor-evoked potentials are produced by rTMS of motor cortex, at 1 and 5 Hz, respectively. rTMS also produces enhanced reactivity of the rat dentate gyrus to electrical stimulation of the perforant path, accompanied by changes in the serotonergic and β-adrenergic modulation of hippocampal activity (67). This effect persists for up to 3 weeks following a 7-day course of rTMS (67), which, together with recently reported effects of rTMS on NMDA binding sites in rats, suggests the involvement of LTP-like mechanisms (68).

Current densities associated with neuroelectromagnetic therapies that we have termed gross are generally of the same order as the baseline intrinsic current density and are most often applied to specific regions within the CNS via indwelling electrodes. For these therapies, the desired outcome is often achieved by adjusting stimulation parameters including intensity, pulse width, and frequency (69,70). Application of DBS in the globus pallidus, thalamus, and subthalamic nucleus produces effects that mimic those produced by lesioning these structures, where it is commonly observed that this blockade is achieved only for stimulation frequencies in excess of 100 Hz. This frequency dependence was long thought to reflect a threshold for a localized depolarization block; however, it now appears that patterned neuronal excitation may also play a major role in damping aberrant activity by desynchronizing neuronal populations within these structures (71). Lower frequency electrical stimulation is typically used when the intent is to activate neuronal pathways or their target structures, as is the case for VNS (73), FES (15), and SCS (14).

The current densities associated with neuroelectromagnetic therapies that we have termed subtle are seemingly negligible relative to the baseline intrinsic current density, and we have therefore proposed that their effects are mediated primarily by the frequency of stimulation. As we have seen, this frequency dependence is not unique to these subtle therapies; however, it is generally the case that these frequency requirements are more exacting than are those for gross or disruptive therapies. This implies that the conditions that must be satisfied for these associated currents to couple within the CNS are similarly exacting. Another way of interpreting this frequency dependence is as a necessary condition for amplification within the CNS of an otherwise insignificant perturbation.

Several lines of evidence suggest that more than one mechanism may be involved in mediating this amplification. For the extreme case in which therapeutic effects have been produced by application of static magnetic fields, which in general impart no energy to the brain, a role for biogenic magnetite has been proposed (30–32). Magnetite is typically found within the mammalian brain in the form of magnetically polarized aggregates called *magnetosomes* (74), which, because of their relatively large magnetic moment, represent an optimal site for direct magnetic coupling. A role for magnetite in cellular physiology has yet to be established however; thus its involvement in regulating any aspect of neuronal function remains entirely speculative.

ICR interactions have been proposed to explain numerous observations that optimal coupling within brain tissue occurs when the alternating electric or magnetic field frequency is precisely tuned in relation to the local static magnetic field intensity (27). The precision of this tuning is exemplified by the fact that relatively subtle variations of these parameters can yield very different therapeutic effects, whereas if the conditions for resonance are not satisfied then no effect is produced (54–56). This form of coupling is postulated to affect the binding and/or transport kinetics of biologically relevant ions in relation to transmembrane and cytosolic proteins (27,75).

Finally, numerous reports have suggested that optimal coupling within brain tissue occurs when the alternating field frequency approximates endogenous oscillatory frequencies associated with particular brain structures (49,51,52,76). These effects appear to be independent of the static magnetic field intensity and, in at least one report, occurred in the complete absence of a static magnetic field. The term *physiological resonance* has been used to describe these interactions and it has been suggested that they reflect coupling within networks of extracellular matrix proteins (77).

It is perhaps not coincidental that many of the effects of neuroelectromagnetic therapies involve structures within the brain in which endogenous oscillations are routinely observed. The network characteristics of these regions, which include the olfactory cortex, hippocampus, and neocortex, facilitate the amplification of very weak endogenous signals, together with resonance interactions, resulting in the synchronous discharge of pyramidal cells and the summation of their resultant dipole potentials to produce the oscillations characteristic of EEG (78). The basic circuit is composed of three types of connections:

1. Pyramidal neurons that receive the primary afferent synapses on their distal dendritic spines and that are the primary source of excitatory output
2. Intrinsic axon collaterals that are reexcitatory to pyramidal neurons over long distances
3. Local interneurons that are activated by afferents to give feedforward inhibition and/or axon collaterals to give lateral inhibition (42)

These circuit elements are organized into lamina in which the pyramidal neurons are aligned parallel to one another and perpendicular to the cortical surface (40,78).

Recent findings suggest that neuronal networks with these circuit characteristics are capable of amplifying weak signals via a stochastic resonance mechanism in a manner requiring only a nonspecific source of noise (above a minimum threshold level), i.e., that associated with the firing patterns of individual neuronal elements (79). Jefferys (80) has proposed that localized neuronal ensembles, consisting of approximately three to seven pyramidal neurons coupled via gap junctions, may initiate such amplification within the hippocampus. This coupling may facilitate synchronization within these ensembles, and the resultant field potentials may then couple to adjoining pyramidal neurons via endogenous field interactions and the induction of subthreshold membrane potential oscillations. Analogous mechanisms have been implicated in olfactory (81) and neocortex as well (46), suggesting that the current density threshold for the initiation of oscillation and synchrony within such structures may be far below the baseline intrinsic current density. These structures might therefore represent a unique context in which currents and/or other periodic perturbations associated with subtle neuroelectromagnetic therapies are similarly amplified to produce their effects, which may include modulation and/or disruption of endogenous oscillations. The larger current densities associated with gross and disruptive therapies might also be expected to couple optimally (though not exclusively) within these structures and might therefore exert some of their effects in the same fashion.

The potential functional significance of endogenous oscillatory states within the brain has only recently been appreciated. As described previously, such states are presently thought to modulate information flow into major processing centers (38,39), to affect changes of state within, and between, neuronal networks with similar resonance characteristics, and to facilitate the binding of distributed processing spread over multiple cortical areas (39,40). As more is learned about signal amplification within the networks that give rise to these oscillations, it seems likely that more nuanced functional characteristics will be similarly revealed. These may include intra- or internetwork interactions that do not require the explicit recruitment of oscillations and/or interactions between these network dynamics and processes associated with learning and memory. As a speculative example, consider the possibility that the α-rhythm, an 8–13 Hz cortical oscillation (see Fig. 1) that emerges in humans and other animals when the eyes are closed, acts to *initiate* the sleep process. This would imply that a oscillations within the thalamocortical networks that generate them also induce the reticular activating system to sleep, without necessarily recruiting equivalent oscillations within the reticular activating system itself. This suggests the possibility that application of signals that mimic the α-rhythm might be used as a treatment for insomnia. It has, in fact, been observed (82) that electrical signals applied directly to the brain can affect sleep. However, the underlying mechanism is presently unknown.

As our understanding of the relationship between signal amplification and oscillatory phenomena in the brain improves, it may be possible to refine existing neuroelectromagnetic therapies to achieve better clinical outcomes. This may be especially true for both subtle and disruptive technologies, where such knowledge may permit a more targeted application including optimization of amplitude and frequency parameters, coil diameter, position and orientation, and exposure duration. Our primary purpose here was to provide a framework for discussing these technologies in terms of their most salient physical characteristics, induced current density, and frequency and to classify them in relation to these variables. In practice, it is likely that our knowledge regarding the mechanisms underlying these therapeutic effects will advance via a reciprocal interaction between empirically derived observations of clinical efficacy and basic research in the neurosciences.

REFERENCES

1. Bassett CAL, Pawluk RJ, Pilla AA. Acceleration of fracture repair by electromagnetic fields: a surgically noninvasive method. In: Liboff AR, Rinaldi RA, eds. Electrically Mediated Growth Mechanisms in Living Systems. Ann NY Acad Sci 1974; 238:242–262.
2. Lavine LS, Lustrin I, Shamos MH, Rinaldi RA, Liboff AR. Electric enhancement of bone healing. Science 1972; 175:1118–1121.
3. Kirsch DL, Smith RB. The use of cranial electrotherapy stimulation in the management of chronic pain: a review. Neurorehabilitation 2000; 14:85–94.
4. Solomon S, Elkind A, Freitag F, Gallagher RA, More K, Swerdlow B, Malkin S. Safety and

effectiveness of cranial electrotherapy in the treatment of tension headaches. Headache 1989; 29:445–450.

5. Stanley TH, Cazalaa JA, Limoge A, Lowville Y. Transcutaneous cranial electrical stimulation increases the potency of nitrous oxide in humans. Anesthesiology 1982; 57:293–297.
6. Reite M, Higgs L, Lebet J-P, Barbault A, Rossell C, Kuster N, Dafni U, Anato D, Pache B. Sleep inducing effect of low energy emission therapy. Bioelectromagnetics 1994; 15:67–75.
7. Lisanby SH, Belmaker RH. Animal models of the mechanisms of action of repetitive transcranial magnetic stimulation (RTMS): comparisons with electroconvulsive shock (ECS). Depression Anxiety 2000; 12:178–187.
8. Limousin P, Krack P, Pollak P, Benazzouz A, Ardouin C, Hoffmann D, Benabid AL. Electrical stimulation of the subthalamic nucleus in advanced Parkinson's disease. N Engl J Med 1998; 339:1105–1111.
9. Dinner DS, Neme S, Nair D, Montgomery EB, Baker KB, Rezai A, Luders H. EEG and evoked potential recording from the subthalamic nucleus for deep brain stimulation of intractable epilepsy. Clin Neurophysiol 2002; 113:1391–1402.
10. Roth RM, Flashman LA, Saykin AJ, Roberts DW. Deep brain stimulation in neuropsychiatric disorders. Current Psychiatry Rep 2001; 3:366–372.
11. Wilder BJ. Vagal nerve stimulation. In: Engle J Jr, Pedley TA, eds. Epilepsy: a Comprehensive Textbook. Philadelphia: Lippincott-Raven, 1997.
12. Sabara J. Inhibition of experimental seizures in canines by repetitive vagal stimulation. Epilepsia 1992; 33:1005–1012.
13. George MS, Nahas Z, Bohning DE, Kozel FA, Anderson B, Chae J-H, Lomarov M, Denslow S, Li X, Mu C. Vagus nerve stimulation therapy: A research update. Neurology 2002; 59:S56–S61.
14. Meyerson BA. Neurosurgical approaches to pain treatment. Acta Anesthesiaol Scand 2001; 45:1108–1113.
15. Holle J, Frey M, Gruber H, Kern H, Stohr H, Thoma H. Functional electrostimulation of paraplegics. Orthop 1984; 7:1145–1155.
16. Rattay F. Ways to approximate current-distance relations for electrically stimulated nerve fibers. J Theor Biol 1987; 125:339–349.
17. Barker AT, Freeston IL, Jalinous R, Jarratt JA. Noninvasive stimulation of motor pathways within the brain using time-varying magnetic fields. Electroencephalogr Clin Neurophysiol 1985; 61:S245.
18. Pasqual-Leone A, Catala MD. Lateralized effect of rapid rate transcranial magnetic stimulation of the prefrontal cortex on mood. Neurology 1996; 46:499–502.
19. Pasqual-Leone A, Rubio B, Pallardo F, Catala MD. Rapid-rise transcranial magnetic stimulation of left dorsolateral prefrontal cortex in drug resistant depression. Lancet 1996; 348: 233–237.
20. Grunhaus L, Dannon P, Schreiber S. Repetitive transcranial magnetic stimulation is as effective as electroconvulsive therapy in the treatment on nondelusional major depressive disorder: an open study. Biol Psychiatry 2000; 47:314–324.
21. Hasey GM. Transcranial magnetic stimulation: using a law of physics to treat psychopathology. J Psychiatry Neurosci 1999; 24:97–101.
22. Seibner HR, Mentschel C, Auer C, Conrad BR. Repetitive transcranial magnetic stimulation has a beneficial effect on bradykinesia in Parkinson's disease. Neuroreport 1999; 10:589–594.
23. Ben-Shachar D, Belmaker RH, Grisaru N, Klein E. Transcranial magnetic stimulation induces alteration in brain monoamines. J Neural Transm 1997; 104:191–197.
24. Ben-Shachar D, Gazawi H, Riboyad-Levin J, Klein E. Chronic repetitive transcranial magnetic stimulation alters β-adrenergic and 5-HT2 receptor characteristics in rat brain. Brain Res 1999; 816:78–83.
25. Devyatkov ND. Influence of the millimeter wavelength range electromagnetic radiation upon biological objects. Soviet Physics Uspekhi 1973; 110:452–454 (in Russian).
26. Logani MK, Anga A, Szabo I, Agelan A, Irizarry AR, Zisken MC. Effect of millimeter waves

on cyclophosphamide induced suppression of the immune system. Bioelectromagnetics 2002; 23:614–621.

27. Liboff AR. Ion cyclotron resonance in biological systems: Experimental evidence. In: Stavroulakis P, ed. Biological Effects of Electromagnet Fields. Berlin: Springer, 2002.

28. Diebert C, McLeod BR, Smith SD, Liboff AR. Ion resonance electromagnetic field stimulation of fracture healing in rabbits with a fibular osteomoty. J Orthopedic Res 1984; 32:878–885.

29. Zhadin MN, Deryugina ON, Pisachenko TM. Influence of combined DC and AC magnetic fields on rat behavior. Bioelectromagnetics 1999; 20:378–386.

30. Dobson JP, Fuller M, Moser S, Wieser HG, Dunn JR, Zoeger J. Evocation of epileptiform activity by weak DC magnetic fields and iron biomineralization in the brain. In: Deeke L, Baumgartner C, Stronik G, Williamson SJ, eds. Advances in Biomagnetism. New York: Plenum Press, 1993.

31. Fuller M, Dobson J, Weiser HG, Moser S. On the sensitivity of the human brain to magnetic fields: evocation of epileptiform activity. Brain Res Bull 1994; 36:155–159.

32. Dobson J, St Pierre TG, Schultheiss-Grassi PP, Weiser HG, Kuster N. Analysis of EEG data from weak-field magnetic stimulation of mesial temporal lobe epilepsy patients. Brain Res 2000; 868:386–391.

33. Kammer T, Beck S, Thielsher A, Laubis-Herrmann U, Topka H. Motor thresholds in humans: a transcranial magnetic stimulation study comparing different pulse waveforms, current densities and stimulation types. Clin Neurophysiol 2001; 112:250–258.

34. Nunez PL. Quantitative states of neocortex. In: Nunez PL, ed. Neocortical Dynamics Human EEG Rhythyms. New York: Oxford Univ Press, 1995:31.

35. Harnalainen M, Hari R, Ilmonierni R, Knuutila J, Lounasmaa O. Magnetoencephalography: theory instrumentation and applications to the noninvasive study of human brain function. Rev Mod Phys 1993; 65:413–497.

36. DeArmond SJ, Fusco MM, Dewey MM. Structure of the human brain: A Photographic Atlas. 3rd ed. New York: Oxford Univ Press, 1989.

37. Ferree TC, Tucker DM. Development of high resolution EEG devices. Intl J Bioelectromagnetism 1999; 1:4–10.

38. Llinas RR. The intrinsic electrophysiological properties of mammalian neurons:insights into central nervous system function. Science 1988; 42:1654–1664.

39. Lisman JE, Idiart MAP. Storage of 7 ± 2 short-term memories in oscillatory subcycles. Science 1995; 267:1512–1515.

40. Singer W. Synchronization of cortical activity and its putative role in information processing and learning. Ann Rev Physiol 1993; 55:349–374.

41. Anderson P, Sears T. The role of inhibition in the phasing of spontaneous thalamo cortical discharge. J Physiol 1964; 173:459–480.

42. Shepherd GM. Neurobiology. New York: Oxford University Press, 1994.

43. Llinas RR. The role of intrinsic electrophysiological properties of central neurons in oscillation and resonance. In: Goldbetter A, ed. Cell to Cell Communication: Experiments to Theoretical Models. London: Academic Press, 1990.

44. Draghun A, Traub RD, Schmitz D, Jefferys JGR. Electrical coupling underlies high-frequency oscillations in the hippocampus in vitro. Nature 1998; 394:189–192.

45. Taylor CP, Dudek FE. Excitation of hippocampal pyramidal cells by an electric field. J Neurophysiol 1984; 52:126–142.

46. Jagadeesh B, Gray CM, Ferster D. Visually evoked oscillations of membrane potential in cells of cat visual cortex. Science 1992; 257:552–554.

47. Berridge MJ. Inositol triphosphate and calcium signaling. Nature 1993; 361:315–325.

48. Heffernan M. The effect of variable microcurrents on EEG spectrum and pain control. Can J Clin Med 1997; 4:4–11.

49. Bell GB, Marino AA, Chasson AL. Frequency-specific responses in the human brain caused by electromagnetic fields. J Neurol Sci 1994; 123:21–32.

50. Jefferys JGR. Influence of electric fields on the excitability of granule cells in guinea-pig hippocampal slices. J Physiol 1981; 319:143–152.

51. Bawin SM, Satmary RA, Jones WR, Adey WR, Zimmerman G. Extremely low frequency magnetic fields disrupt rhythmic slow activity in rat hippocampal slices. Bioelectromagnetics 1996; 17:388–395.
52. Jenrow KA, Zhang X, Renehan WB, Liboff AR. Weak ELF magnetic field effects on hippocampal rhythmic slow activity. Exp Neurol 1998; 153:328–334.
53. Hasey G. Transcranial magnetic stimulation in the treatment of mood disorder: a review and comparison with eletroconvulsive therapy. Can J Psychiatry 2001; 46:720–727.
54. Thomas JR, Schrot J, Liboff AR. Low-intensity magnetic fields alter operant behavior in rats. Bioelectromagnetics 1986; 7:349–357.
55. Lovely RH, Creim JA, Miller DL, Anderson LE. Behavior of rats in a radial arm maze during exposure to magnetic fields: evidence for effect of magnesium ion resonance. 15th Annual Meeting, Bioelectromagnetics Soc., Los Angeles, Abstract E-I-6, 1993.
56. Lyskov E, Chernyshev M, Makarova T, Vasilieava Yu, Michailov V, Sokolov G, Vishnevskiyi A. Behavioral effects of extremely low frequency (ELF) magnetic fields probably depend on the dc component. Proceedings of International Workshop of the European Bioelectromagnetics Association. Russian Academy of Sciences. Moscow Region, Puschino, Russia, 1995.
57. Liboff AR, Cherng S, Jenrow KA, Bull A. Calmodulin-dependent cyclic nucleotide phosphodieserase activity is altered by 20 mT magnetostatic fields. Bioelectromagnetics 2003; 24:32–38.
58. Shuvalova LA, Ostrovskaja MV, Sosunov EA, Lednev VV. Effect of weak magnetic field in the parametric resonance mode on the rate of calmodulin-dependent phosphorylation of myosin in the solution. Doklady Akademii Nauk SSSR (Reports of the Academy of Science of the USSR) 1991; 317:227–230 (in Russian).
59. Liboff AR, Jenrow KA. Physical mechanisms in neuroelectromagnetic therapies. Neurorehabilitation 2002; 17:9–22.
60. Hallett M. Transcranial magnetic stimulation and the human brain. Nature 2000; 406:147–150.
61. Mannheimer J, Lampe G. Clinical Transcutaneous Electrical Nerve Stimulation. Philadelphia: F A Davis, 1984.
62. Schwartz RG. Electric sympathetic block: current theoretical concepts and clinical results. J Back Musculoskel Rehab 1998; 10:31–46.
63. Magnetic Fields, Environmental Health Criteria 69. Geneva: World Health Organization, 1987: 20–21.
64. Fleischmann A, Sternheim A, Etgen AM, Li C, Grisaru N, Belmaker RH. Transcranial megnetic stimulation down-regulates beta-adrenoreceptors in rat cortex. J Neural Transm 1996; 103:1356–1361.
65. McGarvey KA, Zis AP, Brown EE, Nomikos GG, Fibiger HC. ECS-induced dopamine release: effects of electrode placement, anticonvulsant treatment, and stimulus intensity. Biol Psychiatry 1993; 34:152–157.
66. Jennum P, Winkel H, Fuglsang-Frederiksen A. Repetitive magnetic stimulation and motor evoked potentials. Electroencephalogr Clin Neurophysiol 1995; 97:96–101.
67. Levokovitz Y, Marx J, Grisaru N, Segal M. Long-term effects of transcranial magnetic stimulation on hippocampal reactivity to afferent stimulation. J Neurosci 1999; 19:3198–3203.
68. Kole MH, Fuchs E, Zeimann U, Paulus W, Ebert U. Changes in 5-HT1A and NMDA binding sites by a single rapid transcranial magnetic stimulation procedure in rats. Brain Res 1999; 826:309–312.
69. George MS, Nahas Z, Bohning DE, Kozel FA, Anderson FA, Chae J-H, Lomarev M, Denslow S, Li X, Mu C. Vagus nerve stimulation therapy. Neurology 2002; 59:S56–S61.
70. Kiss ZHT, Mooney DM, Renaud L, Hu B. Neuronal response to local electrical stimulation in rat thalamus: physiological implications for mechanisms of deep brain stimulation. Neuroscience 2002; 113:137–143.
71. Benazzouz A, Hallett M. Mechanism of action of deep brain stimulation. Neurology 2000; 55:S13–S16.
72. Chen R, Classen J, Gerloff C, Celnik P, Wassermann EM, Hallett M, Cohen LG. Depression of motor cortex excitability by low-frequency transcranial magnetic stimulation. Neurology 1997; 48:1398–1403.

73. Lomarev M, Denslow S, Nahas Z, Chae JH, George MS, Bohning DE. Vagus nerve stimulation (VNS) synchronized BOLD fMRI suggests that VNS in depressed adults has frequency dependent effects. J Psychiatric Res 2002; 36:219–227.
74. Kirschvink JL, Kobayashi-Kirschvink A, Diaz-Ricci JC, Kirschvink JL. Magnetite in human tissues: a mechanism for the biological effects of weak ELF magnetic fields. Bioelectromagnetics Suppl 1992; 1:101–113.
75. Lednev VV. Possible mechanism of the effect of weak magnetic fields on biosystems. Bioelectromagnetics 1991; 12:71–75.
76. Bell GB, Marino AA, Chesson AL, Struve F. Electrical states in the rabbit brain can be altered by light and electromagnetic fields. Brain Res 1992; 570:307–315.
77. Adey WR. Fields, cell membrane amplification, and cancer promotion. In: Wilson BW, Stevens RG, Anderson LE, eds. Extremely Low Frequency Electromagnetic Fields: The Question of Cancer. Columbus, OH: Battelle Press, 1990.
78. Nunez PL. The Elecric Fields of the Brain: The Neurophysics of EEG. New York: Oxford University Press, 1981.
79. Collins JJ, Chow CC, Imhoff TT. Stochastic resonance without tuning. Nature 1995; 376:236–238.
80. Jefferys JGR. Nopnsynaptic modulation of neuronal activity in the brain: electric currents and extracellular ions. Physiol Rev 1995; 75:689–723.
81. Libet B, Gerard RW. Control of the potential rhythm of the isolated frog brain. J Neurophysiol 1939; 2:153–169.
82. Magora F, Beller A, Aladjemoff L, Magora A, Tannenebaum J. Observations on electrically induced sleep in man. Brit J Anesthesiol 1965; 37:480–491.

15

Is there an Electrical Circulatory System that Communicates Internally and Externally?

Paul J. Rosch

The American Institute of Stress, Yonkers, and New York Medical College, Valhalla, New York, U.S.A.

Björn E.W. Nordenström

Karolinska Institute and Hospital, Stockholm, Sweden

There is evidence of an electrical circulatory system in the body that is reminiscent of ancient Chinese concepts of meridians that conduct Qi (ch'i) energy through prescribed pathways (meridians) in the body in an orderly fashion. In this analogy, the antagonistic and complementary components of yin and yang may be thought of as positive and negative electricity. Similar energy communication conduits may help explain such well acknowledged but poorly understood phenomena as the placebo effect, the power of a strong faith in spontaneous remission of cancer and energy fields that can emanate from chi gong masters and faith healers that appear as auras with Kirlian photography and other imaging techniques.

Dr. Björn Nordenström claims to have found in the human body a heretofore unknown universe of electrical activity that's the very foundation of the healing process and is as critical to well being as the flow of blood. If he's right, he has made the most profound biomedical discovery of the century.

So began the April 1986 cover story in *Discover Magazine* about Björn Nordenström's amazing "cures" of patients with lung and breast tumors based on his theory of biologically closed electrical circuits. It went on to note that some distinguished scientists and physicians believed that if his findings were confirmed by others they would prove to be as important as William Harvey's description of the circulatory system. Some compared his 1983 book (1) explaining his results and theories to Harvey's 1628 treatise on how blood circulates through the body (2). Clinicians who tried to wade through Nordenström's massive tome often had difficulty deciphering the complex electrical schematics and equations that formed the underpinnings of his theory. Others failed to grasp its potential

229

implications. However, the few who did appreciate this as well as the thoroughness of his research were laudatory in their praise and tried to promote his efforts, as evidenced by the following unusual book review by Morton G. Glickman, M.D., Professor of Diagnostic Radiology, Yale University School of Medicine, that appeared in *Investigative Radiology* (Vol. 19. Sept/Oct/ No. 5, 1984):

It has not been the policy of *Investigative Radiology* to publish book reviews. However, the work by Nordenström reviewed below presents such fundamental and far-reaching concepts that a review was deemed desirable in order to call this book to the attention of those who read *Investigative Radiology*. The importance of the concepts presented in Dr. Nordenströms book cannot be overemphasized. Those who are interested in fundamental biological observations will be fascinated by the logical progression of this most imaginative work: *Biologically Closed Electric Circuits*, Björn E. W. Nordenström, MD, 1983 (Nordic Medical Publications, Arsenalsgatan 4, S-1ll 47 Stockholm, Sweden).

This remarkable book introduces a new physiologic concept that could solve many long-standing biologic problems. This far-reaching concept evolved from a series of ingenious experiments that began with the author's search for the explanation of a curious pattern that he observed on a chest x-ray about 30 years ago. His investigations carried him well beyond the original problem and produced original insights into such fundamental processes as wound healing, organ development and differentiation, and extra-cellular fluid dynamics. The primary direction of the book is understanding the interaction of malignant tumors with their surrounding tissues. It leads on the one hand to a possible mechanism of carcinogenesis and on the other to a proposed new mode of therapy of malignancies. Dr. Nordenström has discovered a new circulatory system that is based on spontaneously occurring electrical potentials. Potential gradients have long been known to develop in normal organs as a result of metabolism and in injured or diseased tissue as a result of hemorrhage or necrosis. The investigations detailed in this book reveal that these potentials are more than just a source of error in bioelectric measurements, that, in fact, they drive electric current through what the author calls biologically closed electric circuits (BCEC).

Blood plasma and interstitial fluid are examples of ionic media capable of effectively conducting current. Blood vessel walls and the cells and membranes that surround interstitial spaces insulate these conducting media from their surroundings. Plasma and interstitial fluid are electrically joined across capillary membranes. Thus, blood vessels and interstitial spaces function as insulated electric cables that carry current and transport charged particles over short and long distances. Other BCEC probably also exist, but the book examines this particular circuit in detail, documenting its existence and function with a series of experiments using physical analogs of biologic organs and organ systems, animal models, and tumor and tissue specimens obtained at autopsy or surgical resection. The resultant hypotheses are tested in a series of careful and humane diagnostic experiments and therapeutic trials performed on consenting human volunteers with malignant diseases.

Credit should be given to Dr. John Austin who spent many hours revising the manuscript. The book is written in a lucid, concise prose style and presents its material in approximately chronologic order. Thus, the reader is shown the stepwise development of this complex concept in what must be very close to the way that the author himself arrived at his conclusions. This method of presentation tantalizes the reader as it builds from the proposal of a simple hypothesis to its experimental documentation to the next hypothesis, and gradually but convincingly expands the reader's understanding as the investigations progress to more and more basic levels of biologic insight. Like most significant scientific innovations, the ideas are simple and, once proposed, the reader must wonder why something so obvious took so long to surface. Yet the originality or the hypotheses, the thought processes that led to them, and the experiments that prove them are astounding.

In the mid-1950s Dr. Nordenström observed a peculiar series of radiating and circumferential patterns surrounding a primary carcinoma of the lung on a chest radiograph. He called this pattern corona structures, because of the similarity to the corona of the sun. A prospective study over several years revealed that corona structures were present with considerable frequency around pulmonary malignancies, pulmonary granulomas, and even hamartomas. The book begins the analysis of these structures with a careful description using radiographs of many patients and using serial radiographs of the same patient. The alteration of corona structures with time and the disappearance of some of them with the development of pneumothorax led Dr. Nordenström to postulate that some parts of this radiographic pattern resulted from an unexplained effect of pulmonary masses on distribution of lung water. Thus began a series of experiments that resulted in his conclusion that fluctuating electrical potentials originating within lung masses could alter extracellular fluid dynamics. The author demonstrated that electrical potentials do exist within lung masses by performing a series of measurements in patients undergoing needle biopsy. After preliminary experiments, he succeeded in reproducing corona structures in dogs by implanting artificial "tumors" that produced potential gradients similar to those measured in human pulmonary masses.

The text proceeds to an investigation of the anatomy and physiology of these phenomena and leads to the development of the concept of energy conversion over BCEC. Along the way, explanations of a number of other biologic phenomena are proposed. After demonstrating that electrical potentials are spontaneously generated in organs such as the spleen, and that potentials of this magnitude lead to formation of fibrous tissue at electrical interfaces, the author postulates that organ capsules and other fibrous surfaces such as pleura and peritoneum are formed by BCEC.

Platelets and leukocytes carry a surplus of fixed electronegative surface charges. Thus a spontaneously occurring positive polarity in injured tissue results in accumulation of platelets and then thrombosis of capillaries surrounding a site of injury. This mechanism can also account for attraction of leukocytes to a site of positive electrical potential in injured or diseased tissue.

To test the possibility that BCEC alter the tissue environment around tumors in organs other than the lung, the author undertook a series of experiments with human and animal breast tissue and human breast neoplasms. He demonstrated in a series of mammograms that corona structures similar to those that surround lung masses are present quite commonly around tumors of the breast. Spontaneous electrical potentials occur in breast tumors, just as in lung masses, and have a similar effect on tissue water distribution. However, the abundant fat in breast tissue permitted some even more surprising observations. Histologically normal human breast fat obtained from mastectomy specimens, when subjected to electrophoresis, developed fibrosis similar to the desmoplastic reaction that surrounds breast tumors. Within this desmoplastic tissue, structures developed that were histologically similar to primitive ductal and vascular channels. The author suggests that this may explain the mechanism by which tumor angiogenesis occurs. Similar in vitro experiments produced microcalcifications similar to those found in breast malignancies in previously normal breast fat.

This seminal work opens important new subjects for research and may ultimately explain many heretofore inexplicable biologic phenomena. However, it is more than a scholarly report of a massive research effort. It is an interesting, often exciting account of a brilliant mind in vigorous action. It leaves the reader exhilarated.

A year later, a second article appeared in the *American Journal of Roentgenology*, probably the most prestigious journal in the field. It was a rewrite of one of Nordenström's lectures again accompanied by a comment from the editor who similarly stated that its publication was unconventional and required the following explanation. The work was unique in that unlike the multiauthored papers that such a complex subject usually required, this represented the effort of just one individual, Björn Nordenström. "He alone is responsible for the original concepts, the experiments, the analysis, and the text. Although employing modern terms and instruments, his performance is in the tradition of the pioneer scientist: complete and isolated immersion in the research." While a final judgement on the merit of Nordenström's theory would be premature, the work was "imaginative, experimentally ingenious and provocative" and deserved serious examination by the medical community.

Despite this and other accolades, Gary Taubes, the author of the lengthy *Discover* cover story was surprised to find during his extensive research that few cancer specialists and even radiologists knew anything about Nordenström's research or recognized who he was, much less interested in determining whether he was right or wrong. This, despite the fact that he had pioneered the development of the percutaneous "skinny needle" biopsy technique that all surgeons and interventional radiologists relied on. In addition, Nordenström was Chairman of the Department of Radiology at the prestigious Karolinska Institute and Chairman of the Nobel Assembly that selects the Nobel Laureate in Physiology or Medicine.

Whether Björn Nordenström's BCEC concept is correct, there is little doubt that his treatment protocol based on this can be very effective. I had asked him to chair a session on "Electromagnetic Energy Effects On Psychophysiologic Function" at our 1998 International Congress on Stress in Montreux, Switzerland. It included papers on "The Effect of Electromagnetic Energy on Brain Neurotransmitters" by Norman Shealy and Saul Liss and "The Physiological Effects of Low Energy Emission Therapy" by Boris Pasche, all of whom who have also contributed chapters to this volume. Björn's own presentation on "The Use of Electrical Energies in the Promotion of Healing and Treatment of Cancer" described one patient with a history of ovarian cancer and another with adenocarcinoma of the breast who had subsequently developed metastatic pulmonary lesions. These patients were considered inoperable and one had large lesions in both lungs. Nevertheless following treatment, the tumors gradually disappeared and both were well 8 and 10 years later with no evidence of metastatic disease. Figure 1 shows chest x-rays of the ovarian cancer patient when first seen and 8 months and 2 years following a single painless course of treatment that was completed in 1 day. When last heard from a few years ago, this individual was approximately 90 years old, in good health, and without any evidence of cancer. How could such miraculous results be explained?

According to Nordenström's theory, the body's electrical communication system can be compared to a battery in which the circuit is driven by separation of oppositely charged ions.

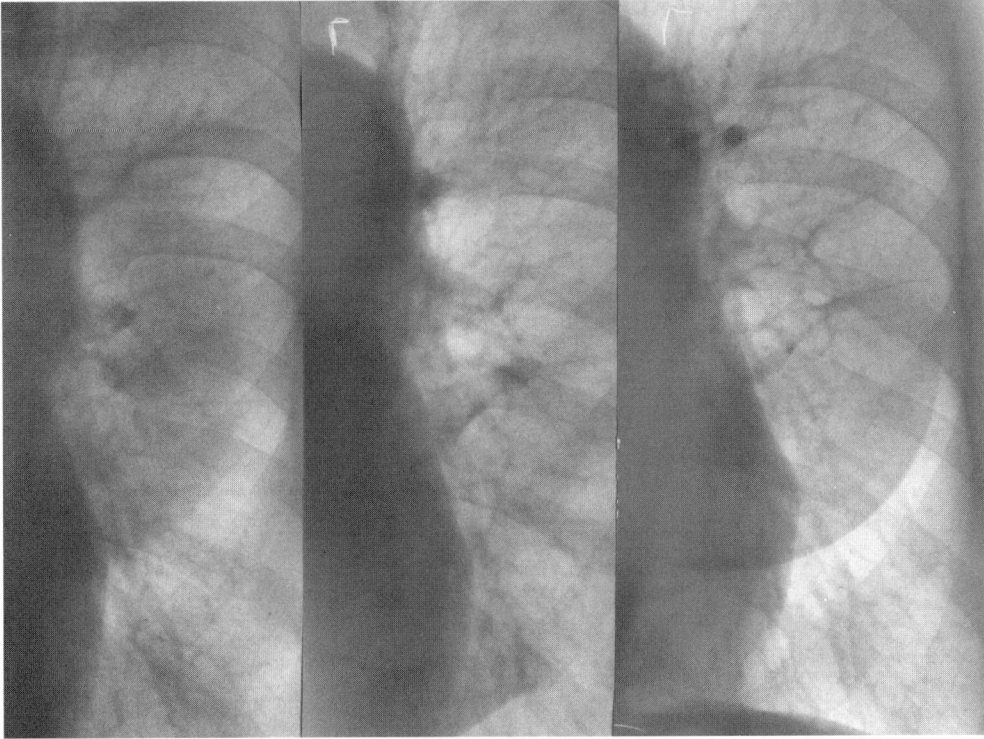

Figure 1 Sixty-six-year-old patient with metastatic ovarian cancer to the lung.

Once the circuit is closed, long distance current flows through the conducting cables and within the battery, ions drift across the permeable barrier as shown in Fig. 2.

When tissue is damaged by injury or malignant growth, there is a buildup of positively charged ions in the affected area, whereas adjacent healthy tissue is negative. As a malignant tumor grows, its inner cells are cut off from the circulatory system and slowly perish. This cell death leads to chemical changes and the production of positive electrical potential in the tumor compared to adjacent tissue as seen in Fig. 3.

This separation of charge sets the stage for the flow of electricity as the tumor's progressive positive charge polarizes nearby tissue, thus turning on the long-distance circuit. Ions flow through blood vessels linked to the tumor as well as percolating throughout the tissue around the tumor as indicated in Fig. 4.

Nordenström's biologically closed electrical circuits are driven by the accumulated charges, which, unlike those in a battery, constantly oscillate between positive and negative. The larger vessels act like insulating cables and the blood plasma functions as a conductor. In permeable tissue around the tumor the fluid between cells conducts ions and capillary membranes function as electrodes, as shown in Fig. 5.

A key component of BCECs are the natural electrodes found in capillary walls. The membranes of the capillary wall cells are known to be charged, causing ions to circulate through the cells via gates and vesicles and between the cells via pores, as shown in Fig. 6. Electrons cross over and enzymes can bridge to close this local circuit. Nordenström discovered that arterial capillaries contract when subjected to an electric field caused by the accumulation of positive charges at a site of tissue injury. As a consequence, the pores and

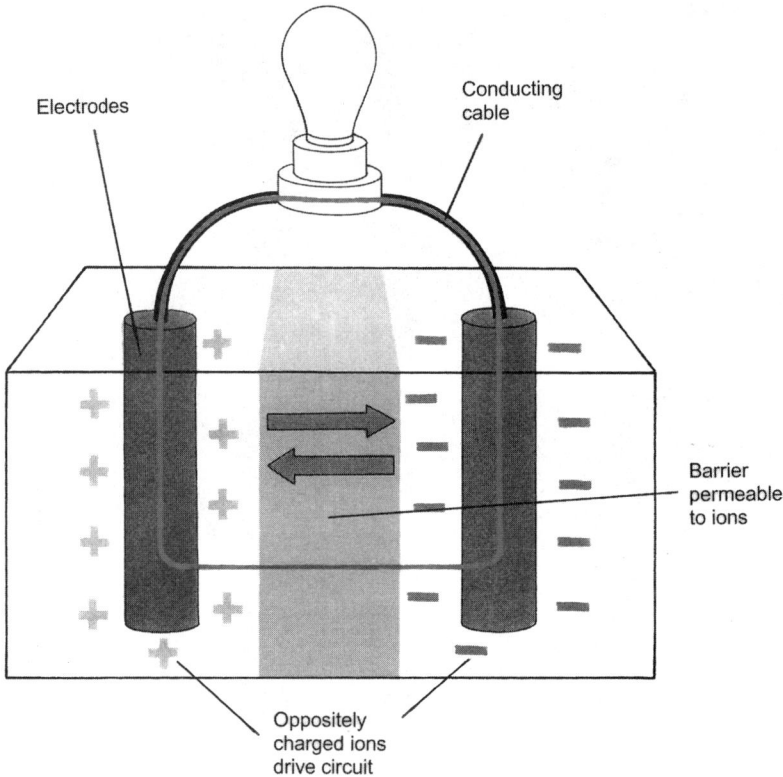

Figure 2 Nordenstrom's biologically closed electrical circuit (BCEC): A biological battery.

gates close, blocking the ionic current and the ions flow through the blood stream and along the capillary walls, thus switching on the long-distance circuit.

In contrast, venous capillaries do not contract in an electrical field. Ions and charged white blood cells that are attracted or repelled by the changes in electrical potential at sites of injury migrate through the pores of adjacent venous capillaries as shown in Fig. 7. This causes an oscillation of electrical potential at injury sites creating an ebb and flow of ions that Nordenström believed was critical for the healing process.

He arrived at these conclusions by initially measuring the electric potential or voltage of lung tumors by using the skinny needles he had introduced as electrodes. A positive electrode was inserted into the tumor and a negative one into adjacent normal tissue as illustrated in Fig. 8. He found that the coronas around malignant tumors seen on x-rays occurred during their electropositive phase; spikes appeared on the surface of the tumor and water moved into the surrounding tissue dehydrating the tumor and forming a series of radiating structures and arches.

By running current into the tumor, Nordenström was able to amplify and prolong the electropositive phase of the existing circuit. He postulated that this would trigger a variety of tumor-fighting effects, including attracting white cells and producing acid at the center of the tumor and the accumulation of water at the negative electrode as shown in Fig. 9.

Since his initial presentation, Björn has provided us with updates on his research at subsequent congresses, and we have become good friends. His results in metastatic lung malignancies and cancer of the breast and other organs have now been confirmed by others in

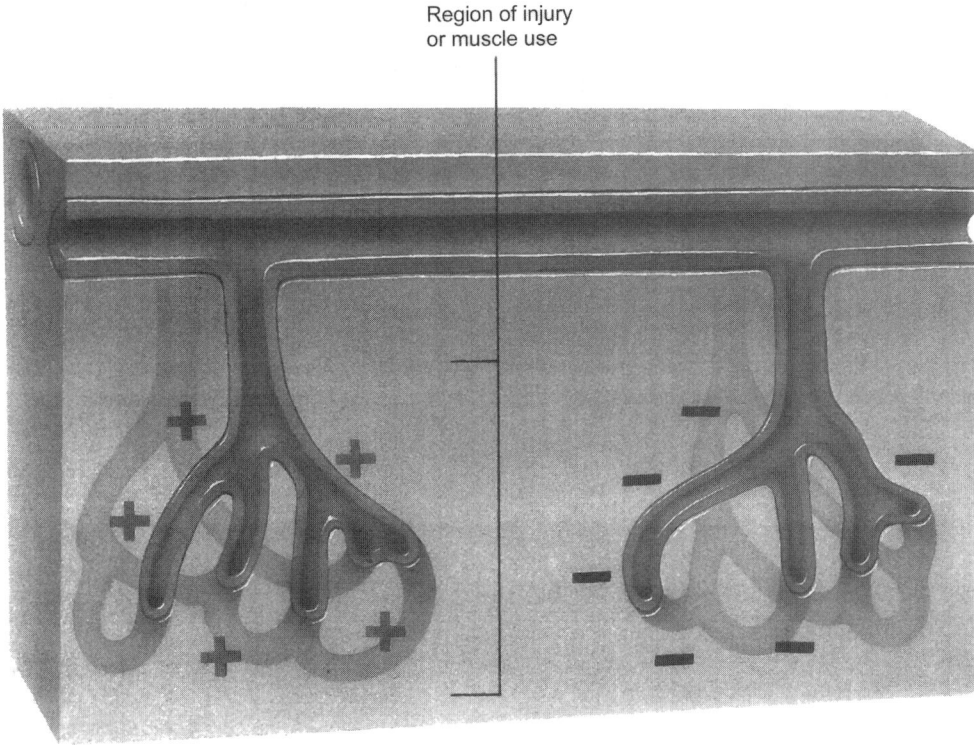

Figure 3 Cancer tissue develops a positive charge.

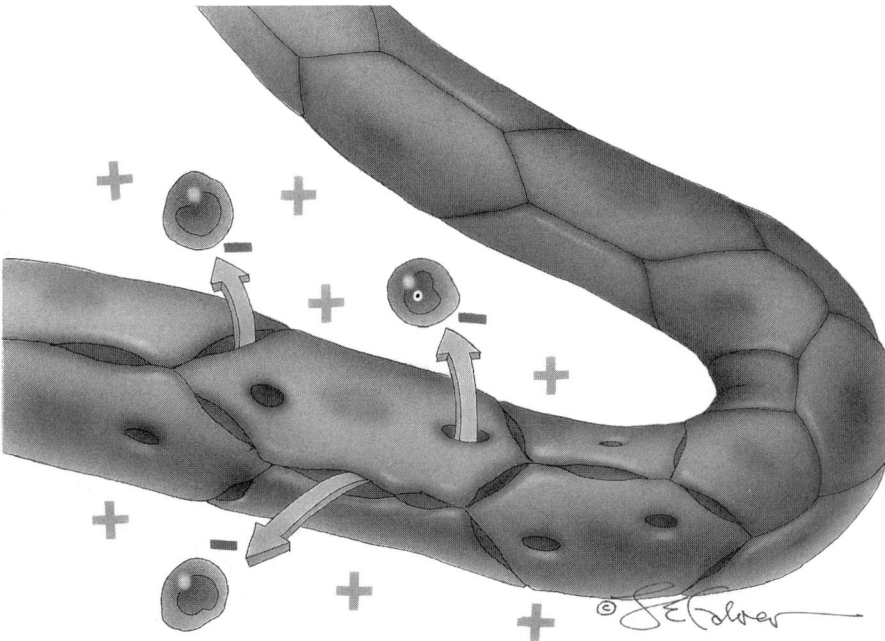

Figure 4 How the biologically closed electrical circuit is activated.

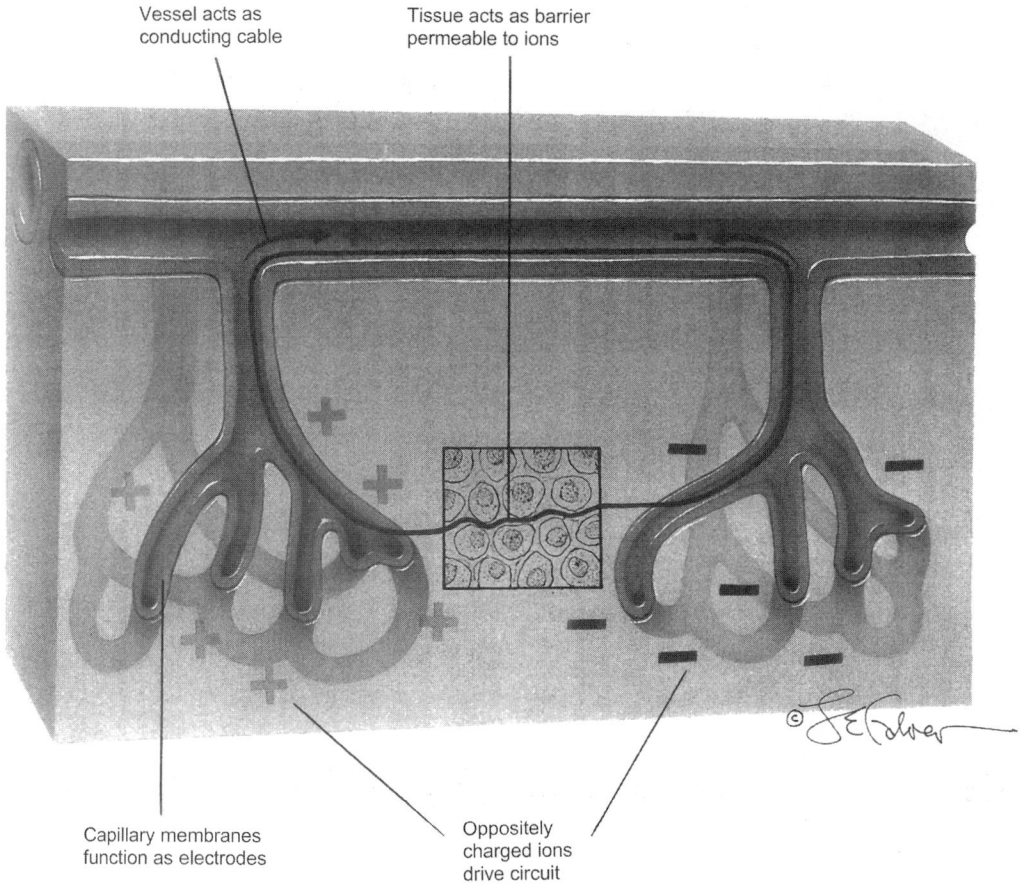

Figure 5 How current flows through the blood stream.

over 10,000 patients. In his 1998 book (3) he explained how the BCEC principle can be utilized to show how biological systems can interact with internal and external electromagnetic fields and asked me to provide a concluding Afterword explaining on how this might relate to ancient concepts of Qi (ch'i), yin, and yang. I had invited him to contribute a chapter to this book but his progressive illness has now made this impossible. Consequently, I have attempted to synopsize some of his recent thoughts and those expressed in my Afterword and have asked Björn to review this for accuracy and to add any additional comments.

I chose to begin my chapter for his last book with this quotation from Claude Bernard: "To be astonished at anything, is the first movement of the mind towards discovery." I felt this was most appropriate since it was his amazement and bewilderment about the curious corona like halos around malignant tumors he had seen on chest x-rays that set Björn off on a quest that has occupied almost five decades of multidisciplinary research. He had published a few papers confirming that the electrical characteristics of lung cancers differed from normal tissue, but there was little response or interest in this. Undaunted, he continued his research, which eventually led him to the conclusion that the body had an additional communication or "electrical" circulatory system not previously appreciated. In 1979, he began writing a book entitled *Biologically Closed Electrical Circuits: Clinical, Experimental and Theoretical Evidence for an Additional Circulatory System* to explain this. The final

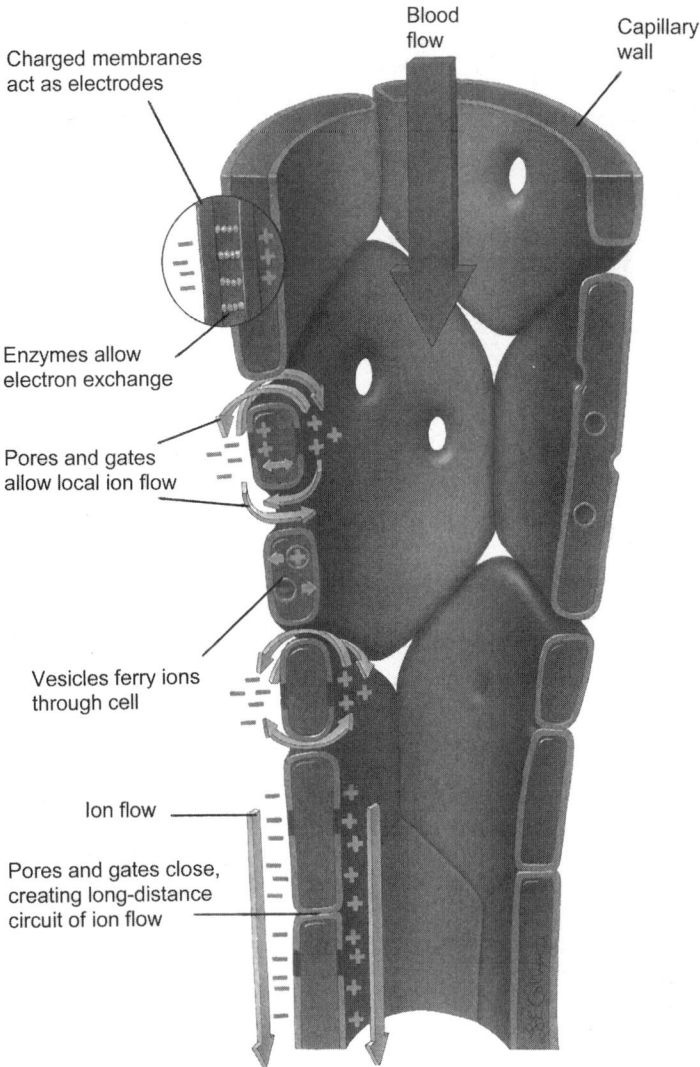

Figure 6 Capillaries close the circuit.

product was a large handsome volume of over 350 pages replete with elaborate art work, diagrams, x-rays, and reproductions of gross and microscopic pathology, many of which were in color. However, the medical publishing houses were not at all interested in this, probably because they thought it would not be profitable, and they were correct. Nordenström had to raise $50,000 to finally publish it himself in 1983, and of the 2000 copies printed, only 200 were sold over the next 2 years. Since then an additional 1000 have been purchased with the majority of the remainder being donated to libraries, institutions, and interested individuals.

My interest in Bjorn's research stemmed from my involvement in studying relationships between stress and cancer. I had been awarded a Fellowship in 1951 to study with Hans Selye, who coined the term *stress* as it is commonly used. Selye had demonstrated in thousands of experiments that when laboratory animals were subjected to severe and

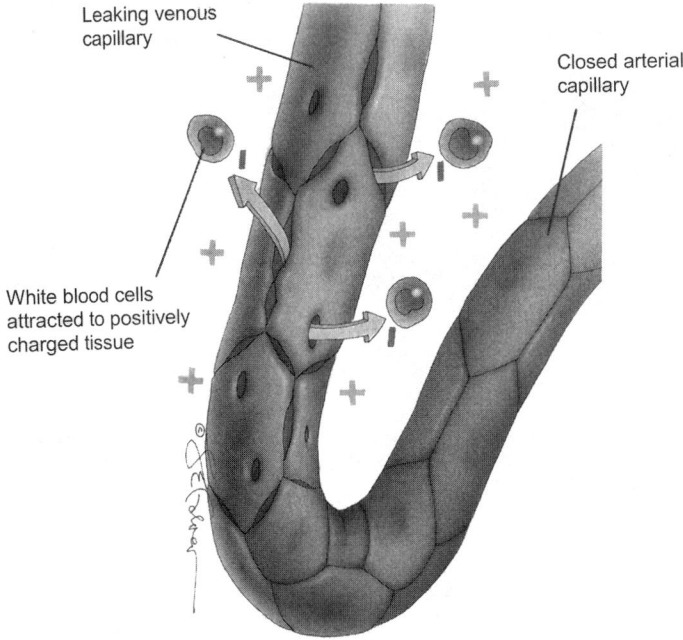

Figure 7 Venous and arterial capillary activities at sites of injury and cancer.

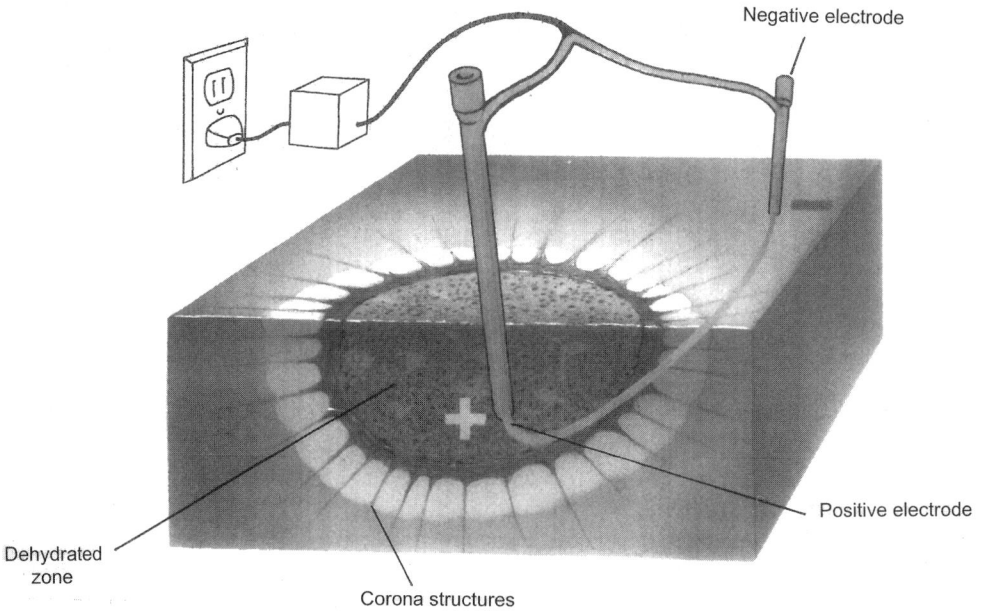

Figure 8 Inserting the electrodes. Using skinny needles inserted into the tumor (positive electrode) and adjacent normal tissue (negative electrode), it was found that the coronas around malignant tumors seen on x-rays occurred during their electropositive phase; spikes appeared on the surface of the tumor, and a series of radiating structures and arches were formed as water moved into the surrounding tissue and the tumor became dehydrated.

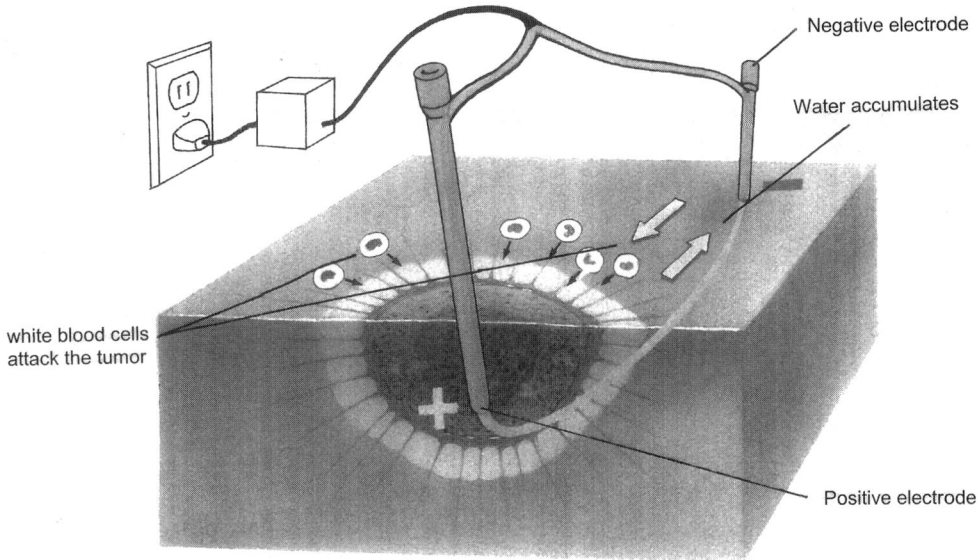

Figure 9 Attacking the tumor. Running current into the cancer prolongs its electropositive phase facilitating a variety of anticancer activities such as attracting tumor-fighting white cells and producing an acidic condition at the center of the tumor as water accumulates at the negative electrode.

prolonged stress there was an immediate activation of the body's defense mechanisms or alarm reaction, followed by a stage of resistance, during which these were maximized, and a final stage of exhaustion, in which defenses diminished and disappeared. He referred to this three staged response as the general adaptation syndrome and observed that during its course, pathologic changes could be seen in tissues and organs indistinguishable from those seen in patients suffering from various diseases, including hypertension, myocardial infarction, nephrosclerosis, peptic ulcers, and rheumatoid arthritis. He suspected that stress could contribute to such disorders in people and referred to them as diseases of adaptation.

Selye and I had developed a close personal and professional relationship and continued to collaborate after I resumed my medical training and entered private practice. However, I was surprised when he invited me to participate in a 1977 conference entitled "Stress, Cancer, and Death," being cosponsored by his International Institute of Stress and the Sloan-Kettering Institute. I explained that although relationships between stress and cancer were of great interest to me, I did not have the background to prepare a proper presentation since I was preoccupied with caring for patients and had not been actively involved in research activities for over 20 years. However, Selye was insistent and reminded me that I had first suggested to him during my fellowship that certain malignancies might also represent diseases of adaptation. While initially skeptical, he now agreed based on a personal experience as well as basic science studies and clinical reports he had assembled and wanted me to review. He promised to put the resources of his institute at my disposal, and a week later I received a very large packet of reprints dealing with various intriguing aspects of this complex subject. The challenge was irresistible and I contributed a paper that was subsequently published in the Sloan-Kettering Cancer Series devoted to the conference (4). In his Preface to this volume, Selye noted, "Perhaps, as Paul Rosch of New York has suggested, cancer might even be an attempt by the human organism to regenerate tissues and organs and even limbs, as lower animals are able to do spontaneously" (5). I had pointed out that the response to physical injury or loss in lower forms of life was purposeful regeneration. Studies in cancer patients showed that the onset of malignancy often followed the death of a spouse or loss of some other important relationship. Perhaps this initiated a similar stimulus to regenerate new tissue that had gone awry and resulted in neoplasia that was now not only no longer purposeful but potentially lethal.

The conference proceedings generated a great deal of interest, and my chapter attracted numerous inquiries and correspondence from researchers with similar views who supplied additional supportive information. The authors were invited to provide an update for an expanded second edition that also included contributions from others on various relevant topics. I had become particularly interested in the unexplained phenomenon of spontaneous remission in cancer and other deadly disorders and the health promoting properties of a firm faith and discussed this in my revised chapter entitled "Some Thoughts on the Endemiology of Cancer" (6). The focus here was not on the role of environmental carcinogens but rather on factors residing in the host that might influence susceptibility to stressful emotional stimuli. The chapter following mine in this 1988 update was by Yujiro Ikemi, a respected Japanese researcher, who had been attempting to integrate Eastern and Western biopsychosocial approaches to understanding and treating disorders, especially those that seemed to be stress related (7). He had thoroughly studied well-documented cases of spontaneous remission in cancer and presented his findings at our 1995 International Congress in Switzerland, where he was honored for his contributions. Ikemi confirmed that the common denominator in these patients was a strong belief system and a very positive expectation of a favorable outcome (8). Others had also reached this conclusion (9), but how were these benefits mediated? What mechanisms were involved?

Research in the flourishing field of *psychoneuroimmunology* had shown that emotional distress could lower immune system resistance to cancer, which seemed an attractive possibility, but this hardly proved that stress could cause cancer. In addition, nobody knew exactly what the immune system consisted of or where it was located, since it had numerous components and could be assessed in various ways. There were rapid humoral responses as well as delayed, cell-mediated processes, each with several markers whose significance was not clear. Immune system *function* or *competency* can be measured by numerous criteria, including different antibodies in blood, saliva, and urine and various cytokines or specialized leukocytes with descriptive names suggesting possible functions, such as "natural killer," "helper," and "suppressor" cells. Others are represented by an "alphabet soup" of confusing letters, numbers, and symbols that are used to monitor immune system competency in AIDS, such as CDF4+ and CDF4+/CDF8+ ratios and NK-associated CD16+ (leu11) leu7− and CD16+(leu11) leu7+ lymphocyte subsets, the inducer subset (CD45RA+CD4+) that activates suppressor–cytotoxic CD8+ cells, etc. During stress varied responses have been observed, including a reduction in cytokines that stimulate both Th1 responses and macrophages (IL-2, IL-12, IFN-(γ) as well as an increase in cytokines that promote the growth and differentiation of Th2 and B-lymphocytes (IL-4, IL-10).

Immune system status is also often measured by older techniques such as macrophage activity by chemiluminescence following stress or responses involving properdin, opsonins, and complement C3. There are assays for interleukins (IL), interferons (IF), tumor necrosis factors (TNF), and transforming growth factors (TGF). Much of the research on the effects of stress is based on the effects of mitogens such as phytohaemagglutinin (PHA) or concanavalin A (ConA) that stimulate T-cell production. However, it is not known whether such in vitro studies accurately reflect changes that have clinical significance or mirror in vivo immune responses. In short, it is quite likely that the same stressor could result in an increase, decrease, or lack of effect on "immune system resistance" depending on the criteria selected. Different types of stressors might have differing effects on the same system and the intensity and duration of the stimulus could also affect responses.

The more I tried to study how stress affected the immune system, the more I confused I became. The traditional explanation of stress-immune system responses as being mediated by activation of the hypothalamic-pituitary-adrenal cortex axis and humoral neuropeptide messengers did not seem to apply since there were no studies to support such a cause–effect relationship between emotional stress and malignant growth. I had wondered whether there might be some other energy communication pathway that might be relevant. In the final analysis, when hormones or small neuropeptides reached their specialized receptor sites on cell walls, the message was ultimately transmitted to the interior of the cell by a feeble electrical stimulus. Thus, EEG waves might not merely reflect the noise of the machinery of the brain but signals being sent to specialized receptor sites in the body through unknown pathways. I postulated this in the concluding chapter entitled "Future Directions in Psychoneuroimmunology: Psychoelectroneuroimmunology?" I was asked to contribute to *Stress, the Immune System and Psychiatry* (10). In his Foreword to this book, my friend Bob Ader, who coined the term *psychoneuroimmunology,* had also emphasized that future progress in this field would require "careful research, new methodologies, and communication between scientists in traditionally distinct fields" (11).

By this time, I had come to the conclusion that cancer was a disease of adaptation to civilization due to faulty communication and lack of a feeling of control. There was abundant support for cancer as a disease of civilization. Dr. Albert Schweizer, the renowned humanitarian, theologian, medical missionary, and Nobel Prize recipient wrote (12):

> On my arrival in Gabon in 1913, I was astonished to encounter no cases of cancer. I cannot, of course say positively that there was no cancer at all; but like other frontier doctors, I can only say that if any cases existed, they must have been quite rare. In the course of the years, we have seen cases of cancer in growing numbers in our region. My observations incline me to attribute this to the fact that the natives are living more and more after the manner of the whites.

The celebrated anthropologist and Arctic explorer, Vilhjalmur Stefansson, in his book, which was actually titled *Cancer; Disease of Civilization?*, emphasized the absence of cancer in the Eskimos during his visits to various North Polar communities but a subsequent increase in the incidence of the disease as closer contact with white civilization was established (13). In *Cancer; A Disease of Either Election or Ignorance*, William Hays commented on this as follows (14):

> A study of the distribution of cancer, among the races of the entire earth, shows a cancer ratio in about proportion to which civilization living predominates; so evidently something inherent in the habits of civilization is responsible for the difference of cancer incidence compared with the uncivilized races and tribes. Climate has nothing to do with this difference as witness the fact that tribes living naturally will show a complete absence until mixture with more civilization, even so does cancer begin to show its head.

One of the most persuasive arguments is to be found in Alexander Berglas' *Cancer; Its Nature, Cause and Cure*. Throughout this book runs the theme that cancer is a disease from which primitive peoples are relatively or wholly free, and that (15)

> We are threatened with death from cancer because of our inability to adapt to present day living conditions. Over the years, cancer research has become the domain of specialists in various fields. Despite the outstanding contributions of

scientists, we have been getting farther away from our goal, the curing of cancer. This specialized work, and the knowledge gained through the study of individual processes, has had the peculiar result of becoming an obstacle to the whole. More than thirty years in the field of cancer research have convinced me that it is not to our advantage to continue along this road of detailed analysis. I have come to the conclusion that cancer may perhaps be just another intelligible natural process whose cause is to be found in our environment and mode of life.

This concept was hardly new and was possibly first proposed in Tanchou's *Memoir on the Frequency of Cancer*, delivered in 1843 to the French Academy of Sciences (16).

M. Tanchou is of the opinion that cancer, like insanity, increases in a direct ratio to the civilization of a country and of the people. And it is certainly a remarkable circumstance, doubtless in no small degree flattering to the vanity of the French savant, that the average mortality rate from cancer in Paris during 11 years was about 0.80 per 1000 living annually, while it is only 0.20 in London! Estimating the intensity of civilization by these data, it clearly follows that Paris is four times more civilized than London!

I was able to cite numerous additional supportive writings in "Stress and Cancer: Disorders of Communication, Control and Civilization" with 254 references that endorsed the other opinions suggested in this title (17).

With regard to being a disorder of communication, Selye had also noted in his Preface to the proceedings of the 1977 conference on stress and cancer that "the ultimate health of the organism, like that of society, appears to depend on how well or appropriately its constituent units communicate with one another" (5). This was essentially a paraphrase of Claude Bernard's dictum that the health of the organism depended on its ability to maintain the constancy of the milieu intrieur (internal environment) (18), which Walter Cannon later described as homeostasis (19). In discussing the importance of communication, Selye had previously written in his best seller, *Stress Without Distress*, "the indispensability of this disciplined, orderly mutual cooperation is best illustrated by its opposite—the development of a cancer, whose most characteristic feature is that it cares only for itself" (20). However, it seemed to me that good health depended not only on good communication within the milieu intrieur but also with the external environment and that this held true for all the hierarchy of living systems ranging upward from a cell, tissue, organ, and person to a family, corporation, nation, or culture. Maintaining good health as well as life itself depends entirely on good communication—both between the components of the system as well as with the external environment.

But exactly how did communication take place within the body? The nervous system relays information by direct contact as adrenergic or cholinergic molecules are released at nerve endings and synapses. Hormones and neurotransmitters are carried via the circulation to specific receptors at sites distant from their point of origin. Much less is known about the immune system, although it is clear that its conversations include both humoral and hardwired connections. However, in the final analysis all of the messages are eventually transmitted by means of weak energy transfers across cell membranes that occur at an atomic rather than molecular level. It had also become clear that the cell membrane was much more than a mere protective shield studded with receptors for antibodies and other small molecules that acted like keys to open special locks. The cell wall had now emerged as a powerful signal amplifier that provides an interactive window through which the cell can sense and respond to environmental changes. Some substances pass freely back and forth through certain channels, whereas the cell wall is an impenetrable barrier for others. When designated molecules fit into special receptor sites, a subtle signal produces a sudden change in the electrical potential between the interior of the cell and its external environment, allowing a new channel to open for a thousandths of a second. During this brief period, although millions of ions may pass back and forth, the total current generated is only a few billionths of an ampere.

As previously proposed, I believe that cell membranes may also have receptor sites for subtle energy signals that react exactly as they would to chemical on molecular stimuli. Electrical stimulation of highly specific areas in the pain pathway produces analgesia and microinjections of morphine at these precise sites have an identical effect. Electrical stimulation or injecting morphine a few millimeters away has no effect. However, combining suboptimal doses of morphine or electrical stimulation that alone are too weak to reduce pain results in a synergistic effect that does provide analgesia. This suggests that for some receptors, the effects of weak electrical stimulation are congruent with those of molecular stimuli. Furthermore, the specific locations at which either chemical or electrical stimulation relieve pain are exactly the sites of action of the opiatelike endorphins, the body's natural pain relievers (21). It seemed highly plausible that these and other receptor sites could readily respond to feeble electromagnetic signals generated internally.

Stress is difficult to define since it is a highly personalized phenomenon that differs for each of us. Things that are distressful for some people may be pleasurable for others, and we also respond to stress differently. Nevertheless, all of our experimental and clinical research confirms that the feeling of having little or no control is always distressful. That also happens to be a good definition of the cancer cell. It is a cell that is out of control because it does not communicate properly with its neighbors or the rest of the organism, as Yamasaki so elegantly demonstrated (22).

> Cancer can be regarded as a rebellion in an orderly society of cells when they neglect their neighbors and grow autonomously over surrounding normal cells. Since intercellular communication plays an important role in maintaining an orderly society, it must be disturbed in the process of carcinogenesis. Evidence suggests that blockage of intercellular communication is important in the promotion process of carcinogenesis.

A domineering, dogmatic determination, firm, forceful faith, fighting spirit; and an aggressive positive attitude all reflect the development of a strong sense of control. They are also common themes in reports of patients who triumphed over seemingly fatal malignancies (23–25). Could this message of control be communicated to cancer cells through unsuspected energy pathways to curb their undisciplined activities?

Anecdotal, but irrefutable reports of cancer cures from shrines, faith healers, laetrile, coffee enemas, acupuncture, macrobiotic diets, and other alternative treatments are difficult to explain. There are numerous reports of cancer regression through the use of various stress reduction or mind altering techniques, including intense meditation, visual imagery, and hypnosis (26–37). Yet, like spontaneous remission, all these cures are extremely rare, and benefits are entirely unpredictable in any given patient. Here again, having a strong faith in anything the individual believes in that provides a sense of control might be the reason. But how are the salutary rewards of faith healing, "therapeutic touch," or the placebo effect mediated? Is there such a thing as psychic healing? How can one explain the well-documented benefits associated with the development of strong social support in patients with cancer and other disorders (38–43)? Conversely, what are the mechanisms involved in the numerous reports of reactivation of dormant cancer following an extremely stressful event, particularly the loss of a loved one (44–47)? No consistent immune, neuroendocrine, or central nervous system changes have been demonstrated in connection with such responses suggesting that they are mediated via other pathways (48,49). Is it possible to harness this subtle energy or to learn how to emulate, simulate, or stimulate it to attain the vast potential for self-healing that resides in all of us?

A related issue is whether communication or signaling exists between people, other forms of life, or Nature through pathways and mechanisms that have not yet been delineated. How does any of this relate to cancer as a disease of communication and control? I believe that Björn Nordenström may have provided a piece of this puzzle. While his 1983 book concentrated on the "vascular-interstitial closed circuit" (VICC), he subsequently demonstrated that there are numerous circuits ranging in size from meters to microns that utilize both ionic and electronic electricity and produce electromagnetic fields with varying frequencies, amplitudes, and wave lengths. He believes that Qi, the energy of life in ancient Chinese medicine is analogous to or perhaps the same as the electromagnetic energy found in biologically closed electrical circuits. Its yin and yang components may be thought of as the positive and negative electrical charges of closed circuit ionic flow. During health, Qi flows through prescribed pathways (meridians) in the body in an orderly fashion, and VICC and other interstitial channels may be thought of as corresponding to these meridians. Qi energy is also believed to project as a corona emanating from the extremities that can be visualized with Kirlian photography.

Nordenström provides other analogies with ancient Oriental concepts of how Qi in nature can affect human health, performance and possibly aging. Lifespan varies greatly in animals, plants, as well as different tissues in humans. It is believed that the life of a cell is genetically predetermined by limiting the number of times it can divide and reproduce. This process of programmed cell death, called *apoptosis*, is specific for each cell. He has described how biomagnetic forces can influence either regression (apoptosis) or proliferation (regrowth and survival) by explaining how a tree preserves its life during the cold winter through altering metabolic activities that sacrifice its leaves in the fall. In the spring, apoptotic regression is replaced by proliferative regeneration, when energy preserved in the tree is activated by heat to again produce the same kind of leaf. He illustrates how even a leaf that is "dead" still has energy in the form of a corona around it that can be seen with Kirlian photography. This repetitive cycle of death and rebirth that is guided by the same energy constantly takes place in other systems. In the Chinese view of nature, they provide balance in the Sheng and Ke cycles of ongoing regeneration and destruction for the five elements as depicted in a diagram I provided for my Afterword chapter (50).

Nordenström believes that although Qi and EMF energies are essentially the same entity that this is not appreciated because of semantic problems. He also believes that these forces flowing in closed biological circuits play a crucial role in the transformation of nonbiological substance into biological matter. However, theories do not have to be correct—only facts do. Some theories prove to be meritorious because of their heuristic value, in that they stimulate others to discover new facts that lead to better theories. Whether Nordenström's theories will prove to provide insights into ancient Oriental concepts of Qi and its flow through meridians remains to be seen. It has been reported that stimulation of an acupuncture point in the foot results in EEG changes that exceed the speed of sound. This and many of the other phenomena described above cannot be explained by any known biological mechanisms but could be consistent with the BCEC concept.

Are the forces or energies in magnetic fields, as well as those involved in faith healing, therapeutic touch, consciousness, intentionality, and BCECs also some manifestation of Qi? Albert Einstein believed that there was an underlying order to the organization and operation of the universe based on mathematical principles. He proposed not only that electromagnetism and gravity were different aspects of the same force but that all the four forms of energy were interrelated, and scientists have been trying to prove this Unified Field Theory ever since. Is Qi a fifth form of energy that will prove to be the glue that binds all of the others together?

The Chinese sage Lao Tsu described Qi as follows:

"Look, it cannot be seen—it is beyond form
Listen, it cannot be heard—it is beyond sound
Grasp, it cannot be held—it is intangible."

Is the human mind capable of comprehending Qi? Or, like infinity, and the lack of distinction between energy and matter at subatomic levels, is it impossible for us to visualize what Qi represents with respect to its composition and the manner in which it functions?

It is now obvious that subtle signals and energies can exert powerful psychophysiologic effects despite the fact that they are nonthermal, which would appear to violate the laws of thermodynamics. Various presentations at our International Congress support the belief that weak energies generated in the brain as well as the heart can have internal as well as external physiologic effects that cannot be explained by known communication pathways. These include energy fields or auras emanating from the hands of healers that were readily visualized with Kirlian and other imaging techniques, but only while they are engaged in their activities. Subjects blinded to the presence of such healers also reported sensations of heat or tingling in different parts of their body corresponding to sites under the healer's hands several inches away. When the position of the healer's hands moved to other areas these sensations consistently shifted to coincide with this. In addition, the ability of certain healers to produce voltage surges of 100 V in the EEG waves of subjects several feet away who were unaware of the purpose of the experiment or the healer's presence was illustrated as had been previously reported (51).

The external force generated by Qigong practitioners, also vividly demonstrated at our congress, is thought to have electromagnetic components. This is supported by studies using a cell free myosin phosphorylation system with high sensitivity to magnetic fields that exhibited the same response to the energies emanating from two Qigong masters (52,53). Clinically, Qigong has been found to be effective in treating reflex sympathetic dystrophy and other complex pain syndromes (54). Similarly, therapeutic touch and other energetic practitioners have demonstrated their ability to relieve pain (55,56), promote wound healing (57), increase hemoglobin levels (58,59) and produce structural changes in DNA and water (60) in addition to other measurable activities (61). As also presented at our congress and discussed elsewhere in this book, Tiller has demonstrated that intentionality can change the pH of a solution and alter the incubation time of fruit fly larvae. Furthermore, this energy can be stored on a computer chip for future use and other applications.

The brain or mind is not the only source of energy. The heart's electromagnetic field is estimated to be 5000 times stronger than that of the brain and can also be measured several feet away from the body with SQUID-based magnetometers (62). Congress presentations by McCraty and co-workers have demonstrated that this field can influence cerebral and cardiovascular function of other individuals in direct physical contact or even a few feet away as assessed by ECG and EEG recordings and as also explained in this volume and elsewhere (63). These observations have been independently confirmed by others (64) who have proposed that the heart actually plays the major role in generating as well as integrating the flow of energy in the body (65).

All of the above is consistent with an emerging paradigm that posits some form of subtle energy communication system in the body that can also detect and respond to external environmental energies or signals. This could help to explain such widely acknowledged but poorly understood phenomena as the placebo effect, faith healing, the power of a strong faith in spontaneous remission in cancer, the salubrious effects of certain olfactory, auditory, visual and tactile stimuli, and certain psychokinetic observations. The proposal that the level or orderly flow of energy in the body determines health and illness and that it is influenced by environmental forces has surfaced over the years as Qi, (ch'i), chakras, prana, archaeus, the aether, animal magnetism, Odic force, orgone, and other constructs in different cultures (66,67). If such forces do indeed exist, is it possible they are being drowned out by man made energies that we are unable to appreciate but are readily detected by FM and AM radio receivers, sonar, radar, and devices that can measure microwaves, electromagnetic fences, and other forces that pollute the atmosphere.

Acupuncture points known since antiquity have electrical properties quite different from sites a few millimeters away even though no distinctions can be seen with electron microscopy. This can be readily demonstrated by injecting radioactive technetium, and these electrical characteristics can be influenced by mental processes (68). The potential to cure disease and enhance health by harnessing such natural energies, as well as similar forces that can be artificially generated, seems enormous. Highly sophisticated technologies may now make it possible to achieve this goal and to integrate ancient Eastern and current Western concepts of health and illness. As also suggested by Mitchell in this volume, quantum physics and quantum mechanics may provide insights into possible mechanisms of action that cannot be explained by newtonian physics.

I have attempted here to provide a brief introduction to some of Bjorn's concepts and regret that his health did not permit him to take a more active role in this presentation. I am very grateful to his son, Professor Jörgen Nordenström, for crafting a chapter entitled "The Paradigm of Biologically Closed Electric Circuits (BCEC) and Its Clinical Applications" consisting of excerpts from some of Björn's publications that provides more detailed information. Professor Xin YuLing and colleagues from China have also contributed a chapter, "Electrochemical Therapy of Tumors," detailing their experience in over 9000 patients with various malignant and benign tumors.

As noted in the *Discover* cover story, some scientists have compared Björn Nordenström's accomplishments to William Harvey's discovery of how blood circulates in the body. In *The Discoverers*, Daniel Boorstin portrayed the state of medicine before Harvey described the circulatory system in 1628 as follows (69):

> Any physician who had labored to learn the academic languages and had become the disciple of some eminent professor of medicine had a heavy vested interest in the traditional lore and accepted dogmas.. . To attack this citadel demanded a willingness to defy the canons of respectability, to uproot oneself from the university community and from the guild.

Boorstin noted that Michael Servetus, who described the pulmonary circulation of the blood in one of his theological tracts, was burned at the stake by Calvin in 1553 for this heresy. However, Harvey led a charmed life. After completing his medical education in Padua, the leading center for anatomical studies, he returned to England in 1602 and married Elizabeth Browne, the daughter of one of the Queen's physicians. Harvey himself obtained a fellowship at the Royal College of Physicians and was appointed as a physician to the court of James I. He later became personal physician to his successor, King Charles I, who not only encouraged but generously supported his research into the circulatory system. Although Harvey's 1628 treatise created an uproar, he was regarded as a respected medical leader and at the time of his death in 1657, his medical and scientific genius were widely celebrated throughout England and Europe.

In contrast, Björn Nordenström has struggled and labored alone for over four decades, personally performing every experiment, with no financial support and at great personal expense. Although renowned for his radiological accomplishments, it seems unlikely that his BCEC concept and its implications will be adequately recognized in his lifetime. As previously indicated (50), he may have also opened the door to a greater understanding of how we can communicate with other living systems to improve health and harmony in nature. He is the epitome of the true scientist, described by Jules Henri Poincar as follows: "The scientist does not study nature because it is useful; he studies it because he delights in it, and he delights in it because it is beautiful. If it were not beautiful, it would not be worth knowing, and if nature were not worth knowing, life would not be worth living."

We would like to express our appreciation to Lewis Calver for permission to reproduce illustrations from the April 1986 *Discover* magazine cover story and to Nordic Medical Publications for material excerpted from Exploring BCEC-Systems (Biologically Closed Electric Circuits), 1998.

REFERENCES

1. Nordenström BEW. Biologically Closed Electric Circuits, Clinical, Experimental and Theoretical Evidence for an Additional Circulatory System. Stockholm: Nordic Medical Publications, 1983.
2. Harvey W. Excercitatio Anatomica de Motu Cordis et Sanguinis in Animalibus. Frankfurt: Anatomical Treatise on the Movement of the Heart and Blood in Animals, 1628.
3. Nordenström BEW. Exploring BCEC-Systems (Biologically Closed Electric Circuits). Stockholm: Nordic Medical Publications, 1998.
4. Rosch PJ. Stress and cancer: a disease of adaptation? In: Taché J, Selye H, Day SB, eds. Cancer, Stress, and Death. New York: Plenum Publishing, 1979:187–212.
5. Selye H. Foreword. In: Taché J, Selye H, Day SB, eds. Cancer, Stress, and Death. New York: Plenum Publishing, 1979:xii.
6. Rosch PJ. Some thoughts on the endemiology of cancer. In: Day SB, ed. Cancer, Stress, and Death. 2d ed. New York: Plenum Publishing, 1986:293–302.
7. Ikemi Y, Nagata K. The introduction of occidental and oriental approaches in biopsychosocial medicine. In: Day SB, ed. Cancer, Stress, and Death. 2d ed. New York: Plenum Publishing, 1986:303–312.
8. Ikemi Y, Nakagawa T, Sugita M. Psychosomatic considerations on cancer patients who have made a narrow escape from death. Dynam Psychiatry 1975; 31:77–92.
9. Cole WH. Spontaneous regression of cancer. The metabolic triumph of the host? Ann NY Acad Sci 1974; 230:111–113.
10. Rosch PJ. Future directions in psychoneuroimmunology: psychoelectroneuroimmunology? In: Leonard B, Miller K, eds. Stress, The Immune System and Psychiatry. Chichester: John Wiley and Sons, 1994:207–232.
11. Ader R. Foreword. In: Leonard B, Miller K, eds. Stress, The Immune System And Psychiatry. Chichester: John Wiley and Sons, 1994:ix–xii.
12. Schweitzer A. Forest Hospital of Lamborene. Oxford: Holt, 1931.
13. Stefansson V. Cancer: Disease of Civilization? New York: Hill and Wang, 1960.
14. Hay WH. Cancer: a disease of either election or ignorance. Am J Cancer 1927; 6:410–422.
15. Berglas A. Cancer: Its Nature, Cause and Cure. Paris: Pasteur Institute, 1957.
16. Statistical researches on cancer. South Med Sur J 1846; 4:273–274. Cited in Le Cont.

17. Rosch PJ. Stress and cancer: Disorders of communication, control and civilization. In: Cooper CL, ed. Handbook of Stress, Medicine, and Health. Boca Raton: CRC Press, 1996:27–50.

18. Bernard C. Introduction to the Study of Experimental Medicine. Paris: Flammarion, 1945. Original edition 1865.

19. Cannon WB. The Wisdom of the Body. New York: Norton, 1932.

20. Selye H. Stress Without Distress. New York: J. B. Lippincott, 1974:65.

21. Rosch PJ. Stress and electromedicine. Med Electron 1989; 19:124–128.

22. Yamasaki H. Abberant expression and function of gap iunctions during carcinogenesis. In: Butterworth BE, Slaga TJ, eds. Nongenotoxic Mechanisms in Carcinogenesis. Cold Spring Harbor, NY: Cold Spring Harbor Laboratory, 1987:279–316.

23. Kobasa S, Maddi S, Kahns S. Hardiness and health: a prospective study. J Personality Soc Psychol 1982; 42:168–177.

24. Achterberg J, Matthews S, Simonton OC. Psychology of the exceptional cancer patient-a description of patients who outlive predicted life expectancies. Psychother Theory Res Practice 1976; 9:1–21.

25. Kune A, Kune S, Watson LF. Perceived religiousness is protective for colorectal cancer; data from the Melbourne Colorectal Cancer Study. J R Soc Med 1993; 86:645–647.

26. Meares A. A form of intensive meditation associated with the regression of cancer. Am J Clin Hypn 1982; 25:114–121.

27. Meares A. Regression of osteogenic sarcoma metastases associated with intensive meditation. Med J Aust 1978; 2:433–434.

28. Meares A. Remission of massive metastasis from undifferentiated carcinoma of the lung associated with intensive meditation. J Am Soc Psychosom Dent Med 1980; 27:40–41.

29. Meares A. Regression of recurrence of carcinoma of the breast at mastectomy site associated with intensive meditation. Aust Fam Physician 1981; 10:218–219.

30. Meares A. Regression of cancer after intensive meditation. Med J Aust 1976; 2:184.

31. Meares A. The quality of meditation effective in the regression of cancer. J Am Soc Psychosom Dent Med 1978; 25:129–132.

32. Meares A. Vivid visualization and dim visual awareness in the regression of cancer in meditation. J Am Soc Psychosom Dent Med 1978; 25:85–88.

33. Bolen JS. Meditation and psychotherapy in the treatment of cancer. Psychic 1973; 4:19–22.

34. Achterberg J, Lawlis GF. Imagery of Cancer. Champaign, IL: Institute for Personality and Ability Testing, 1978.

35. Clawson TA, Swade R. The hypnotic control of blood flow and pain: the cure of warts and the potential for the use of hypnosis in the treatment of cancer. Am J Clin Hypn 1975; 17:160–169.

36. Hall HR. Hypnosis and the immune system: a review with implications for cancer and the psychology of healing. Am J Clin Hypn 1982; 25:92–103.

37. Hedge AR. Hypnosis in cancer. Br J Med Hypn 1960; 12:2–5.

38. Funch DP, Marshall J. The role of stress, social support and age in survival from breast cancer. J Psychosom Res 1983; 27:177–183.

39. Funch DP, Mettlin C. The role of support in relation to recovery from breast surgery. Social Science and Medicine 1982; 16:91–98.

40. Eli K, Nishimoto R, Mediansky L, Mantell J, Hamovitch M. Social relations, social support and survival among patients with cancer. J Psychosom Res 1992; 36:531–541.

41. Bagenal FS, Easton DF, Harris E, Chilvers CED, McElwain TJ. Survival of patients with breast cancer attending Bristol cancer help centre. Lancet 1990; 336:606–610.

42. Spiegel D, Bloom JR, Yalom ID. Group support for patients with metastatic cancer: a randomized prospective outcome study. Arch Gen Psychiatry 1981; 38:527–533.

43. Spiegel D, Bloom JR, Kraemer HC, Gottheil E. Effects of psychosocial treatment on survival of patients with metastatic breast cancer. Lancet 1989; 2:888–891.

44. Ogilvie H. The human heritage. Lancet 1957; ii:42.

45. Gordon-Taylor G. The incomputable factors in cancer prognosis. BMJ 1959; 1, 455.

46. Pendergrass EP. Host resistance and other intangibles in the treatment of cancer. Am J Roentg and Rad Ther 1961; 85:891–898.

47. Miller TR. Psychophysiologic aspects of cancer. Cancer 1977; 39:413–422.
48. Levy SM, Herberman RB, Whiteside T. Perceived social support and tumor estrogen/progesterone receptor status as predictors of natural killer cell activity in breast cancer patients. Psychosom Med 1990; 52:73–85.
49. Rosch PJ. Stress: cause or cure of cancer. In: Goldberg J, ed. Psychotherapeutic Treatment of Cancer Patients. New York: Free Press, 1981:39–57.
50. Rosch PJ. Afterword. In: Nordenström BEW, ed. Exploring BCEC-Systems (Biologically Closed Electric Circuits). Stockholm: Nordic Medical Publications, 1998:98–112.
51. Green EE, Parks PA, Guer BA, Fahrion SL, Coyne L. Anomalous electrostatic phenomena in exceptional subjects. Subtle Energies 1991; 2:69–94.
52. Muehsam DJ, Markov MS, Muehsam PA, Pilla A, Ronger S, Wu I. Static magnetic field modulation of myosin phosphorylation: preliminary experiment. Subtle Energies 1993; 4:1–16.
53. Muehsam DJ, Markov MS, Muehsam PA, Pilla A, Ronger S, Wu I. Effects of Qigong on cell-free myosin phosphorylation: preliminary experiments. Subtle Energies 1994; 5:93–108.
54. Wu W, Bandilla A, Ciccone S, Yang J. Effects of Qigong on late stage complex regional pain syndrome. Altern Ther Health Med 1999; 5:45–54.
55. Keller E. Effects of therapeutic touch on tension headache pain. Nursing Res 1986; 35:101–105.
56. Redner R, Briner B, Snellman L. Effects of a bioenergy healing technique on chronic pain. Subtle Energies 1991; 2:43–68.
57. Wirth DP. The effect of non-contact therapeutic touch on the healing rate of full thickness dermal wounds. Subtle Energies 1990; 1:1–20.
58. Krieger D. The response of in vivo human hemoglobin to an active healing therapy by direct laying on of hands. Human Dimensions 1972; 1:12–15.
59. Krieger D. Healing by the laying on of hands as a facilitator of bio-energetic change: the response of in vivo human hemoglobin. Psychoenergetic Systems 1974; 1:4121–4129.
60. Rein G, McCraty R. Structural changes in water and DNA associated with new physiologically measurable states. J Sci Explor 1994; 8:438–439.
61. Quinn J. Therapeutic touch as an energy exchange: testing the theory. Adv Nursing Sci 1984; 4:42–49.
62. Stroink G. Principles of Cardiomagnetism. In: Williamson SJ, ed. Advances in Biomagnetism. New York: Plenum Press, 1999:47–57.
63. McCraty R. The electricity of touch: Detection and measurement of cardiac energy exchange between people. In: Pribram K, ed. Brain and Values: Is a Biological Science of Values Possible. Mahwah, NJ: Lawrence Erlbaum Associates, Inc., 1998:359–379.
64. Russek L, Schwartz G. Interpersonal heart-brain registration and the perception of parental love: a 42 year follow-up of the Harvard Mastery of Stress Study. Subtle Energies 1994; 5:195–208.
65. Russek L, Schwartz G. Energy cardiology: a dynamical energy systems approach for integrating conventional and alternative medicine. Advances 1996; 12:4–24.
66. Rosch PJ. Stress and subtle energy medicine. Stress Medicine 1994; 10:1–3.
67. Lawrence R, Rosch PJ, Plowden J. Magnet Therapy. Rocklin, CA: Prima Press, 1998.
68. Darras JC. Isotopic and cytolologic assays in acupuncture. Energy Fields in Medicine: A Study of Device Technology Based on Acupuncture Meridians and Chi Energy. Kalamazoo, MI: The John E. Fetzer Foundation, 1989:45–65.
69. Boorstin DJ. The Discoverers. New York: Random House, 1983:365.

16

Magnetic and Electromagnetic Field Therapy: Basic Principles of Application for Pain Relief

Marko S. Markov*

EMF Technologies, Inc., Chattanooga, Tennessee, U.S.A.

The author underlines the similarities and differences between electric current, magnetic fields and electromagnetic fields, and their relation to living tissues. Special attention is devoted to the needs of exact 3-D dosimetry of the applied signals and complete explanation of the physical parameters of the signal. In order for a therapeutical signal to be effective, the target tissue must receive the appropriate stimulation; therefore any dosimetry must be done in respect of the biological target. Based on literature, data, and his own research, the author discusses the possibility selected magnetic fields to be used for pain control.

I. INTRODUCTION

During the second half of 1980s and early 1990s a number of discussions regarding the potential hazard of electromagnetic fields from power lines took place in the news media. Epidemiological studies on the potential hazards of electromagnetic fields (EMF) with respect to the initiation of cancer were the base for controversial opinions (1–3). To help in resolving this issue the congress of the United States allocated $41 million for a 5-year RAPID program designed to investigate the potential of EMF to initiate cancer. After five years this program as well as several other independent panels concluded "there is no convincing evidence to affirm that magnetic fields from power lines are associated with cancer promotion." Neither federal nor state funding was, however, available in the United States for studying the beneficial effects of magnetic and electromagnetic fields for the treatment of various injuries and diseases. The information available for countries from Europe and Asia do not show significant difference in the funding of magnetotherapy.

Current affiliation: Research International, Buffalo, New York, U.S.A.

251

Basically, all innovations, new methods, and instruments are funded by private sponsors or manufacturers of the devices.

The second half of the 1990s marked an increasing interest of the general public toward the use of magnetic fields for pain control. It will be fair to say that there is increasing interest in the therapeutic use of magnetic fields, stimulated in large part by recent advances in alternative and complementary medicine (4,5). The author believes that the widespread use of electromagnetic fields (EMF) or magnetic fields (MF) for therapeutic purposes in the first decade of the new millennium may mark a revolutionary new approach to the treatment of various injuries and diseases.

However, electromagnetic fields are still not widely used in clinical medicine. There are several reasons for this fact. First of all, today western medicine is based mainly on the achievements of chemistry that have been further utilized and expanded by the pharmaceutical industry. Unfortunately, nearly all pharmaceuticals affect not only the target tissues but the entire organism and in many cases cause adverse effects. Second, the education in all medical directions is based upon this chemistry–pharmacology approach and students do not receive proper information for the potential of physical modalities. In a sharp contrast with pharmacological approach, physical medicine in general, and magnetobiology in particular, provides noninvasive, safe, and easily applied methods to directly treat the site of injury, the source of pain and inflammation, or dysfunction. Thus, magnetotherapy has little, if any, side effects, especially having in mind that in order to reach appropriate concentration of pharmacological agent, the patients are pressed to take dosages which are several magnitude larger.

The accumulation of knowledge and critical review of available information has lead to acceptance that the present configuration and functioning of many important systems in living organisms is directed by the electromagnetic interactions. This includes not only nerve conductance or cellular membrane structure but also a whole range of processes that involve ion flow and conformational changes. Today medicine utilizes the electromagnetic nature of life mostly in diagnostic direction. Electrophisiological measurements, electro- and magneto-diagnostics, magnetic resonance imaging, magnetocardiograms, and magnetoencephalograms significantly enlarge the diagnostics instrumentarium (6). (See also the chapter of F. Prato in this book.)

The original approach of ancient physicians was used in China, Japan, and Europe by applying natural magnetic materials for the treatment of various diseases (7). Table 1 summarizes some of the most important events in the history of electromagnetic field therapy. Shortly after Galvani identified "animal electricity" and Volta created the first battery, in 1812, Dr. Birch, a surgeon at St. Thomas Hospital in London, successfully used electric stimulation for slow-healing fractures. Even before any practical applications were possible, Dr. Shaeffer published in Regensburg (today Germany) in 1752 the book *Elektrishe Medizine*. The first book to discuss the healing potential of natural "magnetic stones" was written in 1600 by William Gilbert, *The Magnet and the Big Magnet—the Earth*.

The modern day magnetotherapy originated in Japan immediately after World War II and later attracted the interest of physicians in Asia (China and India) and Europe (mainly Romania and former Soviet Union). During the period 1960–1985 nearly all European countries manufactured and distributed own magnetotherapeutical systems. The first contemporary book on magnetotherapy was written by N. Todorov and published in 1982 in Bulgaria to summarize the author's experience with treatment of 2700 patients with 33 different pathologies (8). Andrew Bassett was the author of the first clinical application of electromagnetic stimulation in the United States in 1974 (9). The method further received FDA label for treatment of nonunion and delayed fractures.

Table 1 Important Events in the History of Magnetobiology and Magnetotherapy

1600	Gilbert, book: "The magnet and the big Magnet - Earth" - London
1752	Shaeffer, book: " Elektrishe Medizin" - Regensburg, Germany
1786	Galvani, frog experiment for "animal electricity," Bologna, Italy
1793	Volta, further developed Galvani's ideas
1812	Birch, first application of electric stimulation for bone healing
1848	Du Bois-Reymond, movement of electrical particles along nerve fiber
1864	Maxwell, created the foundations of modern electromagnetic field theory
1891	Tesla (in USA) and d'Arsonval (France), suggested the use of high-frequency electric current in medicine
1897	French Academy of Sciences, reported large use of high-frequency currents
1907	Nagelschmidt, at medical conference in Dresden demonstrated deep tissue heating by high-frequency currents
1908	Nagelschmidt, introduced DIATHERMY as a method for uniform heating of deep tissues
1913	Jex-Blake, power-frequency electric force can cause destructive effect on living system
1928	Esau, used a vacuum-tube amplifier to generate 100 MHz EMF with several hundred watts of output power
1938	Hollman, microwaves with wavelength of 25 cm could be focused to produce heating of deep tissues without excessive heating of skin
1946	Ratheon Co., provided Mayo Clinic with microwave generators for clinical use.

Numerous publications over the past 25 years suggest that exogenous magnetic and electromagnetic fields may have profound effects on a large number of biological processes, most of which are important for therapy and especially for pain control (8–30). Despite the significant success of Western medicine in the second half of the twentieth century, there are a number of conditions associated with acute or chronic pain for which successful treatments was not established. While acute pain is related mainly to traumatic injuries or swelling and/or inflammation and can be easily controlled, chronic pain represents a serious problem for society. The National Institutes of Health estimate that more than 48 million Americans suffer chronic pain that results in a $65 billion annual loss of productivity and over $100 billion spent on pain care.

Interest in magnetic field therapy in the United States was stimulated in the last decade by the large commercial marketing of permanent magnets (which triggered the interest of the general public) and by the activity of the Office (now Center) of Alternative and Complimentary Medicine. Some of the most enthusiastic users of magnetic field therapy are medical practitioners who already have experience in using acupuncture. While the success rate for EMF therapies is comparable to that produced surgically for delayed and non-union fractures, the cost of this noninvasive therapy is significantly less. This cost decreases substantially when appropriate permanent magnets are applied directly to the site of injury.

It is accepted that pain control occurs via a series of integrated stages, each of which has particular objectives essential to the tissue–system repair processes. During the past 25 years it has been shown that magnetic fields offer an excellent possibility to be a noninvasive method of stimulation for pain management and control. A careful analysis of the successful application of MF for the control of pain with various origins can highlight the cellular and tissue components that may be plausible targets for MF action. Having in mind that the most important clinical principle of injury management is to provide a natural physiological environment for optimum healing, the proper choice of the MF parameters may significantly enhance the healing process.

However, it should be recognized that basic science must create dosimetry and methodology for this type of stimulation. Saying that a patient was "magnetically stimulated" is as nonspecific as saying a patient was given a drug. Space does not permit more than a superficial presentation of evidence here to support the statement that "different MF produce different effects in different targets under differing conditions of exposure" (19).

II. MAGNETS, MAGNETIC FIELDS, ELECTRIC FIELDS, ELECTROMAGNETIC FIELDS

Often even in the scientific literature magnets and magnetic fields are used as synonyms. One thing what everybody must remember is that the magnet itself has no healing capacity. Even the strongest magnets one can find at the market perform their physical actions via the magnetic field they generated. Once again, the magnetic field, not the piece of material, possesses the healing ability.

The next is to distinguish the terms *magnetic field* and *electromagnetic field*. First, should be clarified that an electromagnetic field is a combination of magnetic field and electric field. The basic physics suggests that in each case when the amplitude of magnetic field changes, an electric field is generated and vice versa. Also, any time-varying magnetic field is accompanied with a time-varying electric field.

There are large number of types of commercially available "healing" magnets suggested for pain relief. Because they are permanent magnets, they will deliver to the human body a magnetic field only. (For a review see the chapter of Colbert in this book). If a magnetic field is generated via sinusoidal wave generator, one should expect the effect to be a result of both magnetic and electric field components. This is even more important in a case when superficial tissues are exposed to magnetic field treatment. While magnetic field penetrates the biological tissues, the surface of any physical body, including the human body, acts as a barrier for electric field, and the incident electric field is transferred in an electric current over the body surface.

Today magnetic-field-dependent therapeutic modalities can be categorized into six groups:

1. Permanent magnetic fields are created by various permanent magnets as well as by passing direct current (DC) through a coil.
2. Low-frequency sine waves electromagnetic fields mostly utilize 60 Hz (in the United States and Canada) and 50 Hz (in Europe and Asia) frequency used in distribution lines.
3. Pulsed electromagnetic fields (PEMF) are usually low-frequency fields with very specific shape and amplitude.
4. Pulsed radio-frequency fields (PRF) utilize the selected frequencies in the radio-frequency range: 13.56 MHz, 27.12 MHz, and 40.68 MHz.
5. Millimeter waves have a very high frequency of 30–100 GHz and are mostly used in the former Soviet Union during the last 10–15 years.
6. Transcranial magnetic stimulation is a method of treatment of selected area of the brain with short, but intensive, magnetic pulses.

III. PLANNING MAGNETOTHERAPY

Before discussing the specifics of the choice of magnetic field it should be emphasized the necessity to evaluate the location of the clinical target and the magnetic field this target needs to receive. This is extremely important consideration, and probably most of the failure in reproducing reported effects is due to neglecting the importance of the target dosimetry. It should be taken into account that different types of magnetic field have different characteristics, and even they may have variations in the field characteristics at target site (5,8,12,30–32).

In order to achieve good reproducibility of observed biological and clinical effects, each study should pay special attention to the detailed dosimetry of the study, to the use of a well-established biological and clinical protocol, and to a complete report of the exposure conditions (32). Failure to reproduce the reported effects of a biological or clinical study is, in many cases, due to a failure to explain the exact conditions and/or neglect of some details which appear to be obvious.

A number of studies reported that the stimulation with electric and magnetic fields provides healing effects when other methods have failed (8,12–14). However, there is often confusion among medical practitioners with respect to application of these modalities due to the variety of methods of stimulation, parameters of the applied fields, and lack of a defined biophysical mechanism capable of explaining the observed bioeffects. Animal and human studies demonstrate that the physical parameters and patterns of application can affect both the type of effect and the efficiency in producing a given response.

Another important feature of magnetic and/or electromagnetic stimulation, especially in the relatively low frequency range, is that electric and magnetic field components behave differently. Once an electric field reaches a material surface, it is transferred into electric current along the surface. Conversely, most materials are transparent to the magnetic field component which penetrates deep into the body. The depth of penetration depends on the technique of generating the magnetic field. A common problem when assessing the effects initiated by different devices is that each manufacturer uses its own systems and methods of characterizing the product. Many research and clinical trials have been performed without complete dosimetry of the magnetic field at the site of injury and adequate documentation of the exposure conditions. When the protocol refers, for example, to 15 mT MF, it should be considered that this is the magnetic field at the target site, not at the surface of generating system (32).

It should be noted that when reviewing publications, it is difficult to compare or generalize results obtained at different research or clinical sites. Explanations of experimental protocols even if perfect from a biological or clinical point of view are often incomplete in their characterization of the EMF at the target site.

More details are available elsewhere which indicate that the amplitude, frequency, and exposure pattern windows apparently determine whether a bioeffect will occur and, if it does occur, what its nature will be (5,11,19,20). Therefore a systematic study of EMF action on any particular biological system has to consider the following parameters:

Type of field
Intensity or induction
Gradient (dB/dt)
Vector (dB/dx)
Frequency

Pulse shape

Component (electric or magnetic)

Localization

Time of exposure

Depth of penetration.

It should be taken into account that there are significant differences between electric field and/or current and magnetic field stimulation. Electric stimulation requires electrodes. Electrode size, spacing, and polarity are the most critical factors in the delivery of an adequate stimulating current. Closely spaced, small electrodes generally make the effective area of stimulation rather superficial due to the lower impedance of the current path through proximal tissue. The actual current density at any particular point within the tissue will depend on tissue composition and geometry and will change as these quantities vary during healing. The conduction of electrical current through biological tissues occurs as a result of movement of charges along specific pathways. This charge transfer might result in electro-thermal, electrochemical, and electrophysical effects depending on the type of electrical current and can occur at the membrane, cellular, or tissue level immediately after applying the voltage. The direct response usually results in a multitude of indirect cellular reactions, which subsequently may alter further steps in biochemical and physiological pathways. A further complication of electrodes relates to potentially toxic electrolysis products, particularly if the electrode is placed inside the wound (18).

From that point of view MF stimulation represents a significantly more effective approach to the healing process—it is an easy, inexpensive, and comfortable therapy. MF modalities do not exhibit the complications of contact electrodes because the fields are inductively coupled, i.e., immediate contact is not necessary to achieve the desired dose at the target tissue level. Thus, MF can be applied in the presence of a cast or wound dressing because the MF applicator does not need to contact either the skin or the dressing.

It is well accepted now that when above-mentioned considerations are taken into account, the EMF can provide a practical, exogenous method for inducing cell and tissue modifications that correct selected pathological states (5,8,13,14,20). It should be noted that very little is known about the mechanisms of action, and this limitation has seriously restricted the application of magnetic and electromagnetic fields in clinical practice in the United States. More research and publications can be found in European literature (12,30,33)—more than 2000 papers on the beneficial effects of magnetic and electromagnetic stimulation (5,6,8–10,12–20,22–52). Most of those papers, however, present results of open studies, and only a few have been done as double-blind, controlled studies.

Very frequently the important question is asked: Whether and to what extent magnetic fields may represent a hazard for users? As mentioned earlier, several scientific bodies concluded that there is no evidence that EMF represents a health hazard. It should be clear that hazard issues are based on epidemiological studies that assumed continuous exposure to weak, low-frequency electromagnetic fields (1–3). However, the epidemiological data are inconsistent, and no human cancer has been associated with exposure to electromagnetic fields (53).

In contrast, MF and EMF therapeutic modalities are applied in well-controlled conditions, for a short period of time (mainly 30 min or less), in 10–15 sessions. In order to be therapeutically effective, any applied MF must be orders of magnitude stronger than ambient magnetic fields. However, it appears that long-term follow-up, which may provide adequate information on the possible side effects of the therapeutic application of MF, will be extremely difficult to perform, due to the complexity of the problem and the high cost of such follow-up (5,6,30,31). Based on available evidence worldwide, it is highly unlikely that the therapeutic application of magnetic fields would create a dangerous situation for the patient. Nevertheless, if any hazard exists, the first to be considered is the medical staff, who potentially may be exposed for longer period of time to EMF significantly higher than the ambient levels. There are several documents of the World Health Organization which state that "the available evidence indicate the absence of any adverse effects on human health due to exposure to magnetic fields up to 2 T" (54,55).

IV. SOME IMPORTANT PUBLICATIONS ON CLINICAL APPLICATION OF MF AND EMF

There is a large body of experimental and clinical data that suggest that various exogenous MF at surprisingly low levels can affect a large variety of tissues and processes, most of which are of critical importance for diagnostics and therapy (5,6,8,11–13,19–22,56). The longest clinical applications of magnetic fields in the United States are related to bone unification and the reduction of pain and edema in soft tissues (9,10,13,19,20,22,24,25,28 29,34).

During the past 25 years more than 2 million patients have been treated worldwide for a large variety of injuries, pathologies and diseases. This large number of patients exhibited a success rate of approximately 80%, with virtually no reported complications (13,20,22,30).

Low-frequency sine waves and low-frequency pulsed electromagnetic fields were used for treatment of pain associated with rotator cuff tendinitis, multiple sclerosis, carpal tunnel syndrome, and periathritis. With the exception of periathritis, which reported no difference between treatment and control groups, all other targeted sources of pain received a re-duction in visual analog scale (VAS) pain scores. More importantly, the improvement was observed in 93% of patents suffering carpal tunnel pain, and 83% in rotator cuff tendinitis. It was also reported that 65% of the patient who received daily treatment over 8 weeks for rotator cuff tendinitis were pain free at the end of the study, as well as 70% of the multiple sclerosis patients who received 15 treatments with low-frequency sine wave EMF reported a reduction in spasticity, improvement of bladder control, and improvement in endurance. (See also the chapter of Lipin in this book.)

A number of clinical studies, in vivo animal experiments and in vitro cellular and membrane research suggest that magnetic and electromagnetic field stimulation may accelerate the healing processes (5,8,13–15,20,29). It is now clear that endogenous electro-magnetic and magnetic interactions are associated with many basic physiological processes ranging from ion binding and molecular conformation in the cell membrane to macroscopic alterations in tissues. The investigation of the mechanisms of action of MF on biological systems that are in a state different than their normal physiological one represent the next frontier in electromagnetic biology and medicine. Space does not permit more than a superficial presentation of evidence here to support the statement that "different MF produce different effects in different biotargets under differing conditions of exposure."

Basic science studies suggest that nearly all participants in the healing process (such as fibrinogen, leukocytes, fibrin, platelets, cytokines, growth factors, fibroblasts, collagen, elastin, keratinocytes, osteoblasts, and free radicals) (3,5–8,14,23,37,38,59,62–67) exhibit alterations in their functions as a rcsults of exposure to MF (5,8,12–15,18,26,30,35,36,56–63). Magnetic fields were also shown to affect vasoconstriction and vasodilation, phagocy-tosis, cell proliferation, formation of the cellular network, epithelization, and scar formation (5,12,13,20,23,30,33). Therefore, it is important to evaluate the contribution of MF in the alteration of the basic cellular activities that occur at any one of the distinct stages of tissue repair. The interactions of MF with any structure in the human organism could initiate biophysical and biochemical changes that in turn modify the physiological pathways and accelerate the healing process.

The modality most often employed in the United States for soft tissue applications is pulse radio frequency (PRF), based on the continuous 27.12-MHz sinusoidal diathermy signals that have been employed for decades for deep tissue heating. A question arises: how can this "heating" signal be applied for reduction of pain and edema. The answer is that the pulsed version of this signal (65-μs pulse bursts, 100–600 pulses/s, peak magnetic field of 2 G) allows the target tissue to be exposed to MF and to elicit a nonthermal biological effect. PRF magnetic fields have been applied for the reduction of posttraumatic and postoperative pain and edema in soft tissues, wound healing, burn treatment, ankle sprains, hand injuries, migraine, chronic pelvic pain, neck pain, and whiplash injuries and nerve regeneration (20,63–66).

In parallel with improvement after the injury, the authors reported a reduction in the pain of 35% for patients having migraine, accompanied by a significant reduction of occurrence of headaches. Even more impressive were results for treatment of neck and whiplash injuries. Neck pain was reported to decrease from 7.0 to 4.0 after 3 weeks of daily treatment with PRF and to 2.0 after 6 weeks of treatment. For the whiplash injuries VAS pain scores decreased from 6.75 to 3.75 after 2 weeks, to 2.5 after 4 weeks, and to 1.5 after 12 weeks of daily treatment with PRF. A 50% reduction in use of pain medication was also reported in whiplash patients as result of EMF treatment (3–6).

Therapeutic efficacy depends on the status of the patient (age, general health, and gender) as well as on the stage of pathology and/or disease. It has also been found that there is a distinct relationship between specific diseases and MF parameters that initiate optimal response for these particular pathologies (5,19).

V. TIME-VARYING MAGNETIC FIELDS FOR PAIN CONTROL

Low-frequency sine waves and low-frequency pulsed electromagnetic fields were used for treatment of pain associated with rotator cuff tendinitis, multiple sclerosis, carpal tunnel syndrome, and periathritis (46,50). For example, an improvement was observed in 93% of patients suffering carpal tunnel pain and 83% in rotator cuff tendinitis. It was also reported that 65% of the patients who received daily treatment over 8 weeks for rotator cuff tendinitis were pain free at the end of the study, as well as 70% of the multiple sclerosis patients who received 15 treatments with low frequency sinewave EMF reported a reduction in spasticity, improvement of bladder control, and improvement in endurance (47).

PRF modality was used for treatment of migraine, chronic pelvic pain, neck pain, and whiplash injuries. In parallel with improvement after the injury a reduction in the pain of 35% for patients having migraine, accompanied by a significant reduction in occurrence of headaches was reported. Several chapters in this book are dedicated to the use of time-varying EMF for treatment of multiple sclerosis, migraine, and macular degeneration and for this reason will not be discussed here.

Pulsed signal therapy (PST) has been used for relief of pain and other ostheoarthritis symptoms mainly in Europe and Canada. The system includes a bed, a circular coil of either 11 or 22 in. in diameter that delivers pulses of variable frequencies (in the range of 5–24 pulses/s), and magnetic fields of up to 2 mT. Several double-blind studies report a 88% decrease in pain from knee ostheoarthritis after 18 sessions 30 min daily and the pain relief was present during the next month of follow-up (51,52).

A. Permanent Magnets for Pain Control

Since the middle of the 1990s, permanent magnets have become widely used in the United States for pain relief. Several recent studies report reduction of pain in postpolio patients (up to 76%), fibromyalgia (up to 32%), peripheral neuropathy (up to 33%), and postsurgical wounds (37–65%) (38–42).

These recent studies reported pain management for different etiologies and sites of pain. They demonstrate the potential of a static magnetic field to provide significant pain relief in different disorders. In a double-blind study it was shown that a static magnetic field of 300–500 G significantly decreases the pain score in postpolio pain syndrome patients when compared with a placebo group (38). Another double-blind study demonstrated that sleeping on mattresses in which ceramic permanent magnets are embedded (with magnetic field at the target in the range 200–600 G) provided significant benefits to pain, fatigue, and sleep in patients suffering from fibromyalgia (41). The status of the patients in the real treatment group was improved by more than 30%. In a pilot study a significant improvement in 75% of patients with diabetic neuropathy who used permanent magnetic field stimulation on the soles of their feet was found (39). It appears that the proper choice of magnetic field strength, application site, duration, and frequency of application are of critical importance for the success of the therapy.

It should be noted that several studies failed to obtain any effects when so-called bipolar magnets were used. Reviewing the diverse effects reported recently, we conclude that the failure to find any effect is an obvious result of inaccurate dosimetry and poor planning of the studies.

B. Mechanisms of Action

The main reasons that MF and EMF are still not widely accepted as treatment modalities in the United States could be the absence of agreement about a common mechanism of action for EMF bioeffects and insufficient number of publications in American medical journals. MF are recognized as capable of inducing selective changes in the microenvironment around and within the cell, as well as in the cell membrane which in turn may correct selected pathological states. However, the biophysical mechanism(s) of interaction of weak electric and magnetic fields with biological tissues as well as the biological transductive mechanism(s) remain to be elucidated. The analysis of reported specific reactions to MF and EMF in different biological systems suggests that most of the observed bioeffects strongly depend on the parameters of the applied electromagnetic fields.

To study the biophysical mechanisms of MF interactions one should begin with identification of the desired target to MF action. Then the nature of the initial physico-chemical interaction of EMF with biological systems and the expression of these phys-icochemical changes as a biological response should be investigated. The cell membrane is most often considered the main target for EMF signals (33,67–69). Due to the fact that most of the cellular structures are electrically charged and that the biochemical reactions involve ion transfers, it is easy to assume that MF and EMF possess the potential to influence both the structure and function of the most important biochemical–biophysical processes. Starting from cell size and shape, going through the composition and architecture of the cellular membrane, one can also take into account the different sensitivity of cells based on the above described characteristics. Any change in the electrochemical microenvironment of the cell can cause modifications in the structure of its electrified surface regions by changing the concentration of a specifically bound ion or dipole, which may be accompanied by alterations in the conformation of molecular entities (such as lipids, proteins, and enzymes) in the membrane structure. The role of ions as transducers of information in the regulation of cell structure and function is widely accepted. When cells are organized in a tissue, the expected response should include cell–cell communications. In addition for in vivo experiments the complexity of the animal and human organism and the existence of compensatory mechanisms that work on the organism level must be considered (5,6,12,13,30).

From a clinical point of view it is also difficult to believe that each of these mechanisms might be useful in explaining the beneficial effects of magnetotherapy, especially the significant and rapid pain relief observed in several different studies such as postpolio patients, diabetic neuropathy, postsurgical wounds, and fibromyalgia (38–42).

A series of studies of EMF influence on various biological systems demonstrated the appearance of windows effects (8,11,32,70,71). The windows represent combinations of amplitude and frequency within which the optimal response is observed; outside this range the response is significantly smaller. In other words, this demonstrates the principle "more does not necessarily mean better."

VI. SUMMARY

In summary, the experimental and clinical data demonstrate that exogenous MF and EMF of surprisingly low amplitudes can have a profound effect in healing of a wide variety of pain, injuries, and pathologies. Perhaps the greatest challenge for what we may term *electromagnetic* biology and medicine is to establish the proper dosimetry for modulation of the desired biochemical cascade.

The correct choice of effective electromagnetic stimulation to accelerate healing requires measurement and computation of a variety of parameters, such as amplitude, field frequency and shape, duration of exposure, and site of application. Not only the precise characteristics of the applied or driving field and/or current but also the exact diagnosis and all other clinical data should be considered. Further research in the area of magnetic stimulation should clarify and optimize the choice of the appropriate magnetic field that are optimal for modulation of defined structures and processes that are involved in tissue healing and pain relief. A precise evaluation of electromagnetic field initiated bioeffects becomes increasingly important since the number of electromagnetic technologies and devices used in clinical practice continues to grow.

GLOSSARY

Field   Any physical quantity that takes different values at different points in space

Electric field   A field describing the electrical force on a net electrical charge in space

Magnetic field   A field describing the force experienced by magnetic body or in space electrical charge

Geomagnetic field   The earth's natural magnetic field

Ambient electromagnetic field   The natural and man-made electromagnetic fields surrounding any given body at a given location

Direct current   A continuous unidirectional flow of charged particles due to applied voltage

Permanent magnetic field   A magnetic field created by permanent magnets or by passing a direct current through a coil

Low-frequency sine wave electromagnetic field   A field created by sinusoidal current and/or voltage (50 Hz in USA and Canada, 50 Hz in Europe and Asia)

Pulsed electromagnetic fields   Low-frequency electromagnetic fields with specific wave shapes

Pulsed radio-frequency field   Electromagnetic field in the radiofrequency part of the spectrum (in USA and Canada 13.56 MHz, 27.12 MHz and 40.68 MHz are specified for medical use)

REFERENCES

1. Wartenberg D, Savitz DA. Evaluating exposure cutpoint bias in epidemiological studies of electric and magnetic fields. Bioelectromagnetics 1993; 14:237–245.
2. Deno DW, Carpenter DO. Sources and characteristics of electric and magnetic fields in the environment. In: Carpenter DO, Ayrapetyan S, eds. Biological Effects of Electric and Magnetic Fields. Vol. 1. San Diego: Academic Press, 1994:7–52.
3. Werheimer N, Savitz DA, Leper E. Childhood cancer in relation to indicators of magnetic fields from ground current sources. Bioelectromagnetics 1995; 16:86–96.
4. Rubik B, Becker RO, Flower RG, Hazlewood CF, Liboff AR, Walleczek J. Bioelectromagnetics. Applications in Medicine. Alternative Medicine: Expanding Medical Horizons. Washington DC: US Government Printing Office, 1996:45–65.
5. Markov MS, Colbert A. Magnetic and electromagnetic field therapy. J Back Musculosketal Rehab 2000; 14:1–13.
6. Markov M, Kleinkort J. Magnetic and electromagnetic field—new frontier in biology and medicine. In: Van Paten JJ, ed. Challenges and Opportunities for a New Millennium. Fayetteville: University of Arkansas Press, 1998:184–203.
7. Lawrence R, Rosch PJ, Plowden J. Magnet Therapy. Rocklin, CA: Prima Publishing, 1998:241.
8. Todorov N. Magnetotherapy. Sofia: Meditzina i Physcultura Publishing House, 1982:106.
9. Bassett CAL, Pawluk RJ, Pilla AA. Acceleration of fracture repair by electromagnetic fields (a surgically non-invasive method). Ann NY Acad Sci 1974; 238:242–247.
10. Bassett CAL. Pulsing electromagnetic fields: a new approach to surgical problems. In: Buchwald H, Varco RL, eds. Metabolic Surgery. New York: Grune and Stratton, 1978:255.
11. Markov MS, Todorov NG. Electromagnetic field stimulation of some physiological processes. Studia Biophysica 1984; 99:151–156.
12. Detlavs I, ed. Electromagnetic Therapy in Traumas and Diseases of The Support-motor Apparatus. Riga RMI, 1987:198.
13. Bassett CAL. Fundamental and practical aspects of therapeutic uses of pulsed electromagnetic fields (PEMFs). Critical Review of Biomedical Engineering 1989; 17:451–529.
14. O'Connor ME, Bental RHC, Monaham JC, eds. Emerging Electromagnetic Medicine. New York: Springer Verlag, 1990.
15. Brighton CT, Pollack SR, eds. Electromagnetics in Medicine and Biology. San Francisco: San Francisco Press, 1991:365.
16. Polk C, Postow E, eds. Handbook of Biological Effects of Electromagnetic Fields. Boca Raton, Fl: CRC Press, 1986:618.
17. Blank M, ed. Electromagnetic fields. Biological Interactions and Mechanisms. Washington DC: American Chemical Society, 1975:497.
18. Markov MS. Electric current and electromagnetic field effects on soft tissues. Wounds 1995; 7:94–110.
19. Bassett CAL. Therapeutic Uses of electric and magnetic fields in orthopedics. In: Karpenter D, Ayrapetyan S, eds. Biological Effects of Electric and Magnetic Fields. San Diego: Academic Press, 1994:13–48.
20. Markov MS, Pilla AA. Electromagnetic field stimulation of soft tissues. Wounds 1995; 7:143–151.

21. Dayton PD, Palladino SJ. Electrical stimulation of cutaneous ulcerations. J Am Podiatr Med Assoc 1989; 79:318–321.

22. Pilla AA. State of the art in electromagnetic therapeutics. In: Blank M, ed. Electricity and Magnetism in Biology and Medicine. San Francisco: San Francisco Press, 1993:17–22.

23. Jerabek J. An overview of present research in magnetotherapy. In: Coghil R, ed. Proceedings of First World Congress on Magnetotherapy. Pontypool: Lower Race, 1994:5–78.

24. Bental RH, Cobban RM. Post operative use of radiofrequency emitting spectacles for control of edema and bruising following blepharoplasty. Proc Seventh BEMS Meeting, San Francisco CA, 1985:H-3.

25. Bental RHC. Electromagnetic energy: a historical therapeutic perspective. In: O'Connor ME, Bental RHC, Monaham JC, eds. Emerging Electromagnetic Medicine. New York: Springer Verlag, 1990:1–17.

26. Vodovnik L, Karba R. Treatment of chronic wounds by means of electric and electromagnetic fields. Med Biol Eng Comput 1992; 30:257–266.

27. Detlavs I, Dombrovska I, Klavinsh I, Turauska A, Shkirmante B, Slutskii L. Experimental study of the effect of electromagnetic fields in early stage of wound healing. Bioelectrochem Bioenergetics 1994; 35:13–17.

28. Bassett CAL. Bioelectromagnetics in the service of medicine. Bioelectromagnetics 1992; 13:7–18.

29. Bassett CAL. Bioelectromagnetics in the service of medicine. In: Blank M, ed. Electromagnetic Fields. Biological Interactions and Mechanisms. Washington DC: Amer Chem Soc DC, 1995:261–276.

30. Jerabek J, Pawluk W. Magnetic Therapy in Eastern Europe: A Review of 30 Years of Research. ISBN 0-9664227-0-8

31. Markov MS. Magnetic and electromagnetic fields—a new frontier in clinical biology and medicine. In: Kostarakis P, ed. Proc Millennium International Workshop on Biological Effects of Electromagnetic Fields. Crete, Greece, 2000:365–372, ISBN 960-86733-0-5.

32. Markov M. Biological effects of extremely low frequency magnetic fields. In: Ueno S, ed. Biomagnetic Stimulation. New York: Plenum Press, 1994:91–103.

33. Markov MS. Biophysical aspects of the application of electromagnetic fields in orthopedics and traumatology. In: Detlav I, ed. Electromagnetic Therapy in traumas and diseases of the support-motor apparatus. Riga: Zinatie, 1987:76–86.

34. Polk C. Therapeutic application of low frequency electric and magnetic fields. In: Lin JC, ed. Advances in Electromagnetic Fields in Living Systems. New York: Plenum Press, 1994:129–154.

35. Dunn MG, Doillon CH, Berg RA. Wound healing using a collagen matrix: effect of DC electrical stimulation. J Biomed Mater Res 1988; 22A:191–206.

36. Zukov BN, Lasarovich VG. Magnetotherapy in Angiology. Zdorovie: Kiev, 1989:111.

37. Seaborne D, Quirion-deGirardi C, Rousseau M, Rivest M, Lambert J. The treatment of pressure sores using pulsed electromagnetic energy (PEME). Physiotherapy Canada 1996; 48:131–137.

38. Valbona C, Hazlewood C, Jurida G. Response of pain to static magnetic fields in postpolio patients: a double blind pilot study. Arch Phys Med Rehab 1997; 78:1200–1203.

39. Weintraub M. Chronic submaximal magnetic stimulation in peripheral neuropathy: is there a beneficial therapeutic relationship. Am J Pain Management 1998; 8:12–16.

40. Man D, Man B, Plosker H. The influence of permanent magnetic field therapy on wound healing in suction lipectomy patients: a double-blind study. Plastic and Reconstructive Surgery 1999; 104:2261–2266.

41. Colbert AP, Markov MS, Banerji M, Pilla AA. Magnetic mattress pad use in patients with fibromialgya: a randomized double blind trial. J Back Musculoskeletal Rehab 1999; 13:19–31.

42. Collacott EA, Zimmerman JT, White DW, Rindole JP. Bipolar permanent magnets for the treatment of chronic pain. A pilot study. JAMA 2000; 283:1322–1325.

43. Valbona C, Richards T. Evolution of magnetic therapy from alternative to traditional medicine. Phys Med Rehab Clin NA 1999; 10:729–754.

44. Pilla AA. State of the art in electromagnetic therapeutics. In: Blank M, ed. Electricity and Magnetism in Biology and Medicine. San Francisco: San Francisco Press, 1993:17–22.

45. Pilla AA. State of the art in electromagnetic therapeutics: soft tissue applications. In: Bersani F, ed. Electricity and Magnetism in Biology and Medicine. New York: Kluwer Academic/Plenum Publishing House, 1999:871–874.

46. Battisti E, Fortunato M, Giananneshi F, Rigato M. Efficacy of the Magnetotherapy in idiopathic carpal tunnel syndrome. In: Suminic D, ed. Proc IV EBEA Congress, Zagreb, 1998:34–35.

47. Binder A, Parr G, Hazelman B. Pulsed electromagnetic field therapy of persistent rotator cuff tendinitis. Lancet March 1984; 695–698.

48. Folley-Nolan D, Barry C, Coughan RJ, O'Connor P, Roden D. Pulsed high frequency (27 MHz) electromagnetic therapy for persistent neck pain. Orthopedics 1990; 13(4):445–451.

49. Folley-Nolan D, Moore K, Codd M, Barry C, Coughan RJ, O'Connor P. Low energy high frequency pulsed electromagnetic therapy for acute whiplash injuries. Scand J Rehab Med 1992; 24:51–59.

50. Leclaire R, Bourgoin J. Electromagnetic treatment of shoulder periarthritis: a randomized controlled trial of the efficiency and tolerance of magnetotherapy. Arch Phys Med Rehab 1991; 72:284–287.

51. Trock DH, Bollet AJ, Dyer RH, Fielding LP, Miner WK, Markoll R. A double-blind trial of the clinical effects of pulsed electromagnetic fields in osteoarthritis. J Reumatol 1993; 20:456–460.

52. Trock DH, Bollet AJ, Markoll R. The effect of pulsed electromagnetic fields in the treatment of osteoarthritis of the knee and cervical spine. J Reumatol 1994; 21:1903–1911.

53. Owen RD. MYC mRNA abundance is unchanged in subcultures of HL60 cells exposed to power-line frequency magnetic fields. Radiat Res 1998; 150:23–30.

54. World Health Organization (WHO). Magnetic fields. United Nations Environmental Programme, World Health Organization and The International Radiation Protection Association - Environmental Health Criteria 69, 1987:25–33, 119–127.

55. World Health Organization (WHO). Magnetic fields health and safety guide. United Nations Environmental Programme, World Health Organization and The International Radiation Protection Association - Health and Safety Guide # 27, 1987:7–24

56. Sisken BF, Walker J. Therapeutic aspects of electromagnetic fields for soft tissue healing. In: Blank M, ed. Electromagnetic Fields: Biological Interactions and Mechanisms. Adv Chem Vol. 250. Washington, DC: American Chemical Society, 1995:277–286.

57. Nordenstrom BE. Biologically Closed Electrical Circuits: Clinical, Experimental and Theoretical Evidence for an Additional Circulatory System. Stockholm: Nordic Medical Publications, 1983:358.

58. Bourguignon GL, Bourguignon LYW. Electrical stimulation of protein and DNA synthesis. Med Rehab 1989; 70:624–627.

59. Rodeman HP, Bayreuther K, Pfleiderer G. The differentiation of normal and transformed human fibroblasts in vitro is influenced by electromagnetic fields. Exp Cell Res 1989; 182:610–621.

60. Karba R, Vodovnik L, Jercinovic A, Trontelj K, Benko H, Savrin R. Promotion of wound healing by electrical stimulation. Biomedizinische Technik 1995; 40:20–24.

61. Hudlicka O, Brown M, Cotter M. The effect of long-term stimulation of fast muscle of their blood flow, metabolism, and ability to withstand fatigue. Pfluggers Arch 1977; 369:141–149.

62. Markov M, Pilla AA. Modulation of cell-free myosin light chain phosphorylation with weak low frequency and static magnetic fields. In: Frey AH, ed. On the Nature of Electromagnetic Field Interactions with Biological Systems. Austin TX: R.G.Landes Co., 1994:127–141.

63. Polk C. Electric and magnetic fields for bone and soft tissue repair. In: Polk C, Postow E, eds. Handbook of Biological Effects of Electromagnetic Fields. Boca Raton, FL: CRC Press, 1996:231–246.

64. Ginsberg AJ. Ultrashort radio waves as a therapeutic agent. Med Record 1934; 19:1–8.

65. Wilson DH. Comparison of short-wave diathermy and pulsed electromagnetic energy in treatment of soft tissue injuries. Physiother 1974; 80:309–310.

66. Barclay V, Collier RJ, Jones A. Treatment of various hand injuries by pulsed electromagnetic energy (Diapulse). Physiother 1983; 69:186–188.

67. Ross Adey W. Nonlinear electrodynamics in cell membrane transductive coupling. In: Aloia RC, Curtain CC, Gordon LM, eds. Membrane Transport and Information Storage. Vol. 4 New York: Wiley-Liss, 1990:1–27.

68. Tenforde TS. Biological interactions of extremely low frequency electromagnetic fields. In: Ueno S, ed. Biological Effects of Magnetic and Electromagnetic Fields. New York: Plenum Press, 1996:23–35.

69. Blank M. Electric and magnetic field signal transduction in the membrane Na^+-K^+ adenosinetriphosphatase. In: Blank M, ed. Electromagnetic Field: Biological Interactions and Mechanisms. Washington DC: Amer Chem Soc, 1995:339–348.

70. Bawin SM, Adey WR. Sensitivity of calcium binding in cerebral tissue to weak environmental electric fields oscillating at low frequency. Proc Natl Acad Sci USA 1976; 73: 1999–2003.

71. Markov MS, Todorov SI, Ratcheva MR. Biomagnetic effects of the constant magnetic field action on water and physiological activity. In: Jensen K, Vassileva Yu, eds. Physical Bases of Biological Information Transfer. New York: Plenum Press, 1975:441–445.

17

Deep Brain Stimulation for Parkinson's Disease and Movement Disorders

E. Oscar Richter

University of Florida, Gainesville, Florida, U.S.A.

Andres M. Lozano

University of Toronto, Toronto Western Hospital Research Institute, Toronto, Ontario, Canada

Signs and symptoms of Parkinson's disease and other movement disorders appear to be related to abnormal firing of dopamine deficient neurons that disrupt cortical and brainstem areas controlling movement. Destroying these areas via surgical ablation can provide improvement but is often associated with adverse side effects. Electrical stimulation of these targets can mimic the effects of ablation with far fewer compilations. This approach has produced striking improvement in patients with movement disorders like Parkinson's disease, dystonia, and essential tremors not responsive to medication.

I. INTRODUCTION

For poorly understood reasons, the dopamine-producing cells in the substantia nigra of patients with Parkinson's disease die. When patients lose approximately 50% of their dopamine-producing cells, they develop the signs and symptoms of Parkinson's disease, that is, tremor, rigidity, akinesia (slowness of movements), and postural and gait abnormalities (1). How the dopamine deficiency leads to these signs and symptoms is not fully understood, but it is becoming clear that groups of neurons in the circuits that are deprived of dopamine start behaving abnormally. It is thought that these abnormally firing neurons cause disruption in the cortical and brainstem areas that control movements (2).

The discovery that destroying certain of these malfunctioning brain areas (also known as *ablation surgery*) in patients with Parkinson's disease can lead to improvements in motor function (3–5) has lead to a variety of surgical interventions. Unfortunately, when these neurons are destroyed, there can be undesirable side effects. This is particularly true if patients have symptoms on both sides and require bilateral operations (6).

Passing high-frequency electrical stimulation through the target can mimic the effects of ablation. By stimulating these areas intraoperatively, it is possible to produce acute improvements in motor function (7). This technique has been extended to the chronic delivery of electrical stimulation with striking improvements in tremor, rigidity, and akinesia in patients with Parkinson's disease (8,9). Chronic electrical stimulation of neural structures has now become a mainstay of treatment for patients with movement disorders like Parkinson's disease (9), dystonia (10), and essential tremor (11), which continue to be disabled despite the best available medical therapy.

There are three primary targets for surgical intervention in movement disorders. They are the thalamus, the globus pallidus, and the subthalamic nucleus.

II. THE THALAMUS

The ventral intermediate (Vim) nucleus of the thalamus is a preferred target for patients with certain tremor disorders (12). The most common is essential tremor (11). Neurons in the Vim nucleus of the thalamus fire in synchrony with the patient's tremor (7). The close temporal relationship between the peripheral tremor and the activity in these neurons suggests that these neurons could be performing a pacemaker function (13), responsible for driving the tremor. Indeed, destroying these neurons or interfering with their activity with chronic electrical stimulation is very effective for tremor control (14). Specific adverse effects that are encountered with deep brain stimulation in the ventral intermediate nucleus include speech, corticospinal, and ataxic symptomatology and paresthesias related to current spread to the adjacent tactile ventrocaudal nucleus (Vc). Because these effects are related to spread of the current to adjacent white matter tracts or nuclear structures, in many cases the stimulation parameters can be adjusted to reduce these adverse effects (15), though sometimes at the expense of a less than total control of tremor.

The target is chosen on the basis of several physiologic findings (16). First, neurons in Vim fire at tremor frequency; second, the Vim neurons are anterior to the tactile relay nucleus Vc; third, neurons in Vim respond to kinesthetic or joint movements; and fourth, stimulation within the Vim complex produces tremor arrest. When these findings have been confirmed, the target is identified. The clinical effectiveness of Vim stimulation varies from one tremor disorder to another. In general, tremor is very well treated with Vim stimulation, but it does little or nothing for the akinesia, rigidity, and gait disturbance of Parkinson's disease, and for this reason Vim is not the preferred target for patients with Parkinson's disease. Patients with essential tremor can obtain approximately an 80% reduction in tremor (17,18). The benefits of thalamic procedures for patients with other disorders, such as posttraumatic tremor or tremors associated with MS can be more variable depending on the exact pathophysiology in these patients. Often, the effects are of lesser magnitude and shorter lived (19).

III. THE GLOBUS PALLIDUS

The internal segment of the globus pallidus (GPi) is used in the treatment of both Parkinson's disease (9,20) and dystonia (21). The GPi is a large structure, and some of the variability in the clinical effects may be related to the position of the lesion or electrode within the GPi complex (22–25). The benefits of pallidal DBS are similar to those of pallidotomy (creating lesions in the globus pallidus) (26). Again, particularly when patients require bilateral procedures, the safety profile of DBS makes it clearly advantageous over lesion surgery (6,26).

It is important in globus pallidus targeting are to identify the sensorimotor territory of the GPi, that is, the portion of the GPi that is populated by kinesthetic neurons (neurons that respond to peripheral movements). It is also important to identify the optic tract and the corticospinal tract. These can be identified by electrical stimulation, which produces phosphenes when in the optic tract and motor contractions when in the corticospinal tract (23,27). While the effects of pallidal lesions and pallidal DBS in Parkinson's disease can be immediate, in patients with dystonia there is often a delay of several days or weeks between initiation of therapy (lesion placement or turning the stimulator on) and an apparent benefit (28–30). The reasons why the benefit in patients with dystonia is delayed and often progressive are not fully understood. It remains controversial whether the target for Parkinson's disease is the optimal target for dystonia within the pallidal complex or not.

IV. THE SUBTHALAMIC NUCLEUS

The subthalamic nucleus (STN) is currently the most popular target for the treatment of patients with medication refractory symptoms of Parkinson's disease. Major improvements are seen in tremor, rigidity, akinesia, and gait disturbances. Drug-induced involuntary movements can also be greatly ameliorated by interventions at the level of the STN because medications can often be reduced or in some cases even eliminated (31–44).

The objectives during surgery are to identify the sensorimotor territory in the subthalamic nucleus and to avoid adverse side affects related to important adjacent structures such as the fibers of the third cranial nerve (medial to the subthalamic nucleus), the corticospinal tract (anterior and lateral), and the fibers of the medial lemniscus (posterior). These structures are identified by microelectrode recordings and by intraoperative stimulation (45). Stimulation in the third nerve produces eye deviations, and stimulation of the medial lemniscus produces paresthesias.

V. GENERAL FEATURES

Stereotactic procedures to implant electrodes can be divided into the following five stages:

1. Stereotactic imaging
2. Electrophysiologic mapping
3. Electrode implantation
4. Pulse generator implantation
5. Programming

Electrode implantation is performed through a small hole in the skull, and the electrode gently passed directly to the chosen anatomic target. To do this requires precise control of the position of the electrode without visualization. Stereotaxis is the process whereby the anatomic position based on neuroimaging studies is described in terms of a three-dimensional coordinate system, and a device is used to control the surgical instruments, keeping them at specific coordinates. There are a large variety of such systems, but chronic stimulation and ablative surgeries have traditionally been performed by the use of head frames rigidly attached through the skin to the patient's skull (Fig. 1). An imaging study is

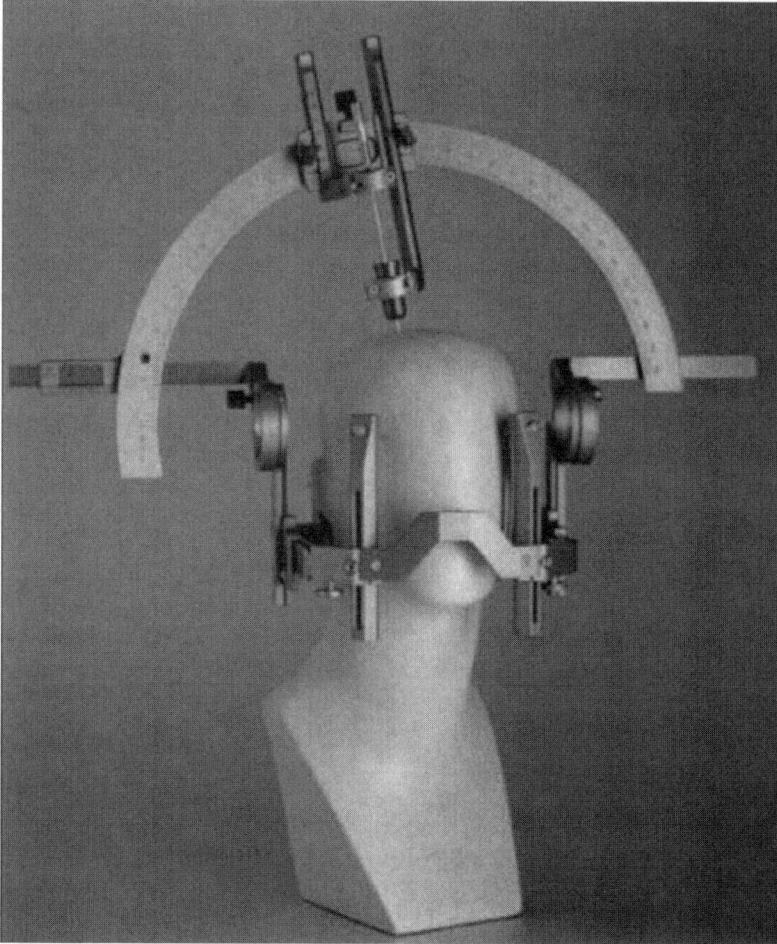

Figure 1 A stereotactic head frame system. Traditional stereotactic systems use a frame rigidly fixed to the patient's skull. During surgery, instruments are attached to this frame by an assembly such as the arc complex shown here, which restricts the position of the instruments to the chosen three-dimensional coordinates. (Picture by courtesy of Elekta.)

then obtained that allows the calculation of the coordinates of any point in the brain relative to the rigid external frame.

After the reference coordinate system is established, the patient is taken to the operating room for electrophysiologic mapping. This is done with microelectrodes; for example, Parylene-C insulated tungsten plated with gold and platinum, with tip lengths around 30 µm and impedance on the order of 0.5 MΩ. The amplified, filtered output is fed to an audio

Figure 2 Radiologic verification of electrode placement. The accuracy of the final electrode placement is verified by intraoperative x-ray (a) once the final(physiologically determined) target has been selected. Postoperatively, the anatomic placement of the electrodes can be verified with MRI (b, different patient).

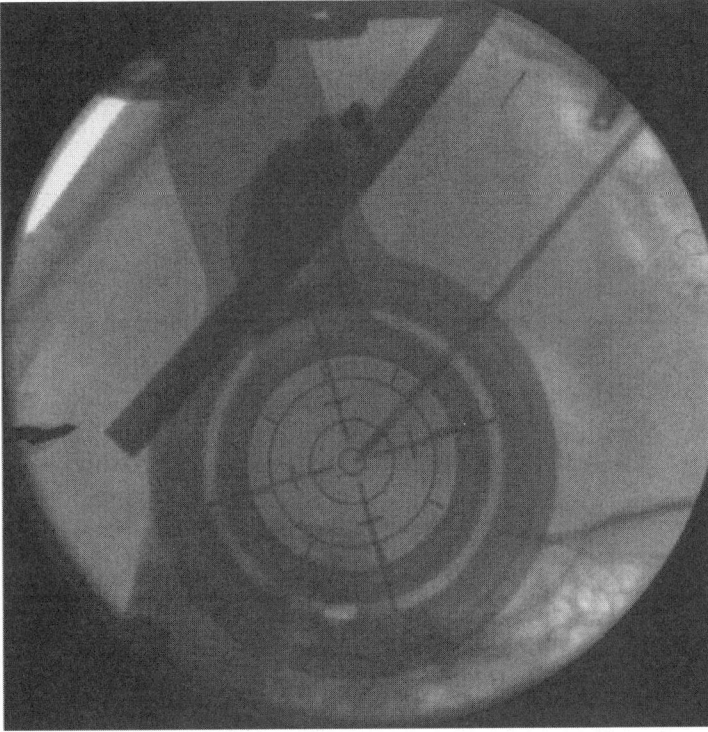

(a)

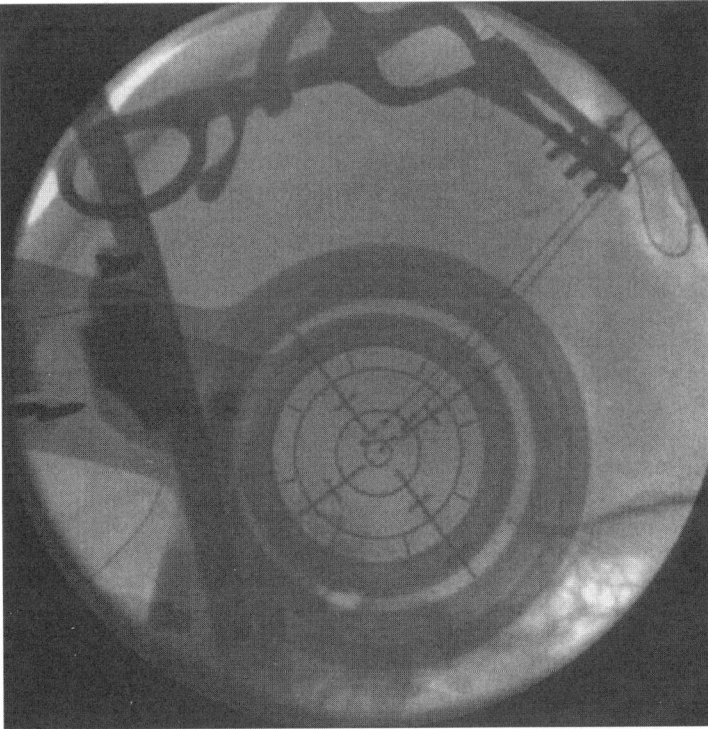

(b)

monitor and an oscilloscope, and a window discriminator determines discharge frequency (45). The specific neuronal characteristics that identify the optimal location vary by target.

The mapping results in an adjusted set of target coordinates specific to that patient. The electrode is then placed at that location, and accurate positioning relative to the frame is usually verified by intraoperative x-ray (Fig. 2). The pulse generator may be implanted in a subcutaneous pocket (Fig. 3) at this time, or a percutaneous extension cable may allow continued test stimulation prior to implantation. Programming to find the optimal stimulation parameters is an ongoing process.

Deep brain stimulating electrodes currently in use are quadripolar, with four cylindrical contacts made of platinum and iridium (Medtronic 3387 or 3389, Minneapolis Minnesota). The four contacts are spaced either 1.5 or 2.5 mm apart (Fig. 4) and are positioned so as to span the desired target. The electrode is connected to a handheld pulse generator for intraoperative and postoperative testing through a percutaneous extension cable. Once the electrode producing the most therapeutic benefit is identified, it can be connected to an

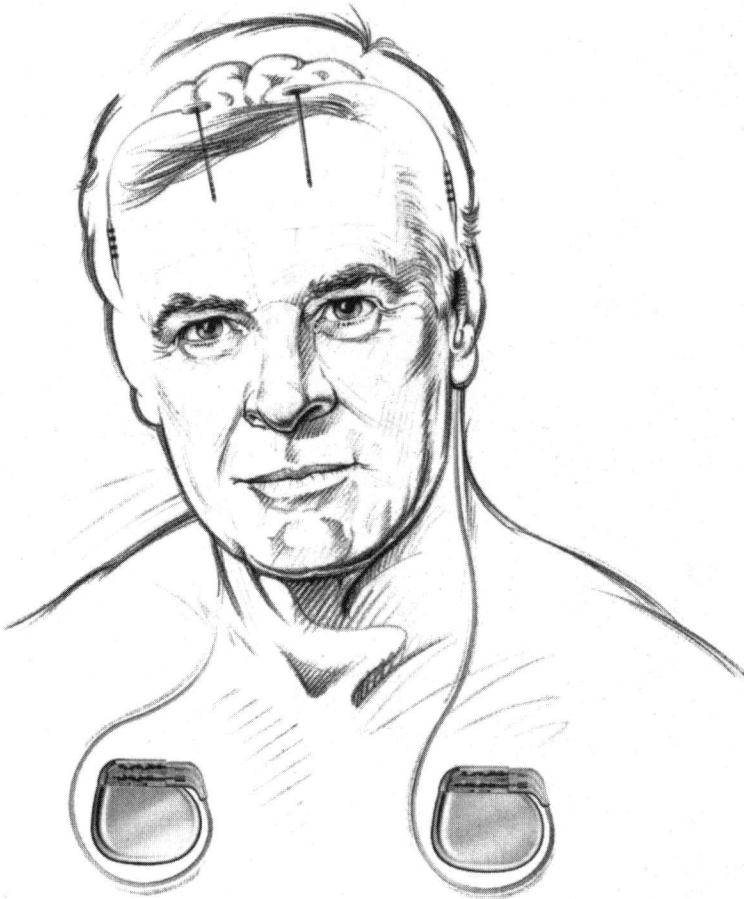

Figure 3 An artist's schematic representation of a fully implanted bilateral stimulator system. The electrodes are seen implanted through bilateral holes in the skull, and the cables are tunneled under the scalp and connected to extension cables, which extend to the IPG implanted in a subclavicular subcutaneous pocket. (Illustration courtesy of Medtronic, Inc.)

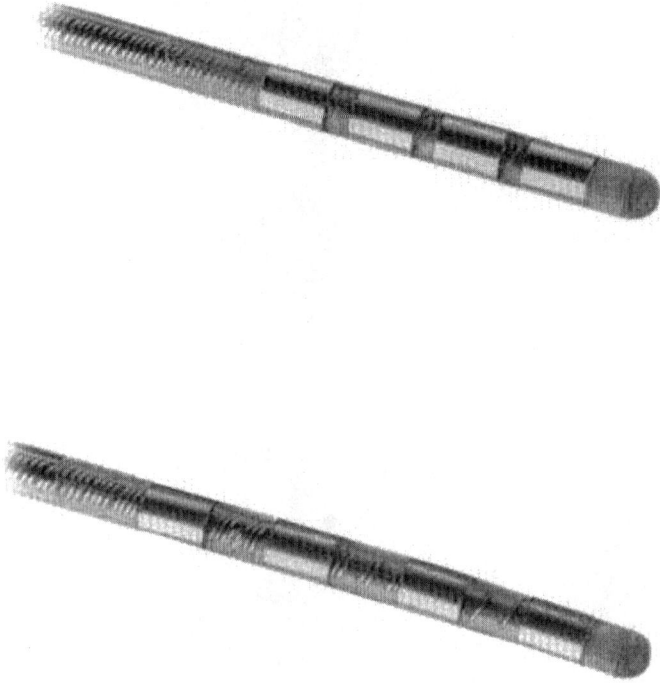

Figure 4 The two most common models of deep brain stimulating electrodes. They are both quadripolar, with cylindrical contacts. The difference between the two leads is the distance between the contacts. (Illustration courtesy of Medtronic, Inc.)

internal pulse generator (Fig. 5). Such generators have lithium batteries and are capable of delivering continuous pulses of stimulation for 5 to 6 years. Typical stimulation parameters depend on the choice of target. The STN or GPi usually requires stimulation in the range of 3 V and a 60- to 90-μs pulse width at 130 to 185 Hz to produce good clinical effects (8,40). In most cases patients leave their stimulating electrodes on 24 h/day.

Each contact may be designated independently to be anode, cathode, or off. Stimulation may be unipolar, with the case of the IPG functioning as ground, or bipolar. There are 29 frequency settings from 2 to 185 Hz (pps), 10 pulse width settings from 60 to 450 μs and 106 voltage settings from 0 to 10.5 V. The large number of possible combinations of stimulation parameters greatly increases the adaptability of the stimulation, but also contributes to the complexity of choosing the optimal stimulation parameters. Indeed, several efforts are now under way to try to test a large number of stimulation parameter combinations in an efficient manner.

VI. HOW DOES DBS WORK?

Although DBS has been clearly shown to be clinically beneficial, its mechanism of action has not yet been fully elucidated. To date, clinical decisions regarding its application have been largely based on the assumption that high frequency chronic stimulation will mimic the effects of a lesion of the same location, albeit with reversible and adjustable properties. This assumption originally arose from the similarity of clinical outcome in thalamotomy

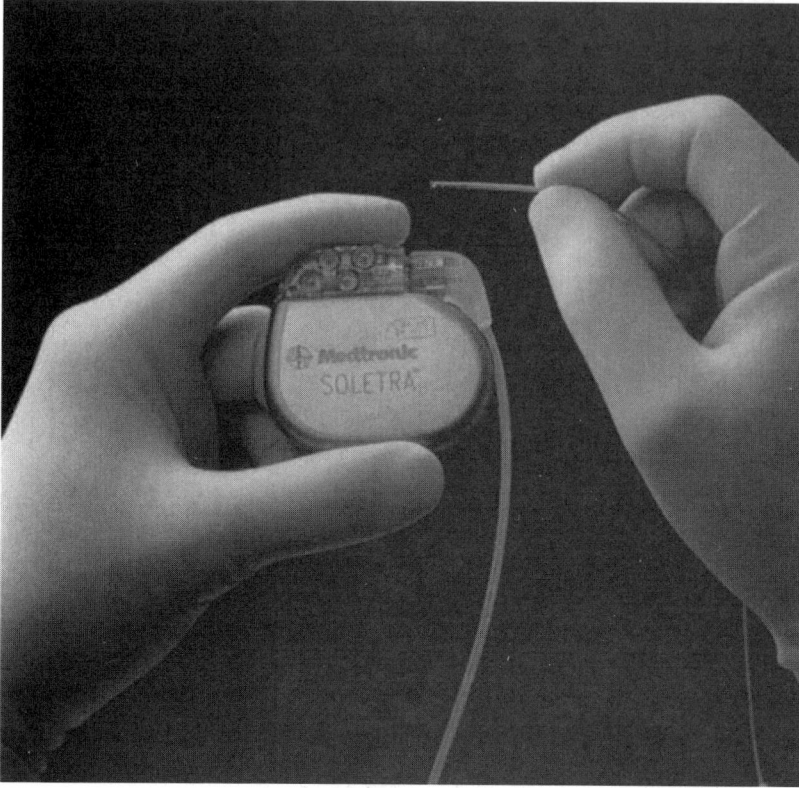

Figure 5 Implantable pulse generator with attached quadripolar electrode. (Photo courtesy of Medtronic, Inc.)

and thalamic DBS (46). The underlying mechanism, however, remains a topic of much discussion (47–49).

A given target nucleus is composed of neuronal cell bodies, dendrites, presynaptic nerve terminals, axons arising from the cell bodies, and axons of passage. These elements are connected in a precise and spatially complex pattern. Each element will respond to the externally applied field and the currents it induces in a different fashion. Axons are the most sensitive to stimulation, and neuronal bodies more resistant (50). It is important to note that when stimulated to threshold, axons send an action potential in both directions (31). Although cortical potentials have been demonstrated with STN stimulation (51), the effects of antidromic stimulation are not understood and are likely complex. An antidromic action potential would also be expected, upon reaching a point of collateral branching to propagate along it in an orthodromic fashion to influence any collateral targets. Whether an action potential activated a collateral branch would be affected by a number of factors, including the types and density of channels in the membrane, the degree of myelination, and the relative diameters of the two branches. The interaction between elements in this network may be frequency dependent and may also involve nonsynaptic mechanisms over longer time courses (31,48). Many portions of the central nervous system are organized according to a well-described center-surround pattern (52–54). It is possible that synchronous activation of all fibers in an excitatory axon bundle could fail to have an overall excitatory influence on its target network secondary to a center-surround organization of the target structure.

The mechanisms that might contribute in varying degrees to the clinical success of DBS include the following (48): modification of a feedback loop, activation of inhibitory structures included in a more complex network, inactivation of membrane ion channels (55), depolarization blockade (56), synaptic exhaustion, induction of early genes, vascular effects, effects on glia, changes in ion concentrations (56), or forms of neural plasticity. There is evidence that in pallidal DBS inhibition of pallidal neurons is due to activation of inhibitory projections onto those cells (47,57).

VII. FUTURE DIRECTIONS

There are continuing efforts to produce computer models of the effects of electrical stimulation on nervous tissue. Previous efforts have accurately reproduced some electrophysiologic results (58–62). The eventual goal is patient-specific modeling of current densities as a function of stimulation parameters and subsequent correlation with clinical outcome. This would facilitate the development of a rational approach to the selection of stimulation parameters, which to date has been entirely trial and error. The importance of such an advance becomes obvious when one realizes that a Medtronic IPG in basic square wave mode has pulse amplitude settings from 0 to 10.5 V in 0.1-V increments, 28 rate settings from 2 to 185 Hz, and 10 pulse width settings from 60 to 450 μs. Each of these can be varied independently at each of four contacts that are set as anode, cathode, or off, resulting in a very large number of possible combinations of stimulation parameters.

Because of the striking improvement seen with DBS in movement disorders, the possibility of applying DBS to other neurologic conditions is being explored. There is work suggesting that DBS can also benefit such varied disorders such as pain (63), epilepsy (10), and based on success with ablative procedures (64–67), even psychiatric disease (68). As we understand more about the pathophysiology of these conditions and the selection of which brain areas to target, and as we have a greater understanding of how DBS works, the role of deep brain stimulation for treating a variety of neurologic conditions will continue to expand. Other forms of electrical stimulation of the nervous system are also reaching clinical use, such as sheets of electrodes placed on the surface of the brain for pain control (69), or stimulation of the vagus nerve for epilepsy (70–73). Much work remains to be done in understanding and improving these techniques in order to improve the lives of patients with neural disorders.

REFERENCES

1. Lang AE, Lozano AM. Parkinson's disease. First of two parts. N Engl J Med 1998; 339(15): 1044–1053.
2. Lang AE, Lozano AM. Parkinson's disease. Second of two parts. N Engl J Med 1998; 339(16): 1130–1143.
3. Meyers R. The modification of alternating tremor, rigidity and festination by surgery of the basal ganglia. Res Publ Assoc Nerv Ment Dis 1941; 21:602.
4. Meyers R. A surgical procedure for the alleviation of postencephalitic tremor, with notes on the physiology of the premotor fires. Arch Neurol Psychiatry 1940; 44:445–459.
5. Cooper IS. Ligation of the anterior choroidal artery for involuntary movements of parkinsonism. Psychiatr Q 1953; 27:317–319.

6. Hariz M. Complications of movement disorder surgery and how to avoid them. In: Lozano A, ed. Movement disorder surgery. Karger: Basel, 2000:256–265.

7. Pahapill PA, Levy R, Dostrovsky JO, et al. Tremor arrest with thalamic microinjections of muscimol in patients with essential tremor. Ann Neurol 1999; 46(2):249–252.

8. Benabid A. Subthalamic nucleus deep brain stimulation. In: Lozano A, ed. Movement Disorder Surgery. Karger: Basel, 2000:196–226.

9. Pollak P, Fraix V, Krack P, et al. Treatment results: Parkinson's disease. Mov Disord 2002; 17(suppl 3):S75–S83.

10. Benabid AL, Koudsie A, Benazzouz A, et al. Deep brain stimulation of the corpus luysi (subthalamic nucleus) and other targets in Parkinson's disease. Extension to new indications such as dystonia and epilepsy. J Neurol 2001; 248(suppl 3):Iii37–47.

11. Pahwa R, Lyons KE, Wilkinson SB, et al. Comparison of thalamotomy to deep brain stimulation of the thalamus in essential tremor. Mov Disord 2001; 16(1):140–143.

12. Lozano AM. Vim thalamic stimulation for tremor. Arch Med Res 2000; 31(3):266–269.

13. Lenz FA, Tasker RR, Kwan HC, et al. Single unit analysis of the human ventral thalamic nuclear group: correlation of thalamic "tremor cells" with the 3–6 Hz component of parkinsonian tremor. J Neurosci 1988; 8(3):754–764.

14. Schuurman PR, Bosch DA, Bossuyt PM, et al. A comparison of continuous thalamic stimulation and thalamotomy for suppression of severe tremor. N Engl J Med 2000; 342(7):461–468.

15. Tasker RR. Deep brain stimulation and thalamotomy for tremor compared. Acta Neurochir Suppl (Wien) 1997; 68:49–53.

16. Lozano A. Thalamic deep brain stimulation for the control of tremor. In: Rengachary S, Wilkins R, eds. Neurosurgical Operative Atlas. Chicago: American Association of Neurological Surgeons, 1998:125–133.

17. Benabid AL, Pollak P, Gao D, et al. Chronic electrical stimulation of the ventralis intermedius nucleus of the thalamus as a treatment of movement disorders. J Neurosurg 1996; 84(2):203–214.

18. Koller W, Pahwa R, Busenbark K, et al. High-frequency unilateral thalamic stimulation in the treatment of essential and parkinsonian tremor. Ann Neurol 1997; 42(3):292–299.

19. Shahzadi S, Tasker RR, Lozano A. Thalamotomy for essential and cerebellar tremor. Stereotact Funct Neurosurg 1995; 65(1–4):11–17.

20. Bakay RAE. Rational basis for pallidotomy in the treatment of parkinson's disease. In: Lozano AM, ed. Movement Disorder Surgery. Karger: Basel, 2000:118–131.

21. Vercueil L, Krack P, Pollak P. Results of deep brain stimulation for dystonia: a critical reappraisal. Mov Disord 2002; 17(suppl 3):S89–S93.

22. Gross RE, Lombardi WJ, Lang AE, et al. Relationship of lesion location to clinical outcome following microelectrode-guided pallidotomy for Parkinson's disease. Brain 1999; 122(pt 3):405–416.

23. Lozano A, Hutchinson W, Kiss Z, Tasker R, Davis K, Dostrovsky J. Methods for micro-electrode-guided posteroventral pallidotomy. J Neurosurg 1996; 84(2):194–202.

24. Bejjani B, Damier P, Arnulf I, et al. Pallidal stimulation for Parkinson's disease. Two targets? Neurology 1997; 49(6):1564–1569.

25. Krack P, Pollak P, Limousin P, et al. Opposite motor effects of pallidal stimulation in Parkinson's disease. Ann Neurol 1998; 43(2):180–192.

26. Kumar R. Pallidotomy and deep brain stimulation of the pallidum and subthalamic nucleus in advanced Parkinson's disease. Mov Disord 1998; 13(suppl 1):73–82.

27. Kirschman DL, Milligan B, Wilkinson S, et al. Pallidotomy microelectrode targeting: neuro-physiology-based target refinement. Neurosurgery 2000; 46(3):613–622.

28. Tronnier VM, Fogel W. Pallidal stimulation for generalized dystonia. Report of three cases. J Neurosurg 2000; 92(3):453–456.

29. Kumar R, Dager A, Hutchinson WD, Lang AE, Lozano AM. Globus pallidus deep brain stimulation for generalized dystonia: clinical and PET investigation. Neurology 1999; 53(4):871–874.

30. Volkmann J, Benecke R. Deep brain stimulation for dystonia: patient selection and evaluation. Mov Disord 2002; 17(suppl 3):S112–S115.

31. Lozano AM. Deep brain stimulation for parkinson's disease. Parkinsonism & Related Disorders 2001; 7:199–203.

32. Thobois S, Mertens P, Guenot M, et al. Subthalamic nucleus stimulation in Parkinson's disease: clinical evaluation of 18 patients. J Neurol 2002; 249(5):529–534.

33. Simuni T, Jaggi JL, Mulholland H, et al. Bilateral stimulation of the subthalamic nucleus in patients with Parkinson disease: a study of efficacy and safety. J Neurosurg 2002; 96(4):666–672.

34. Voges J, Volkmann J, Allert N, et al. Bilateral high-frequency stimulation in the subthalamic nucleus for the treatment of Parkinson disease: correlation of therapeutic effect with anatomical electrode position. J Neurosurg 2002; 96(2):269–279.

35. Yokoyama T, Sugiyama K, Nishizawa S, et al. Subthalamic nucleus stimulation for gait disturbance in Parkinson's disease. Neurosurgery 1999; 45(1):41–47.

36. Burchiel KJ, Anderson VC, Favre J, Hammerstand JP. Comparison of pallidal and subthalamic nucleus deep brain stimulation for advanced Parkinson's disease: results of a randomized, blinded pilot study. Neurosurgery 1999; 45(6):1375–1382.

37. Krack P, Pollak P, Limousin P, et al. Subthalamic nucleus or internal pallidal stimulation in young onset Parkinson's disease. Brain 1998; 121(pt 3):451–457.

38. Kumar R, Lozano AM, Kim YJ, et al. Double-blind evaluation of subthalamic nucleus deep brain stimulation in advanced Parkinson's disease. Neurology 1998; 51(3):850–855.

39. Vingerhoets FJG, Villemure JG, Temperli P, Pollo C, Pralong E, Ghika J. Subthalamic DBS replaces levodopa in Parkinson's disease: two-year follow-up. Neurology 2002; 58(3):396–401.

40. Volkmann J, Allert N, Voges J, Weiss PH, Freund HJ, Sturm V. Safety and efficacy of pallidal or subthalamic nucleus stimulation in advanced PD. Neurology 2001; 56(4):548–551.

41. Limousin P, Krack P, Pollak P, et al. Electrical stimulation of the subthalamic nucleus in advanced Parkinson's disease. N Engl J Med 1998; 339(16):1105–1111.

42. Houeto JL, Damier P, Bejjani PB, et al. Subthalamic stimulation in Parkinson disease: a multidisciplinary approach. Arch Neurol 2000; 57(4):461–465.

43. Molinuevo JL, Valldeoriola F, Tolosa E, et al. Levodopa withdrawal after bilateral subthalamic nucleus stimulation in advanced Parkinson disease. Arch Neurol 2000; 57(7):983–988.

44. Fraix V, Pollak P, Van Blercom N, et al. Effect of subthalamic nucleus stimulation on levodopa-induced dyskinesia in Parkinson's disease. Neurology 2000; 55(12):1921–1923.

45. Rezai A, Hutchinson W, Lozano A. Chronic subthalamic nucleus stimulation for parkinson's disease. In: Rengachary S, Wilkins R, eds. Neurosurgical Operative Atlas. The American Association of Neurological Surgeons: Chicago, 1999:195–207.

46. Benabid A, et al. Subthalamic nucleus deep brain stimulation. In: Lozano A, ed. Movement Disorder Surgery. Karger: Basel, 2001:196–226.

47. Dostrovsky JO, Lozano AM. Mechanisms of deep brain stimulation. Mov Disord 2002; 17(suppl 3):S63–S68.

48. Benabid AL, Benazzous A, Pollak P. Mechanisms of deep brain stimulation. Mov Disord 2002; 17(suppl 3):S73–S74.

49. Vitek JL. Mechanisms of deep brain stimulation: excitation or inhibition. Mov Disord 2002; 17(suppl 3):S69–S72.

50. Ranck JB Jr. Which elements are excited in electrical stimulation of mammalian central nervous system: a review. Brain Res 1975; 98(3):417–440.

51. Ashby P, Paradiso G, Saint-Cyr JA, et al. Potentials recorded at the scalp by stimulation near the human subthalamic nucleus. Clin Neurophysiol 2001; 112(3):431–437.

52. Bastian J, Chacron MJ, Maler L. Receptive field organization determines pyramidal cell stimulus-encoding capability and spatial stimulus selectivity. J Neurosci 2002; 22(11):4577–4590.

53. Nambu A, Tokuno H, Takada M. Functional significance of the cortico-subthalamo-pallidal 'hyperdirect' pathway. Neurosci Res 2002; 43(2):111–117.

54. Kaji R. Basal ganglia as a sensory gating devise for motor control. J Med Invest 2001; 48(3–4):142–146.

55. Beurrier C, Bioulac B, Audin J, Hammond C. High-frequency stimulation produces a transient

blockade of voltage-gated currents in subthalamic neurons. J Neurophysiol 2001; 85(4):1351–1356.

56. Bikson M, Lian J, Hahn PJ, Stacey WC, Sciortino C, Durand DM. Suppression of epileptiform activity by high frequency sinusoidal fields in rat hippocampal slices. J Physiol 2001; 531(pt 1): 181–191.

57. Lozano A, Dostrovsky J, Chen R, Ashby P. Deep brain stimulation for parkinson's disease: disrupting the disruption. Lancet Neurol 2002; 1(4):225–231.

58. Richardson AG, McIntyre CC, Grill WM. Modeling the effects of electric fields on nerve fibres: influence of the myelin sheath. Med Biol Eng Comput 2000; 38(4):438–446.

59. McIntyre CC, Grill WM. Modeling of thalamic DBS: cellular and network effects. In: Neuromodulation 2002: Defining the Future. France: Aix-Les-Bains, 2002.

60. McIntyre CC, Grill WM. Selective microstimulation of central nervous system neurons. Ann Biomed Eng 2000; 28(3):219–233.

61. McIntyre CC, Grill WM. Finite element analysis of the current-density and electric field generated by metal microelectrodes. Ann Biomed Eng 2001; 29(3):227–235.

62. McIntyre CC, Richardson AG, Grill WM. Modeling the excitability of mammalian nerve fibers: influence of afterpotentials on the recovery cycle. J Neurophysiol 2002; 87(2):995–1006.

63. Tasker RR, Vilela Filho O. Deep brain stimulation for neuropathic pain. Stereotact Funct Neurosurg 1995; 65(1–4):122–124.

64. Price BH, Baral I, Cosgrove GR, et al. Improvement in severe self-mutilation following limbic leucotomy: a series of 5 consecutive cases. J Clin Psychiatry 2001; 62(12):925–932.

65. Feldman RP, Alterman RL, Goodrich JT. Contemporary psychosurgery and a look to the future. J Neurosurg 2001; 95(6):944–956.

66. Montoya A, Weiss AP, Price BH, et al. Magnetic resonance imaging-guided stereotactic limbic leukotomy for treatment of intractable psychiatric disease. Neurosurgery 2002; 50(5):1043–1049.

67. Dougherty DD, et al. Prospective long-term follow-up of 44 patients who received cingulotomy for treatment-refractory obsessive-compulsive disorder. Am J Psychiatry 2002; 159(2):269–275.

68. Nuttin B, et al. Electrical stimulation in anterior limbs of internal capsules in patients with obsessive-compulsive disorder. Lancet 1999; 354(9189):1526.

69. Garcia Larrea L, et al. Functional imaging and neurophysiological assessment of spinal and brain therapeutic modulation in humans. Arch Med Res 2000; 31(3):248–257.

70. Zamponi N, et al. Intermittent vagal nerve stimulation in paediatric patients: 1-year follow-up. Childs Nerv Syst 2002; 18(1–2):61–66.

71. Sucholeiki R, et al. fMRI in patients implanted with a vagal nerve stimulator. Seizure 2002; 11(3):157–162.

72. Bernard EJ, et al. Insertion of vagal nerve stimulator using local and regional anesthesia. Surg Neurol 2002; 57(2):94–98.

73. Cramer JA, Ben Menachem E, French J. Review of treatment options for refractory epilepsy: new medications and vagal nerve stimulation. Epilepsy Res 2001; 47(1–2):17–25.

18

Noninvasive Pulsed Electromagnetic Therapy for Migraine and Multiple Sclerosis

Martha S. Lappin

Energy Medicine Developments, Burke, Virginia, U.S.A.

There is a striking similarity in neurotransmitter and neuroendocrine mechanisms involved in migraine, multiple sclerosis, and depression. Depression is very common in MS and is typically correlated with MS fatigue, while migraineurs have a four-fold increase in the risk of major depression and often show biological markers of depression. Cranioelectrical stimulation approaches such as repetitive transcranial magnetic stimulation and vagal and deep brain stimulation have proven effective for the treatment of drug resistant depression. We have also found that specific weak, pulsating EMFs can significantly reduce the frequency and severity of migraine attacks and improve fatigue, bladder control, and spasticity in patients with MS.

I. INTRODUCTION

Following FDA approval of pulsed electromagnetic field (EMF) therapies for nonunion bone fractures in 1979, evidence supporting the effectiveness of these treatments for a variety of orthopedic conditions has accumulated at an impressive rate (1). Double-blind placebo controlled trials have demonstrated that weak, pulsed EMFs can alleviate the pain and disability associated with osteoarthritis and musculoskeletal pain (2). The serendipitous discovery that diagnostic transcranial magnetic stimulation (TMS) had mood altering effects in some patients (3) led to further research in this area. Shealy and co-workers confirmed a decrease in serotonin in depressed patients and demonstrated that transcranial electrical stimulation could improve depression and restore serotonin levels to normal (4). More recently it has been shown that repetitive transcranial magnetic stimulation (rTMS) using 10 to 20 Hz magnetic fields targeted to the left prefrontal cortex can alleviate drug resistant depression (5). Similar results have been obtained with vagal nerve stimulation (6) and deep brain stimulation of the ventrointermediate nucleus of the thalamus (7).

This chapter addresses the effects of weak, pulsating EMFs in patients with migraine and multiple sclerosis (MS). Clinical trials and outcome studies on the effects of weak, pulsed

EMFs are reviewed, and mechanisms through which EMFs might provide benefits in these disorders are discussed. There is considerable overlap between the documented neuro-chemical and electrophysiological effects of pulsed EMFs and the specific neurochemical and electrophysiological dysfunctions involved in the pathophysiology of migraine and MS, particularly the fatigue often associated with MS. While such associations do not prove a causal linkage, they do provide a starting point for plausible hypotheses about possible mechanisms of action.

Our own studies on migraine and MS have been conducted using a small, portable pulsed electromagnetic field generator called the *Enermed* (Energy Medicine Developments, Vancouver, B.C.) as described below.

II. THE ENERMED TREATMENT

The Enermed is a small, portable device slightly over 1 in. in diameter powered by a 3-V lithium battery that emits a 50–100 mG electromagnetic field generated by a solenoid coil. The input waveform is a 1-ms positive square wave that that can be pulsed between 1 and 25 Hz. This device differs from most EMF generators in that it can be programmed to emit multiple and patient-specific frequencies. While the frequencies used in most EMF thera-pies, including rTMS, fall into the 1 to 25 Hz range, the selection of specific treatment frequencies is often a trial-and-error process based on empirical observations. As yet, there is little theory or research to guide the selection of specific frequencies in clinical applications, even though frequency-specific biological (8) and electrophysiological (9,10) effects high-light the importance of matching field parameters (e.g., frequency and strength) to their "biotargets" (11).

The selection of Enermed treatment frequencies is based on guidelines emerging from clinical experience and analyses of individual bioelectromagnetic profiles. The profile analysis is based on an innovative application of the electromagnetic sensitivities of piezo-electric quartz crystals. Subtle electromagnetic signals emanating from the crown of the head are detected by passing a beam of light through a piezoelectric crystal. Modulations in the light signal caused by the bioelectromagnetic field are amplified and sent to a computer for analysis. The time domain signal is Fourier transformed and displayed as a spectrum with a range of 1 to 25 Hz. Low-amplitude signals within the frequency ranges that clinical ex-perience suggests are helpful for different symptom profiles are identified for each individual. Typically four frequencies are programmed into the device, and each is "on" for 12.7 s in a continuously repeating pattern.

Although most EMF therapies require office visits for treatment, once the Enermed is programmed, patients can use it at home. The device is designed to be worn continuously, 12 to 24 h a day, either attached to the upper chest area (typically over the brachial plexus) with an adhesive tape or worn on a cord around the neck. In clinical trials, effects are evaluated after 1 to 3 months, although some patients continue to report improvements even after the first few months. When patients stop using the device, effects typically wear off in 1 to 2 weeks.

III. DETECTION AND MECHANISM OF ACTION OF WEAK EMFs

The magnetic field emitted by the Enermed (50 to 100 mG or 5 to 10 μT) is slightly weaker than the earth's magnetic field. This is similar in strength to devices often used to treat osteoarthritis, but about 100,000 times weaker than the 0.5 to 1-T fields typically used in rTMS. rTMS fields are strong enough to induce electrical currents and neuron depolarization in underlying tissue; however, magnetic fields in the microTesla range are not. As Ross Adey, one of the leading pioneers in this field has emphasized, the effects of very weak electromagnetic fields "cannot be explained by traditional equilibrium models of cellular excitation based on depolarization of the membrane potential and on associated massive changes in ionic equilibria across cell membranes" (see Ref. 12, p. 411). How very weak EMFs are detected by the central nervous system is still not entirely clear, but various models have been proposed. Speculation about mechanisms of action in this review will be limited to identifying those influences that might be pertinent to or possibly explain our results in migraine and MS.

IV. PULSED EMF MIGRAINE RESEARCH

A. Migraine Characteristics and Prevalence

Migraine is a common, episodic headache disorder characterized by severe unilateral or pulsating pain usually accompanied by nausea and extreme light and/or sound sensitivity. In about one fourth of the cases the headache is preceded by a characteristic aura consisting of disturbances of the visual system (e.g., appearance of jagged lights, blind spots) and occasionally sensory or motor symptoms. It is estimated that 6% of all men, and 18% of all women between the ages of 12 and 80 experience at least one migraine a year and that 5% of the general population will experience at least 18 migraine attacks annually (13,14).

Current migraine treatments focus on alleviating pain with general analgesics or narcotics, aborting attacks with sumatriptan or newer drugs in the triptan family, and/or attempting to prevent migraine attacks with beta blockers, calcium channel blockers, antidepressants, or antiepileptics. However, not all patients respond to these medications or side effects limit their use and there is an urgent need for effective and safer alternatives (15).

B. Early Enermed Migraine Research

The first systematic study of an EMF treatment for migraine was an uncontrolled outcome study (16). Fifty-four chronic migraine patients were tracked for three months after receiving individually programmed 50–100-mG prototypes of the present Enermed device. Headache diaries indicated that migraine frequency dropped from an average of 1.2 to.6 per week, a 50% reduction, and significant diminution in severity and duration were also reported.

In a second study, one page questionnaires asking for pre- and posttreatment symptom ratings were mailed to just over 1000 people who had purchased early versions of the Enermed in Great Britain in the mid1990s (17). The overall survey response rate was 42% including 262 individuals who were treated specifically for migraines. Nearly all of the migraine patients (94%) reported severe pretreatment symptoms (ratings in the 7 to 10 range, where 10 = extremely bad), while only 21% reported severe problems after treatment. Almost two-thirds (63%) of posttreatment ratings were in the 1 to 4 range (1 being perfectly well), typically reflecting improvements of five points or more on the 10-point scale.

C. Double-Blind, Placebo Controlled Migraine Trial

Although the preliminary, uncontrolled studies described above are of limited scientific value, they did provide the impetus for a subsequent, NIH funded, double-blind, placebo controlled trial. In this study (not yet published), 21 subjects with confirmed migraine diagnoses received the typical clinical treatment—an active Enermed individually programmed with four frequencies between 4 and 15 Hz. The control group received either inactive place-bo devices ($n = 11$) or devices preprogrammed to emit a single, 2-Hz frequency field ($n = 9$).

Participants were randomly assigned to treatment groups and both subjects and investigators remained blinded to treatment conditions throughout the study. Diaries were used to record migraine frequency during the 4- to 8-week baseline period and the three month treatment period. Preliminary analyses revealed no significant differences between the placebo and 2-Hz control groups so they were combined into a single control group for the final evaluation. In the active treatment group, the average number of migraines per month fell from 7.2 to 4.8, while the mean for the control group remained unchanged at 6.7 migraines per month. Active vs. control group differences were significant using both parametric (t test) and nonparametric (Mann-Whitney U test) analyses.

In terms of percentages, one fourth of the control group and just over half (52%) of the active group saw a 25% or greater reduction in the number of migraine days they ex-perienced. Post hoc analyses suggested an interesting age and gender effect on treatment effectiveness. There were five postmenopausal women 55 years of age or older in the active group, none of whom experienced a substantial (25% or more) reduction in headache frequency. In the remainder of the active group (six men of varying ages and 10 women under the age of 55), 69% reported substantial improvements. One possible explanation for this disparity may be the well-known relationship between hormonal fluctuations and headaches in female migraineurs (18).

D. Other EMF Migraine Studies

The only other published study involving a pulsed EMF treatment for migraine utilized the Diapulse device, a high-powered, high-frequency (27.12 MHz) instrument originally developed for healing nonunion fractures. This study was initiated after a VA Hospital patient reported that she stopped having migraines once she started Diapulse treatments for an orthopedic condition. A preliminary open study employing the same treatment protocol (placing the unit on the upper thigh for 1 h a day, 5 days a week for 2 to 4 weeks) in 23 chronic migraine sufferers showed a marked reduction in headache frequency that lasted several months (19). This pilot study was followed by a double-blind, placebo controlled trial in which 42 subjects received 10 1-h active or sham treatment sessions over the course of 2 weeks (20). At the end of the treatment period headaches were tracked for another month and compared to baseline measures. In the posttreatment month, 67% of those receiving EMF stimulation versus 20% of those in the placebo group showed improvements of 20% or more on at least two of five outcome variables. These results improved when non-responders to the first 2 weeks of treatment received 2 additional weeks of treatment at the end of the first month.

Since migraineurs who learn to raise their finger temperature by increasing peripheral blood flow using biofeedback (21,22) also show reduced headache activity, the authors suggested that improvement might be due to a resultant increase in peripheral blood flow. No data were presented to support this hypothesis, nor would this explain why weaker EMF treatments produced similar benefits. Other possible explanations will be discussed follow-ing the review of EMF research on multiple sclerosis.

V. PULSED EMF MULTIPLE SCLEROSIS (MS) RESEARCH

A. Characteristics and Prevalence of MS

MS is a demyelinating disease of the central nervous system affecting between 250,000 and 300,000 people in the United States and, like migraine, is three to four times more likely to afflict women (23). MS signs and symptoms include gait problems, spasticity, fatigue, cognitive impairments, and bladder and bowel dysfunction. Although fatigue is often the most prevalent and disabling complaint there has been relatively little research on fatigue specific treatments (24,25). Fatigue was a primary focus of the multicenter Enermed study, and the results suggest that pulsed EMFs may be a promising treatment option.

B. Enermed MS Pilot Study

A team headed by Dr. Todd Richards, a neurophysicist at the University of Washington, conducted an exploratory, double-blind, placebo controlled study of the effects of the Enermed on 30 MS patients in 1996 (26). The primary outcome measure, the MS perform-ance scale (MSPS), is a summed composite of disability ratings in eight areas: bladder control, cognitive functioning, fatigue, hand function, mobility, sensory symptoms, spas-ticity, and vision (27). After a 2-month treatment period, subjects randomly assigned to the active treatment group showed statistically significant improvements on the MSPS relative to the control group. Furthermore, out of the eight individual symptoms assessed in the MSPS, six improved relative to baseline scores in the active group compared to only three in the placebo group. The symptoms that appeared most responsive to treatment were fatigue, bladder control, and spasticity.

C. Multicenter Double-Blind, Placebo Controlled Enermed Study

The positive results of the pilot study led to a second, much larger study, funded by the Multiple Sclerosis Association of America (28). This study used validated, multi-item mea-sures of fatigue, bladder control, spasticity, and pain from the MS Quality of Life Inventory (MSQLI), a well-validated instrument developed by the Consortium of MS Centers Health Services Research Subcommittee (29). Secondary outcome measures included the MSPS and daily diary ratings of spasticity and bladder control problems.

Research sites included centers in Seattle, New Jersey, and Virginia. The study used a crossover design in which each subject received four weeks of active and four weeks of sham treatment in randomized order separated by a 2-week washout period. A total of 117 subjects (82% of those initially enrolled) completed both phases of the study. Most withdrawals occurred early in the study and did not appear to be related to the treatment. Results were assessed using paired t tests after subtracting baseline scores from active and placebo treatment scores. Although daily ratings of bladder and spasticity problems did not change across treatment sessions, two of the four MSQLI scales (fatigue and spasticity) showed significant improvement. A Quality of Life composite from the MSQLI (fatigue, spasms, pain) also showed significant treatment benefits. Post hoc analyses indicated that neither the type nor the duration of the disease affected the results, but disease severity as assessed by a mobility index did appear to influence prognosis. Moderately disabled subjects showed the strongest effects, while those largely confined to a wheelchair because of severe disability had no treatment effects. This may be due to greater nerve damage in the severely disabled group or to limitations in the fatigue scale since this measure focused primarily on physical activities, which are obviously limited in patients with severe mobility disabilities.

D. The Enermed Patient Survey

The most recent Enermed study was a 1999 patient survey examining long-term treatment outcomes of all patients treated in Canada over the previous four years (30). A total of 158 of the 253 patients who received the questionnaires returned them, for a 62% response rate. The results for the 134 MS patients were very positive with 45% indicating that the therapy was very effective (ratings of 7 to 10 on a 10-point effectiveness scale) in alleviating their symptom. Less than a fourth of respondents reported no benefit from the treatment, while 22% rated the therapy moderately effective (ratings of 4 to 6). Increased energy or reduced fatigue was the most frequently mentioned benefit.

Taken together these three studies lend strong support to the hypothesized positive effects of the Enermed on MS symptoms. The effects are best detected with quality-of-life-oriented measures, and the symptom most frequently improved is fatigue. This could have important implications for MS patients because severe fatigue is one of the most common and debilitating consequences of this disease.

E. Other MS Studies Using Pulsed EMFs

The Gyuling-Bordacs device developed in Hungary consists of a coil that generates a 5- to 7-mT field consisting of a 300-Hz sine wave pulsed at 2 to 50 Hz (31). In a small double-blind trial, 7 of 10 subjects improved in the active treatment group in contrast to only 2 of 10 placebo controls. Improvement was judged by the Expanded Disability Status Scale (EDSS) (32) and subjective assessments of clinical status. In an open trial, 80% of the 104 MS patients reported at least some improvement, primarily with respect to bladder control, spasticity, and fatigue. A "pico Tesla" device developed in the United States has also been reported to provide improvement in a variety of MS complaints, but only anecdotal information is available (33).

VI. NEUROCHEMICAL EFFECTS OF PULSED EMFs AND THEIR RELEVANCE TO MIGRAINE AND MS

A variety of animal and clinical studies have shown that weak (0.5–2 mT) 60-Hz EMFs can affect important neurotransmitters, including the endorphins (34,35), melatonin (36–38), and serotonergic and dopaminergic systems (39–41). Animal and human TMS studies show that strong EMFs pulsed at 20 to 25 Hz also affect serotonergic and dopaminergic systems (42–45). Considerable evidence supports the important role of serotonin in the pathophysiology of migraine (46) and PET imaging studies confirm abnormalities in serotonin synthesis (47). Dysregulation of dopaminergic systems has also been reported (48–52) and apomorphine, a dopamine receptor agonist, has been shown to reduce the frequency of migraine attacks (53). Melatonin levels may be decreased in migraineurs (54,55) especially women whose migraines are associated with monthly hormonal fluctuations (18). These findings suggest that the clinical benefits of pulsed EMFs in migraine may be due to intermediate effects on relevant neurotransmitters, a possibility also proposed to explain the positive effects of TMS on depression. The four-fold increase in the risk of major depression in migraine patients (56) suggests that migraine and depression probably share one or more underlying neurotransmitter (57) or central regulatory dysfunctions (58) and thus may respond to the same treatments.

Pulsed EMFs also affect the neuroendocrine system, specifically the functions of the hypothalamic–pituitary–adrenocortical (HPA) axis. Long-term (6 days and 8 weeks) 20-Hz TMS produced significantly attenuated HPA responses to stress (reduced ACTH, corticosterone, and cortisol levels) in rats (59,60) and effects on cortisol levels and thyroid stimulating hormone have been demonstrated in humans (61,62). This is important since one of the most consistent findings with respect to neurochemical abnormalities in MS is the dysregulation of the HPA system. MS patients typically show elevated baseline plasma cortisol levels and an exaggerated increase in plasma cortisol concentrations during dexamethasone suppression tests (63,64). Moreover, elevated cortisol is associated with greater cognitive impairment, neurologic disability, depression, and inflammatory disease activity (65–67). The attenuated stress responses associated with exposure to pulsed EMFs may underlie the clinical effects of weak EMFs observed in MS, and perhaps migraine as well since many migraine sufferers also show elevated cortisol levels (68).

VII. ELECTROPHYSIOLOGICAL EFFECTS OF PULSED EMFs AND THEIR RELEVANCE TO MIGRAINE AND MS

The TMS literature clearly demonstrates that strong, pulsing EMFs can have electrophysiological effects on the human brain. These effects can be excitatory or inhibitory depending on the stimulation frequency and the prestimulation level of cortical arousal. Evoked potential studies demonstrate that short-term, low-frequency (1 Hz) stimulation typically reduces motor cortex excitability while high-frequency (20 Hz) stimulation generally increases cortical arousal (69–73). However, these effects are not uniform. In patient populations characterized by abnormal levels of cortical arousal (e.g., patients suffering from chronic fatigue, depression, or migraine), opposite response patterns to high- and low-frequency stimulation have been observed (74–78).

Studies of weak, pulsed EMFs have focused on the effects of .01- to 1-G (1 to 100 μT) stimulation on EEG frequencies. Both slow (1.5 Hz) and mid-range (10 Hz) stimulation frequencies have been shown to alter activity in the corresponding EEG frequencies during very brief (2 s) stimulation periods (79). A follow-up study showed that a 10-s exposure to 10-Hz stimulation typically decreased EEG activity in the stimulated frequency in the 1-min poststimulation interval (80). Another laboratory found an overall slowing effect of 3-Hz stimulation resulting in increased EEG power in the theta band (3.5–7.5) and decreased power in the beta band (12.5–25 Hz) during a 20-min stimulation period (81).

Like TMS effects, frequency specific effects of very weak fields on the brain may depend on baseline or prestimulation characteristics. In one study, Bell and colleagues found that stimulating rabbit brains at a frequency dominant in the EEG selectively reinforced brain wave activity at that frequency, while stimulation at a nondominant frequency had little or no effect on brain wave activity (82). Additional research is required to determine how baseline arousal levels and dominant frequencies moderate the effects of weak EMF stimulation; however, both variables have been shown to be important determinants of the effects of photic stimulation (flashing lights) on brain wave activity (83,84).

Enermed research provides further evidence of the effects of weak EMFs on brain wave activity in specific frequency ranges (26,85). In a study with 20 MS patients, subjects exposed to either active or placebo devices were assessed using quantitative electroencephalography (qEEG) both before and treatment. There were two test conditions: variable frequency photic stimulation using goggles fitted with four red LEDs, and a language task requiring subjects to silently generate a verb after hearing a noun. EEG analyses showed a significant difference between active and placebo groups in alpha production in the test conditions, but not in resting eyes open and eyes closed conditions. During the language task (performed after devices were removed at the end of the 3-month treatment period), subjects who had received the active devices showed significant pre- to posttreatment increases in alpha power at 6 of 19 electrode sites, whereas no significant pre- to posttreatment changes were observed in the placebo group. In the photic stimulation condition, active device subjects showed increased alpha at all 19 electrode sites both during and after stimulation, and after correcting for multiple comparisons, significant active-vs.-placebo differences were observed at three sites. Treatment frequencies for those in the active Enermed group were varied; each subject received four individually programmed frequencies, but all were in the 4 to 15 Hz range, and most were in the alpha range of frequencies.

The electrophysiological effects of pulsed EMFs are relevant to both migraine and MS. Migraine is characterized by interictal abnormalities in electrophysiological excitability and habituation. In healthy normal subjects, the amplitudes of evoked potentials produced by visual, auditory, and response contingent stimuli decrease over time. This habituation to external stimuli is a primitive, learned response, presumably designed to facilitate selective attention to novel or important information in the environment, and to protect the brain against overstimulation (86). This process is impaired in migraineurs. Visual evoked potential (VEP) studies show that migraine patients do not habituate to repeated presentations of visual stimuli and may even become more sensitive to the stimulus after repeated trials. (87–89). Auditory evoked potentials (AEP) show a similar phenomenon—a heightened sensitivity to stimulus intensity and deficient habituation over time (90–92). Research on contingent negative variation (CNV)—an event related slow negative cortical potential provides further evidence of cortical hypersensitivity and deficient habituation in migraine subjects (93–95). It is unclear whether these abnormal responses are a function of especially low or high preactivation levels of cortical arousal (96), but both models confirm that cortical excitability is abnormal and threshold regulation is impaired in migraine. Evidence that amplitude and habituation abnormalities generally peak right before a migraine then normalize during the attack (94,97–100) suggests that a migraine episode may represent a protective, self-regulatory mechanism designed to "reset" the brain, or restore homeostasis after overstimulation (98,100).

Pulsed EMFs may prevent migraine attacks either by normalizing baseline arousal levels through stimulation at appropriate frequencies or by facilitating habituation to repetitive external and perhaps internal stimuli. Support for this hypothesis comes from a study examining the effects of 1-Hz and 10-Hz TMS on visual evoked potentials (74). Short-term 10-Hz TMS normalized electrophysiological responses of migraine patients, producing a significant increase in initial VEP responses and normal habituation in subsequent stimulation blocks. No effect was seen with 1-Hz stimulation. This positive, normalizing effect of 10-Hz stimulation in migraine and the corresponding absence of any response to 1-Hz stimulation is intriguing in light of the results of the unpublished Enermed migraine study described earlier. One of the control conditions in this trial was constant low-frequency (2 Hz) stimulation. Subjects in this group showed no clinical improvements, in fact, several appeared to get worse, while there were significant reductions in migraine frequency in the group receiving multiple-frequency, mid-range stimulation (5 to 15 Hz). This suggests that stimulation at the proper mid-range frequencies may not need to be strong to normalize cortical arousal and habituation in migraine and, through this mechanism, reduce the frequency of migraine attacks.

Like migraine sufferers, MS patients also show abnormal responses to visual and auditory stimuli. Typically, VEP and AEP response amplitudes are reduced in MS relative to healthy controls, and it is noteworthy that these reductions appear to be confined to the alpha range frequencies (101,102). This suggests that alpha blocking may be extended or exaggerated in MS, just as it is in migraine patients (94). As noted previously, Enermed treatment resulted in significant posttreatment increases in alpha power in a group of MS patients who also showed concomitant clinical improvement (26,85). Similar increases in alpha activity during remissions following intensive immunosuppresive therapy have also been reported (103,104). These findings suggest that the positive effects of the Enermed on MS fatigue may be related to the ability of weak, predominantly alpha frequency EMFs to increase alpha production when the brain is challenged or stimulated.

MS is also characterized by hypoactivity in the prefrontal cortex. Relative to healthy controls, MS patients show reduced prefrontal glucose metabolism (105) and significantly increased theta power in the frontotemporal-central regions of the brain (106). Moreover, the level of hypoactivity is correlated with MS fatigue (105), cognitive impairment (106), and overall disability (104). Daily sessions of 10- or 20-Hz prefrontal stimulation have been shown to increase regional cerebral blood flow (rCBF) (107,108) in addition to exciting cortical neurons. Weak EMFs pulsed in the 10 to 20 Hz range could have similar excitatory effects on cortical arousal and thus alleviate MS fatigue by normalizing prefrontal hypoactivity.

In summary, the EMF literature indicates that both strong and weak EMFs can affect the state of arousal and electrophysiological response of the brain. Abnormal preactivation levels of cortical arousal are implicated in both migraine and MS, and suggest one mechanism through which appropriately pulsed EMFs may produce clinical benefits. Dysregulation of threshold levels and habituation is also characteristic of migraine, and it is possible that simply being exposed to repetitive stimuli in the form of pulsed EMFs could strengthen habituation processes. In MS, evoked potentials are characterized by reduced power in the alpha range of frequencies. Evidence that long-term exposure to the Enermed can increase alpha in certain conditions suggests that this may also be a route through which pulsed EMFs could produce clinical improvements.

With respect to treatment of any clinical condition, the pulsed EMF literature highlights the need to select those stimulation frequencies most likely to address the underlying dysfunction. Although mid- to high-frequency stimulation generally has excitatory effects and low-frequency stimulation typically has inhibitory effects, there are important exceptions, especially in diverse clinical populations. The TMS literature points to the importance of baseline levels of cortical arousal in selecting appropriate treatment frequencies, while photic stimulation and weak EMF studies suggest that dominant frequencies or the overall level of activity in a specific frequency band may be an important consideration. The positive effects of the Enermed therapy in migraine and MS may be related to the ability to program unique combinations of treatment frequencies for individual patients. Although it is not clear how the bioelectromagnetic profile used in the Enermed therapy is related to EEG parameters, the concept of basing treatment frequencies on relevant individual differences has solid empirical and theoretical support.

VIII. SUMMARY AND CONCLUSIONS

This review has attempted to draw parallels between the factors involved in the pathogenesis of migraine and MS and the observed neurochemical and electrophysiological effects of pulsed electromagnetic fields. Processes ranging from disturbances in critical neurotransmitter systems, dysregulation of the HPA axis, and abnormal cortical activation and inhibition patterns have all been implicated in the etiology and symptomatology of both migraine and MS fatigue. The research reviewed above suggests several possible mechanisms of action that might explain the clinical benefits we have observed with weak pulsed EMFs.

First, weak electromagnetic fields have been shown to affect dopamine and serotonin, both of which can have abnormal activity patterns in migraine and MS. Clinical improvement following exposure to weak pulsed EMFs might be mediated by effects on these and other relevant neurotransmitters. Second, there is strong evidence that the HPA axis is compromised in MS, and TMS research shows that pulsed EMFs can affect this system. The

HPA axis might be a pathway through which EMF therapies can alleviate MS symptoms like depression, fatigue, and cognitive impairments. Finally, both migraine and MS are characterized by abnormal resting EEGs and unusual electrophysiological responses to stimulation. There is a good deal of evidence that even short-term exposure to pulsed electromagnetic fields can influence such responses, and long-term exposure to the weak, mid-range frequency fields emitted by the Enermed has been shown to produce clinically relevant changes in alpha brain wave activity.

Although much additional research will be required before we fully understand the mechanisms of action of pulsed EMFs, the clinical possibilities suggested by the research conducted to date are exciting. As the neurochemical and electrophysiological effects of pulsed EMFs in specific patient populations are explored, we will acquire the information and insights needed to optimize treatment parameters and maximize the clinical potential of bioelectromagnetics. At the same time, bioelectromagnetic research will continue to deepen our understanding of the human body as an intricately organized electromagnetic system that both sends and responds to subtle energy signals.

REFERENCES

1. Bassett CA. Therapeutic uses of electric and magnetic fields in orthopedics. In: Carpenter DO, Ayrapetyan S, eds. Biological Effects of Electric and Magnetic Fields: Beneficial and Harmful Effects. New York: Academic P, 1994:14–48.
2. Markoll R. Pulsed signal therapy: a practical guide for clinicians. In: Weiner R, ed. Pain Management: A Practical Guide for Clinicians. Boca Raton: CRC Press, 2001:715–728.
3. Bickford RG, Guidi M, Fortesque P, Swenson MR. Magnetic stimulation of human peripheral nerve and brain: response enhancement by combined magnetoelectrical technique. Neurosurgery 1987; 20:110.
4. Shealy CN, Cady RK, Wilkie RG, Cox RH, Liss S, Closson W. Depression: a diagnostic neurochemical profile and therapy with cranial electric stimulation (CES). J Neurol Orthoped Med Surg 1989; 10:319–321.
5. Pascual-Leone A, Rubio B, Pallardo F, Catala MD. Rapid-rate transcranial magnetic stimulation of left dorsolateral prefrontal cortex in drug-resistant depression. Lancet 1996; 348:233–237.
6. Rush AJ, George MS, Sackeim HA, Marangell LB, Husain MM, Giller C, Nahas Z, Haines S, Simpson RK Jr, Goodman R. Vagus nerve stimulation (VNS) for treatment-resistant depressions: a multicenter study. Biol Psychiatry 2000; 47:276–286.
7. Lozano A. Deep brain stimulation: challenges to integrating stimulation technology with human neurobiology, neuroplasticity, and neural repair. J Rehabil Res Dev 2001; 38:x–xix.
8. Goodman R, Henderson AS. Effects of electric and magnetic fields on transcription. In: Carpenter DO, Ayrapetyan S, eds. Biological Effects of Electric and Magnetic Fields: Beneficial and Harmful Effects. New York: Academic, 1994:157–176.
9. Fierro B, Piazza A, Brighina F, La Bua V, Buffa D, Oliveri M. Modulation of intracortical inhibition induced by low- and high-frequency repetitive transcranial magnetic stimulation. Exp Brain Res 2001; 138:452–457.
10. Modugno N, Nakamura Y, MacKinnon CD, Filipovic SR, Bestmann S, Berardelli A, Rothwell JC. Motor cortex excitability following short trains of repetitive magnetic stimuli. Exp Brain Res 2001; 140:453–459.
11. Bassett CA. Beneficial effects of electromagnetic fields. J Cell Biochem 1993; 51:387–393.
12. Adey WR. Biological effects of electromagnetic fields. J Cell Biochem 1993; 51:410–416.
13. Ferrari MD. The economic burden of migraine to society. Pharmacoeconomics 1998; 13:667–676.
14. Stewart WF, Lipton RB, Celentano DD. Prevalence of migraine headache in the United

States: Relation to age, income, race and other sociodemographic factors. JAMA 1992; 267:64–69.

15. Ferrari MD. Migraine. Lancet 1998; 351:1043–1051.

16. Young S, Davey R. Pilot study concerning the effects of extremely low frequency electromagnetic energy on migraine. Int J Alt Complement Med, October 1993.

17. Lappin MS. Research on the Utility of the Medigen Device as a Treatment for Migraines. Vancouver, BC: Energy Medicine Developments, 1995.

18. Benedetto C, Allais G, Ciochetto D, De Lorenzo C. Pathophysiological aspects of menstrual migraine. Cephalalgia 1997; 17(suppl 20):32–34.

19. Sherman RA, Robson L, Marden LA. Initial exploration of pulsing electromagnetic fields for treatment of migraine. Headache 1998; 38:208–213.

20. Sherman RA, Acosta NM, Robson L. Treatment of migraine with pulsing electromagnetic fields: a double-blind, placebo controlled study. Headache 1999; 39:567–575.

21. Baumann RJ. Behavioral treatment of migraine in children and adolescents. Paediatr Drugs 2002; 4:555–561.

22. Reid GJ, McGrath PJ. Psychological treatments for migraine. Biomed Pharmacother 1996; 50:58–63.

23. Goodin DS. Survey of multiple sclerosis in northern California. Northern California MS Study Group. Multiple Sclerosis 1999; 5:78–88.

24. Branas P, Jordan R, Fry-Smith A, Burls A, Hyde C. Treatments for fatigue in multiple sclerosis: a rapid and systematic review. Health Technol Assess, 2000, 4.

25. Comi G, Leocani L, Rossi P, Colombo B. Physiopathology and treatment of fatigue in multiple sclerosis. J Neurol 2001; 248:174–179.

26. Richards TL, Lappin MS, Acosta-Urquidi J, Kraft GH, Heidi BS, Lawrie FW, Merrill BS, Melton GB, Cunningham CA. Double-blind study of pulsing magnetic field effects on multiple sclerosis. J Alt Complement Med 1997; 3:21–29.

27. Schwartz CE, Vollmer T, Lee H. Reliability and validity of two self-report measures of impairment and disability for MS North American Research Consortium on Multiple Sclerosis Outcomes Study Group. Neurology 1999; 52:63–70.

28. Lappin M, Richards T, Lawrie F, Kramer E. Effects of a pulsed electromagnetic therapy on multiple sclerosis fatigue and quality of life: A double-blind, placebo controlled crossover trial. Altern Ther Health Med 2003; 9:38–48.

29. Rivto PG, Fischer JS, Miller DM, Andrews H, Paty DW, LaRocca NG. Multiple Sclerosis Quality of Life Inventory: A User's Manual. New York: National Multiple Sclerosis Society, 1997.

30. Lappin MS. Enermed Patient Survey Results. Vancouver, BC: Energy Medicine Developments, 1998.

31. Guseo A. Pulsing electromagnetic field therapy of multiple sclerosis by the Gyuling-Bordacs device: Double-blind, crossover and open studies. J Bioelectricity 1987; 6:23–35.

32. Kurtzke JF. Rating neurologic impairment in multiple sclerosis: An expanded disability status scale (EDSS). Neurology 1983; 33:1444–1452.

33. Sandyk R. Therapeutic effects of alternating current pulsed electromagnetic fields in multiple sclerosis. J Altern Complement Med 1997; 3:365–386.

34. Kavaliers M, Ossenkopp KP. Magnetic field inhibition of morphine-induced analgesia and behavioral activity in mice: evidence for involvement of calcium ions. Brain Res 1986; 379:30–38.

35. Kavaliers M, Ossenkopp KP. Magnetic fields differentially inhibit mu, delta, kappa and sigma opiate-induced analgesia in mice. Peptides 1986; 7:449–453.

36. Levine RL, Dooley JK, Bluni TD. Magnetic field effects on spatial discrimination and melatonin levels in mice. Physiol Behav 1995; 58:535.

37. Reiter RJ. Electromagnetic fields and melatonin production. Biomed Pharmacotherapy 1993; 47:439–444.

38. Reiter RJ. Static and extremely low frequency electromagnetic field exposure: reported effects on the circadian production of melatonin. J Cell Biochem 1993; 51:394.

39. Chance WT, Grossman CJ, Newrock R, Bovin G, Yerian S, Schmitt G, Mendenhall C. Effects
     of electromagnetic fields and gender on neurotransmitters and amino acids in rats. Physiol
     Behav 1995; 58:743–748.

40. Massot O, Grimaldi B, Bailly JM, Kochanek M, Deschamps F, Lambrozo J, Fillion G.
     Magnetic field desensitizes 5-HT(1B) receptor in brain: pharmacological and functional studies.
     Brain Res 2000; 858:143–150.

41. Seegal RF, Wolpaw JR, Dowman R. Chronic exposure of primates to 60-Hz electric and
     magnetic fields: II. Neurochemical effects. Bioelectromagnetics 1989; 10:289–301.

42. Ben-Shachar D, Belmaker RH, Grisaru N, Klein E. Transcranial magnetic stimulation induces
     alterations in brain monoamines. J Neural Transm 1997; 104:191–197.

43. Ben-Shachar D, Gazawi H, Riboyad-Levin J, Klein E. Chronic repetitive transcranial magnetic
     stimulation alters beta-adrenergic and 5-HT2 receptor characteristics in rat brain. Brain Res
     1999; 816:78–83.

44. Keck ME, Sillaber I, Ebner K, Welt T, Toschi N, Kaehler ST, Singewald N, Philippu A, Elbel
     GK, Wotjak CT, Holsboer F, Landgraf R, Engelmann M. Acute transcranial magnetic
     stimulation of frontal brain regions selectively modulates the release of vasopressin, biogenic
     amines and amino acids in the rat brain. Eur J Neurosci 2000; 12:3713–3720.

45. Strafella AP, Paus T, Barrett J, Dagher A. Repetitive transcranial magnetic stimulation of the
     human prefrontal cortex induces dopamine release in the caudate nucleus. J Neurosci 2001;
     21:RC157.

46. Diamond S, Wenzel R. Practical approaches to migraine management. CNS Drugs 2002;
     16:385–403.

47. Chugani DC, Niimura K, Chaturvedi S, Muzik O, Fakhouri M, Lee ML, Chugani HT.
     Increased brain serotonin synthesis in migraine. Neurology 1999; 53:1473.

48. Del Zompo M. Dopaminergic hypersensitivity in migraine: clinical and genetic evidence.
     Funct Neurol 2000; 15:163–170.

49. Fanciullacci M, Alessandri M, Del Rosso A. Dopamine involvement in the migraine attack.
     Funct Neurol 2000; 15:171–181.

50. Nappi G, Costa A, Tassorelli C, Santorelli FM. Migraine as a complex disease: heterogeneity,
     comorbidity and genotype-phenotype interactions. Funct Neurol 2000; 15:87–93.

51. Ophoff RA, van den Maagdenberg AM, Roon KI, Ferrari MD, Frants RR. The impact of
     pharmacogenetics for migraine. Eur J Pharmacol 2001; 413:1–10.

52. Peroutka SJ. Dopamine and migraine. Neurology 1997; 49:650–656.

53. Lai M, Loi V, Pisano MR, Del Zompo M. Therapy of migraine by modulating dopamine
     hypersensitivity: its effect on mood and pain. Int J Clin Pharmacol Res 1997; 17:101–103.

54. Brun J, Claustrat B, Saddier P, Chazot G. Nocturnal melatonin excretion is decreased in
     patients with migraine without aura attacks associated with menses. Cephalalgia 1995; 15:136–
     139.

55. Claustrat B, Loisy C, Brun J, Beorchia S, Arnaud JL, Chazot G. Nocturnal plasma melatonin
     levels in migraine: a preliminary report. Headache 1989; 29:241–244.

56. Breslau N, Schultz LR, Stewart WF, Lipton RB, Lucia VC, Welch KM. Headache and major
     depression: is the association specific to migraine? Neurology 2000; 54:308–313.

57. Silberstein SD, Lipton RB, Breslau N. Migraine: association with personality characteristics
     and psychopathology. Cephalalgia 1995; 15:337–369.

58. Othmer S, Othmer SF, Kaiser DA. EEG Biofeedback: An Emerging Model for its Global
     Efficacy. In: Evans J, Abarbanel A, eds. Introduction to Quantitative EEG and Neurofeed-
     back. New York: Academic P, 1999.

59. Keck ME, Engelmann M, Muller MB, Henniger MS, Hermann B, Rupprecht R, Neumann ID,
     Toschi N, Landgraf R, Post A. Repetitive transcranial magnetic stimulation induces active
     coping strategies and attenuates the neuroendocrine stress response in rats. J Psychiatr Res
     2000; 34:265–276.

60. Keck ME, Welt T, Post A, Muller MB, Toschi N, Wigger A, Landgraf R, Holsboer F,
     Engelmann M. Neuroendocrine and behavioral effects of repetitive transcranial magnetic

stimulation in a psychopathological animal model are suggestive of antidepressant-like effects. Neuropsychopharmacology 2001; 24:337–349.

61. Evers S, Hengst K, Pecuch PW. The impact of repetitive transcranial magnetic stimulation on pituitary hormone levels and cortisol in healthy subjects. J Affect Disord 2001; 66:83–88.

62. George MS, Wassermann EM, Williams WA, Steppel J, Pascual-Leone A, Basser P, Hallett M, Post RM. Changes in mood and hormone levels after rapid-rate transcranial magnetic stimulation (rTMS) of the prefrontal cortex. J Neuropsych Clin Neurosci 1996; 8:172–180.

63. Grasser A, Moller A, Backmund H, Yassouridis A, Holsboer F. Heterogeneity of hypothalamic-pituitary-adrenal system response to a combined dexamethasone-CRH test in multiple sclerosis. Exp Clin Endocrinol Diabetes 1996; 104:31–37.

64. Kumpfel T, Then Bergh F, Friess E, Uhr M, Yassouridis A, Trenkwalder C, Holsboer F. Dehydroepiandrosterone response to the adrenocorticotropin test and the combined dexamethasone and corticotropin-releasing hormone test in patients with multiple sclerosis. Neuroendocrinology 1999; 70:431–438.

65. Fassbender K, Schmidt R, Mossner R, Kischka U, Kuhnen J, Schwartz A, Hennerici M. Mood disorders and dysfunction of the hypothalamic-pituitary-adrenal axis in multiple sclerosis: association with cerebral inflammation. Arch Neurol 1998; 55:66–72.

66. Heesen C, Gold SM, Raji A, Wiedemann K, Schulz KH. Cognitive impairment correlates with hypothalamo-pituitary-adrenal axis dysregulation in multiple sclerosis. Psychoneuroendocrinology 2002; 27:505–517.

67. Then Bergh F, Kumpfel T, Trenkwalder C, Rupprecht R, Holsboer F. Dysregulation of the hypothalamo-pituitary-adrenal axis is related to the clinical course of MS. Neurology 1999; 53:772–777.

68. Peres MF, Sanchez del Rio M, Seabra ML, Tufik S, Abucham J, Cipolla-Neto J, Silberstein SD, Zukerman E. Hypothalamic involvement in chronic migraine. J Neurol Neurosurg Psychiatry 2001; 71:747–751.

69. Fitzgerald PB, Brown TL, Daskalakis ZJ, Chen R, Kulkarni J. Intensity-dependent effects of 1 Hz rTMS on human corticospinal excitability. Clin Neurophysiol 2002; 113:1136–1141.

70. Muellbacher W, Ziemann U, Boroojerdi B, Hallett M. Effects of low-frequency transcranial magnetic stimulation on motor excitability and basic motor behavior. Clin Neurophysiol 2000; 111:1002–1007.

71. Romero JR, Anschel D, Sparing R, Gangitano M, Pascual-Leone A. Subthreshold low frequency repetitive transcranial magnetic stimulation selectively decreases facilitation in the motor cortex. Clin Neurophysiol 2002; 113:101–107.

72. Gangitano M, Valero-Cabre A, Tormos JM, Mottaghy FM, Romero JR, Pascual-Leone A. Modulation of input-output curves by low and high frequency repetitive transcranial magnetic stimulation of the motor cortex. Clin Neurophysiol 2002; 113:1249–1257.

73. Maeda F, Gangitano M, Thall M, Pascual-Leone A. Inter- and intra-individual variability of paired-pulse curves with transcranial magnetic stimulation (TMS). Clin Neurophysiol 2002; 113:376–382.

74. Bohotin V, Fumal A, Vandenheede M, Gerard P, Bohotin C, Maertens De Noordhout A, Schoenen J. Effects of repetitive transcranial magnetic stimulation on visual evoked potentials in migraine. Brain 2002; 125:912–922.

75. Brighina F, Piazza A, Daniele O, Fierro B. Modulation of visual cortical excitability in migraine with aura: effects of 1 Hz repetitive transcranial magnetic stimulation. Exp Brain Res 2002; 145:177–181.

76. Samii A, Wassermann EM, Ikoma K, Mercuri B, George MS, O'Fallon A, Dale JK, Straus SE, Hallett M. Decreased postexercise facilitation of motor evoked potentials in patients with chronic fatigue syndrome or depression. Neurology 1996; 47:1410–1414.

77. Shajahan PM, Glabus MF, Gooding PA, Shah PJ, Ebmeier KP. Reduced cortical excitability in depression. Impaired post-exercise motor facilitation with transcranial magnetic stimulation. Br J Psychiatry 1999; 174:449–454.

78. Speer AM, Kimbrell TA, Wassermann EM, J DR, Willis MW, Herscovitch P, Post RM.

Opposite effects of high and low frequency rTMS on regional brain activity in depressed patients. Biol Psychiatry 2000; 48:1133–1141.

79. Bell GB, Marino AA, Chesson AL. Frequency-specific responses in the human brain caused by electromagnetic fields. J Neurol Sci 1994; 123:26–32.

80. Bell GB, Marino AA, Chesson AL. Frequency-specific blocking in the human brain caused by electromagnetic fields. Neuroreport 1994; 5:510–512.

81. Heusser K, Tellschaft D, Thoss F. Influence of an alternating 3 Hz magnetic field with an induction of 0.1 millitesla on chosen parameters of the human occipital EEG. Neurosci Lett 1997; 239:57–60.

82. Bell G, Marino A, Chesson A, Struve F. Electrical states in the rabbit brain can be altered by light and electromagnetic fields. Brain Res 1992; 570:307–315.

83. Pigeau RA, Frame AM. Steady-state visual evoked responses in high and low alpha subjects. Electroencephalogr Clin Neurophysiol 1992; 84:101–109.

84. Rosenfeld J, Rienhart A, Srivastava S. The effects of alpha (10 Hz) and beta (22 Hz) "entrainment" stimulation on the alpha and beta EEG bands: individual differences are critical to prediction of effects. Appl Psychophysiol Biofeedback 1997; 22:3–20.

85. Richards T, Acosta-Urquidi J. Pulsing magnetic field effects on brain electrical activity in multiple sclerosis. Biologic Effects of Light Conference. Basel, Switzerland. Boston: Kluwer Academic Publishers, 1998:337–342.

86. Gerber WD, Schoenen J. Biobehavioral correlates in migraine: the role of hypersensitivity and information-processing dysfunction. Cephalalgia 1998; 18(suppl 21):5–11.

87. Afra J, Cecchini AP, De Pasqua V, Albert A, Schoenen J. Visual evoked potentials during long periods of pattern-reversal stimulation in migraine. Brain 1998; 121:233–241.

88. Afra J, Proietti Cecchini A, Sandor PS, Schoenen J. Comparison of visual and auditory evoked cortical potentials in migraine patients between attacks. Clin Neurophysiol 2000; 111:1124–1129.

89. Schoenen J. Deficient habituation of evoked cortical potentials in migraine: a link between brain biology, behavior and trigeminomuvascular activation? Biomed Pharmacother 1996; 50:71–78.

90. Ambrosini A, De Pasqua V, Afra J, Sandor PS, Schoenen J. Reduced gating of middle-latency auditory evoked potentials (P50) in migraine patients: another indication of abnormal sensory processing? Neurosci Lett 2001; 306:132–134.

91. Wang W, Timsit-Berthier M, Schoenen J. Intensity dependence of auditory evoked potentials is pronounced in migraine: an indication of cortical potentiation and low serotonergic neurotransmission? Neurology 1996; 46:1404–1409.

92. Wang W, Schoenen J. Interictal potentiation of passive "oddball" auditory event-related potentials in migraine. Cephalalgia 1998; 18:261–265. discussion 241.

93. Kropp P, Gerber WD. Is increased amplitude of contingent negative variation in migraine due to cortical hyperactivity or to reduced habituation? Cephalalgia 1993; 13:37–41.

94. Siniatchkin M, Gerber WD, Kropp P, Voznesenskaya T, Vein AM. Are the periodic changes of neurophysiological parameters during the pain-free interval in migraine related to abnormal orienting activity? Cephalalgia 2000; 20:20–29.

95. Siniatchkin M, Kirsch E, Kropp P, Stephani U, Gerber WD. Slow cortical potentials in migraine families. Cephalalgia 2000; 20:881–892.

96. Siniatchkin M, Hierundar A, Kropp P, Gerber WD, Stephani U. Self-regulation of slow cortical potentials in children with migraine: an exploratory study. Applied Psychophysiology and Biofeedback 2000; 25:13–32.

97. Judit A, Sandor PS, Schoenen J. Habituation of visual and intensity dependence of auditory evoked cortical potentials tends to normalize just before and during the migraine attack. Cephalalgia 2000; 20:714–719.

98. Kropp P, Gerber WD. Contingent negative variation during migraine attack and interval: evidence for normalization of slow cortical potentials during the attack. Cephalalgia 1995; 15:123–128. discussion 178–129.

99. Kropp P. Prediction of migraine attacks. Cephalalgia 1999; 19:477.

100. Siniatchkin M, Kropp P, Gerber WD, Stephani U. Migraine in childhood—are periodically occurring migraine attacks related to dynamic changes of cortical information processing? Neurosci Lett 2000; 279:1–4.

101. Basar-Eroglu C, Warecka K, Schurmann M, Basar E. Visual evoked potentials in multiple sclerosis: frequency response shows reduced alpha amplitude. Int J Neurosci 1993; 73:235–258.

102. Schurmann M, Warecka K, Basar-Eroglu C, Basar E. Auditory evoked potentials in multiple sclerosis: alpha responses are reduced in amplitude, but theta responses are not altered. Int J Neurosci 1993; 73:259–276.

103. Brau H, Ulrich G. Electroencephalographic vigilance dynamics in multiple sclerosis during an acute episode and after remission. Eur Arch Psychiatry Neurol Sci 1990; 239:320–324.

104. Colon E, Hommes OR, de Weerd JP. Relation between EEG and disability scores in multiple sclerosis. Clin Neurol Neurosurg 1981; 83:163–168.

105. Roelcke U, Kappos L, Lechner-Scott J, Brunnschweiler H, Huber S, Ammann W, Plohmann A, Della S, Maguire RP, Missimer J, Radu EW, Steck A, Leemders KL. Reduced glucose metabolism in the frontal cortex and basal ganglia of multiple sclerosis patients with fatigue: a 18F-fluorodeoxyglucose positron emission tomography study. Neurology 1997; 48:1566–1571.

106. Leocani L, Locatelli T, Martinelli V, Rovaris M, Falautano M, Filippi M, Magnani G, Comi G. Electroencephalographic coherence analysis in multiple sclerosis: correlation with clinical, neuropsychological, and MRI findings. J Neurol Neurosurg Psychiatry 2000; 69:192–198.

107. Conca A, Peschina W, Konig P, Fritzsche H, Hausmann A. Effect of chronic repetitive transcranial magnetic stimulation on regional cerebral blood flow and regional cerebral glucose uptake in drug treatment-resistant depressives. A brief report. Neuropsychobiology 2002; 45:27–31.

108. Mottaghy F, Keller C, Gangitano M, Ly J, Thall M, Parker J, Pascual-Leone A. Correlation of cerebral blood flow and treatment effects of repetitive transcranial magnetic stimulation in depressed patients. Psychiatry Res 2002; 115:1.

19

Repetitive Transcranial Magnetic Stimulation (rTMS) for Depression and Other Indications

**Mark S. George*, Ziad Nahas, F. Andrew Kozel*,
Xingbao Li, Kaori Yamanaka, Alexander Mishory,
Sarah Hill, and Daryl E. Bohning**

*The Brain Stimulation Laboratory (BSL), Psychiatry Department,
and the Center for Advanced Imaging Research (CAIR),
Medical University of South Carolina (MUSC), Charleston, South Carolina, U.S.A.*

Repetitive transcranial magnetic stimulation (rTMS) differs from other cranio-electrical stimulation techniques in that it constantly converts electrical fields into electromagnetic fields and vice versa to stimulate a specific area of the brain known to be involved in depression. The evolution of rTMS, its possible mechanism of action, and studies demonstrating its efficacy and safety in treating depression are reviewed, and possible applications for other mental and neurologic disorders are discussed.

I. INTRODUCTION

Transcranial Magnetic Stimulation (TMS) can noninvasively and relatively painlessly focally stimulate the brain of awake individuals (1). When TMS pulses are delivered in a periodic repeating pattern, it is referred to as repetitive TMS (rTMS). rTMS is sometimes modified by the adjectives *fast*, to describe stimulation frequencies greater than 1 Hz, or *slow*, frequencies of 1 Hz or less (2). Fast rTMS is currently limited to very brief runs with frequencies of 25–30 Hz. Stimulation frequencies faster than this have an increased seizure risk, and most modern capacitors cannot keep delivering the needed energy before depleting (3).

---

*George and Kozel also work at the Ralph H. Johnson VA Medical Center, Charleston.

TMS is able to focally and painlessly stimulate the cortex by creating a time-varying magnetic field generated by the brief but powerful electrical currents passed through the coil (4). This localized pulsed magnetic field over the surface of the head depolarizes underlying superficial neurons (5,6), which then induces electrical currents in the brain (7). High-intensity current is rapidly turned on and off in the electromagnetic coil through the discharge of capacitors. The end result of TMS is thus electrical stimulation of the brain, and some refer to TMS as *electrodeless electrical stimulation* (see Fig. 1). The magnetic fields produced by TMS are thus the trick to get energy across the skull. Figure 1 shows how the electrical energy stored in a capacitor discharges and creates about 3000 A. Through Maxwell's equations and Faraday's law, this creates a powerful magnetic field, on the order of 2 T. This rapidly changing magnetic field (~ 30 kT/s) then travels across the scalp and skull and induces an electric field within the brain (~ 30 V/m). This induces current to flow in the brain by creating a transmembrane potential (for a thorough discussion see Ref. 8).

TMS, which produces powerful but brief magnetic fields that in turn induce electrical currents in the brain, therefore differs from most of the techniques discussed elsewhere in this book where direct electrical or magnetic energy is applied to the brain or body (9). TMS also radically differs from the currently popular use of low-level static magnetic fields as alternative therapies. The chapters in the rest of this book describe how constant exposure to static magnetic fields can have biological effects. However, TMS does not produce magnetic fields for very long (microseconds), and they are relatively weak except directly under the TMS coil. Most TMS researchers assume that TMS produces its behavioral effects solely through the production of electrical currents in the cortex of the brain. However, this assumption has not been proved. Although direct transcutaneous applications of electricity can influence brain function, this is extremely painful (10). Moreover, as the skull acts as a large resistor, it is difficult to focus the electricity to specific brain regions.

The magnetic field induced by TMS declines rapidly with distance away from the coil. Thus, with current technology, TMS coils are only able to directly electrically stimulate the superficial cortex, and are not able to produce direct electrical stimulation deep in the brain (8). Although this limited depth of penetration is a limitation of present technology, deeper brain structures can be influenced by cortical TMS, due to the cortex's massive interconnections, and redundant cortical-subcortical loops (11) (see Fig. 2). Moreover, there are several groups working on novel TMS coil designs that might be able to reach deeper into the brain without overwhelming superficial cortical structures. The studies combining TMS with functional imaging (PET, SPECT, fMRI), have now convincingly shown that TMS applied to the cortex can activate cortical-limbic loops. Whether secondarily transmitted TMS signals are involved in therapeutic mechanisms of action remains unclear.

The amount of electricity needed to cause changes in the cortex varies from person to person and also from one brain region to the next (12). One commonly used method for standardizing and adjusting the amount of electricity delivered and induced by TMS across different individuals is to determine each person's motor threshold (MT). The MT is commonly defined as the minimum amount of electricity needed to produce movement in the contralateral thumb, when the coil is placed optimally over the primary motor cortex. MT can be determined either by using EMG recordings (13) or, with less precision, by using visible movement (14).

TMS was originally used over the prefrontal cortex to treat depression because of the potential for activating cortical-limbic loops. Imaging studies such as in Fig. 2 show that this assumption was likely correct and that the prefrontal cortex is a window to stimulating subcortical and limbic sites. Future work is needed to determine the optimum cortical sites

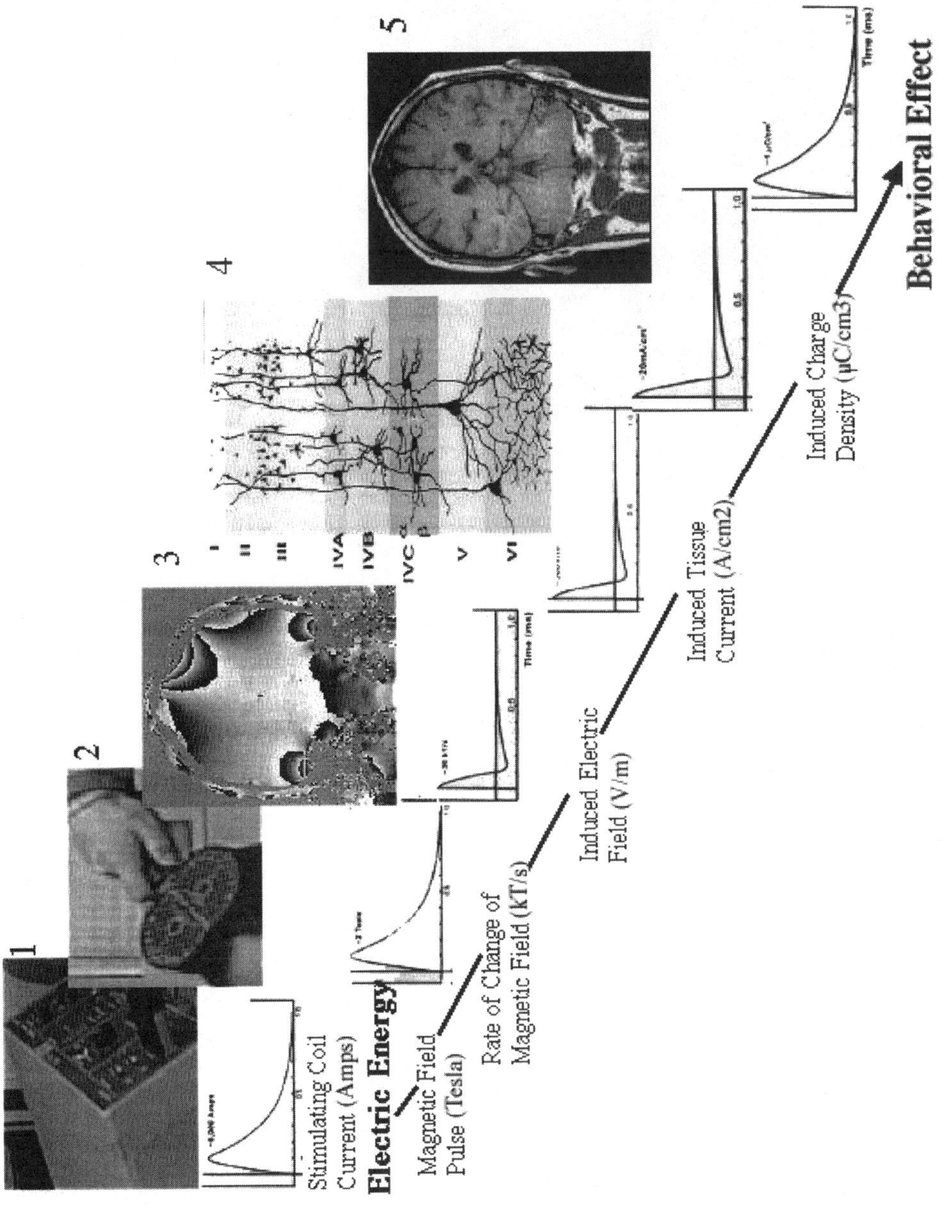

Figure 1   The cascade of events that occur following a TMS pulse. (Modified from George and Belmaker, 2000.)

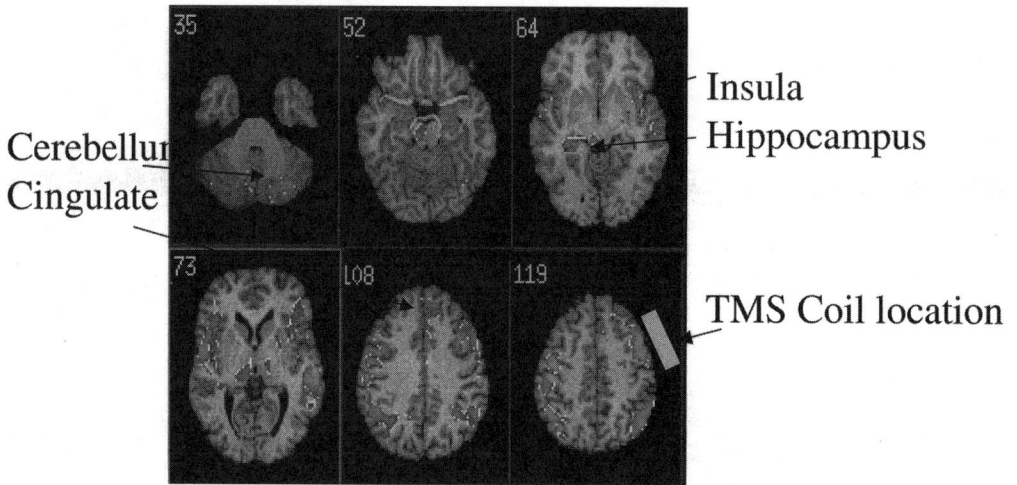

Figure 2 fMRI Demonstrates the Secondary Brain Effects of Prefrontal TMS. Shown in color are the brain regions that are significantly activated compared to rest ($p < 0.01$, extent $p < 0.05$) in six adults with clinical depression during left prefrontal TMS at 1 Hz and 110% MT for 20 s. The differences are projected on a common brain (Talairach). The arrow depicts the TMS coil position, which follows the algorithm developed in 1994 for probabilistically finding the prefrontal cortex based on relative distance from the motor cortex. (From work in progress, MUSC Brain Stimulation Laboratory and Center for Advanced Imaging Research, Dr. Li).

for maximal clinical effectiveness, and whether there are general rules for finding this across individuals or should be individually guided based on structural or functional imaging.

II. TMS MECHANISMS OF ACTION

TMS' mechanisms of action can be grouped according to the time course of their effects: immediate (seconds), intermediate (minutes), and long term (days). TMS has been shown to produce *immediate effects (within seconds)*, such as the movement of the thumb, or direct inhibition of another TMS pulse followed shortly in time. These immediate effects are thought to result from direct excitation of inhibitory or excitatory neurons. There is some evidence to suggest that TMS at different intensities, frequencies, and coil angles excites different elements (cell bodies, axons) of different neuronal groups (interneurons, neurons projecting to other parts of the cortex, U fibers) (3,15,16). This is further complicated by the complex six-layer arrangement of human neocortex, along with the varying gyral folds, which place some aspects of the brain very close to the surface, and others far away in sulcal folds.

A quick jerky movement or a flash of light are about the only easily observable short-term effects that have been produced with TMS. This is somewhat disappointing given the rich literature of complex smells, sounds, and memories produced in epilepsy patients with direct electrical stimulation (17). Why does TMS not produce the same immediate behavioral effects as does direct electrical stimulation? A full discussion of this most interesting question is beyond this chapter (see Ref. 18). An important method for studying immediate TMS effects is through a process called *paired-pulse TMS* (ppTMS). This technique involves delivering two TMS pulses to the same region with varying interpulse intervals (usually milliseconds long) and intensities (13). Depending on the relative strength of the first pulse to the second, and the interpulse interval, the first pulse can either inhibit or enhance the second pulse. Paired pulse TMS (ppTMS) over the motor area can be used to assess natural brain inhibitory and excitatory systems, both at rest in individuals with different disorders (19) and following the administration of different centrally active compounds or other treatments (20). Because it uses a motor evoked potential (MEP) as the endpoint variable, paired-pulse TMS can only make statements about the motor cortex. In an exciting new development, Dr. Daryl Bohning at MUSC has recently demonstrated the feasibility of doing paired-pulse TMS within an MRI scanner, using blood flow as the endpoint (21). This would then allow one to do ppTMS over any brain region, to determine if there might be focal abnormalities in brain inhibition or excitation.

One of the most easily demonstrated immediate effects of TMS is *speech arrest*, where high frequency TMS, placed precisely over the Broca's area, can immediately and transiently block fluent speech (22). TMS, used in studies like this, can produce what are sometimes referred to as *virtual lesions*. Importantly, none of these temporary lesion effects have been demonstrated to persist beyond the time of active TMS administration. Thus, the lesions are truly virtual and temporary. It is unclear what is happening at a neurobiologic level during speech arrest. It is likely that the TMS pulses are interfering with normal brain function, prohibiting that brain region from participating in coordinated circuit behavior. Early theories that the region was 'jammed' are not likely true, as speech arrest can be achieved with frequencies as low as 4 Hz. Recent modeling and experimental work with deep brain stimulation (DBS) has shown that even at frequencies of >100Hz, information is still flowing through a stimulated region (23), albeit of a highly regular and nonphysiologic nature.

The *intermediate effects of TMS* (seconds to several minutes) likely arise from transient changes in local pharmacology, such as GABA or glutamate. Much attention has been focused on whether and to what degree different frequencies of TMS might have divergent intermediate-term biological effects. For example, repeated stimulation of a single neuron at low frequency in culture produces long-lasting inhibition of cell-cell communications (called *long-term depression*, or LTD) (24,25). Conversely, repeated high-frequency stimulation can improve cell-cell communication (called *long-term potentiation*, or LTP) (26). Scientists have wondered whether TMS, exciting hundreds or thousands of neurons in a pulse, can produce sustained inhibitory or excitatory effects in a way analogous to single cell electrical stimulation (27). Supporting this concept, several studies have now shown that chronic low-frequency stimulation of the motor cortex can produce inhibitory *intermediate term effects* (lasting for several minutes) following stimulation (28). There is also some evidence that high frequency stimulation can produce intermediate term excitatory effects (29). However, more work is needed in this important area.

Many investigators have used TMS to influence brain functions at this immediate or intermediate time domain to explore how the brain works. These studies have investigated movement (30), visual perception (31), memory (32), attention, speech (33), and mood (34). A full review is beyond the scope of this chapter (see Refs. 35 and 36).

Longer-term effects of TMS are those that occur over days to weeks. The antidepressant effects of TMS fit under this category. Less is known about the neurobiologic mechanisms involved in this class of effects, although new studies are being published monthly. As discussed below, TMS causes changes in cortical-limbic loops, and function in these circuits is changing over time. There is also some evidence that TMS might have long-term anticonvulsant effects.

A. Animal Models

Numerous animal studies have been important in trying to understand the modes of action of TMS. TMS studies with intracranial electrodes in rhesus monkeys have provided information about the nature and spatial extent of the rTMS-induced electric field (37). Corticospinal tract development, aspects of motor control, and medication effects on corticospinal excitability have been studied fairly extensively in nonhuman primates using single-pulse TMS (38–44). Such work has yielded information about TMS neurophysiological effects, such as the observation that TMS evoked motor responses result from direct excitation of corticospinal neurons at or close to the axon hillock (44).

Rodent rTMS studies have reported antidepressant-like behavioral and neurochemical effects. In particular, rTMS enhances apomorphine-induced stereotypy and reduces immobility in the Porsolt swim test (45). rTMS has been reported to induce electroconvulsive-shock (ECS)-like changes in rodent brain monoamines, beta-adrenergic receptor binding, and immediate early gene induction (46). The effects of rTMS on seizure threshold are variable and may depend upon the parameters and chronicity of stimulation (47). Within the past year, Pope and Keck have completed a series of studies using more focal TMS in rat models (48). They have largely replicated earlier TMS animal studies using less focal coils. Even with the attempt at focal rat stimulation, the effects involve an entire hemisphere and cannot readily be extrapolated to what is happening in human TMS using focal coils (49). Several groups are now considering performing analogous TMS animal studies using a diffuse electrical stimulation, assuming that the induced electrical stimulation is actually what conveys the biological activity of TMS. However, creating electrodes that match the TMS field is a challenge and is subject to questions of comparative validity.

B. Combining TMS with Functional Imaging

A critically important area that will ultimately guide clinical parameters is to combine TMS with functional imaging to directly monitor TMS effects on the brain and to thus understand the varying effects of different TMS use parameters on brain function. Since it appears that TMS at different frequencies has divergent effects on brain activity, combining TMS with functional brain imaging will better delineate not only the behavioral neuropsychology of various psychiatric syndromes, but also some of the pathophysiologic circuits in the brain. In contrast to imaging studies with ECT which have found that ECT shuts off global and regional activity (50), most studies using serial scans in depressed patients undergoing TMS have found increased activity in the cingulate and other limbic regions (51,52). However, two studies have now found divergent effects of TMS on regional activity in depressed patients, determined both by the frequency of stimulation and the baseline state of the patient (53,54). That is, for patients with global or focal hypometabolism, high-frequency prefrontal stimulation has been found to increase brain activity over time, with the opposite happening as well. Conversely, patients with focal hyperactivity have been shown to have reduced activity over time following chronic daily low-frequency stimulation. However, these two small sample studies have numerous flaws. They simultaneously show the potential, and the complexity, surrounding the issue of how to use TMS to change activity in defined circuits. They also point out an obvious difference with ECT, where the net effect of the ECT seizure is to decrease prefrontal and global activity (50).

Several recent studies combining TMS with other neurophysiological and neuroimaging techniques have helped to elucidate how TMS achieves its effects. Our group at MUSC has pioneered and perfected the technique of interleaving TMS with blood-oxygen-level-dependent (BOLD) fMRI, allowing for direct imaging of TMS effects with high spatial (1–2 mm) and temporal (2–3 s) resolution (55–59). Another group in Germany has now succeeded in interleaving TMS and fMRI in this manner, partially replicating the earlier MUSC work (60). Work with this technology has shown that prefrontal TMS at 80% motor threshold (MT) produces much less local and remote blood flow changes than does 120% MT TMS (61). Strafella and Paus (2001) used PET to show that prefrontal cortex TMS causes dopamine release in the caudate nucleus (62) and has reciprocal activity with the anterior cingulate gyrus (63). Our group at MUSC (51), as well as in Scotland (52) and Australia (54), have all shown that lateral prefrontal TMS can cause changes in the anterior cingulate gyrus and other limbic regions in depressed patients. It is thus clear that TMS delivered over the prefrontal cortex has immediate effects in important subcortical limbic regions (see Fig. 2). The initial TMS effect on cortex and the secondary synaptic changes in other regions likely differs as a function of mood state, cortical excitability, and other factors that would change resting brain activity. Combining TMS with functional imaging will likely continue to be an important method for understanding TMS mechanisms of action. Combinational TMS–imaging will likely also evolve to be an important neuroscience tool for researching brain connectivity (64,65).

III. AN UPDATE ON THERAPEUTIC USES OF TMS

A. Depression

Although there is controversy, and much more work is needed, certain brain regions have consistently been implicated in the pathogenesis of depression and mood regulation (66–74). These include the medial and dorsolateral prefrontal cortex, the cingulate gyrus, and other regions commonly referred to as *limbic* (amygdala, hippocampus, parahippocampus, septum, hypothalamus, limbic thalamus, insula) and *paralimbic* (anterior temporal pole, orbitofrontal cortex). A widely held theory over the last decade has been that depression results from a dyregulation of prefrontal cortical and limbic regions (71,74–76).

The original uses of TMS as an antidepressant were not influenced by this regional neuroanatomic literature, and stimulation was applied over the vertex (77–79). However, working within the prefrontal cortical limbic dysregulation framework outlined above and realizing that theories of ECT action emphasize the role of prefrontal cortex effects (80), one of us (MSG) in 1995 performed the first open trial of prefrontal TMS as an antidepressant (81), followed immediately by a cross over double-blind study (82). The theory behind this work was that chronic, frequent, subconvulsive stimulation of the prefrontal cortex over several weeks might initiate a therapeutic cascade of events both in the prefrontal cortex as well as in connected limbic regions, thereby alleviating depression symptoms (83). The imaging evidence previously discussed now shows that this hunch was correct—prefrontal TMS sends direct information to important mood-regulating regions like the cingulate gyrus, orbitofrontal cortex, insula, and hippocampus (see Fig. 2). Thus, beginning with these prefrontal studies, modern TMS was specifically designed as a focal, nonconvulsive, circuit-based approach to therapy. TMS was conceived of and launched to bridge from functional neuroimaging advances in circuit knowledge to the bedside as a focal, noninvasive treatment.

Since the initial studies, there has been continued high interest in TMS as an antidepressant treatment. Multiple trials have been conducted from researchers around the world. In general, there is not a large industry sponsoring or promoting TMS as an antidepressant (or therapy for other disorders), and the funding for these trials has largely come from foundations and governments. The sample sizes in these antidepressant trials are thus small (in all, less than 100 per trial) compared to industry-sponsored pharmaceutical trials of antidepressants. A thorough review of all of these trials is beyond the scope of this update. However, the overwhelming majority of approximately 20 studies have found modest antidepressant effects that take several weeks to build. Not all TMS antidepressant treatment studies have been positive (84).

B. Meta-Analyses of TMS Antidepressant Effect

One way of understanding the state of the art of TMS as an antidepressant is to perform meta-analyses on the published trials. There have now been five independent meta-analyses of the published or public TMS antidepressant literature, each differing in the articles included and the statistics used (85–89). Their results are the same—daily prefrontal TMS delivered over several weeks has antidepressant effects greater than sham treatment. For example, Burt and colleagues examined 23 published comparisons for controlled TMS prefrontal antidepressant trials and found that TMS had a combined effect size of 0.67, indicating a moderate to large antidepressant effect (87). A subanalysis was done on those studies directly comparing TMS to ECT. The effect size for TMS in these studies was greater than in the studies comparing TMS to sham, perhaps reflecting subject selection bias. The authors suggested that perhaps TMS works best in patients who are also clinical candidates for ECT. The meta-analysis conducted by Kozel and George (86) was confined to published double-blind studies with individual data using TMS over the left prefrontal cortex. The summary analysis using all 10 studies that met criteria revealed a cumulative effect size of 0.53 (Cohen's D) (0.31 to 0.97) with the total number of subjects studied being 230. A funnel plot technique assesses whether there is a publication bias in the literature to date and whether this bias might affect the results of the meta-analysis. (This technique assumes that with small sample studies, there is a large chance of both erroneous positive and negative results. As the sample size of studies increases, the effect sizes should begin to converge, resembling a funnel.) The funnel plot indicated that a publication bias is likely and that there are more positive small sample studies in the TMS antidepressant literature than should occur by chance. These authors then employed techniques to determine how large this publication bias would have to be in order to change the results of the meta-analysis. The fail-safe results indicated that there would have to be 56 nonsignificant unpublished studies of approximately the same average sample size as the published studies, in order to change the cumulative meta-analysis effect to a nonsignificant result (56 studies with Rosenthal's method, 22 with Orwin's method). The most critical meta-analysis of the TMS antidepressant field was recently conducted using the guidelines put forth in the Cochrane library (89). However, even this stringent meta-analysis included 14 trials suitable for their analysis and found that left prefrontal TMS at 2 weeks produced significantly greater improvements in the Hamilton Rating Scale than did sham (89). *In summary, all five meta-analyses of the TMS published literature concur that repeated daily prefrontal TMS for 2 weeks has antidepressant effects greater than sham.*

Although there is general consensus that TMS has statistically significant antidepressant effects, a more important question is whether these effects are clinically significant. The meta-analyses above concur on an effect size of Cohen's D of 0.65, which is a moderate effect, in the same range as the effects of antidepressant medications. For example, small to medium effect sizes (0.31–0.40) are common in randomized controlled trials of novel antidepressants (90). Thus, with respect to whether or not TMS has clinical significance, an important clinical issue is whether TMS would be clinically effective in patients referred for ECT. This question has been addressed in a series of studies in which ECT referrals were randomized to receive either ECT or rTMS. In an initial study, Grunhaus et al. compared 40 patients who presented for ECT treatment and were randomized to receive either ECT or TMS (91). ECT was superior to TMS in patients with psychotic depression, but the two treatments were not statistically different in patients without psychotic depression. This same group recently replicated this finding in a larger and independent cohort with an improved design (92). Recently, Janicak and colleagues reported a similar small series, finding near equivalence between TMS and ECT (93). The major differences between these studies and the rest of the controlled studies of TMS efficacy are the patient selection (suitable for ECT), the length of treatment (3–4 weeks), the lack of a blind, and the lack of a sham control. Unfortunately, none of the studies explicitly measured differences in cognitive side effects, although presumably TMS has no measurable cognitive side effects, while ECT has several. In a similar but slightly modified design, Pridmore (2000) recently reported a study comparing the antidepressant effects of standard ECT (3 times/week) and one ECT/week followed by TMS on the other 4 weekdays (94). At 3 weeks they found that both regimens produced similar antidepressant effects. Unfortunately, detailed neuropsychological testing was not performed, but one would assume that the TMS and ECT group had less cognitive side effects than the pure ECT group. Finally, the Israeli group recently published that relapse rates in the 6 months following ECT or rTMS were similar (95). In sum, the studies to date suggest that TMS clinical antidepressant effects are in the range of other antidepressants and persist as long as the clinical effects following ECT.

C. Unresolved Issues

Although the literature suggests that prefrontal TMS has an antidepressant effect greater than sham and that the magnitude of this effect is at least as large as other antidepressants, many issues are not resolved. For example, it is unclear how best to deliver TMS to treat depression. Most, but not all (96), studies have used focal coils positioned over the left prefrontal cortex. It is still not known whether TMS over one hemisphere is better than another, or whether there are better methods for placing the coil. For the most part, the coil has been positioned using a rule-based algorithm to find the prefrontal cortex, which was adopted in the early studies (81). However, this method was shown to be imprecise in the particular prefrontal regions stimulated directly underneath the coil, depending largely on the subject's head size (87). Additionally, most studies have stimulated with the intensity needed to cause movement in the thumb (called the *motor threshold*, or MT). There is now increasing recognition that higher intensities of stimulation are needed to reach the prefrontal cortex, especially in elderly patients, where prefrontal atrophy may outpace that of motor cortex, where the motor threshold is measured (98–101). There is also emerging data that TMS therapeutic effects likely take several weeks to build. Consequently, many of the initial trials, which lasted only 1–2 weeks, were likely too brief to generate maximum clinical antidepressant effects. There is only limited data on using TMS as a maintenance treatment in depression (102). At MUSC recently, seven treatment resistant bipolar depressed patients who had responded to an acute treatment were entered into a maintenance study. TMS was performed 1 day per week over the left prefrontal cortex at 110% motor threshold, 5 Hz for 8 s for 40 trains. During this follow-up period, four subjects dropped out of the maintenance study and were labeled nonresponders (average 25 weeks of treatment). Three subjects completed 1 full year of weekly TMS without a depression relapse. These data suggest that TMS might eventually be used as a maintenance tool in depression, and that one treatment per week might be a good first attempt at a maintenance schedule. Much more work is needed however.

D. TMS to Treat Mania

Grisaru and colleagues in Israel delivered right or left prefrontal TMS to a series of BPAD patients admitted to their hospital for mania (103). TMS was given daily in addition to the standard treatment for mania. After 2 weeks, the group receiving right-sided TMS was significantly more improved than the group that had received left sided TMS. The authors concluded that TMS might be useful as an antimanic agent. However, although subjects were assigned to the two groups at random, the left-sided group was more ill than the right-sided group on several measures. Further work is needed.

E. Current State of TMS Clinical Practice for Depression

In summary, TMS is a promising tool for treating depression acutely. It likely can also induce mania or hypomania in BPAD patients or susceptible patients. Its antimanic properties remain to be explored. Although it is approved in Canada and Israel as a treatment, it is still considered investigational in the United States by the FDA. Despite the body of work showing antidepressant efficacy, prefrontal TMS is not an approved treatment from the standpoint of the FDA. The FDA treats the data from each TMS manufacturer separately, precluding consideration of the meta-analyses above. Additionally, with no use patent on the procedure, it has been difficult to garner industry interest in sponsoring a large-scale clinical trial designed for FDA approval. However, there is continued activity in this area, and the NIMH is also considering funding a multisite trial, the results of which could also be used for pivotal FDA approval, if positive. A small number of U.S., Canadian, and European psychiatrists are using TMS in clinical practice to treat depression, under their general license to practice.

F. A Review of Potential Antidepressant Mechanisms

How does TMS act to improve depression? Work done to date has shown *clear evidence that prefrontal TMS produces immediate* (61–63,104,105) *and longer term* (51) *changes in mood-regulating circuits.* Thus, the original hypothesis about its antidepressant mechanism of action is still the most likely explanation. What remains unclear is which specific prefrontal or other brain locations might be the best for treating depression and whether this can be determined with a group algorithm or needs individual imaging guidance. Much work remains to understand the optimum dosing strategy for the antidepressant effect of TMS. It is unlikely that the initial combinations of intensity, frequency, coil shape, scalp location, number of stimuli, or dosing strategy (daily, twice daily) are the most effective for treating depression. Finally, it is not understood how electrical stimulation of these circuits over time results in improvement of depression symptoms. The translational cascade of events remains undefined. It is clear that determining these answers using clinical trials alone would be a slow and expensive process. Work with animal models and functional imaging will hopefully streamline this research area.

Some behavioral evidence from treatment trials is consistent with the functional imaging data above showing repeated subtle changes in mood-regulating circuits. Szuba and colleagues initially discovered that there is a very subtle but statistically significant improvement in self-rated mood within each day over the 20 min of a daily TMS session (and that this is greater than with sham TMS) (106,107). We recently found a trend consistent with this idea in an independent study in bipolar depression (108). A more recent clinical trial has found this as well (109), and suggest that these subtle within subject, within session effects might predict eventual response. These three studies suggest that during each treatment session, the mood regulating circuit is being activated and slightly normalized. This gradual daily improvement then sums over several weeks when genuine clinical antidepressant effects emerge. Moreover, if they are important in eventual clinical response, one could consider dose-finding studies of different use parameters designed to find the parameters that maximally produced within-day changes. These would be hypothesized to also be the most potent for eventual full treatment.

There is less data to suggest that TMS works to improve depression through activating normal anticonvulsant regulating systems—a widely held theory about the antidepressant mechanisms of action of ECT (110). An appealing notion is that the brain 'interprets' TMS induced currents as potential seizures, with resultant activation of anticonvulsant cascades, which are tied to antidepressant efficacy. In support of this hypothesis, several animal studies have found that TMS has ECS-like anticonvulsant effects (111–113). However there is only scant evidence to suggest that TMS has anticonvulsant effects in depressed patients. An initial open study found that the motor threshold (MT) slightly increased over two weeks of TMS (114). However, the MT does not always correlate with seizure threshold, and this was an open study with only small effects. Operator bias can influence MT determination, particularly with respect to coil location and angle. In a recent double-blind study, we examined for and failed to find a significant change in MT over the course of a TMS treatment trial (108). Moreover, if TMS antidepressant efficacy were linked to its ability to initiate anticonvulsant cascades, then the TMS use parameters closest to producing seizures would be predicted to be the most efficacious. However, there is no clear advantage of higher frequency TMS (115,116), even though it is clearly more likely to provoke seizures. Further work, perhaps using surrogate markers like MR spectroscopy measured GABA, is needed to explore this hypothesized antidepressant mechanism of action.

IV. TMS AS A TREATMENT FOR OTHER CONDITIONS

TMS has also been investigated as a possible treatment for a variety of neuropsychiatric disorders. In general, the published literature in these conditions is much less extensive than for TMS as an antidepressant, and therefore conclusions about the clinical significance of effects must remain tentative until large sample studies are conducted.

A. Movement Disorders

Some initial studies found positive effects in Parkinson's Disease (117); however, one of these early results failed to replicate (118), and some of the methods described were actually not credible. Moreover, a recent study found that TMS delivered over the supplementary motor area (SMA) actually worsened PD symptoms (119). However, a recent study (120), as well as a study from Japan using TMS over the prefrontal cortex, at very low frequencies and doses (121), report that TMS may improve effects in PD. Remember that Strafella and colleagues demonstrated in healthy adults that prefrontal TMS can change dopamine activity in the caudate (62). Thus, it should be remembered that only a small portion of the combinations of use parameters, brain regions, and dosing schedules have been tried. Further studies are needed.

There are two small positive studies showing that TMS can benefit *writer's cramp*, a form of focal dystonia (122). Following a positive small abstract, two groups have used TMS to investigate and possibly treat Gilles de la Tourette syndrome (123). One study found modest and transient beneficial effects on tics when applied over prefrontal cortex (personal communication, M. Trimble). Another study at MUSC also found positive effects on tics, and OCD symptoms (123). Further work is needed in this promising area.

The TMS motor threshold is reduced in patients with untreated epilepsy (124), hinting at widespread problems in cortical excitability. Therapeutically, there is one report of potential beneficial effects of slow rTMS in action myoclonus (125). Additionally, TMS has been used to examine cortical excitability and inhibition in Tourette syndrome (GTS), dystonia, and obsessive-compulsive disorder (OCD) (126). Reduced intracortical inhibition has been reported in all three illnesses.

B. Schizophrenia

Several studies have used TMS to investigate schizophrenia, without consistent replications of early findings which were compounded by medication issues (127). A 1-day prefrontal TMS challenge study by Nahas and colleagues at MUSC failed to find significant effects on negative symptoms (128). Hoffman and colleagues have used low frequency TMS over the temporal lobes to treat hallucinations in patients with schizophrenia (129).

C. Anxiety Disorders

In a randomized trial of left and right prefrontal and mid-occipital 20-Hz stimulation in 12 patients with obsessive compulsive disorder (OCD), Greenberg et al. (130) found that a single session of right prefrontal rTMS decreased compulsive urges for 8 h. Mood was also transiently improved, but there was no effect on anxiety or obsessions. Using TMS probes, the same group reported decreased intracortical inhibition in patients with OCD (131), which has also been noted in patients with Tourette's disorder (126). Somewhat surprisingly, OCD patients had a lowered MEP threshold in one study (132), unrelated to intracortical inhibition, and which appears to replicate (E.M. Wassermann, personal communication). Only two other studies have examined possible therapeutic effects of rTMS in OCD. A double-blind study using right prefrontal slow (1 Hz) rTMS and a less-focal coil failed to find statistically significant effects greater than sham (133). In contrast, a recent open study in a group of 12 OCD patients, refractory to standard treatments, who were randomly assigned to right or left prefrontal fast rTMS, found that clinically significant and sustained improvement was observed in a third of patients (134). Clearly, further work is warranted testing TMS as a potential treatment for OCD.

McCann et al. (135) reported that two patients with PTSD improved during open treatment with 1 Hz rTMS over the right frontal cortex. Grisaru et al. similarly stimulated 10 PTSD patients over motor cortex and found decreased anxiety (136). Grisaru and colleagues also reported a positive TMS study in PTSD patients (N. Grisaru, Personal Communication, May, 2001). Further work is needed.

V. SAFETY ISSUES ASSOCIATED WITH TMS

Despite the initial safety concerns about TMS, it continues to have a good safety record. Inadvertent seizures can occur, but they have not happened over the past 4 years when researchers have been following the safety guidelines (137). It is important to realize that this TMS safety table was developed in a small subject sample using a surrogate endpoint for a seizure—spread of TMS induced motor evoked potentials (MEP) beyond the target area of stimulation. Thus, the safety table exists only for stimulation of motor cortex and cannot readily be applied to using TMS over other brain regions. Further, although the intensity and frequency of stimulation were examined, the intertrain interval was not. One of the inadvertent seizures was induced with stimulation trains that were within the safety guidelines but were administered with an excessively short intertrain interval (138). A general rule of thumb is that one should have an intertrain interval at least as long as the period of stimulation. A known seizure disorder, history of epilepsy, or intracranial abnormality such as a prior stroke can all increase the risk of a TMS induced seizure (139). Although an inadvertent seizure is the main safety hazard associated with TMS, there have been only 12 reported cases since 1985, when cranial TMS began. It is, in fact, not easy to intentionally use TMS to produce a seizure, even in patients with epilepsy (140). For example, an attempt to use TMS to intentionally produce a seizure in a patient with a focal epilepsy was not successful (140). In addition, in a study exploring rTMS as a method to induce therapeutic seizures, stimulation parameters far above the published safety thresholds had to be used to reliably induce seizures (141). There do not appear to be any deleterious cognitive side effects of TMS even when used in high doses for several days (142). A muscle tension type headache and discomfort at the site of stimulation are less serious but relatively common side effects of TMS. In the United States, fast rTMS is an experimental procedure that requires an investigational device exemption (IDE) from the FDA for research. As mentioned before, modern TMS did not begin until 1985 (1), and the total number of subjects or patients to receive TMS is likely still less than 10,000. However, substantial experience to date suggests that at least in the short term (<10 years), TMS at moderate intensity has no other evident lasting adverse effects in adults.

VI. SUMMARY AND CONCLUSIONS

TMS is thus a powerful new brain stimulation tool, with extremely interesting research and one confirmed and several putative therapeutic potentials. TMS is unique among the new class of brain stimulation techniques because of its noninvasiveness and positive safety and side effect profile. It clearly has the ability to engage subcortical-limbic circuits and to produce immediate, intermediate, and long-term effects. Further understanding of the ways by which TMS changes neuronal function, especially as a function of its use parameters, will improve its ability both to answer neuroscience questions as well as to treat diseases.

ACKNOWLEDGEMENTS AND DISCLOSURE

The authors' work with TMS has been supported in part by research grants from NARSAD, the Stanley Foundation, the Borderline Personality Disorders Research Foundation (BPDRF), the Dana Foundation (Bohning), NINDS grant RO1- AG40956, and the Defense Advanced Research Projects Agency (DARPA). Drs. George, Nahas, Kozel, and Bohning hold several TMS-related patents, either alone or in combination. These are not in the area of TMS therapeutics but rather are for new TMS machine designs as well as combining TMS with MRI.

REFERENCES

1. Barker AT, Jalinous R, Freeston IL. Non-invasive magnetic stimulation of the human motor cortex. Lancet 1985; 1:1106–1107.
2. Wassermann EM. Risk and safety of repetitive transcranial magnetic stimulation: report and suggested guidelines from the International Workshop in the Safety of Repetitive Transcranial Magnetic Stimulation, June 5–7, 1996. Electroencephalogr Clin Neurophysiol 1998; 108:1–16.

3. Roth BJ, Saypol JM, Hallett M, Cohen LG. Theoretical calculation of the electric field induced in the cortex during magnetic stimulation. Electroencephalo Clin Neurophysiol 1991; 81:47– 56.

4. Faraday M. Effects on the production of electricity from magnetism (1831). In: Williams LP, ed. Michael Faraday. New York: Basic Books, 1965:531.

5. George MS, Belmaker RH. Transcranial magnetic stimulation in neuropsychiatry. In: George MS, Belmaker RH, eds. Washington, DC: American Psychiatric Press, 2000.

6. George MS, Lisanby SH, Sackeim HA. Transcranial magnetic stimulation: applications in neuropsychiatry. Arch Gen Psychiatry 1999; 56:300–311.

7. Barker AT, Freeston IL, Jarratt JA, Jalinous R. Magnetic stimulation of the human nervous system: an introduction and basic principles. In: Chokroverty S, ed. Magnetic Stimulation in Clinical Neurophysiology. Boston: Butterworths, 1989:55–72.

8. Bohning DE. Introduction and overview of TMS physics. In: George MS, Belmaker RH, eds. Transcranial Magnetic Stimulation in Neuropsychiatry. Washington, DC: American Psychiatric Press, 2000:13–44.

9. Council NR. Possible Health Effects of Exposure to Residential Electric and Magnetic Fields. Washington, DC: National Academy Press, 1996.

10. Ajmone-Marsan C. Focal electrical stimulation. In: Purpura DP, Penry JK, Tower DB, Woodbury DM, Walter RD, eds. Experimental Models of Epilepsy. New York: Raven Press, 1972:147–172.

11. Alexander GE, DeLong MR, Strick PL. Parallel organization of functionally segregated circuits linking basal ganglia and cortex. Annu Rev Neurosci 1986; 9:357–381.

12. Stewart LM, Walsh V, Rothwell JC. Motor and phosphene thresholds: a transcranial magnetic stimulation correlation study. Neuropsychologia 2001; 39:415–419.

13. Ziemann U, Hallett M. Basic neurophysiological studies with TMS. In: George MS, Belmaker RH, eds. Transcranial Magnetic Stimulation in Neuropsychiatry. Washington, DC: American Psychiatric Press, 2000:45–98.

14. Pridmore S, Filho JAF, Nahas Z, Liberatos C, George MS. Motor threshold in transcranial magnetic stimulation: a comparison of a neurophysiological and a visualization of movement method. J ECT 1998; 14:25–27.

15. Amassian VE, Eberle L, Maccabee PJ, Cracco RQ. Modelling magnetic coil excitation of human cerebral cortex with a peripheral nerve immersed in a brain-shaped volume conductor: the significance of fiber bending in excitation. Electroencephalo Clin Neurophysiol 1992; 85:291–301.

16. Davey KR, Cheng CH, Epstein CM. Prediction of magnetically induced electric fields in biologic tissue. IEEE Trans Biomed Eng 1991; 38:418–422.

17. Penfield W, Jasper H. Epilepsy and the Functional Anatomy of the Human Brain. Boston: Little, Brown and Company, 1954.

18. George MS, Nahas Z, Lisanby SH, Schlaepfer T, Kozel FA, Greenberg BD. Transcranial magnetic stimulation. Neurosurg Clin N Am 2003. In press.

19. Greenberg BD, Ziemann U, Harmon A, Murphy DL, Wassermann EM. Reduced intracortical inhibition in obsessive-compulsive disorder on transcranial magnetic stimulation. Lancet 1998; 352:881–882.

20. Ziemann U, Steinhoff BJ, Tergau F, Paulus W. Transcranial magnetic stimulation: its current role in epilepsy research. Epilepsy Res 1998; 30:11–30.

21. Bohning DE, Walker JA, Mu Q, Li X, Denslow S, George MS. Interleaved Paired Pulse TMS and BOLD fMRI [abstract]. Magn Res Med 2003.

22. Epstein CM, Lah JJ, Meador K, Weissman JD, Gaitan LE, Dihenia B. Optimum stimulus parameters for lateralized suppression of speech with magnetic brain stimulation. Neurology 1996; 47:1590–1593.

23. Grill WM, McIntyre CC. Extracellular excitation of central neurons: implications for the mechanisms of deep brain stimulation. Thalamus & Related Systems 2001; 1:269–277.

24. Bear MF. Homosynaptic long-term depression: a mechanism for memory? Proceedings of the

National Academy of Sciences of the United States of America Aug 17, 1999; 96(17):9457–9458.

25. Stanton PK, Sejnowsky TJ. Associative long-term depression in the hippocampus induced by hebbian covariance. Nature 1989; 339:215–218.

26. Malenka RC, Nicoll RA. Long-term potentiation: a decade of progress? Science Sep 17, 1999; 285(5435):1870–1974.

27. Wang H, Wang X, Scheich H. LTD and LTP induced by transcranial magnetic stimulation in auditory cortex. NeuroReport 1996; 7:521–525.

28. Chen R, Classen J, Gerloff C. Depression of motor cortex excitability by low-frequency transcranial magnetic stimulation. Neurology 1997; 48:1398–1403.

29. Wu T, Sommer M, Tergau F, Paulus W. Lasting influence of repetitive transcranial magnetic stimulation on intracortical excitability in human subjects. Neuroscience Letters 2000; 287:37–40.

30. Desmurget M, Epstein CM, Turner RS, Prablanc C, Alexander GE, Grafton ST. Role of the posterior parietal cortex in updating reaching movements to a visual target. Nature Neurosci 1999; 2:563–567.

31. Epstein CM, Verson R, Zangaladze A. Magnetic coil stimulation suppresses visual perception at an extra-calcarine site. J Clin Neurophysiol 1996; 13:247–252.

32. Grafman J, Wassermann E. Transcranial magnetic stimulation can measure and modulate learning and memory. Neuropshcologia 1999; 37(2):159–167.

33. Flitman SS, Grafman J, Wassermann EM. Linguistic processing during repetitive transcranial magnetic stimulation. Neurology 1998; 50:175–181.

34. George MS, Wassermann EM, Williams W. Changes in mood and hormone levels after rapid-rate transcranial magnetic stimulation of the prefrontal cortex. J Neuropsychiatry Clin Neuro 1996; 8:172–180.

35. Grafman J. TMS as a primary brain mapping tool. In: George MS, Belmaker RH, eds. Transcranial Magnetic Stimulation (TMS) in Neuropsychiatry. Washington, DC: American Psychiatric Press, 2000:115–140.

36. George MS, Lisanby SH, Sackeim HA. Transcranial magnetic stimulation - Applications in neuropsychiatry. Arch Gen Psychiatry 1999; 56:300–311.

37. Lisanby SH, Luber B, Finck D. Primate models of transcranial magnetic stimulation. Biological Psychiatry 1998; 41:76s.

38. Amassian VE, Quirk GJ, Stewart M. A comparison of corticospinal activation by magnetic coil and electrical stimulation of monkey motor cortex. Electroencephalo Clin Neurophysiol 1990; 77:390–401.

39. Edgley SA, Eyre JA, Lemon RN, Miller S. Excitation of the corticospinal tract by electro-magnetic and electrical stimulation of the scalp in the macaque monkey. J Physiol (London) 1990; 425:301–320.

40. Lemon RN, Johansson RS, Wrestling G. Modulation of corticospinal influence over hand muscles during gripping tasks in man and monkey. Canadian J Physiol Pharmacol 1996; 74:547–558.

41. Baker SN, Olivier E, Lemon RN. Task-related variation in corticospinal output evoked by transcranial magnetic stimulation in the macaque monkey. J Physiol 1995; 488:795–801.

42. Ghaly RF, Stone JL, Aldrete A, Levy W. Effects of incremental ketamine hydrochloride doses on motor evoked potentials (MEPs) following transcranial magnetic stimulation: a primate study. J Neurosurg Anesthesiol 1990; 2:79–85.

43. Stone JL, Ghaly RF, Levy WJ, Kartha R, Krinsky L, Roccaforte P. A comparative analysis of enflurane anesthesia on primate motor and somatosensory evoked potentials. Electro-encephalo Clin Neurophysiol 1992; 84:180–197.

44. Baker SN, Olivier E, Lemon RN. Recording an identified pyramidal volley evoked by transcranial magnetic stimulation in a conscious macaque monkey. Experimental Brain Res 1995; 99:529–532.

45. Fleischmann A, Sternheim A, Etgen AM, Li C, Grisaru N, Belmaker RH. Transcranial

magnetic stimulation downregulates beta-adrenoreceptors in rat cortex. J Neural Transm 1996; 103:1361–1366.

46. Ben-Sachar D, Belmaker RH, Grisaru N, Klein E. Transcranial magnetic stimulation induces alterations in brain monoamines. J Neural Transm 1997; 104:191–197.

47. Jennum P, Klitgaard H. Effect of acute and chronic stimulations on pentylenetetrazole-induced clonic seizures. Epilepsy Res 1996; 23:115–122.

48. Pope A, Keck ME. TMS as a therapeutic tool in psychiatry: what do we know about neurobiological mechanisms? J Psychiatr Res 2001; 35:193–215.

49. Weissman JD, Epstein CM, Davey KR. Magnetic brain stimulation and brain size: relevance to animal studies. Electroencephalo Clin Neurophysiol 1992; 85:215–219.

50. Nobler MS, Oquendo MA, Kegeles LS. Decreased regional brain metabolism after ECT. Am J Psychiatry 2001; 158:305–308.

51. Teneback CC, Nahas Z, Speer AM. Two weeks of daily left prefrontal rTMS changes prefrontal cortex and paralimbic activity in depression. J Neuropsychiatry Clin Neurosci 1999; 11:426–435.

52. Shajahan PM, Glabus MF, Steele JD. Left dorso-lateral repetitive transcranial magnetic stimulation affects cortical excitability and functional connectivity, but does not impair cognition in major depression. Progress in Neuropsychopharmacology and Biological Psychiatry 2002; 26:945–954.

53. Speer AM, Kimbrell TA, Wasserman EM. Opposite effects of high and low frequency rTMS on regional brain activity in depressed patients. Biological Psychiatry 2000; 48(23):1133–1141.

54. Mitchel P. 15 Hz and 1 Hz TMS have different acute effects on cerebral blood flow in depressed patients. Int J Neuropsychopharmacol 2002; 5:S7 (s.08.02).

55. Shastri A, George MS, Bohning DE. Performance of a system for interleaving transcranial magnetic stimulation with steady state magnetic resonance imaging. Electroencephalo Clin Neurophysiol Suppl 1999; 51:55–64.

56. Bohning DE, Shastri A, Nahas Z. Echoplanar BOLD fMRI of brain activation induced by concurrent transcranial magnetic stimulation (TMS). Invest Radiol 1998; 33(6):336–340.

57. Bohning DE, Shastri A, McConnell K. A combined TMS/fMRI study of intensity-dependent TMS over motor cortex. Biological Psychiatry 1999; 45:385–394.

58. Bohning DE, Shastri A, Wassermann EM. BOLD-fMRI response to single-pulse transcranial magnetic stimulation (TMS). J Magnetic Resonance Imaging 2000; 11:569–574.

59. Bohning DE, Shastri A, McGavin L. Motor cortex brain activity induced by 1-Hz transcranial magnetic stimulation is similar in location and level to that for volitional movement. Invest Radiol 2000; 35(11):676–683.

60. Baudewig J, Siebner HR, Bestmann S. Functional MRI of cortical activations induced by transcranial magnetic stimulation (TMS). NeuroReport 2001; 12:3543–3548.

61. Nahas Z, Lomarev M, Roberts DR. Unilateral left prefrontal transcranial magnetic stimulation (TMS) produces intensity-dependent bilateral effects as measured by interleaved BOLD fMRI. Biological Psychiatry 2001; 50(9):712–720.

62. Strafella AP, Paus T, Barrett J, Dagher A. Repetitive transcranial magnetic stimulation of the human prefrontal cortex induces dopamine release in the caudate nucleus. J Neurosci 2001; 21:RC157.

63. Paus T, Castro-Alamancos MA, Petrides M. Cortico-cortical connectivity of the human mid-dorsolateral frontal cortex and its modulation by repetitive transcranial magnetic stimulation. European J Neurosci 2001; 14:1405–1411.

64. George MS, Bohning DE. Measuring brain connectivity with functional imaging and transcranial magnetic stimulation (TMS). In: Desimone B, ed. Neuropsychopharmacology, Fifth Generation of Progress. New York: Lipincott, Williams and Wilkins, 2002:393–410.

65. Paus T, Jech R, Thompson CJ, Comeau R, Peters T, Evans AC. Transcranial magnetic stimulation during positron emission tomography: a new method for studying connectivity of the human cerebral cortex. J Neurosci 1997; 17:3178–3184.

66. Kimbrell TA, Ketter TA, George MS. Regional cerebral glucose utilization in patients with a range of severities of unipolar depression. Biological Psychiatry 2002; 51:237–252.

67. George MS, Huggins T, McDermut W, Parekh PI, Rubinow D, Post RM. Abnormal facial emotion recognition in depression: serial testing in an ultra-rapid-cycling patient. Behavior Mod 1998; 22:192–204.

68. George MS. An introduction to the emerging neuroanatomy of depression. Psychiatr Ann 1994; 24:635–636.

69. George MS, Ketter TA, Parekh PI. Regional brain activity when selecting a response despite interference: an H215O PET study of the stroop and an emotional stroop. Human Brain Mapping 1994; 1:194–209.

70. George MS, Ketter TA, Parekh PI, Horwitz B, Herscovitch P, Post RM. Brain activity during transient sadness and happiness in healthy women. Am J Psychiatry 1995; 152:341–351.

71. George MS, Ketter TA, Post RM. What Functional Imaging Studies Have Revealed About the Brain Basis of Mood and Emotion. In: Panksepp J, ed. Advances in Biological Psychiatry. Greenwich, Conn: JAI Press, 1996:63–113.

72. George MS, Ketter TA, Parekh PI. Blunted left cingulate activation in mood disorder subjects during a response interference task (The Stroop). J Neuropsychiatry Clin Neuro 1997; 9:55–63.

73. Ketter TA, Andreason PJ, George MS. Anterior paralimbic mediation of procaine-induced emotional and psychosensory experiences. Arch Gen Psychiatry 1996; 53:59–69.

74. George MS, Ketter TA, Post RM. Prefrontal cortex dysfunction in clinical depression. Depression 1994; 2:59–72.

75. George MS, Post RM, Ketter TA, Kimbrell TA. Neural mechanisms of mood disorders. Current Review of Mood and Anxiety Disorders 1997; 1:71–83.

76. Mayberg HS, Liotti M, Brannan SK. Reciprocal limbic-cortical function and negative mood: converging PET findings in depression and normal sadness. Am J Psychiatry May 1999; 156(5): 675–682.

77. Beer B. Uber das Auftretten einer objectiven Lichtempfindung in magnetischen Felde. Klinische Wochenzeitschrift 1902; 15:108–109.

78. Kolbinger HM, Hoflich G, Hufnagel A, Moller H-J, Kasper S. Transcranial Magnetic Stimulation (TMS) in the treatment of major depression—a pilot study. Human Psychopharmacol 1995; 10:305–310.

79. Grisaru N, Yarovslavsky U, Abarbanel J, Lamberg T, Belmaker RH. Transcranial magnetic stimulation in depression and schizophrenia. European Neuropsychopharmacol 1994; 4:287–288.

80. Nobler MS, Sackeim HA, Prohovnik I. Regional cerebral blood flow in mood disorders, III. Treatment and clinical response. Arch Gen Psychiatry 1994; 51:884–897.

81. George MS, Wassermann EM, Williams WA. Daily repetitive transcranial magnetic stimulation (rTMS) improves mood in depression. NeuroReport 1995; 6:1853–1856.

82. George MS, Wassermann EM, Williams WE. Mood improvements following daily feft prefrontal repetitive transcranial magnetic stimulation in patients with depression: a placebo-controlled crossover trial. Am J Psychiatry 1997; 154:1752–1756.

83. George MS, Wassermann EM. Rapid-rate transcranial magnetic stimulation (rTMS) and ECT. Convulsive Therapy 1994; 10(4):251–253.

84. Loo C, Mitchell P, Sachdev P, McDarmont B, Parker G, Gandevia S. A double-blind controlled investigation of transcranial magnetic stimulation for the treatment of resistant major depression. Am J Psychiatry 1999; 156:946–948.

85. Holtzheimer PE, Russo J, Avery D. A meta-analysis of repetitive transcranial magnetic stimulation in the treatment of depression. Psychopharmacol Bull 2001; 35:149–169.

86. Kozel FA, George MS. Meta-analysis of left prefrontal repetitive transcranial magnetic stimulation (rTMS) to treat depression. J Psychiatr Practice 2002; 8:S56–S61.

87. Burt T, Lisanby SH, Sackeim HA. Neuropsychiatric applications of transcranial magnetic stimulation. Int J Neuropsychopharmacol 2002; 5:73–103.

88. McNamara B, Ray JL, Arthurs OJ, Boniface S. Transcranial magnetic stimulation for depression and other psychiatric disorders. Psychological Medicine 2001; 31:1141–1146.

89. Martin JLR, Barbanoj MJ, Schlaepfer TE. Transcranial magnetic stimulation for treating depression (Cochrane Review). The Cochrane Library. Oxford: Update Software, 2002.

90. Thase ME. The need for clinically relevant research on treatment-resistant depression. J Clin Psychiatry 2001; 62:221–224.

91. Grunhaus L, Dannon PN, Schreiber S. Repetitive transcranial magnetic stimulation is as effective as electroconvulsive therapy in the treatment of nondelusional major depressive disorder: an open study. Biological Psychiatry 2000; 4(47):314–324.

92. Grunhaus L, Schreiber S, Dolberg OT, Polack D, Dannon PN. Randomized controlled comparison of ECT and rTMS in severe and resistant non-psychotic major depression. Biological Psychiatry 2003; 53(4):324–331.

93. Janicak PG, Dowd SM, Martis B. Repetitive transcranial magnetic stimulation versus electroconvulsive therapy for major depression: preliminary results of a randomized trial. Biological Psychiatry 2002; 51:659–667.

94. Pridmore S. Substitution of rapid transcranial magnetic stimulation treatments for electro-convulsive therapy treatments in a course of electroconvulsive therapy. Depress Anxiety 2000; 12(3):118–123.

95. Dannon PN, Dolberg OT, Schreiber S, Grunhaus L. Three and six-month outcome following courses of either ECT or rTMS in a population of severely depressed individuals-preliminary report. Biological Psychiatry 2002; 51:687–690.

96. Klein E, Kreinin I, Chistyakov A. Therapeutic efficacy of right prefrontal slow repetitive transcranial magnetic stimulation in major depression: a double-blind controlled study. Arch Gen Psychiatry 1999; 56:315–320.

97. Herwig U, Padberg F, Unger J, Spitzer M, Schonfeldt-Lecuona C. Transcranial magnetic stimulation in therapy studies: examination of the reliability of "standard" coil positioning by neuronavigation. Biological Psychiatry 2001; 50(1):58–61.

98. McConnell KA, Nahas Z, Shastri A. The transcranial magnetic stimulation motor threshold depends on the distance from coil to underlying cortex: a replication in healthy adults comparing two methods of assessing the distance to cortex. Biological Psychiatry 2001; 49(5):454–459.

99. Mosimann UP, Marre SC, Werlen S. Antidepressant effects of repetitive transcranial magnetic stimulation in the elderly: correlation between effect size and coil-cortex distance. Arch Gen Psychiatry 2002; 59:560–561.

100. Padberg F, Zwanzger P, Keck ME. Repetitive transcranial magnetic stimulation (rTMS) in major depression: Relation between efficacy and stimulation intensity. Neuropsychopharmacology 2002; 27:638–645.

101. Kozel FA, Nahas Z, DeBrux C. How the distance from coil to cortex relates to age, motor threshold and possibly the antidepressant response to repetitive transcranial magnetic stimulation. J Neuropsychiatry Clin Neurosci 2000; 12:376–384.

102. Nahas Z, Oliver NC, Johnson M. Feasibility and efficacy of left prefrontal rTMS as a maintenance antidepressant. Biological Psychiatry 2000, (abstract) 57.

103. Belmaker RH, Grisaru N. Antibipolar potential for transcranial magnetic stimulation. Bipolar Disord 1999; 1(2):71–72.

104. Li X, Teneback CC, Nahas Z. Lamotrigine inhibits the functional magnetic resonance imaging response to transcranial magnetic stimulation in healthy adults. Biological Psychiatry 2002; 51:8S (#567).

105. George MS, Stallings LE, Speer AM. Prefrontal repetitive transcranial magnetic stimulation (rTMS) changes relative perfusion locally and remotely. Human Psychopharmacol 1999; 14:161–170.

106. Szuba MP, O'Reardon JP, Rai AS. Acute mood and thyroid stimulating hormone effects of transcranial magnetic stimulation in major depression. Biological Psychiatry 2001; 50:22–57.

107. Szuba MP, Rai A, Kastenberg J. Rapid mood and endocrine effects of TMS in major depression. Proceedings of the American Psychiatric Association Annual Meeting. 1999:201.

108. Nahas Z, Kozel FA, Li X, Anderson B, George MS. Left prefrontal transcranial magnetic stimulation (TMS) treatment of depression in bipolar affective disorder: a pilot study of acute safety and efficacy. J Bipolar Disorders. Under review.

109. Grunhaus L, Dolberg OT, Polak D, Dannon PN. Monitoring the response to rTMS in depression with visual analog scales. Human Psychopharmacol 2002; 17:349–352.

110. Sackeim HA, Decina P, Malitz S, Resor SR, Prohovnik I. Anticonvulsant and antidepressant properties of electroconvulsive therapy: a proposed mechanism of action. Biological Psychiatry 1983; 18:1301–1310.

111. Fujiki M, Steward O. High frequency transcranial magnetic stimulation mimics the effects of ECS in upregulating astroglial gene expression in the murine CNS. Molecular Brain Res 1997; 44:301–308.

112. Belmaker RH, Grisaru N. Magnetic stimulation of the brain in animal depression models responsive to ECS. J ECT 1998; 14(3):194–205.

113. Ebert U, Ziemann U. Altered seizure susceptibility after high-frequency transcranial magnetic stimulation in rats. Neurosci Lett 1999; 273:155–158.

114. Triggs WJ, McCoy KJ, Greer R. Effects of left frontal transcranial magnetic stimulation on depressed mood, cognition, and corticomotor threshold. Biological Psychiatry 1999; 45:1440–1446.

115. Padberg F, Haag C, Zwanzger P. Rapid and slow transcranial magnetic stimulation are equally effective in medication-resistant depression: a placebo-controlled study. CINP Abstracts 1998; 21st Congress:103-st0306.

116. George MS, Nahas Z, Molloy M. A Controlled trial of daily transcranial magnetic stimulation (TMS) of the left prefrontal cortex for treating depression. Biological Psychiatry 2000; 48(10):962–970.

117. Pascual-Leone A, Valls-Sole J, Brasil-Neto JP, Cohen LG, Hallett M. Akinesia in Parkinson's disease. I Shortening of simple reaction times with focal, single-pulse transcranial magnetic stimulation. Neurology 1994; 44:884–891.

118. Ghabra MB, Hallett M, Wassermann EM. Simultaneous repetitive transcranial magnetic stimulation does not speed fine movement in PD. Neurology 1999; 52:768–770.

119. Boylan LS, Pullman SL, Lisanby SH, Spicknall KE, Sackeim HA. Repetitive transcranial magnetic stimulation to SMA worsens complex movements in Parkinson's disease. Clin Neurophysiol 2001; 112:259–264.

120. Mally J, Stone TW. Therapeutic and "dose-dependent" effect of repetitive microelectroshock induced by transcranial magnetic stimulation in Parkinson's disease. J Neurosci Res 1999; 57(6):935–940.

121. Shimamoto H, Morimitsu H, Sugita S, Nakahara K, Shigemori M. Therapeutic Effect of repetitive transcranial magnetic stimulation in Parkinson's disease. Rinsho Shinkeigaku 1999; 39:1264–1267.

122. Siebner HR, Tormos JM, Ceballos-Baumann AO. Low frequency repetitive transcranial magnetic stimulation of motor cortex in patients with writer's cramp. Neurology 1999; 52:529–537.

123. Chae JH, Nahas Z, Wassermann EM. Pilot study using rTMS to probe the functional neuroanatomy of tics in Tourette syndrome. Neuropsychiatry Neuropsychol Behavioral Neurol 2003.

124. Reutens DC, Puce A, Berkovic SF. Cortical hyperexcitability in progressive myoclonus epilepsy: a study with transcranial magnetic stimulation. Neurology 1993; 43:186–192.

125. Wedegaertner F, Garvey M, Cohen LG, Hallett M, Wassermann EM. Low frequency repetitive transcranial magnetic stimulation can reduce action myoclonus. Neurology 1997; 48:A119.

126. Ziemann U, Paulus W, Rothenberger A. Decreased motor inhibition in Tourette's disorder: evidence from transcranial magnetic stimulation. Am J Psychiatry 1997; 154:1277–1284.

127. Feinsod M, Sreinin B, Chistyakov A, Klein E. Preliminary evidence for a beneficial effect of low-frequency, repetitive transcranial magnetic stimulation in patients with major depression and schizophrenia. Depression Anxiety 1998; 7:65–68.

128. Nahas Z, McConnell K, Collins S. Could left prefrontal rTMS modify negative symptoms and attention in schizophrenia? Biological Psychiatry 1999; 45:37S #120.

129. Hoffman R, Boutros N, Berman R, Krystal J, Charney D. Transcranial magnetic stimulation and hallucinated 'voices'. Biological Psychiatry 1998; 43:93s. #310.

130. Greenberg BD, George MS, Dearing J. Effect of prefrontal repetitive transcranial magnetic stimulation (rTMS) in obsessive compulsive disorder: a preliminary study. Am J Psychiatry 1997; 154:867–869.

131. Cora-Locatelli G, Greenberg BD, Harmon A. Cortical excitability and augmentation strategies in OCD. Biological Psychiatry 1998; 43:77s (#258).

132. Greenberg BD, Ziemann U, Cora-Locatelli G. Altered cortical excitability in obsessive-compulsive disorder. Neurology 2000; 54:142–147.

133. Alonso P, Pujol J, Cardoner N. Right prefrontal TMS in OCD: a double-blind, placebo-controlled study. Am J Psychiatry 2001; 158:1143–1145.

134. Sachdev PS, McBride R, Loo CK, Mitchell PB, Malhi GS, Croker VM. Right versus left prefrontal transcranial magnetic stimulation for obsessive-compulsive disorder: a preliminary investigation. J Clin Psychiatry 2001; 62:981–984.

135. McCann UD, Kimbrell TA, Morgan CM. Repetitive transcranial magnetic stimulation for posttraumatic stress disorder (letter). Arch Gen Psychiatry 1998; 55:276–279.

136. Grisaru N, Amir M, Cohen H, Kaplan Z. Effect of transcranial magnetic stimulation in posttraumatic stress disorder: a preliminary study. Biological Psychiatry 1998; 44:52–55.

137. Wassermann EM. Report on risk and safety of repetitive transcranial magnetic stimulation (rTMS): suggested guidelines from the International Workshop on Risk and Safety of rTMS (June 1996). Electroencephalo Clin Neurophysiol 1997; 108:1–16.

138. Wassermann EM, Cohen LG, Flitman SS, Chen R, Hallett M. Seizures in healthy people with repeated safe trains of transcranial magnetic stimuli. Lancet 1996; 347:825–826.

139. Lorberbaum JP, Wassermann EM. Safety concerns of transcranial magnetic stimulation. In: George MS, Belmaker RH, eds. Transcranial Magnetic Stimulation in Neuropsychiatry. Washington, DC: American Psychiatric Press, 2000:141–162.

140. Jennum P, Winkel H. Transcranial magnetic stimulation. Its role in the evaluation of patients with partial epilepsy. Acta Neurol Scand Suppl 1994; 152:93–96.

141. Lisanby SH, Schlaepfer TE, Fisch HU, Sackeim HA. Magnetic seizure therapy for major depression. Arch Gen Psychiatry 2001; 58:303–305 (let).

142. Little JT, Kimbrell TA, Wassermann EM. Cognitive effects of 1 and 20 Hz repetitive transcranial magnetic stimulation in depression: Preliminary report. Neuropsychiatry Neuropsychol Behavioral Neurol 2000; 13:119–124.

20

Repetitive Transcranial Magnetic Stimulation for Tinnitus

Paul J. Rosch

The American Institute of Stress, Yonkers, and New York Medical College, Valhalla, New York, U.S.A.

The varied types of electrical stimulation for the treatment of tinnitus over the past 200 years are reviewed, and the difficulties involved in proving their efficacy are emphasized. Part of the problem is that few plausible mechanisms of action have been proposed, and it is difficult to rule out placebo effects because of the lack of objective measurement parameters. Repetitive transcranial magnetic stimulation (rTMS) has very recently been shown to provide promising results in a pilot study. The success of rTMS in drug resistant depression has sparked research efforts to delineate mechanisms of action that may lead to more effective use of this exciting modality in tinnitus patients.

Many multiauthored medical texts such as this have a lag time of 2 years or more between inception and publication so that recent advances occurring during this period can not be included. Dekker not only agreed to publish this volume within 6 months of receipt of approved manuscripts but has also been able to accommodate late-breaking contributions not originally anticipated, such as the chapter on radio-frequency coblation for low back pain. As of this writing, I am still unaware of any article on this technique that has been published in a peer-reviewed journal. Another example is rTMS (repetitive magnetic stimulation) for the treatment of tinnitus. When the comprehensive review on this rapidly emerging modality was submitted by Mark George there was nothing in the literature on its potential use for tinnitus. Such a report has just been published but the authors were unable to submit a brief chapter in time to meet the publication deadline. I believe it is very important to present their observations since it provides an opportunity to review other electromagnetic stimulation approaches that illustrate the tremendous interest in this topic as well as a potential breakthrough for alleviating this disorder, which is notoriously resistant to treatment.

Different forms of electrical stimulation have been used to treat deafness and tinnitus for over 200 years (1,2) as illustrated in Fig. 1.

It is not likely that such approaches would have persisted and proliferated in recent years if they did not provide some benefits. However, the mechanisms of action that might be responsible for relief of tinnitus have not been delineated and may be difficult to determine until more is known about the varied causes and therefore pathophysiology of this disorder. Various theories have been proposed for specific types of tinnitus. Although many patients also suffer from deafness tinnitus is not always accompanied by hearing loss and the precise prevalence of this association is difficult to determine for several reasons (3).

The significantly increased incidence of cochlear damage has led many to suggest that tinnitus arises in this organ (4,5). When cochlear implants became available, it was noted that patients frequently reported improvement in their tinnitus as well as hearing (6). One possible explanation was acoustical masking of the tinnitus by the ambient sounds that the cochlear implant now provided (7). It was also suggested that tinnitus might have been suppressed by the electrical impulses sent through the auditory nerve by the implant and that external stimulation of the implant might provide additional benefits. Several studies using sundry electrical stimulation techniques reported improvement (8–15) ranging from 22% (11) to 87% (15) depending on the degree of severity, presumed etiology, type and duration of therapy, criteria used to rate benefits, and other factors. Most reported success rates between 50–70% (9,11,12) and in one trial, patients with noise induced hearing loss did not do as well as others without this history, and those in the post skull trauma group did the worst. The best results were seen in patients with tinnitus accompanied by disturbances in the vertebro-basilar artery who reported a 64% improvement, including 28% who had complete relief (1). In one small trial in which patients had the ability to induce electrical stimulation when desired on an outpatient basis, tinnitus lessened in all and half reported an improvement in hearing and sleeping (16).

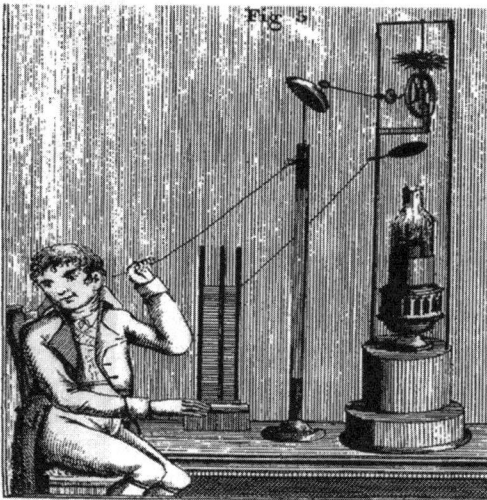

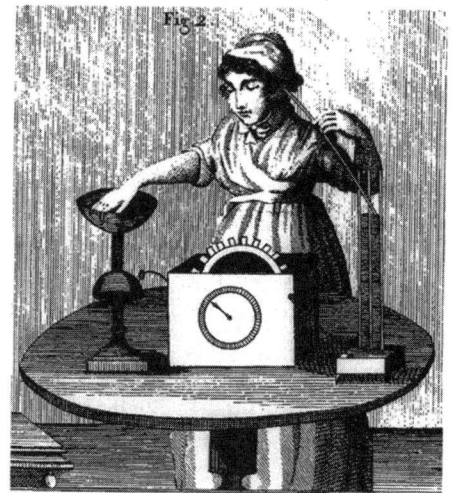

Figure 1 From Aldini, J. Essai theorique et expérimental sur le galvanisme, avec une série, d'expériences faites en presence des commisaires de l'Institut national de France, et en divers amphithéatres anatomiques de Londres Paris, 1804 (2). (Courtesy of the Bakken Library.)

It was proposed that electrical stimulation provided additional benefits by increasing acoustical masking since relief was also noted on the contralateral side (17). Others postulate that positive DC produces a hyperpolarization of nerve fibers that inhibits spontaneous discharge rates (15,18) or that electrostimulation changes the basal membrane potential since better results were obtained with low frequency stimulation (19). One study concluded that the underlying mechanism was a synchronization of auditory nerve fiber discharges following electrical stimulation (20). In another, negative DC increased autoacoustic emission while positive DC reduced it (21). This is consistent with the view that electrical stimulation with positive DC can change the spontaneous activity of cochlear nerve fibers and that some of the benefits are "due to increased microcirculation in part of the auditory pathways as a reflex effect" (1). This would especially apply to early treatment of tinnitus due to noise-induced hearing loss since increased oxygenation could not only provide improvement in hearing but might suppress or abolish tinnitus (22). In addition to cochlear stimulation, transcutaneous nerve stimulation was reported to improve 81% of patients in one study (23) but only 53% (24) and 27% in others (25). Deep brain stimulation has produced variable results (26,27). Low-power (60 mW) transmeatal laser irradiation had no effect in one trial (28) but alternating current (62 Hz to 8000 Hz) applied to the eardrum via a special probe was reported to reduce tinnitus in five of 10 patients (29). Another study found that pulsed electromagnetic stimulation applied to the mastoid bone resulted in improvement in 45% of patients with long-standing tinnitus compared to only 9% of controls in a double-blind, placebo controlled study (30) and this approach is being pursued. Patients with TMJ and cervical spine disorders can present with tinnitus as a primary or secondary complaint (31–34), and although it was assumed that any relief experienced was due to concomitant improvement in craniocervical mandibular pathology, no such consistent correlation has been demonstrated. Because severe tinnitus and chronic pain share so many common characteristics, it has been suggested that pain relief therapies might also benefit tinnitus patients (35,36). As will be seen, the recent report that prompted this review provides some support for this.

The problem is that tinnitus is more of a description than a diagnosis since it is not a discrete disease but rather a symptom of some underlying disorder that usually involves the ear, auditory nerve, or other portion of the brain. The term derives from the Latin word *tinnire*, which means "to ring." Tinnitus may be defined as a ringing, buzzing clicking, popping, blowing or other constant or intermittent sound in one or both ears of varying pitch and intensity. It is essential to differentiate between objective tinnitus, in which the patient hears real sounds and subjective tinnitus, which is much more common and difficult to treat since it has many more causes (34). The pulsatile sounds reported by 4% of tinnitus patients are usually caused by vibrations from turbulent blood flow that reach the cochlea (37), whereas clicking or low pitched sounds often indicate palatal myoclonus or contractions of the tensor tympani or stapedius muscle (38). In general, the term usually refers to subjective tinnitus, or the false perception of sound in the absence of any known acoustic stimulus. The cause and therefore the pathophysiology of subjective tinnitus is usually obscure, which helps to explain why most therapies are ineffective.

Tinnitus occurs in all age groups but seems to increase as we grow older until the age of 70, when it starts to taper off. It is more common in men than women and is present in 12% of men aged 65–74. The incidence is higher in married individuals and although whites are affected more often than blacks, the prevalence in southern states is almost double that reported from northern U.S. regions (3,39). Surveys show that an estimated 13% of children with normal hearing test scores have experienced transient tinnitus, although spontaneous complaints are rare (40). According to the American Tinnitus Association up to 50 million

Americans have probably experienced tinnitus at some time and its persistence or severity cause 12 million to seek medical attention because of interference with sleep, ability to concentrate, job performance, or social interactions (41). Almost three out of four patients are depressed (42) and an estimated 2 million are disabled by the disorder (43).

In evaluating tinnitus therapies it is important to note that adverse effects tend to be greatest in patients who "report physical immobility, sleeplessness, and pain and among those who are depressed or irritable, who are socially isolated, or who have psychiatric symptoms" (44). Special questionnaires have been devised to assess these issues (45). Correcting such problems may cause patients to perceive that they are improved despite the fact that there has been no alteration of the underlying pathophysiology (45,46). As with other subjective complaints, it is always difficult to rule out a placebo effect, especially when the nature of the therapeutic intervention precludes a double-blind study, which is often the case. A recent comprehensive review in the *New England Journal of Medicine* covered various causes of tinnitus, differential diagnostic considerations including the use of sophisticated imaging studies as well as the various treatment options available (3). Although it was emphasized that most cases do not respond to therapy, there was no reference to any electrical stimulation approaches, which reflects the lack of familiarity with this emerging modality.

That is likely to change as a result of the study that prompted this review, which was stimulated by the research showing that tinnitus can persist after ablation of the cochlea and auditory nerve (47,48). As previously noted, stress and emotional factors can influence the patient's perception of the severity of symptoms, as can attentional states (49). These observations suggest that higher centers may be involved in the pathophysiology of tinnitus so that maladaptive cortical reorganization might play an important role (50). In particular, certain similarities with phantom limb pain has led to the concept of *auditory phantom perception* (51,52) and the proposal that chronic tinnitus, like chronic pain, stems from extensive maladaptive attempts at cortical reorganization due to peripheral injury (53). Support for this comes from magnetencephalography studies demonstrating that chronic tinnitus patients exhibit reorganization activities in cortical auditory areas (54) as well as functional imaging investigations showing activation of the temporoparietal cortex specifically during tinnitus pereception (55,56).

In some instances, such as tinnitus associated with various drugs, high or low blood pressure, anemia, diabetes and other endocrine disorders and possibly zinc deficiency, relief is often obtained when the underlying cause is corrected (3,57). However, when tinnitus has persisted for a long time it may affect higher cortical centers that tend to make it self-perpetuating even when the cause is corrected, including removal of an acoustic neuroma (47). All long standing tinnitus may thus be perpetuated by a common pathway and referred to as central tinnitus, "despite the fact that it is initiated by cochlear hearing loss or is localized to the hearing loss ear" (58). Since studies have demonstrated an irregular activation of the temporoparietal cortex (54–56), it was postulated that if this reflected a functionally relevant process responsible for the perception of tinnitus, temporarily blocking this should result in transient reduction or relief.

To test this hypothesis that abnormal brain activity is creating the illusion of sound in the absence of acoustic stimuli, researchers applied 10-Hz repetitive transcranial magnetic stimulation to eight scalp and four control positions in 14 right-handed patients complaining of chronic tinnitus for more than a year (59). Tinnitus was bilateral in 12 patients and left-sided in two patients. Three patients had normal hearing thresholds and the remainder had varying degrees of hearing loss. All patients were blinded to the 3-s stimulation procedure. Tinnitus was temporarily reduced in most of the patients only when the left temporoparietal cortex was stimulated. This supports the theory that this site, which contains several auditory association areas, may be critical for tinnitus perception as suggested by other studies (56–58,60–62). The authors emphasize that this is a preliminary report and that further studies to determine whether different types of stimulation such as rTMS at 1 Hz for several minutes might produce longer inhibition of tinnitus as has been shown for other disorders that respond to this modality (63).

An equally important issue is whether all of the relevant functional areas responsible for tinnitus perception have been targeted. This seems unlikely in view of the small depth of penetration and the sites selected since portions of the auditory cortex are located deep in the Sylvian fissure. Indeed, a very recent study suggests that functional auditory pathways exist in the entire superior temporal gyrus and large portions of the parietal, prefrontal, and limbic lobes, some of which overlap previously identified visual areas (64). Researchers believe that as in the visual system, these may contain separate pathways for processing stimulus quality, location, and motion. The fact that favorable results were obtained by jamming abnormal electrical activity with focused stimulation to only one area is very encouraging. Targeting other sites and changing the parameters of delivery should significantly improve results that may benefit numerous tinnitus patients who are currently told by frustrated physicians to "go home and learn to live with it" (65).

Since this chapter was written, an additional report on the successful treatment of tinnitus with rTMS has also been published (Eichhammer P, Langguth B, Marienhagen J, Kleinjung T, Hajak G. Neuronavigated repetitive transcranial magnetic stimulation in patients with tinnitus: A short case series. Biol Psychiatry 2003 Oct 15; 54: 862).

REFERENCES

1. Konopka W, Zalewski P, Olszewski J, Olszewska-Ziaber A, Pietkiewicz P. Tinnitus suppression by electrical promontory stimulation (EPS) in patients with sensorineural hearing loss. Auris Nasus Larynx 2001 Jan; 28(1):35–40.
2. Aldini J. Essai theorique et expérimental sur le galvanisme, avec une série d'expériences faites en presence des commisaires de l'Institut national de France, et en divers amphithéatres anatomiques de Londres Paris, De l'Impr. de Fournier, 1804.
3. Lockwood AH, Salvi RJ, Burkard RF. Tinnitus. N Engl J Med 2002; 347:904–910.
4. Zenner HR, Ernst A. Cochlea-motor, transduction and sdignal-transfer tinnitus: models for three types of cochlear tinnitus. Eur Arch Otorhinolaryngol 1993; 249:447–454.
5. Eggermont JJ. On the pathophysiology of tinnitus: a review and a peripheral model. Hear Res 1990; 48:111–124.
6. Ito J, Sakakihara J. Suppression of tinnitus by cochlear implantation. Am J Otolaryngol 1994 Mar–Apr; 15(2):145–148.
7. Vernon JA. Masking of tinnitus through a cochlear implant. J Am Acad Audiol 2000 Jun; 11(6):293–294.
8. Sakajiri M, Imamura T, Hirata Y, Izumi T, Ifukube T, Matsushima J. A method for suppressing tinnitus by electrical stimulation to cochlea and remedial value. Journal of the Acoustical Soc Japan 1993; 14(6):453–455.
9. Matsushima JI, Fujimura H, Sakai N, Suganuma T, Hayashi M, Ifukube T, Hirata Y, Miyoshi S. A study of electrical promontory stimulation in tinnitus patients. Auris Nasus Larynx 1994; 21(1):17–24.
10. House JW. Therapies for tinnitus. Am J Otol 1989; 10(3):163–165. Ito J, Sakahikara J. Tinnitus suppression by electrical stimulation of the cochlear wall and by cohclear implantation. Laryngoscope 1994;104(6):752–754.
11. Balkany T, Banti H. Direct electrical stimulation of the inner ear for the relief of tinnitus. Am J Otol 1987; 8(3):207–1212.

12. Okusa M, Shiraishi T, Kubo T, Matsunaga T. Tinnitus suppression by electrical promontory stimulation in sensorineural deaf patients. Acta Otolaryngol 1993; 501:54–58.

13. Hazell JW, Meerton LJ, Conway MJ. Electrical tinnitus suppression (ETS) with a single channel cochlear implant. J Laryngol Otol 1989; 18:39–44.

14. Zwolan TA, Kileny PR, Souliere CR JR, Kemink H. Tinnitus suppression following cochlear implantation. In: Aran J-M, Dauman R, eds. Tinnitus 91: Proceedings of the Fourth International Tinnitus Seminar. The Netherlands. Amsterdam: Kugler Publications, 1992:417–442.

15. Portman M, Casals Y, Negrevergne M, Aran JM. Temporary tinnitus suppression in man through electrical stimulation of the cochlea. Acta Otolaryngol 1979; 87:294–299.

16. Matsushima J, Sakai N, Sakajiri M, Miyoshi S, Uemi N, Ifukube T. An experience of the usage of electrical tinnitus suppressor. Artificial Organs 1996; 20(8):955–958.

17. Battner RD, Heerman R, Laszig R. Suppression of tinnitus by electric stimulation in cochlear implant patients. HNO 1989; 37(4):148–152.

18. Casals Y, Negrevergne M, Aran JM. Electrical stimulation of the cochlea in man: hearing introduction and tinnitus suppression. J Am Audiol Soc 1978; 3:209–213.

19. Hazell JW, Jastreboff PJ, Meerton LE, Conway MJ. Electrical tinnitus suppression: frequency dependence of effects. Audiology 1993; 32(1):68–77.

20. Watanabe K, Okawara D, Baba S, Yagi T. Electrocochleographic analysis of the suppression of tinnitus by elecgrical promontory stimulation. Audiology 1997; 36(3):147–154.

21. Roddy J, Hubard AE, Mountain DC, Xue S. Effects of electrical biasing on electrically-evoked otoacoustic emissions. Hear Res 1994; 73(2):148–154.

22. Vavrina J, Muller W. Therapeutic effect of hyperbaric oxygenation in acute acoustic trauma. Rev Laryngol Otol Rhinol 1995; 116(5):377–380.

23. Engelberg M, Bauer W. Transcutaneous electrical stimulation for tinnitus. Laryngoscope 1985; 95(10):1167–1173.

24. Steenerson RL, Cronin GW. Treatment of tinnitus with electrical stimulation. Otolaryngol Head Neck Surg 1999 Nov; 121(5):511–513.

25. Rahko T, Kotti V. Tinnitus treatment by transcutaneous nerve stimulation (TNS). Acta Otolaryngol Suppl 1997; 529:88–89.

26. Shi Y-B, Martin WH. Deep brain stimulation for tinnitus. Neurology 2000; 54(7 suppl 3):A169.

27. Soussi T, Otto SR. Effects of electrical brainstem stimulation on tinnitus. Acta Otolaryngol 1994; 114(2):135–140.

28. Nakashima T, Ueda H, Misawa H, Suzuki T, Tominaga M. Transmeatal low-power laser irradiation for tinnitus. Otol Neurotol May 2002; 23(3):296–300.

29. Kuk FK, Tyler RS, Rustad N, Harker LA, Tye-Murray N. Alternating current at the eardrum for tinnitus reduction. J Speech Hearing Res 1989; 32(2):393–400.

30. Roland NJ, Hughes JB, Daley MB, Cook JA, Jones AS, McCormick MS. Electromagnetic stimulation as a treatment of tinnitus: a pilot study. Clini Otolaryngol 1993; 18:278–281.

31. Gelb H, Gelb ML, Wagner ML. The relationship of tinnitus to craniocervical mandibular disorders. Cranio 1997 Apr; 15(2):136–143.

32. Vernon J, Griest S, Press L. Attributes of tinnitus that may predict temporomandibular joint dysfunction. Cranio 1992 Oct; 10(4):282–287. Discussion 287–288.

33. Vernon J, Griest S, Press L. Attributes of tinnitus associated with the temporomandibular joint syndrome. Eur Arch Otorhinolaryngol 1992; 249(2):93–94.

34. Marsot-Dupuch K. Pulsatile and nonpulsatile tinnitus. Semin Ultrasound 2001; 22:250–270.

35. Moller AR. Similarities between chronic pain and tinnitus. Am J Otol 1997 Sep; 18(5):577–585.

36. Moller AR. Similarities between severe tinnitus and chronic pain. J Am Acad Audiol 2000 Mar; 11(3):115–124.

37. Stoufler JL, Tyler RS. Characteristics of tinnitus by tinnitus patients. J Speech Hear Disord 1990; 55:439–453.

38. Fox GN, Baer MT. Palatal myoclonus and tinnitus in children. West J Med 1991; 154:98–102.

39. Adams PE, Hendershot GE, Marano MA. Current Estimates from the National Health Inventory Survey, 1996. Hyatsville Md.: National Center for Health Statistics, 1999.

40. Baguley DM, McFerran DJ. Tinnitus in childhood. Int J Pediatr Otorhinolaryngol 1999; 49:99–105.
41. Sanders BT. There is something you can do about tinnitus (www.healthyhearing.com).
42. Recent tinnitus surveys (www.ata.com).
43. Voss M. Tinnitus. In: Jafek B, ed. ENT Secrets. Philadelphia, Pa: Hanley & Belfus, 1996:58–61.
44. Holgers KM, Erlandsson ST, Barrenas Ml. Predictive factors for the severity of tinnitus. Audiology 2000; 39:284–291.
45. Sullivan M, Katon W, Russo J, Dobie R, Sakal C. A randomized trial of nortriptyline for severe chronic tinnitus:effects on depression, disability and tinnitus symptoms. Arch Int Med 1993; 153:2251–2259.
46. Folmer RG, Griest SG, Meikle MB, Martin WH. Tinnitus severity, loudness and depression. Otolaryngol Head Neck Surg 1999; 121:48–51.
47. Matthies C, Samii M. Management of 1000 vestibular schwannomas (acoustic neuromas): clinical presentation. Neurosurgery 1997; 40:1–9.
48. Lenarz T, Schreiner C, Snyder RL. Neural mechanisms of tinnitus. Eur Arch Otorhinolaryngol 1993; 249:441–446.
49. Newman CW, Wharton JA, Jacobson GP. Self-focused and somatic attention in patients with tinnius. J Am Acad Audiol 1997; 8:143–149.
50. Rauschecker JP. Auditory cortical plasticity: a comparison with other sensory systems. Trends Neurosci 1999; 22:74–80.
51. Jastreboff PJ. Phantom auditory perception (tinnitus): mechanisms of generation and perception. Neurosci Res 1990; 8:221–254.
52. Folmer RL, Griest SE, Martin WH. Chronic tinnitus as phantom auditory pain. Otolaryngol Head Neck Surg 2001; 124:394–400.
53. Moller AR. Similarities between severe tinnitus and chronic pain. J Am Acad Audiol 2000; 11:115–124.
54. Muhlmickel W, Ebert T, Taub E. Reorganization of auditory cortex in tinnitus. Proc Soc Nat Acad Sci USA 1998; 95:10340–10343.
55. Giraud AL, Chery CS, Fischer G. A selective imaging of tinnitus. Neuroreport 1999; 10:1–5.
56. Mirz F, Pederson B, Ishizu K. Positron emission tomography of cortical centers of tinnitus. Hear Res 1999; 134:133–144.
57. Ochi K, Kinoshita H, Kenmochi M, Nishino H, Ohashi T. Zinc deficiency and tinnitus. Auris Nasus Larynx 2003; 30:25–28.
58. Eggermont JJ. Central tinnitus. Auris Nasus Larynx 2003; 30:7–12.
59. Plewnia C, Bartels M, Gerloff C. Transient suppression of tinnitus by transcranial magnetic stimulation. Ann Neurol 2003; 53:263–266.
60. Arnold W, Bartenstein P, Oestricher E. Focal metabolic activation in the predominant left auditory cortex in patients with suffering from tinnitus: a PET study with [18F]deoxyglucose. ORL (Basel) 1996; 58:195–199.
61. Andersson G, Lyttkens L, Hirvela C. Regional cerebral blood flow during tinnitus: a PET case study with lidocaine and auditory stimulation. Acta Otolaryngol 2000; 120:967–972.
62. Gardener A, Pagani M, Jacobson H. Differences in resting state regional cerebral blood flow assessed with 99mTc-HMPAO SPECT and brain atlas matching between depressed patients with and without tinnitus. Nucl Med Commun 2002; 23:429–439.
63. Siebner HR, Tormos JM, Ceballos-Baumann AO. Low frequency repetitive magnetic stimulation of the motor cortex in writer's cramp. Neurology 1999; 52:529–537.
64. Poremba A, Saunders RC, Crane M, Cooke M, Sokoloff L, Mishkin M. Functional mapping of the primate auditory system. Science 2003; 299:568–572.
65. Brody J. New hope for quieting the roaring in the ears. New York Times 2002 October 29; F7.

21

Low-Energy Emission Therapy: Current Status and Future Directions

Boris Pasche and Alexandre Barbault

Symtonic S.A., Renens, Switzerland

Low energy emission therapy (LEET) is a novel approach that noninvasively administers very low levels of electromagnetic energy to the hypothalamic pituitary-area via an intrabuccal electrode. Polysomnography studies at leading sleep centers demonstrating significant increases in total sleep time have confirmed its clinical efficacy, as demonstrated in double-blind insomnia trials. Other double-blind studies using different clusters of amplitude modulated electromagnetic fields have also shown efficacy and safety in the treatment of anxiety disorders. Long-term follow-up reveals no adverse side effects, rebound, or addictive tendencies.

Low-energy emission therapy (LEET) is a new method to administer low levels of electromagnetic energy. It consists of amplitude-modulated electromagnetic fields delivered intrabuccally by means of an electrically conducting mouthpiece in direct contact with the oral mucosa. The LEET device is a battery-powered device emitting a carrier frequency of 27.12 MHz, which is modulated at specific frequencies between 0.1 and 300 Hz.

LEET therapeutic efficacy relies on two major advances in the field of bioelectromagnetics:

1. A safe and user-friendly method to administer well-defined levels of electromagnetic energy to humans
2. The discovery of specific clusters of modulation frequencies with therapeutic effects in insomnia and anxiety disorders

The treatment of chronic psychophysiological insomnia presents a challenge that has not been met using currently available pharmacotherapy. LEET has been initially developed as a potential alternative for this disorder.

The first evidence of LEET's clinical effects was demonstrated on 104 healthy volunteers at two different centers who received 15 min of either active of inactive LEET treatment.

Electroencephalographs obtained during the 15-min period following LEET treatment showed decreased sleep latency and a deeper sleep than following placebo treatment (1,2). LEET treatment was also associated with objective and subjective feelings of relaxation (3).

The effects of LEET on chronic insomnia were assessed with polysomnography (PSG) on a total of 106 patients at two different centers (4). Active or inactive LEET was administered for 20 min in late afternoon three times a week for a total of 12 treatments. There was a significant increase in total sleep time as assessed by PSG between baseline and posttreatment values for the active treatment group (76.0 ± 11.1 minutes, $p = 0.0001$). The increase for the inactive group was not statistically significant. There was also a significant decrease in sleep latency as assessed by PSG between baseline and posttreatment values for the active treatment group (-21.6 min ± 5.9 min, $p = 0.0006$), whereas the decrease noted for the inactive treatment group was not statistically significant. Interestingly, the number of physiological sleep cycles per night increased by 30% after active treatment ($p = 0.0001$) but was unchanged following inactive treatment. Subjects did not experience rebound insomnia, and there were no significant side effects. Hence, LEET was able to effectively improve the sleep of chronic insomniacs by increasing the number of sleep cycles without altering the percentage of the various sleep stages during the night. The therapeutic action of LEET differs from that of currently available therapies in that the sleep pattern noted in insomniacs following LEET treatment more closely resembles nocturnal physiological sleep.

Studies of LEET for the treatment of anxiety are in progress. LEET was tested in an open label pilot study performed on ten patients suffering from chronic anxiety. The patients received a 15-min treatment in the morning and a 30-min treatment in the evening every day for 6 weeks. Recent results show that the anxiety level as measured with the Hamilton Anxiety Scale (HAM-A) improved by more than 50% in 61% of the patients at the end of the first week and in 90% of the patients by the end of the third week. A double-blind study conducted on 30 patients showed a trend towards significant HAM-A improvement favoring the active treatment group and a significant improvement of the clinical global impression (CGI).

LEET is an efficacious new therapy for chronic insomnia and shows promising potential for anxiety disorders.

The medical use of radiofrequency (RF) electromagnetic fields (EMF) has become more common in recent decades. Magnetic resonance imaging (MRI) devices that emit amplitude modulated frequencies between 20 and 100 MHz have become standard diagnostic tools, and even such procedures as the ablation of abnormally conducting pathway in the heart rely on RF EMF (5).

Empirical and scientific data on the ability of electromagnetic fields to interact with and influence biological systems dates back to the 1920s, but the first effort to convert theory to practical application occurred when we assembled a small multidisciplinary team of physicians, engineers, and physicists in 1982 to investigate the biological effects of very low levels of radio-frequency electromagnetic (RFEM) fields. We hypothesized that the human body may be able to sense low level of amplitude-modulated electromagnetic fields. We hypothesized that the biological effects of low levels RFEM are likely mediated by yet undiscovered receptor mechanisms. The initial application approach was the stimulation of the nasal mucosa by means of magnetic, electric, or photonic energy. We then developed an intrabuccal probe allowing the homogeneous administration of very low levels of amplitude-modulated RFEM; the concept of low energy emission therapy (LEET) was born. Interest was further stimulated by the discovery of studies conducted by Dr. Ross Adey and coworkers suggesting that very low levels of amplitude-modulated electromagnetic fields could both modify the electroencephalographic activity and increase the release of ions and neurotransmitters from nerve cells when applied to the brain of different species of animals (6).

The Symtonic research team decided to initiate tests on healthy volunteers in Switzerland as early as 1983 with levels of RFEM fields exposure far below the limits of international safety standards. In collaboration with the Swiss Federal Institute of Technology in Zurich, the team also improved over the years its technology for the delivery of RFEM fields by means of an intrabuccal antenna to achieve minimal interpatient variability with respect to the absorption of RF EMF. The researchers began to experiment with both the individual RFEM variables (amplitude, frequencies, etc.) and the means to deliver the treatment. The result was the Symtonic LEET device which serves as both the energy source and the controller of the treatment (Fig. 1). The method consists in the administration of electromagnetic fields by means of an electrically conducting mouthpiece in direct contact with the oral mucosa (Fig. 2). During that time the team undertook the development of a proprietary technology which enabled the researchers to identify the frequencies of modulation most likely to induce a sleep-restoring or anti-anxiety effect. Using this method we identified several modulation frequencies comprised between 0.5 and 300 Hz and tested them in a series a pilot studies conducted on healthy subjects. A preliminary report on a prototype of the present device was presented by Dr. Paul Rosch at a 1984 conference on Electromagnetic Fields and Neurobehavioral Function in Corsendonk, Belgium (7) and at the First International Montreux Congress on Stress sponsored by the American Institute of Stress and Biotonus Clinic in Montreux, where some early clinical studies had been conducted (8).

We validated these findings in double-blind crossover studies performed again on healthy subjects. The sleep electroencephalogram (EEG) of a 15-min treatment with a single frequency was tested in two separate double-blind crossover studies performed in the United States and in Switzerland (1,2). In each study 52 healthy volunteers were exposed to both

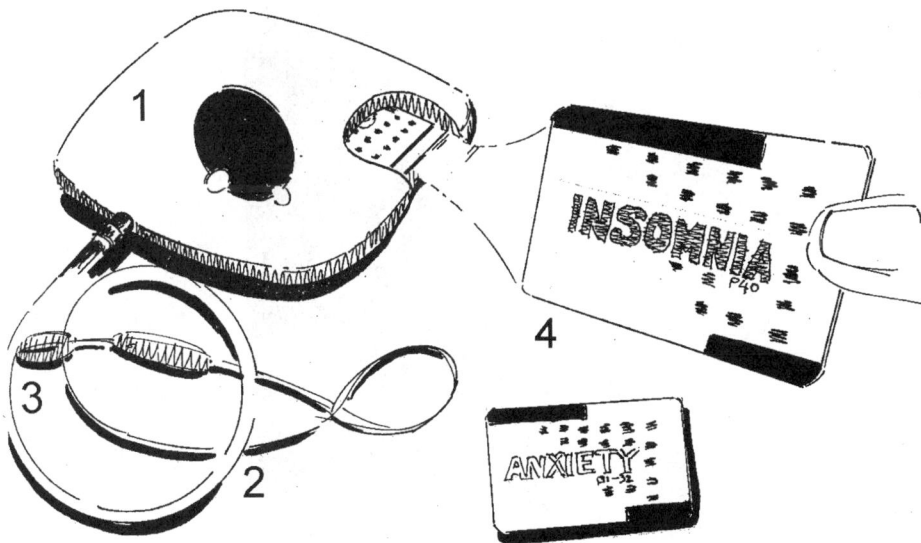

Figure 1   The Symtonic LEET device consists of (1) an emitting box connected to (2) a coaxial cable, which ends with (3) a spoonlike metallic mouthpiece. Different combinations of frequencies (programs) are used to treat (4) insomnia and anxiety.

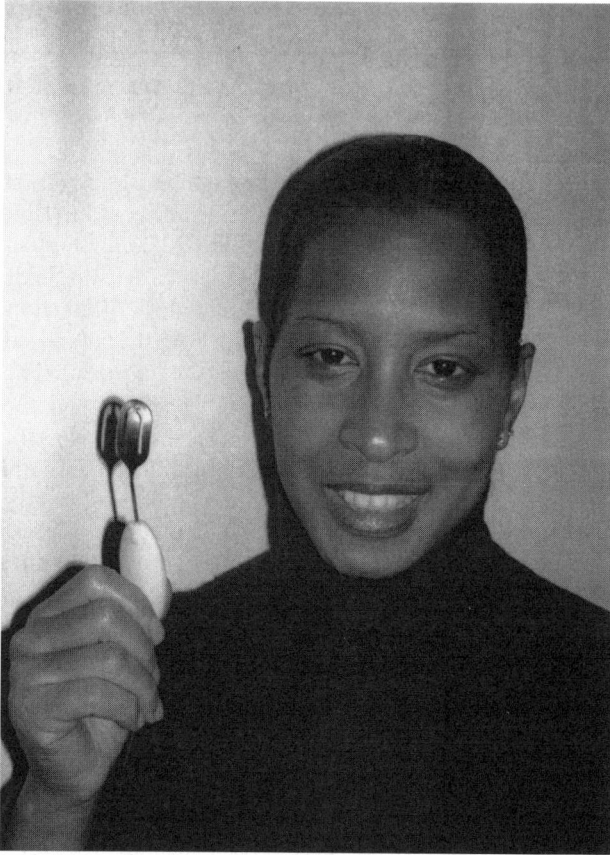

(a)

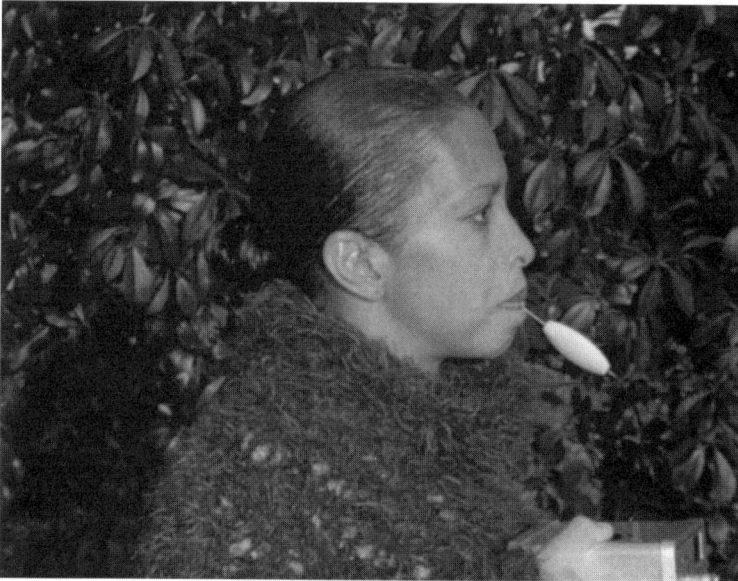

(b)

Figure 2 Patient receiving Symtonic LEET treatment: (a) Patient holds mouthpiece in hand prior to treatment and (b) patient holds mouthpiece in mouth during treatment.

active and inactive LEET treatment sessions, with a minimum interval of 1 week between the 2 sessions. Baseline EEGs where obtained, and 15-min posttreatment EEGs were recorded and analyzed according to the Loomis classification.

In the first study a significant decrease in sleep latency two stage B2 (-1.78 ± 5.57 min, $p = 0.013$) and an increase in the total duration of stage B2 (1.15 ± 2.47 min, $p = 0.0008$) were observed on active treatment as compared with inactive treatment. The deepest sleep state achieved (B1 to D) following active treatment was also significantly higher than that following inactive treatment ($p = 0.040$). In the second study, a significant increase in the duration of stage B1 sleep (0.58 ± 2.42 min, $p = 0.046$), decreased latency to the first 10 s epoch of sleep (-1.23 ± 5.32 min, $p = 0.051$) and decreased latency to sleep stage B2 (minus 1.21 ± 5.25 min, $p = 0.052$) were observed after active treatment. A combined analysis of these two studies showed that LEET had a significant effect on afternoon sleep induction and maintenance with shorter sleep latencies, an increased duration of stage B2, an increase in the total duration of sleep, and a more prominent establishment of slow waves with progression to a deeper sleep stage. Analysis of these two studies concluded that the intermittent 42.7-Hz amplitude modulations of 27.12-MHz electromagnetic fields results in electroencephalographic changes consistent with shorter sleep latencies, longer sleep duration, and deeper sleep in healthy subjects (2).

This single-frequency treatment was further tested on patients with chronic physiological insomnia. Two double-blind studies failed to confirm any significant changes in total sleep time or sleep latency between the active and inactive treatment group (data on file, Symtonic S.A.). This prompted the design a new treatment program (P40) made of the four most promising frequencies for insomnia, including 42.7 Hz. This combination of frequencies was first tested on a group of 30 patients (9), then in a double-blind, randomized, multicenter study on a total of 106 patients suffering from chronic psychophysiological insomnia (4). Active or inactive LEET was administered for 20 min in late afternoon three times a week for a total of 12 treatments.

Primary efficacy endpoints evaluating the results were changes from baseline in PSG-assessed total sleep time and sleep latency. Secondary endpoints were changes in sleep efficiency, sleep stages, and subjective reports of sleep latency and total sleep time. There was a significant increase in total sleep time as assessed by polysomnography between baseline and posttreatment values for the active treatment group (76.0 ± 11.1 min, $p = 0.0001$). The increase for the inactive treatment group was not statistically significant. The total sleep time improvement was significantly greater for the active group when compared to the inactive group (adjusted for baseline total sleep time; $p = 0.020$, $R^2 = 0.20$). There was a significant decrease in sleep latency as assessed by polysomnography between baseline and posttreatment values for the active treatment group (-21.6 ± 5.9 min, $p = 0.0006$), whereas the decrease noted to the inactive treatment group was not statistically significant. The difference in sleep latency between the two treatment groups was marginally significant (adjusted for baseline sleep latency and center; $p = 0.068$, $R^2 = 0.60$). The number of sleep cycles per night increased by 30% after active treatment ($p = 0.0001$) but was unchanged following inactive treatment. Subjects did not experience rebound insomnia, and there was no significant side effects.

This study showed that LEET was safe and well tolerated and effectively improved the sleep of chronic insomniacs given at 12 treatments over a 4-week period by increasing the number of sleep cycles without altering the percentage of the various sleep stages during the night. It was concluded that the therapeutic action of LEET differs from that of currently available drug therapies in that the sleep pattern noted in insomniacs following LEET treatment more closely resembles nocturnal physiological sleep. This study indicated that

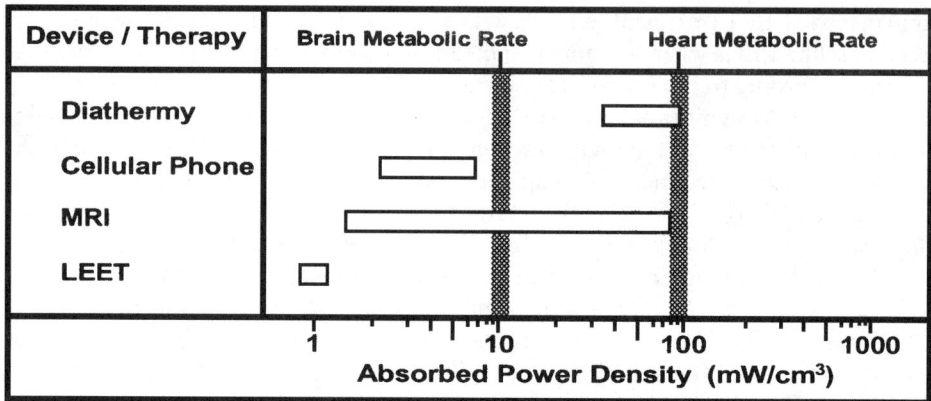

Figure 3 Comparison of power density ranges for diathermy, cellular phones, MRI, and LEET. Estimated absorbed power density ranges for therapeutic diathermy, cellular phones, and magnetic resonance imaging (MRI), as compared to low-energy emission therapy (LEET). Incident power density for MRI is highly dependent on frequency and pulse characteristics. The range shown here is for a 100-MHz device. Approximate brain and heart metabolic rates are shown for comparison. This plot is on a log scale.

LEET may offer an attractive alternative therapy for chronic insomnia (4). Analysis of sleep rating forms showed that the average user of LEET experiences subjective sleep improvement only after several treatment sessions, suggesting that the primary indication of this therapy might be chronic insomnia (10).

Studies of LEET for the treatment of anxiety are in progress. LEET was tested in an open label pilot study performed on 10 patients suffering from chronic anxiety. The patients received a 15-min treatment in the morning and a 30-min treatment in the evening every day for 6 weeks. Recent results show that the anxiety level as measured with the Hamilton Anxiety Scale (HAM-A) improved by more than 50% in 61% of the patients at the end of the first week and in 90% of the patients by the end of the third week. Preliminary analysis of a double-blind study conducted on 30 patients showed a trend towards significant HAM-A improvement favoring the active treatment group and a significant improvement of the Clinical Global Impression (CGI) (data on file, Symtonic S.A.).

LEET results in levels of absorbed electromagnetic energy in the brain that are approximately 100 to 1000 times lower than those generated by handheld cellular phones (Fig. 3). Retrospective analysis of more than 400 patients treated with LEET over several years does not indicate any increased risk of either cancer or cardiovascular disease (11). The only noticeable side effect reported in several studies has been increased dreaming (data on file, Symtonic S.A.).

LEET is emerging as a promising safe and effective new therapy for insomnia. Ongoing studies on patients with generalized anxiety disorders will determine its potential usefulness in this area.

ACKNOWLEDGMENTS

This work was supported by Symtonic S.A., Avenue des Baumettes 9, CH-1020-Lausanne, Switzerland. Disclaimer: Dr. Pasche and Dr. Barbault own Symtonic S.A. stocks.

REFERENCES

1. Reite M, Higgs L, Lebet JP, Barbault A, Rossel C, Kuster N, Dafni U, Amato D, Pasche B. Sleep inducing effect of low energy emission therapy. Bioelectromagnetics 1994; 15:67–75.
2. Lebet JP, Barbault A, Rossel C, Tomic Z, Reite M, Higgs L, Dafni U, Amato D, Pasche B. Electroencephalographic changes following low energy emission therapy. Ann Biomed Eng 1996; 24:424–429.
3. Higgs L, Reite M, Barbault A, Lebet J-P, Rossel C, Amato D, Dafni U, Pasche B. Subjective and objective relaxation effects of low energy emission therapy. Stress Med 1994; 10:5–13.
4. Pasche B, Erman M, Hayduk R, Mitler M, Reite M, Higgs L, Dafni U, Amato D, Rossel C, Kuster N, Barbault A, Lebet JP. Effects of low energy emission therapy in chronic psychophysiological insomnia. Sleep 1996; 19:327–336.
5. Lesh MD. Interventional electrophysiology—state-of-the-art 1993. Am Heart J 1993; 126:686–698.
6. Adey WR. Biological effects of electromagnetic fields. J Cell Biochem 1993; 51:410–416.
7. Rosch P. J. Electromagnetic waves and neurobehavioral function: comments from clinical medicine. In: O'Connor ME, Lovely H, eds. Electromagnetic Fields and Neurobehavioral Function. New York: Alan R. Liss, 1988:377–388.
8. Pasche B. The physiological effects of low energy emission therapy (LEET). First International Montreux Congress on Stress, 1988.
9. Pasche B, Erman M, Mitler M. Diagnosis and management of insomnia. N Engl J Med 1990; 323:486–487.
10. Koziol JA, Erman M, Pasche B, Hajdukovic R, Mitler MM. Assessing a changepoint in a sequence of repeated measurements with application to a low-energy emission therapy sleep study. J Applied Statistics 1993; 20:393–400.
11. Amato D, Pasche B. An evaluation of the safety of low energy emission therapy [published erratum appears in Compr Ther 1994; 20(12):681]. Compr Ther 1993; 19:242–247.

22

Vagus Nerve Stimulation for the Treatment of Epilepsy

Steven C. Schachter

Harvard Medical School, Boston, Massachusetts, U.S.A.

Vagus nerve stimulation (VNS) is the first non-pharmacological treatment to be approved by the FDA as safe and effective for the treatment of partial-onset seizures resistant to drug treatment. Mechanisms of action, neuroimaging studies, and long-term results are discussed, as well as the efficacy of VNS for other types of epilepsy and associated complaints such as depression.

I. INTRODUCTION

The 1990s witnessed an unprecedented release of new antiepileptic drugs (AEDs) for the treatment of epilepsy, a disorder characterized by recurrent seizures that occurs in 0.5–1% of the population. Nonetheless, a sizable proportion of patients with epilepsy, specifically those whose seizures arise from a focal area of the brain (called *partial-onset seizures*), have not benefited from new pharmacological treatments and continue to have medically refractory epilepsy (1,2). Prior to 1997, the available nonpharmacological approaches for such patients included surgical excision of the seizure-generating brain tissue (epilepsy surgery) (3), electrical stimulation of the cerebellum (4) or thalamus (5), and a high-fat, low-carbohydrate diet (the ketogenic diet). However, some patients refuse intracranial surgery and others are not good candidates based on test results, the efficacy, and safety of deep brain stimulation is not proven, and adults do not generally respond to the ketogenic diet.

In 1997, the VNS Therapy System (Cyberonics, Inc), formerly known as the Neurocybernetic Prosthesis, was approved by the FDA as adjunctive therapy for adults and adolescents over 12 years of age whose partial-onset seizures were refractory to AEDs. Vagus nerve stimulation (VNS) thus became the first nonpharmacological epilepsy treatment to be recognized by the FDA as safe and effective. VNS therapy is also approved in numerous European Union countries for use in reducing the frequency of seizures in patients whose epileptic disorder is dominated by partial seizures, and in Canada for similar patients who do not have adequate seizure control with AED therapy. This chapter reviews the relevant anatomy of the vagus nerve, the mechanism of action of VNS, pre-clinical experiments, and the results of clinical trials in patients with epilepsy.

II. RELEVANT ANATOMY AND PHYSIOLOGY

The vagus nerve is a mixed nerve consisting of about 80% sensory fibers that provide the brain with visceral sensation from the head, neck, thorax, and abdomen. The right vagus innervates the cardiac atria more so than the left vagus nerve, whereas the left vagus nerve provides predominant innervation of the ventricles (6). Consequently, stimulation of the left vagus would be predicted to be less likely to cause deleterious cardiac effects. This prediction is borne out by clinical experience.

The nodose ganglion contains the cell bodies of the sensory axons in the vagus nerve. These cell bodies relay sensory information to the nucleus of the solitary tract (NTS), which in turn relays the information via three main pathways (7). Of greatest potential importance to the action of VNS in patients with epilepsy is the pathway that ascends to the forebrain by means of the parabrachial nucleus, which is in the dorsal pons lateral to the locus coeruleus (7). The parabrachial nucleus also provides direct input to several components of the thalamus, including the ventroposterior parvocellular nucleus, which acts as a relay for visceral sensation to the insular cortex (8), an area often affected by partial-onset seizures.

The parabrachial nucleus also projects to the intralaminar nuclei of the thalamus (9). This pathway possibly has more widespread effects on cortical activity, because the intralaminar nuclei project widely into the cerebral cortex. Other projections from the parabrachial nucleus and the NTS provide visceral sensation to the hypothalamus, amygdala, and basal forebrain; the latter two regions are often involved in partial-onset seizures. Finally, both the lateral hypothalamus and basal forebrain contain neurons that project diffusely to the cerebral cortex, and these pathways also have the potential to influence overall cortical activity (10).

The brain circuitry that is activated during VNS has been mapped using c-fos expression as a marker (11). Other work has suggested that the locus coeruleus is critically involved in the anticonvulsant effects of VNS, possibly through the release of norepinephrine (12).

III. MECHANISM OF ACTION

A. Neurophysiological Studies

Early experiments in animals showed that repetitive vagus stimulation could synchronize or desynchronize the electroencephalogram (EEG), depending on stimulus frequency and current strength (i.e. which in turn determined the fiber types in the vagus nerve that were recruited) (13–15). Specifically, high-intensity, high-frequency (>70 Hz) vagus stimulation produced desynchronization of the cortical EEG in cats, but lower intensity stimulation at the same rate caused synchronization. These studies suggested a possible benefit of VNS against seizures, because desynchronization is generally viewed as having an anticonvulsant effect, and prompted study in animal models of epilepsy.

More recent work has focused on cortical neurophysiology. In rats, low-intensity trains of VNS (100 μA, 30 Hz, 500 μs, 20 s on time) hyperpolarize pyramidal neurons of the parietal association cortex (16). Interestingly, stimulus intensities that predominantly activate myelinated fibers are more effective in inducing long-lasting inhibitory effects than higher stimulus intensities that also activate nonmyelinated vagus afferents. These findings are consistent with the observation that VNS suppressed pentylenetetrazol-induced seizures in rats pretreated with capsaicin, an agent that produces selective excitotoxic lesions of afferent C fibers (17).

Whereas previous studies in humans failed to find an effect of VNS on EEG background rhythms, Olejniczak and colleagues found that VNS affected interictal epileptiform activity (patterns of electrical activity associated with epilepsy) (18). They studied a patient with left temporal lobe-onset seizures who underwent depth electrode monitoring. Reduced interictal epileptiform activity was seen from the left hippocampus with 30-Hz stimulation of the left vagus nerve, while 5-Hz stimulation was associated with increased activity from the same site.

B. Neuroimaging Studies

The effects of VNS on activation of human CNS structures have been studied using positron-emission tomography (PET) scanning. Reports of changes in regional blood flow during VNS have been inconsistent: one study noted increased flow in the ipsilateral anterior thalamus and cingulate cortex (19), and another noted increased flow in the contralateral thalamus and temporal cortex and ipsilateral putamen and cerebellum (20) However, of five patients in one study, two had electrographic seizures during image acquisition (19). Whether the stimulator was activating the same fiber subset in all patients is not certain. Also, the possibility exists that VNS alters cerebral blood flow in ways that are different from changes in local neuronal activation (21,22) Anatomic localization with PET is primitive relative to the small structures examined.

Ring and colleagues obtained SPECT with particular attention to thalamic and insular regions in seven subjects treated for at least 6 months with VNS (23). Rapid cycling stimulation (7 s on, 12 s off) was associated with decreased regional cerebral blood flow (rCBF) in the medial thalamic regions bilaterally. Vonck et al. also found evidence on SPECT scans of thalamic hypoperfusion with stimulation, and noted that the degree of rCBF changes did not correlate with seizure reduction (24). By contrast, Henry et al found relationships using PET scans between bilateral thalamic changes and reductions in seizure frequency (25), as well as between stimulation parameters and both chronicity of stimulation and the volumes of activation and deactivation sites (26,27).

Bohning et al have demonstrated the feasibility of recording VNS-synchronized fMRI (28). In a cohort of nine patients enrolled in a depression protocol, they found blood oxygenation level-dependent responses to VNS in bilateral orbitofrontal and parieto-occipital cortices, left temporal cortex, the hypothalamus, and the left amygdala. Further studies in patients with epilepsy should take advantage of this technique.

IV. EFFICACY OF VNS IN ANIMAL MODELS OF EPILEPSY

VNS was studied in several animal models of epilepsy, typically just before or after seizures occurred (29–32). In other studies, the relationship between VNS and the extent of stimulation and the temporal persistence of anticonvulsant effects was evaluated (33,34), which is of particular relevance to human epilepsy. For example, right VNS was administered at the onset of each spontaneous seizure or at least every 3 h for 40 s in an alumina-gel monkey model of spontaneous partial and secondarily generalized seizures (33). In two of four monkeys, seizures were completely controlled; in the other two, the frequency of seizures was reduced. In all animals, the prophylactic anticonvulsant effect continued after cessation of the applied stimulus to the vagus nerve. In another study, Takaya and colleagues (34) demonstrated a relationship between the cumulative duration of VNS and its anticonvulsant effect.

V. VNS EFFICACY STUDIES IN PATIENTS WITH EPILEPSY

Proof of principle trials began in 1988 (35). The first pivotal trial of VNS was the E03 study (36–39) and the second pivotal clinical study was the E05 study (40). In 1991, a compassionate-use trial enrolled 124 patients with all types of intractable seizures (the E04 study) (41).

The E03 and E05 studies were multicenter, blinded, randomized, active-control trials that compared two different VNS stimulation protocols for the treatment of medically refractory partial-onset seizures: high stimulation (30 Hz, 30 s on, 5 min off, 500-μs pulse width) and low stimulation (1 Hz, 30 s on, 90–180 min off, 130-μs pulse width). The hypothesis was that the low-stimulation treatment was less effective than the high-stimulation treatment. Study candidates had their seizure frequencies monitored prospectively for 12–16 weeks. They then underwent implantation with the VNS therapy system. Two weeks later, study patients were randomized to receive either high or low stimulation. Over the next 2 weeks, those patients randomized to the high-stimulation group had their generator output current increased as high as could be tolerated, whereas those randomized to the low-stimulation group had the current increased only to the point that stimulation could be perceived. The effect of VNS on seizure frequency was then measured during the remaining 12 weeks of the treatment phase. At the conclusion of the study, patients were eligible to enter long-term open studies.

A. Enrollment Information

Patients enrolled in the E03 and E05 studies were at least 12 years of age, had at least six seizures per month, and were taking one to three AEDs at the time the study began. In the E05 study, patients had to have partial seizures with alteration of consciousness (called *complex partial seizures*) to enroll. In the E03 study, 125 patients were enrolled; 114 completed the prospective baseline and were implanted. The average duration of epilepsy was 23 years for patients in the high-stimulation group ($n = 54$) and 20 years for the low-stimulation group ($n = 60$). Patients in both groups were taking a mean of 2.1 AEDs at study entry. In the E05 study, 254 patients were entered, including 55 who were discontinued from baseline for failing protocol eligibility, and 199 patients were implanted. The demographics for patients in the high-stimulation group ($n = 95$) and those in the low-stimulation (n = 103) were consistent with the E03 study.

B. Results During the Three-Month Blinded Treatment Phase

In both studies, the primary measure of efficacy was the percentage change in seizure frequency during VNS treatment compared to the preimplantation baseline. Changes in seizure frequencies in the high- and low-stimulation groups were then compared in each study. In the E03 study, the high-stimulation group had a mean reduction in seizure frequency of 24.5%, versus 6.1% for the low-stimulation group ($P = 0.01$). In the E05 study, the corresponding decreases were 28 and 15% for the high- and low-stimulation groups, respectively ($P = 0.039$). Thus both studies showed that high-stimulation was more effective than low-stimulation. Other efficacy analyses confirmed the primary measure. In the E03 study, 31% of patients receiving high-stimulation had at least 50% reduction in seizures compared to 13% of patients in the low-stimulation group ($P = 0.02$). In the E05 study, 11% of patients in the high-stimulation group had at least a $>75\%$ reduction of seizures compared to baseline versus 2% of patients in the low-stimulation group ($P = 0.01$).

C. Long-Term Efficacy

The results of several studies suggest that seizure control further improved after the initial blinded, 3-month treatment period for patients who completed the E03 and E05 studies (38,42,43) Because VNS treatment was then unblinded, and stimulation parameters and AED dosages could be adjusted as clinically necessary, these results are not conclusive.

One study compared seizure frequencies for the first year following the conclusion of the E05 study to the preimplantation baseline (44). The median seizure reductions at 3 and 12 months were 34% and 45%, respectively ($P = 0.0001$, 12 vs. 3 months). In addition, 20% of patients had at least 75% reduction in seizure frequency at 12 months. An attempt to correlate changes in the stimulation parameters during the year with seizure control showed no significant correlation (45).

Another prospective study (21 patients; mean duration of epilepsy of 17 years, mean 2.8 AEDs) followed VNS-treated patients for an average of 13 months. In 15 patients (71%), number or dosages of AEDs were reduced without loss of seizure control (46,47). This finding is interesting because many patients with medically refractory seizures have AED-related side effects that impact quality of life negatively.

D. VNS Efficacy in Other Seizure Types and in Children and the Elderly

Adjunctive VNS may have potential for patients with generalized seizures, which are generally believed to originate deep in the brain and affect both cerebral hemispheres synchronously (41,48). VNS also appears to be a promising treatment modality in epileptic children (49). Among 12 children aged 4 to 16 with medically and surgically refractory seizures who were implanted with the VNS, five patients had $>90\%$ reduction in seizure frequency and four patients were able to reduce the number of AEDs used (50). Other series have shown similar results, including improvements in developmentally disabled or mentally retarded patients with epilepsy and children with a particularly devastating form of epilepsy called *Lennox-Gastaut syndrome* (LGS) (51–59).

Epilepsy in the elderly is a growing problem because of the aging population. Sirven and colleagues evaluated the efficacy, safety and tolerability of VNS for medically refractory seizures in 45 patients aged 50 or older (60). After 3 months of treatment, 12 patients had a $>50\%$ decrease in seizure frequency; at 1 year, 21 of 31 patients had $>50\%$ reduction. Side effects were mild and transient, and quality-of-life measurements improved significantly during the first year of treatment.

VI. EFFICACY IN CONDITIONS THAT ARE OFTEN SEEN IN PATIENTS WITH EPILEPSY

Patients with epilepsy frequenty complain about poor memory. Based on findings that memory storage in rats was enhanced by posttraining stimulation of the vagus nerve (61), Clark et al. studied word recognition memory in patients with epilepsy (62). After reading paragraphs that contained highlighted words, patients then received either VNS or sham stimulation. Retention of verbal learning (word recognition) was significantly enhanced by VNS but not sham stimulation. Another study evaluated the effects of 4.5 minutes high-intensity VNS (>1mA) on material-specific memory and decision times in patients with medically refractory epilepsy (63). The results indicated reversible worsening of figural but not verbal memory, and a trend of accelerated decision times during VNS. The effect of standard VNS stimulation on memory in epileptic patients with memory complaints has not yet been evaluated.

Up to 40% of patients with epilepsy have clinically significant depression. Two studies have measured the effect of VNS on mood in patients with long-standing, poorly controlled partial-onset seizures (64,65) While improvement in mood was found, it did not correlate with seizure reduction or stimulation parameters. Another study of epileptic patients found improvements in tenseness, negative arousal and dysphoria—but not of depression—associated with VNS (66). Two reports of children with developmental disabilities and epilepsy noted increased independent behavior, mood improvements, and fewer symptoms of pervasive developmental disorders (67,68).

One of the potential side effects of many AEDs is impaired cognitive function. Dodrill and Morris (69) evaluated cognition in 160 patients enrolled in the E05 study. Overall, there were no statistically significant changes in cognition comparing the baseline to treatment period between the high- and low-stimulation treatment groups. Similarly, another study evaluated cognition in 36 adult patients before and at least 6 months after implantation and found no evidence of cognitive worsening (70). Sleep studies suggest that VNS may improve sleep quality in some epileptic patients and reduce daytime sleepiness (71).

VII. SAFETY AND TOLERABILITY OF VNS IN PATIENTS WITH EPILEPSY

A. The E03 and E05 Studies

While high-frequency stimulation may theoretically be associated with tissue damage (72), there is no evidence that the stimulation settings used clinically to treat epilepsy damage the vagus nerve (73,74).

Double-blind studies provide the most reliable assessment of safety and tolerability. In the E03 study (described above), the side effects that occurred in at least 5% of patients in the high-stimulation group during treatment were hoarseness (37%), throat pain (11%), coughing (7%), dyspnea (shortness of breath, 6%), paresthesia (tingling, 6%), and muscle pain (6%). Hoarseness was the only side effect that occurred significantly more often with high stimulation than with low stimulation.

In the E05 study, there were no serious side effects attributed to VNS. The implantation procedure caused temporary left vocal cord paralysis in two patients, lower facial muscle paralysis in two patients, and pain and fluid accumulation over the generator requiring aspiration in one patient. The surgical procedure also produced temporary neck pain (29%), coughing (14%), voice alteration (13%), chest pain (12%), and nausea (10%). Following randomization, the side effects reported by patients in the high-stimulation group at some time during treatment were similar to those seen in the E03 study. The only two side effects that occurred significantly more often in the high-stimulation group than in the low-stimulation group were dyspnea and voice alteration. No significant changes in heart rhythm (as measured by Holter monitoring) or pulmonary function were found. No deaths occurred during either study, and no changes in blood tests (such as AED serum concentrations, blood counts or liver function tests) were observed in either study.

B. Other Studies of Safety and Tolerability

Because the treatment of epilepsy is usually chronic, long-term side effects of seizure therapies are of interest. Among 444 patients who continued VNS after participating in a clinical study, the most commonly reported side effects at the end of the first year were voice alteration (29%) and paresthesia (12%); at the end of 2 years, voice alteration (19%) and cough (6%); and at 3 years, dyspnea (3%) (75). Thus there appears to be diminishment of side effects over time. Notably absent with VNS stimulation therapy are the typical central nervous system side effects of AEDs, such as sedation, lack of coordination, and double vision.

The overall impact of seizure treatment can be assessed using quality-of-life (QOL) batteries. Studies of VNS treatment generally show improved QOL scores beyond reduction in seizures (76,77).

Patients with severe epilepsy are at risk for dying suddenly and unexpectedly. The mortality rates for patients treated with VNS are comparable with those of age-matched adults with refractory seizures who are not treated with VNS (78). Interestingly, the rate of sudden, unexpected death is significantly less after 2 years of VNS treatment.

Transient asystole lasting up to 20 s has been reported in nine patients (0.1% of all implantations) during the implantation procedure in association with the lead test (79–81). The lead test is performed intraoperatively and assesses stimulator functioning and system integrity by turning on the generator briefly at 1.0 mA, 500 µs and 20 Hz. Five patients were implanted and chronically stimulated without further. There were no serious consequences in any of the patients. Other studies have found no consistent clinically relevant effects of VNS on cardiorespiratory function (82,83).

Other isolated, transient side effects attributed to VNS are the subject of case reports or small series (84–89). Children with severe mental and motor retardation who are dependent on assisted feeding may be at increased risk for aspiration while being fed during vagus stimulation (90,91). The manufacturer of the VNS therapy system has cautioned patients treated with VNS not to undergo short-wave diathermy, microwave diathermy or therapeutic ultrasound diathermy because of the theoretical possibility that the generator or lead could cause thermal tissue damage. There are no documented cases of this complication in VNS-treated patients.

The potential for birth defects from AEDs is a major concern for epileptic women of childbearing potential. Eight VNS-treated women who became pregnant were reported (92). Five of the pregnancies concluded with full-term, healthy infants. There was one spontaneous abortion, one unplanned pregnancy was terminated by an elective abortion, and another pregnancy ended with an elective abortion because of abnormal fetal development that was attributed to seizure medications. These numbers are too small to draw any firm conclusions about the safety of VNS for developing fetuses.

VIII. CLINICAL USE OF VAGUS NERVE STIMULATION FOR EPILEPSY

Over 22,000 patients have been treated with the VNS therapy system worldwide. As opposed to the relative simplicity of writing prescriptions for AEDs, the successful implementation of a VNS program requires a team of health care providers to provide patient education, perform the surgical implantation, and implement programming changes (93).

Because VNS is the first nonpharmacological therapy approved for epilepsy, and owing to its initial high cost, which may be offset by later cost savings, clinicians have actively debated its role in the treatment of epilepsy (94–96). Today VNS treatment is generally offered to patients with medically refractory partial-onset seizures who are either opposed to intracranial surgery or are not candidates. Similarly, VNS may be recommended to patients with medically refractory generalized seizures, though data to support this recommendation comes only from open, uncontrolled studies at the present time. Typical stimulation parameters used in clinical practice are shown in Table 1.

Table 1 Typical Stimulation Parameters

Parameter	Setting
Output current	Up to 3.5 mA
Frequency	30 Hz
Pulse width	500 μs
On time	30 s
Off time	5 min

mA = milliamperes; Hz = Hertz; μs = microseconds; s = seconds; min = minutes.

IX. CONCLUSIONS

Trial results and clinical experience show that VNS is effective, safe, and well tolerated in patients with long-standing, refractory partial-onset seizures patients who are not good candidates for intracranial brain surgery or who refuse brain surgery (97). Evidence of benefit for other seizure types, and in children and the elderly, is promising. Side effects occur during stimulation in the minority of patients, are usually mild to moderate in severity and diminish with time or reduction in stimulation intensity. Caution should be exercised when considering VNS for patients with sleep apnea and cardiac conduction disorders. Surgical complications are infrequent (98) and likely to decline with further enhancements in surgical techniques and postoperative care (99–102). There has been no indication of tolerance to therapeutic effect in long-term, open studies.

The era of proven nonpharmacological treatment of seizures began with the introduction of VNS (103,104). Further controlled studies are needed to understand its role in patients with generalized seizures, to explore the optimum stimulation settings, and to determine whether patients who benefit from VNS can be identified prospectively.

REFERENCES

1. Lhatoo SD, Wong IC, Polizzi G, Sander JW. Long-term retention rates of lamotrigine, gabapentin, and topiramate in chronic epilepsy. Epilepsia 2000; 41:1592–1596.
2. Fisher RS, Vickrey BG, Gibson P, Hermann B, Penovich P, Scherer A, Walker SG. The impact of epilepsy from the patient's perspective II. Views about therapy and health care. Epilepsy Res 2000; 41:53–61.
3. Kemeny AA. Surgery for epilepsy. Seizure 2001; 10:461–465.
4. Loddenkemper T, Pan A, Neme S, Baker KB, Rezai AR, Dinner DS, Montgomery EB, Luders HO. Deep brain stimulation in epilepsy. J Clin Neurophysiol 2001; 18:514–532.
5. Velasco M, Velasco F, Velasco AL. Centromedian–thalamic and hippocampal electrical stimulation for the control of intractable epileptic seizures. J Clin Neurophysiol 2001; 18:495–513.
6. Saper CB, Kibbe MR, Hurley KM, Spencer S, Holmes HR, Leahy KM, Needleman P. Brain natriuretic peptide-like immunoreactive innervation of the cardiovascular and cerebrovascular systems in the rat. Circ Res 1990; 67:1345–1354.
7. Saper CB. The central autonomic system. In: Paxinos G, ed. The Rat Nervous System. 2d ed. San Diego: Academic, 1995:107–131.
8. Cechetto DF, Saper CB. Evidence for a viscerotopic sensory representation in the cortex and thalamus in the rat. J Comp Neurol 1987; 262:27–45.
9. Fulwiler CE, Saper CB. Subnuclear organization of the efferent connections of the parabrachial nucleus in the rat. Brain Res Rev 1984; 7:229–259.
10. Saper CB. Diffuse cortical projection systems: anatomical organization and role in cortical

function. In: Plum F, ed. Handbook of Physiology. The Nervous System V. Bethesda: American Physiological Society, 1987:169–210.

11. Naritoku DK, Terry WJ, Helfert RH. Regional induction of fos immunoreactivity in the brain by anticonvulsant stimulation of the vagus nerve. Epilepsy Res 1995; 22:53–62.

12. Krahl SE, Clark KB, Smith DC, Browning RA. Locus coeruleus lesions suppress the seizure-attenuating effects of vagus nerve stimulation. Epilepsia 1998; 39:708–714.

13. Chase MH, Sterman MB, Clemente CD. Cortical and subcortical patterns of response to afferent vagal stimulation. Exp Neurol 1966; 16:36–49.

14. Chase MH, Nakamura Y, Clemente CD, Sterman MB. Afferent vagal stimulation: neurographic correlates of induced EEG synchronization and desynchronization. Brain Res 1967; 5:236–249.

15. Chase MH, Nakamura Y, Clemente CD, Sterman MB. Cortical and subcortical EEG patterns of response to afferent abdominal vagal stimulation: neurographic correlates. Physiol Behav 1968; 3:605–610.

16. Zagon A, Kemeny AA. Slow hyperpolarization in cortical neurons: a possible mechanism behind vagus nerve simulation therapy for refractory epilepsy? Epilepsia 2000; 41:1382–1389.

17. Krahl SE, Senanayake SS, Handforth A. Destruction of peripheral C-fibers does not alter subsequent vagus nerve stimulation-induced seizure suppression in rats. Epilepsia 2001; 42:586–589.

18. Olejniczak PW, Fisch BJ, Carey M, Butterbaugh G, Happel L, Tardo C. The effect of vagus nerve stimulation on epileptiform activity recorded from hippocampal depth electrodes. Epilepsia 2001; 42:423–429.

19. Garnett ES, Nahmias C, Scheffel A, Firnau G, Upton ARM. Regional cerebral blood flow in man manipulated by direct vagal stimulation. Pacing Clin Electrophysiol 1992; 15(10 Pt 2):1579–1580.

20. Ko D, Heck C, Grafton S, Apuzzo MLJ, Couldwell WT, Chen T, Day JD, Zelman V, Smith T, DeGiorgio CM. Vagus nerve stimulation activates central nervous system structures in epileptic patients during PET H2^{15}O blood flow imaging. Neurosurgery 1996; 39(2):426–431.

21. Ferris EB, Capps RB, Weiss S. Carotid sinus syncope and its bearing on the mechanism of the unconscious state and convulsions. Medicine 1934; 14:377–453.

22. Reis DJ, Iadecola C, Nakai M. Control of cerebral blood flow and metabolism by intrinsic neural systems in brain. In: Plum F, Pulsinelli W, eds. Cerebrovascular Diseases. New York: Raven Press, 1985:1–25.

23. Ring HA, White S, Costa DC, Pottinger R, Dick JPR, Koeze T, Sutcliffe J. A SPECT study of the effect of vagal nerve stimulation on thalamic activity in patients with epilepsy. Seizure 2000; 9:380–384.

24. Vonck K, Boon P, Van Laere K, D'Have M, Vandekerchhove T, O'Connor S, Brans B, Dierckx R, De Recuk J. Acute single photon emission computed tomographic study of vagus nerve stimulation in refractory epilepsy. Epilepsia 2000; 41:601–609.

25. Henry TR, Votaw JR, Pennell PB, Epstein CM, Bakay RAE, Faber TL, Grafton ST, Hoffman JM. Acute blood flow changes and efficacy of vagus nerve stimulation in partial epilepsy. Neurology 1999; 52:1166–1173.

26. Henry TR, Bakay RAE, Votaw JR, Pennell PB, Epstein CM, Faber TL, Grafton ST, Hoffman JM. Brain blood flow alterations induced by therapeutic vagus nerve stimulation in partial epilepsy: I. Acute effects at high and low levels of stimulation. Epilepsia 1998; 39:983–990.

27. Henry TR, Votaw JR, Bakay RAE, Pennell PB, Epstein CM, Faber TL, Grafton ST, Hoffman JM. Vagus nerve stimulation-induced cerebral blood flow changes differ in acute and chronic therapy of complex partial seizures [abstr]. Epilepsia 1998; 39(suppl 6):92.

28. Bohning DE, Lomarev MP, Denslow S, Nahas Z, Shastri A, George MS. Feasibility of vagus nerve stimulation-synchronized blood oxygenation level-dependent functional MRI. Invest Radiol 2001; 36:470–479.

29. McLachlan RS. Suppression of interictal spikes and seizures by stimulation of the vagus nerve. Epilepsia 1993; 34:918–923.

30. Woodbury DM, Woodbury JW. Effects of vagal stimulation on experimentally induced seizures in rats. Epilepsia 1990; 31(suppl 2):S7–S19.

31. Woodbury JW, Woodbury DM. Vagal stimulation reduces the severity of maximal electroshock seizures in intact rats: use of a cuff electrode for stimulating and recording. Pacing Clin Electrophysiol 1991; 14:94–107.

32. Zabara J. Inhibition of experimental seizures in canines by repetitive vagal stimulation. Epilepsia 1992; 33:1005–1012.

33. Lockard JS, Congdon WC, DuCharme LL. Feasibility and safety of vagal stimulation in monkey model. Epilepsia 1990; 31(suppl 2):S20–S26.

34. Takaya M, Terry WJ, Naritoku DK. Vagus nerve stimulation induces a sustained anticonvulsant effect. Epilepsia 1996; 37:1111–1116.

35. Penry JK, Dean JC. Prevention of intractable partial seizures by intermittent vagal stimulation in humans: preliminary results. Epilepsia 1990; 31(suppl 2):S40–S43.

36. Ben-Menachem E, Manon-Espaillat R, Ristanovic R, Wilder BJ, Stefan H, Mirza W, Tarver WB, Wernicke JF. Vagus nerve stimulation for treatment of partial seizures: 1. A controlled study of effect on seizures. Epilepsia 1994; 35:616–626.

37. Ramsay RE, Uthman BM, Augustinsson LE, Upton ARM, Naritoku D, Willis J, Treig T, Barolat G, Wernicke JF. Vagus nerve stimulation for treatment of partial seizures: 2. Safety, side effects, and tolerability. Epilepsia 1994; 35:627–636.

38. George R, Salinsky M, Kuzniecky R, Rosenfeld W, Bergen D, Tarver WB, Wernicke JF. Vagus nerve stimulation for treatment of partial seizures: 3. Long-term follow-up on first 67 patients exiting a controlled study. Epilepsia 1994; 35:637–643.

39. The Vagus Nerve Stimulation Study Group. A randomized controlled trial of chronic vagus nerve stimulation for treatment of medically intractable seizures. Neurology 1995; 45:224–230.

40. Handforth A, DeGiorgio CM, Schachter SC, Uthman BM, Naritoku DK, Tecoma ES, Henry TR, Collins SD, Vaughn BV, Gilmartin RC, Labar DR, Morris GL, Salinsky MC, Osorio I, Ristanovic RK, Labiner DM, Jones JC, Murphy JV, Ney GC, Wheless JW. Vagus nerve stimulation therapy for partial-onset seizures: a randomized active control trial. Neurology 1998; 51:48–55.

41. Labar D, Murphy J, Tecoma E. Vagus nerve stimulation for medication-resistant generalized epilepsy. E04 VNS Study Group. Neurology 1999; 52:1510–1512.

42. Michael JE, Wegener K, Barnes DW. Vagus nerve stimulation for intractable seizures: one year follow-up. J Neurosci Nurs 1993; 25:362–366.

43. Salinsky MC, Uthman BM, Ristanovic RK, Wernicke JF, Tarver WB. Vagus nerve stimulation for the treatment of medically intractable seizures. Results of a 1-year open-extension trial. Arch Neurol 1996; 53:1176–1180.

44. DeGiorgio CM, Schachter SC, Handforth A, Salinsky M, Thompson J, Uthman B, Reed R, Collins S, Tecoma E, Morris GL, Vaughn B, Naritoku DK, Henry T, Labar D, Gilmartin R, Labiner D, Osorio I, Ristanovic R, Jones J, Murphy J, Ney G, Wheless J, Lewis P, Heck C. Prospective long-term study of vagus nerve stimulation for the treatment of refractory seizures. Epilepsia 2000; 41:1195–1200.

45. DeGiorgio CM, Thompson J, Lewis P, Arrambide S, Naritoku D, Handforth A, Labar D, Mullin P, Heck C. Vagus nerve stimulation: analysis of device parameters in 154 patients during the long-term XE5 study. Epilepsia 2001; 42:1017–1020.

46. Tatum WO. Vagus nerve stimulation and drug reduction: reply. Neurology 2001; 57:938–939.

47. Tatum WO, Johnson KD, Goff S, Ferreira JA, Vale FL. Vagus nerve stimulation and drug reduction. Neurology 2001; 56:561–563.

48. Rafael H, Moromizato P. Vagus nerve stimulation (VNS) may be useful in treating patients with symptomatic generalized epilepsy. Epilepsia 1998; 39:1018.

49. Hornig G, Murphy JV. Vagal nerve stimulation: updated experience in 60 pediatric patients [abstr]. Epilepsia 1998; 39(suppl 6):169.

50. Murphy JV, Hornig G, Schallert G. Left vagal nerve stimulation in children with refractory epilepsy. Preliminary observations. Arch Neurol 1995; 52:886–889.

51. Lundgren J, Amark P, Blennow G, Stromblad LG, Wallstedt L. Vagus nerve stimulation in 16 children with refractory epilepsy. Epilepsia 1998; 39:809–813.

52. Parker AP, Polkey CE, Binnie CD, Madigan C, Ferrie CD, Robinson RO. Vagal nerve stimulation in epileptic encephalopathies. Pediatrics 1999; 103:778–782.

53. Helmers SL, Al-Jayyousi M, Madsen J. Adjunctive treatment in Lennox-Gastaut syndrome using vagal nerve stimulation [abstr]. Epilepsia 1998; 39(suppl 6):169.

54. Murphy JV, Hornig G. Chronic intermittent stimulation of the left vagal nerve in nine children with Lennox-Gastaut syndrome [abstr]. Epilepsia 1998; 39(suppl 6):169.

55. Frost M, Gates J, Helmers SL, Wheless JW, Levisohn P, Tardo C, Conry JA. Vagus nerve stimulation in children with refractory seizures associated with Lennox–Gastaut syndrome. Epilepsia 2001; 42:1148–1152.

56. Murphy JV. Left vagal nerve stimulation in children with medically refractory epilepsy. J Pediatr 1999; 134:563–566.

57. Hosain S, Nikalov B, Harden C, Li M, Fraser R, Labar D. Vagus nerve stimulation treatment for Lennox–Gastaut syndrome. J Child Neurol 2000; 15:509–512.

58. Patwardhan RV, Stong B, Bebin EM, Mathisen J, Grabb PA. Efficacy of vagal nerve stimulation in children with medically refractory epilepsy. Neurosurgery 2000; 47:1353–1358.

59. Andriola MR, Vitale SA. Vagus nerve stimulation in the developmentally disabled. Epilepsy Behav 2001; 2:129–134.

60. Sirven JI, Sperling M, Naritoku D, Schachter S, Labar D, Holmes M, Wilensky A, Cibula J, Labiner DM, Bergen D, Ristanovic R, Harvey J, Dasheiff R, Morris GL, O'Donovan CA, Ojemann L, Scales D, Nadkarni M, Richards B, Sanchez JD. Vagus nerve stimulation therapy for epilepsy in older adults. Neurology 2000; 54:1179–1182.

61. Clark KB, Smith DC, Hassert DL, Browning RA, Naritoku DK, Jensen RA. Posttraining electrical stimulation of vagal afferents with concomitant vagal efferent inactivation enhances memory storage processes in the rat. Neurobiol Learn Mem 1998; 70:364–373.

62. Clark KB, Naritoku DK, Smith DC, Browning RA, Jensen RA. Enhanced recognition memory following vagus nerve stimulation in human subjects. Nat Neurosci 1999; 2:94–98.

63. Helmstaedter C, Hoppe C, Elger CE. Memory alterations during acute high-intensity vagus nerve stimulation. Epilepsy Res 2001; 47:37–42.

64. Elger G, Hoppe C, Falkai P, Rush AJ, Elger CE. Vagus nerve stimulation is associated with mood improvements in epilepsy patients. Epilepsy Res 2000; 42:203–210.

65. Harden CL, Pulver MC, Ravdin LD, Nikolov B, Halper JP, Labar DR. A pilot study of mood in epilepsy patients treated with vagus nerve stimulation. Epilepsy Behav 2000; 1:93–99.

66. Hoppe C, Helmstaedter C, Scherrmann J, Elger CE. Self-reported mood changes following 6 months of vagus nerve stimulation in epilepsy patients. Epilepsy Behav 2001; 2:335–342.

67. Aldenkamp AP, Van de Veerdonk SHA, Majoie HJM, Berfelo MW, Evers SMAA, Kessels AGH, Renier WO, Wilmink J. Effects of 6 months of treatment with vagus nerve stimulation on behavior in children with Lennox–Gastaut syndrome in an open clinical and nonrandomized study. Epilepsy Behav 2001; 2:343–350.

68. Murphy JV, Wheless JW, Schmoll CM. Left vagal nerve stimulation in six patients with hypothalamic hamartomas. Pediatr Neurol 2000; 23:167–168.

69. Dodrill CB, Morris GL. Effects of vagal nerve stimulation on cognition and quality of life in epilepsy. Epilepsy Behav 2001; 2:46–53.

70. Hoppe C, Helmstaedter C, Schermann J, Elger CE. No evidence for cognitive side effects after 6 months of vagus nerve stimulation in epilepsy patients. Epilepsy Behav 2001; 2:351–356.

71. Malow BA, Edwards J, Marzec M, Sagher O, Ross D, Fromes G. Vagus nerve stimulation reduces daytime sleepiness in epilepsy patients. Neurology 2001; 57:879–884.

72. Terry RS, Tarver WB, Zabara J. The implantable neurocybernetic prosthesis system. Pacing Clin Electrophysiol 1991; 14:86–93.

73. Agnew WF, McCreery DB. Considerations for safety with chronically implanted nerve electrodes. Epilepsia 1990; 31(suppl 2):S27–S32.

74. Tarver WB, George RE, Maschino SE, Holder LK, Wernicke JF. Clinical experience with a helical bipolar stimulating lead. Pacing Clin Electrophysiol 1992; 15:1545–1556.

75. Morris GL, Mueller WM. Long-term treatment with vagus nerve stimulation in patients with refractory epilepsy. Neurology 1999; 53:1731–1735.

76. Cramer JA. Exploration of changes in health-related quality of life after 3 months of vagus nerve stimulation. Epilepsy Behav 2001; 2:460–465.

77. Morrow JI, Bingham E, Craig JJ, Gray WJ. Vagal nerve stimulation in patients with refractory epilepsy. Effect on seizure frequency, severity and quality of life. Seizure 2000; 9:442–445.

78. Annegers JF, Coan SP, Hauser WA, Leestma J. Epilepsy, vagal nerve stimulation by the NCP system, all-cause mortality, and sudden, unexpected, unexplained death. Epilepsia 2000; 41: 549–553.

79. Asconape JJ, Moore DD, Zipes DP, Hartman LM, Duffell WH. Bradycardia and asystole with the use of vagus nerve stimulation for the treatment of epilepsy: a rare complication of intra-operative device testing. Epilepsia 1999; 40:1452–1454.

80. Tatum WO, Moore DB, Stecker MM, Baltuch GH, French JA, Ferreira JA, Carney PM, Labar DR, Vale F. Ventricular asystole during vagus nerve stimulation for epilepsy in humans. Neurology 1999; 52:1267–1269.

81. Andriola MR, Rosenzweig T, Vlay S. Vagus nerve stimulator (VNS): induction of asystole during implantation with subsequent successful stimulation [abstr]. Epilepsia 2000; 41(suppl 7):223.

82. Frei MG, Osorio I. Left vagus nerve stimulation with the Neurocybernetic Prosthesis has complex effects on heart rate and on its variability in humans. Epilepsia 2001; 42:1007–1016.

83. Binks AP, Paydarfar D, Schachter SC, Guz A, Banzett RB. High strength stimulation of the vagus nerve in awake humans: a lack of cardiorespiratory effects. Respir Physiol 2001; 127:125–133.

84. Sanossian N, Haut S. Chronic diarrhea associated with vagal nerve stimulation. Neurology 2002; 58:330.

85. Kim W, Clancy RR, Liu GT. Horner syndrome associated with implantation of a vagus nerve stimulator. Am J Ophthalmol 2001; 131:383–384.

86. Leijten FSS, Van Rijen PC. Stimulation of the phrenic nerve as a complication of vagus nerve pacing in a patient with epilepsy. Neurology 1998; 51:1224–1225.

87. Malow BA, Edwards J, Marzec M, Sagher O, Fromes G. Effects of vagus nerve stimulation on respiration during sleep: a pilot study. Neurology 2000; 55:1450–1454.

88. Blumer D, Davies K, Alexander A, Morgan S. Major psychiatric disorders subsequent to treating epilepsy by vagus nerve stimulation. Epilepsy Behav 2001; 2:466–472.

89. Prater JF. Recurrent depression with vagus nerve stimulation. Am J Psychiatry 2001; 158:816–817.

90. Schallert G, Foster J, Lindquist N, Murphy JV. Chronic stimulation of the left vagal nerve in children: effect on swallowing. Epilepsia 1998; 39:1113–1114.

91. Lundgren J, Ekberg O, Olsson R. Aspiration: a potential complication to vagus nerve stimulation. Epilepsia 1998; 39:998–1000.

92. Ben-Menachem E, Ristanovic R, Murphy J. Gestational outcomes in patients with epilepsy receiving vagus nerve stimulation [abstr]. Epilepsia 1998; 39(suppl 6):180.

93. Doerksen K, Klassen L. Vagus nerve stimulation therapy: nurses role in a collaborative approach to a program. Axone 1998; 20:6–9.

94. McLachlan RS. Vagus nerve stimulation for treatment of seizures? Maybe. Arch Neurol 1998; 55:232–233.

95. Boon P, Vonck K, D'Have R, O'Connor S, Vandekerckhove T, De Reuck J. Cost benefit of vagus nerve stimulation for refractory epilepsy. Acta Neurol Belg 1999; 99:275–280.

96. Ben-Menachem E. Vagus nerve stimulation for treatment of seizures? Yes. Arch Neurol 1998; 55:231–232.

97. DeGiorgio CM, Amar A, Apuzzo MLJ. Surgical anatomy, implantation technique, and operative complications. In: Schachter SC, Schmidt D, eds. Vagus Nerve Stimulation. London: Martin Dunitz, 2001:31–50.

98. Patil A-A, Chand A, Andrews R. Single incision for implanting a vagal nerve stimulator system (VNSS): technical note. Surg Neurol 2001; 55:103–105.

99. Vaughn BV, Bernard E, Lannon S, Mann B, D'Cruz OF, Shockley W, Passanante A. Intraoperative methods for confirmation of correct placement of the vagus nerve stimulator. Epileptic Disord 2001; 3:75–78.

100. Ortler M, Luef G, Kofler A, Bauer G, Twerdy K. Deep wound infection after vagus nerve stimulator implantation: treatment without removal of the device. Epilepsia 2001; 42:133–135.

101. Liporace J, Hucko D, Morrow R, Barolat G, Nei M, Schnur J, Sperling M. Vagal nerve stimulation: adjustments to reduce painful side effects. Neurology 2001; 57:885–886.

102. Chadwick D. Vagal-nerve stimulation for epilepsy. Lancet 2001; 357:1726–1727.

103. Binnie CD. Vagus nerve stimulation for epilepsy: a review. Seizure 2000; 9:161–169.

104. Schmidt D. Vagus nerve stimulation for the treatment of epilepsy. Epilepsy Behav 2001; 2:S1–S5.

23

Electrical Stimulation of the Internal Globus Pallidus in Advanced Generalized Dystonia

Laura Cif, Nathalie Vayssiere, Simone Hemm, Monique Azais, Cédric Monnier, Eric Hardouin, Amandine Gannau, and Philippe Coubes

Service de Neurochirurgie B, Centre Gui de Chauliac, CHU Montpellier, Montpellier, France

Michel Zanca

Service de Médecine Nucléaire, Centre Gui de Chauliac, CHU Montpellier, Montpellier, France

Electrical stimulation of the globus pallidus for the treatment of disabling dystonia is based on the results obtained with pallidotomy and the efficacy of deep brain stimulation in Parkinson's disease. A description of the procedure, discussion of mechanisms of action and the results of functional magnetic resonance imaging studies are presented, as well as evidence of long-term efficacy of this novel, reversible, and highly adaptable approach.

General dystonia is a movement disorder characterized by tonic, involuntary contractions of one or several muscle groups (Fig. 1). On the basis of results obtained with bilateral pallidotomy for treating the most severe forms of primary generalized dystonia (PGD) and the well-established efficiency of deep brain stimulation in Parkinson disease (1–5), we treated 60 eight patients with severely disabling generalized dystonia with bilateral, chronic electrical stimulation of the globus pallidus internus. We are reporting on the long-term efficacy and safety of this new, reversible, and adaptable therapy. This treatment consists of a current drain delivery (electrical neuromodulation) to a deep located brain structure called *internal globus pallidus*. This stimulation is applied after neurosurgical stereotactical implantation of electrodes secondarily connected to subcutaneously implanted pulse generators. The parameters for stimulation are selected using a radio-frequency method-

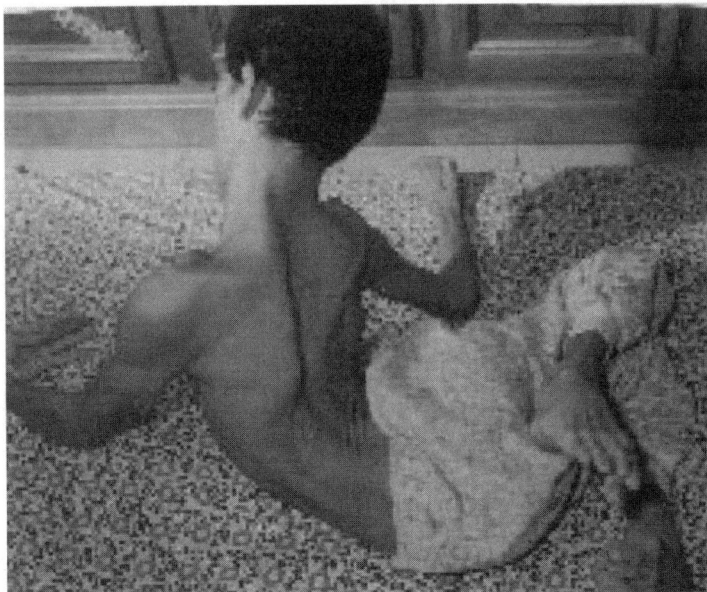

Figure 1 Patient with a primary generalized dystonia.

ology enabling the physician to adapt the current drain characteristics to the clinical evolution of movement disorders.

I. CLINICAL EXPERIENCE

A. The Surgical Procedure

In our center, considering the young age, the poor general condition, and the permanent restless situation of most patients presenting movement disorders, especially children, we developed a stereotactic procedure under general anesthesia to be completed during a 1-day single session. It is based solely on 3D-MR imaging for target localization without intra-operative microelectrode recordings or clinical control allowing the procedure to be shortened to 1 h per electrode. General anesthesia was induced before affixing the MR-compatible stereotactic frame (Leksell G frame; Elekta Instruments, Stockholm, Sweden) to the patient's head in the operating room. The patient was then immediately transported to the MR imaging unit, and surgical planning was completed while the patient was prepared and draped for the operation.

In the operating room, the stereotactic electrode-guiding device was installed and a 14-mm burr hole was made at the level of the predetermined trajectory. Dural opening and cortical incision were performed under direct visual control. No microelectrode recording was used in these patients. Electrode implantation was achieved under real-time strict-profile radioscopic control to prevent any modification of the electrode position until the end of the procedure. The implanted electrode was an MR-compatible quadripolar device on which the contacts were numbered as follows: lower contact, 0; upper contact, 3 (model 3389; Medtronic, Rueil-Malmaison, France). The upper border of contact 1 was strictly aligned with the target position (Fig. 2). Immediately after surgery, the patient was again

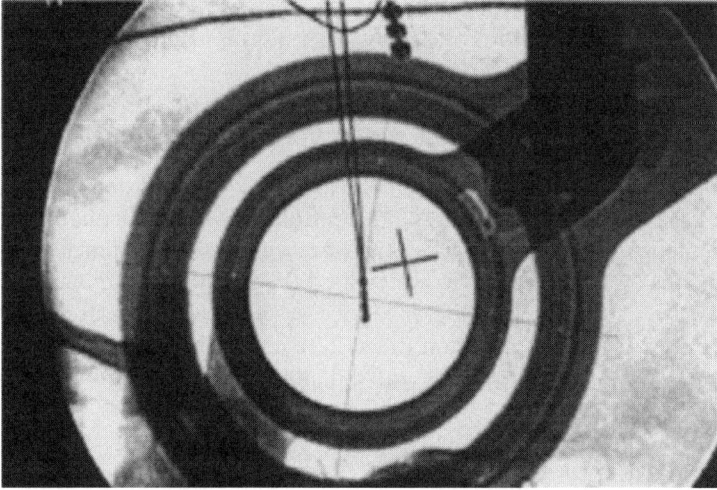

Figure 2 MRI selected target and radioscopic control.

transported to the MR imaging unit and a control MR image (with the stereotactic frame in place) was obtained, which allowed us to check the electrode position and detect any error caused by MR imaging distortions (6).

B. Magnetic Resonance Image Acquisition

Magnetic resonance image acquisition was performed with a 1.5-T magnet. Control studies used to assess the homogeneity of the main magnetic field and the calibration of the gradients were obtained the day before the stereotactic operation. All these control studies were performed according to European standards. The procedure included a control with a quality assessment phantom and Quick Shim software under the responsibility of the maintenance department. The MR images were acquired with the head frame in place. The performed sequence consisted of a 3D fast-transformed volume of contiguous transverse axial sections. The parameters used for T1-weighted images were: slice thickness 1.5 mm, TE 6 msec, TR 15 ms, tilt angle 25°, and one excitation.

C. Target and Trajectory Determination for 3D-MR Imaging

The neurosurgeon selected the target by using a 3D cursor, following visual recognition of the GPi boundaries on the 1.5-mm-thick transverse axial section including the inferior border of the anterior commissure. On this slice, the GPi appears as an ellipse whose long axis can be divided in four equal parts. From the front, the third quarter was selected whose center was the target. The coordinates were then automatically calculated. We used the stereotactic software developed by the departments of neuroradiology (Pr. Cordoliani, Pr Derosier) and neurosurgery (Pr. Desgeorges) in the Val de Grâce hospital, Paris (7). This software allowed simultaneous visualization of the three orthogonal sections and the position of the cursor in all directions. The software also added the trace of a vector linked to the point that defined the trajectory. The best electrode trajectory was selected after varying the planes and orientations. The corresponding line was then displayed point by point in the cerebral volume. Importantly, it appeared crucial to display slices orthogonally to the electrode trajectory to anticipate precisely the relative position of each contact with the surrounding GPi boundaries. The procedure was repeated until an optimal electrode position was obtained.

D. Distortion Control at the Periphery of the Field of View (FOV)

The frame and localizer were designed to fit the head coil closely. In this way the fiducial markers were visible at the periphery of the FOV. Using the G-frame localizer as a phantom, we checked that 3D-MR imaging of the localizer was consistent with the actual dimensions (120–190 mm) and shape (square) of the FOV. We calculated the mean distance between fiducial markers before and after surgery. The differences observed between measured and theoretical distances were not statistically significant ($|t| < 2.2$), indicating that distortions at the periphery of the field were not detectable and did not modify the geometrical characteristics of the localizer (6).

E. Distortion Control at the Center of the FOV

The white anterior and posterior commissures, AC and PC are commonly used as essential landmarks in stereotactic surgery because of their mesial, deep location as well as their fixed position in the brain. To calculate the error caused by distortion in the center of the FOV, the coordinates of the AC and PC, as well as the AC-PC distance (distance between the corresponding midpoints), were calculated pre- and postoperatively for each patient. The results indicate that distortions at the center of the field were not significant and did not modify the geometrical representation of the brain (6).

F. Control of Electrode Position

Immediately after surgery the patient was transported to the MR imaging unit, where a control MR image was obtained with the stereotactic frame in place (Fig. 3). The coordinates of the final position of the electrode ($P_2[x_2, y_2, z_2]$) upper border of contact 1 were calculated and compared with those of the preoperative selected target ($P_1[x_1, y_1, z_1]$). There was no statistical difference between pre- and postoperative coordinates when considered as distinct sets, in both the x and y directions and on both the left and right

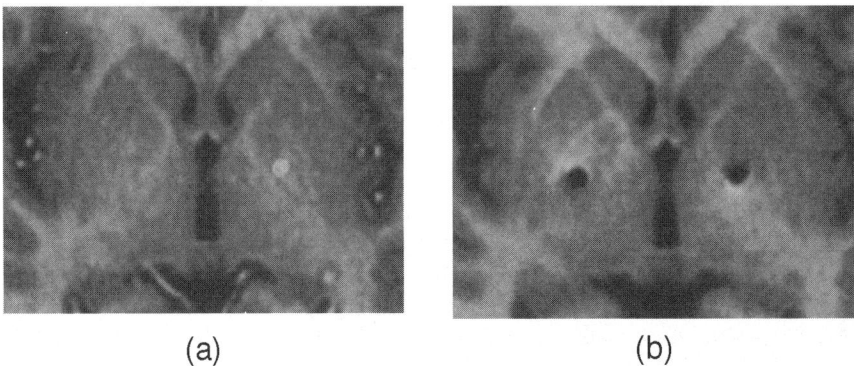

(a)   (b)

Figure 3 (a) Preoperative calculation of target coordinates (white circle) on an axial transverse image (MRI) with the Leksell's stereotactic frame. (b) Immediate post operative control image with the Leksell's stereotactic frame: the correct positioning of the electrode is controlled. Its diameter appears overestimated due to the artifact generated by the metallic component.

sides ($p < 0.05$). This indicated that the electrode was exactly positioned in the selected target (Fig. 3).

G. Electrical Settings

The pulse generator can be programmed by telemetry for electrical stimulation settings, contact (cathode or anode), voltage (0 to 10.5 V), rate (2 to 185 Hz), pulse width (60 to 450 µs), and timing (cyclic or continuous stimulation). The physician selected the electrical settings after surgery and at each follow-up examination. The patient cannot modify the stimulation himself. The following settings were first implemented: contact 1 as cathode, stimulator as anode, rate: 130 Hz, pulse width: 450 µs, voltage: 0.8 V continuous bilateral stimulation. The settings were then adapted by increasing progressively the voltage in adaptation to the clinical evolution of each patient to reach a mean value of 1.6 V. After 6 weeks, if necessary, the volume to be stimulated was increased by activating an additional contact (usually contact 2). It is recommended not to modify the medical treatment at the initial phase of stimulation in order not to interfere with the evaluation of dystonia.

H. Surgical Experience

Between November 1996 and April 2002, 68 patients (32 men and 36 women) from 6 to 63 years of age (average age, 21.13 years) underwent bilateral electrode implantation for continuous stimulation of the GPi. For precise assessment of therapeutic efficacy, each patient was evaluated using the Burke-Marsden-Fahn's dystonia rating scale (BMFDRS) (8,9) pre- and postoperatively, at given intervals, and at the latest follow-up.

1. Selection

The following criteria can be proposed for selecting the patients for surgery: a primary dystonia, DYT 1 mutation present, PKAN mutation present, preserved motor pattern, prominent quick (ballistic) component, no permanent hypertonia, pain, and before skeleton deformities.

2. Classification

The current classification for etiology divides the dystonia into two major categories, namely idiopathicand symptomatic (10). The first group of idiopathic dystonia, group 1, could be divided into two subgroups, group 1A of idiopathic dystonia with the DYT1 mutation (11–13) and group 1B of idiopathic dystonia without identified mutation. Group 1A (patients with the DYT1 mutation), comprised 12 children and 7 adults, the mean age at surgery was 19 years 5 months (8–49 years), the mean follow-up was 32.3 months (1–54 months). Group 1B (patients without identified mutation), comprised 9 children and 20 adults, mean age at surgery was 21 years 6 months (6–63 years), the mean follow-up was 26.6 months (1–67 months). Three of them did not accepted the follow up program and were excluded of the study.

The second group, Group 2, of symptomatic dystonia comprised patients with an identified etiology and multifocal brain lesions. It regrouped three patients with the PANK2 mutation (14) (group 2A), eight with a post anoxia (group 2B), one tyrosinemia, two posttrauma, two mitochondrial cytopathy, one rhesus incompatibility, one diabitus melitus, one postsurgical, and one Gougerot syndrom. In this group nine children and 11 adults have been included, mean age at surgery was 28 years 3 months (5–51 years) and the mean follow-up was 25.3 months (5–52 months). At the time of surgery, all patients were severely disabled in performing daily activities. All patients were under pharmaceutical treatment with various medications (benzodiazepine, anticholinergic drugs, L-dopa). All patients or their guardians

Table 1 Clinical Scores (BMFDRS) for Group 1 Patients

Follow-up	< 1 Year	1 Year	2 Years	> 3 Years
DYT1+ (19)	80% $n = 19$	85% $n = 16$	79% $n = 10$	87% $n = 5$
no mutation (26)	60% $n = 26$	59% $n = 23$	64% $n = 13$	78% $n = 7$

gave written informed consent. The protocol was approved by the French National Ethical Committee (reference number 98.07.02).

3. Complications

We observed three cases of delayed unilateral infection around the device (*Staphylococcus epidermidis*). The whole system should be explanted under general anesthesia in one patient, and only the IPG for the two others. The patients were reoperated 6 months later with subsequent excellent clinical improvement. We observed, in one patient, a head trauma with a posttraumatic fracture of both electrode and extension due to a direct shocking of the connector which was visible in the wound. In another case, a reoperation was performed to anticipate on a skin opening after a skin erosion having been detected during the monthly control. No electrode migration was noticed especially in the pediatric population. No surgery-related hemorrhage and no case of hardware malfunction were found. The most frequent software complication was the unexpected and unexplained IPG switch off resulting in every case in a quick worsening of the dystonic symptoms.

I. Clinical Results

The evolution of the clinical score of the Burke–Marsden–Fahn dystonia rating scale (BMFDRS) is reported for the 65 patients separated in the groups previously described. In each group, the improvement is highly significant ($P < 0.01$) (Tables 1 and 2). We did not find a significant difference of the overall improvement in children when compared to adults for the clinical one ($p = 0.87$).

II. STUDY OF MECHANISMS OF ACTION OF DBS

A. Stimulator Management

In the previous chapter we showed that patients are successfully treated by DBS in our center. However the clinical response varies from patient to patient depending on several factors, including etiology, extent, and severity of dystonia (15–17). Based on this data, we supposed the existence of individual factors influencing the response of the brain to electrical stimulation. The calculation of in vivo impedance and current values is a basic requirement for a better understanding of the electrical field distribution around the electrode and for the

Table 2 Clinical Scores (BMFDRS) for Group 2 Patients

Follow-up	< 1 Year	1 Year	2 Years	> 3 Years
PKAN+ (3)	49% $n = 3$	52.5% $n = 1$	62% $n = 1$	
Postanoxia (8)	35% $n = 6$	32% $n = 3$	40% $n = 2$	
Secondary (20)	44% $n = 17$	32% $n = 15$	38% $n = 11$	32% $n = 10$

3D modeling of the electrical current delivery. Such an approach is susceptible to improve our knowledge on the mechanism of action of deep brain stimulation and to assist the physician for selecting the stimulation setting. In an in vivo study, we investigated whether electrical brain impedance and current drain could be one of these factors.

1. Patients

Twenty-four dystonic patients suffering from generalized dystonia, treated in our center by bilateral continuous electrode stimulation of the globus pallidus internus, were consecutively included in this study. The 24 patients were divided into two groups: patients in whom the clinical condition has been improved and stabilized for at least three 3 and patients still being in the initial test period. The group of stable patients was subdivided into two groups: (1) patients with an excellent result (BMFDS improvement $\geq 80\%$) (2) patients with remaining symptoms (BMFDS improvement $< 80\%$).

2. Protocol for Impedance and Current Measurements

During the course of high-frequency chronic stimulation, impedance and current measurements were performed using the internal pulse generator's software and the console programmer (Medtronic). We distinguished between two different conditions for a given contact referring to the fact that the contacts were never activated all together:

Measurements were first performed for the currently selected electrical setting.

Measurements were performed on each contact (activated or not) using the same "standardized" pulse characteristics (pulse width: 450 μs, frequency: 130Hz, amplitude: 1.0 V)

As a function of time, we examined short time variations for the current electrical setting and long time variations for each contacts' impedance (standardized conditions). For the stable patients, impedance and current mean values were compared:

Under standardized conditions

With the current electrical setting

3. Results

   a. *Impedance and Current as a Function of Time.*   Short Time Variations—Current Electrical Setting.   In all patients, we noticed that a change of the stimulation parameters always causes variations of the total impedance Z and current drain I, especially in the first hours (Fig. 4). The delay before impedance and current drain reach a steady state is variable.

   Long Time Variations (Three Months)—Standardized Conditions.   The current stimulation parameters have been identified as factors influencing impedance and current values. In all patients, a great difference in impedance (ΔZ) was found between the (negatively or positively) stimulated versus the nonstimulated contacts. The results reflect a completely reversible impedance decrease: The contact's impedance decreases during stimulation and increases when it is deactivated. A raise of the pulse amplitude is followed by an impedance decrease as well, an increase of this amplitude by an impedance decrease. Figure 5 shows a typical evolution of each contacts' impedance.

   b. *Impedance and Current as a Function of the Clinical Outcome.*   Mean Values for the Activated Contacts Under Standardized Conditions.   In patients in whom the clinical condition has been improved and stabilized for at least three months, we did not find any significant difference in impedance and current between the group of patients with an excellent result (ΔBMFDRS $\geq 80\%$) and the group B with remaining symptoms (ΔBMFDRS $< 80\%$) (Table 3).

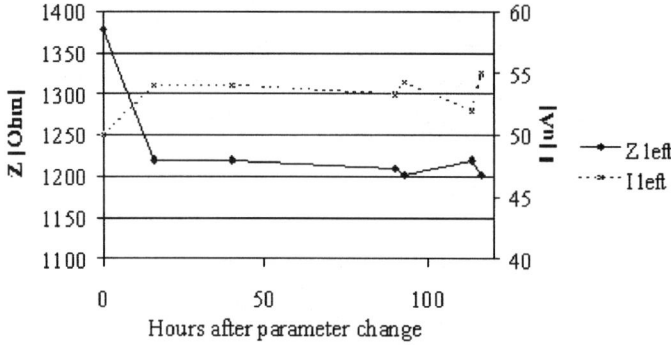

Figure 4 Evolution of impedance and current with time. Activation of contact 0 replacing contact 1 maintaining the same pulse characteristics [case positive, 130-Hz frequency, 450-μs pulse width, 1-V amplitude].

Mean Values for Current Stimulation Parameters. Comparing the total impedance and current mean values of the patient group with an improvement of at least 80% and the group with remaining symptoms, we did not find a significant difference ($p(Z) = 0.85$, $p(I) = 0.74$) (Table 4).

4. Discussion

By recording impedance and current values, we expected to explain the different responses of patients to DBS. Furthermore, we looked for indications on the stimulation mechanism of action on the brain. For this purpose, the relationship between impedance and current values versus different factors susceptible to influence the efficacy of DBS (current stimulation setting, time course and clinical outcome) was studied. The clinical outcome is not statistically correlated with impedance and current mean values. The fact that for a given current drain, impedance values differ between patients made us conclude that the

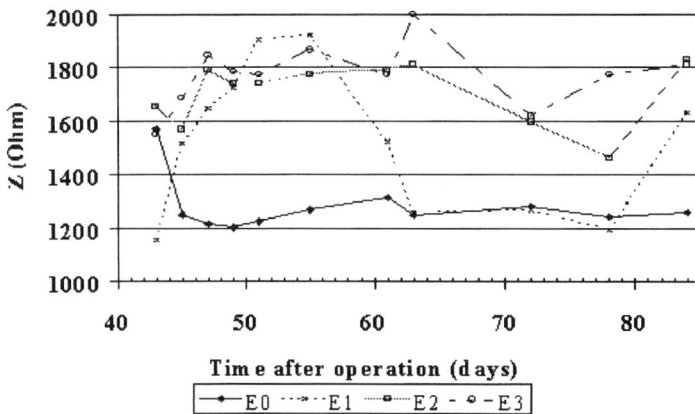

Figure 5 Example of one patient's left electrode: Impedance variations of each contact (E) under the standardized conditions.

Table 3 Impedance and Current of the Activated Contacts Compared to the Clinical Outcome

	Impedance (OHM) mean (SD)	Current (μA) mean (SD)
Improvement ≥ 80%	1378 (222)	63 (16)
Improvement < 80%	1366 (299)	66 (14)
p (Student)	0.88	0.14

electrical brain impedance is an individual factor. Nevertheless, we obtained mean values for in vivo brain impedance and optimal current drain that are now used in our center as an in vivo reference, as well for model description as for clinical practice. Especially the current drain measurement appears to be probably the most relevant criterion to be used for the follow-up of the patients (lower standard deviation). Nevertheless, the calculated mean values (especially, the current drain) are a very helpful basis for the follow-up of each patient. It reflects a correct delivery of electrical stimulation to the targeted structures. This can be useful in case of incomplete clinical results and when the good function of the system can be questioned.

Based on the results of this study, a special protocol based on impedance and current drain has been designed to regularly check the stimulation level and the good functioning of the stimulator. The observed reversible decrease of electrical brain impedance and, as a consequence, the facilitation of the current delivery in the short term as well as in the long term follow-up clearly indicates an adaptive mechanism. This cannot be explained at the moment but is probably in close relationship with the mechanism of action of electrical modulation of the pallidum (GPi) in dystonic patients. Despite the wide use of this technique, this has not yet been elucidated. The reversible decrease of impedance probably reflects a plasticity phenomenon. It implies an electrically induced reorganization of neuronal networks within or without the pallidum. Based on this data, it appears that the delay observed before reaching the steady state cannot be predicted depending on each patient. This make us recommend not to change the parameter setting too quickly during the test period because one important result of this study is to demonstrate that a delay is necessary to obtain the optimal conditions for deep brain stimulation.

B. Electric Field

Based on the obtained impedance and current mean values, a theoretical model of the stimulation system was developed (collaboration with Gérard Mennessier, physics depart-

Table 4 Impedance and Current of the Current Setting Compared to the Clinical Outcome

		Impedance (OHM) Mean (SD)	Current (μA) mean (SD)
Improvement ≥ 80%	1 contact	1283 (215)	80 (19)
	2 contacts	885 (118)	115 (45)
Improvement < 80%	1 contact	1355 (209)	79 (26)
	2 contacts	1027 (335)	128 (23)

ment, University of Science, Montpellier). With the help of this model, we calculated the stimulated volume for several parameter configurations and several voltages. To get an idea of the electric field distribution around the electrode, the different, mostly used electrode configurations have been visualized by 2D modeling (Fig. 6).

C. Study of the Electrical Stimulation of the Internal Globus Pallidus by Functional Magnetic Resonance Imaging

In order to improve the comprehension of the mechanism of action of stimulation of the internal globus pallidus, we have studied by fMRI a motor activation paradigm, on reference subjects and on dystonic patients with their stimulator on and off. Five references subjects and four dystonic patients (2 DYT1 positive patients) suffering from generalized dystonia and treated by deep brain stimulation of the GPi were tested by fMRI during the realization of a simple fingertip paradigm. All data were obtained on a 1.5-T research MRI scanner. Fast multislice echoplanar imaging with a gradient echo sequence was used to acquire data. The imaging parameters for the acquisition of 15 slices of 8 mm thickness were field of view 256×256 mm, matrix size 128×128. Slices were positioned parallel to the AC-PC line. Statistical comparison allowed showing activated areas with a threshold of 5%, 1%, and 0.1%. The fMRI of the five reference subjects presented a cerebral activation correlated with the paradigm at the level of the

Supplementary motor area (AC-PC $+62$ and $+46$ mm)
Primary motor and sensitive areas (AC-PC $+62$, $+54$ and $+46$ mm)
Pre- and postcentral gyri (AC-PC $+22$ and $+30$ mm)
Cerebellum (AC-PC -18 mm)

For the four dystonic patients, the pre- and postcentral gyri (AC-PC $+22$ and $+30$ mm) were not activated without stimulation. On the other hand, when the stimulation was switched on, these areas were activated. We can suppose facilitation in the motor cortex by

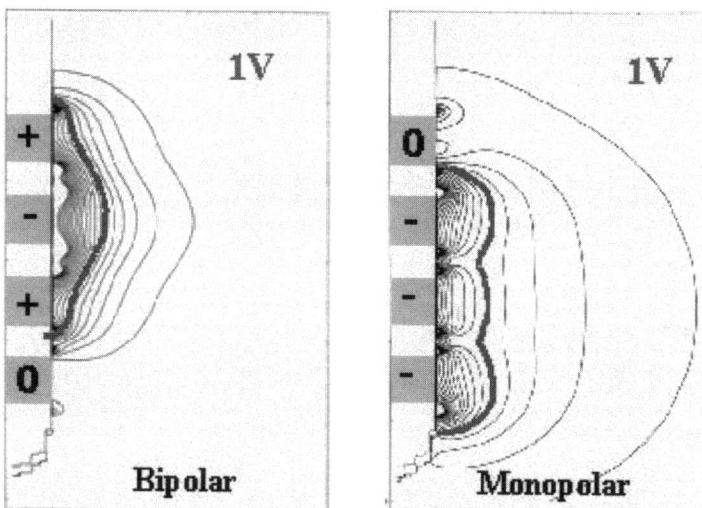

Figure 6 Comparison of the stimulated volume in the monopolar and the bipolar stimulation mode.

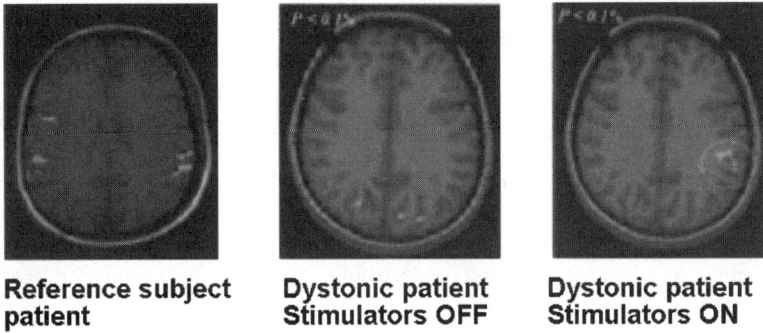

Reference subject   **Dystonic patient**   **Dystonic patient**
patient   **Stimulators OFF**   **Stimulators ON**

Figure 7   Motor facilitation by the electrical stimulation of internal pallidum.

the electrical stimulation of GPi. DBS allows an activation of cortical areas normally activated for healthy subjects and not activated for dystonic subjects without electrical stimulation (IPG off) (Fig. 7).

D.   Growth and Puberty in Children with Genetic Dystonia Treated by Deep Brain Stimulation of the Internal Globus Pallidus

The purpose of this study was to confirm that GPi stimulation has no negative impact on the development parameters of dystonic children. The existence of neuronal connections (indirect and direct) between the GPi and the hypothalamus could emphasize the involvement of the GPi in the hypothalamus's functioning and, subsequently, in puberty and growth of the children.

In 25 dystonic children (14 girls and 11 boys, mean age 13.1 ± 2.7 years), we have studied before and after stimulation:

Growth parameters curves (height and weight)

Dosages of hormonal secretions (growth hormones, gonadotrophins and sexual hormones)

Radiographic results (hand, elbow, pelvis)

The development's stage of puberty has been defined on the basis of these results and after the clinical evaluation. For the statistical analysis we have used a Fisher test with and without Yates correction. Twenty three patients showed an increase in height and weight. Eighty percent of patients had a normal height and 76% a normal weight. We found no significant difference for all parameters before and after operation ($p > 0.05$).

In conclusion there was no negative impact of DBS on the growth and the development of dystonic children. Furthermore, the subsequent neurological improvement allowed a compensation of the developmental retardation in most cases.

REFERENCES

1.   Laitinen LV. Brain targets in surgery for Parkinson's disease. Results of a survey of neurosurgeons. J Neurosurg 1985; 62(march):349–351.
2.   Laitinen LV, Bergenheim AT, Hariz MI. Ventroposterolateral pallidotomy can abolish all parkinsonian symptoms. Stereotact Funct Neurosurg 1992; 58(1–4):14–21.

3. Benabid AL, Pollak P, Louveau A, Henry S, de Rougemont J. Combined (thalamotomy and stimulation) stereotactic surgery of the VIM thalamic nucleus for bilateral Parkinson disease. Appl Neurophysiol 1987; 50(1–6):344–346.
4. Benabid AL, Benazzouz A, Hoffmann D, Limousin P, Krack P, Pollak P. Long-term electrical inhibition of deep brain targets in movement disorders. Mov Disord 1998; 13(suppl 3):119–125.
5. Limousin P, Pollak P, Benazzouz A, Hoffmann D, Le Bas JF, Broussolle E, Perret JE, Benabid AL. Effect of parkinsonian signs and symptoms of bilateral subthalamic nucleus stimulation. Lancet 1995; 345(8942):91–95.
6. Vayssiere N, Hemm S, Zanca M, Picot MC, Bonafe A, Cif L, Frerebeau P, Coubes P. Magnetic resonance imaging stereotactic target localization for deep brain stimulation in dystonic children. J Neurosurg 2000; 93(5):784–790.
7. Derosier C, Buee C, Ledour O, Horf F, Desgeorges M, Cosnard G. MRI and stereotaxis. Choice of an approach route on an independent console. J Neuroradiol 1991; 18(4):333–339.
8. Burke R, Fahn S, Marsden C. Validity and reliability of a rating scale for the primary torsion dystonia. Neurology 1985; 35:73–77.
9. Burke RE. Idiopathic torsion dystonia. Mov Disord 1992; 7(4):387–388.
10. Fahn S. Concept and classification of dystonia. Adv Neurol 1988; 50(2):1–8.
11. Kramer PL, de Leon D, Ozelius L, Risch N, Bressman SB, Brin MF, Schuback DE, Burke RE, Kwiatkowski DJ, Shale H. Dystonia gene in Ashkenazi Jewish population is located on chromosome 9q32–34. Ann Neurol 1990; 27(2):114–120.
12. Ozelius LJ, Hewett JW, Page CE, Bressman SB, Kramer PL, Shalish C, de Leon D, Brin MF, Raymond D, Corey DP, Fahn S, Risch NJ, Buckler AJ, Gusella JF, Breakefield XO. The early-onset torsion dystonia gene (DYT1) encodes an ATP-binding protein. Nat Genet 1997; 17(1):40–48.
13. Fletcher NA. The genetics of idiopathic torsion dystonia. J Med Genet 1990; 27(7):409–412.
14. Zhou B, Westaway SK, Levinson B, Johnson MA, Gitschier J, Hayflick SJ. A novel pantothenate kinase gene (PANK2) is defective in Hallervorden- Spatz syndrome. Nat Genet 2001; 28(4):345–349.
15. Hemm S, Cif L, Monnier C, Diakonova N, Hardouin E, Ganau A, Vayssiere N, Roubertie A, Azais M, Tuffery S, Mansour M, Claustres M, Echenne, B. P. C. Dystonies généralisées primitives: traitement par stimulation électrique chronique du globus pallidus interne. Mouvements 2001; 8:4–13.
16. Coubes P, Cif L, Azais M, Roubertie A, Hemm S, Diakonoya N, Vayssiere N, Monnier C, Hardouin E, Ganau A, Tuffery S, Claustre M, Echenne B. Traitement des syndromes dystoniques par stimulation électrique chronique du globus pallidus interne. Arch Pediatr 2002; 9(suppl 2):84s–86s.
17. Coubes P, Roubertie A, Vayssiere N, Hemm S, Echenne B. Treatment of DYT1-generalised dystonia by stimulation of the internal globus pallidus. Lancet 2000; 355(9222):2220–2221.

24

Peripheral Stimulation for Pain Control and the Development of Modern Transcutaneous Stimulation for Pain

Donlin M. Long
Johns Hopkins Hospital, Baltimore, Maryland, U.S.A.

Norman Hagfors
St. Paul, Minnesota, U.S.A.

The origin of transcutaneous and peripheral nerve electrical stimulation for the treatment of pain is reviewed as well as the development of spinal cord stimulation that has led to modern implantable electrodes. Mechanisms of action and clinical applications for a variety of pain syndromes are discussed as well as.

Transcutaneous stimulation of the nervous system using electricity applied through the skin has been used empirically for pain control since dependable sources of electricity have been available. Benjamin Franklin experimented with electrical stimulation for the treatment of trigeminal neuralgia. During the nineteenth century, an enormous array of portable and office electrical devices were marketed throughout the world for treatment of disease and relief of pain. The claims for many were absurd, but one consistent theme was relief of pain. One of the largest and most expensive of these devices provided electricity for fulguration of the hemorrhoids at one end of the spectrum and application to the skin for pain control on the other (27).

The modern era of neuroaugmentation began when Wall and Sweet observed control of pain with transcutaneous electrical stimulation of the trigeminal system (41,43). This was the first practical application of the justly famous gate-control theory of pain perception and modulation (33). Before publication of the gate-control theory by Melzack and Wall, neurosurgical involvement in pain had been primarily destructive. Shealy was the first to apply the basic concepts of the theory and the human observations of Sweet and Wall to control pain by modification of nervous system function, rather than destruction of pain pathways. The development of spinal cord stimulation first proposed by Shealy is described in greater detail in Chapter 7. After his first scientific publication (1967) and the oral presentation at the annual meeting of the American Association of Neurological Surgeons that followed, an interested group of neurosurgeons joined together to form a study group to investigate the feasibility of spinal cord stimulation for control of chronic pain.

As with any new technology, the first step was to plan clinical trials to determine the effectiveness of spinal cord stimulation. One of the immediate issues was a screening technique that might predict with greater accuracy patients who would respond to electrical stimulation. Shealy had already employed a device that has been available for years and could be purchased in many drug stores, the Electreat (personal observation). It was a battery-powered roller with ports for pad electrodes. The roller and pads provided electrical stimulation to the area to be treated, but the stimulation received was variable and the hand and arm applying the electrical signal got about as much stimulation as the area to be stimulated. Still, this was the best device available and most of the physicians involved in the early evaluation of stimulation of the nervous system for pain control employed it in the hope that it would provide screening for patients who would best respond to spinal cord stimulation (29) (Fig. 1).

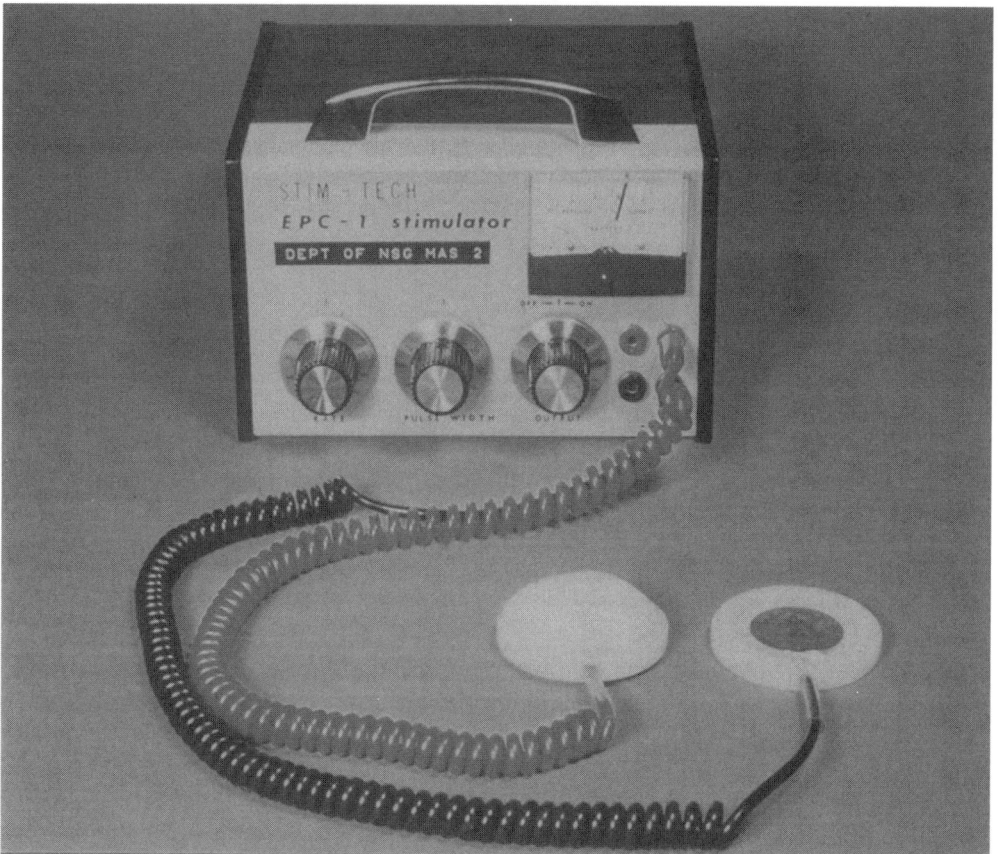

Figure 1 An early version of the EPC-1 with controls for rate, pulse width, and amplitude. The electrodes were covered with disposable, moistened sponge.

There was some evidence that transcutaneously applied electrical stimulation could be valuable alone. One anecdote in the medical literature described a patient in England with obvious neuropathic pain who relieved it by leaning against an electrical fence for a short period of time, stimulating above the area of nerve injury. When we began to apply transcutaneous electrical stimulation as a diagnostic screening tool to people with chronic pain of many types, we discovered that some received such satisfactory pain control that no additional therapy was required (26,29). We also noted that this was most likely to occur in patients with obvious peripheral nerve injuries. Pain relief was obtained when stimulation over the injured nerve trunk was carried out proximate to the injury and pain was usually worsened when stimulation was applied distal to the injury. These observations led to two separate lines of technology development: transcutaneous electrical stimulation and implantable stimulation of peripheral nerves for nerve injury pain.

I. TRANSCUTANEOUS ELECTRICAL STIMULATION

Shortly after the self-styled Dorsal Column Study Group was formed, sponsored by Medtronics and under my chairmanship, to investigate spinal cord stimulation, I met Mr. Norman Hagfors. Mr. Hagfors was an engineer who had been involved in the early development of a practical spinal cord stimulator for the Medtronics company with Dr. Shealy. He had established his own company and had already considered the development of a well-designed, variably controllable transcutaneous electrical stimulator (Fig. 2). He and I discussed the principles of design and the practical considerations of what clinicians and patients would require. Mr. Hagfors began the development and shortly after, brought me the EPC-1, the first reliable transcutaneous electrical stimulator (27). We began a series of clinical trials after much personal experience with the device. My wife and children still talk about sitting in our family room with Mr. Hagfors and I applying different electrical parameters to them and recording their responses to differing waveform, intensity, and frequency. We spent hours applying these stimulations to ourselves, concentrating on areas over major peripheral nerves to determine the effects.

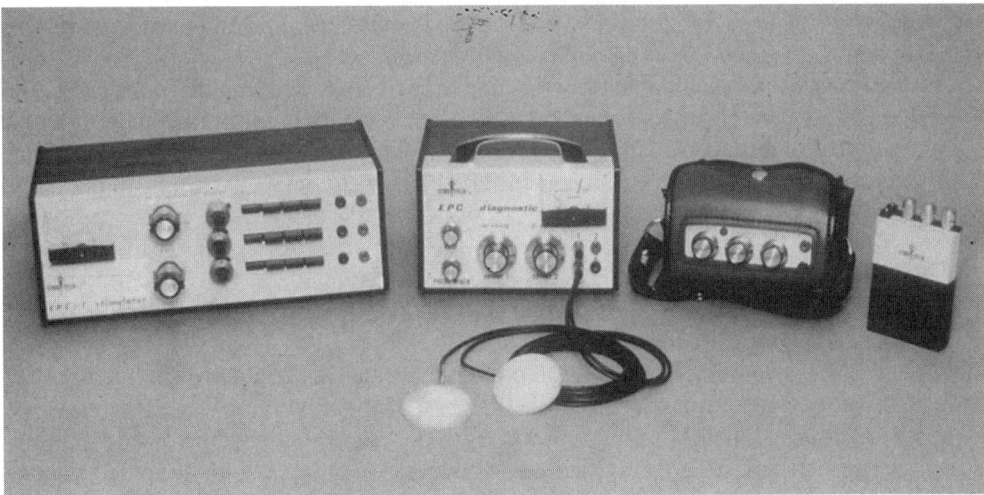

Figure 2 The family of stimulators (from L to R): our testing device, the EPC-1, the first personal stimulator, the first miniature version for patient use.

I have notebooks full of these acute observations, along with examinations of the effect of duration of stimulation. One anecdote comes to mind. In the course of all of this, I had to have hernia repair; so Mr. Hagfors arranged to make sterile electrodes which could be applied on either side of the skin incision after closure. I then amused myself for several days after surgery comparing the analgesic effect of different waveforms and intensities and comparing electrical stimulation with parental narcotics. I observed that the electrical stimulation, when applied continuously, gave excellent analgesia and was as effective as any parenteral narcotic that I utilized. Once we were convinced of safety, we began an observational study in patients to determine efficacy across a broad spectrum of chronic pain states. Our goal at this point was to understand more about which groups of patients might be benefited among the heterogeneous array of patients complaining of pain who confront the pain physician (26,27,29).

In the course of these early studies, we determined that central pain states were never helped and usually worsened by stimulation, while peripheral nerve injury patients were uniformly found transcutaneous stimulation helpful when the intact nerve proximal to the injury could be stimulated effectively. The majority of patients suffering from chronic pain have low back pain, and we determined that a significant number of them would be benefited by local electrical simulation alone or as a part of an active rehabilitation program. These observational studies were reported as early as 1973, and we then undertook specific, placebo-controlled clinical trials to examine the value of electrical stimulation in more specifically diagnosed pain groups (27). We determined the transcutaneous stimulation was of no value as a predictor of the success of percutaneous or implanted stimulation techniques, except for patients with peripheral nerve injury pain problems. Transcutaneous stimulation was found to be of greatest value in these patients with peripheral nerve injury and of least value in pain states where no significant cause could be demonstrated. Postincisional pain could be predictably relieved in a significant number of patients with low back and/or joint pain benefitted by direct electrical stimulation.

Once these principles of stimulation had been established, our major efforts were devoted to improving the technology for patient use. Mr. Hagfors played an important role in the miniaturization of stimulators to allow them to be used effectively by patients. Of course, this work was not unique, though we were the first, and there were many other physicians and engineers, predominantly at the Medtronics company in the early days who were pursuing very much the same objectives in the same ways.

There were some key factors in transforming the principles of stimulation defined in the research phase to devices suitable for clinical use. The availability of proven materials and manufacturing techniques, which we developed for earlier medical devices, proved very valuable in designing a reliable product. In the late 1950s we developed a totally implantable pacemaker for use clinically in treating patients with heart block. As we learned how to overcome the hostile environment of the body, the longevity and reliability of pacemakers were increased to the point where they are no longer an issue.

With the improved pacemaker technology available, we worked with Seymour Swartz on a device to stimulate the carotid sinus nerve for the treatment of essential hypertension. A key issue was the development of an implantable electrode that could be used to stimulate the nerve bundle on a continuous basis. We designed a bipolar cuff electrode that encircled the nerve providing a uniform stimulation current. The electrodes on which the nerves were seated were made of platinum, and the body of the electrode was made of molded silicone rubber. From our experience, we had modified the cuff electrode to use malleable platinum strips for the nerve contacts in the electrode. This allowed shaping of the electrode to accommodate varying sizes of nerve bundles. The leads consisted of a pair of stainless steel coil springs insulated in bilumen silicone rubber tubing, which connected to the implanted pulse generator or receiver. The dorsal column stimulator and peripheral nerve stimulator were designed using the technology developed for the carotid sinus nerve stimulator. The pulse generator consisted of an external RF transmitter with on–off switch and adjustable stimulation parameters coupled to an implanted passive receiver. For the dorsal column stimulator, we designed a bipolar electrode consisting of two platinum contacts, each approximately 5 mm square, arranged longitudinally and molded into a thin silicone rubber patch. This electrode assembly was sutured to the dura 1 to 3 mm from the dorsal column. The peripheral nerve stimulators used the RF coupled pulse generator and implanted receiver in conjunction with the bipolar nerve electrode.

II. TRANSCUTANEOUS ELECTRICAL NERVE STIMULATION

The transcutaneous electrical nerve stimulation (TENS) system consisted of a battery-powered stimulator and two or more surface electrodes. The first electrodes used a wet sponge for electrical contact with the skin. The sponge electrodes were typically about 5 cm in diameter and were moistened with tap water. These electrodes were backed by a nonconductive nylon shell and could be moved by the physician or patient to locate the site of best pain relief. With the development of other longer term surface electrodes, the sponge electrodes were often used for site evaluation.

Silicone, impregnated with carbon for electrical conductivity, was developed for molding stimulating electrodes to be worn for extended use. They were applied to the skin surface with conductive gels and held in place with adhesive patches. These electrodes were typically 3 to 5 cm wide and 5 to 20 cm long. They had a connector for attaching the lead wires.

The greatest problems with the early electrodes were lack of convenient attachment to the patient and skin irritation from long-term continuous use. To solve these problems, conductive adhesive gel electrodes were developed that provided self-adhesion when applied. Karaya gum was the first of these adhesive gels. It had been used in a variety of stoma seals for a number of years. With the success of this approach, a variety of electrically conductive polymers were developed for these electrodes, providing good contact with the irregularities of the skin surface and a more uniform current density at the electrode dermal interface. The result has been the development of self-adhesive electrodes that can be used for extended periods with minimal skin irritation.

A variety of stimulator packages were developed; however, the electrical characteristics were similar. Typically they provided a biphasic nonsymmetrical pulse of 0 to 50 mA in amplitude, a pulse duration of 0.05 to 0.150 ms, and a pulse repetition rate of 40 to 150 pulses/s. Some units provided pulse bursts of 1 to 10 bursts/s as a way of reducing battery power consumption and providing a greater variety of stimulation sensations for the patient. Rechargeable batteries that were easily replaced along with the use of microcircuits contributed to the design of small-sized devices that were convenient for the patient to wear.

III. PERCUTANEOUS AND IMPLANTABLE STIMULATION FOR THE PERIPHERAL NERVE INJURY PAIN

The observation that transcutaneous stimulation was effective for peripheral nerve injury pain was duplicated by nearly everyone working in the field, and this led to the development of the first implantable peripheral nerve stimulator by the Medtronics company and several of their engineers, principally Lincoln Ong and Don Maurer. To begin this investigation, I (DML) decided to carry out percutaneous nerve stimulation on myself. I had much data on transcutaneous stimulation applied over major nerve trunks, principally the ulnar nerve at the elbow and the median nerve at the wrist, but I thought we should have more direct stimulation data before attempting implantable stimulation on humans. Therefore, I inserted insulated percutaneous cordotomy electrodes onto or in the vicinity of my left ulnar nerve in the ulnar groove at the elbow. I then recorded the motor and sensory effects of a variety of waveforms, frequencies, and intensity parameters upon neurological function. Once I had determined the safety of the stimulation and established that a square wave pulse of perceptible intensity in frequencies between 60 and 120 seemed to provide safe, reliable stimulation, I began to employ the percutaneous technique for diagnosis in patients with neuropathic pain from peripheral nerve injury.

I first attempted stimulating the nerves proximal to the injury and then examined the effects of stimulation at other sites and especially stimulation of peripheral nerve distal to the site of injury. In doing this, I was able to determine that stimulation of an injured nerve proximal to the site of injury predictably completely relieved pain and associated trophic changes which were transitory temporarily during and shortly after stimulation. With this information, the existing dorsal column stimulator was modified by Medtronics engineers, and together, we developed a series of cuff electrodes to go around peripheral nerves of different sizes.

We began a clinical study and demonstrated the effectiveness of peripheral nerve stimulation. An interesting sidelight was the application of peripheral nerve stimulation for sciatica when the electrode was placed distal to the level of injury. In these patients, the problem was injury to the nerve in the course of a lumbar surgical procedure. Stimulation of the distal sciatic nerve provided immediate relief in the majority of patients, but the relief was short lived and pain recurred within 6 months in nearly all (27).

IV. THE CLINICAL USE OF TRANSCUTANEOUS ELECTRICAL STIMULATION

Shortly after the introduction of transcutaneous electrical stimulation, controlled evaluations began to appear. Fox and Melzak demonstrated that more than half of patients complaining of low back pain were benefitted temporarily (31,32). Long examined 300 patients subjected to random trials of TENS, subliminal stimulation, and treatment with a batteryless unit. One third of those treated continued with actual TENS to achieve satisfactory pain relief at 1 year, while there were no long-term successes in patients who received sham stimulation. Fourteen patients with peripheral nerve injury achieved long-term control (28). Jeans carried out a double-blind placebo controlled trial and found stimulation was significantly better than placebo for pain control (22). In 1983 Myerson reviewed the published data on electrical stimulation, pointing out the methodological problems of many published papers. He concluded that acute pain states were relieved satisfactorily and that approximately 30% among selected patients complaining of chronic pain could achieve long-term benefit from electrical stimulation (34).

Since that time, a number of papers have reported the effect in diverse painful states. It is now well-accepted that peripheral nerve injury pain is uniformly benefited by stimulation proximal to the site of injury (13,27). More than 50% of patients with isolated arthropathy obtain pain control. Excellent results have been achieved with dysmenorrhea and angina

(30). Similar benefits have been demonstrated in extremities painful because of vascular disease. All of these conditions have been investigated through controlled studies. Uncontrolled reports of relief of pain have appeared in the irritable bowel syndrome, interstitial cystitis, the arthropathy of hemophilia, and repeatedly with angina. There is general agreement that headache is rarely benefited (4,7,11,12,14,18,30).

Early studies indicated that TENS was a satisfactory way to control postoperative pain (19,40). I realize this is an anecdote, but I should repeat details of my own experience. I was to undergo an inguinal hernia repair at about the time that we were beginning serious examinations of postoperative pain control. Mr. Hagfors created a multipotential stimulator with many wave forms and variable parameters of stimulation (Figs. 3–6). I then used the device for pain control in the first 48 h after surgery comparing stimulation with narcotics with 4-h intervals. I found the stimulation was effective as narcotic at rest and more effective with ambulation.

Some studies suggested that TENS was of value in the control of labor pain. Between 40% and 70% of patients found TENS alone to be satisfactory for delivery analgesia (4,18).

The technique has been remarkably free of complications. The major issue was skin reaction to the electrodes, gels, and perhaps the electrical current. Muscle cramping can be produced, and prolonged stimulation over a nerve trunk can lead to both weakness and hypalgesia, which are transitory.

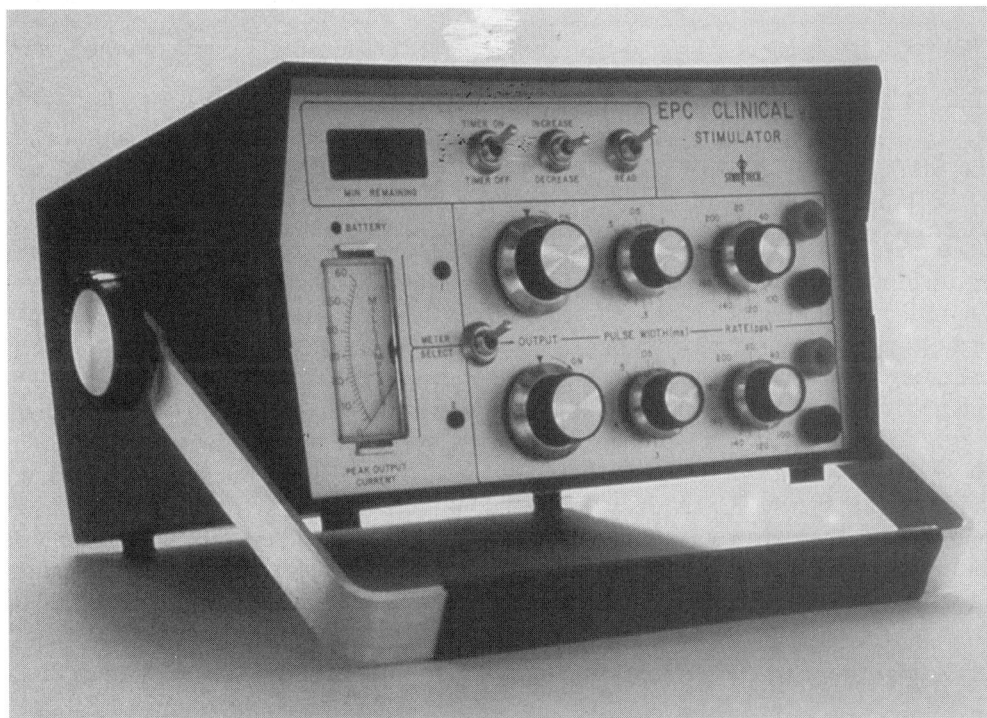

Figure 3   The clinical testing device used for transcutaneous and percutaneous testing. Practice parameter control was available.

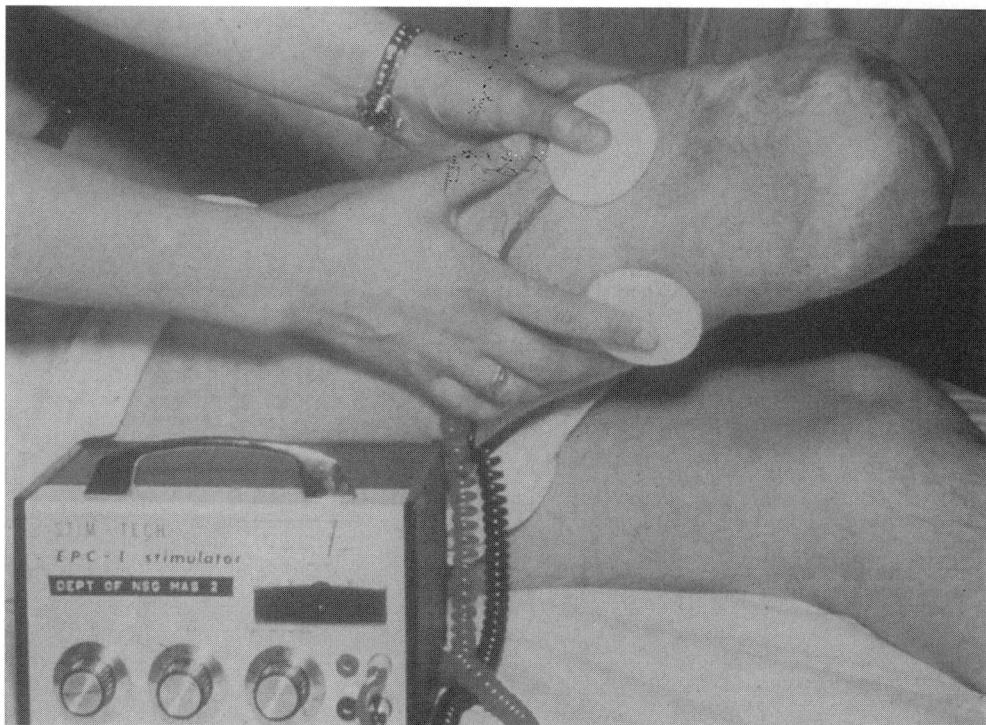

Figure 4 Stimulation for stump-neuroma pain: University of Minnesota Pain Treatment Center, 1971.

V. PHYSIOLOGICAL EFFECTS OF TRANSCUTANEOUS ELECTRICAL STIMULATION

There have been several studies which demonstrate increase in pain threshold to experimental induced pain following transcutaneous electrical stimulation (2,5,6). Why these changes in pain threshold occur is less clear. There is additional information that determines that changes in parameters of stimulation can modify the effects (10,15,20,24,34). Much more has been done with parameter change with internal stimulators than with transcutaneous stimulation. The original stimulators provided a range of 60–100 Hz. Short bursts appear to be as effective as prolonged stimulation and square waves are usually employed. However, many different wave forms have been tested and seem to be effective. Effects are not parameter specific (10,13,15,20,21,24,34).

There is also controversy about whether the effects of TENS are reversible by naloxone. In our own work, we were unable to determine any effect of naloxone. Other investigators have shown that low-frequency stimulation pain relief is reversible by naloxone (1,8,17,39).

VI. MECHANISMS OF ACTION

Transcutaneous electrical stimulation was originally based upon the general concept enunciated by Melzak and Wall in their justly famous gate-control theory (33). The hypothesis was that the stimulation of peripheral receptors would block or modify pain transmission from nociceptors probably at the spinal cord level and thus reduce pain. Several variations

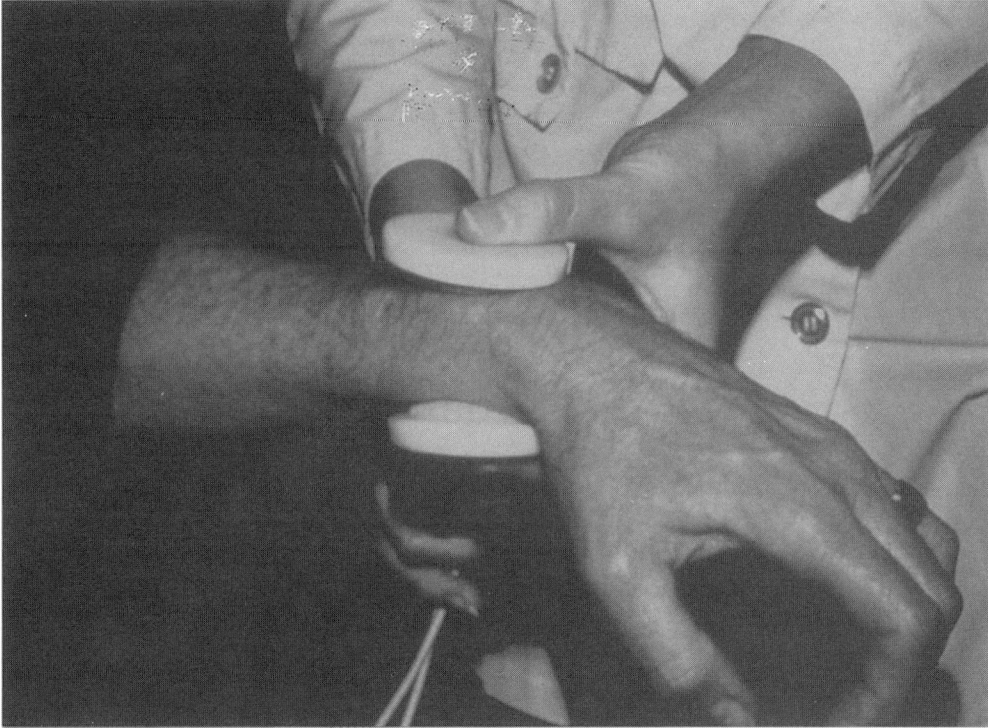

Figure 5 Stimulation for neuropathic pain of chronic median nerve injury: University of Minnesota Pain Treatment Center, 1971.

on this theme have been presented. It has been suggested that the block may be local at the receptor level or involve peripheral nerves (41). The stimulation may activate an inhibitory system at the level of the dorsal horn, or it may activate a descending inhibitory tract originating principally from thalamus and brainstem (9,34).

A placebo response has also been invoked. There are enough controlled studies that compare TENS with sham simulation, subliminal stimulation, and other kinds of sham therapies to demonstrate that the effect of stimulation is beyond what can be explained by placebo (23,28).

While very little direct research has been done on the possible effects of TENS, there is much material from pain in literature that provides additional information about possible modes of action. There are accepted causes of pain, which include acute tissue injury, peripheral nerve injury, peripheral nerve compression, or spinal instability. All activate nociceptors (42). There are theoretical causes of pain for which there is strong experimental evidence. Nociceptors may be activated by chemical agents, such as might be derived from a degenerated disk. Nociceptors sensitization after injury is a well-accepted event, and associated mechanosensitivity, such as occurs in types 2 and 3 neurons, has also been demonstrated (42). There is definite evidence that sensitization of a c-fiber nociceptors, which is usually confined at the site of the injury, is a first event in pain perception. Central sensitization of A nociceptors, which occurs in the site of injury and the surround, is also known to occur and sensitization of AB non-nociceptors, which produces allodynia, has also been demonstrated. The possibility that electrical stimulation modifies the sensitization

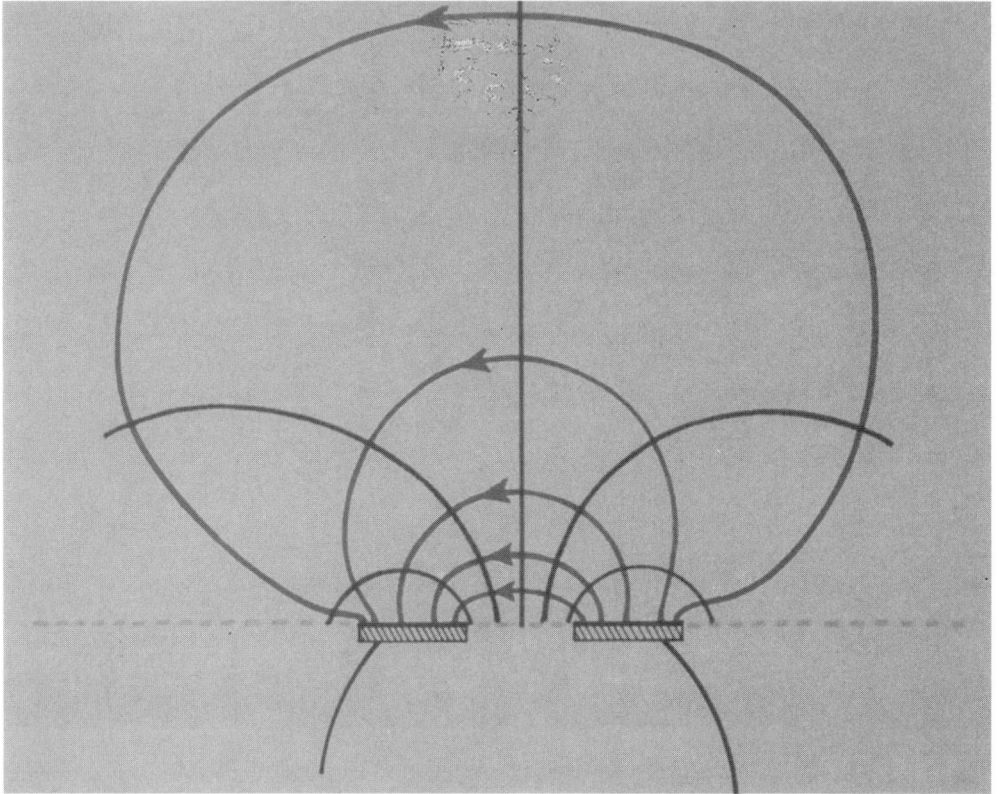

Figure 6 Early current-flow-intensity diagram from experimental data of Mr. Norman Hagfors, used to model electrode placement. Mr. Hagfors produced similar data for all electrode configurations and placements.

process either through its local effects or at the level of the dorsal horn is a reasonable supposition. An experimental model that is used to investigate peripheral nerve injury also indicates that much of the perceived pain is mediated through adjacent uninjured nerves. A blocking effect preventing this spread of the pain signal is certainly possible (42).

Central facilitation of the reduction of pain threshold is known to occur. This central facilitation is reduced by pain-relieving procedures, and this is another possible explanation of the effects of electrical stimulation of the nervous system. The central inhibition may also be an important phenomenon. The central inhibition is impaired when pain is continuous and reappears when pain is controlled. Increasing the effectiveness of central inhibition is another possible explanation (3,35,42).

VII. PRACTICAL USE OF TRANSCUTANEOUS ELECTRICAL STIMULATION

I still employ transcutaneous electrical stimulation as one of several ways to provide relief for patients with chronic neuropathic or neuromuscular pain. It will be sufficient as the only therapy for some and a useful adjunct for pain relief in many others. The key to successful use is an appropriate diagnosis. Pain is a common complaint that is frequently modified by psychological, behavioral, and socioeconomic factors (23,27,29). It is unlikely that transcutaneous stimulation or any other form of pain relief will affect these aspects of the pain syndrome. Even when transcutaneous stimulation is effective for pain relief, it should be supplemented by appropriate education about body mechanics in an exercise program to provide muscle strengthening and increase range of motion all patients where these are issues. Supplementation with analgesic medications may make the technique even more effective and the stimulation allows smaller doses of medication to be used. TENS is not a panacea for chronic pain, but simply one tool available to the pain therapist for management of the complaint (27).

The skill of the therapist is also an important issue. Patients must be educated in how to use the device, and there must be someone available to them to answer questions and coach them about continuing appropriate use. Most busy physicians do not have time to do this, so it's important to have technical assistance from someone who is skilled in the use of stimulation. Patient education is an extremely important issue. When the patient is simply given the devices, failure is almost certain (27).

VIII. SUMMARY

The unscientific use of electrical stimulation for pain control has a long history over the last 200 years or more (27). In the early 1970s, well-engineered controllable devices were developed and since that time, many well-controlled studies have indicated the value of the technique (26,28,29). There are many applications for which stimulation is a reasonable alternative to other symptomatic methods of pain control. Many other poorly designed and uncritical reports are in the literature describing transcutaneous electrical stimulation which has been inexpertly applied to patients. When an appropriate diagnosis has been made and the patient educated in the use of the technique, it remains a valuable adjunct in pain management that will provide satisfactory relief to many.

REFERENCES

1. Abraham SE, Reynolds AC, Cusick JF. Failure to naloxonee to reverse analgesia from transcutaneous electrical stimulation in patients with chronic pain. Anesth Analg 1981; 60:81–84.
2. Anderson SA, Holmgren E. Pain threshold effects of peripheral conditioning stimulation. In Bonica JJ, Albe-Fesard DG, eds. Advances in Pain Research and Therapy. Proc. First World Congr Pain. Vol 1. New York: Raven Press, 1976:761–768.
3. Arendt-Nielsen L, Bjerring P. Long-term effect of low and high frequency TNS on pain related cortical responses. Pain 1987; 4(suppl):S366.
4. Augustinsson L-E, Bohlin P, Bundsen P, Carlsson CA, Forssman I. Pain relief during delivery by transcutaneous electrical nerve stimulation. Pain 1977; 4:59–65.
5. Callaghan M, Sternback RA, Nyquist JK, Timmermans G. Changes in somatic sensitivity during transcutaneous electrical analgesia. Pain 1978; 5:115–128.
6. Campbell JN, Taub A. Local analgesia from percutaneous electrical stimulation: A peripheral mechanism. Arch Neurol 1973; 28:347–350.
7. Carlsson CA, Augustinsson L-E, Lund S, Roupe G. Electrical transcutaneous nerve stimulation for the relief of itch. Experientia 1975; 31:191.
8. Chapman CR, Benedetti C. Analgesia following transcutaneous electrical stimulation and its partial reversal by a narcotic antagonist. Life Sci 1977; 21:1645–1648.

9. Cheng RSS, Pomeranz B. Electracupuncture analgesia could be mediated by at least two pain-relieving mechanisms: Endorphin and non-endorphin systems. Life Sci 1979; 25:1957–1962.

10. Finch L, Melzak R, Birks RI, Davis MWL. Comparison of conventional versus short burst TENS. Pain 1987; 4(suppl):S365.

11. Ekblom A, Hansson P. Extrasegment transcutaneous electrical nerve stimulation and mechanical vibratory stimulation as compared to placebo for the relief of acute oro-facial pain. Pain 1985; 23:223–229.

12. Fall M. Conservative management of chronic interstitial cystitis: transcutaneous electrical nerve stimulation and transurethral resection. J Urol 1985; 133:774–777.

13. Fields HL, Adams JE, Hosobuchi Y. Peripheral nerve and cutaneous electrohypalgesia. Adv Neurol 1974; 4:749–754.

14. Finsen V, Persen L, Lovlien M, Veslegaard EK, Simensen M, Gasvann AK, Benum P. Transcutaneous electrical nerve stimulation after major amputation. J Bone Joint Surg 1988; 70B:109–112.

15. Golding JF, Ashton H, Marsh R, Thomson JW. Transcutaneous electrical nerve stimulation produces variable changes in somatosensory evoked potentials, sensory perception and pain threshold: clinical implications for pain relief. J Neurol Neurosurg Psychiatry 49:1397–1406.

16. Hagfors NR, Schwartz SI. Implantable Electronic Carotid Sinus Nerve Stimulators for Reducing Hypertension. Proceedings of the Nineteenth Annual Conference on Engineering in Medicine and Biology 1966; 8:36.

17. Hansson P, Ekblom A, Thomsson M, Fjellner B. Influence of naloxonee on relief of acute oro-facial pain by transcutaneous electrical nerve stimulation (TENS) or vibration. Pain 1986; 24:323–329.

18. Harrison RF, Woods T, Shore M, Mathews G, Unwin A. Pain relief in labour using transcutaneous electrical nerve stimulation (TENS). A TENS/TENS placebo controlled study in two parity groups. Br J Obstet Bynaecol 1986; 93:739–746.

19. Hymes AC, Raab DE, Yonehiro EG, Nelson G, Printy A. Electrical surface stimulation for control of acute postoperative pain and prevention of ileus. Surg Forum 1973; 24:447–449.

20. Ignelzi RJ, Nyquist JK. Direct effect of electrical stimulation on peripheral nerve evoked activity: implications in pain relief. J Neurosurg 1976; 45:159–165.

21. Ignelzi RJ, Nyquist JK. Excitability changes in peripheral nerve fibers after repetitive electrical stimulation. J Neurosurg 1979; 51:824–833.

22. Jeans ME. Relief of chronic pain by brief, intense transcutaneous electrical stimulation—a double-blind study. In: Bonica JJ, Liebeskind JC, Albe-Fessard DG, eds. Advances in Pain Research and Therapy. Vol 3. New York: Raven Press, 1979:601–606.

23. Johansson F, Almay BGL, von Knorring L. Personality factors related to the outcome of treatment with transcutaneous nerve stimulation. Psychiatr Clin North Am 1981; 14:96–104.

24. Linzer M, Long DM. Transcutaneous neural stimulation for relief of pain. IEEE Trans Biomed Eng 1976; 23:341–345.

25. Loewenstein WR. Modulation of cutaneous mechanoreceptors by sympathetic stimulation. J Physiol 1956; 132:40–60.

26. Long DM. External electrical stimulation as a treatment of chronic pain. Minn Med 1974; 57:195–198.

27. Long DM. Fifteen years of transcutaneous electrical stimulation for pain control. Stereotactic Funct Neurosurg 1991; 56:2–19.

28. Long DM, Campbell JN, Guver G. Transcutaneous electrical stimulation for relief of chronic pain. In: Bonica JJ, Liebeskind JC, Albe-Fessard DG, eds. Advances in Pain Research and Therapy. Vol 3. New York: Raven Press, 1979:593–599.

29. Long DM, Hagfors N. Electrical stimulation in the nervous system: The current status of electrical stimulation of the nervous system for relief of pain. Pain 1975; 1:109–123.

30. Mannheimer C, Augustinsson L-E, Carlsson C-A, Manhem K, Wilhelmsson C. Epidural spinal electrical stimulation in severe angina pectoris. Br Heart J 1988; 59:56–61.

31. Melzak R. Prolonged relief of pain by brief intense transcutaneous stimulation. Pain 1975; 1:357–373.
32. Melzak R, Vetere P, Finch L. Transcutaneous electrical nerve stimulation for low back pain. Phys Ther 1983; 63:489–493.
33. Melzak R, Wall PD. Pain mechanism: a new theory. Science 1965; 150:971–979.
34. Meyerson BA. Electrostimulation procedure: effects, presumed rationale, and possible mechanisms. In: Bonica JJ, Lindblom U, Iggo A, eds. Advances in Pain and Research and Therapy. Proceedings of Third World Congress on Pain. Vol. 5. New York: Raven Press, 1983:495–534.
35. Satran R, Goldstein MN. Pain perception: modification of threshold of intolerance and cortical potentials by cutaneous stimulation. Science 1973; 180:1201–1202.
36. Schwartz SI, Griffith LSC, Neistadt A, Hagfors N. Chronic carotid sinus nerve stimulation in the treatment of essential hypertension. Am J Surg 1967; 114:5–15.
37. Shealy CN, Maurer D. Transcutaneous nerve stimulation for control of pain: a preliminary technical note. Surg Neurol 1974; 2:45–47.
38. Shealy CN, Mortimer JT, Hagfors NR. Dorsal column electroanalgesia. J Neurosurg 1970; 32:560–564.
39. Sjolund B, Eriksson M. The influence of natoxone analgesia from peripheral conditioning stimulation. Brain Res Sep 14, 1979; 173(2):295–301.
40. Solomon RA, Viernstein MC, Long DM. Reduction of postoperative pain and narcotic use by transcutaneous electrical nerve stimulation. Surgery 1980; 87:142–146.
41. Sweet WH, Wepsic JG. Treatment of chronic pain by stimulation of fibers of primary different neurons. Trans Am Neurol Assoc 1968; 93:103–107.
42. Treede R-D, Rolke R, Andrews K, Magerl W. Pain elicited by blunt pressure: neurobiological basis and clinical relevance. Pain 2002; 98:235–240.
43. Wall PD, Sweet WH. Temporary abolition of pain in man. Science 1967; 155:108–109.

25

Low-Frequency Electromagnetic Field Effects on Lymphocytes: Potential for Treatment of Inflammatory Diseases

Gabi Nindl, Mary T. Johnson, and Walter X. Balcavage
Indiana University School of Medicine, Terre Haute Center for Medical Education, Terre Haute, Indiana, U.S.A.

The authors propose a new approach for the treatment of inflammatory diseases: the use of electromagnetic fields (EMFs), which exert anti-inflammatory effects by eliminating inflammatory T cells. The authors briefly review the process of inflammation and describe a T lymphocyte cell model that is useful in studying the role of EMFs as a therapeutic agent. It is suggested that EMF therapy may be most efficacious when used in conjunction with other more conventional therapies (which might induce cells into a metastable metabolic state amenable to EMF therapy. The authors' ideas are based on a review of the pertinent EMF literature, and their own work on EMF effects on lymphocytes.

I. PERSPECTIVES ON THE IMPACT OF EMFs FOR TREATMENT OF INFLAMMATORY DISEASES

For centuries, claims have been made that EMFs from natural sources such as loadstones or EMFs from man-made static and time-varying sources have therapeutic efficacy. Such fields have been used to treat almost every conceivable human illness or malady, and it is not surprising to find amongst them many inflammatory diseases such as arthritis or psoriasis. Likewise, EMF therapy has always been associated with pain reduction and accelerated healing, and it is possible that EMFs might exert these effects by regulating processes involved in inflammation and autoimmune diseases. Inflammation is a cascade of physiological processes instigated by the body to repair cellular damage in vascularized tissues and to restore the tissue to its normal function.

The characteristic signs and symptoms that accompany inflammation include redness generated by increased blood flow, heat generated by the metabolism of leucocytes and macrophages recruited to the damage site, swelling due to edema, and pain caused by the production of pro-inflammatory prostaglandins. While inflammation is a necessary and beneficial process, its intensity during the initial acute phase can be pathologically exaggerated and it often persists longer than necessary developing into chronic inflammation. Chronic inflammation is generally associated with dysfunction of one or more immune system components and leads to the ongoing tissue damage found in diseases like tendinitis, arthritis or psoriasis. Recently, chronic inflammation also has been implicated in the etiology of cancer and Alzheimer's disease, illnesses that traditionally have not been associated with inflammation (1). Inflammation is the net result of a cascade of biological processes that is generated and supported by the interaction of a number of immune cell types including lymphocytes, macrophages, and neutrophils with other cell types such as fibroblasts, endothelial cells, and vascular smooth muscle cells playing a regulatory role in the cascade. These cells and the metabolic pathways they employ to generate inflammation provide numerous targets for therapies aimed at controlling inflammation in the acute phase and in preventing progression to chronic inflammation.

In this chapter, we review evidence for interaction of nonionizing, low-frequency, alternating electromagnetic fields (EMFs) with lymphocytes and discuss the potential of EMFs to provide an anti-inflammatory, noninvasive therapy for eliminating lymphocytes. Due to space constraints, we do not discuss the evidence on static magnetic fields indicating their potential to modulate cell replication and apoptosis of lymphocytes. Inflammation can be initiated by many causes, and the nature of the precipitating event is important in designing therapeutic interventions for inflammatory diseases (2). In bacterial infections, early infiltration of the affected site by polymorphonuclear neutrophils (PMNs) is followed by the arrival of T cells that upregulate PMN-dependent processes, an event that is requisite to bacterial death. In cases like this, eliminating inflammatory T cells might be counterproductive to healing. Conversely, in trauma-induced injury, T cells are less important for resolving tissue damage, and may even be harmful if present for prolonged periods. In these cases, early elimination of T cells in the acute phase of inflammation could minimize the unwanted side effects of inflammation, accelerate healing, and reduce the risk of chronic inflammatory disease. In chronic inflammatory diseases such as rheumatoid arthritis, psoriasis, and chronic tendinitis, maintenance of the disease state is dependent upon the presence of T cells. Again, killing T cells would be viewed as a favorable method of therapy for these and similar chronic diseases.

Many models have been used to study the impact of EMFs on cells and metabolic pathways involved in the inflammation cascade. In this laboratory, we use Jurkat cells, a $CD4^+$ T lymphocyte cell line to study EMF effects at the cellular level. We are also developing a rat model of tendinitis to study the effects of EMFs on inflamed tissues (3,4). Using our T-cell model, we have discovered that EMFs can induce apoptotic cell death in T lymphocytes. Since T cells are a major regulator of the inflammatory cascade, our discovery led us to hypothesize that EMFs might be used as a noninvasive treatment for inflammatory diseases such as tendinitis or psoriasis (4,5). In this chapter we present results from our laboratory where we used Jurkat cell cultures as a T cell model to evaluate the effects of EMFs on normal and inflammatory T lymphocytes. We place them in the context of recent EMF studies on lymphocytes and other inflammatory cells to evaluate the potential of EMF therapy for treatment of inflammatory diseases.

II. EFFECT OF POWER FREQUENCY EMFs ON LYMPHOCYTES AND IMMUNE FUNCTIONS

The recent upsurge of interest in the biological effects of EMFs evolved and grew from epidemiological reports of the late eighties and early nineties that linked powerline (50 and 60

Hz) EMF exposure to negative health effects such as childhood leukemia (6,7), a cancer of bone marrow cells. In leukemia, abnormal white blood cells are present in peripheral blood and infiltrate other immune organs such as liver, spleen, and lymph nodes. And so the patients' immune system and their ability to fight infections are impaired. Governments throughout the world reacted to concerns that EMFs could promote leukemia and perhaps other forms of cancer and funded studies to determine if powerline EMFs have carcinogenic effects. Many of these studies are important to review here since they reveal valuable insight into potential interactions of EMFs with lymphocytes. All of the final reports emanating from the governmentally funded programs agree that low-intensity, 50- and 60-Hz EMFs associated with electrical power distribution systems do not pose a significant risk of leukemia or otherwise negatively affect human health.

Although we have not performed studies to assess the possibility that EMFs pose a risk to human health, our EMF research experience with cells and animals leads us to agree with the developing consensus that it is unlikely that EMFs associated with power distribution systems pose a substantial health risk. However, we do not agree with the criticism on the validity and expense of the health assessment programs (8). As a result of the concern over the safety of environmentally encountered EMFs, numerous changes have been made in the design and construction of electrical devices ranging from changes in power-line transmission construction to the configuration of heating wires in electric blankets. In various countries standards have been developed for EMF emissions from devices that use electricity in the workplace and in residences. Extended programs are underway to investigate the impact of radio-frequency, cell-phone-frequency, and microwave-frequency EMFs used in communications and data transfer on health. The knowledge accumulated from all these studies significantly contributes to our understanding of how to safely use electricity in our daily life and how to expand the use of electricity for diagnostics and therapy.

We also do not agree with the even more extreme position that EMFs, including 50 and 60 Hz power frequency EMFs, can have no substantial effect on biological systems. The rationale for our position on this issue stems from our own research with T lymphocytes, which we will review below, and the fact that numerous reputable investigators have reported substantial biological outcomes from experiments conducted to test the effect of a wide range of EMFs. The fact that many of these reports could not be replicated, sometimes even in the same laboratory, does not necessarily mean that the original observations were wrong or inaccurate, but rather, that the conditions necessary to replicate the experiments were unrecognized. The latter is not surprising since without understanding the mechanism(s) by which EMFs influence biological systems it is virtually impossible to assure that the correct controls are used in experimental protocols.

Many of the studies we allude to, including those from our group, were performed in order to try to uncover the primary EMF sensitive cellular site(s), or more descriptively the "biological antenna(e)," and how these entities connect to metabolic pathways. Although the EMF sensitive sites remain unknown their downstream effects on signal transduction pathways and connected physiological endpoints like cell proliferation or cell death can now be readily documented. With this information in hand, it is possible to optimize EMF effects in model systems and design studies to evaluate the therapeutic efficacy of EMFs. In our laboratory, in contradistinction to many investigators in the field, we early developed the hypothesis that if weak EMFs could modulate lymphocyte biology such as appeared to be the case in childhood leukemia, then the underlying mechanisms, once understood, could be turned to therapeutic advantage while avoiding oncogenic side effects. We have consistently maintained this as our guiding research philosophy and as a filter that we use to view the literature in this area.

A. EMF Effects on T Lymphocyte Signaling

In studies aimed at linking EMFs with signal transduction pathways Korzh-Sleptsova et al. (9) presented data that 50-Hz, 0.15-mT EMFs increased the level of inositol triphosphate (IP_3) in Jurkat cells, the same cells that we use as our T-cell model. The appearance of IP_3 depends on signal transduction through CD45, a major transmembrane glycoprotein in all lymphocytes. CD45's cytosolic domain is a tyrosine phosphatase and its extracellular domain is heavily O-glycosylated. Cells with native CD45 and those with modified extracellular domains responded to EMFs with increased IP_3, while cells with a modified cytosolic domain, and thus lacking tyrosine phosphatase activity, were unresponsive to EMFs (10). These results indicated that the primary EMF target was involved in activating CD45 and thus located very early in the T-cell signaling pathway. In studies published in 1998, the same investigators found that Jurkat clones lacking the alpha and beta subunits of the T-cell receptor (TCR) had diminished EMF sensitivity as assayed by intracellular calcium oscillations (11). In continuing investigations Lindstroem et al. traced the influence of EMFs through the signal transduction pathway consisting of CD45, the downstream tyrosine kinase Lck, the zeta chains of the TCR, and protein kinase C (PKC) (12). They found that modification of any component in this pathway eliminated the sensitivity of cells to EMFs. Thus, these investigators have built a strong chain of evidence implicating EMFs in activation of an important signal transduction pathway that can induce T-cell death or cell replication depending on other extracellular signals. Other laboratories also reported EMF effects on PKC. For instance, Holian et al. (13) found an EMF-dependent (60 Hz electric field, 330 mV/cm) decrease of cytosolic PKC activity in the HL60 human leukemia cell line. The same laboratory confirmed this result in H9 human leukemia cells but found no effect at higher or lower electric field intensities (14).

When we first considered research in the area of bioelectromagnetics, we reviewed the mechanisms that had been proposed to account for EMF effects and concluded, in agreement with most investigators, that there was no consensus in favor of any mechanism that had been proposed. However, to broaden our own perspectives on how EMFs might impact biological systems and to introduce new ideas into the area of theoretical bioelectromagnetics, we developed a model based on the classical Hall effect. Applied to biological systems, our model in its simplest form states that EMFs could perturb ion flow through voltage-gated ion channels including those for Na^+, K^+, and Ca^{2+} (15). In turn, we calculated that these events could trigger conformation changes in membrane proteins leading to altered functional states of the ion channels and subsequent intracellular events such as those initiated by CD45. The mechanism we proposed remains a viable alternative to explain how ion modulated processes, e.g., Ca-calmodulin regulated pathways, could be modified by EMFs.

Since it was known that there is a tight coupling between activation of the TCR and increased intracellular free Ca^{2+}, we hypothesized that EMFs might alter Ca^{2+} flux in cells stimulated by TCR-activating ligands like anti-CD3, an antibody against the CD3 subunit of the TCR. In collaboration with Liburdy and Eckert (16), we also studied EMF-dependent anti-CD3 binding as a prelude to planned studies on EMF-dependent Ca^{2+} flux. Essentially identical to the results of Liburdy's group we found a substantial increase in anti-CD3 bound to Jurkat cells when the binding reaction was performed in a 60-Hz, 0.1-mT field (17). A typical Scatchard plot from our experiments is illustrated in Fig. 1. In these experiments log phase Jurkat cells were exposed to either 0.1-mT, 60-Hz fields developed by a vertically oriented solenoid plus the local geofield (horizontal component about 0.04 mT), or to the geofield alone (controls).

After correcting the results shown in Fig. 1 for low-affinity, nonspecific binding we calculate that EMF exposure induced a 41.7% increase in B_{max}. Please note that B_{max}

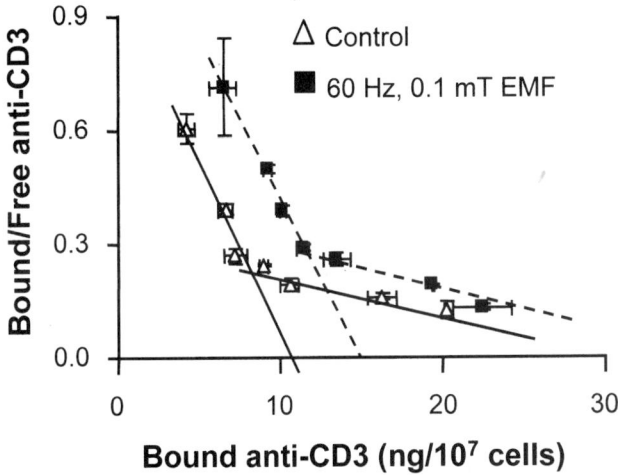

Figure 1 Representative scatchard analysis showing increased ligand binding (B_{max}) to the Jurkat T cell receptor by 60-Hz, 0.1-mT EMFs. Nanogram quantities of FITC-labeled anti-CD3, an antibody to the gamma subunit of the T cell receptor, were incubated at 25°C with 10^7 Jurkat cells in the presence of EMFs supplied by a solenoid or controls exposed to the earth's geofield only. For details of these assays see Ref. 17. Error bars represent ± one standard deviation. Thirteen similar experiments were performed and these results are summarized in Table 1.

represents the relative number of high-affinity anti-CD3 binding sites per 10^7 cells and does not stand here for maximal magnetic field flux. In these experiments B_{max} is determined as the x intercept of the linear regression lines. B_{max}, the number of high-affinity anti-CD3 binding sites per 10^7 cells, was estimated by extrapolating the linearized binding isotherms to the abscissa, as shown in the Fig. 1. K_d, the dissociation constant for the binding reaction, is proportional to the reciprocal of the slope of the lines. Data points represent the average of triplicate assays. We repeated this experiment 13 times and present the corrected results of all those experiments in Table 1. In more than half the experiments the EMF exposure produced statically significant increases in the B_{max} of anti-CD3 binding, ranging from 9.9% to 65.2%, with only minor effects on the K_d of the binding reaction (determined as the negative reciprocal of the slope). In the remaining experiments there was no statistically significant difference between experimental and control data sets. When we combined the data from all 13 experiments, we calculated a mean B_{max} of 12.3 binding sites per 10^7 cells for controls (90% confidence interval of 1.7), while the mean B_{max} for cells exposed to 0.1-mT EMFs was 14.9 binding sites per 10^7 cells (90% confidence interval of 2.5). This 21% mean increase in ligand binding induced by the EMF exposure suggests that the EMF fields have a significant effect on the apparent B_{max} for anti-CD3 binding to the Jurkat TCR.

In spite of these statistically impressive results, we had a substantial number of experiments where there was little or no EMF effect. Although we work hard to control the homeostatic state of the cells that we use in our experiments, we suspect that the variable results are due to subtle differences in the cells, which we do not yet adequately control. This is a finding that has accompanied our work throughout the years and leads us to conclude that only distinct metastable cell states are EMF sensitive. In the following sections, we add further evidence for this hypothesis that, if true, has important implications for EMF therapy.

Table 1 Summary of 13 Experiments[a]
Illustrating the Effect of EMFs on Anti-CD3
Binding to the Jurkat T Cell Receptor

Control	EMF	% Diff.
8.85	11.30	27.7
12.48	16.82	34.8
12.38	13.60	9.9
7.12	10.09	41.7
13.30	21.97	65.2
13.62	20.65	51.6
21.80	26.77	22.8
8.78	9.23	5.1
13.07	13.80	5.6
12.85	13.35	3.9
11.99	12.01	0.2
12.84	12.74	−0.8
11.29	10.01	−11.3

[a] The 13 experiments summarized in the table
were performed exactly as described in Fig. 1.
The number of high affinity binding sites
(B_{max}) was evaluated after subtracting low-
affinity and nonspecific ligand binding. In
seven of 13 experiments EMFs produced an
average increase of 36% in high affinity anti-
CD3 binding (B_{max}) with only minor effects
on K_d. In the remaining six experiments there
was no significant difference between experimental and control data sets. When the
results of all the experiment were averaged,
the net effect was a 20% increase in high
affinity anti-CD3 binding induced by 60-Hz,
0.1-mT EMFs.

B. EMF Effects on B Lymphocyte Signaling

In a series of studies like those from Lindstroem's laboratory (9–12) with T cells, Uckun et al.
(18) studied the effects 1-mT, 60-Hz EMFs on signal transduction in a human B-cell line. In
the B-cell signal transduction pathway antigen binding of the B-cell receptor activates LYN,
and LYN phosphorylates the cytosolic domain of the B-cell receptor (a regulatory process
that is reminiscent of phosphorylation of the TCR by LCK). The phosphorylated receptor
then serves as a site that sequesters the cytosolic tyrosine kinase SYK, a regulatory process
again reminiscent of T-cell regulation where TCRs phosphorylated by LCK control protein
tyrosine kinases, such as Zap-70. Both, T- and B-cell pathways, culminate in PKC activation.
In their early studies using the human B-cell line NALM-6, Uckun et al. (18) showed that
EMFs stimulated the production of PKC. In continuing studies using a second human B-cell
line (DT 40), they showed that EMFs stimulate the activity of LYN and SYK and that the
appearance of these activities is followed by the appearance of activated PKC, PLC-
gamma2, and IP$_3$, all important downstream regulators of B-cell receptor signaling pathways (19). When this group tested B cells deficient in Bruton's tyrosine kinase (BTK), an

intermediate in the signal transduction pathway located between LYN and PLC, they found that EMF exposure did not lead to PLC activation in deficient cells but that transgenic restoration of BTK activity restored the EMF effect on PLC (20). These interesting results are in accord with and support the earlier work of this group. Similarly, cells made deficient in LYN, SYK, or PLC-gamma2 became EMF unresponsive, and the EMF effect could be restored when the genes for the signaling molecules were reconstituted to their native state (18). Since B-cell receptor and T-cell receptor signaling pathways follow similar patterns, it is very exciting to see data accumulating that point towards a cellular pathway used by EMFs to exert biologically relevant long-term effects. Other investigators have extended these findings by demonstrating modifications in the morphology and cytoskeletal arrangement of a human lymphoid cell line when exposed to 50-Hz, 2-mT EMFs (21).

C. The Question of Reproducibility

The reports outlined above appear to provide important support for our hypothesis that EMF therapy can be used to regulate the activity of inflammatory T cells and B cells and thereby provide a noninvasive tool to treat inflammatory diseases. Unfortunately, when attempts were made to test the reproducibility of many of the EMF effect in T and B cells, other researchers were unable to obtain similar positive EMF results in their laboratories. Two groups tried unsuccessfully to confirm EMF effects in the B-cell lines (22,23). One of the two groups further tested the EMF-dependent regulation of signaling molecules from the NF-kappaB and AP-1 pathways in another leukemia cell line. They could not find any effect of magnetic fields up to 1.3 mT (24). The EMF effects reported by the other B-cell investigators we cited (18–20) should have been apparent since these protooncogene pathways include BTK, PLC, and PKC, the molecules that previously were observed to be activated by 60-Hz EMFs. So challenged, Dibirdik et al. published a new study in which they confirmed and extended their original findings (25). In this study, they showed that in seven of 13 experiments there was a significant effect of EMFs on IP_3 production. In the same report they also showed that in seven separate experiments EMFs activated BTK in all cases. Interestingly, the variable incidence of positive EMF effects in the IP_3 experiments is very much like the variation that we found in our TCR anti-CD3 binding studies that were described above (17).

From the results of the experiments of Dibirdik et al. (25), it might be hypothesized that EMF-dependent biological effects are most robustly observed in assays that probe events close to the EMF interaction site and that the farther the endpoint assay is from the EMF interaction site the weaker and more variable the biological outcome. This hypothesis rests on the observation that signal transduction and metabolic pathways contain an immense number of downstream feedback regulators that act to restore cellular homeostasis and that the more distal the endpoint is from the site of pathway stimulation, the more likely the biological system is to be stabilized or buffered by feedback signals. There are several important cases where this kind of complex feedback regulation has been observed and authenticated. In Jurkat cells, transitory activation of the TCR was shown to cause substantial activation of Ca-calmodulin kinase IV. However, within 5 minutes after removing the TCR-activating signal, the activated kinase returned to control levels as a consequence of feedback-induced deactivation (26). In fibroblasts, it was recently shown that the biological consequence of stimulating the mitogen-activated protein kinase (MAPK) cascade strongly depended on the subtle differences in the physiological history of the cells (27). The investigators concluded that in these cells there are two metastable physiological states and that the response to extracellular signals is related to which state the cell is in when the signal arrives.

Another important factor that often diminishes experimental reproducibility is that cell cultures are usually composed of a number of subpopulations whose physicochemical sensitivity and reactivity can vary significantly from time to time and from laboratory to laboratory. In most cases the subpopulations are simply different cell (28) or cell cycle (29,30) states, but in other cases cultures can be composed of different cell types, especially when the cultures are directly cloned from tissue samples by the investigators. More insidious is the fact that many laboratories harbor unrecognized intracellular parasites that infect experimental cultures and markedly affect their metabolic state by stressing the host cells (31). Evidence for population diversity in EMF experiments comes from single-cell studies. For example, Mattsson et al. reported that 60-Hz, 0.15-mT EMFs caused intra-cellular Ca^{2+} oscillations in 27 of 53 (51%) of the Jurkat cells they tested (32). The basis for the variability reported by Mattsson et al. is not known but is characteristic not only for experiments within one laboratory but also for the results of the 20-year history of EMF effects on Ca^{2+} or Ca^{2+}-dependent processes in lymphocytes. These studies have been reviewed on several occasions (30,33). Despite many negative results on EMF regulation of intracellular Ca^{2+} in lymphocytes, several recent, thoroughly controlled studies report EMF-dependent changes of this important intracellular messenger. For instance, McCreary et al. found significant changes in intracellular Ca^{2+} of Jurkat cells exposed to either 60-Hz, 0.1-mT EMFs or to 0.078 mT DC or to the combination of both fields, when compared to controls kept at zero alternating and static magnetic fields (30).

While the general lack of reproducibility encountered in EMF studies is disturbing, there seem to be a sufficient number of robustly positive experimental results to affirm the idea that some investigators observe real effects of low-intensity, low-frequency EMFs on biological systems. When we place this observation against a real-world background in which biologists, untrained in the engineering principals, build and deploy their own EMF delivery systems and physicists and/or engineers, not well trained in biological method-ologies, carry out biological experiments in their well-designed EMF delivery systems, it is not surprising to find the discrepancies that are all too abundant in the field.

To be clear about the basis of the irreproducibility problem, we can be certain that some of us measure artifacts arising from bad EMF delivery systems, certainly many of us perform cell culture experiments that yield variable results because there are unrecognized metabolic differences in the cultures we employ, and certainly many of us are hampered in designing appropriate controls by our lack of insight into the mechanism of EMF action in our experimental systems. For example, it is possible that EMFs have a large impact on cellular electron transfer reactions so that the robustness of the EMF effect is a reflection of the net rate of these reactions as suggested by Blank and Soo (34) and implicit in our earlier theoretical model (15). If this were true then it would be very difficult to find reproducible results since no EMF research group does report controlling for this metabolic aspect. Likewise, Bentsman et al. (35) suggest that EMF effects depend on the cellular redox potential, another factor that has rarely been controlled in EMF studies. EMFs could interact with cellular systems in a nonlinear and/or chaotic way as suggested by Wallezcek (36) and Marino et al. (37). In this case, appropriate analytic tools have to be used to properly study nonlinear reaction processes. However the final truth unfolds, we currently see that there are too many good experiments, too many fractures healed, and too much pain eased to explain all EMF effects as artifactual or the result of placebo effects.

D. EMF Long-Term Effects on Lymphocytes

The study of reactions and processes proximal to the site of interaction between EMFs and cells gives the most promise of finding a mechanism of action, the holy grail of the basic theoretical scientist. More pragmatic, medically oriented scientists and engineers like those who discovered and promoted aspirin are often more interested in practical outcomes of therapies than in mechanisms. In this laboratory we have both kinds of investigators. Thus, when we found that EMFs increase the binding of anti-CD3 to the TCR in Jurkat cells (see Fig. 1), we considered the long-term consequences and speculated that EMFs might induce apoptosis in Jurkat cells, which at that time was a suggested effect of anti-CD3-induced TCR activation. We proceeded to obtain detailed baseline information on downstream effects of anti-CD3 in our Jurkat cell model and then asked if EMFs are synergistic or additive to TCR activation in Jurkat cells. In control experiments, with anti-CD3 alone, we observed a delayed but progressive loss of cells from the cycling population as measured by flow cytometry, cell counts, and [^{3}H]thymidine incorporation into DNA. By 24–48 h almost all cells in the culture had progressed through an irreversible metabolic step, which resulted in 70–80% inhibition of cell growth at 48 and 72 h after stimulation. When we tested the effect of 60-Hz, 0.1-mT EMFs on cells coexposed to anti-CD3, we found a further 40% inhibition of [^{3}H]thymidine incorporation into DNA (Fig. 2). We obtained a similar effect when we employed a therapeutic 1.8-mT bone-healing EMF provided by Electro Biology Inc. (EBI, Parsippany, NJ). EMF treatment alone, either the 60-Hz field or the EBI field inhibited [^{3}H]thymidine incorporation by a small (10–20%) but significant amount compared to unexposed cells. Generally, the EMF inhibitory effect was most apparent several cell generations after EMF exposure (48 and 72 h) and then the EMF effect seemed to disappear. These results indicate that the effects of EMFs are additive or synergistic to anti-CD3.

To investigate if anti-CD3 and EMFs achieve their inhibition of cell growth by inducing apoptosis, we studied the appearance of apoptotic DNA fragments. Figure 3 shows agarose gel electrophoresis pictures of genomic DNA and a bar graph showing quantitative image analysis of the relative intensity of the 3-nucleosome sized DNA band. Anti-CD3 treated cells exhibited some evidence of DNA fragmentation, 72 h after treatment, which was clearly enhanced when cultures were coexposed to anti-CD3 and 60-Hz, 0.1-mT EMFs. These experiments confirmed that EMFs augment the anti-CD3 effect in inducing significant long-lasting changes in the metabolic fate of Jurkat cells. We confirmed these observations with flow cytometry studies from which we concluded that treatment with anti-CD3 caused an early restriction in G2-M. This induced a secondary block in G0-G1 from which cells exited the cell cycle and underwent apoptosis. With flow cytometry, apoptotic cells are defined as those containing less than a diploid complement of DNA (generally referred to as sub-G1 cells). Cultures treated with anti-CD3 showed a significant proportion (21.9%) of apoptotic, sub-G1 cells, and this proportion was consistently higher in cultures cotreated with anti-CD3 plus 60-Hz, 0.1-mT EMFs (38). Taken together, these results indicate that both anti-CD3 and EMFs induce downstream effects through similar pathways resulting in growth inhibition and apoptosis.

In work progressing toward EMF studies with animals we questioned if EMF effects observed in Jurkat cells were the same in isolated normal peripheral blood lymphocytes (PBLs). Unlike transformed Jurkat cells that down regulate DNA synthesis and undergo apoptosis in response to anti-CD3, human or rat PBLs are known to respond to anti-CD3 by proliferating. This dramatic difference is due to the fact that in addition to T cells, PBL cultures contain B cells, monocytes, and macrophages. These accessory cells provide a complex array of complimentary extracellular signals to the T cells when they are activated at the TCR by anti-CD3 in vitro. Thus, when we tested PBLs, it was not surprising to find that anti-CD3 stimulated proliferation of T cells and that 60-Hz, 0.1-mT EMFs increased cell proliferation induced by anti-CD3 (17,39). While there may be other ramifications of this observation, it strongly supports the notion that EMFs augment long-term downstream

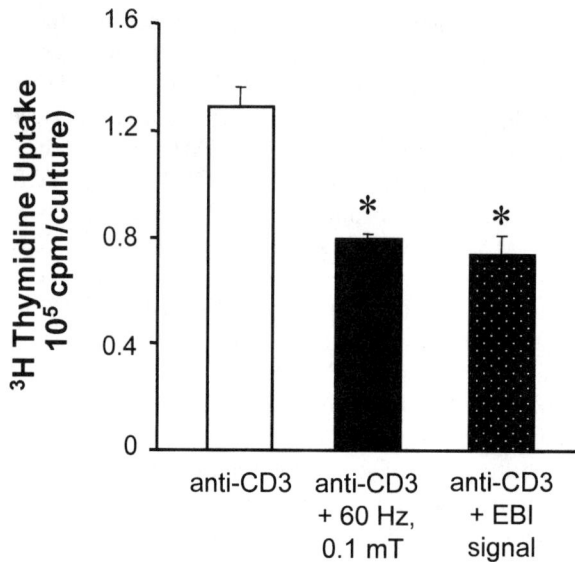

Figure 2 Inhibition of DNA synthesis in Jurkat cells cotreated with anti-CD3 and EMFs. Jurkat cells growing in log phase were transferred to 96 well-cultured plates coated with anti-CD3 (50 μl of a 10 μg/ml solution) and immediately exposed for 20 min to 0.1-mT, 60-Hz EMFs generated by a 3-coil Merrit coil system or to a commercial bone-healing EMF generated by a Helmholtz coil (EBI, Parsippany, NJ) maintained at 37°C (±0.5°C). Control cultures containing anti-CD3 were treated similarly but received exposure to the earth's geofield only. For details of the DNA synthesis assay, see Ref. 28. Compared to untreated controls, anti-CD3 alone causes a 70–80% inhibition of [^{3}H]thymidine incorporation into DNA, 48 and 72 h later (data not shown). This is the normal response of T cells stimulated only at the TCR. In cells cotreated with anti-CD3 plus EMFs an additional 38% inhibition of [^{3}H]thymidine incorporation into DNA was observed (black bars) compared to cells stimulated with anti-CD3 alone (white bar), $P < 0.001$, Student's t-test. The maximum EMF effect was most apparent several cell generations after EMF exposure usually appearing between 48 and 72 h after treatment. Compared to untreated controls EMFs alone caused a 17% inhibition of DNA synthesis, 48 h after treatment. (data not shown, $P < 0.005$). The data shown here is representative of five identical experiments. Bars represent the average of four replicates. Error bars represent one standard deviation.

events that are initiated at the TCR and that the EMF effect is closely associated with events that occur at the TCR. Indeed, the results obtained in the intact Jurkat and PBL cell studies may be caused by additional EMF-induced ligand binding at the TCR as shown in Fig. 1. In accord with these results we also found that costimulation of PBLs using anti-CD3 plus the EBI EMF leads to the same effect as the 60-Hz field and that the EBI field and 60-Hz fields also augment proliferation in human or rat PBLs treated with the T-cell mitogen Concanavalin A (17,39).

In initial animal studies we performed experiments parallel to the latter PBL studies in which we exposed rats to 60-Hz, 0.1-mT EMFs or to sham fields, 4 h/day for 21 or 28 days, isolated PBLs and tested their response to anti-CD3. We anticipated that we might find that mitogenic stimulation was compromised in these cells and might lead to apoptosis, but we found no difference in the proliferative capacity of mitogen-stimulated PBLs from either sham or EMF treated animals [unpublished observation]. In retrospect, we might have more

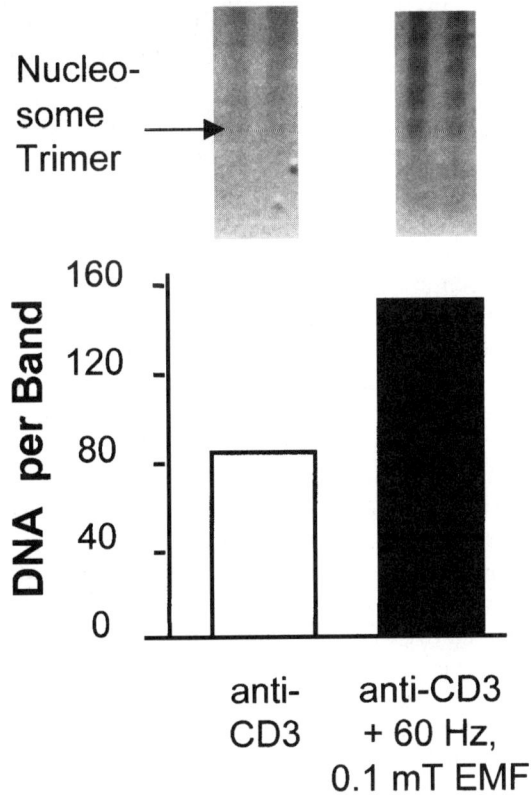

Figure 3 Agarose gel electrophoresis of DNA illustrating induction of apoptotic DNA in Jurkat cells cotreated with anti-CD3 plus EMFs. Cells were exposed to anti-CD3 or EMFs plus anti-CD3 exactly as described in Fig. 2. After 72 h cells were isolated and their DNA isolated as described earlier (5). The pictures above their respective bars show a weak apoptotic DNA banding pattern for the anti-CD3 treated controls and a much more prominent set of bands from the EMF cotreated cells. The two lanes in each picture represent DNA extracts from replicate cultures. The bars represent the results of quantitative densitometric analysis of the 3-nucleosome-size bands from each set of electrophoretigrams. Cells treated with anti-CD3 plus EMFs show enhanced apoptotic DNA fragmentation compared to cells treated with anti-CD3 alone. A similar result was obtained from analysis of DNA isolated from cultures harvested 96 hours after stimulation with anti-CD3 and EMFs (data not shown). Treatment with EMFs alone did not induce apoptotic fragmentation (data not shown).

profitably compared the number of T cells in the two animal populations, and we will do that in the near future, but there have been numerous studies with healthy animals and humans where that has been done and no differences have been found (40,41). However, there is some evidence that EMF effects on lymphocytes may be different in stressed animals and that EMF-damaged cells may undergo rapid repair when removed from the animal. Thus, compared to matched controls, Skyberg et al. (42) found increased numbers of DNA lesions in PBL cultures from individuals exposed to EMFs plus additional stressors (like smoking or breathing oil mists and vapors) and attributed the lesions to the environmental EMF exposures. It is important to understand that this difference was only observed when DNA repair was prevented after blood samples were obtained indicating that environmentally damaged PBLs rapidly revert to ther native state when they are placed in cell culture conditions.

III. EFFECT OF THERAPEUTIC EMFs ON LYMPHOCYTES AND IMMUNE FUNCTIONS

A. Pulsed EMFs

The net result from power-frequency studies discussed in Sec. II indicates that EMFs can influence lymphocyte metabolism but that the initial cellular changes are often weak and counteracted by rapid repair and homeostatic feedback loops. Thus the objective of therapeutic EMFs is to overcome these counteracting forces by optimizing the EMFs so that exposure will lead to long-lasting therapeutically relevant outcomes including regulation of lymphocyte proliferation. There are currently many commercial EMF devices in clinical use and a number of them are promoted for treatment of inflammatory diseases (e.g., Ref. 43). A common characteristic of many commercial EMF devices delivering time-varying magnetic fields is that the EMFs are delivered in pulses. Pulsed signals were originally designed to mimic piezo electric signals that emanate from stressed bone (44) and Pilla et al. (45) maintains that interrupted trains of these signals, described as pulse burst signals, deliver a low frequency EMF to cells and tissues most efficiently. The authors suggested that while directly delivered low-frequency fields can produce biological effects in test systems comprised of isolated enzymes and regulatory proteins, they are less effective in cell, tissue, and animal studies because of the markedly different electrical properties of these biosystems. Instead, pulse-burst-modulated high-frequency fields seem to deliver low-frequency signal components to EMF-sensitive sites in tissues much more effectively and can therefore yield improved therapeutic outcomes in clinical settings. Our limited observations with Jurkat cells support this idea because when we compared the pulsed EBI bone healing field with sinusoidal power frequency EMFs, we found similar or improved effects with the bone healing field. Inspired by the clinical acceptance and efficacy of the devices approved for bone healing and spine fusion, other therapeutic devices delivering a wide variety of pulsed EMFs surfaced. Pulsed EMF therapies are currently more widely employed in medical practices of Eastern European countries (e.g., Refs. 46 and 47) than they are in the United States and other Western countries where they are considered an alternative therapy.

In our Jurkat cell model, we tested the effect of two pulsed EMF devices from EBI Inc., and some of those results are presented above. Recently, we began testing a pulsed EMF device that is currently under development by EMF Therapeutics Inc. (Chattanooga, TN) and described in detail in Chapter 39 of this book. The field that we have evaluated is a complex 120 pps signal with each pulse separated by a 1.4-ms static signal component. We first evaluated the safety of the field using our normal proliferating Jurkat cells as a model of circulating nonactivated T lymphocytes in a healthy organism. In these studies we tested the EMF Therapeutics field using flux densities from 5 to 25 mT and found no effects on cell proliferation or cell death (48). We interpret these Jurkat cell data to mean that this field is unlikely to induce inflammation in healthy tissue by activating normal circulating T lymphocytes. Likewise, using anti-CD3 activated Jurkat cells, which resemble aberrantly activated T cells in vivo, we found that the pulsed EMF Therapeutics field does not cause biologically significant effects, suggesting that physiologically normal T cell selection is most likely not impaired by EMF therapy (48).

Conversely, Jurkat cells activated with anti-CD3 plus a second signal such as phorbol myristic acid (PMA) are often used as a model for inflammatory T cells. Inflammatory T cells produce variable quantities of interleukin-2 (IL-2), which at low rates of production act as autocrine and paracrine hormones, stimulating T-cell proliferation and regulating the activity of other cells in inflamed tissue. However, in situ, and in Jurkat cells, IL-2 at high concentration acts as an apoptosis-inducing autocrine factor. Jurkat cells that are activated with anti-CD3 plus PMA to produce IL-2 respond to pulsed EMFs delivered by the EMF Therapeutics device by producing under certain conditions up to threefold the amount of IL-2 produced by control cultures. Figure 4 shows the EMF effect on IL-2 production of Jurkat cells from 10 independent experiments using Jurkat cells from different metabolic states. The different results of those 10 experiments leads us to the same conclusion that we acquired from the power-frequency studies presented in Sec. II and that we will further discuss in the following paragraph: The metabolic state, or the *metabolic bias*, of cells seems to be critically important in dictating the result of weakly stimulating signal transduction such as the result after EMF stimulation.

To explain the latter statement with the results of Fig. 4, let us first clearly explain the only difference between the 10 otherwise identical experiments. Jurkat cells in log phase growth were harvested, resuspended in fresh complete culture medium at 10^6 cells per ml and incubated at 37°C and 5% CO_2/95% air for the time periods indicated on the abscissa of the graph. The incubation period was aimed at allowing the cells to recover from the stress induced by cell handling. After the equilibration periods, cells were treated with anti-CD3 and PMA, (which stimulates IL-2 production) or with anti-CD3 and PMA plus the EMF

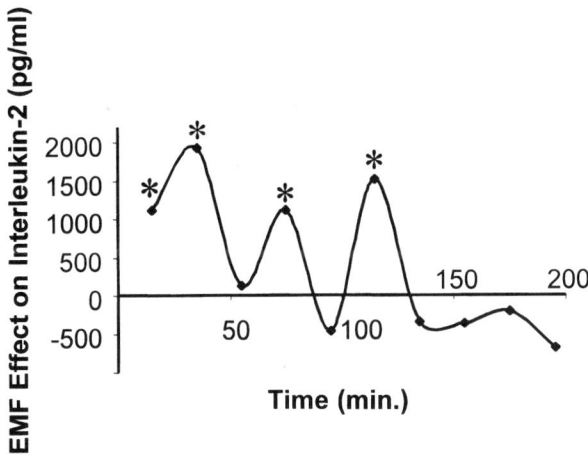

Figure 4 Ten separate experiments showing an oscillating sensitivity of stressed Jurkat cells to a 15-mT EMF (EMF Therapeutics Inc., Chattanooga, TN) and revealing the existence of two metabolic states differing in EMF sensitivity. The data shown represent the difference in IL-2 secretion obtained by subtracting the control IL-2 levels from the EMF coexposed IL-2 levels. We interpret the figure to indicate that as cells recover from the stress induced by cell handling, they oscillate between two metabolic states. One state responds to EMFs with increased IL-2 production, one state is relatively EMF insensitive. Data points represent the mean of four replicate cultures. $P < 0.01$, Student's t-test.

Therapeutics' field. Anti-CD3 was as described in Fig. 2, PMA was 50 ng/ml. The cells were then equilibrated to 37°C and 5% CO_2 for 5 min in a tissue culture incubator before being exposed to EMFs for 10 min in a 37°C warm room. Controls were simultaneously incubated in the same room at a place, where the DC was equal to the DC measured inside the coil in standby mode. IL-2 was measured in the culture supernatant, 48 h after exposure, using an enzyme-linked immunosorbent assay (ELISA).

Most cultured cells are stressed by simple manipulation of the cultures and Jurkat cells are no exception. Thus, in order to evaluate the effect of handling artifacts on EMF-induced cell activity like IL-2 production, we stimulated cells with mitogens plus a sham field or mitogens plus the EMF Therapeutics field at various times after handling. We then compared the IL-2 production of the two treatment sets after a 48-h incubation period. In Fig. 4, the difference in IL-2 production between the control and experimental sets is plotted as a function of time after cell handling. We found that there is great temporal variation in cytokine production by Jurkat cells. While the oscillatory pattern of IL-2 production is striking, there is little doubt that it will ultimately be explainable as the result of positive and negative feedback regulation and feedforward regulation in a complex metastable network of biological reactions (26,27).

When we tested the effects of 15 mT EMFs on the oscillatory IL-2 release, we found mainly two outcomes that could be explained with Jurkat cells in two main physiological states induced by cell handling stress. In one state the cells responded to EMFs with greatly increased IL-2 production (indicated in Fig. 4 by asterisks), and in the second state they were virtually refractory to EMFs. From a practical standpoint, if we had not tested cultures at the time points represented by the three oscillatory peaks, then we could easily have concluded that the EMF Therapeutics device had no effect on IL-2 production and thus no effect on proliferation or apoptosis in inflammatory T cells, and no beneficial effect on inflammation in animals.

The effects with the pulsed EMFs from EMF Therapeutics Inc. are highly significant and the EMF-stimulated production of IL-2 is the most prominent EMF effect that we have encountered in all of our EMF studies. However, it is important to caution that further studies will be required to determine if the fields delivered by this device also induce IL-2 production in vivo and if IL-2 produced in response to EMFs has a beneficial inflammation-modulating effect in the animal. IL-2 producing Jurkat cells undergo apoptosis and the EMF-dependent increase in IL-2 production is also evident as increased subsequent apoptosis (data not shown). These findings are consistent with our hypothesis that EMFs have an anti-inflammatory potential due to their ability to induce apoptosis in inflammatory T lymphocytes.

There are other studies on EMF modulation of the immune system and autocrine and paracrine transcellular communication that are not reviewed here in detail. Especially investigators in Italy have a long history of studying pulsed and low-frequency EMFs on human leukocytes and their cytokine production in basic science and therapeutic settings. These studies have been summarized on several occasions (e.g., Ref. 49) and were the basis for some therapeutic applications as presented in Chapter 26. Consistent with our results on Jurkat cells, Pessina and Aldinucci reported several years ago that mitogen-stimulated PBLs exposed for 12 h to EMFs (50-Hz square wave, 3 mT, 0.5 duty cycle) responded with increased IL-2 (50). Control cells without mitogen and cells exposed to EMFs for shorter time periods were not sensitive to the EMFs (in Ref. 50). Cossarizza et al. (51,52) reported that exposure to pulsed EMFs enhanced utilization of IL-2 by lymphocytes from older donors and donors affected by Down syndrome. These data extend our conclusions that

EMFs seem to be therapeutically most effective in metastable systems from cell-based experiments to clinically more relevant studies.

B. EMF Intensity and Frequency

While clinical results using pulsed EMFs seem promising, the significance of the intensity and frequency of the pulse has yet to be discovered. Most clinical EMF therapeutic devices deliver fields with magnetic flux densities higher than 0.1 mT, a fact that seems to be based on empirical observations. FDA-approved devices for bone healing have peak intensities up to a few milliTesla, while devices for pain reduction such as the EMF Therapeutics device described above emit fields about 10 times greater than bone-healing fields. Increasing the magnetic field intensity seems to be an obvious way to optimize EMF effects based on the rationale that more energetic EMFs will overwhelm the potential negative feedback regulation discussed earlier leading to persistent long-term biological effects. However, the general outcomes of animal and human studies testing the impact of power-frequency EMFs at intensities higher than 0.1 mT are as mixed as the results from studies with lower intensities.

For instance, while Fam and Mikhail (53) report an increased incidence of lymphomas in mice exposed for three generations to 25-mT EMFs, Mandeville et al. (54) found no carcinogenic influence on a large cohort of rats exposed to 2-mT EMFs for 2 years. Discrepancies like these support the idea that there are EMF intensity "windows" and there are several cell-based studies that corroborate this notion (e.g., Ref. 55). Recently, nonlinear models that help explain how such amplitude windows occur have been developed (56). Taken together, all the studies on magnetic flux density indicate that simply raising the flux density of EMFs is not the way to develop EMFs that can be reliably used in a therapeutic application. In our Jurkat T-cell model, we have not yet systematically tested the impact of varying EMF intensities. However, when we tested sinusoidal 60-Hz and 100-Hz EMF effects on DNA synthesis of Jurkat cells, using ultraviolet B (UVB) light as a costressor, we found 1-mT EMFs to be significantly more effective in inducing apoptosis than 0.1-mT EMFs (5).

In addition to having elevated flux density, therapeutic devices produce EMFs with complex time-varying waveforms that are comprised of different frequencies with combinations of alternating and static magnetic fields. Many investigators who tested the impact of different EMF frequencies on biological systems report a nonlinear relationship between EMF frequency and the biological response studied (i.e., frequency windows). While these windows are reported to be quite narrow for bone cell cultures (57), for lymphocytes the effective frequency windows seem to be broader. Lindstroem et al. (58) tested the effect of EMFs from 5 to 100 Hz, 0.15 mT on intracellular Ca^{2+} flux in Jurkat cells and found that most frequencies modulated Ca^{2+} flux, but that 50 Hz EMFs had the greatest effect. Broad, low-frequency windows, like the latter were predicted by Pilla et al. (45) who propose that these low-frequency effects can be amplified at the EMF-sensitive coupling site (the biological antenna) by delivering the EMFs as pulse bursts of high-frequency fields (e.g., 27.12 MHz). Belyaev and Alipov (59) tested EMF-dependent chromatin conformation changes in human lymphocytes and found the cells from some donors to be affected by EMFs around 8 and 58 Hz when combined with a parallel 43-μT static magnetic field. These data support another proposed EMF mechanism since they show consistencies with models that hypothesize ion cyclotron resonance (60) or ion parametric resonance (61). Other authors report EMF effects at 13.6 Hz, 0.02 mT on calcium uptake of a murine leukemia cell line (62) and a transient decrease of the level of ras proto-oncogene p21 in lymphoblastoid cells when exposed to pulsed 72 Hz EMFs for 6 to 16 h (63).

In our work to develop EMF therapeutic devices we take advantage of the oft-reported observation that we have already highlighted several times in this chapter: EMF interactions with cells are most prominent when the cells are already stressed and in a metastable state. Thus, we found that EMFs potentiate apoptosis in Jurkat cells coexposed to EMFs and UVB, which is used to treat inflammatory skin diseases like psoriasis (5). In Fig. 5 we present results from these studies showing that 1-mT EMFs are additive or synergistic to UVB in inhibiting cell proliferation and that a 100-Hz sinusoidal 1-mT EMF is more efficacious than a 60-Hz, 1-mT EMF. Our observations suggest that in a clinical setting UVB and 100-Hz EMFs may be therapeutically combined to substantially lower the periodic UVB exposure used to control psoriasis, one of the most common skin diseases in the world. If these expectations are fulfilled in clinical studies, then the benefits of UVB therapy will be greatly prolonged for psoriatic patients without a concomitantly increased risk for skin cancer. Since we have not exhaustively studied this problem, it remains likely that fields with other frequencies, waveforms, and intensities may be more efficacious than those few we have studied to date. For instance, interferential currents, amplitude-modulated 4000-Hz EMFs, have been shown in a small clinical trial to beneficially affect healing of psoriasis (64). Our current operating hypothesis is that there are likely to be specific optimal combinations of intensities, frequencies, and waveforms that will modulate one or another physiological process in mammalian cells. Once identified, the optimal combination of field characteristics should be useful for treating diseases associated with aberrations in specific physiological processes. Thus, there is an opportunity for investigators willing to exhaustively evaluate

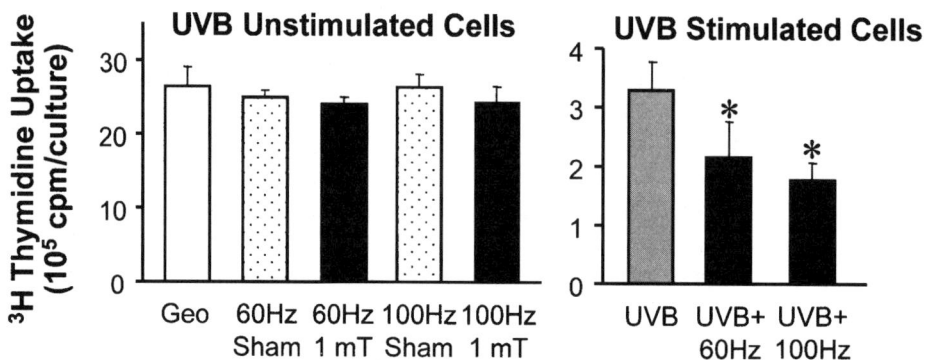

Figure 5 Inhibition of DNA synthesis in Jurkat cells cotreated with ultraviolet B light (UVB) and EMFs. Jurkat cells were exposed to sinusoidal 60- or 100-Hz, 1-mT EMFs for 10 min, to therapeutic UVB (500 J/m^2, emission peak at 316 nm) for 10 min, or to EMFs and UVB simultaneously for 10 min. EMFs were generated by a 4-coil Merritt coil system with an integrated UVB exposure system [for details see (72,73)]. To assay DNA synthesis, we used a 3-h [^{3}H]thymidine pulse-labeling period, 48 h after UVB/EMF exposures (5). DNA synthesis was not affected in cultures exposed to the geofield, the sham field, or 60 and 100 Hz EMFs (left panel labeled UVB unstimulated cells). As shown in the right panel, UVB alone inhibited [^{3}H]thymidine uptake by about 83% (note the ordinate difference in the left and right panels). Cells exposed to UVB plus EMFs exhibited significantly increased inhibition of DNA compared to cells irradiated with UVB alone with 100-Hz EMFs being more effective than 60-Hz EMFs. Bars represent the average of 20 replicate cultures. Error bars represent one standard deviation. $P < 10^{-5}$, Student's t test.

pulsed EMFs from a therapeutic standpoint with the aim of developing "designer EMFs" capable of inexpensive noninvasive therapy for a wide variety of human diseases.

IV.   FUTURE PERSPECTIVES ON EMF THERAPY FOR INFLAMMATORY DISEASES

In our EMF based studies with Jurkat cells or PBLs from rats and humans, we observe only minor biological changes in cells as a consequence of interactions between a variety of EMFs and normal proliferating cells. However, when the stable homeostatic state of cells is changed and made metastable by submaximal interactions with strong stimulatory factors, then we often see an impact of EMFs on cell cultures. We have observed these "costimulatory" EMF effects with a variety of agents including cytokines, ligands to the TCR, and physical agents such as UVB as discussed above.

Other investigators have reported results of EMF studies that lead to the same conclusions. In in vitro studies, Hintenlang (65) showed that 60-Hz EMFs potentiate radiation-induced lymphocyte death while EMFs alone had no effect. Narita et al. (66) found that 60-Hz, 45-mT EMFs induced apoptosis in leukemia cell lines while normal PBLs were unaffected. Robinson et al. (67) reported 60-Hz, 0.15-mT EMF–dependent protection from apoptosis in leukemia and lymphoma cell lines, while Maes et al. (68) found protection from mutagenic death by 50-Hz, 0.5-mT fields in human PBLs cultures stresed by handling, and increased death of x-ray-treated PBLs by 50-Hz, 0.088-mT EMFs.

In clinical studies, mainly from Eastern Europe there are numerous reports on beneficial effects of EMFs where the EMFs can be interpreted as acting in a costimulatory way. Many, but not all of these studies were recently reviewed (47), and we will not review them in detail here. However it is important to note that improved outcomes of EMF therapy include edema reduction and pain reduction, both outcomes that could be related to an anti-inflammatory action of the therapies. In addition, often, general improvements for inflammatory disease symptoms are described (69,70). Especially interesting in the context of our hypothesis that metastable cells are most EMF sensitive are studies showing augmentation of conventional treatments like laser phototherapy, antibiotic infusion, and surgical manipulation through the use of specific intensity and frequency EMFs (69,71).

There are important implications of all these observations to the development of EMF therapy. For example, these observations could mean that EMF therapy will specifically target cells that are metastable as a consequence of disease or metastable as a consequence of other ongoing therapy. Thus, EMF therapy may become an important cotherapy in many diseases including cancer, psoriasis, wound healing, and bacterial infections. A marked advantage of this kind of outcome would be that normal homeostatically stable cells would remain unaffected by EMFs but effects from other treatments on diseased tissue might be potentiated without proportional increases in the side effects. In chronic inflammatory diseases cells are characteristically maintained in metastable states as a consequence of cytokine secretions and other stressors associated with the disease. In these cases, EMF therapy could work as a stand-alone therapy. The challenge to successfully implement EMF therapy will be to better understand the biophysical interaction between cells and EMFs and to develop the knowledge base to use EMFs to direct target cells down one or another preferred metabolic pathway.

In summary, we presented evidence from our own and other laboratories on the interaction of nonionizing, low-frequency alternating electromagnetic fields (EMFs) with lymphocytes. We mainly presented data from Jurkat cells that we use as a model for T lymphocytes, and from this series of studies we are confident that, at least in the cell cultures we studied, weak, low-frequency EMFs induce apoptosis in activated T-cell cultures and that this effect is reproducible with normal PBLs. We presented evidence that EMF effects are seen mainly in metabolically metastable cells where the weak effects of EMFs can tip the balance on directing cells down one or another metabolic pathway. We finished with our views on the future course that development of EMF therapy should take, and we are confident that EMF therapy will become an important tool in modern clinical medicine, especially as an anti-inflammatory therapy.

DEDICATION

The authors would like to dedicate this paper to the memory of Margarete Heß, beloved mother of Gabi Nindl, who passed away while this paper was in press. With her unlimited love, Margarete has touched countless lives in a major way. Thank you.

REFERENCES

1. Propovic M, Caballero-Bleda M, Puelles L, Popovic N. Importance of immunological and inflammatory processes in the pathogenesis and therapy of Alzheimer's disease. Int J Neurosci 1998; 95(3–4):203–236.
2. Winkler JD. Apoptosis in Inflammation. Basel, Boston: Birkaeuser Verlag, 1999.
3. Jasti AC, Wetzel BJ, Aviles H, Vesper DN, Nindl G, Johnson MT. Effect of a wound healing electromagnetic field on inflammatory cytokine gene expression in rats. Biomed Sci Instrum 2001; 37:209–214.
4. Wetzel BJ, Nindl G, Swez JA, Vesper DN, Johnson MT. Quantitative characterization of rat tendinitis to evaluate the efficacy of therapeutic interventions. Biomed Sci Instrum 2002; 38:157–162.
5. Nindl G, Hughes EF, Johnson MT, Spandau DF, Vesper DN, Balcavage WX. Effect of ultraviolet B radiation and 100 Hz electromagnetic fields on proliferation and DNA synthesis of Jurkat cells. Bioelectromagnetics 2002; 23:455–463.
6. Wertheimer N, Leeper E. Electrical wiring configurations and childhood cancer. Am J Epidemiol 1979; 109:273–284.
7. Feychting M, Ahlbohm A. Magnetic fields and cancer in children residing near Swedish high-voltage power lines. Am J Epidemiol 1993; 138:467–481.
8. Adair RK. Static and low-frequency magnetic field effects: health risks and therapies. Rep Prog Phys 2000; 63:415–454.
9. Korzh-Sleptsova IL, Lindstroem E, Hansson Mild K, Berglund A, Lundgren E. Low frequency MFs increased inositol 1,4,5-triphosphate levels in the Jurkat cell line. FEBS Lett 1995; 359:151–154.
10. Lindstroem E, Berglund A, Mild KH, Lindstroem P, Lundgren E. CD45 phosphatase in Jurkat cells is necessary for response to applied ELF magnetic fields. FEBS Lett 1995; 370:118–122.
11. Lindstroem E, Hansson Mild K, Lundgren E. Analysis of the T cell activation signaling pathway during ELF magnetic field exposure, p56^{lck} and [Ca^{2+}]$_i$-measurements. Bioelectrochem Bioenerg 1998; 46:129–137.
12. Lindstroem E, Still M, Mattsson M-O, Hansson Mild K, Luben RA. ELF magnetic fields initiate protein tyrosine phosphorylation of the T cell receptor complex. Bioelectrochem 2000; 53:73–78.
13. Holian O, Astumian RD, Lee RC, Reyes HM, Attar BM, Walter RJ. Protein kinase C activity is altered in HL60 cells exposed to 60 Hz AC electric fields. Bioelectromagnetics 1996; 17(6):504–509.
14. Walter RJ, Shtil AA, Roninson IB, Holian O. 60-Hz electric fields inhibit protein kinase C activity and multidrug resistance gene (MDR1) up-regulation. Radiat Res 1997; 147:369–375.
15. Balcavage WX, Alvager T, Swez JA, Goff CW, Fox MT, Abdullyava S, King MW. A mechanism

for action of extremely low frequency electromagnetic fields on biological systems. Biochem Biophys Res Comm 1996; 222:374–378.

16. Liburdy RP, Eckert V. Preliminary evidence for receptor-ligand binding during calcium signal transduction as an interaction site for ELF magnetic fields. Annual review of research on biological effect of electric and magnetic fields. From the generation delivery & use of electricity, Albuquerque, NW, 1994:67.

17. Nindl G, Balcavage WX, Vesper DN, Swez JA, Wetzel BJ, Chamberlain JK, Fox MT. Experiments showing that electromagnetic fields can be used to treat inflammatory diseases. Biomed Sci Instrum 2000; 36:7–13.

18. Uckun FM, Kurosaki T, Jin J, Jun X, Morgan A, Takata M, Bolen J, Luben R. Exposure of B-lineage lymphoid cells to low energy electromagnetic fields stimulates lyn kinase. J Biol Chem 1995; 270:27666–27670.

19. Dibirdik I, Kristupaitis D, Kurosaki T, Tuel-Ahlgren L, Chu A, Pond D, Tuong D, Luben R, Uckun FM. Stimulation of Src family protein-tyrosine kinases as a proximal and mandatory step for SYK kinase-dependent phospholipase Cγ2 activation in lymphoma B cells exposed to low energy electromagnetic fields. J Biol Chem 1998; 273:4035–4039.

20. Kristupaitis D, Dibirdik I, Vassilev A, Mahajan S, Kurosaki T, Chu A, Tuel-Ahlgren L, Tuong D, Pond D, Luben R, Uckun FM. Electromagnetic field-induced stimulation of Bruton's tyrosine kinase. J Biol Chem 1998; 273(20):12397–12401.

21. Santoro N, Lisi A, Pozzi D, Pasquali E, Serafino A, Grimaldi S. Effect of extremely low frequency (ELF) magnetic field exposure on morphological and biophysical properties of human lymphoid cell line (Raji). Biochim Biophys Acta 1997; 1357:281–290.

22. Miller SC, Furniss MJ. Bruton's tyrosine kinase activity and inositol 1,4,5-triphosphate production are not altered in DT40 lymphoma B cells exposed to power line frequency magnetic fields. J Biol Chem 1998; 273(49):32618–32626.

23. Woods M, Bobanovic F, Brown D, Alexander DR. Lyn and syk tyrosine kinases are not activated in B-lineage lymphoid cells exposed to low-energy electromagnetic fields. FASEB J 2000; 14:2284–2290.

24. Miller SC, Haberer J, Venkatachalam U, Furniss MJ. NF-κB or AP-1-dependent reporter gene expression is not altered in human U937 cells exposed to power-line frequency magnetic fields. Radiat Res 1999; 151:310–318.

25. Dibirdik I, Bofenkamp M, Skeben P, Uckun F. Stimulation of Bruton's tyrosine kinase (BTK) and inositol 1,4,5-triphosphate production in leukemia and lymphoma cells exposed to low energy electromagnetic fields. Leuk Lymph 2000; 40(1–2):149–156.

26. Westphal RS, Anderson KA, Means AR, Wadzinski BE. A signaling complex of Ca^{2+}-calmodulin-dependent protein kinase IV and protein phosphatase 2A. Science 1998; 280:1258–1261.

27. Bhalla US, Ram PT, Iyengar R. MAP kinase phosphatase as a locus of flexibility in a mitogen-activated protein kinase signaling network. Science 2002; 297:1018–1023.

28. Nindl G, Swez JA, Miller JM, Balcavage WX. Growth stage dependent effect of electromagnetic fields on DNA synthesis of Jurkat cells. FEBS Lett 1997; 414:501–506.

29. Loeschinger M, Thumm S, Haemmerle H, Rodemann HP. Induction of intracellular calcium oscillations in human skin fibroblast populations by sinusoidal extremely low-frequency magnetic fields (20 Hz, 8 mT) is dependent on the differentiation state of the single cell. Radiat Res 1999; 151:195–200.

30. McCreary CR, Thomas AW, Prato FS. Factors confounding cytosolic calcium measurements in Jurkat E6.1 cells during exposure to ELF magnetic fields. Bioelectromagnetics 2002; 23:315–328.

31. Hackstadt T. Redirection of host vesicle trafficking pathways by intracellular parasites. Traffic 2000; 1:93–99.

32. Mattsson M-O, Lindstroem E, Still M, Lindstroem P, Hansson Mild K, Laudgren E. $[Ca^{2+}]_i$ rise in Jurkat E6-1 cell lines from different sources as a response to 50 Hz magnetic field exposure is a reproducible effect and independent of poly-L-lysine treatment. Cell Biol Internat 2001; 25(9):901–907.

33. Walleczek J. Electromagnetic field effects on cells of the immune system: the role of calcium signaling. FASEB J 1992; 6:3177–3185.

34. Blank M, Soo L. Electromagnetic acceleration of electron transfer reactions. J Cell Biochem 2001; 81(2):278–283.

35. Bentsman J, Dardynskaya IV, Shadyro O, Pellegrinetti G, Blauwkamp R, Gloushonok G. Mathematical modeling and stochastic H(infinity) identification of the dynamics of the MF-influenced oxidation of hexane. Math Biosci 2001; 169(2):129–151.

36. Wallezcek J. Self-organized biological dynamics and nonlinear control. Cambridge: Cambridge University Press, 2000.

37. Marino AA, Wolcott RM, Chervenak R, Jourd'heuil F, Nilsen E, Frilot II C. Nonlinear dynamical law governs magnetic field induced changes in lymphoid phenotype. Bioelectromagnetics 2001; 22:529–546.

38. Nindl G, Miller JM, Voehringer P, Balcavage WX. Electromagnetic 60 Hz fields increase apoptosis of lymphocytes—a new area for possible therapeutic employment of EMFs. Twenty-first annual meeting of the Bioelectromagnetics Society, Long Beach, CA, June, 1999.

39. Johnson MT, Vanscoy-Cornett A, Vesper DN, Swez JA, Chamberlain JK, Seaward MB, Nindl G. Electromagnetic fields used clinically to improve bone healing also impact lymphocyte proliferation in vitro. Biomed Sci Instrum 2001; 37:215–220.

40. Thun-Battersby S, Westermann J, Loscher W. Lymphocyte subset analyses in blood, spleen and lymph nodes of female Sprague-Dawley rats after short or prolonged exposure to a 50-Hz 100-μT magnetic field. Radiat Res 1999; 152(4):436–443.

41. Selmaoui B, Bogdan A, Auzeby A, Lambrozo J, Touitou Y. Acute exposure to 50 Hz magnetic field does not affect hematologic or immunologic functions in healthy young men: a circadian study. Bioelectromagnetics 1996; 17(5):364–372.

42. Skyberg K, Hansteen IL, Vistnes AI. Chromosomal aberrations in lymphocytes of employees in transformer and generator production exposed to electromagnetic fields and mineral oil. Bioelectromagnetics 2001; 22(3):150–160.

43. Trock DH. Electromagnetic fields and magnets. Investigational treatment for musculoskeletal disorders. Rheum Dis Clin North Am 2000; 26(1):51–62.

44. Bassett CA, Pawluk RJ, Pilla AA. Augmentation of bone repair by inductively coupled electromagnetic fields. Science 1974; 184:575–577.

45. Pilla AA, Muehsam DJ, Markov MS, Sisken BF. EMF signals and ion/ligand binding kinetics: predictions of bioeffective waveform parameters. Bioelectrochem Bioenerg 1999; 48:27–34.

46. Jerabek J. Pulsed magnetotherapy in Czechoslovakia-a review. Rev Environ Health 1994; 10:127–134.

47. Zhadin MN. Review of Russian literature on biological action of DC and low-frequency AC magnetic fields. Bioelectromagnetics 2001; 22:27–45.

48. Nindl G, Johnson MT, Hughes EF, Markov MS. Therapeutic electromagnetic field effects on normal and activated Jurkat cells. Proceedings of the Second International Workshop on Biological Effects of Electromagnetic Fields. Rhodes, Greece, October 7–11, 2002. In press.

49. Chiabrera A, Cadossi R, Bersani F, Franceschi C, Bianco B. Electric and magnetic field effects on the immune system. In: Carpenter DO, Ayrapetyan S, eds. Biological Effects of Electric and Magnetic Fields. London: Academic Press, 1994:121–145.

50. Pessina GP, Aldinucci C. Pulsed electromagnetic fields enhance the induction of cytokines by peripheral blood mononuclear cells challenged with phytohemagglutinin. Bioelectromagnetics 1998; 19(8):445–451.

51. Cossarizza A, Monti D, Bersani F, Paganelli R, Montagnani G, Cadossi R, Cantini M, Franceschi C. Extremely low frequency pulsed electromagnetic fields increase interleukin-2 (IL-2) utilization and IL-2 receptor expression in mitogen-stimulated human lymphocytes from old subjects. FEBS Lett 1989; 248(1–2):141–144.

52. Cossarizza A, Monti D, Bersani F, Scarfi MR, Zanotti M, Cadossi R, Franceschi C. Exposure to low-frequency pulsed electromagnetic fields increases mitogen-induced lymphocyte proliferation in Down's syndrome. Aging (Milano) 1991; 3(3):241–246.

53. Fam WZ, Mikhail EL. Lymphoma induced in mice chronically exposed to very strong low-frequency electromagnetic field. Cancer Lett 1996; 105(2):257–269.

54. Mandeville R, Franco E, Sidrac-Ghali S, Paris-Nadon L, Rocheleau N, Mercier G, Desy M, Gaboury L. Evaluation of the potential carcinogenicity of 60 Hz linear sinusoidal continuous-wave magnetic fields in Fischer F344 rats. FASEB J 1997; 11(13):1127–1136.

55. Berg H. Problems of weak electromagnetic field effects in cell biology. Bioelectrochem Bioenerget 1999; 48:355–360.

56. Binhi VN, Goldman RJ. Ion-protein dissociation predicts 'windows' in electric field-induced wound-cell proliferation. Biochim Biophys Acta 2000; 1474:147–156.

57. Fitzsimmons RJ, Ryaby JT, Magee FP, Baylink DJ. Combined magnetic fields increased net calcium flux in bone cells. Calcif Tissue Internat 1994; 55(5):376–380.

58. Lindstroem E, Lindstroem P, Berglund A, Lundgren E, Mild KH. Intracellular calcium oscillations in a T-cell line after exposure to extremely-low-frequency magnetic fields with variable frequencies and flux densities. Bioelectromagnetics 1995; 16:41–47.

59. Belyaev IY, Alipov ED. Frequency-dependent effects of ELF magnetic field on chromatin conformation in *Escherichia coli* cells and human lymphocytes. Biochim Biophys Acta 2001; 1526:269–276.

60. Liboff AR, McLeod BR, Smith SD. Resonance transport in membranes. In: Brighton CT, Pollack SR, eds. Electromagnetic in Biology and Medicine. San Francisco: San Francisco Press, 1991:67–77.

61. Blanchard JP, Blackman CF. Clarification and application of an ion parametric resonance model for magnetic field interactions with biological systems. Bioelectromagnetics 1994; 15:217–238.

62. Lyle DB, Wang X, Ayotte R, Sheppard A, Adey WR. Calcium uptake by leukemic and normal T-lymphocytes exposed to low frequency magnetic fields. Bioelectromagnetics 1991; 12:145–156.

63. Phillips JL, Haggren W, Thomas WJ, Ishida-Jones T, Adey WR. Effect of 72 Hz pulsed magnetic field exposure on ras p21 expression in CCRF-CEM cells. Cancer Biochem Biophys 1993; 13(3):187–193.

64. Philipp A, Wolf GK, Rzany B, Dertinger H, Jung EG. Interferential current is effective in palmar psoriasis: an open prospective trial. Europ J Dermatol 2000; 10(3):195–198.

65. Hintenlang DE. Synergistic effects of ionizing radiation and 60 Hz magnetic fields. Bioelectromagnetics 1993; 14:545–551.

66. Narita K, Hanakawa K, Kasahara T, Hisamitsu T, Asano K. Induction of apoptotic cell death in human leukemic cell line, HL-60, by extremely low frequency electric magnetic fields: analysis of the possible mechanisms in vitro. In Vivo 1997; 11(4):329–335.

67. Robinson JG, Pendleton A, Monson KO, Murray BK, O'Neill K. Decreased DNA repair rates and protection from heat induced apoptosis mediated by electromagnetic field exposure. Bioelectromagnetics 2002; 23:106–112.

68. Maes A, Collier M, Vandoninck S, Scarpa P, Verschaeve L. Cytogenic effects of 50 Hz magnetic fields of different magnetic flux densities. Bioelectromagnetics 2000; 21(8):589–596.

69. Iashchenko LV, Chistiakov IV, Gakh LM, Ostapiak ZN, Siurin SA. Low-frequency magnetic fields in the combined therapy of inflammatory lung diseases. Probl Tuberk 1988; 3:53–56.

70. Gerasimenko MY. Effect of red laser and alternative magnetic field on repair process after palatoplasty. Vopr Kurortol Fizioter Lech Fiz Kult 1993; 4:34–35.

71. Alyshev VA, Viaznikov AL, Gertsen IG, Krylov NL, Rutskii VV, Roizin VL, Serdiuk VV, Ushakov AA, Sheliakhovskii MV. Magnetotherapy in the complex treatment of patients with suppurative wounds and osteomyelitis. Vestn Khir 1988; 140(4):141–143.

72. Vesper DN, Swez JA, Nindl G, Fox MT, Sandrey MA, Balcavage WX. Models of the uniformity of electromagnetic fields generated for biological experiments by Merritt Coils. Biomed Sci Instrum 2000; 36:409–415.

73. Vesper DN, Nindl G, Johnson MT, Spandau DF, Swez JA, Balcavage WX. A system for simultaneous ultraviolet light and electromagnetic field exposure in in vitro experiments. Biomed Sci Instrum 2001; 37:221–226.

26

Orthopaedic Clinical Application of Biophysical Stimulation in Europe

Ruggero Cadossi
Research and Development, Igea, Capri, Italy

Gian Carlo Traina
Department of Biomedical Sciences, Orthopaedic Clinic, University of Ferrara, Ferrara, Italy

The chapter starts with an explanation of the appearance of electric fields in bones as a response to mechanical deformation. Further, the authors review European experiences in the use of biophysical methods for osteogenesis enhancement. Detailed consideration of these methods includes directly applied electric current via faradic systems and inductive and capacitive systems for inducing electric current in the targeted tissues. The authors discuss application of these methods for treatment of delayed and fresh fractures. Finally, the rationale for clinical use of biophysical stimulation of endogenous bone repair is given.

The employment of physical energy to modulate osteogenetic response and, ultimately, to enhance fracture healing is a topic widely researched in Europe. Interest in the relation between biological systems and electrical energy can be dated back as far as the studies by Galvani (1) and by Matteucci (1811–1868) who, already in the nineteenth century, had identified the lesion currents and had perceived their role in repair processes.

In the last century the studies performed by Fukada and Yasuda (2) and by Bassett and Becker (3) identified the relationship between mechanical loading and electrical activity in the bone, wherein lie the scientific origins of the electrical, magnetic, and mechanical stimulation of osteogenesis.

These methods have been approved for clinical use by the U.S. Food and Drug Administration and are employed in many countries to promote and reactivate the formation of bone tissue. The electrical, magnetic and mechanical stimulation of osteogenesis belongs to bioengineering and biophysics.

The above studies have clearly identified the relationship between bone tissue, mechanical deformation, and electric potentials. Since then it has become clear that bone generates two types of electric signal: one in response to mechanical deformation, the other in the absence of deformation.

I. ELECTRICAL SIGNAL IN THE PRESENCE OF MECHANICAL DEFORMATION

Structural deformation following the application of a load to the bone, not necessarily vital, generates an electrical signal that can be ascribed to a dual origin:

Direct Piezoelectric Effect. The signal measured on the bone surface deformed by a load can be attributed to the piezoelectric properties of the collagen matrix only when the bone is dehydrated. The signal is generated by the asymmetric redistribution of the molecular charges resulting from mechanical deformation (4,5).

Electrokinetic Phenomenon of the Flow Potential. In physiological conditions, the electrical signal induced by mechanical deformation can be imputed to the electrokinetic phenomenon occurring when ion flow occurs within haversian and endocanalicular spaces (5–8).

Independently of the mechanism, piezoelectric or electrokinetic, by which it is generated, the electrical signal induced by the mechanical deformation, containing the information of site, direction, and amplitude necessary to modulate the bone remodeling, has been considered to be the transducer of a physical force in a cell response. It is, indeed, intelligible from the cells, as is proved by the cellular effects that can be activated by exogenous electrical signals similar to the endogenous ones (9). The aforesaid electrical signal has thus been taken to be the mechanism that determines the continuous adaptation of the mechanical competence of bone, according to the Wolff's law (10).

II. ELECTRICAL SIGNAL IN THE ABSENCE OF MECHANICAL DEFORMATION

In the absence of mechanical stress, the vital bone generates an electrical signal detectable in vivo as surface *stationary bioelectric potential* and ex vivo as *stationary electric (ionic) current* that can be measured.

Stationary bioelectric potential, measured in vivo, in intact bone, displays a characteristic distribution with an electrically negative area in the metaphyseal site (11–14) and epiphyseal growth cartilage (12). When the bone is fractured, the fracture immediately alters the typical distribution of the bioelectric potentials, inducing an electrically negative area at the site of the lesion (11,15). It is thought that the lesion generates an electrical signal because it alters the different ion distribution between endocanalicular fluid and systemic extracellular fluid. The electrical signal at the site of the lesion has been ascribed to the endosteal cell layer (16). Nevertheless, the electrical contribution from the concomitant muscular lesions (16) and cutaneous lesions (15) cannot be disregarded.

Stationary electric (ionic) current is detectable ex vivo on bones immersed in a physiological solution. The ionic current induced by a transcortical lesion enters in the site of the lesion (17,18). The fracture exposes the endocanalicular ionic fluid to the external plasma environment, and thus the cellular system deputed to maintaining the bone–plasma ion gradients is activated (17,19).

Despite the different experimental conditions of detection, both the electrical signals induced by mechanical deformation and those generated by vital bone have been interpreted as local control factors of bone remodeling and/or modeling and reparative osteogenesis. Ever since the first detection of these signals it has therefore been held that inducing them in bone by means of external generators could be of clinical importance particularly in situations where repair processes have remained incomplete (9,11,17,20–23).

In the research sector involved in the histophysiology of bone tissue, the above observations regarding the relation between bone tissue and electric potentials have aroused great interest in the possibility of active intervention, with physical stimuli (exogenous electrical, magnetic, and mechanical stimulation), on bone cell metabolic activity, in particular that of preosteoblasts and osteoblasts. A number of experimental studies have shown how and to what extent, in various animal models, it is possible to enhance endogenous bone repair by applying physical stimuli. The effectiveness of biophysical stimulation is already well documented and rests on solid scientific bases, as is proved by the results of in vitro (24–29) and in vivo (23,30–34) studies. It has, indeed, been possible to quantify the effect of electrical stimulation on the mineral apposition rate, which increases by 80% (35,36).

Today, electrical, magnetic, or mechanical stimulation must be framed within a more extensive sector of orthopaedic therapy, clinical biophysics, which deals with the study of the nonthermal effects of nonionizing radiation—effects mediated by a specific interaction of the physical agent with the structures of the cell membrane. Even though the final effects are the increase of osteogenetic activity, the pathways of the cell membrane through which this effect is achieved differ according to the energy employed: voltage-gated calcium channels for capacitive coupling, intracellular calcium stores for inductive coupling, and finally inositol phosphate for mechanical stimulation (26).

In humans, electrical, magnetic, and mechanical stimulation is used to speed fracture healing and to finalize bone repair in failed unions, such as delayed unions and pseudoarthroses. Research performed up to now has enabled evaluation of:

1. The different effectiveness of methods of applying electrical, magnetic, and mechanical stimulation to the bone tissue.
2. Modalities, times, and doses needed to obtain a positive influence on osteogenesis.

In Europe research on the possible application of physical energy to bone repair processes has been ongoing throughout the past century: study has been made of the effects of electrical current directly applied (faradic) to the fracture site, of the employment of magnetic fields (inductive) and electrical fields (capacitive), and of the use of ultrasound to produce mechanical stimulation.

III. ANALYSIS OF THE METHODS

There are various mechanisms of action by which osteogenesis is enhanced through application of biophysical stimuli with the four methods described above.

A. Directly Applied Electric Current: Faradic Systems

The direct action of continuous electric current manifests both with purely electrical phenomena, which affect the dynamic of the ions at the site of the fracture, and with chemical-type phenomena, which lead to a reduction in the local tension of oxygen and a small increase in pH. Furthermore, the positioning of the electrode, by means of a small surgical intervention, determines a mechanical stimulus that may, however, interfere with the osteogenetic processes. With the faradic systems the electrical tensions applied to the bone tissue are of various entities (37) but greater than those applied with inductive or capacitive systems.

The therapeutic effectiveness of the continuous electric current depends on its intensity. Values of electric current ranging from 2 to 20 $\mu A/cm^2$ are considered optimal for stimulation of osteogenesis. As regards application, the current is utilized 24 h/day; the negative pole must be positioned very precisely in the site of the fracture where stimulation of the osteogenetic response is desired; the positive pole is placed in contact with the soft tissues, far from the site.

Values of applied current below 2 $\mu A/cm^2$ are ineffective, while currents of over 50 $\mu A/cm^2$ may cause necrosis of the tissue. For this reason the apparatus employed in clinical practice is limited in tension (typically below 2.3 V) (37).

As refers to the European experience, Traina and Gulino (38) proposed using as cathode an endomedullar nail covered with insulating material excluding the part near the fracture site, with the anode placed on the skin. The method was first tested on animals and was then employed on some patients, but further developments were limited, if not hindered, by technical problems connected with the difficulty of soldering the electric cable to the endomedullary nail.

Again in the context of faradic stimulation, Jorgensen (39) suggested using the pins of the external fixators as electrodes, the proximal and distal ones respectively nearer to the fracture site. Statistical analysis reveals 30% acceleration in healing in the electrically treated group. Healing required 3.6 months in the control group and 2.4 months in the stimulated one ($p < 0.001$). Nevertheless, the method leaves open problems of a theoretical kind in relation to its working, for the administration of the electric current to the pins (which are electrically insulated with respect to the frame of the external fixator) should be mainly distributed to the soft tissues, in consideration of the greater electrical resistance offered by the bone tissue.

Zichner (40) developed an implanted stimulator (FKS), with implant of the cathode in the fracture site and the anode in soft tissue or medullary cavity, the battery being housed in a capsule also implanted. Fifty-three patients out of 57 suffering from nonunion healed in 5.3 months in average.

In Europe, unlike in the United States, faradic techniques have never had much following, nor have they been applied beyond small series generally performed for purposes of research.

B. Alternating Electric Current Induced by Electromagnetic Fields: Inductive Systems

As regards pulsed electromagnetic fields (PEMFs) inductive method, the biological activity may occur both by means of the magnetic component varying in time and by means of the electrical component, i.e., the induced electric field. These are signals with a complex wave form, whose predominant spectral content ranges between a few tenths to a few ten thousandths of hertz. To explain the biological effects of electromagnetic fields, mathematical models have been proposed: cyclotronic resonance, ligand-receptor interaction, and stochastic resonance. The first two have received most attention and appear to be compatible with experimental results (24,41). The cell membrane is the main site of interaction of PEMFs, and the most favoured candidates are the membrane receptors and Ca^{2+} channels (25,26). Experiments in vitro have shown that PEMF exposure increases the proliferation of lymphocytes, osteoblast, and chondrocytes (28,42,43). Furthermore, it has been described that electromagnetic stimulation of human bone cells recovered from a nonunion site increases the expression and release of TGFβ1 (27). In vivo, authors have observed an increase in the formation of bone tissue (29) and a shorter healing time of experimental fractures and/or bone lesions (33–35,44).

All authors agree that there exists a direct link between the specificity of the electromagnetic signals and the effects observed in bone tissue.

For both clinical and experimental applications, use has been made of signals with frequency of repetition rate ranging from 2 to 100 Hz, with spectral content up to 100 kHz with intensity between 0.1 and 30 G of magnetic induction (10 G = 1 mT), and with induced electric field from 0.01 to 10 mV/cm. More limited findings have been reported with magnetic fields of greater intensity, up to 200 G.

Application of an inductive technique to human pathology was first made in 1972 in Garmish by Kraus and Lechner (45), who were the first to report the effect of an electromagnetic field on the healing of failed unions. The technique involved the implant in the fracture site of an electrical circuit. The method entailed three variables: surgical operation to implant the receiving circuit, an internal synthesis device to stabilize the fracture site, and the external time-varying electromagnetic field used to induce an electrical current in the implanted circuits. In the outcome, it never became clear which of these factors was responsible for the healing.

The 1980s witnessed widespread development throughout Europe of the totally non-invasive methods of stimulation. Interest in the inductive systems had also been aroused by the results of studies performed by Bassett in the United States, contributing to the collection of a vast clinical experience of undoubted scientific value (46).

On the one hand, some clinicians have enlarged the American experience by developing a series of investigations by utilizing the EBI method. On the other, new and effective signals have been studied and clinically validated in Italy, the United Kingdom, and the Netherlands.

C. Alternating Electric Current Induced by Electrical Fields: Capacitive System

With this non invasive method the biological effects are linked with the sole presence of the time-varying electric field. The literature on these systems (47) is certainly not as abundant as for the inductive systems. The site of interaction of the electric field lies at the level of the cell membrane; an increase in Ca^{2+} transport across voltage-gated channels is observed followed by an increase in cell proliferation. Furthermore, the exposure to electric field of osteoblastlike primary cells increases the synthesis of bone matrix and favours their proliferation and differentiation (26, 48). In vivo, in experimental fractures produced on rabbit fibula, a significant shortening of healing time has been observed (31).

The method foresees the use of electrodes placed in contact of the skin by means of conductive gel. The voltage applied ranges between 1 and 10 V at frequencies from 20 to 200 kHz. Optimal values lie, however, between 50 and 100 kHz. The electric field within the tissue ranges from 1 to 100 mV/cm. The density of the electric current produced in the tissue varies between 0.5 and 50 $\mu A/cm^2$ (31).

More recently, though in much more limited form, clinical experiments using the capacitive systems have been performed also in Europe along the lines of those of Brighton in the United States. Of late, the technique has been further developed in Italy and applied with good results to patients with failed union.

D. Mechanical Vibration Induced by Ultrasound: Ultrasound System

Ultrasound is a mechanical vibration with a frequency higher than 20 kHz. It propagates through a medium by the movement of mutual interaction of the particles. The method is based on the assumption that the mineral component of the bones, in response to a mechanical vibration, converts it into an electrical signal that enhances the osteogenesis.

Ultrasound irradiation at optimal dosage of 30 mW/cm^2 has been used to enhance fracture healing (49–51). Ultrasounds are used at a frequency of 1.5 MHz and are delivered in pulse burst of 200 μs at 1 kHz. Exposure length does not exceed 30 min/day. Mechanical vibration interacts with the cell membrane affecting Ca^{2+} transport and on the inositol-phosphate cascade, thus promoting cell proliferation. In vivo, ultrasound stimulation was able to shorten the healing time of osteotomies in rabbits and rats and to promote experimental nonunion healing in rats (52).

The employment of ultrasound was originally put forward as far back as the 1950s by Corradi and Cozzolino (53), who reported the positive effect of applying ultrasound in the fracture site in order to enhance healing—findings that remained long neglected. The ultrasound method has lately been reappraised in various European countries, both to accelerate the healing of recent fractures and to treat failed union.

With all the above bone growth stimulator technologies, original research has been carried out in several European countries, extending knowledge and clinical experience in the employment of electrical stimulation. The latter has undoubtedly been favoured by the absence of legislation prescribing prior approval by EU authorities of these methods before they are used on patients. Unlike the United States, where entry of apparatus on the market is regulated by the FDA, there is no norm in Europe regarding the use of nonionizing radiation in humans. While this has favoured the development of new technologies, it has also meant the proliferation of systems of treating patients with no scientific basis or study demonstrating their effectiveness. Patients may actually undergo treatments potentially able to hinder the repair process. This deficiency will certainly need to be remedied by the authorities responsible in the matter.

IV. CLINICAL EXPERIENCES WITH BIOPHYSICAL STIMULATION IN EUROPE

In the following section, we summarize the results of clinical studies in the different bone pathologies; within each of these we look at the results obtained with the stimulation methods described above.

Table 1 reports the results of the main European clinical experiences with reference to the particular method employed, the pathology treated, and especially the clinical protocol used, i.e., studies with control group or double blind.

A. Stimulation of Reparative Osteogenesis in Congenital Pseudoarthrosis

Congenital pseudoarthrosis is a rare abnormality; almost all authors agree that the most common sequence of events leading to pseudoarthrosis occurs in a tibia of an infant in whom there are either stigmata of neurofibromatosis, particularly café-au-lait spots, or a family history of neurofibromatosis. Either the tibia alone or the tibia and fibula may be affected; more rarely it may affect the forearm. An exstensive review of the treatment of congenital pseudoathrosis with PEMFs was prepared by Sharrard (54). The European experience is limited to the use of the inductive systems, and the only clinical series have been reported in the United Kingdom (55,56) and in Italy (57).

All clinical studies underline the importance of a correct orthopaedic procedure to be associated with the electrical stimulation (58–60). The treatment should aim not only at bone

Table 1 Clinical Studies Regarding Demonstration of the Osteogenetic Effect of Electrical, Magnetic, and Mechanical Stimulation

Author	Method	Pathology	Protocol
Fontanesi et al. 1986 (44)	Inductive	Recent tibia fractures	Control
Borsalino et al. 1988 (77)	Inductive	Femur osteotomies	Double blind
Traina et al. 1989 (94)	Inductive	Pseudoarthrosis	Control
Sharrard et al. 1990 (64)	Inductive	Tibia delayed union	Double blind
Mammi et al. 1993 (78)	Inductive	Tibia osteotomies	Double blind
Capanna et al. 1994 (79)	Inductive	Osteotomies + bone grafts	Double blind
Hinsenkamp et al. 1984 (74)	Inductive	Recent fracture with external fixators	Control
Scott et al. 1994 (69)	Capacitive	Tibia pseudoarthrosis	Double blind
Emami et al. 1999 (76)	Ultrasound	Tibial fractures	Double blind

union but also at preventing refracture and at protecting the failure of the osteosynthesis devices utilized to maintain alignment. The success rate with inductive systems reaches 80% when associated with endomedullary nailing. A study on a group of congenital pseudo-arthrosis of tibia has shown that employment of stimulation in support of surgical intervention with endomedullar synthesis is able to limit dysmetry of limbs and protect the patient from the risk of refracture (61).

B. Stimulation of Reparative Osteogenesis in Failed Union

The expression *failed union* comprises both delayed union and pseudoarthroses. Various studies refer to delayed union for fractures failing to consolidate in 6–9 months following trauma, whereas the pseudoarthroses are those fractures failing to consolidate at least 9 months from trauma. It should, however, be emphasized that the distinction based on time alone is nowadays felt to be insufficient, such that the FDA has recently suggested that any fracture failing to heal at more than 6 months after trauma be considered pseudoarthrosis.

The European clinical studies have mainly addressed the employment of the inductive techniques and, to a much lesser extent, the other methods. Regarding the faradic techniques, as was said above, there have been no significant European clinical series.

For inductive method in 1982 Hinsenkamp et al. (46) reported the results of a European multicenter study, with success percentages above 70%. The same positive outcome was obtained in France by Sedel et al. (62). In Italy Marcer et al. (63) reported the results of a series of 147 patients treated with external fixation and PEMFs, the overall healing rate was 73%, the humerus being the least successful site. Sharrard in 1990 demonstrated the efficacy of PEMF stimulation in a double-blind study involving patients suffering from delayed union (64). In the United Kingdom Dehaas et al. (65) in 1980 and Watson (66) in 1983 reported positive results (80% success) in the treatment of pseudoarthrosis with an inductive system at frequencies in the range 1–11 Hz and magnetic fields of intensity ranging between 20 and 500 G that they developed originally. Figure 1 shows the waveform of the induced electric field employed in these clinical studies.

Vast experience has been collected in Europe with the inductive technique developed in Italy; Fig. 2 shows the waveform of signal employed. Success rate in various series has always exceeded 75%. Dal Monte et al. (57) reported a success rate of 84% in a clinical series of 248 patients, average time to healing was 4.3 months. The presence of infection did not influence the outcome of the treatments. Figure 3 shows examples of successful treatment in this clinical series. In Spain, a multicenter study, including 1710 patients suffering from

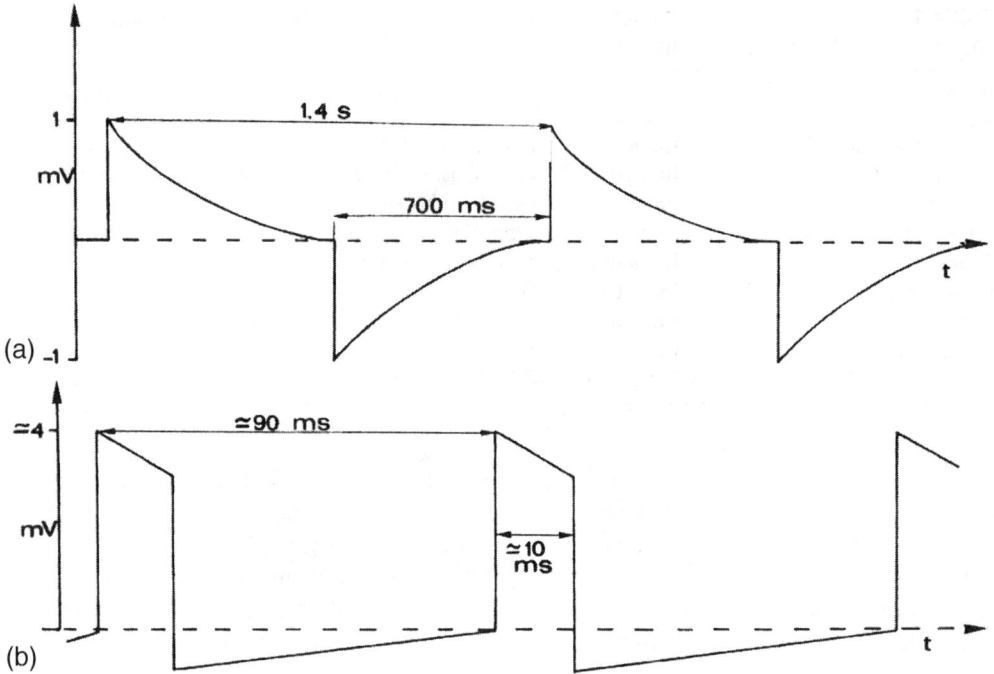

Figure 1 Waveform of the induced electric field used in U.K. experience to treat patients suffering from nonunions: (a) (top) Dehaas (65), (b) (bottom) Watson (66).

nonunion, reported positive results with an average treatment time of 4.8 months. Vaquero (67), in a retrospective study on the effect of PEMF on nonunions, reported a success rate of 74%; among the factors influencing the results were the age of the patient ($p = 0.048$), the site of fracture ($p < 0.001$), the type of nonunion ($p = 0.02$), and the presence of infection ($p = 0.01$).

In the Netherlands, using high-frequency electromagnetic fields, Fontijne and Konings (68) reported a positive experience with 85% success. Figure 4 shows the waveform used in the system as reported by Pienkowsky et al. (32).

The European experience with the capacitive system for the treatment of nonunions is extremely limited and only two series have been reported. Scott and King (69) conducted a prospective double blind study in a group of 21 patients suffering from established nonunion, using the Orthopak. Sixty percent healing was achieved in an active group, while none of the patients healed in the placebo group ($p = 0.004$). This is the only double-blind study reported in the literature for nonunions. Mattei et al. (70) reported a success rate of 89% with the use of capacitive system in patients suffering from nonunions in Italy. Figure 5 shows the characteristics of the signal used.

All authors report that electrical and magnetic stimulation with inductive and capacitive systems is particularly indicated in cases of infected lesions. The infection of the bone tissue or the surrounding soft tissues does not affect the outcome of the treatment. Employment of electrical and magnetic stimulation is able to promote healing in short times of large lesions of the soft tissues associated with very serious traumas. Figure 6 shows an example of a successful stimulation of an infected nonunion of the tibia with an inductive system.

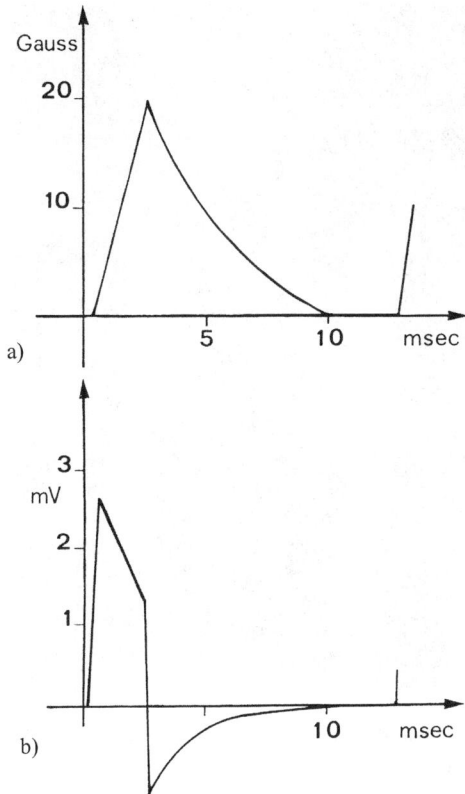

Figure 2 Waveform of the signal used by Igea inductive method: (a) magnetic field and (b) wave-form of the electric field induced in a standard coil probe (44).

Mechanical stimulation by means of ultrasound has collected a fairly ample experience in Europe, in particular in Germany and Italy. The authors have reported a success rate above 75% in the treatment of nonunions (71,72).

All authors concur on the need to employ electrical, magnetic, and mechanical stimulation in combination with correct orthopaedic treatment, and in particular it has been observed that the possible diastasis of the fracture stumps must not exceed half the diameter of the skeletal segment site of the failed union to guarantee a succesful outcome of the treatment.

C. Stimulation of Reparative Osteogenesis in Recent Fractures

1. Post-Traumatic

Biophysical stimulation has been shown to be able to accelerate healing of recent fractures, fractures of the leg treated with plaster and/or external splinting, or complex fractures with serious damage to the soft tissues and ample exposure of the bone tissue. In all cases, stimulation succeeded in shortening the average time of healing. None of the authors suggest a generalized use of the therapy in all fractures; however, in those cases where the site, type of exposure, morphology of the fracture, or conditions of the patient foreshadow difficulties in the repair process, biophysical stimulation is rightly indicated (44,73–75).

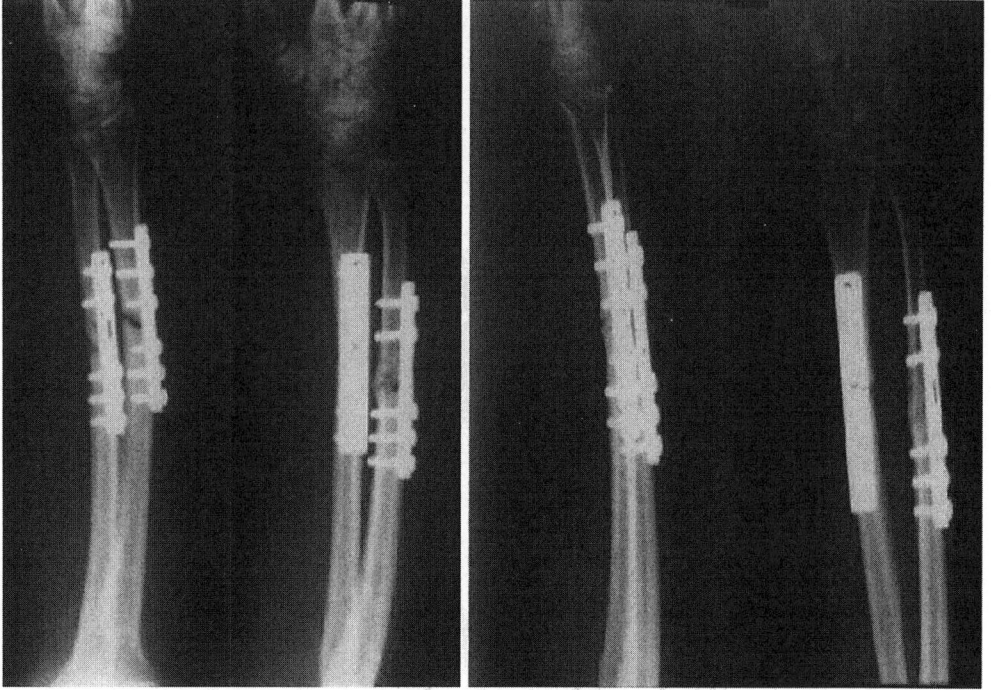

Figure 3 Female aged 38. Left: Pseudoarthrosis of radio and ulna 10 months from trauma. Right: Complete healing after 4 months of inductive stimulation.

Fontanesi et al. (44), in a controlled study of 40 tibia recent fractures treated with plaster, remarked how the effect of stimulation is evidenced through a reduction in average healing times. Stimulated fractures healed in 85 days compared to 109 for control group ($p < 0.005$); nevertheless, no fractures are seen to heal before 70 days. This observation demonstrates how in optimal conditions, i.e., of rapid healing, the repair process cannot be further accelerated. Hinsenkamp et al. (74) too noted a shortening in the time to union of

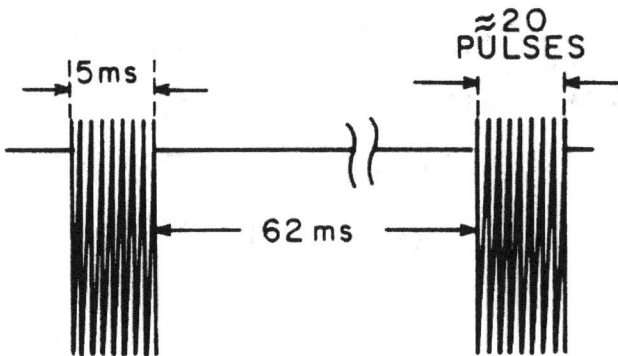

Figure 4 Schematic illustration of asymmetrical PEMF (32) used in a clinical series in The Netherlands (68).

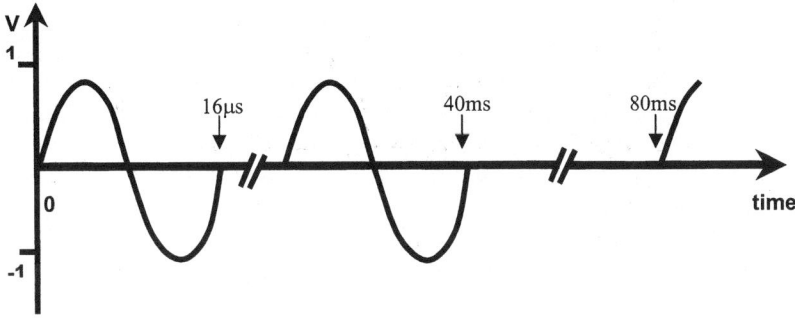

Figure 5   Waveform of the signal of Igea capacitive method: sine wave at 60 kHZ (16.6 μs period). Burst length 40 ms at 12.5 Hz.

stimulated tibial recent fractures treated with external fixation. The author reports a significant but relatively important shortening in healing time for delayed healing, similar to what described by Fontanesi et al. (44).

Benazzo et al. (73), however, using capacitive coupling stimulation, observed earlier recovery in athletes with stress fracture. The authors seem to rule out as inappropriate the use of stimulation on all recent fractures as against fractures that might present problems of union.

Ultrasound stimulation has been used to enhance the healing of forearm and tibia fractures with good results (51) in the United States. Nevertheless, in Sweden, Emami used ultrasound in a double-blind study (76) in patients with tibia fractures treated with endomedullary nailing but did not observe any positive effect of the ultrasound. The effects of this endomedullary synthesis device on ultrasound stimulation has still to be clarified.

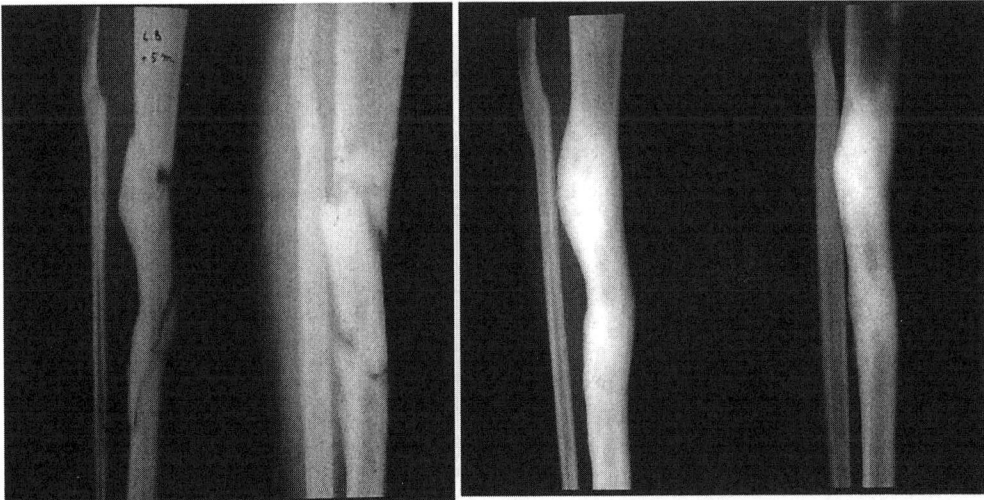

Figure 6   Male aged 42. Left: Infected pseudoarthrosis of the tibia 12 months after the trauma. Healing was obtained after 3 months of stimulation. Right: X-ray image at 36 months of follow-up.

2. Osteotomies

The study of electromagnetic stimulation on osteotomies represents an original approach in an attemp to quantify the effects of PEMF. Three double-blind studies have been performed: human femoral intertrochanteric osteotomies (77), tibial osteotomies (78), and osteotomies in patients undergoing massive bone graft (79).

The osteotomies of tibia and femur showed how the application of electromagnetic stimulation favors rapid healing of the osteotomic line and, in the case of femur osteotomy, an early mineralization of the bone callus demonstrated by computer analysis of the x-ray films. As regards the effects on massive bone grafts, a significant shortening of the healing time from 9 to 6 months was observed for patients not undergoing chemotherapy after the operation.

Electromagnetic stimulation was also tested in two European studies in which after the osteotomies the patients underwent limb lengthening. The first one, performed in the United Kingdom, with the EBI technique, noted and quantified with DEXA a positive effect on osteoporosis occurring distally in the lengthened limb (80). The other one, conducted in Spain with the IGEA method in patients undergoing bilateral limb lengthening, showed that in the limb subjected to stimulation the external fixator was removed 30 days earlier versus the controlateral nonstimulated limb (75).

D. Stimulation of Reparative Osteogenesis in Vertebral Arthrodesis or in Presence of Bone Grafts

Various clinical experiences have also shown the validity of associating bone grafts (used to bridge an excessive bone gap) with stimulation for treating pseudoarthrosis. The ability of electrical stimulation to enhance healing of bone grafts in vertebral arthrodesis was demonstrated first on animal models, then in clinical studies (81–83). In Europe, two clinical studies have shown how the use of stimulation with electromagnetic fields immediately following operation for vertebral arthrodesis, with no internal synthesis devices, can favor the maturation of the bone callus according to the classification of Dawson (82,83). The literature reports no experience in Europe with other methods of stimulation.

E. Stimulation of Reparative Osteogenesis in Avascular Necrosis of the Femoral Head

The avascular necrosis of the femoral head is an infrequent disease mostly affecting young males. Bone necrosis is observed in the femoral head as a consequence of the sudden deficit in the vascular supply. In most instances the origin of the deficit is unknown, but it has also been associated to the use of steroid, dyalisis, and metabolic diseases. In consequence of the osteonecrosis an early appearance of osteoarthrosis is observed leading to the need of hip replacement. The diagnosis and the progression of the disease can be determined by x-rays, nuclear magnetic resonance, and computer tomography. The severity of the disease can be quantified according to Ficat staging (84).

The use of electromagnetic stimulation was initially proposed by Bassett et al. (85). In stages I, II, and (with reservation) III of the Ficat staging, stimulation with inductive systems has proved effective in arresting the progress of the lesion, thus limiting recourse to surgical intervention or replacement with hip prosthesis. The inductive systems have been demonstrated to be useful in treating avascular necrosis in association with core decompression (86). The European experience (86–89) has confirmed the observations conducted in the

United States (90). The indication for employing bone stimulation with electromagnetic fields is especially important when one considers that, thanks to the introduction of nuclear magnetic resonance, it is now possible to reach a very early diagnosis. In the initial stages of the disease, the use of PEMFs can justly be considered the treatment of choice for avascular necrosis of the head of the femur. Figure 7 shows an example of the treatment of avascular necrosis of Ficat I stage.

There is no experience reported in Europe concerning capacitive and faradic system in the treatment of avascular necrosis, nevertheless, the information available for U.S. experience has not demonstrated that these methods are indicated for the treatment of avascular necrosis (91,92).

F. Stimulation of Reparative Osteogenesis in the Presence of a Prosthesis

Biophysical stimulation has proven useful to favor experimental bone ingrowth (93). For the orthopaedic surgeon, the possibility to stimulate osteogenetic activity in the presence of a primitive prosthetic implant—and most importantly in revision arthroplasty—represents an important therapeutic possibility. Some studies indicate that electrical and magnetic stimulation in the short term may resolve pain in subjects with mobilized, painful prostheses (94,95). Nevertheless, the available clinical information is still limited and further studies are needed.

G. Indication for Use

In Table 2 we report the biophysical treatments that have proven to be effective in different bone pathologies we discussed above.

H. Rationale for Clinical Use of Biophysical Stimulation of Endogenous Bone Repair

The clinical use of biophysical stimulation, as proposed by Bassett, initially entailed immobilization in plaster of the bone to be treated and subsequent application of the

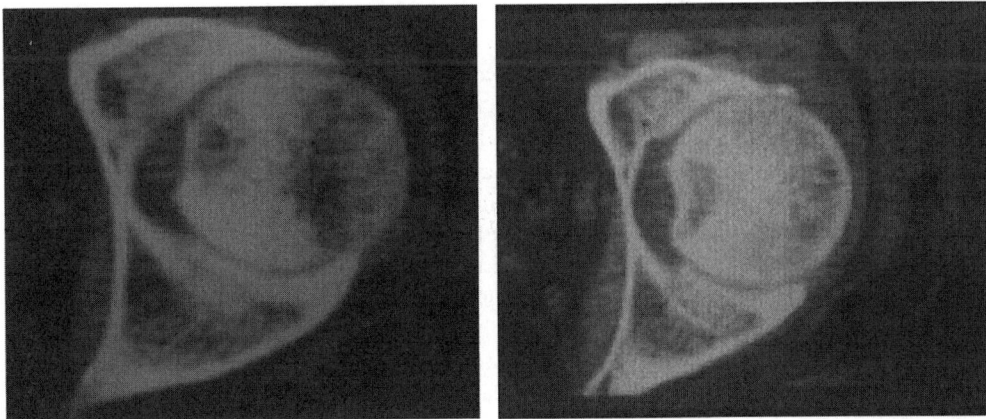

Figure 7 Male aged 45. Left: Computed tomography of the right femoral head showing an osteonecroisis area that does not alter the femoral head shape: Ficat I stage. Right: Complete healing after 6 months stimulation and 1 year follow-up.

Table 2 Indications for Use of the Different Modalities of Application of Electrical, Magnetic, and Ultrasound Stimulation for the Various Pathologies of Orthopaedic-Traumatologic Concern

Pathology	Modality of application of therapy			
	Faradic	Inductive	Capacitive	Ultrasound
Congenital pseudoarthrosis	Yes	Yes	No	No
Pseudoarthosis	Yes	Yes	Yes	Yes
Delayed union	Yes	Yes	Yes	Yes
Fracture at risk	No	Yes	No	Yes
Recent fracture	No	Yes	No	Yes
Bone grafts	Yes	Yes	Yes	No
Vertebral arthrodesis	Yes	Yes	Yes	No
Avascular necrosis	No	Yes	No	No
Limb lengthening	No	Yes	No	Yes

stimulator to be maintained until healing; some patients underwent treatment even for 9–12 months and beyond.

This approach has never been considered adequate by European orthopaedists, who have preferred to develop a rationale able to guide the surgeon in choosing or rejecting biophysical stimulation as a means of treatment. In particular, it has been observed how not all failed unions should be considered as potentially elegible for stimulation. In addition, the time needed to heal should not be considered a secondary factor since in modern orthopaedics and traumatology the healing time is not a negligible parameter.

In Europe it has been felt necessary to pose the problem of the differential diagnosis, i.e. to identify the causes underlying the failed union, in a prejudicial way (96). Following the observations of Frost (22), it can be recognized that in 50% of cases pseudoarthrosis is due to a mechanical failure—that is, the conditions of stability, alignment, and contact of the stumps are not satisfied—20% of failed union is due to a biological failure, namely inadequate activation and finalization of the reparative osteogenetic process; while in the remaining 30% of cases the failed union is accounted for by combined problems of mechanical and biological order.

While mechanical failure has for many years been defined as inadequate alignment, contact, and immobilization, it remains to be defined what is meant by biological failure. Firstly, the failed union can be ascribed to a biological failure when, even in presence of adequate mechanical conditions, the fracture does not consolidate: owing to infection, serious local osteoporosis, patient's age, presence of systemic diseases that inhibit the repair processes, or an idiopathic anergy of the bone tissue.

With these premises, differential diagnosis enables us to adopt the best solution and/or therapy. Identification of the causes underlying the failed union directs toward the choice of a surgical solution in the case of mechanical failure, of a noninvasive solution by stimulation in the case of biological failure, and the adoption of both (surgery and stimulation) in the case where, as well as a biological deficiency, there is a mechanical condition of instability at the fracture site capable of hindering healing.

A clinical study based on these principles observed how the percentage of union obtainable with surgery (used to correct inadequate mechanical conditions) or with stimulation (when the failed union can be attributed to a biological deficiency only) is exactly the same 87% for noninfected pseudoarthroses. In presence of infection, the percentage of success of surgery falls to 40%, whereas infection does not impair the good result of stimulation. It is clear that in presence of infection and unsatisfactory mechanical conditions, we face a case of combined (biological and mechanical) failure in which the association of surgery and stimulation can offer the best results (97).

In view of all these observations we are led to develop a further concept that has been gaining ground in Europe in recent years, namely fractures at risk. Sensitivity to the biological environment in which healing takes place certainly represents a fairly new aspect in orthopaedics. Once the surgical technique has achieved an optimal level, there remains in the common experience the observation that some fractures in any case show difficulties to heal, perhaps for reasons connected with the patient's state of health, type and site of fracture, and local complications. All these considerations have led orthopaedists to employ biophysical stimulation at earlier times—that is, in an aim to prevent the onset of failed union. In particular, if after 45–60 days the x-ray film shows no formation of bone callus, stimulation should be used to finalize osteogenetic activity and to obtain union.

Today, the orthopaedic surgeon has available various physical and chemical (growth factors) methods able locally to enhance endogenous repair. The orthopaedist needs to develop an increasing sensitivity toward the biological environment in which the repair activity of a fracture takes place, bearing in mind that while mechanical instability may impede union, in every case the healing of a fracture cannot but be the result of the local cellular activity.

The availability of chemical and physical methods capable of maximizing and finalizing endogenous osteogenetic response represents a further possibility for the orthopaedist in order to reduce healing times and enable swifter functional and working recovery by the patient.

REFERENCES

1. Galvani L. De viribus electricitatis in motu muscolari commentaries. Bologna: Instit. Scient., 1791.
2. Fukada E, Yasuda I. On the piezoelectric effect of bone. J Phys Soc Japan 1957; 12:121–128.
3. Bassett CAL, Becker RO. Generation of electric potentials in bone in response to mechanical stress. Science 1962; 137:1063–1064.
4. Black J. Electrical Stimulation. New York: Praeger, 1987.
5. Guzelsu N. Piezoelectric- and electrokinetic effects in bone tissue—review. Electro and Magnetobiol 1993; 12(1):51–82.
6. Green J, Kleeman CR. Role of bone in regulation of systemic acid-base balance. Kidney Int 1991; 39:9–26.
7. Otter MW, Vincent R, Palmieri VR, Dadong DWu, Seiz KG, Mac Ginitie LA, Cochran GVB. A comparative analysis of streaming potentials in vivo and in vitro. J Orthopaedic Res 1992; 10:710–719.
8. Pollack SR. Bioelectrical properties of bone. Endogenous electrical signals. Orthop Clin North Am 1984; 15:3–14.
9. Behari J. Electrostimulation and bone fracture healing. Biomed Eng 1992; 18:235–254.
10. Wolff J. Das Gesetz der Transformation der Knochen. Berlin: Hirschwald, 1892.
11. Friedenberg ZB, Brighton CT. Bioelectric potentials in bone. J Bone Joint Surg 1966; 48A:915–923.
12. Friedenberg ZB, Dyer R, Brighton CT. Electro-osteograms of long bones of immature rabbits. J Dent Res 1971; 50:635–640.

13. Friedenberg ZB, Harlow MC, Heppenstall R, Brighton CT. The cellular origin of bioelectric potentials in bone. Calcif Tissue Res 1973; 13:53–62.

14. Rubinacci A, Brigatti L, Tessari L. A reference curve for axial bioelectric potentials in adult rabbit tibia. Bioelectromagnetics 1984; 5:193–202.

15. Chakkalakal DA, Wilson RF, Connolly JF. Epidermal and endosteal sources of endogenous electricity in injured canine limbs. IEEE Trans Biomed Eng 1988; 35:19–29.

16. Lokietek W, Pawluk RF, Bassett CAL. Muscle injury potentials: a source of voltage in the undeformed rabbit tibia. J Bone Joint Surg 1974; 56B:361–369.

17. Borgens RB. Endogenous ionic currents traverse intact and damaged bone. Science 1984; 225:478–482.

18. De Ponti A, Villa I, Boniforti F, Rubinacci A. Ionic currents at the growth plate of intact bone: occurrence and ionic dependence. Electro- MagnetoBiol 1996; 15(1):37–48.

19. Rubinacci A, De Ponti A, Shipley A, Samaja M, Karplus E, Jaffe LF. Bicarbonate dependence of ion current in damaged bone. Calcif Tissue Int 1996; 58:423–428.

20. Becker RO, Murray DG. The electrical control system regulating fracture healing in amphibians. Clin Orthop Rel Res 1970; 73:169–209.

21. Chiabrera A, Grattarola M, Parodi G, Marcer M. Interazione tra campo elettromagnetico e cellule. Le Scienze 1984; 192:78–94.

22. Frost HM. The biology of fracture healing: an overview for clinicians. Part I and II. Clin Orthop Rel Res 1989; 248:283–309.

23. O'Sullivan ME, Chao EY, Kelly PJ. The effects of fixation on fracture-healing. J Bone Joint Srug 1989; 71-A:306–310.

24. Bianco B, Chiabrera A. From the Longevin-Lorentz to the Zeeman model of em effects on ligand-receptor binding. Bioelectrochem Bioenerg 1992; 28:355–365.

25. Varani K, Gessi S, Merighi S, Iannotta V, Cattabriga E, Spisani S, Cadossi R, Borea PA. Effect of low frequency electromagnetic fields on A_{2A} adenosine receptors in human neutrophils. Brit J Pharmacol 2002; 136:57–66.

26. Brighton CT, Wang W, Seldes R, Zhang G, Pollack SR. Signal transduction in electrically stimulated bone cells. J Bone Joint Surg Am 2001; 83:1514–1523.

27. Guerkov HH, Lohmann CH, Liu Y, Dean DD, Simon BJ, Heckman JD, Schwartz Z, Boyan BD. Pulsed electromagnetic fields increase growth factor release by nonunion cells. Clin Orthop 2001; 384:265–279.

28. Cadossi R, Bersani F, Cossarizza A, Zucchini P, Emilia G, Torelli G, Franceschi C. Lympho-cytes and low-frequency electromagnetic fields. FASEB J 1992; 6:2667–2674.

29. Aaron RK, Ciombor MD, Jolly G. Stimulation of experimental endochondral ossification by low-energy pulsing electromagnetic fields. J Bone Miner Res 1989b; 4:227–233.

30. Bassett CAL, Valdez MG, Hernandez E. Modification of fracture repair with selected pulsing electromagnetic fields. J Bone Joint Surg 1982a; 64A:888–895.

31. Brighton CT, Hozcack WJ, Brager MD, Windsor RE, Pollack SR, Vreslovic EJ, Kotwick JE. Fracture healing in rabbit fibula when subjected to various capacitively coupled electrical fields. J Orthop Res 1985a; 3:331–340.

32. Pienkowski D, Pollack SR, Brighton CT, Griffith NJ. Comparison of asymmetrical and sym-metrical pulse waveforms in electromagnetic stimulation. J Orthop Res 1992; 10:247–255.

33. Bassett CAL, Pawluk RJ, Pilla AA. Augmentation of bone repair by inductively coupled electromagnetic fields. Science 1974; 184:575–577.

34. Canè V, Botti P, Farneti D, Soana S. Electromagnetic stimulation of bone repair: a histo-morphometric study. J Orthop Res 1991; 9:908–917.

35. Canè V, Botti P, Soana S. Pulsed magnetic fields improve osteoblast activity during the repair of an experimental osseous defect. J Orthop Res 1993; 11:664.

36. Canè V, Zaffe D, Botti B, Cavani F, Soana S. Correlation between PEMF exposure time and new bone formation. IV Congresso Nazinale Società Italiana Chirurgia Veterinaria, Napoli, Maggio: 1997.

37. Friedenberg ZB, Andrews ET, Smolenski BI, Pearl BW, Brighton CT. Bone reaction to varying amounts of direct current. Surg Gynecol Obstet 1970; 131:894–899.

38. Traina GC, Gulino G. Medullary rods as electrical conductors for osteogenic stimuli in human bone. In: Brighton CT, Black J, Pollack S, eds. Electrical Properties of Bone and Cartilage. New York: Grune and Stratton, 1979:567–579.

39. Jorgensen TE. Electrical stimulation of human fracture healing by means of a slow pulsating asymmetrical direct current. Clin Orthop 1977; 124:124–127.

40. Zichner L. Repair of nonunions by electrically pulsed current stimulation. Clin Orthop 1981; 161:115–121.

41. Liboff AR, Parkinson WC. Search for ion-cyclotron resonance in an Na^+-transport system. Bioelectromagnetics 1991; 12:77–83.

42. Sollazzo V, Massari L, Caruso A, De Mattei M, Pezzetti F. Effects of low-frequency pulsed electromagnetic fields on human osteoblast-like cells in vitro. Electro MagnetoBiol 1996; 15:75–83.

43. Pezzetti F, De Mattei M, Caruso A, Cadossi R, Zucchini P, Carinci F, Traina GC, Sollazzo V. Effects of pulsed electromagnetic fields on human chondrocytes: an in vitro study. Calcif Tissue Int 1999; 65:396–401.

44. Fontanesi G, Traina GC, Giancecchi F, Tartaglia I, Rotini R, Virgili B, Cadossi R, Ceccherelli G, e Marino AA. La lenta evoluzione del processo riparativo di una frattura puo' essere prevenuta? G.I.O.T. 1986; XII(3):389–404.

45. Kraus W, Lechner F. Die Heilung von Pseudarthrosen und Spontanfrakturen durch strukturbildende elektrodynamische Potentiale. Munchen Mudizinische Woch 1972; 114:1814–1817.

46. Hinsenkamp M, Ryaby J, Burny F. Treatment of nonunion by pulsing electromagnetic field: European multicenter study of 308 cases. Reconstr Surg Traumatol 1985; 19:147–156.

47. Brighton CT, Pollack SR. Treatment of recalcitrant nonunion with a capacitively coupled electric field. J Bone Joint Surgery 1985; 67A:577–585.

48. Hartig M, Joos U, Wiesmann HP. Capacitively coupled electric fields accelerate proliferation of osteoblast-like primary cells and increase bone extracellular matrix formation in vitro. Eur Biophys J 2000; 29:499–506.

49. Wang SJ, Lewallen DG, Bolander ME, Chao EY, Ilstrup DM, Greenleaf JF. Low intensity ultrasound treatment increases strength in a rat femoral fracture model. J Orthop Res 1994; 12:40–47.

50. Jingushi S, Azuma V, Ito M, Harada Y, Takagi H, Ohta T, Komoriya K. Effect of noninvasive pulsed low-intensity ultrasound on rat femoral fracture. Proceedings of the Third World Congress of Biomechanics. 1998; 140.

51. Rubin C, Bolander M, Ryaby JP, Hadjiargyrou M. The use of low-intensity ultrasound to accelerate the healing of fractures. J Bone Joint Surg Am 2001; 83:259–270.

52. Takikawa S, Matsui N, Kokubu T, Tsunoda M, Fujioka H, Mizuno K, Azuma Y. Low-intensity pulsed ultrasound initiates bone healing in rat nonunion fracture model. J Ultrasound Med 2001; 20:197–205.

53. Corradi C, Cozzolino A. The action of ultrasound on the evolution of an experimental fracture in rabbits. Minerva Ortop 1952; 55:44–45.

54. Sharrard WJW. Treatment of congenital and infantile pseudoarthorsis with pulsing electromagnetic fields. Othop Clin North Am 1984; 15(1):143–162.

55. Sharrard WJW. Treatment of congenital and infantile pseudoarthorsis of the tibia with pulsing electromagnetic fields. Biological Effects of Nonionizing Electromagnetic Radiation. 1985; IX(3):42.

56. Sutcliffe ML, Goldberg AAJ. The treatment of congenital pseudoarthrosis of the tibia with pulsing electromagnetic fields. A survey of 52 cases. Clin Orthop Rel Res 1982; 166:45–52.

57. Dal Monte A, Fontanesi G, Giancecchi F, Poli G, Cadossi R. Treatment of congenital pseudarthorsis and acquired nonunion with pulsing electromagnetic fields (PEMFs). Orthop Trans JBJS 1986; 10(3):452.

58. Bassett CAL, Schinkascani M. Long-term pulsed electromagnetic field results in congenital pseudoarthrosis. Calcif Tissue Int 1991; 49:3–12.

59. Kort J, Schink MM, Mitchell SN, Bassett CAL. Congenital pseudarthrosis of the tibia: Treatment with pulsing electromagnetic fields. The international experience. Clin Orthop Rel Res 1982; 165:124–137.

60. Lavine LS, Lustrin I, Shamos MH. Treatment of congenital pseudoathrosis of the tibia with direct current. Clin Orthop Rel Res 1977; 124:69–74.

61. Poli G, Verni E, Dal Monte A. A double approach to the treatment of congenital pseudoarthrosis: Endomedullary nail fixation and stimulation with low frequency pulsing electromagnetic fields (PEMFs). Bioelectrochem Bioenerget 1985; 14:151.

62. Sedel L, Christel P, Duriez J, Duriez R, Evard J, Ficat C, Cauchoix J, Witvoet J. Resultats de la stimulation par champ electromagnetique de la consolidation des pseudarthroses. Rev Chir Orthop Traum 1981; 67:11–23.

63. Marcer M, Musatti G, Bassett CAL. Results of pulsed electromagnetic fields (pemfs) in ununited fractures after external skeletal fixation. Clin Orthop Rel Res 1984; 190:260–265.

64. Sharrard WJW. A double-blind trial of pulsed electromagnetic field for delayed union of tibial fractures. J Bone Joint Surg 1990; 72B:347–355.

65. DeHaas WG, Watson J, Morrison DM. Non-invasive treatment of ununited fracture of the tibia using electrical stimulation. J Bone Joint Surg 1980; 62B:465–470.

66. Watson J. A battery-operated portable orthopaedic stimulator. San Francisco: BRAGS 3, 1983:55.

67. Vaquero DH. Resultados y factores pronósticos de la electrestimulación en los trasftornos de la consolidación ósea, ATTI VII corso internazionale sulla stimolazione biofisica della riparazione endogena nel tessuto osseo e cartilagineo, Pescatina, 2001:8–9.

68. Fontijne WPJ, Konings PC. Botgroeistimulatie met PEMF bij gestoorde fractuurgenezing. Ned Tijoschr Traum 1998; 5:114–119.

69. Scott G, King JB. A prospective double blind trial of electrical capacitive coupling in the treatment of non-union of long bones. J Bone Joint Surg 1994; 76A:820–826.

70. Mattei A, Spurio Pompili GF, Impagliazzo A. Experience with the treatment of delayed unions and pseudoarthrodesis with capacitive coupled electric fields. Seventh International course, Biophysical Stimulation of Endogenous Repair in Bone and Cartilage. 2001:14.

71. Mayr E, Wagner S, Ecker M, Ruter A. Treatment of non unions by means of low-intensity ultrasound. Unfallchirurg 1997; 268:958–962.

72. Romanò C, Messina J, Meani E. Low-intensity ultrasound for the treatment of infected nonunions. In: Agazzi M, ed. Quaderni di Infezioni Otseoarticolari. Milan: Masson, 1999:83–93.

73. Benazzo F, Mosconi M, Beccarisi G, Galli U. Use of capacitive coupled electric fields in stress fractures in athletes. Clin Orthop Rel Res 1995; 310:145–149.

74. Hinsenkamp M, Bourgois R, Bassett C, Chiabrera A, Burny F, Ryaby J. Electromagnetic stimulation of fracture repair. Influence on healing of fresh fracture. Acta Orthop Belg 1978; 44:671–698.

75. Luna GF, Arevalo RL, Labajos UV. La EEM en las elongaciones y transportes oseos. In: Vaquero H, Stern L, eds. La Estimulacion Electromagnetica en la Patologia Osea. Madrid: San Martin IG, 1999:236–246.

76. Emami A, Petren-Mallmin M, Larsson S. No effect of low-intensity ultrasound on healing time of intramedullary fixed tibial fractures. J Orthop Trauma 1999; 13:252–257.

77. Borsalino G, Bagnacani M, Bettati E, Fornaciari G, Rocchi R, Uluhogian S, Ceccherelli G, Cadossi R, Traina G. Electrical stimulation of human femoral intertrochanteric osteotomies: double blind study. Clin Orthop Rel Res 1988; 237:256–263.

78. Mammi GI, Rocchi R, Cadossi R, Traina GC. Effect of PEMF on the healing of human tibial osteotomies: a double blind study. Clin Orthop Rel Res 1993; 288:246–253.

79. Capanna R, Donati D, Masetti C, Manfrini M, Panozzo A, Cadossi R, Campanacci M. Effect of electromagnetic fields on patients undergoing massive bone graft following bone tumor resection: a double-blind study. Clin Orthop Rel Res 1994; 306:213–221.

80. Eyres KS, Saleh M, Kanis JA. Effect of pulsed electromagnetic-fields on bone-formation and bone loss during limb lengthening. Bone 1996; 18:505–509.

81. Guizzardi S, Di Silvestre M, Govoni P, Scandroglio R. Pulsed electromagnetic field stimulation on posterior spinal fusions: a histological study in rats. J Spinal Disord 1994; 7(1):36–40.

82. Savini R, Di Silvestre M, Gargiulo G, Bettini N. The use of pulsing electromagnetic fields in posterolateral lumbosacral spinal fusion. J Bioelectricity 1990; 9:9–17.

83. Mammi GI, Rocchi R, Di Silvestre M. Effect of PEMF on spinal fusion: a prospective study with a control group. In: Blank M, ed. Electricity and Magnetism in Biology and Medicine. San Francisco Press, 1993:800–803.

84. Ficat RP. Idiopathic bone necrosis of the femoral head: early diagnosis and treatment. J Bone Joint Surg 1985; 67(B):3–9.

85. Bassett CAL, Schink-Ascani M, Lewis SM. Effects of pulsed electromagnetic fields of Steinberg ratings of the femoral head osteonecrosis. Clin Orthop Rel Res 1989; 246:172–185.

86. Santori FS, Vitullo A, Manili M, Montemurro G, Stopponi M. Necrosi avascolare della testa del femore: l'associazione dei CEMP al trattamento chirurgico di decompressione e innesti ossei autoplastici, Impiego dei Campi Elettromagnetici Pulsati In Ortopedia e Traumatologia, Walberti Editore, Ferrara 12 Maggio 1995 e Roma 20 Maggio 1995:75–83.

87. Hinsenkamp M, Hauzeur JP, Sintzoff S. Preliminary results in electromagnetic field treatment of osteonecrosis. Bioelectrochem Bioenergetics 1993; 30:229–235.

88. Hinsenkamp M, Hauzeur JP, Sintzoff S. Long term results in electromagnetic fields (EMF) treatment of osteonecrosis. In: Schoutens A, ed. Bone Circulation and Vascularization in Normal and Pathological Conditions. New York: Plenum Press, 1993:331–336.

89. Garcia-Andrade G, Esteban DI, Lluch CB, Stern LD. La EEM en el tratamiento de la necrosis avascular de la cabeza femoral. In: Vaquero H, Stern L, eds. La Estimulacion Electromagnetica en la Patologia Osea. Madrid: San Martin I.G., 1999:219–235.

90. Aaron RK, Lennox D, Bunce GE. The conservative treatment of osteonecrosis of the femoral head: a comparison of core decompression and PEMF. Clin Orthop Rel Res 1989; 249:209–218.

91. Steinberg ME, Brighton CT, Corces A, Hayken GD, Steinberg DR, Strafford B, Tooze SE, Fallon M. Osteonecrosis of the femoral head. Results of core decompression and grafting with and without electrical stimulation. Clin Orthop Rel Res 1989; 249:199–208.

92. Steinberg ME, Brighton CT, Bands RE, Hartman KM. Capacitive coupling and adjunctive treatment for avascular necrosis. Clin Orthop Rel Res 1990; 261:11–18.

93. Fini M, Cadossi R, Canè V, Cavani F, Giavaresi G, Krajewsti A, Martini L, Nicoli Aldini N, Ravaglioli A, Rimondini L, Torricelli P, Giardino R. The effect of PEMFs on the osteointegration of HA implants in cancellous bone: a morphogenetic and microstructural in vivo study. JOR 2002; 20:756–763.

94. Rispoli FP, Corolla FM, Mussner R. The use of low-frequency pulsing electromagnetic fields inpatients with painful hip prosthesis. J Bioelectricity 1988; 7:181–187.

95. Pipino F, Molfetta L, Losito A, Capozzi M. Sui risultati della stimolazione con campi elettromagnetici in ortopedia e traumatologia, ATTI I Corso Avanzato di Bioelettricita', Venezia, April 1990:91–98.

96. Fontanesi G, Giancecchi F, Rotini R, e Cadossi R. Terapia dei Ritardi di Consolidazione e Pseudoartrosi con Campi Elettromagnetici Pulsati a Bassa Frequenza. G.I.O.T. 1983; IX:319–333.

97. Traina GC, Fontanesi G, Costa P, Mammi GI, Pisano F, Giancecchi F, Adravanti P. Effect of electromagnetic stimulation on patients suffering from nonunion. A retrospective study with a control group. J Bioelectricity 1991; 10:101–117.

27

Electromagnetic Stimulation in Orthopaedics: Biochemical Mechanisms to Clinical Applications

James T. Ryaby

OrthoLogic Corp, and Arizona State University,
Tempe, Arizona, U.S.A.

Dr. Ryaby starts this chapter with discussion on the concept evolving mechanoelectrical signals in the development of therapeutical devices primarily for bone repair. Three different techniques are discussed: capacitive coupling, direct current, and pulsed electromagnetic/combined magnetic fields. Cellular studies and preclinical and clinical models are shown as a basis for randomized, double-blind studies on the effects of electromagnetic stimulation in bone repair and spinal fusion.

I. INTRODUCTION

The development of electrical and electromagnetic technologies for use in orthopaedics is based on the discovery of the electrical properties of bone tissue in the 1950s and 1960s. The first report by Fukada and Yasuda on bone piezoelectric properties appeared in 1954 (1). These investigators measured an electric potential upon deformation of dry bone and compared this effect to electret material. Following up on these important results was the work of Andy Bassett's group at Columbia University and Carl Brighton's group at the University of Pennsylvania, among others, who both reported the generation of electrical potentials in wet bone upon mechanical deformation (2–5). These observations were then extended to other tissues including collagen and cartilaginous tissues subject to mechanical deformation (6–8).

The concept that evolved from these studies was mechanoelectrical signals originating during loading of bone and other connective tissue(s) were stimulatory and provided a biophysical signal generation basis for Wolff's law. Current thinking predicts that the main stimulatory or regulatory component of applied load is probably the mechanical component (9). However, even if a secondary component in loading-induced responses, effects of electric

411

fields (EF) and electromagnetic fields (EMF) (on EF/EMF) on cells and tissues have been well-documented and recently reviewed (10,11).

The application of these concepts led to development of EF/EMF therapeutic devices focused primarily on bone repair. The first therapeutic device used implanted electrode based direct current techniques, which was followed by the development of noninvasive technologies using electrical and electromagnetic fields. Clinical evaluation of these technologies in orthopaedics was based on well-designed human clinical trials that resulted in FDA-approved applications for treatment of fractures (nonunions and fresh fractures) and spine fusion (12). Clinical trials for additional orthopaedic indications have also been conducted for treatment of osteonecrosis (13,14), tendonitis (15), osteoporosis (16,17), and osteoarthritis (18,19). Applications of EMF for therapeutic treatment of osteoarthritis will not be covered herein as this is the subject of a separate chapter in this monograph. FDA approval for these other orthopaedic indications has not been granted in the United States to date.

The spectrum of clinical conditions that respond positively to therapeutic EF/EMF stimulation clearly demonstrates the effectiveness of these stimulation devices to enhance musculoskeletal tissue healing. This chapter will summarize the scientific basis for these technologies and the key prospective clinical trials demonstrating their clinical efficacy and utility.

II. ELECTRICAL AND ELECTROMAGNETIC FIELD STIMULATION

Electrical fields (EF) and electromagnetic fields (EMF) have been developed for the past 30 years as therapeutic, noninvasive stimulation techniques for fracture healing, spine fusion, and bone repair. The physical mechanism(s) of interaction of electric and magnetic fields remains an active field of inquiry, probably due to the low level of EF/EMF used and its nonthermal characteristics (10). It should be emphasized that from a physical perspective each electrical and electromagnetic field system is unique in their respective signal parameters. Following is a brief synopsis of work performed in the past several years on cell- and tissue-level mechanisms of EF/EMF stimulation.

Three different techniques are used for therapeutic EF/EMF stimulation in FDA-approved applications in orthopaedics. These three techniques are capacitive coupling, direct current, and electromagnetic stimulation. Capacitive coupling (CCEF) uses 60-kHz sinusoidal electrical fields, which induce electrical fields of approximately 7 μA/cm^2 at the skin surface. Direct current (DC) uses implanted electrodes delivering a current of approximately 20 μA. There are two types of inductively coupled devices approved for use in the United States, these are the pulsed electromagnetic field (PEMF) and combined magnetic field (CMF) technologies. The first technology developed and approved for clinical use by the FDA uses PEMF, which induce an electrical field in tissue of approximately 20 μA/cm^2. This complex field is believed to act by the induced electrical field, which is the subject of a recent review by Otter et al. (20). This field is pulsed using frequency modulation at 15 Hz. The second inductive coupling technique, combined magnetic fields (CMF), uses a specific combination of DC and AC magnetic fields that are believed to couple specifically to ion transport processes (21).

Over the past 10 years, cellular and animal studies have discovered effects of electromagnetic fields on both signal transduction pathway(s) and growth factor biosynthesis. Fitzsimmons and Ryaby, in several publications, have proposed a model for combined magnetic field (CMF) action(s) on bone repair. The resulting working model from these studies is CMF stimulates secretion of growth factors (i.e., insulinlike growth factor-II) after a short duration CMF stimulus of 30 min. The clinical CMF effect on bone repair is proposed to be due to this upregulation of growth factor production. In other words, short-term CMF exposure acts as stimulus, triggering mechanism(s) that couple to the normal molecular regulation of bone repair. The studies underlying this working model have shown effects of CMF in osteoblasts on calcium ion transport (22), cell proliferation (23), IGF-II release (24), and IGF-II receptor expression (25), as well as effects of CMF on rat fracture callus (26). The role of growth factors in transduction of CMF in cells and tissues and the link to the observed clinical benefit of CMF requires further inquiry.

In accordance with the model above, Aaron and Ciombor (27) have reported on stimulation of transforming growth factor beta (TGF-β) mRNA with PEMF in a bone induction model in the rat. These results show that the increase in growth factor production by PEMF may be related to the induction of cartilage differentiation. These authors have also shown that the responsive cell population is most likely mesenchymal cells (28), which are recruited early in the PEMF stimulus to enhance early cartilage formation. Recent studies by Boyan and colleagues (29,30) have also demonstrated upregulation of TGF-β mRNA by PEMF both in the human osteoblastlike cell line MG-63 and in cells derived from human nonunion tissue. Significant increases in TGF-β1 were noted with PEMF stimulation. The conclusion drawn from the above studies is growth factor upregulation is the culmination of the stimulation of signaling events in EMF interaction(s) with cells and tissues.

The upregulation of growth factor production has also emerged as a common denominator in the tissue level mechanisms underlying the capacitively coupled electrical stimulation technologies. Brighton's group (31,32) showed an increase in both TGF-β1 mRNA and protein in osteoblast cultures after CCEF exposure. Using specific inhibitors, these authors have provided data to suggest that CCEFs act through a calmodulin-dependent pathway. However enticing, more work needs to be performed to fully understand the role of growth factors in transduction of biophysical stimuli and the clinical relevance. The proposed working model for EF/EMF stimulation of growth factor production in fracture nonunions is depicted in Fig. 1.

There has been extensive research on PEMF effects on bone and cartilage using preclinical animal models. For example, Cane, Cadossi, and colleagues have used a transcortical defect model for the past 10 years to address basic histomorphometric and molecular aspects of EMF stimulation. The model used by these investigators is the bilateral cortical hole defect model in the metacarpal bones in horses, with quantitative histomorphometric methods employed to quantify differences between treated and control limbs. The first study reported in 1991 (33) that PEMF-treated defects showed a statistically significant increase in the amount of new bone formation at 60 days of treatment in diaphyseal defects. The follow-up study (34) showed a significant increase in bone formation and mineral apposition rate with PEMF treatment. Useful information on EF/EMF effects has also been derived from in vivo studies on osteopenic animal models (Fig. 2) (35–38).

In summary, these studies emphasize that EF/EMF can couple to cellular signal transduction pathways, leading to an increase in local growth factor production. These studies provide a potential tissue level mechanism for observed EF/EMF effects in orthopaedic clinical applications.

A. Clinical Studies

The application of EF/EMF for the treatment of fracture nonunions is the therapeutic application with the longest FDA approved regulatory history in the United States, with the

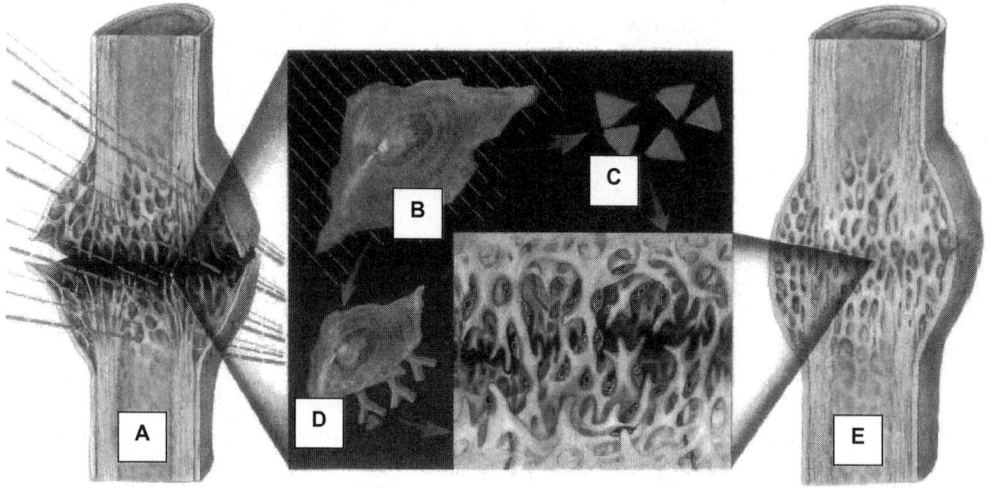

Figure 1 Model for EMF growth-factor-dependent regulation of bone repair in fracture nonunion. (A) Magnetic fields pass through the fracture site. (B) Cells in fracture site sense EMF stimulation. (C) Cells produce regulatory molecules (i.e., growth factors) and also increase growth factor cellular receptors (D). (E) This EMF stimulation of the normal biological regulation processes controlling bone repair leads to healing of fracture nonunion.

initial approval of PEMF occurring in 1979. Currently there are four FDA-approved devices in use for EF/EMF treatment of nonunions; these devices have specific signal parameters, device configurations, and widely variable daily prescribed treatment times from 30 min/day to 24 h/day (12). Capacitive coupling stimulation using electrodes placed on the skin (noninvasive, manufactured by Biolectron/EBI) was developed by the groups of Brighton and Pollack at University of Pennsylvania. Direct current stimulation using implanted electrodes (invasive, EBI) was developed by Patterson and colleagues in Australia. Three electromagnetic stimulation technologies using inductive coupling (non-

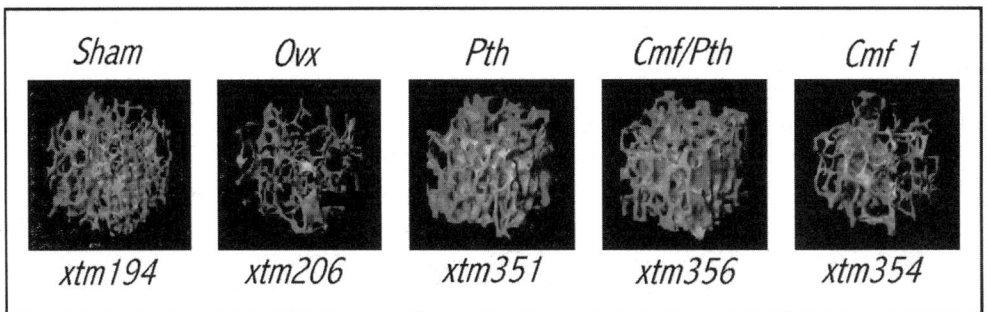

Figure 2 Three-dimensional renderings of representative trabecular bone cubes taken from the rat proximal tibial metaphysis using synchrotron-based x-ray tomography. Ovariectomized rats were allowed to lose bone for 6 weeks, then therapeutic intervention was initiated with either combined magnetic fields (CMF), parathyroid hormone (PTH), or combined CMF/PTH. Controls were sham or OVX. (Adapted from Ref. 37 and 38.)

invasive) are in use today. These are pulsed electromagnetic fields (PEMF, EBI, and Orthofix) and combined magnetic fields (CMF, OrthoLogic).

As stated previously, evaluation of the clinical benefit of these devices for orthopaedic conditions were based on prospective clinical trials conducted under a FDA investigational device exemption. The first system developed for clinical treatment of nonunions was direct current stimulation with implanted electrodes. This technique produces a localized electrical current (E field) between electrodes inserted at the fracture site and is predominantly used clinically today for augmentation of spine fusion. This technique was developed concurrently by Friedenberg and Brighton in the United States (39) and Patterson (40) in Australia. The relative success rates for nonunion treatment in these prospective clinical studies ranged from 78 to 86%, respectively. Reasons for the limited clinical acceptance of the implanted technology for nonunion treatment were the subsequent availability of noninvasive methods of EF/EMF treatment, limited electric field exposure metrics, and complication rate.

The first noninvasive system approved by the U.S. FDA uses pulsed electromagnetic fields (PEMF). This technique was developed by Bassett, Pilla, and Ryaby (the author's father) (41) and uses an external coil to produce a complex asymmetric signal of pulses repeating at 15 Hz. In one prospective series by Bassett (42), 127 tibial diaphyseal delayed unions or nonunions were exposed to PEMF for 10 h/day. At the study conclusion, 87% were healed with a median healing time of 5.2 months. The follow-up study by Heckman et al. (43) showed a lower success rate of 64% in a series of 149 patients with PEMF treatment. More rigorous entry criteria in the Heckman study may have led to this decrease in efficacy. Clinical studies using PEMF are the subject of comprehensive reviews by Bassett (44) and Gossling et al. (45).

Noninvasive capacitive coupling (CCEF), developed by Brighton and Pollack (46), uses disk electrodes coupled to the skin via a conductive gel. The device produces a 60-kHz symmetrical sine wave with a recommended daily treatment time of 24 h/day. The first nonunion study reported an overall efficacy of 77%, with a mean time to healing of 23 weeks in a series of 22 nonunions. The most recent FDA-approved technology using combined magnetic fields was first evaluated as a treatment for fracture nonunions in the mid-1990s (47). The CMF device uses an external pair of coils oriented parallel to one another, with an alternating sinusoidal magnetic field of 76.6 H and amplitude of 40 μT peak to peak and a static field of 20 μT. Eighty-four nonunions were evaluated in the clinical trial, with one 30-min treatment per day with the CMF device until healed or for a maximum of 9 months. The results noted by the blinded radiographic review panel showed 51 nonunions healed (61%), with tibial nonunions showing an efficacy of 76% (Fig. 3). The conclusion drawn from these above studies is EF/EMF is effective for the treatment of fracture nonunions.

B. Randomized, Double-Blind Studies

The use of EF/EMF for nonunion treatment does not have universal acceptance in the orthopaedic community. The following double-blind, placebo controlled trials were designed to use the most rigorous criteria possible for assessment of the beneficial effects of EF/EMF on bone healing (Table 1). The first successful prospective, randomized, double-blind, placebo controlled trial for bone repair was performed by Borsalino et al. (48) in Italy. This was followed by the study of Mammi et al. (49), who reported on the treatment of tibial osteotomies with PEMF. These authors showed that use of the active PEMF device increased the percentage of patients at late stage healing (3/4). The use of PEMF in orthopaedics in Italy is the subject of a chapter in this monograph by Cadossi.

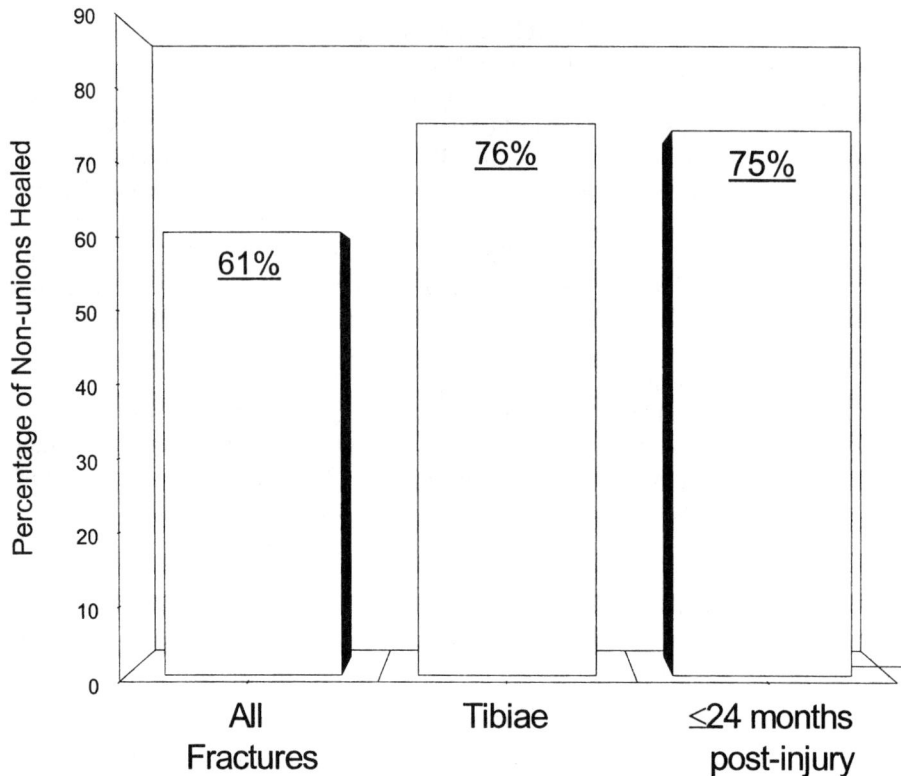

Figure 3 Graph showing the percentage of fractures healed at completion of the CMF nonunion clinical trial conducted by OrthoLogic Corp (see Table 2).

The first placebo controlled, double blind, randomized trial on fracture healing (tibial delayed unions) was reported by Sharrard in 1990 (50). Fifty-one patients were enrolled in this trial, and both an orthopaedic surgeon and a musculoskeletal radiologist performed blinded radiographic assessment. Results of this study showed a significant effect of the active device on healing, with the surgeon's assessment more favorable than the radiologist. The only prospective, randomized, double-blind, placebo controlled study on nonunions, which is the FDA-approved indication, was reported by Scott and King in the United Kingdom (51). Capacitively coupled electrical fields (CCEF) were used on long bone nonunions for 24 h/day for a maximum of 6 months. Sixty percent of the active CCEF device patients healed with a mean time of 21 weeks compared to none in the placebo device group. Finally, Brighton et al. (52) have published on a logistic regression model investigating the clinical factors that govern whether a given nonunion is responsive to EF/EMF stimulation. These authors show that age of nonunion and number of prior failed procedures correlate with responsiveness to EF/EMF stimulation.

C. Spine Fusion

Three randomized, double-blind, placebo controlled clinical trials have been performed addressing the use of bone growth stimulation technologies as an adjunct to spine fusion. These trials form the basis for FDA approval of these technologies as adjunctive stimulation

Table 1 Randomized and Randomized, Double-Blind, Placebo Controlled Trials Performed to Assess Safety and Efficacy of EF and EMF Stimulation Techniques

Author	Year	Technology	Trial design	Indication	Ref.
Binder et al.	1984	PEMF	Randomized, double blind	Tendinitis	15
Borsalino et al.	1988	PEMF	Randomized, double blind	Femoral Osteotomies	48
Aaron et al.	1989	PEMF	Randomized	Avascular necrosis	13
Steinberg et al.	1989	CCEF	Randomized	Avascular necrosis	14
Sharrard	1990	PEMF	Randomized, double blind	Delayed Union	49
Mooney	1990	PEMF	Randomized, double blind	Spine Fusion	54
Mammi et al.	1993	PEMF	Randomized, double blind	Tibial Osteotomies	50
Scott and King	1994	CCEF	Randomized, double blind	Non-union	51
Trock et al.	1994	EMF	Randomized, double blind	Osteoarthritis	18
Zizik et al.	1995	EF	Randomized, double blind	Osteoarthritis	19
Goodwin et al.	2000	CCEF	Randomized, double blind	Spine Fusion	55
Linovitz et al.	2002	CMF	Randomized, double blind	Spine Fusion	56

devices for the enhancement of spine fusion. The first randomized trial was the study by Kane in 1989, who utilized an implantable direct current (DC) stimulator (53). This device uses electrodes that are surgically placed lateral to the fusion site that is powered by a battery pack to deliver a current of 20 μA/cm^2. Fifty-nine patients were enrolled in this study, with 81% of the EF-stimulated group healed compared to 54% in the control group, a statistically significant increase. The major limitation of in this study was the lack of a placebo control.

The first randomized, double-blind evaluation of a noninvasive electromagnetic technology for adjunctive stimulation was the study by Mooney, who reported on the use of pulsed electromagnetic fields (PEMF) for stimulation of interbody fusions in 1990 (Orthofix SpinalStim) (54). This was a prospective, randomized, double-blind, placebo controlled clinical trial and analysis was ultimately performed on 195 patients with a mean age of 38 years. Patients were instructed to use the electromagnetic device for a minimum of 8 h/day for 12 months. This trial used a confirmatory reading of fusion success by a blinded radiologist. The data was stratified into consistent (≥8 h/day) and inconsistent users (<4 h/day). In the 117 patients who were consistent users, the active device patients achieved a fusion success rate of 92%, compared to the placebo success rate of 68%, a statistically significant difference. Patients who used the device inconsistently had the same success rate in the active and placebo groups, 65 and 61%, respectively. This study was the first to show a dose response for a PEMF-based noninvasive electromagnetic treatment.

The second noninvasive technology for stimulation of spine fusion is capacitively coupled electrical fields (CCEF, Biolectron, SpinalPak) as recently reported by Goodwin in 1999 (55). The study design was a multicenter, prospective, randomized, double-blind, placebo controlled trial that reported on 179 patients with a mean age of 43 years (Table 2). The daily device treatment time was 24 h/day, and efficacy was determined using a blinded radiographic and clinical review panel with the study end-point at 9 months. The results showed that 85% of the active device patients fused compared to 65% of the placebo patients, a statistically significant difference. Posterolateral fusion patients comprised this group, as the anterio- and posteriolateral interbody fusion groups did not reach statistical significance due to low patient numbers.

Table 2 Comparison Table of FDA-Approved EF and EMF Technologies for Fracture Nonunion Treatment[a]

	EBI	Orthofix	Bioelectron/EBI	Orthologic
Technology	Pulsed electromagnetic fields (PEMF)	Pulsed electromagnetic fields (PEMF)	Capacitively coupled electrical fields (CCEF)	Combined magnetic fields (CMF)
Study population	Nonunion	Nonunion	Nonunion	Nonunion
Clinical trial	Prospective	Prospective	Prospective	Prospective
No. patients	115	120	79	84
No. investigators	20	70?	16	16
Enrollment criteria verification	Investigator	Investigator	Investigator	Panel
Efficacy evaluation	Investigator	Investigator/panel	Investigator/panel	Panel
Efficacy rate (%)	63.5	72	50	61
Long-term follow-up	Yes	Yes	Yes	Yes
Change after long-term follow-up	Downgraded	Downgraded	Downgraded	No change
FDA approval date	1979	1986	1986	1994
Daily treatment time	8–10 hours	Minimum 3 h	Recommended 24 h	30 min

[a] All technologies were evaluated in prospective clinical trials conducted under an FDA IDE and PMA approval date is provided.

The third noninvasive technology for adjunctive stimulation of spine fusion is combined magnetic fields, as reported by Linovitz et al. (56). The clinical study conducted was a prospective, randomized, double-blind, placebo controlled trial on primary, uninstrumented lumbar spine fusion, which is the only spine trial performed to date on a uniform surgical procedure. The combined magnetic field device uses a single posterior coil, centered over the fusion site, with one 30-min treatment per day for 9 months. The primary endpoint was assessment of fusion at nine months based on evaluation by a blinded panel consisting of the treating physician, a musculoskeletal radiologist, and a spine surgeon. This is the largest study to date, with 201 patients evaluated. There was a significant effect observed based on both the total patient population and in female patients. Active device patients healed at 64% compared to 43% of placebo device patients. This was the first study to stratify by gender, with the results showing 67% of active-device females fused compared to 35 percent of placebo device females. For the overall patient population, generalized estimating equations analysis showed a significant time by treatment interaction, indicating acceleration of healing.

At present no clinical studies have been performed on any of the EF/EMF technologies using an outcome instrument such as the Oswestry score. Regardless, the above studies, based on rigorous randomized double-blind trials do provide compelling data in support for the adjunctive use of EF/EMF in spine fusion patients.

III. POTENTIAL ADDITIONAL CLINICAL APPLICATIONS

One recent paper describe effects of CMF treatment on Charcot neuroarthropathy by Hanft and colleagues (57). The trial was a prospective, randomized pilot study on acute, phase 1 Charcot patients. The study design initially was randomized, then statistical analysis showed a statistical benefit for the CMF treatment group. Subsequently, an additional ten patients were added to the CMF treatment group. The final results showed that treatment with the CMF device decreased the time to consolidation to 11.1 weeks, compared to 23.2 weeks in the control group, a statistically significant difference ($p < 0.001$). There was no statistically significant difference in entry criteria between the control and CMF groups, and the authors concluded that the CMF treatment "significantly accelerated" the process of consolidation in this study.

IV. DISCUSSION AND CONCLUSION

The development of additional clinical applications of EF/EMF stimulation is predicated on large, multicenter clinical trials conducted under FDA guidelines. The major constraint is identification of clinical need and justification for financial support for these trials. This is the biggest challenge facing the field of EF/EMF stimulation in orthopaedics. The second challenge is the ever more demanding reimbursement environment. As such, many of the open, unanswered questions in the clinical application(s) of EF/EMF remain to be solved.

To answer these remaining questions, several approaches could be widely used to design future clinical studies. The first would be to conduct additional double-blind clinical trials to determine if biophysical stimulation can affect the healing rate and outcome for the intended orthopaedic indication. Secondly, outcome studies could be performed, randomizing patients in two- or three-arm clinical trials comparing different treatment regimes to biophysical stimulation. Thirdly, well-designed registry studies may be useful in expansion of clinical indications where there already exist FDA-approved indications. This might include an expansion of indication to all spine fusion, not the current limitation of lumbar fusion only.

In conclusion, electrical, electromagnetic, and ultrasonic devices have been demonstrated to positively affect the healing process in fresh fractures, delayed and nonunions, osteotomies, and spine fusion. These outcomes have been validated by well-designed and statistically powered double-blind clinical trials. The FDA-approved indications for these biophysical stimulation devices are limited at present to these indications. Based on these findings, biophysical stimulation technologies provide an additional arm to current treatment management strategies for these conditions. Future delineation of additional clinical indication(s) for musculoskeletal conditions awaits further basic scientific, preclinical, and clinical research.

REFERENCES

1. Fukada E, Yasuda I. On the piezoelectric effect of bone. J Phys Soc Japan 1957; 12:121–128.
2. Bassett CAL, Becker RO. Generation of electric potentials in bone in response to mechanical stress. Science 1962; 137:1063–1064.
3. Friedenberg ZB, Brighton CT. Bioelectric potentials in bone. J Bone Joint Surg 1966; 48A:915–923.
4. Shamos MH, Lavine LS. Piezoelectricity as a fundamental property of biological tissues. Nature 1967; 212:267–268.
5. Williams WS, Perletz L. P-n junctions and the piezoelectric response of bone. Nature 1971; 233:58–59.
6. Anderson JC, Eriksson C. Electrical properties of wet collagen. Nature 1968; 227:166–168.
7. Bassett CAL, Pawluk RJ. Electrical behavior of cartilage during loading. Science 1974; 814:575–577.
8. Grodzinsky AJ, Lipshitz H, Glimcher MJ. Electromechanical properties of articular cartilage during compression and stress relaxation. Nature 1978; 275:448–450.
9. Duncan RL, Turner CH. Mechanotransduction and the functional response of bone to mechanical strain. Calcif Tissue Intl 1995; 57:344–358.
10. Pilla AA, Markov MS. Bioeffects of weak electromagnetic fields. Rev Environ Health 1994; 10:55–69.
11. Donahue HJ. Gap junctions and biophysical regulation of bone cell differentiation. Bone 2000; 26:417–422.
12. Ryaby JT. Clinical effects of electromagnetic and electrical fields on fracture healing. Clin Orthop 1998; 355S:205–215.
13. Aaron RK, Lennox D, Bunce GE, Ebert T. The conservative treatment of osteonecrosis of the femoral head. A comparison of core decompression and pulsing electromagnetic fields. Clin Orthop 1989; 249:209–218.
14. Steinberg ME, Brighton CT, Corces A, Hayken GD, Steinberg DR, Strafford B, Tooze SE, Fallon M. Osteonecrosis of the femoral head. Results of core decompression and grafting with and without electrical stimulation. Clin Orthop 1989; 249:199–208.
15. Binder A, Parr G, Hazelman B, Fitton-Jackson S. Pulsed electromagnetic field therapy of persistent rotator cuff tendinitis: a double-blind controlled assessment. Lancet 1984; 1:695–697.
16. Tabrah F, Hoffmeier M, Gilbert F, Batkin S, Bassett CAL. Bone density changes in osteoporosis-prone women exposed to pulsed electromagnetic fields (PEMFs). J Bone Min Res 1990; 5:437–442.
17. Garland DE, Adkins RH, Matsuno NN, Stewart CA. The effect of pulsed electromagnetic fields on osteoporosis at the knee in individuals with spinal cord injury. J Spinal Cord Med 1999; 22:239–245.
18. Trock DH, Bollet AJ, Markoll R. The effect of pulsed electromagnetic fields in the treatment of

osteoarthritis of the knee and cervical spine. Report of randomized, double blind, placebo controlled trials. J Rheumatol 1994; 21:1903–1911.

19. Zizic TM, Hoffman KC, Holt PA, Hungerford DS, O'Dell JR, Jacobs MA, Lewis GC, Deal LC, Caldwell JR, Cholewczyinski JG, Free SM. The treatment of osteoarthritis of the knee with pulsed electrical stimulation. J Rheumat 1995; 22:1757–1761.

20. Otter MW, McLeod KJ, Rubin CT. Effects of electromagnetic fields in experimental fracture repair. Clin Orthoped 1998; 355S:90–104.

21. McLeod BR, Liboff AR. Cyclotron resonance in cell membranes: the theory of the mechanism. In: Blank MJ, Findl E, eds. Mechanistic Approaches to Interactions of Electromagnetic Fields with Living Systems. New York: Plenum, 1987:97–108.

22. Fitzsimmons RJ, Ryaby JT, Magee FP, Baylink DJ. Combined magnetic fields increase net calcium flux in bone cells. Calcif Tissue Int 1994; 55:376–380.

23. Fitzsimmons RJ, Baylink DJ, Ryaby JT, Magee FP. EMF-stimulated bone cell proliferation. In: Blank MJ, ed. Electricity and Magnetism in Biology and Medicine. San Francisco: San Francisco Press, 1993:899–902.

24. Fitzsimmons RJ, Ryaby JT, Mohan S, Magee FP, Baylink DJ. Combined magnetic fields increase IGF-II in TE-85 human bone cell cultures. Endocrinology 1995; 136:3100–3106.

25. Fitzsimmons RJ, Ryaby JT, Magee FP, Baylink DJ. IGF-II receptor number is increased in TE-85 cells by low-amplitude, low-frequency combined magnetic field (CMF) exposure. J Bone Min Res 1995; 10:812–819.

26. Ryaby JT, Fitzsimmons RJ, Khin NA, Culley PL, Magee FP, Weinstein AM, Baylink DJ. The role of insulin-like growth factor in magnetic field regulation of bone formation. Bioelectrochem Bioenerg 1994; 35:87–91.

27. Aaron RK, Wang S, Mck.Ciombor D. Upregulation of basal TGFb1 levels by EMF coincident with chondrogenesis—implications for skeletal repair and tissue engineering. J Orthop Res 2002; 20:233–240.

28. Aaron RK, Mck.Ciombor D. Acceleration of experimental endochondral ossification by biophysical stimulation of the progenitor cell pool. J Orthop Res 1996; 14:582–589.

29. Lohmann CH, Schwartz Z, Liu Y, Guerkov H, Dean DD, Simon B, Boyan BD. Pulsed electromagnetic field stimulation of MG63 osteoblast-like cells affects differentiation and local factor production. J Orthop Res 2000; 18:637–646.

30. Guerkov HH, Lohmann CH, Liu Y, Dean DD, Simon BJ, Heckman JD, Schwartz Z, Boyan BD. Pulsed electromagnetic fields increase growth factor release by nonunion cells. Clin Orthop 2001; 180:265–279.

31. Zhuang H, Wang W, Seldes RM, Tahernia AD, Fan H, Brighton CT. Electrical stimulation induces the level of TGF-B1 mRNA in osteoblastic cells by a mechanism involving calcium/calmodulin pathway. Biochem Biophys Res Comm 1997; 237:225–229.

32. Brighton CT, Wang W, Seldes R, Zhang G, Pollack SR. Signal transduction in electrically stimulated bone cells. J Bone Joint Surg 2001; 83A:1514–1523.

33. Cane V, Botti P, Farnetti P, Soana S. Electromagnetic stimulation of bone repair: a histomorphometric study. J Orthop Res 1991; 9:908–917.

34. Cane V, Botti P, Soana S. Pulsed magnetic fields improve osteoblast activity during the repair of an experimental osseous defect. J Orthop Res 1993; 11:664–670.

35. Brighton CT, Katz MJ, Goll SR, Nichols CE III, Pollack SR. Prevention and treatment of sciatic denervation disuse osteoporosis in the rat tibia with capacitively coupled electrical stimulation. Bone 1985; 6:87–97.

36. McLeod KJ, Rubin CT. The effect of low frequency electrical fields on osteogenesis. J Bone Joint Surg 1992; 74A:920–929.

37. Ryaby JT, Jurischk E, Haupt DL, Kinney JH. Combined magnetic fields reverse osteopenia and restore strength in a rodent model of osteoporosis. Proceedings of the Third International Congress on Bioelectricity 2000; 3:153–154.

38. Ryaby JT, Jurischk E, Haupt DL, Kinney JH. Reversal of experimental osteopenia with combined magnetic field treatment. 2002. Submitted for publication.

39. Brighton CT, Friedenberg ZB, Mitchell EI, Booth RE. Treatment of nonunion with constant direct current. Clin Orthop 1977; 124:106–123.

40. Patterson D. Treatment of nonunion with a constant direct current: a totally implantable system. Orthop Clin North Am 1984; 15:47–59.

41. Brighton CT, Pollack SR. Treatment of recalcitrant nonunion with a capacitively coupled electric field. J Bone Joint Surg 1985; 67A:577–585.

42. Bassett CAL, Pawluk RJ, Pilla AA. Augmentation of bone repair by inductively coupled electromagnetic fields. Science 1974; 184:575–577.

43. Bassett CAL, Mitchell SN, Gaston SR. Treatment of ununited tibial diaphyseal fractures with pulsing electromagnetic fields. J Bone Joint Surg 1981; 63A:511–523.

44. Heckman JD, Ingram AJ, Lloyd RD, Luck JV, Mayer PW. Nonunion treatment with pulsed electromagnetic fields. Clin Orthop 1981; 161:58–66.

45. Bassett CAL. Fundamental and practical aspects of therapeutic uses of pulsed electromagnetic fields (PEMFS). CRC Crit Rev Biomed Eng 1989; 17:451–529.

46. Gossling HR, Bernstein RA, Abbott J. Treatment of ununited tibial fractures: a comparison of surgery and pulsed electromagnetic fields. Orthopedics 1992; 16:711–717.

47. Longo JA. The management of recalcitrant nonunions with combined magnetic field stimulation. Orthop Trans 1998; 22:408–409.

48. Borsalino G, Bagnacani M, Bettati E, Fornaciari F, Rocchi R, Uluhogian S, Ceccherelli G, Cadossi R, Traina GC. Electrical stimulation of human femoral intertrochanteric osteotomies: double-blind study. Clin Orthop 1988; 237:256–263.

49. Sharrard WJW. A double-blind trial of pulsed electromagnetic fields for delayed union of tibial fractures. J Bone Joint Surg 1990; 72B:347–355.

50. Mammi GI, Rocchi R, Cadossi R, Traina GC. Effect of PEMF on the healing of human tibial osteotomies: a double blind study. Clin Orthop 1993; 288:246–253.

51. Scott G, King JB. A prospective double blind trial of electrical capacitive coupling in the treatment of nonunion of long bones. J Bone Joint Surg 1994; 76A:820–826.

52. Brighton CT, Shaman P, Heppenstall RB, Esterhai JL Jr, Pollack SR, Friedenberg ZB. Tibial nonunion treated with direct current, capacitive coupling, or bone graft. Clin Orthop 1995; 321:223–234.

53. Kane WJ. Direct current electrical bone growth stimulation for spinal fusion. Spine 1988; 13:363–365.

54. Mooney V. A randomized double blind prospective study of the efficacy of pulsed electromagnetic fields for interbody lumbar fusions. Spine 1990; 15:708–715.

55. Goodwin CB, Brighton CT, Guyer RD, Johnson JR, Light KI, Yuan HA. A double blind study of capacitively coupled electrical stimulation as an adjunct to lumbar spinal fusions. Spine 1999; 24:1349–1357.

56. Linovitz RJ, Pathria M, Bernhardt M, Green D, Law MD, McGuire RA, Montesano PX, Rechtine G, Salib RM, Ryaby JT, Faden JS, Ponder R, Muenz LR, Magee FP, Garfin SA. Combined magnetic fields accelerate and increase spine fusion: a double-blind, randomized, placebo controlled study. Spine 2002; 27:1383–1389.

57. Hanft JR, Goggin JP, Landsman A, Surprenant M. The role of combined magnetic field bone growth stimulation as an adjunct in the treatment of neuroarthropathy/Charcot joint: an expanded pilot study. J Foot Ankle Surg 1998; 37:510–515.

28

Application of Electromagnetic Fields in Traumatology and Orthopaedics

Imants Detlavs

Medical-Scientific Center "ELMA-LA", Riga, Latvia

One of the leading scientists in the former Soviet Union in the application of magnetic fields in traumatology and orthopedics, Dr. Detlavs reviews the use of magnetic fields as therapeutic modality not only in Latvia and the former Soviet Union, but worldwide. The analysis of basic science and clinical data of magnetic field effects in soft tissues is followed by an extensive review of the use of static, time-varying, and modulated magnetic fields as well as millimeter waves in traumatology and orthopedics. This part of the paper represents the author's specific area of interests, and explains the use of magnetoelastic materials as an easy-to-apply source of magnetic fields for the treatment of superficial problems.

I. INTRODUCTION

Traumatology and orthopaedics is a branch of medical science which applies methods of magnetotherapy widely on its patients. During the last 30–40 years the experience and results of active research and proactive application have been vast—there is ample literature on theoretical and applied issues of magnetotherapy. Due to limited space of the chapter, it will not be possible to deal with all aspects of magnetotherapy. Considering the fact that Eastern European countries have widely applied magnetotherapy and have developed much literature which is mainly published in Russian, and thus many Western magnethologists have not had a possibility to acquaint themselves with it, the editors of the given publication asked me to devote most of the space to literature published in Russian. It is clear that only a small part of the published literature could be discussed in this chapter. The author hopes for the readers' understanding concerning the incomplete and missing analysis of some publications.

When the researcher reads this chapter he will notice that authors from the former Soviet Union do not mention double-blind trials in their research. It should be stated that this type of research was actually impossible. The comparative control groups and experiments and wide application of magnetotherapy allowed them to develop different methods of magnetotherapy.

II. MAGNETIC FIELDS AND SOFT TISSUE

Presently, it is widely accepted that electric and electromagnetic fields may effectively stimulate the wound healing process. It was shown that electromagnetic fields (EMF) in the nonionizing frequency range enhance the production of collagen during wound repair and that pulsing extremely low frequency (PELF) and extremely high frequency (EHF) EMF accelerate healing of soft-tissue incisions and long-bone fractures (1–4). From the point of view of a clinician, it is important to select the best kinds of static magnetic field (SMF) and EMFs in order to use them in the treatment of wounds and bone fractures. Coordination of the cellular invasion and extracellular matrix deposition phases is of great importance in the normal healing response. Wound healing, in particular the development of granulation fibrous tissue (GFT), is very difficult to measure quantitatively.

The experimental model we developed of a dermal wound with epithelization prevented artificially (5) proved suitable for study of the biochemical peculiarities of GFT and its regulation. Biochemical parameters of granulation-fibrous tissue developing for 7 days in incised full thickness circular dermal wounds in rats were studied. The wounded regions of experimental animals were exposed to different EMF (6) or SMF (7,8) for 5 consecutive days after the operation. The extremely high frequency EMF of 53.53 and 42.19 GHz (wave lengths 5.6 and 7.1 mm respectively, without frequency modulation) inflicted a significant lowering of components of glycoproteins macromolecules—hexosamines, hexoses, and, especially, sialic acids. Taking into account that in early phase of wound healing glyco-proteins are mainly constituents of inflammatory exudate, these results may be interpreted as a manifestation of exudative inflammatory reaction inhibition of uncomplicated wound healing. As a consequence the collagen accumulation, evaluted by hydroxyproline concen-tration, was restarted, but the properties of collagenous structures were not deteriorated as judged from unchanged hydroxylysine/hydroxyproline coefficient. On the contrary, the EHF EMF of 42.19 GHz frequency with frequency modulation band within 200 MHz induced an increase of glycoprotein concentrations, indicating an activation of the inflam-matory reaction. This activation is accompanied by pronounced (by 29% in comparison with control animals) elevation of collagen concentration, showing stimulation of wound scar maturation. The relation hydroxylysine/hydroxyproline was also elevated.

We suppose that different influence of millimeter (mm) waves is due to the presence of frequency modulations in the EMF used, since other EMFs tested in our experiment, though different in other physical parameters but having in common the absence of frequency modulations, exerted an opposite effect, namely an anti-inflammatory one, particularly diminishing the exudative component of inflammation. Both directions of mm waves EMF influence on the wound healing process and the development of the GFT could be successfully used in clinical practice, the choice being dependent on peculiarities of the healing process.

Our experimental data show clearly that biochemical changes of the wound granula-tion-fibrous tissue are directed differently in depending on peculiarities of EMF. It was noted that one of the important factors in this aspect is the presence or absence of frequency modulation. The fact that EHF EMF can influence the proliferative—reparative connective tissue reaction in opposite directions, either inhibiting or stimulating its inflammatory stage and GFT development—is of great practical significance, since it opens a possibility to choose a kind of EMF for wound and ulcera treatment in dependence with a clinical healing course.

SMF induced a highly significant augmentation of colagen gene expression. A strong SMF increases the accumulation of total and acid-soluble collagen in the GFT developing in rats in open wound defects (7). However, the structural stability of collagen accumulated in the early stage of wound healing did not fully reach the control level (8). The degree of maturity of glucosaminoglycans was lowered under influence of the SMF. In our opinion these peculiarities of the extracellular matrix of the GFT developing in experimental conditions are dependent on the fact that the SMF used only partly stimulated expression of inflammatory glycoproteins; this is in contrast to the effect of some EHF EMF that intensify the inflammatory exudation (9), the latter being a necessary enhancing factor of collagen maturity in GFT.

Scientists from the United States (10) stress the SMF positive reduction of pain, oedema, and inflammation in soft-tissue treating. The increased blood flow to the site of surgery which is pooling oxygen and nutrients, thereby accelerating the overall healing process, is very important.

Our studies confirm the perspectiveness of using these physical factors in treatment of wounds and trophic ulcers, taking into account that SMF and EMF with different parameters may induce different reaction of the GFT (8,9,11). Regarding the mechanisms of the observed effect, we could admit the possibility of direct action of EHF EMF, ELF EMF, and SMF upon the cells participating in the production of the GFT matrix and healing process, since our study characterized its early stage when the blood vessels and nerves have not yet developed in the GFT. SMF was applied for the treatment of kelloid scar, hypertrophic scars, and contractur (12,13). The duration of treatment was from 3 to 6 weeks, in the result that relapse of kelloid scar was prevented. Histological research testifies to the influence of SMF on the displacement of collagen fibrous—they were displaced in parallel with SMF lines of strength (14). The determination of cohesion (strength) of post-operation scar showed that under the influence of a magnetic field with intensity of 264 kA/m, which is necessary for a break (tensile test), it increases in comparison with the control.

We have investigated the influence of PEMF on the muscle mitochondria (15). We applied PEMF generated by our elaborated device Pulsar, which contained an exponentially shaped pulse with a duration of 0.8–1 ms, a repetition frequency of 50 Hz, and a field magnetic flux density between 0.25 and 1.0 mT. This experiment was conducted on 30 adult white rats (both intact specimens and those with surgically created defect in the femur), whose back extremities had been exposed to PEMF 4 h/day, 5 times per week, for a total of 20 sessions. Ten animals served as a control group. The enzymes in the mitochondria of muscles biceps femoris, succinic dehydrogenase (SDH), and nicotinamide-adenine dinucleotide (NAD) were investigated upon the completion of this experiment. The levels of these oxidative enzymes were reduced in animals that had undergone the femur operations. In the PEMF exposed animals, the levels of SDH and NAD were elevated as compared to both animals from the control group and animals that had been operated on but received no PEMF exposure. The results suggest that the type of the field employed by the authors over the course of this research has an effect on the dynamics of the tricarboxylic acid cycle, i.e., on the foremost bioenergy processes. These results indicate the promising nature of PEMF use for improving the efficiency of intact muscles or enhancing the compensatory mechanism to a damaged locomotor system.

Our observations of positive influence of PEMF on the injured muscles coincide with the results of other authors (16) who investigated the oxygen pressure (pO_2) in the muscles and observed that pO_2 is remarkably diminished—7.48 mm Hg in injured extremities but 29.6 mm Hg in the intact extremities. In the testing group, treated by alternating EMF (AEMF) 14 days after operation pO_2 22,97 mm Hg was higher than in the control groups. A similar ratio was also observed after 21 days, but after 30 days this difference had disappeared. These investigations prove that AEMF influence oxygenization becomes normal much more rapidly than in the control group. It shows that peripheric blood circulation as well as the tissue trofic improves.

III. MAGNETOTHERAPY IN TRAUMATOLOGY

A. Application of Electromagnetic Fields

For the improvement of reparative regeneration, SMF, low-frequency AEMF, and PEMF are used. In Western countries the attention mainly has been on PEMF, less to static fields, but in Eastern block countries the opposite is true. Bassett together with a group of scientists demonstrated the influence of low-frequency PEMF on bone regeneration (17). Soon it was proved with patients suffering from pseudoarthrosis (18–21) and nonunion (18, 22, 23). A group of patients with 147 ununited bone fractures were treated with external skeletal fixation combined with PEMFs. Consolidation of ununited fractures in the femur observed 81% and in the tibia 75%. Patients with humerus fractures were less successful, with only 5 of 13 humeri united (24).

Since 1965 Russian scientists (25) along with Western scientists attempted to find possibilities of effective action on the reparative regeneration. The electrophysiological parameters of bone tissue both in norm and pathology were studied. The effect of SMF, PEMF, and low-frequency AEMF on the consolidation of bone was studied. Since 1972 electromagnetic stimulation was used with success by the authors in 92 patients in operative treatment of fractures (58 patients) and pseudoarthroses (34 patients). The electromagnetic stimulation was used in buried metal osteosynthesis in 55 patients and extrafocal transosseous osteosynthesis in 28 patients. Union of bone fragments within short terms was observed in all patients with a follow-up from 3 months up to 2 years.

Further positive influences of PEMF and AEMF were observed while treating the patients with fresh bone fractures as well as with congenital pseudoarthrosis and those of nonunion fractures (26–29).

The influence of MF on the human body has not been sufficiently investigated yet. Some authors have mentioned the dependence of the results of EMF on frequencies of the applied field (30). Garland et al. (31) reported that patients with nonunions who used PEMF therapy less than an average of 3 h a day had a success rate of 35.7%, while those who used the field treatment in excess of 3 h daily had an 80% success rate. The success rate of PEMF treatment for nonunion repair demonstrated no statically significant change over a long-term follow-up. The improvement of blood circulation and microcirculation after the application of EMF plays an important role (16,31–34). Some experiments with animals showed that application of PEMF is useful in the early stages of fresh fracture treatment to significantly reduce the healing time (35). PEMF enhances the early vascular reaction, stimulated chondrogenesis, and bone formation. Prolonged PEMF treatment may be deleterious, enhancing chondrogenesis beyond a point observed in normal repair and thus disturbing normal subsurface trabeculation.

Some authors have published positive results influenced by low-energy AEMF combined in parallel with SMF (36). In experiments full-thickness plugs of articular cartilage harvested from young adult bovine knee joints were used. The results of this work indicate that combined magnetic fields have the ability to stimulate the metabolism of resting or steady-state articular cartilage. M. A. Meskens et al. (37) observed positive results by PEMF in 67.7% of fracture nonunions. Their observation showed that the disability time had no effect on the success rate.

Magnetotherapy is useful in bone lengthening in an external fixation system. Fifty patients with pseudoarthrosis of the tibia underwent a complex treatment with external skeletal fixation (Ilizarov's apparatuses) and PEMF (apparatus Pulsar, Latvia) (38). One week after the operation, the injured region was stimulated with PEMF. The stimulation lasted for 3 weeks. After a year of treatment 46 patients suffering from pseudoarthrosis were healed (92%).

Twenty-eight patients with bone lengthening in external skeletal fixation (apparatus Kalnberza) were treated by PEMF (10 patients), AEMF (14 patients), and SMF (4 patients) (34). Patients reported that after the magnetotherapy course the postoperation pain diminished, as well as the pain in distraction time, using the compression-distraction apparatus. Diminishing of oedema caused by operation after the application of MF was also observed. No patient developed inflammation on the operated segment. For two patients the operation was made in order to prolong the extremities from (10 to 15 cm) in compression-destruction apparatus. Before electromagnetotherapy the regeneration of bones was not observed for a long time. After the application of PEMF the process of regeneration began and consolidation was observed.

Eyres et al. (39) reported on double-blind studies of 13 patients who had limb lengthening in external fixation system combined with PEMF therapy. The authors did not observe any difference in the rate or amount of new bone formation between the control and treated groups. The authors observed that PEMF significantly reduced the bone loss in the segments of bone distal to the lengthening sites. The authors agree on the possibility to prevent or reverse disuse osteoporosis.

B. Application of Static Magnetic Field

Many authors have reported positive effects of SMF with induction from 10 to 20 mT for treating patients with bone fractures (33,40–42). The scientists of our institute began to work on this problem during the 1970s (43). It was observed in experiments that during the first weeks after trauma the concentration of DNA and RNA in bone tissue increased under the influence of SMF, but on the third week the concentration of calcium and phosphorus increased too. This means that the process mineralization takes place more rapidly. In our hospital we observed 478 patients with bone fractures and concluded that when applying SMF on the patients with fresh injuries the pain syndrome, oedema, and inflammation diminish (34).

Habirova (44) studied the effect of SMF on the tissues of joint in the intraarticular injuries and the effect on the reparative osteogenesis in experiments on 164 rats. SMF was found to remove the posttraumatic oedema and the aseptic inflammatory process. A stimulating effect was exerted on the state of nervous apparatuses of the articular capsule and on the reparative osteogenesis. SMF was applied with a positive clinical effect on treatment of 106 patients with the intraarticular injuries.

Gurbo and Nikitenko (45) reported treatment of 114 patients suffering from closed injured knee joint using AEMF therapy of Poljus-1 together with a medicine complex. The field induction was from 10 to 25 mT, with exposure from 10 to 20 min. The treating course consisted of 5 to 15 exposures. In 72 patients the symptoms of traumatic arthritis disappeared completely (72.8%). Degen treated 25 patients suffering from traumatic oedema (1 month to 3 years after trauma) with SMF. After completion of the course, the oedema disappeared in 18 and markedly decreased in six patients. In one case the effect was insignificant (46).

In order to study the influence of magnetoelasts, which generate SMF, on the revascularization of bone fragments a number of authors made experiments on animals.

Bone tissue (having a high metabolic level) needs a sufficient arterial blood circulation for reparative osteogenesis, especially in the period of cell differentiation. The experiment (32) was made on 20 rabbits. Under local anesthesia a segmented resection of radius was made from 7 to 10 mm and a plaster was dressed. In the experimental group (10 animals) the plates of magnetoelasts with SMF induction 10–15 mT were placed on the resection region. On the third day in the control group cortical layer of bone fragments was practically avascular, but in the experimental group separate blood vessels appeared in the bone fragments and there was a more intensive vascularization in periosteum. On the seventh day in the experimental group vascularization of fragments in the form of thick blood vessel net was observed. The formation of a blood vessel system in the depth of regenerate was marked, and it greatly differed from weak revascularization in the control group. On the twenty-first day in the experimental group thick blood vessel system of the bone tissue and regeneration tissue was observed, and an avascular zone was not stated. In the control group, as before, there was less expressed blood vessel concentration in the bone fragments and the center of regenerate avascular region was tested. Results of the experiment show that a local application of magnetoelasts with induction 10–15 mT promotes a faster and more active revascularization of bone fragments as well as of the forming regenerate.

Fjodorova (47) applied elastic magnets on 900 patients with induction 30–35 mT, exposition time 40–45 min for 20 days, to carry out as complex treatment of gunshot fractures and prophylaxis of wound infection. The treatment significantly diminished pain syndrome, decreased local oedema of tissues, improved the wound healing and regeneration of bone, prevented posttraumatic vascular insufficiency, and helped to normalize coagulation of blood system in a short time.

Nikolsky et al. (48) used elastic magnets with induction of 35–50 mT in treatment of 70 patients after operations on the spine. The course of therapy consisted of 10 to 20 procedures of 30–40 min daily, and a conclusion is made that SMF has a positive influence on the course of the postoperative period, producing an anti-inflammatory, analgesic, spasmolytic effect, the posttraumatic oedema decreases, and the blood coagulant function normalizes.

A similar study (40) of SMF influence on the fresh bone fracture was made in an experiment with two groups of rats: 30 control group rats, and 30 experimental group rats. After the end of the treatment course (42 days) it was observed that bone regenerate is more mature in the experimental group than in the control one.

Strokov (49) treated 71 patients who suffered from long tubular bone fractures applying magnetoelasts with induction of 20 mT, twice a day, exposition time 1 h, for 15–20 days. The control group consisted of 30 patients with analogous fractures but without magneto-therapy treatment. After the magnetotherapy application to patients, the pain syndrome and oedema diminished, the regional blood circulation as well as the natural resistance of organism normalized (lisocim from 5.7 mkg/ml, to 4.53 mkg/ml) in the control group (beta lizin from 50% to 40.5% $P < 0.05$). The last results were a good prognosis in treatment.

Lately interest has increased in Western countries to SMF generated by flexible magnetic fields, referred to as *plastilloy* and *hard materials* which include ceramic or exotic metal magnets (50). In the United States there are two research centers that study the biological responses to relatively weak (less than 1000 G) magnetic fields (51). In the former Soviet Union in 1970–1980 such flexible elastic magnets were manufactured and widely applied. There are many reports in Eastern European countries that, like the above-mentioned experiments, confirm the efficiency of magnetoelasts in treatment of patients with support-motor apparatus diseases. Markov (50) reminds that there are two types of

SMF "unipolar" and "bipolar" magnets that are thin, with repeatable north–south polarity on the same side of the material. The other type are unipolar magnets. The depth of penetration of unipolar magnets is 3–4 times larger than for bipolar magnets, and the influence of unipolar magnets is more pronounced than that of bipolar one on the given target. The magnetoelasts in the Soviet Union usually were bipolar. Our above-mentioned studies from Eastern countries, as the further experience in a more than 30-year period, confirm the bipolar efficiency in treating patients with soft tissue and bone-joint pathology. They prove our opinion that unipolar magnets, slaced in opposite sides of the pathological process, will be more effective.

We (34) observed 13 patients with traumatic osteomyelitis, four of them with closed form of osteomyelitis. Nine patients were suffering from wound inflammation. Magnetotherapy applied to the patients caused an increase of inflammation during the first days, but further on a remarkable diminishing of inflammation was observed. However, such an improvement was observed in patients with fistulas. For two patients the application of MF caused pain because of the absence of fistulas, and that is why the application of magnetotherapy was interrupted. On 16 patients suffering from tissue inflammation, magnetotherapy was applied around needles. After the application of SMF or AEMF, the inflammation disappeared.

IV. MAGNETOTHERAPY IN ORTHOPAEDICS

A. Magnetic Fields and Rheumatic Diseases

Electromagnetic therapy was applied (52) on 260 patients suffering from rheumatic diseases: rheumatoidarthritis, 260, spondilarthritis, 35; system sklerodermia, 25; and rheumatic poliarthritis, 14 patients. The AEMF was applied every day from 10 to 15 min with induction 18–25 mT when treating the pathological regions of patients. Under the influence of magnetotherapy the majority of observed patients showed improvement of clinical symptoms together with positive hormonal and neurohormonal changes: the increase of neurohormonal level, and a partial increase of cateholamins and steroids in blood and daily urine, which was lowered before treatment.

Fifty-five patients suffering from rheumatic arthritis underwent treatment by AEMF (53). Not only was clinical improvement observed, but blood circulation was also improved. Investigation of blood microcirculation proved that the greater part of patients suffering from rheumatic arthritis at the beginning of the course had some disturbance of blood circulation-spastic or atonic vessel changes, aneurisma of venulas, and perivascular oedema. Aggregation of eritrocites was observed in medium or small artheria and in venulas. With some patients the same phenomenon was observed in blood macrocirculation. At the end of the treatment course positive dynamic was observed in spastic-atonic changes of blood vessel as well as perivascular oedema, and aggregation of eritrocites diminished or disappeared completely.

SMF application was used in treatment patients with carpal tunnel syndrome. One hundred-nineteen hands of 71 patients were treated for decreasing pain, oedema, and increasing microcirculation (54). The results recommend this method in initial stages of this syndrome with pain and paresthesia but do not recommend it for patients with movement disturbances as no positive effect was obtained on patients.

Italian scientists (55) applied sinusoidaly modulated magnetic field (induction 1–5 G, 100 Hz) for treating idiopathic carpal tunnel syndrome. They observed, like the above-mentioned authors, positive results and concluded that this therapy is effective only in the early phases, when the degenerative process of the axon have not yet started.

We (34) have treated 10 patients with SMF suffering from carpal tunnel syndrome, which was the result of dislocation of bone fragments after fracture of distal metaepiphysis of forearm bones (five patients 2 to 3 months, the other five patients 0.5 to 2 years after trauma). SMF with induction 20–30 mT was used. In five patients pain and numbness diminished, but in the case of the other five patients pain and numbness disappeared completely. Improvement of patients was proven by the investigation of vibration sensitivity.

B. Magnetotherapy of Degenerative Dystrophic Process of Spine

Many authors have demonstrated the therapeutic effect of SMF, PEMF, and AEMF on degenerative-dystrophic process of the spine (56–59).

This present report shows our 30 years of experience in treating more than 5000 patients aged 20 to 80 with degenerative-dystrophic process of the spine (56). We have used SMF with an induction of 10–40 mT with 0.12 mT/cm gradient on the spine, AEMF of 15 mT, and PEMF of 5–10 mT. The course lasted for 3–4 weeks. In some magnetosensitive people the therapeutic effect was achieved in 7–10 days, which enabled us to reduce the course of treatment. Some patients showed improvement after the first or second exposition of EMF. Half of the patients complained of aggravation of pain (for 2–3 days) at the end of the first week with a subsequent gradual improvement afterward. There were a few patients who did not experience any noticeable improvement during the course of magnetotherapy, but owing to the aftereffect improvement ensued in 3–6 months after the completion of magnetotherapy.

Estimating the effectiveness of treatment, the dynamics of subjective and objective symptoms were taken into consideration, together with the data of a number of clinical-laboratory studies. Marked positive dynamics were noted in the majority (80%) of patients with spondylosis and osteochondrosis. The best therapeutic effect of treatment with the magnetic field was observed patients with reflex-pain syndrome and with syndrome of vertebral artery. Our observations show that not only does the degree of degenerative-dystrophic process of the spine determine the effectiveness of magnetotherapy but also the individual reaction of the organism. According to our data it is possible to eliminate reflex-pain syndrome and improve the blood circulation not only in acute but also in severe chronic pathological changes of the spine. The results of treatment do not depend on the intensity of the pain syndrome: we have observed patients with a pronounced pain syndrome who felt evident improvement after a few expositions, and vice versa, some patients with a subacute pain syndrome felt only a slight improvement. The analysis of our results shows that the best results are patients with acute and less improvement patients with long duration of diseases.

Nikitenko et al. (59) treated 158 patients with low back pain. All patients had suffered from the disease 3 years or even longer. SMF therapy with induction 15–25 mT, exposition 15–20 min was applied to all of them for 20 days. Seventy-four patients recovered completely after the treatment and returned to their job. Twenty-two patients after the treatment did not have significant improvement, but after 2–3 months their pain syndrome diminished and the movements were rehabilited. They could return to their job.

C. Joint Pathology and Magnetic Fields

There are many reports about the application of magnetic fields in patients with joint osteoarthrosis. Authors observed improvement of health after applying SMF (60–62), AEMF

(57), and PEMF (57,63–65). The application of magnetotherapy results in decrease of pain increase of movement amplitude, lessening of oedema, and improvement of blood micro- and macrocirculation, metabolism, and the immunobiological conditions. Some patients after three to five exposures reported that pain in tissues decreased. Together with decrease of the pain syndrome, the movement amplitude in joints increased. During the first week of treatment, some patients complained that pain become more acute. However, after this, all patients had improvement. The treatment course lasted for 3–4 weeks. At the end of the course 20–30% of patients reported a considerable 75–80% improvement.

It has been observed that after application of SMF the antibodies against cartilage and collagen decrease (64). One of the most important parts of the joint that is disturbed in the case of osteoarthritis is cartilage. Cartilage has the inability to repair itself after injury. In some patients this leads to degeneration and secondary oateoarthritis. Several reports have suggested that articular cartilage may have the ability to generate a repair response if subjected to appropriate stimuli. It is shown (66) that PEMF may be useful in treating cartilage diseases in humans. PEMF can stimulate proteoglycan synthesis and increased GAG concentration in human osteoarthritic cartilage. Matrix restoration was observed in cartilage with a milder degree of involvement. In seriously damaged cartilage that is very fibrillated, response is less expressed. It is one of the reasons why the improvement after EMF therapy is not sufficient in patients with serious osteoarthritis.

Hip joint arthrosoarthritis or femoral head osteonecrosis is one of the more serious joint pathologies. Magnetic resonance investigation and histology studies have helped to understand the pathogenesis of the femoral head osteonecrosis and to choose the right treatment method. Bone necrosis is the end result of severe and prolonged ischaemia. A number of authors had applied PMF for treating these pathologies: pain decreased and movement amplitude increased (61,64,67).

Bassett et al. (68) treated 95 patients with femoral head osteonecrosis with PEMFs from 1979 to 1985. In stage 0-II (Steinberg classification) of osteonecrosis none showed progression of lesions and grading improvement was observed in 9 of 15. Stage IV and V lesions after treatment progressed and none improved. Hinsenkamp et al. (69) reported results of PEMF therapy (by Bassett) of 23 patients having 35 osteonecroses of femoral heads. Clinical evaluation after a mean period treatment of 36 months showed improvement in all Ficat II and 46% Ficat III; 2 patients with Ficat IV improved after 32 months.

Aaron et al. (70) reported that about 52% of the PEMF treated patients (Ficat II and III) exhibited clinical improvement and rentgenographic stabilization. Authors concluded that PEMF reduced the incidence of clinical and rentgenographic progression of osteonecrosis of the femoral head and prevented its collapse. Many patients have had as long as 5 years of improved functions.

Golubenko (71) investigated intraosseous pressure in 26 patients with idiopathic aseptic necrosis of the femoral head. Intraosseous pressure in these patients was increased (up to 3–4 kPa) in comparison with healthy subjects (0.3–1.2 kPa). The patients were treated with AMF of 35 mT (Poljus-1) or PEMF with an induction 6 and 20 mT and 100 kHz frequency (Alimp-1). After a whole course of magnetotherapy (15 min for 15 days) the most reduction of intraosseous pressure was obtained by a PEMF field with an induction of 6 mT in 50% cases, with an induction of 20 mT in 40% cases, and after alternating magnetic field of 35mT in 17% cases. Magnetotherapy is also useful for treatment of patients with hip protheses in the postoperative period for decreasing the pain and oedema as well as in later periods for patients with loosening (72,73).

D. Application of Extremely High Frequency Electromagnetic Field

Several authors have also applied millimetric wave therapy in traumatology and orthopaedics. It has been reported that EHF EMF affects regeneration of soft tissues and bones
(74,75).

Millimeter-wave EMF was used over 10 years in treatment of more than 1000 patients
with diseases and traumata of the bone–muscle system (74). Authors indicate the positive
influence of EMF as a stabilizer of pathological process and the further elimination of
damages. The authors stress that this therapy does not give results in the tissue with
structural injuries. The reverse process of pathological changes is very important for
achieving positive results.

Devjatkov (76) reported that the improvement of healing laser wounds under the
influence of mm waves improves the inflammation stage and stimulates growth and
maturation of granulation tissue. The scar of the wound after the application of mm waves
develops without kelloid signs. In two patients who suffered from chronic osteomyelitis in
lower extremities and acute pain syndrome, opened fistulas were treated with mm waves
(wave length 7.1 mm) complex with surgical methods. After magnetic therapy with mm
waves, signs of osteomyelitis were not observed during 5 years of observation (77).

There are reports (78) about the application of EMF mm-wave radiation having an
effect on biologically active points with frequency 55–65 GHz and intensity 0.1–1 W/cm. The
exposition lasted from 15–60 min/day for 10–12 days and depending on clinical indications
repeated from two to five exposures daily. One hundred and six patients were treated: spinal
osteohondrosis, 115, infantile cerebral paralysis, 12, Pertesa disease, 26 patients.

Millimeter-wave therapy was applied to 38 children, among them 12 children with
infantile cerebral paralysis, and 12 children with Pertesa disease. An improvement of health
was observed in all treated children. Spasticity diminished in infantile cerebral paralysis
patients. Radiographical and clinical stabilization and improvement patients with Pertesa
disease was observed.

It is reported from the Ukraine (79) about the application of EHF EMF for treating
patients suffering from hemophilic arthopathy. The apparatus Electronika-KVCH-101 was
applied with the frequency band 61 ± 4 GHz with output power 10 mW/cm^2. The advantage
of this treatment over the classical methods is the following:

1. Pain diminishing in points already after the first treating expositions.
2. Possibility to diminish the intraarticular dose of hormonal medicine.
3. The diminishing of hemartrouse recidive.
4. Antihemophylic factor increased in blood from two to three times after the
   treatment (reaching the stability zone of spontaneous bleeding).

E. Modulated EMF in Traumatology and Orthopaedics

We applied complicated modulated EMF generated by the therapeutic device VIOFOR
(Poland). Every atom, molecule, and human cell that exist have a vibration, generating
personal electromagnetic waves. Most of them have a frequency range from 0.3 to 1000 Hz.
Frequencies of diseased tissues and organs are destroyed. In treating the patient with EMF it
is necessary to ensure influence with a full package of personal frequencies that support the
body to perform its own functions. For this purpose the apparatus generates waves with
wide-scale frequencies. VIOFOR uses sawtooth-shaped waves. This shape of waves seems to
create an optimum level on ion transport. These waves are arranged in various groups; the
groups formed series with various intervals between them. The directions of waves (polarity)

periodically change. The electromagnetic stimulation was exposed on the whole body (big applicator) or localized on a part of body (small, pillowlike applicator). The amplitudes of pulsating field of the big applicatior were 0.15–8.1 μT, and the pillowlike applicator 0.63–24 μT. The exposure lasted for 12 min one to two times per day. The course lasted for 10–20 days.

Our data showed that the majority of patients had both a subjective and objective improvement after VIOFOR exposure (80). After exposure we observed the increase of skin temperature from 0.2 to 3.0°C on the finger. The increase of temperature was more significant in patients with lower temperature before exposure, thus demonstrating different transfer of blood enlargement after exposure of the VIOFOR. We should like to pay attention to the influence of the magnetostimulation on the changed muscular tonus and contractures.

We have observed a decrease of muscle tone and improvement of joint and limb movement amplitudes 3–4 years after cerebral infarct (four patients), in a 4-year-old boy suffering from infantile cerebral paralysis, and seven patients with humeros-scapular periarthrosis. Two patients 3 months after trauma had very hard posttraumatic disturbances—Zudech syndrome after 1 week treatment showed remarkable improvement.

We have observed decrease of pain, oedema, muscular hypertonus, and improvement of movements in patients with diseases of support-motor apparatus (arthrosis, spondylosis, spondylarthrosis). Thus our preliminary observations showed that a complicated modulated EMF generated by apparatus VIOFOR has a positive influence in the treatment of patients with diseases of support-motor apparatus, and in some diseases they are more effective than earlier results.

V. CONCLUSION

Our experience and analysis of many other authors' reports allow us to conclude that the application of SMF or various EMF is useful in treatment and prophylaxis of many diseases and traumata of the support-motor apparatus. The grade of influence on how the patient's health improves depends on the field parameters and the biological state of the organism. In future in order to obtain the best, most optimal results of magnetotherapy, research by clinical doctors, physicists, biologists should be continued to find out the most effective signal configurations, dose regimens in different forms and stages of diseases, and individual reactions of the patients.

REFERENCES

1. Bassett CAL, Pawluk RJ, Pilla AA. Acceleration of fracture repair by electromagnetic fields: a surgically non-invasive method. Ann NY Acad Sci 1974; 238:242–261.
2. Delport F, Cheng N, Mulier JC. Clinical analysis of 90 patients with pulsed electromagnetics fields. In: Bone Healing with Electrical and Electromagnetical Stimulation. Dresden Symposium. Dresden, 1984: 73–74.
3. Mitbreit IM, Lavrishcheva GI, Manjahin VD, Mihailovska LH. Reparative regeneration of bones under the influence of alternating magnetic field. Orthop Traumatol, 1978:55–64. In Russian.
4. Shaposhnikov JG, Devjatkov ND, Kamenev JF. Clinical evaluation of application of millimetric radiation of low intensity to patients suffering from wound infection of extremities. Millimeter waves in Medicine and Biology. IRE AN SSSR, Moscow, 1989:16–20. In Russian.
5. Slutskii LI, Sevastjanova NA, Ozolanta IL, Kuzmina IV, Dombrovska LE. Reactogenicity of biomaterials as studied by biochemical, morphological and ultrastructural techniques. Cells Mater 1992; 2:119–134.

6. Detlavs I, Dombrovska I, Klavinsh I, Turauska A, Shkirmante B, Slutskii L. Experimental study of the effect of electromagnetic fields in the early stage of wound healing. Bioelectrochem Bioenergetics 1994; 35(1):13–17.

7. Liepa ME, Slutskii LJ, Dombrovska LZ. Peculiaritics of the influence of static magnetic field in the healing process of wound and bone fractures depending on intensity and application time. Application of magnetic fields in clinic. Theses of reports of Kuibishev regional conference, Kuibishev, June 1976:54–55. In Russian.

8. Detlavs I, Dombrovska L, Turauska A, Slutskii L. The influence of a static magnetic field (SMF) on biochemical parameters of granulation-fibrous tissue (GFT) in wound defects. Abstracts Book of Third International Congress of European Bioelectromagnetic Association in Nancy, France, February 29–March 3, 1996; 7:140.

9. Detlavs I, Dombrovska L, Turauska A, Shkirmante B, Slutskii L. Experimental study of the effects of radiofrequency electromagnetic fields on animals with soft tissue wounds. The Science of the Environment 1996; 180:35–42.

10. Man D, Plosker H, Markov M. Application of tectonic permanent magnets for treatment of surgical flaps. Proceedings of the Fourth EBEA Congress, Zagreb, November 19–21, 1998:30–31.

11. Detlavs I, Dombrovska L, Shkirmante B, Turauska A, Slutskii L. Effects of radiofrequency electromagnetic fields on granulation-fibrous tissue. Abstracts Book of COST 244 Workshop in Kuopio, Finland, September 3–4, 1995:17.

12. Degen IL. Possibilities and perspectives (prospects) of magnetic therapy. Materials of III All-Union Symposium:The influence of magnetic fields to the biological objects. Kaliningrad 1975:167–168. In Russian.

13. Bruvele MS, Junson RK, Liepa ME, Slutskii LI. The application of static magnetic fields for treatment of kelloid cicatrix. Materials of III Congress of Traumatologists and Orthopaedists of Estonia, Latvia, Lithuania. Tallin, 1978:135–136. In Russian.

14. Liepa ME, Dombrovska LE, Sluckii LI. The influence of SMF to the cohesion of skin scar and to the break (tensileted) and chemical contents of granulated fiber tissue. Materials of the III All-Union Symposium: The Influence of Magnetic Fields to the Biological Objects. Kaliningrad, 1975:180. In Russian.

15. Detlav IE, Aboltina MJ, Turauska AV, Erdmanis JV. The influence of constant and pulsing electromagnetic fields on muscle oxidation in experimental animals. In: Detlav IE ed. Electromagnetic Therapy in Traumas and Diseases of the Support-Motor Apparatus, Riga: RMI, 1987:12–16. In Russian.

16. Mitbreit IM, Dirin HA. Oxygenization of muscles of injured extremities of animals in the process of reparative regeneration of bones under the influence of low frequency magnetic field. Magnetic biology and magnetic therapy in the field of medicine. Report from the all-union scientific-practical conference in Vitebsk, September 1-3, 1980:218–219. In Russian.

17. Bassett CAL, Pawluk RJ, Pilla AA. Augmentation of bone repair by inductively-coupled electromagnetic fields. Science 1974; 184:575–577.

18. Bassett CAL, Pilla AA, Pawluk RJ. A non operative salvage of surgically-resistant pseudoarthrosis and non-unions by pulsing electromagnetic field. Clin Orthop 1977; 124:128–143.

19. Cadossi R, Fontanesi G, Rinaldi E. Non invasive treatment of pseudo-arthrosis with low frequency pulsing electromagnetic fields. A multicenter study. Evidence of periosteal bone callus formation. Bone Healing with Electrical and Electromagnetical Stimulation. Dresden Symposium, Dresden, 1984:72.

20. Giancecchi F, Poli G, Cadossi R. Use of low frequency pulsing electromagnetic fields for treatment of congenital and acquired pseudarthrosis. In: Detlav IE, ed. Electromagnetic Therapy in Traumas and Diseases of the Support-Motor Apparatus, Riga: RMI, 1987:124–134.

21. Nahoda J, Koudela K, Freyova J. Heilung von Pseudarthrosen der langen Röhrenknochen mit Hilfe eines pulsierenden elektromagnetischen Feldes. In: Detlav IE, ed. Electromagnetic Therapy in Traumas and Diseases of the Support-Motor Apparatus, Riga: RMI, 1987:135–145.

22. Bassett CAL, Mitchell SN, Schink MM. Treatment of therapeutically resistant non-unions with bone grafts and pulsing electromagnetics fields. J Bone Joint Surg 1982; 64-A(8):1214–1220.

23. Hinsenkamp M, Ryaby J, Burny F. Treatment of non-union by pulsing electromagnetic field: European multicenter study of 308 cases. Reconstr Surg Traumat 1985; 19:147–151.

24. Marger M, Musatti G, Bassett CAL. Results of Pulsed Electromagnetic Fields (PEMFs) in Ununited Fractures After External Skeletal Fixation. Clin Orthop Rel Res 1984; 190:260–265.

25. Tkachenko SS, Rutzky VV. Basis and experience in use of electromagnetic stimulation in operative treatment of fractures and pseudarthroses. Orthop Traumatol Prosthetics 1975; 1:6. In Russian.

26. Hinsenkamp M, Bourgois R, Bassett CAL. Electromagnetic stimulation of fracture repair. Influence on healing of fresh fractures. Acta Orthop Belg 1978; 44(5):672–698.

27. Wahlström O. Stimulation of fresh fracture healing with electromagnetic fields of extremely low frequency. In: Detlav IE, ed. Electromagnetic Therapy in Traumas and Diseases of the Support-Motor Apparatus, Riga: RMI, 1987:146–150.

28. Mitbreit IM, Manjahin VD. The influence of low frequency magnetic field to the reparative regeneration of bone. The application of magnetic fields in medicine, biology and agriculture, Saratov: Publ. Saratov's University, 1978:139–140. In Russian.

29. Saveljev VN, Muravjov MF. Electromagnetic stimulation in the consolidation process of ununion fractures and pseudoarthrosis of long tubular bones. Application of magnetic fields in clinic. Theses of reports of Kuibishev regional conference, Kuibishev, June 1976:151–152. In Russian.

30. Bassett CAL, Valdes MG, Hernandez E. Modification of fracture repair with selected pulsing electromagnetic fields. J Bone Joint Surg July, 1982; 64-A(6):888–895.

31. Garland DE, Moses B, Salyer W. Long-term follow-up of fractures nonunions treated with PEMFs. Contemp Orthop 1991; 22(3):295–302.

32. Stosh NV, Harlampovich SI, Artjomov GS, Levdikova SS. Revascularization of bone fragments and forming regenerate in reparative osteogenesis after SMF therapy. Application of magnetic fields in clinic. Theses of reports of Kuibishev regional conference, Kuibishev, June 1976:79–80.

33. Demetskaja NA, Nadgerijeva VM, Kameneva JF. Clinical aspects of the use of electromagnetic therapy in the treatment of patients with closed fractures of long tubular bones. In: Detlav IE ed. Electromagnetic Therapy in Traumas and Diseases of the Support-Motor Apparatus, Riga: RMI, 1987:102–109. In Russian.

34. Detlav IE, Blaus AP, Naudinja IJ, Turauska AV. Magnetic therapy in the treatment of long tubular bone fractures and lengthening of extremities. In: Detlav IE, ed. Electromagnetic Therapy in Traumas and Diseases of the Support-Motor Apparatus, Riga: RMI, 1987:110–123. In Russian.

35. Grande DA, Magee FP, Ryaby JT, Weinstein AM, Mcleod B. The effect of ion specific magnetic fields on articular cartilage metabolism. First Congress EBEA. Brussels, January 23–25, 1992.

36. Ryaby JT, Cai FF, DiDonato JA. Combined magnetic fields inhibit IL-1α and TNF-α dependent NF-κB activation in osteoblast-like cells. Trans Third Congress EBEA, Nancy, 1996.

37. Meskens WA, Stuyck JAR, Feys H, Mulier JC. Treatment of non-union using pulsed electromagnetic fields: A retrospective follow-up study. Acta Orthop Belg 1990; 2(56):483–488.

38. Anisimov AN, Karpcov VI, Jemeljanov VG. Application of electromagnetic fields of sound range frequences to optimize osteoregeneration. Actual problems associated with application of magnetic and electromagnetic fields in medicine. Theses from Reports of All-Union Conference, Leningrad, 1990: 49–50. In Russian.

39. Eyres KS, Saleh M, Kanis JA. Effect of pulsed electromagnetic fields on bone formation and bone loss during limb lengthening. Bone 1996; 18(6):505–509.

40. Artjomov GS, Fedosjutkin BF, Goljahovskij VJ, Stosh NV. The influence of local and continuous SMF to the reparative osteogenesis. Application of magnetic fields in clinic. Theses of reports of Kuibishev regional conference, Kuibishev, June, 1976:143–145. In Russian.

41. Kuchemenko AE, Shevchuk VJ. The application of magnetoelasts in traumatology and orthopaedics. Application of magnetic fields in clinical medicine and in the experiment. Theses of report of 2. Povolshkij Conference, Kuibishev, 1979:71–72. In Russian.

42. Nikolsky MA, Aleksejev AP. The influence of static magnetic fields on the consolidation of fractures in after operation period in the experiment and in clinics. Clinical application of magnetic fields. Theses of reports of all-union scientific-practical conference, Izhevsk, 1977: 61–62. In Russian.

43. Liepa ME, Slutskii LI, Dombrovska LE. Peculiaritics of the influence of static magnetic field in the healing process of wound and bone fractures depending on intensity and application time. Application of magnetic fields in clinic. Theses of reports of Kuibishev regional conference, Kuibishev, June, 1976:54–55.

44. Habirova GF. Use of magnetic field in the therapy of intraarticular injuries. Orthop Traumatol Prosthetics 1978; 12:53–57. In Russian.

45. Gurbo SA, Nikitenko IK. Magnetic therapy in complex treatment of knee joint traumatic arthritis. Actual problems associated with application of magnetic and electromagnetic fields in medicine. Theses from reports of all-union conference, Leningrad, 1990:57–58. In Russian.

46. Degen IL. Treatment of traumatic oedema with magnetic field. Orthop Traumatol Prosthetics 1970; 11:47–49.

47. Fjodorova RI, Zheleznjak VA, Nikolsky MA. Antiinflammation influence of SMF of elastic magnets on treating wounds, traumatic oedema in experiment and clinic. Magnetobiology and magnetotherapy in medicine. Theses of reports of all-union scientific-practical conference, Vitebsk 1980:50–51. In Russian.

48. Nikolsky MA, Demetzky AM. Static magnetic field of elastic magnetics in the complex therapy of patients in operative interventions on the spine. Orthop Traumatol Prosthetics 1980; 4:22–25. In Russian.

49. Strokov VI. The application of SMF for healing fractures of long tubular bones. Theses of report of region scientific-practical conference in traumatology and orthopaedics, Orenburg 1982:24–26. In Russian.

50. Markov MS. Clinical application of permanent magnets:dosimetry. Proceedings of the Fourth EBEA Congress, Zagreb, Croatia, November 19–21, 1998:99–100.

51. Markov MS. Clinical application of permanent magnets: USA experience. Proceedings of the Fourth EBEA Congress, Zagreb, Croatia, November 19–21, 1998:20–21.

52. Ibragimova AG, Nikonova LV, Baigildejeva FM, Ledovskih NM. Magnetotherapy in clinics of rheymatic diseases. Theses of reports of regional scientific-practical conference, Kuibishev, November 1984:24–29. In Russian.

53. Nikonova LV. Microcirculation of patients suffering from rheumatic arthritis undergoing a course of treatment of alternating low frequency magnetic field. Application of magnetic fields in medicine, biology, agriculture, Russia: Saratov University, 1978:148. In Russian.

54. Dumbere RT, Liepa ME. The use of constant magnetic field in the treatment of carpal tunnel syndrome. In: Detlav IE, ed. Electromagnetic Therapy in Traumas and Diseases of the Support-Motor Apparatus, Riga: RMI, 1987:179. In Russian.

55. Battisti E, Fortunato M, Ginanneschi F, Rigato M. Eficacy of the magnetotherapy in idipathic carpal tunnel syndrome. Proceedings of the Fourth EBEA Congress, Zagreb, Croatia, November 19–21, 1998:34–35.

56. Detlav IE, Ivashenko MV, Naudinja IJ, Turauska AV. Magnetotherapy in the treatment of osteochondrosis of the spine. Theses from reports of all-union congress of traumatology and orthopaedics, Moscow 1988; 1:165–166.

57. Imamaliev AS, Askerov LD, Gnetetskaja LN, Stepnova NV. The "Travelling" impulse magnetic field (TIMF) in the treatment of orthopaedic patients. Abstracts of Second International school. Electromagnetic Fields and Biomembranes, Pleven, October 2–8, 1989:102.

58. Savchenko AP, Mitbreit IM. Low-frequency magnetic field in the complex treatment of the patients with spine osteochondrosis. Application of Magnetic Fields in Clinical Medicine and Experiments, Kuibishev, 1979:99. In Russian.

59. Nikitenko IK, Zhilnikov VM. The treatment of spine osteochondrosis with a constant magnetic field. Application of Magnetic Fields in Medicine, Biology and Agriculture. Saratov, 1978:147–148. In Russian.
60. Strokov VN, Safronov AA, Vlasenko IV. The application of constant magnetic field in treating of arthritis and synovits of knee joint. Theses from reports of regional scientific-practical conference of traumatology. Orenburg, 1984:27–28. In Russian.
61. Detlav IE, Turauska AV, Grase AA. The application of constant magnetic field in treatment of patients with coxarthrosis. Theses of reports of regional scientific-practical conference, Kuibishev, November 1984:100–103. In Russian.
62. Arishenskaja AM, Osipov VV, Vershcher EL, Jagodzinska VV. The indications of applying SMF in treatment infectious non-specific poliarthritis. Application of magnetic fields in clinic. Theses of reports of Kuibishev regional conference, Kuibishev, June 1976:147–148. In Russian.
63. Aaron Rk, Ciombor DMcK. Therapeutic effects of electromagnetic fields in the stimulation of connective tissue repair. J Cell Biochem 1993; 52:42–46.
64. Harrison MH, Bassett CA. The results of a double-blind trial of pulsed electromagnetic frequency in the treatment of Perthes' disease. J Pediatr Orthop 1997; 17(2):264–265.
65. Trock DH, Bollet AJ, Dyer RH, Fielding LP, Miner WK, Markoll R. A double-blind trial of the clinical effects of pulsed electromagnetic fields in osteoarthritis. J Rheumatol 1993; 20:456–460.
66. Ciombor KJ, Ciombor DMcK. Stimulation of proteoglycan synthesis in human osteoarthritic cartilage by PEMF. Abstract Book of BEMS Sixteenth Annual Meeting, Copenhagen, Denmark, June 1994; 40:12–17.
67. Grigorjeva VL, Parfis PG, Gerasimova VN. Application of alternative magnetic field in treating patients with osteochondrosis deformies. Theses of report of all-union scientific-practical conference, Vitebsk, 1980:204.
68. Bassett CAL, Schink-Ascani M, Lewis SM. Effects of Pulsed Electromagnetic Fields on Steinberg Ratings of Femoral Head Osteonecrosis. Clin Orthop Rel Res 1989; 246:172–183.
69. Hinsenkamp M, Hauzeur JP, Sintzoff S. Preliminary results electromagnetic field treatment of osteonecrosis. Bioelectrochem Bioenergetics 1993; 30:229–235.
70. Aaron RK, Lennox D, Bunce GE, Ebert T. The Conservative Treatment of Osteonecrosis of the Femoral Head. Clin Orthop Rel Res 1989; 249:209–218.
71. Golubenko GN. The influence of low frequency magnetic field on the intra-osseous microcirculation in patients with idiopathic aseptic necrosis of the femoral head in adults (preliminary announcement). In: Detlav IE, ed. Electromagnetic Therapy in Traumas and Diseases of the Support-Motor Apparatus, Riga: RMI, 1987:162–163. In Russian.
72. Kennedy WF, Roberts CG, Zuege RC, Dicus WT. Use of pulsed electromagnetic fields in the treatment of loosened hip prostheses. In: Brighton CT, Pollack SR, eds. Electromagnetics in medicine and biology, San Francisco: San Francisco Press, 1991:313–322.
73. Konrad K, Sevcic K, Foldes K, Piroska E, Molnar E. Therapy with pulsed electromagnetic fields in aseptic loosening of total hip protheses: a prospective study. Clin Rheumatol 1996; 15(4):325–328.
74. Kamenev YF, Shitikov VA, Baptenov ND, Kozhakmatova GS. Clinical methods of mm wave application and the principles of increasing their therapeutic potency in traumatology and orthopaedics. Digest paepers 11 Russian symposium millimeter waves in medicine and biology, Moscow, April 21–24, 1997:31–32. In Russian.
75. Kamenev JF, Sarkisjan AG, Urazgiljdejevs ZI. The application of millimetric waves for treating complicated infections of injured extremities. Millimeter waves in Medicine and Biology, Moscow: IRE AN SSSR, 1989:21–23. In Russian.
76. Devjatkov ND. The possibility of application EMF mm range for treatment laser wounds. Millimeter waves in Medicine and Biology, Moscow: IRE AN SSSR, 1989:5–9. In Russian.
77. Polyak EV, Shitikov VA, Lyalin LL. Experience of application of EHF-Therapy in the complex treatment of the sick at chronic osteomyelitis. Millimeter waves in Medicine and Biology, Moscow. 1994; 4:46–48. In Russian.

78. Shevchenko SD, Makolinets VI, Kiselyov VK, Gruntovsky 6ch, Grashchenkova TN. Experience in treatment of some orthopaedic diseases with low intensity electromagnetic radiation of mm-band. Digest of Papers 11 Rusian symposium millimeter Waves in Medicine and Biology, Moscow, April 21–24, 1997:32–35.

79. Aleshchenko VV, Pisanko OI. EHF-Therapy of hemophilic arthropathy and hemoarthritis of knee joints. Millimeter waves in Medicine and Biology. Digest of Papers 10 Russian Symposium, Moscow, April 24–26 1995:61–63. In Russian.

80. Detlavs I, Turauska A. The application of modulated electromagnetic field therapy. Proceedings of the Latvian Academy of Sciences. In press.

29

Neurorehabilitation of Standing and Walking After Spinal Cord Injury

Tadej Bajd

University of Ljubljana, Ljubljana, Slovenia

Dr. Bajd summarizes the achievement of Slovenian scientists in development of functional eletrical stimulation (FES) to provide restoration of mobility in patients with complete or incomplete spinal cord injury. This neurorehabilitation system consists of three components: actuation, sensory, and cognitive systems. The author discusses all these components while paying special attention to cognitive feedback. The importance of the feedback system in re-education for standing and walking is demonstrated. It is amazing to see paralyzed people standing, walking, and even climbing stairs as results of FES developed and used in Ljubljana.

Neurorehabilitation systems for restoration of standing and walking in patients with complete and incomplete injury to the spinal cord are presented. A neurorehabilitation system consists from three components: actuation, sensory, and cognitive system. As actuation, functional electrical stimulation of paralyzed muscles was used. Artificial sensors such as goniometers, accelerometers, gyroscopes, inclinometers, and pressure shoe insoles were used to assess standing and walking parameters. After processing this sensory information, the cognitive feedback was delivered to the patient through visual display, audio signal, or sensory electrical stimulation.

Functional electrical stimulation (FES) is a rehabilitation technology that uses electrical currents applied to the peripheral nerves. FES provides restoration of movement or function, such as standing or walking by a person with complete or incomplete spinal cord injury (1,2).

An FES rehabilitative system generally consists of a control unit, pulse generator, and electrodes. The control unit determines the intensity of electrical stimuli applied to the patient through the electrodes. The pulse generator provides the electrical stimuli. When a stimulating current is applied to the electrodes placed on the skin overlaying a muscle, an electric field is established between the electrodes. Within the tissue the current is carried by the ions. The ionic flow across the nerve influences the transmembrane potential and generates an action potential. The action potential propagates along the nerve causing contraction of the muscle. The muscle responds to the artificially initiated action potential just as it would to a natural signal. The magnitude of the effect of the electrical stimulation depends on the number of nerve fibers that are activated by the electrical current.

I. STANDING EXERCISE IN COMPLETELY PARALYZED SCI PATIENTS

A. Problems Associated with FES Standing

Prolonged immobilization, such as occurs after the spinal cord injury (SCI), results in several physiological problems. It has been demonstrated that standing exercise can ameliorate many of these problems. Bone loss occurs in both healthy and traumatized individuals during prolonged bed-rest immobilization. Disuse of large masses of bone and muscle produces abnormal losses of bone calcium, reduced bone density, and hypercalciuria. Passive standing therapy (3 h/day) proved to be sufficient to induce a slow decline of the elevated calcium excretion (3). Urinary tract infections occur in more than half of persons with SCI. It was shown that bladder pressure is for about three times higher in the standing posture than in the supine position. Urine is drained more completely during micturition in the standing position, reducing in this way the incidence of bladder infections. The limitation of range of motion caused by contractures has serious impact on mobility and independence for the individual with SCI. It was demonstrated that patients can maintain the range of motion solely through passive standing. Passive standing has been shown to produce significant decreases in muscular tone in patients with spasticity (4). Following 30 min of standing with the feet in dorsiflexed position, there was observed a 30% decrease in resistance to passive stretch. Due to loss of sympathetic vascular tone and the skeletal muscle pump, patients with SCI have problems maintaining blood pressure and cardiac output. It is well accepted that repeated and progressive standing can lead to cardiovascular system adaptation producing functional circulation (5). Pressure sores are important medical complication after SCI. Regular standing allows sustained periods of relief to the sacral and ischial high-pressure areas of the buttocks.

In addition to stationary standing frames and long-leg braces, standing exercise can be performed also by the help of functional electrical stimulation. An overview of the early applications of FES for the standing exercise can be found in Vodovnik et al. (6) and Kralj and Bajd (1). The first application of FES to a paraplegic patient was reported by Kantrowitz in 1963 (7). The quadriceps and glutei muscles of a T-3 paraplegic subject were stimulated using surface electrodes. The patient's erect standing was achieved for a few minutes. The next similar trial was performed by implanted FES at Rancho Los Amigos Hospital in California in 1970 (8). They have implanted stimulators to both femoral and gluteal nerves with the aim to obtain contraction of knee and hip extensors. A T-5 female paraplegic patient was able to stand with the aid of FES, crutches, and short leg-ankle braces. The stimulation frequency was set between 20 and 25 Hz, while 0.3-ms pulse duration was chosen. First continuous FES standing exercise program was reported in Ljubljana in 1979 (9) and is lasting up to nowadays. It was shown by our group that standing for therapeutic purposes can be achieved by a minimum of two channels of FES delivered to both knee extensors through two pairs of large surface electrodes. The patients must make use also of the arm support usually provided by a walker, parallel bars, or simple standing frame. The stimulation frequency of 20 Hz and the pulse duration of 0.3 ms are used.

Through the use of two stimulation channels and the arm support some paraplegic persons can stand for an hour and even more.

The following are the advantages of FES-assisted standing training as compared to passive standing accomplished by the supporting frames and mechanical orthoses (10,11):

Patient's own muscles are used together with their own metabolic energy.

Atrophied paralyzed muscle restrengthening is achieved.

Improved reduction in spasticity and increase in muscle and skin blood flow are achieved.

FES orthosis has a favorable appearance, is quickly and easily applied to the extremity, has no attachments to cause pressure spots or decubiti, does not depend on extremity size to fit, and costs less than mechanical orthosis.

Approximately 500 SCI patients were admitted to the Rehabilitation Institute in Ljubljana in the 10-year period from 1983 to 1993 (12). According to our criteria 94 were recognized as candidates for functional application of electrical stimulation. The applied indications for FES standing were the following:

Upper motor neuron lesion

No joint contractures

No major skin problems

Adequate upper extremity function

Adequate physiological status

Motivated and cooperative

The 94 paraplegic patients selected were trained to use FES and 83 were capable of performing the standing exercise when leaving the rehabilitation center. At the end of the 10 years period some of our first patients were visited at their homes. Two of such cases are presented in Fig. 1. The upper two photographs show our first patient (9) after being trained and able to stand for 45 min. The patient was living alone and was not motivated enough to exercise standing regularly. Strong contractures, which are specially evident in his hip joints, are preventing standing posture 10 years after (Fig. 1b). In contrary, the second patient, shown in Figs. 1c and 1d, had strong moral support from the side of his family. It can be observed that he was capable of the same well aligned posture after 10 years of daily use of FES.

B. Biomechanics of FES Standing

A study was undertaken to demonstrate that biomechanical parameters are important for efficient standing exercise (13). The patients were standing with one leg on the force plate. The balance was provided by the help of arm support while FES was delivered to both knee extensors. The markers were attached to approximate centers of hip, knee, and ankle joint rotation. The torques were calculated in the three joints from the force plate data and photographic presentation of the lower extremity during FES-assisted standing.

The selected paraplegic subjects (all with thoracic spinal cord lesion) were not equally successful in performing FES-assisted standing. From the upper diagram in Fig. 2 it can be observed that the first three SCI subjects were able to stand for about 15 min (T_{max}), while the subjects 4 and 5 could stand for over 1 and even 2 h. In the next diagram of Fig. 2 the hip joint torques (M_H) are presented. Rather large positive values were obtained in subjects 2, 4, and 5. These patients were assuming the characteristic "C" posture with hyperextended hip

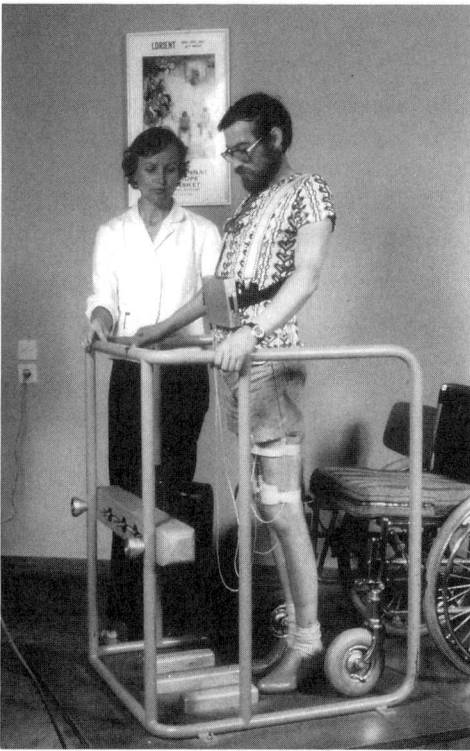
(a)

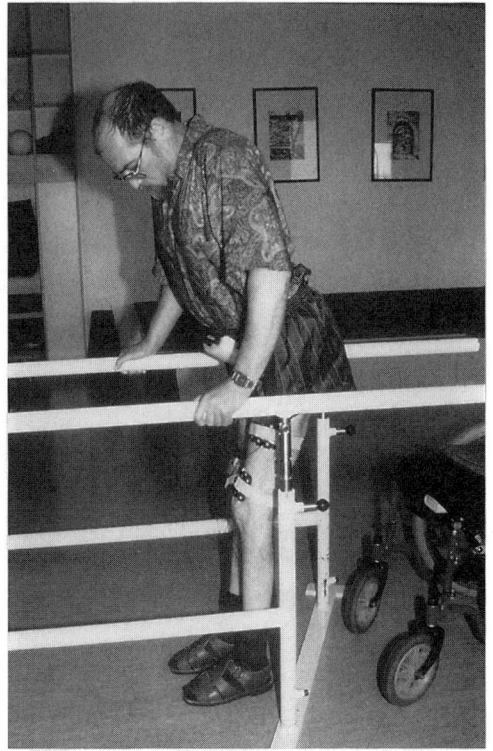
(b)

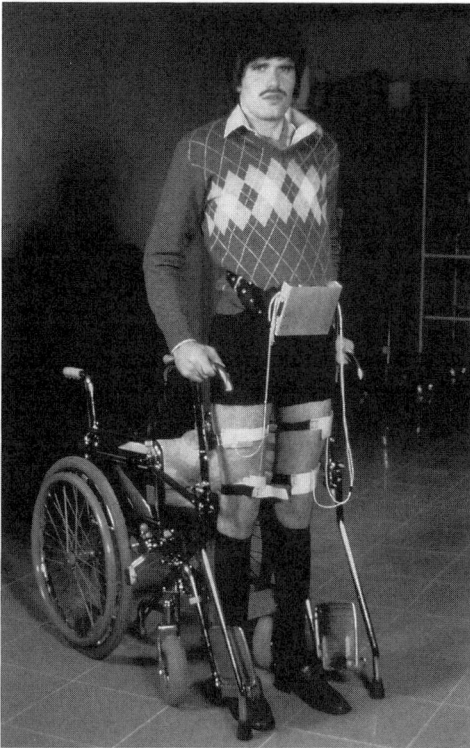
(c)

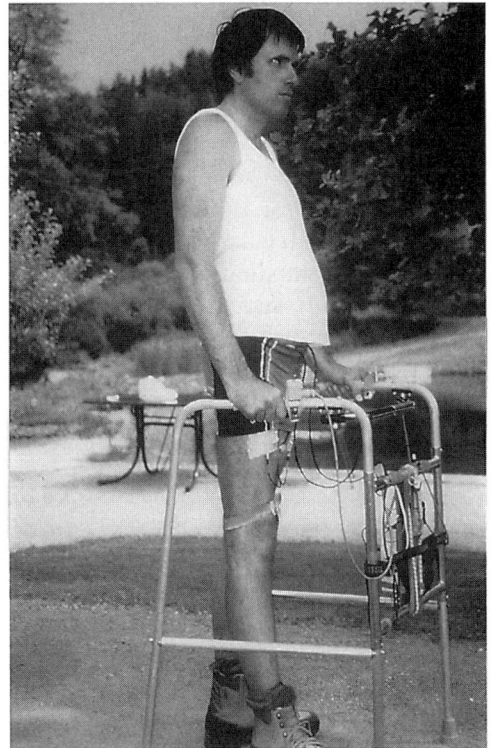
(d)

Figure 1 FES-assisted standing in two paraplegic persons shown soon after the accident (a and c) and 10 years after (b and d). The first SCI patient (a and b) omitted use of FES, while the second patient (c and d) is still regularly training with FES (from Bajd et al., Ref. 13).

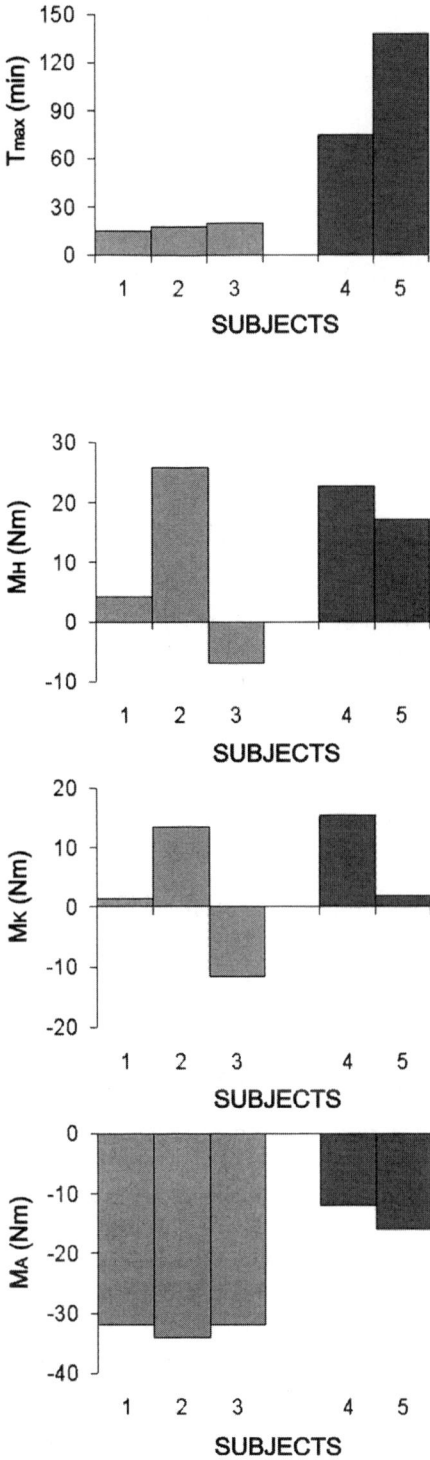

Figure 2 Maximal durations of FES-standing together with hip, knee, and ankle joint torques assessed during standing of five paraplegic subjects.

joints where the body weight vector was passing behind the axis of the hip joints rotation. In this way the hip joints were passively locked during standing. Low hip joints torque values were found in patients 1 and 3, which is also the main characteristic of the knee joint torques (M_K) assessed in all five SCI persons. This is a necessary condition for FES-assisted standing as electrically stimulated knee extensors cannot counteract large external joint moments. The highest correlation was found between the maximal standing time and the ankle joint moments (M_A) presented in the lower diagram of the Fig. 2. Large ankle joint torques (over 30 Nm) were found in paraplegic persons who were able to stand for only about 15 min, while rather low ankle torques were assessed in subjects who were able to perform long lasting standing exercise.

The static ankle joint torque is a sum of two components, the first is produced by the vertical component and the second by the horizontal component of the ground reaction force. The part of the ankle joint torque appertaining to the horizontal ground reaction force represents less than 10% of the total ankle joint moment. The component belonging to the vertical reaction force is therefore crucial for the efficacy of FES assisted standing. It is a product of the vertical reaction force and the lever represented by the horizontal distance between the ground reaction vector and the center of the ankle joint. For an adequate standing exercise we wish that as much as possible of the body weight is carried by the legs. To minimize the ankle joint torque, the lever belonging to the vertical reaction force should be decreased. The length of this lever was around 10 cm in the subjects who were able to stand for about 15 min and around 5 cm in the patients who were performing standing exercise more efficiently (13). Good alignment of the posture, not only in the knees but also in the ankle joints, is a prerequisite for efficient FES assisted and arm supported standing exercise.

C. Cognitive Feedback

The standing balance is influenced by the sensory signals from vestibular organ, eyes, muscle, tendon, and joint receptors. The completely paralyzed SCI persons have vision and vestibular organ preserved, while no sensory information arrives from the lower extremities. Cognitive feedback was introduced in order to improve the balancing exercise (1). A precision pendulum was attached to the sacral part of a paraplegic patient. The amplified signal from the sensor was split into positive and negative part, representing forward and backward leaning of the body. The voltage proportional to the angle of the leaning was transformed into sinusoidal signals of different frequencies which were led to two loudspeakers. When the standing person was leaning forward the loudspeaker placed in front was loud, when leaning backward the loudspeaker placed behind was active. The frequency of the tone was proportional to the angle of leaning. In the beginning the subjects were able to stand for several seconds by the help of one arm support. After 2 weeks of training with cognitive feedback the standing time increased to several minutes.

Fatiguing of electrically stimulated paralyzed muscles is a major factor limiting the duration of the FES-assisted standing exercise. Fatiguing can be significantly delayed by changing the posture (1). Standing by FES-stimulated knee extensors is not the only possible standing posture. When the body weight line is passing in front of the knee joints (when the subject is leaned slightly forward) standing can be achieved by stimulating the ankle plantar flexors only. Fatiguing of a stimulated muscle is considerably decreased when applying cyclical rather than continuous FES. By switching between the posture with stimulated knee extensors and the posture with activated ankle plantar flexors, the total standing time can be significantly increased.

As the completely paralyzed SCI persons are not aware of the position and orientation of their legs, a cognitive system was developed providing the information about the posture in the sagittal plane (14). The center of the pressure (COP) under the feet was assessed by a shoe insole measuring system. The acquired signals were transformed into electrotactile sensory input. Three pairs of concentric surface electrodes were symmetrically placed with respect to both sides of the upper body. The range of the COP signal was divided into anterior, middle, and posterior regions of the foot. The location of the COP in the anterior, middle, and posterior region corresponded to stimulation pair at the shoulders, lateral back skin, and medial back skin, respectively. The subjects were asked to incline in the anterior and posterior directions to different extent. The target posture, that a standing subject had to reach, was provided to the patient through a visual display. If the time when the current posture matched the target posture exceeded 50% of the total trial duration (10 s), the trial was judged as successful. The results of the tracking experiment have demonstrated the ability of each participating subject to accurately relate the current and target posture when using electrocoutaneous cognitive feedback system. The success of the subjects without feedback was considerably poorer. It was, therefore, shown that the residual sensory system was not sufficient to track different postures consistently when the cognitive feedback was withheld.

II. WALKING EXERCISE IN COMPLETELY PARALYZED SCI PATIENTS

A. Problems Associated with FES Walking

A minimum of four channels of FES were used in Ljubljana Rehabilitation Institute for synthesis of a simple reciprocal gait pattern in completely paralyzed paraplegic subjects. During reciprocal walking, the stimulator must be controlled through three different phases of walking: right swing phase, double stance phase, and left swing phase. This is achieved by two hand push buttons that are built into the handles of walker or crutches. When neither of the push buttons is pressed, both knee extensors are stimulated providing support to the body. On pressing the push button in the right hand, the right leg is stimulated to flex. The same is true for the left leg (15).

When the pushbutton is pressed, the stimulation is delivered to the ipsilateral peroneal nerve resulting in synergistic flexion response. The stimulated leg is in the swing phase of walking. The stimulation is delivered through two small round electrodes. By placing the electrodes close to the peroneal nerve, the largest of the lower threshold afferent fibers are excited. Simultaneous flexion of the hip and the knee and dorsiflexion of the ankle are thus obtained by single channel of electrical stimulation. The stimulation frequency used is 50 Hz and the pulse duration 0.3 ms. The flexion response may be altered by increasing or decreasing the stimulation amplitude. The subject remains in the swing phase of walking as long as the subject is pressing the push button. When the walking subject releases the hand push button, the peroneal stimulation is discontinued and the stimulation of the ipsilateral knee extensors is started making the contact of the stimulated leg with the ground. The stimulation frequency of the knee extensors is 20 Hz, the pulse duration 0.3 ms, and the amplitude of stimuli up to 150 V. The electrical stimulation is applied through large (6 × 4 cm) sheet-metal electrodes covered with water-soaked gauze.

The Ljubljana FES walking system consists of two small two-channel stimulators attached to each leg. Only three electrodes are applied to single leg in order to produce knee extension and flexion response. As both activities never occur simultaneously, the distal electrodes placed over knee extensor represents the common electrode for both stimulation channels. In the year 1990 we had 28 paraplegic patients who were able to walk by the help of a walker. Twelve patients could walk also when using crutches (16). The energy efficiency of FES-assisted walking in completely paralyzed SCI persons was rather low. Considerable body weight was, specially during the leg or crutch transfer, supported by the arms. Four-channel FES gait pattern was also for about 10 times slower than normal walking.

The Cleveland approach differed considerably from the minimal FES gait pattern proposed by the Ljubljana researchers. Complex lower extremity motions were synthesized by activating 48 leg and trunk muscles (17). Electrical stimuli were delivered with chronically indwelling fine-wire intramuscular percutaneous electrodes. In this way muscles were activated that are inaccessible with surface FES. In 1994, 13 paraplegic persons were using such FES systems enabling them to walk for short periods. Their walking speed was for about five times higher than in Ljubljana patients. The rehabilitative FES system provided also the mobility functions such as one-handed reaching, forward-, side-, and backstepping, and stair ascent and descent. The Cleveland FES system used preprogrammed sequences of stimulation to produce each leg movement trajectory. The preprogrammed stimulation patterns were derived from trial-and-error experimentation, starting with what is known of electromyographic muscle activity in normal gait (18).

The studies using percoutaneous electrodes were essential to proceeding with trials of implanted FES technology (19). Eight and sixteen-channel FES systems were surgically implanted in complete thoracic or incomplete low-cervical injured subjects. Epimysial and intramuscular electrodes were used. The implanted systems enabled standing, transfers, and short-distance mobility. FES standing and walking exercise may be an effective mechanism to improve fitness in completely paralyzed SCI persons and may provide health benefits similar to regular exercise in able-bodied individuals.

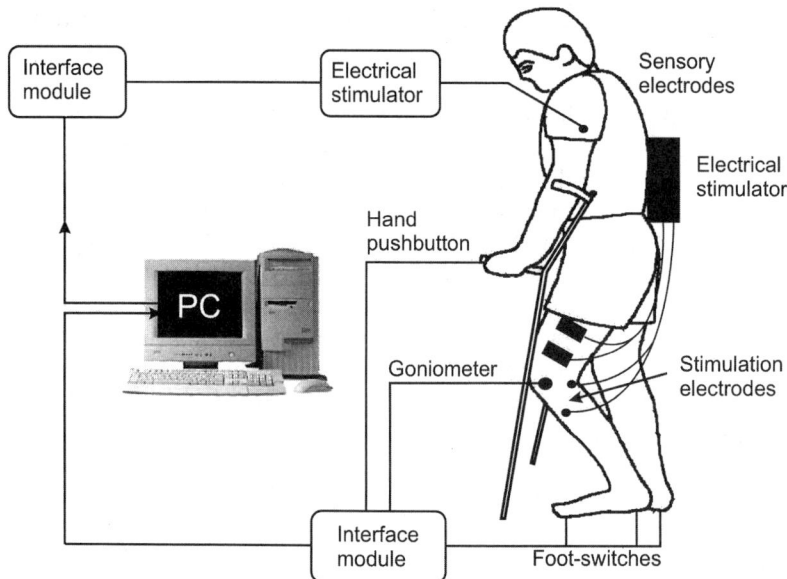

Figure 3 Sensory integrated feedback system for training of walking in completely paralyzed paraplegic subjects (from Bajd et al., Ref. 2).

B. Sensory Integrated Feedback System

Walking of a SCI person relies primarily upon the visual information about the position of the paralyzed extremity. Frequent inappropriate looking down to the legs is resulting in rather slow walking. This is specially noticeable during the foot contact phase when the patient is checking whether the leg which comes into the contact with the ground will provide reliable support to the body. The aim of the developed FES sensory integrated feedback system was to provide to the patient simple and efficient information based on sensory integration (20). Information, provided in the form of sensory stimulation, was delivered to the skin of the patient's nonparalyzed upper arm in order to reward the patient for successful progression from the swing phase into the double-support phase.

The following sensors were connected to the FES sensory integrated feedback system: crutch push buttons, knee goniometers, and foot-switches (Fig. 3). Hand push buttons were built into the handles of the crutches and were primarily used for voluntary control of a four-channel FES gait pattern. The signals from the pushbutton were also used for recognition of the desired phase of walking. The knee angle was measured by the use of flexible goniometer. This goniometer was easily attached to the knee joint and caused only small errors due to the

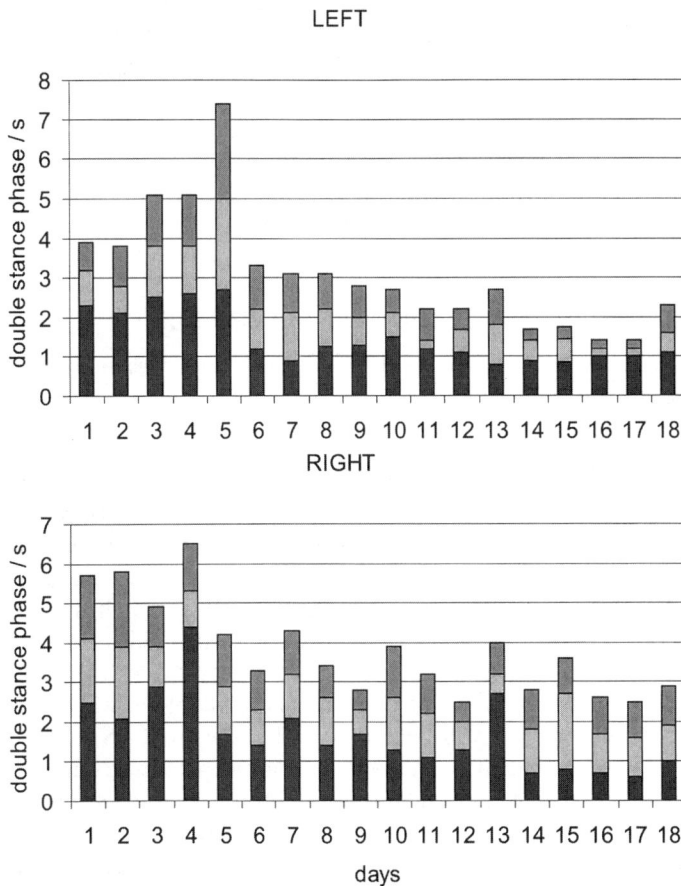

Figure 4 Influence of gait training with the sensory integrated feedback system on the duration of the double-stance phase (from Bajd et al., Ref. 20).

skin movement. The foot switches were attached under the heel. The described sensors were applied bilaterally. Two additional stimulation channels provided sensory stimulation feedback. The sensory stimulation was delivered to the patient through a pair of electrodes placed over the skin of the ipsilateral upper arm. The stimulation frequency was 50 Hz, pulse duration 0.3 ms, and the amplitude between 30 and 40 V. This sensory signal lasted for a predetermined time interval of 0.2 s and was generated in the beginning of the double-support phase when the stimulated leg made the contact with the ground. From the control algorithm point of view, the double-support phase started after the patient voluntarily released the crutch push button. During this phase the patient must make a contact with the ground having the leg extended. The successful foot contact was recognized when the knee angle was lesser than the maximal allowed knee flexion and the heel switch was in the *on* state. In this situation the *reward* sensory signal was generated.

Testing of the proposed sensory integrated feedback system was performed in SCI patients (20) having complete thoracic spinal cord lesion. Bilateral stimulation of knee extensors and peroneal nerve was used in all three subjects. The purpose of this investigation was to demonstrate that the improvements in walking occur as a consequence of applying the sensory feedback system. The gait measurements lasted for a month. During the first week the average values and variability of basic gait parameters were assessed when walking with FES but without sensory feedback. In the next 3 weeks the basograms were measured while training the patient to walk by the help of the described sensory feedback. The aim of the FES sensory feedback system was to increase the speed of walking. In this respect it is of utmost importance to make the double stance phase as short as possible. The average values and standard deviations of the double support time appertaining to the right and left leg are shown in Fig. 4. Comparing the gait data at the beginning and at the end of the investigation it can be concluded that the patient with T-12 spinal cord lesion (14 months after the accident) adopted new and considerably faster technique of walking.

III. FES-ASSISTED WALKING IN INCOMPLETELY PARALYZED SCI PATIENTS

A. Prognosis of Ambulation

In the last few decades advances in traffic control and motor vehicle engineering together with more efficient first aid and improved transport to the emergency center have resulted in a reduction in the number of complete SCI patients. As a consequence, more incomplete cases are arriving in spinal units. There are more incomplete tetraplegic than paraplegic cases. About one-half of the incomplete SCI patients recover and need no orthotic aid. In these patients FES can be used as therapeutic treatment in the early posttrauma phase (21). Some incomplete SCI patients are candidates for use of FES rehabilitative aids also after release from the rehabilitation center (22,23).

Soon after the accident many of the incomplete SCI patients are unable to walk. It is therefore of interest to predict which patients will be able to walk after the FES rehabilitation process completed. It was found that early recovery of quadriceps muscle strength post spinal injury is a useful predictor of future ambulation (24). Motor incomplete spinal-cord injured patients who recovered to a quadriceps strength greater than 3/5 by 2 months postinjury had an excellent prognosis for subsequent ambulation by half a year postinjury. No relationship was found between age and ambulatory status. Also, no relationship between the level of injury and recovery of ambulation was observed. This is in accordance with the data presented in a study (25) where no significant differences in motor recovery were related to the type of injury and type of spinal fracture. In another study (26) all subjects with an early quadriceps muscle grade greater than 0/5 ambulated.

The same examinators also noticed that somatosensory evoked potentials did not offer any additional prognostic value over that provided by the clinical examination. However, the prognostic value of preserved sensation was proven in the study. The preservation of pinprick sensation between the level of the injury and the sacral dermatomes was the best prognostic indicator for useful motor recovery with the patients regaining the ability to walk (27). The relationship between neurocontrol patterns evoked by lower limb movement in the supine position and the assistive device used for ambulation in chronic incomplete SCI patients was also evaluated (28). Marked decreases in motor unit output and/or loss of motor organization were found in the nonambulatory group of patients. Coactivation of proximal muscles, poor timing of muscle activity, and radiation of activity into contralateral muscles were also noted in subjects who required a walker or crutches.

Our purpose was primarily to develop a diagnostic procedure which will soon after the accident predict which incomplete SCI patients are candidates for use of FES walking aid.

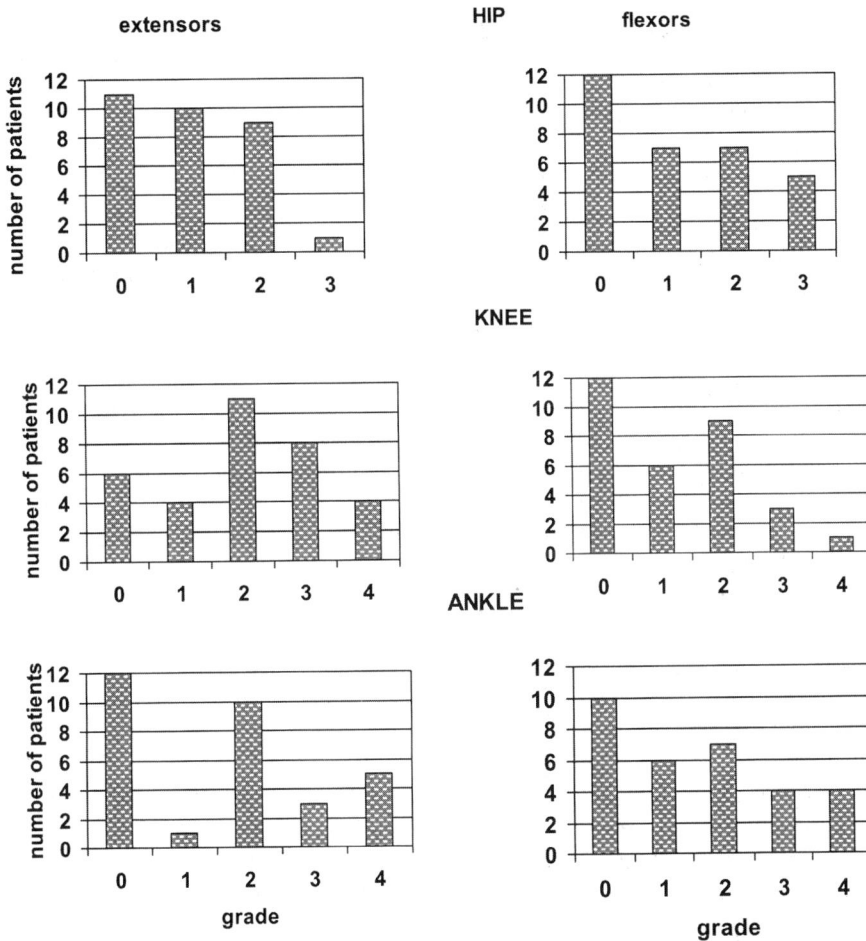

Figure 5 Distribution of the muscle strength in agonist and antagonist muscles of the hip, knee, and ankle joint as assessed in a group of incomplete SCI persons.

On every incomplete SCI patient manual muscle tests were performed by physiotherapists at the arrival of the patient to the rehabilitation unit. The muscle groups governing the hip movement (extensors and flexors), knee movement (extensors and flexors), and ankle joint movement (dorsal and plantar flexors) were evaluated. In the manual muscle test the responses to voluntary control were estimated by nine grades (0, 1, −2, 2, −3, 3, −4, 4, 5). It was observed that both hip and ankle antagonists were rather severely affected in most of the subjects (Fig. 5). The strongest muscle group was knee extensors. Significant nonsymmetry between the strength of the right and left paralyzed leg was often observed in the group of incomplete SCI persons. The data appertaining to the severely handicapped extremity were taken into consideration for further computer analysis. General patient's data have been gathered: year of birth, sex, date of accident, level of spinal cord lesion, and cause of accident or disease. Thirty-one incomplete SCI patients with central (thoracic or cervical) SCI were included into the study. Twenty-three incomplete SCI patients had cervical lesion to the spinal cord, while 8 patients had thoracic lesion. Twenty-five were males and six females. Eighteen spinal cord lesions resulted from accident and 13 from different diseases. Only the patients who were unable to walk on the day of examination were taken into account.

Apart from regular therapeutic treatment, cyclic electrical stimulation for restrengthening of disuse atrophied muscles was delivered to the patients during several months of their stay in the rehabilitation center. The therapeutic electrical stimulation program consisted of cyclic stimulation of partially paralyzed knee extensor muscles where stimulation trains of 4 s and pauses of equally 4 s alternately followed one another. The electrical pulses used were rectangular and monophasic. A stimulation frequency of 20 Hz, a pulse duration of 0.3 ms, and a stimulation amplitude of sufficient intensity to bring the legs into full extension were used. During the training, the patients were positioned supine with both lower extremities semiflexed to approximately 30° by a pillow under the knees. The FES session lasted for half-hour a day (1). Another FES therapeutic treatment was aimed to decrease the spasticity in patients lower extremities. Knee extensor spasticty can be efficiently influenced through cutaneous stimulation of selected dermatome (29). The electrodes are placed over L-3,4 dermatome, one medially below the knee and the other laterally above it, with the aim to decrease the spasticity of the knee extensors (innervated from the same spinal cord level as the dermatome). A stimulation frequency of 100 Hz and a pulse duration of 0.3 ms are used. The electrical stimulation is not causing any muscle contraction. The FES session lasted for 20 min. In some patients FES for standing and walking was also applied (1). At the release from the rehabilitation center the patients were divided into four different classes regarding their locomotor capabilities:

Wheelchair users (nineteen patients)

Users of FES and crutches (four patients)

Users of mechanical brace and crutches (two patients)

No orthotic aid (six patients)

One-channel electrical stimulators were given to the patients for further exercise after release from the rehabilitation center. One channel FES was delivered to the peroneal nerve resulting in flexion response of the lower extremity (30). In this way simultaneous hip and knee flexion and ankle dorsiflexion were obtained enabling swing phase of walking.

The decision tree prognosing the ambulation abilities of incomplete SCI persons, as obtained through the machine learning (31) approach, is shown in Fig. 6. At the root of the tree the strength of the ankle dorsiflexors is tested. This is quite in accordance with the FES rehabilitative method as peroneal stimulation predominantly results in improved ankle

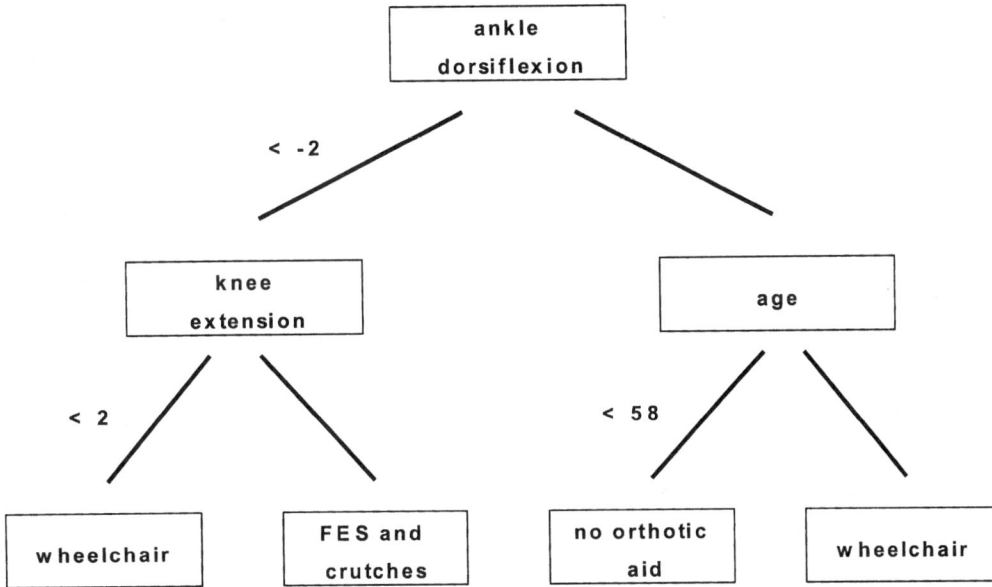

Figure 6   The decision tree predicting walking capabilities of incomplete SCI subjects.

dorsiflexion. In patients with inadequate voluntary ankle dorsiflexion (lesser than 2), the strength of the knee extensors must be evaluated. This finding is in agreement with the observation of other authors (24,26). Patients with sufficiently strong knee extensors (over 2) are candidates for the use of peroneal electrical stimulator and crutches. Patients with weak knee extensors are bound to the wheelchair. It is interesting to note that in patients with adequate ankle dorsiflexion (above −2), the voluntary strength of the knee extensors contraction has not to be tested. These patients are divided on the basis of their age. Older patients are wheelchair users, while younger can walk without any orthotic aid.

B. Peroneal FES

When more effects of the FES training are expected, the incomplete SCI patient may be a candidate for the application of an FES orthotic system after release from the rehabilitation center. Simple peroneal stimulator can turn several of them into community walkers, effectively using the stimulator throughout the day. It was our observation that the peroneal nerve stimulation was found useful in at least 10% of incomplete SCI patients. Here it must be also noted that significant nonsymmetry of the neuromuscular properties of the right and left paralyzed legs was often observed in incomplete SCI patients. In this way the peroneal stimulation was most often applied unilaterally.

It was our further observation that the incomplete SCI patients who are candidates for permanent use of the peroneal stimulator are all crutch users (32). In this respect we found more appropriate to use the hand push button built into the handle of the crutch to trigger the electrical stimulation than the more often used heel switch. The heel switch is a source of frequent malfunctions of the peroneal stimulator. In addition, moderate to high degree of extensor spasticity was usually observed in the lower extremities of the incomplete SCI persons. This extensor responses increased when loading the leg during standing posture or during the stance phase of walking. The extensor response is useful from the point of view of supporting the body, but is quite cumbersome during the transition from the stance into the swing phase. The patients have difficulties breaking the spontaneous extensor activity in order to be able to lift the heel and thus start the peroneal stimulation.

Interconnecting wires between the crutches and the stimulator are inconvenient in daily activities. They hinder a patient when standing up or sitting down. The wire connection was found particularly inappropriate in situations when patients, while sitting, wish to discard the crutches. To overcome these problems, a telemetry system was developed providing reliable and interference resistant wireless control of FES-assisted walking (33). The crutch push-button signals are coded and transferred from the transmitter placed in the crutch to the receiver which is part of the stimulator and is firmly attached to the patient's lower leg. Another important achievement of the telemetric system is the improved appearance, since the stimulator can be hidden under the clothing of the patient. The single-channel stimulator (Fig. 7) was developed in compliance with the EC requirements for safety. It is controlled by an 8-bit microprocessor and built in surface mount technology. A constant voltage output stage provides biphasic, asymmetric and charge balanced output pulses of up to 135-V peak output voltage. The voltage is adjusted manually with the only potentiometer available on the stimulator casing. The stimulator enables also cyclic electrical stimulation for muscle restrengthening. An external module enables the adjustment of the other FES parameters, such as frequency, pulse width, and on–off period of cyclic stimulation.

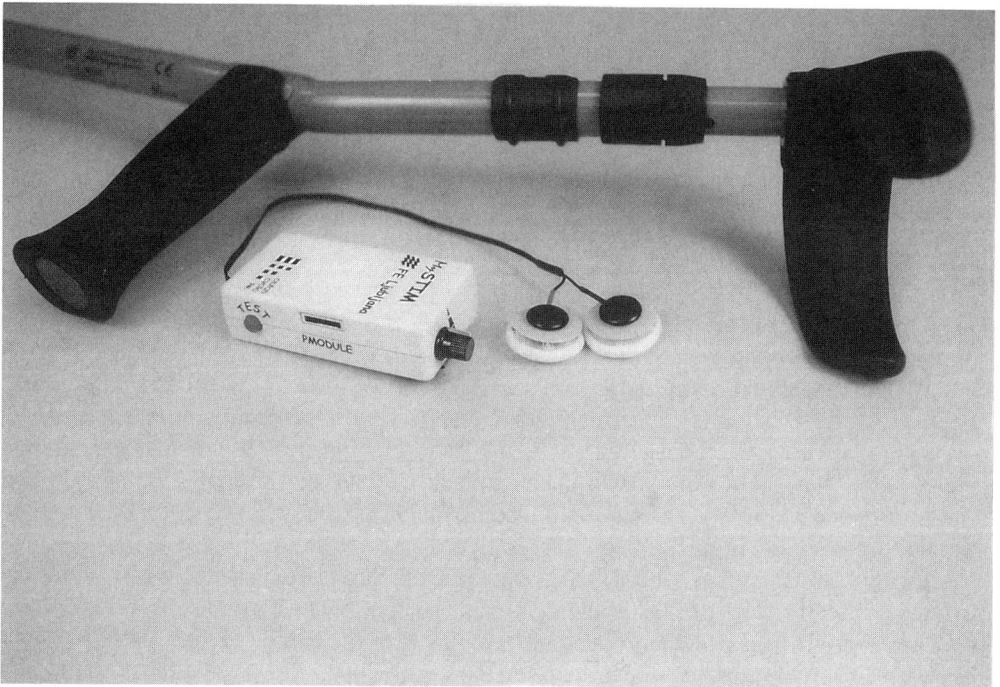

Figure 7   Peroneal stimulator together with hand pushbutton and transmitter built into the handle of the crutch.

The influence of the peroneal stimulation on gait efficiency and energy consumption was investigated. Gait performance of an incomplete SCI subject was compared to a healthy person's walking. The patient was a 48 year-old male. The level of injury, which took place 4 years ago, was C3–C4. The patient was using the peroneal stimulator in everyday life. Two already established gait evaluation methods were used: measurement of oxygen consumption and heart rate analysis. The metabolic energy expenditure was calculated from the difference between oxygen consumption during walking and rest and was expressed by the net energy physiological cost index (EPCI). The heart rate was recorded by a system for physiological measurements. Average heart rate and physiological cost index (PCI) were calculated (34). The expired air collection and heart rate monitoring took place during the last two minutes of resting and walking. The patient walked first without any orthotic aid and afterwards by using the peroneal stimulator. Both assessment approaches showed major difference between the gait of the normal subject and the patient. The results illustrate that the patient's gait is energy less efficient than the gait of the normal subject (Fig. 8). Performance of patient's gait with the use of FES is much improved as compared to the gait without FES. It is evident that the peroneal stimulation can significantly reduce energy consumption and improve incomplete SCI patient's gait efficiency. In the period 1983–2000 (35) 57 peroneal stimulators were given to incomplete spinal-cord injured persons in Ljubljana Institute of Rehabilitation. Thirty-five were tetraparetic and 22 paraparetic patients. A questionnaire evaluating the home use of FES and its influence on the quality of life was sent to the SCI persons. Thirty-two patients used FES for walking and the rest for muscle strengthening only. Nine patients were able to walk outdoors, while 24 used FES only at home.

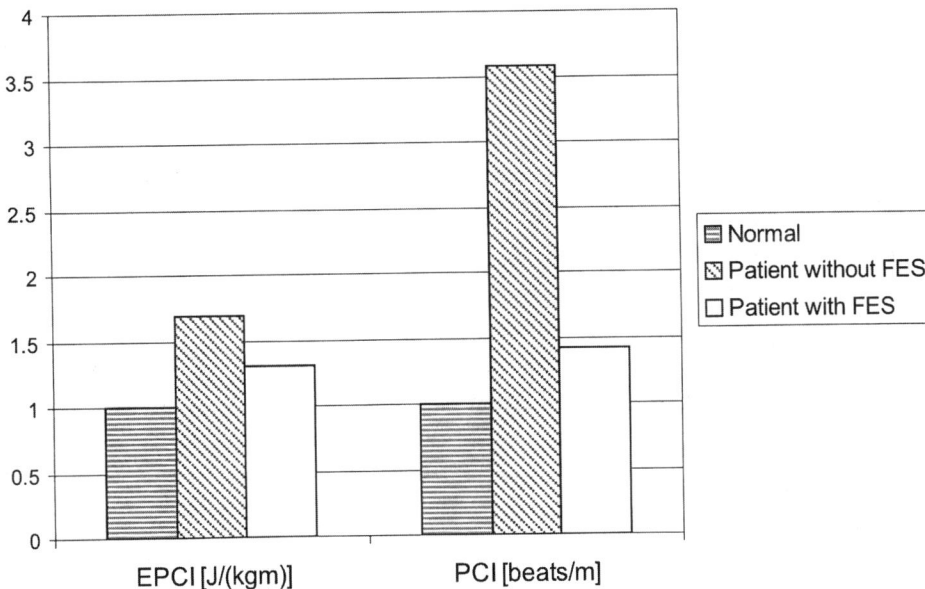

Figure 8 Energy efficiency of incomplete SCI patient's walking with and without FES based on oxygen consumption (EPCI) and heart rate (PCI). The values are normalized to the results of healthy subjects (from Bajd et al., Ref. 20).

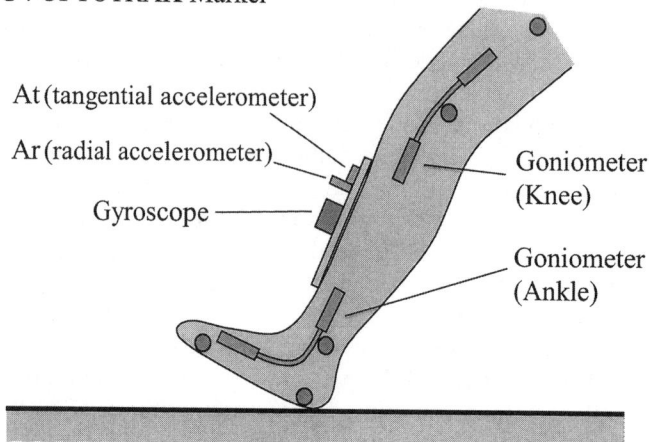

Figure 9 Multisensory system including the knee and ankle goniometers, two pairs of accelerometers, and gyroscope. The position of Optotrak markers is also shown.

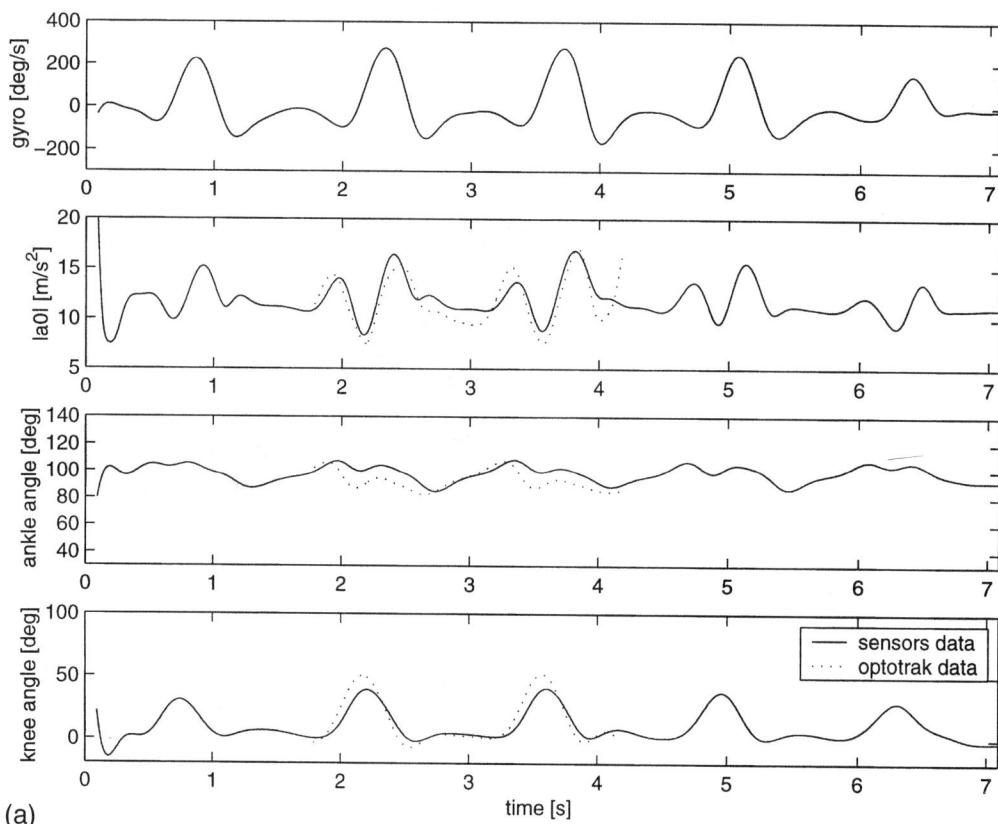

Figure 10 Time courses of gyroscope signal, absolute value of calf acceleration, knee and ankle joint goniogram during level walking of healthy (a) and incomplete SCI person (b).

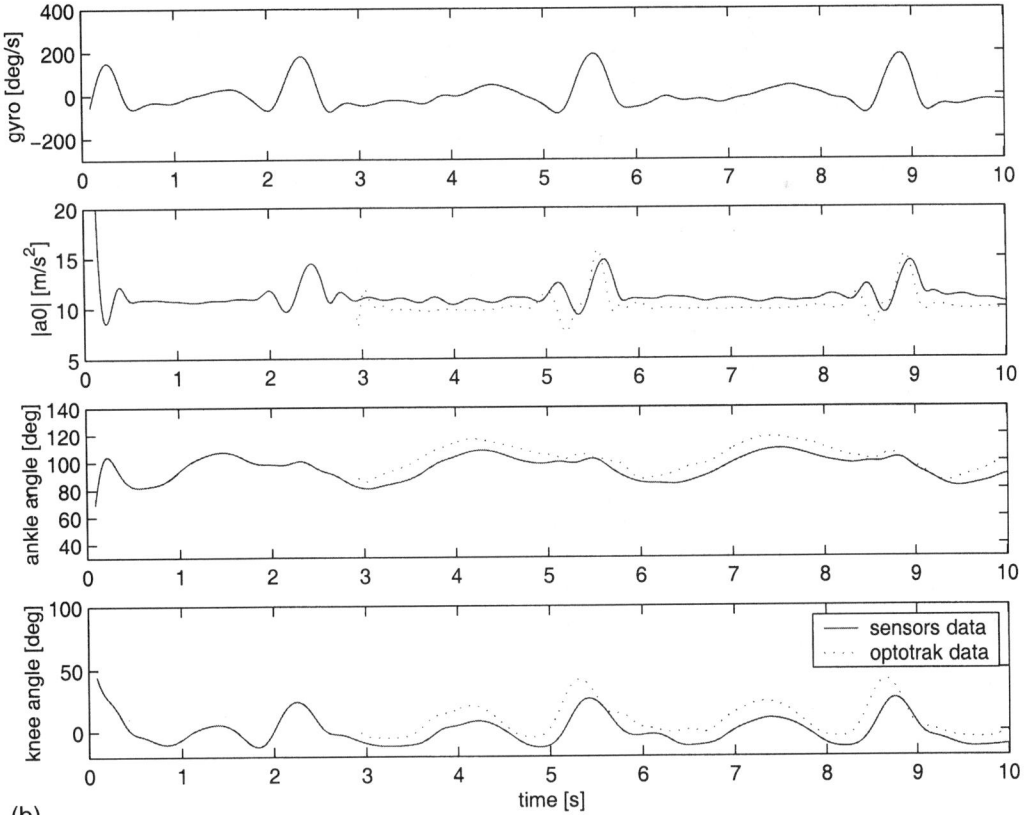

(b)

Figure 10 Continued.

C. Reeducation of FES Walking

The aim of an FES rehabilitative system for reeducation of walking is not only to deliver electrical stimulation to the paralyzed muscles but also to assess the sensory information from the paralyzed limb. The sensory information is fed back to the patient and not to the stimulator control unit. The FES rehabilitation system for reeducation of walking is intended to be used in incomplete SCI patients soon after the accident or onset of disease. The system is to be used within the rehabilitation centers and applied by therapists. Use of surface electrical stimulation is therefore appropriate.

The concept of transmitting the sensory stimulation directly to the patient is not new. According to the author's knowledge it was first described by Norbert Wiener. In the introduction to his famous *Cybernetics* he is discussing the loss of cutaneous and kinesthetic sensations in an amputated patient (36). He is stating as follows:

He has no adequate report of the position and motion of the articulated limb, and this interferes with his sureness of step on an irregular terrain. There does not seem to be any difficulty in equipping the artificial joints and the sole of the artificial foot with strain or pressure gauges, which are to register electrically or otherwise, say through vibrators, on intact areas of skin.

The intriguing idea of the genial Norbert Wiener had to wait for the advent of miniature and reliable sensors that can be easily attached to the patient's paralyzed extremity.

There exists a great variety of the sensors, which can be applied to walking: foot switches, pressure shoe insoles, goniometers, accelerometers, gyroscopes, and inclinometers. There are also different possibilities how to transfer the sensory information to the patient. Vibration, mentioned by Wiener, is just one of the options. Sensory electrical stimulation of different skin areas can be used. Voice control using an earphone also appears to be a promising solution. A haptic interface, transforming the sensory signal into force, is another possible approach to transferring the information to the paralyzed person (37).

We are developing a FES gait reeducation system based on estimation of the quality of the swing phase (38). In incomplete SCI patients one leg is usually considerably more affected than the other one. The aim of the proposed gait reeducation system is therefore to make the swinging movement of the more affected leg similar to the movement of the less affected leg. We developed a multisensor system employing two goniometers, single-axial gyroscope, and two pairs of single-axial accelerometers. Two goniometers are used to measure the ankle and knee joint angle. Accelerometers are mounted on a small aluminum plate and positioned perpendicularly in pairs. They are measuring the tangential and radial acceleration components of the swinging movement. The gyroscope is mounted on a board together with analog bandpass filter and amplifier and placed in the middle of the plate (Fig. 9). It is used to measure the angular velocity of the shank. The plate is attached to the shank of the patient's leg by the Velcro straps. All sensory signals are low pass filtered. Personal computer with acquisition board is used to assess the gait data. The gyroscope signal is used for swing phase detection. The cognitive feedback signal is based on the correlation between the acceleration and angular signals belonging to the right and left extremity.

In order to test the developed multisensor system, the contactless optical measuring system Optotrak was used. The measuring results acquired by the Optotrak were compared with the data assessed by the sensory system. Time course of the gyroscope signal, knee and ankle goniograms, and absolute value of the ankle joint acceleration are presented in Fig. 10. Healthy subjects and incomplete SCI persons participated in the experiment. Based on the measurements in both groups of subjects we can conclude that the multisensor system developed provides sufficiently reliable data.

In order to foster the gait reeducation process, the electrical stimulation should be voluntarily controlled by the patient. The following control transducers can be used: hand push buttons, crutch control lever (37), foot switches, and EMG signals from the non-paralyzed part of the body. Finally, one must select the appropriate FES according to the patient's gait deficits. It is our belief that only simple FES systems are interesting from the clinical point of view. Electrical stimulation of spinal neural circuits, rather than direct activation of motoneurons, will simplify generation of complex motor behaviours. When accomplishing the swing phase of walking the peroneal stimulation should be considered, along with ankle plantar flexors stimulation (32), or dermatome stimulation (39). The described gait reeducation system is inexpensive, simple for donning and doffing, simple to operate, can be easily adjusted to the patient's needs, and is not encumbering patient's walking. It is our belief that the FES gait reeducation systems will find their way into the clinical environment.

In summary, a neurorehabilitation system for reeducation of a lost movement or functional activity of a paralyzed limb has two purposes: therapy and evaluation. Its intended use is in patients with the damage to the central nervous system. The system is to be used and applied by therapists within a rehabilitation center soon after the accident or onset of disease. Its aim is not only to provide actuation but also to assess the sensory information from the paralyzed extremity. This sensory information can be used in three ways. First, it can be used for evaluation of patient's performance. The results measured are compared to the results assessed on previous days, compared with parameters of nonaffected contralateral limb, or compared with parameters obtained from a healthy person. Second, the sensory information can be, in a form of cognitive feedback, sent back to the patient who voluntarily controls the actuation system. Finally, the sensory information can directly influence the actuation system.

Functional electrical stimulation can be efficiently used as the actuation system in the patients with an upper motor neuron lesion. Different kinds of motors can also help to restore the lost movement. When using a chain of motors actuating several joints of a paralyzed extremity, we are speaking about the rehabilitation robots.

Goniometers, gyroscopes, and accelerometers can assess kinematics of movement. Contact-less optical methods can be also used. Forces during walking can be measured by pressure shoe insoles or force plates. Different strain-gauge-based devices can assess gripping forces. Here, it is important to stress that the integration of sensory information must be performed, as only simple form of cognitive feedback can be delivered to the patient.

There are different possible means of transferring the sensory information to the patient. Sensory electrical stimulation or vibration of different skin areas can be used. Voice control using an earphone also appears to be a promising solution. A haptic interface, transforming the sensory signal into force, is another possible approach to transferring the information to the paralyzed person. Visual feedback, using computer screen together with tracking methods of movement assessment, is another challenging approach.

Neurorehabilition system for reeducation of movement or lost function can be used for therapy and evaluation of various daily activities such as standing and balancing, standing up or sitting down, walking, arm manipulation, and gripping. In the chapter neurorehabilitation systems for reeducation of standing and walking in completely and incompletely paralyzed SCI patients were presented.

REFERENCES

1. Kralj A, Bajd T. Functional Electrical Stimulation: Standing and Walking after Spinal Cord Injury. Boca Raton: CRC Press, 1989.
2. Popović D, Sinkjaer T. Control of Movement for the Physically Disabled. London: Springer, 2000.
3. Issekutz B, Blizzard NC, Rodhal K. Effect of prolonged bed rest on urinary calcium output. J Applied Physiol 1966; 21:1013–1020.
4. Odeen I, Knutsson E. Evaluation of the effects of muscle stretch and weight load in patients with spastic paraplegia. Scand J Rehab Med 1981; 13:117–121.
5. Krebs M, Ragnarsson K, Tuckman J. Orthostatic vasomotor response in spinal man. Paraplegia 1983; 21:72–80.
6. Vodovnik L, Bajd T, Gračanin F, Kralj A, Strojnik P. Functional electrical stimulation for control of locomotor systems. CRC Critical Rev Bioeng 1981; 6:63–131.
7. Kantrowitz A. Electronic Physiologic Aids. A report of the Maimondies Hospital, Brooklyn, NY1960.
8. Wilemon WK, Mooney V, McNeal D, Reswick J. Surgically Impanted Peripheral Neuroelectric Stimulation. Rancho Los Amigos Hospital internal report, Downey, CA, 1970.
9. Kralj A, Bajd T, Turk R, Benko H. Paraplegic patients standing by functional electrical stimulation. XII International Conference on Medical and Biological Engineering, Jerusalem, Israel, Aug 19–24, 1979.

10. Bajd T, Kralj A, Šega J, Turk R, Benko H, Strojnik P. Use of a two-channel electrical stimulator to stand paraplegic patients. Phys Ther 1981; 61:526–527.

11. Triolo RJ, Reilley BWB, Freedman W, Betz RR. The functional standing test. IEEE Eng Med Biol Mag 1992; 11:32–34.

12. Kralj A, Bajd T, Turk R. Enhancement of gait restoration in spinal injured patients by functional electrical stimulation. Clin Orthop 1988; 233:34–43.

13. Bajd T, Munih M, Kralj A. Problems associated with FES-standing in paraplegia. Techn Health Care 1999; 7:301–308.

14. Matjačić Z, Jensen PL, Riso RR, Voigt M, Bajd T, Sinkjaer T. Development and evaluation of a two-dimensional electrocutaneous cognitive feedback system for use in paraplegic standing. J Med Eng Technol 2000; 24:215–226.

15. Bajd T, Kralj A, Turk R, Benko H, Šega J. The use of a four-channel electrical stimulator as an ambulatory aid for paraplegic patients. Phys Ther 1983; 63:1116–1120.

16. Kralj AR, Bajd T, Munih M, Turk R. FES gait restoration and balance control in spinal cord-injured patients. Progress in Brain Research 1993; 97:387–396.

17. Kobetic R. Advancing step by step. IEEE Spectrum 1994; 32:27–31.

18. Chizeck HJ, Kobetic R, Marsolais EB, Abbas JJ, Donner IH, Simon E. Control of functional neuromuscular stimulation systems for standing and locomotion in paraplegics. Proc IEEE 1988; 76:1155–1165.

19. Triolo RJ, Bogie K. Lower extremity applications of functional electrical stimulation after spinal cord injury. Top Spinal Cord Inj Rehabil 1999; 5:44–65.

20. Bajd T, Cikajlo I, Šavrin R, Erzin R, Gider F. FES rehabilitative systems for re-education of walking in incomplete spinal cord injured persons. Neuromodulation 2000; 3:167–174.

21. Bajd T, Kralj A, Turk R, Benko H, Šega J. Use of functional electrical stimulation in the rehabilitation of patients with incomplete spinal cord injuries. J Biomed Eng 1989; 11:96–102.

22. Granat MH, Ferguson ACB, Andrews BJ, Delargy M. The role of functional electrical stimulation in the rehabilitation of patients with incomplete spinal cord injury — observed benefits during gait studies. Paraplegia 1993; 31:207–215.

23. Stein RB, Belanger M, Wheeler G, Wieler M, Popović DB, Prochazka A, Davis LA. Electrical systems for improving locomotion after incomplete spinal cord injury: an assessment. Arch Phys Med Rehabil 1993; 74:954–959.

24. Crozier KS, Cheng LL, Graziani V, Zorn G, Herbison G, Ditunno JF. Spinal cord injury: prognosis for ambulation based on quadriceps recovery. Paraplegia 1992; 30:762–767.

25. Waters RL, Ien S, Adkins RH, Yakura JS. Injury pattern effect on motor recovery after traumatic spinal cord injury. Arch Phys Med Rehabil 1995; 76:440–443.

26. Jacobs SR, Yeaney NK, Herbison GJ, Ditunno JF. Future ambulation prognosis as predicted by somatosensory evoked potentials in motor complete and incomplete quadriplegia. Arch Phys Med Rehabil 1995; 76:635–641.

27. Katoh S, El Masry WS. Motor recovery of patients presenting with motor paralysis and sensory sparing following cervical spinal cord injuries. Paraplegia 1995; 33:506–509.

28. Tang SFT, Tuel SM, Mc Kay BW, Dimitrijević MR. Correlation of motor control in the supine position and assistive device used for ambulation in chronic incomplete spinal cord-injured persons. Am J Phys Med Rehabil 1994; 73:268–274.

29. Bajd T, Gregorič M, Vodovnik L, Benko H. Electrical stimulation in treating spasticity resulting from spinal cord injury. Arch Phys Med Rehabil 1985; 66:515–517.

30. Štefančič M, Kralj A, Turk R, Bajd T, Benko H, Šega J. Neurophysiological background of the use of functional electrical stimulation in paraplegia. Electromyogr Clin Neurophysiol 1986; 26:423–435.

31. Breiman L, Friedman JH, Olshen RA, Stone CJ. Classification and regression trees. Belmont: Wadsworth Int. Group, 1984.

32. Bajd T, Kralj A, Štefančič M, Lavrač N. Use of FES in the lower extremities of incomplete SCI patients. Artif Organs 1999; 23:403–409.

33. Matjačić Z, Munih M, Bajd T, Kralj A. Voluntary telemetry control of functional electrical stimulators. J Med Eng Technol 1996; 20:11–15.

34. MacGregor J. The evaluation of patient performance using long-term ambulatory monitoring technique in the domiciliary environment. Physiotherapy 1981; 67:30–33.
35. Benko H, Obreza P, Burger H. FES as an orthotic aid in patients with spinal injury. In: Marinčhler Č, Knops H, Andrich R, eds. Assistive Technology-Added Value to the Quality of Life. Amsterdam: IOS Press, 2000:518 521.
36. Wiener N. Cybernetics or Control and Communication in the Animal and the Machine. Paris: Herman & C^{1e} Editeurs, 1948.
37. Cikajlo I, Bajd T. Use of telekinesthetic feedback in walking assisted by functional electrical stimulation. J Med Eng Technol 2000; 24:14–19.
38. Cikajlo I, Bajd T. Swing phase estimation in paralyzed persons walking. Technol Health Care. In press.
39. Bajd T, Munih M, Šavrin R, Benko H, Cikajlo I. Dermatome electrical stimulation as a therapeutic ambulatory aid for incomplete spinal cord injured patients. Artif Organs 2002; 26:260–262.

30

Electromagnetic Linkages in Soft Tissue Wound Healing

Harvey N. Mayrovitz

College of Medical Sciences, Nova Southeastern University,
Ft. Lauderdale, Florida, U.S.A.

Starting with an overview of the wound healing process, the author explains the requirements for designing a proper strategy for wound healing and an adequate choice of magnetic/electromagnetic stimulation. The chapter demonstrates the successful use of this modality for treatment of venous, arterial-ischemic, diabetes-related, and pressure ulcers. Finally, possible mechanisms of action and potential physiological targets for EMF therapy are discussed.

I. INTRODUCTION

The concept underlying electric current therapy (ET) or electromagnetic field therapy (EMFT) for soft tissue wound healing is that the fields and/or currents beneficially affect functional aspects of cells and processes involved in tissue repair. For soft-tissue wound healing, the most relevant application is for patients with wounds that are chronic, non healing or slow healing, or otherwise recalcitrant to standard therapy. The rationale for its use has multiple historical bases, most notably its therapeutic efficacy in bone healing. Extensions to soft-tissue wound or ulcer healing have evolved with their own plausible rationales, which in part stem from the body's natural bioelectric system (1,2) and early observed relationships between electrical events and wound repair (3). At the macroscopic level, naturally occurring current loops of about 10 μA have been measured in the legs of humans (4), and at the microscopic level, membrane function is largely determined by intrinsic electrical processes. Because dermal wounds interrupt normal transepithilial potentials at injury sites, the electric field and injury current that develop are postulated to play an important role in the healing process (5,6). Central to this concept is the fact that cells involved in wound healing are electrically charged, so that endogenous bioelectricity may facilitate cellular migration to the wound area, and might be involved with angiogenesis (7) and other wound healing processes.

461

The extension of this concept is that if wound healing becomes stalled, external electrical stimulation may mimic one or more of the bioelectric effects and help to trigger a renewed healing progression. It has also been suggested that externally applied EMF may interact directly with the wound currents or with related signal transduction processes (8), thereby restimulating retarded or arrested wound healing. Wound-healing acceleration via direct currents in the range of 200–800 μA, applied via a portable unit, may be an example of such a process (9). Research indicating potential benefits of both electric current and electro-magnetic fields on a variety of cellular or other processes involved in wound repair are available: Reviews (8,10) indicate effects that include edema reduction, neutrophil and macrophage attraction, growth factor receptor upregulation, fibroblast and granulation tissue proliferation, epidermal cell migration, and increased blood flow, all of which are important for wound healing. However, many findings are only suggestive of beneficial outcomes for clinical wounds, and require verification in a clinical setting. Such studies in humans are made difficult by the complexity of the wound-healing process itself and by logistical and practical aspects of clinically based wound research. In spite of these intrinsic difficulties, clinical research with ET and EMFT continues, with a number of promising findings and an increasing amount of direct and indirect evidence of benefits.

To date, wound studies have typically involved skin ulcers caused by arterial or venous dysfunction, diabetes related ulcers, pressure ulcers, and surgical and burn wounds. Human testing has provided some evidence that some therapies help to trigger the healing of "stalled" soft-tissue ulcers or wounds. Human studies showing a positive benefit of EMFT range from those on a single subject with multiple experimental wounds (11) through (a limited number of) randomized controlled trials. Many experiments on animals have also shown positive connections between ET or EMFT and wound healing. But most, if not all, of these are based on wound models that diverge in one or more important aspects from human "chronic" wounds, those in which repair is stalled and difficult to manage. Yet these are precisely the types of wounds that would most likely benefit from such adjunctive treatments. However, many EMFT-related effects on cells, tissues, and processes involved in tissue repair have been convincingly shown to occur, as will subsequently be described.

A meta-analysis of studies on combined chronic wound types and therapies revealed that ET was associated with an overall weekly healing rate of 22% compared with 9% for controls (12). Extrapolation of these figures would indicate that those with ET would heal fully in less than 5 weeks compared to about 10 weeks without stimulation. In another meta-analysis, which included 613 wound patients, a significant favorable effect of ET or EMFT was concluded (13). However, many published clinical reports do not meet the rigorous inclusion criteria associated with the high level of confidence required to validate medical efficacy. Experimental protocols that control and adequately characterize patient, wound, and treatment variables are logistically difficult and very expensive of both time and money. However, the importance of this has been emphasized (14) and is being increasingly recognized, so it is likely that more well designed "randomized, controlled clinical trials" will be forthcoming.

The scientific case for an electrical or electromagnetic connection in soft tissue wound repair processes is neither complete nor fully validated, but based on many specific clinical, experimental, and cellular observations, a clear linkage between EMFT and wound healing is strongly suggested. In July of 2002, the accumulated background of information led the U.S. Centers for Medicare and Medicaid Services to finally approve coverage for electrical stimulation as adjunctive therapy for stage III and stage IV pressure ulcers, arterial ulcers, diabetic ulcers, and venous ulcers, providing that improvement had not occurred after 30 days of standard wound treatment. Despite this implicit acknowledgment of efficacy, much is yet to be learned about the factors involved, mechanisms of action, specific targets, optimal dosing and patterns, and temporal strategies for treatment. These aspects require further targeted research and exploration.

II. OVERVIEW OF THE WOUND HEALING PROCESS

Normal Healing is characterized by three broad phases: inflammation, proliferation, and remodeling. These normally proceed in a well-ordered, functionally overlapping sequence, the outcome of which depends upon interactions among many cell types, growth factors, and processes. Vascular, (platelets, macrophages, mast, neutrophils, monocytes, endothelial, and smooth muscle), epidermal (keratinocytes, melanocytes, and Langerhans cells), and dermal (fibroblasts and myofibroblasts) cells are involved (15). As part of the repair process, cells release and/or interact with many components including structural proteins, growth factors, cytokines (16), chemokines (17), adhesion molecules (18), nitric oxide (19), trace elements (20), and proteases. Any participant or interaction could, in theory, be a target for adjunctive electromagnetic field-related therapy.

In terms of the sequence and functional aspects of wound healing events, the initial inflammatory process serves to limit blood loss (via clotting), to promote entry of antibodies and fibrin into interstitial spaces (via increased vascular permeability), and to deliver needed blood flow to the affected area via vasodilation. This initial hyperemia increases oxygen delivery, which supports the antibacterial (and other) actions of accumulating neutrophils. Activated macrophages, attracted to the wound area by chemotactic and/or galvanotactic signals associated with inflammation, release substances important for angiogenesis, for the development of granulation tissue, and for the proliferation of fibroblasts and epithelial cells. Angiogenesis involves endothelial cell proliferation and new capillary formation that serves to supply ischemic regions of the wound and represents an important phase of granulation tissue development. It is stimulated by angiogenic factors released from macrophages in response to low oxygen in the wound (21) and by growth factors from fibroblasts and endothelial cells. Nitric oxide, present in the wound (22) affects macrophage and fibroblast functions and also affects the keratinocytes (23). Fibroblasts migrate to the wound site and subsequently proliferate. Collagen synthesis is triggered by fibroblast-stimulating growth factors from macrophages and continues at a rate that is linked to the adequacy of local blood flow to deliver oxygen and nutrients for protein synthesis. These nutrients include amino acids and, interestingly, ferrous iron. Epithelialization of dermal open wounds depends on an initial migration of epithelial cells, triggered by epidermal growth factor released from both macrophages and platelets, and subsequently on the proliferation of epithelial cells.

Epithelialization can take days to months depending on wound related factors and depends on keratinocyte proliferation, migration, stratification, and differentiation (24) and on features of the extracellular matrix (25). Wound closure occurs as a result of active contractile forces developed within myofibroblasts, which in turn depends on adequate blood flow to provide energy substrates. Wound closure does not end the wound healing process, and wound remodeling may continue for months to years. In the remodeling phase, wound strength is increased via collagen cross-linking, excess collagen within the wound is eliminated, and many of the capillaries developed during early wound healing are resorbed.

Retarded Wound Healing may be due to many factors. A wound is an added "metabolic organ", and appropriate progression of healing depends on the abilities of the body as a whole to supply the demands of this "temporary organ." Delay of wound healing beyond about 3 months is a criterion sometimes used to characterize a wound as *chronic* or *nonhealing*, the causes of which may be of systemic or local origin. Some of the factors that impede wound healing include infection, inadequate blood flow, tissue hypoxia (due to inadequate O_2 delivery or to increased O_2 demand by white blood cells or other exudate components), and inadequate nutrient availability to support tissue building metabolic processes. Certain conditions such as diabetes have further implications: Hyperglycemia and impaired insulin signaling may directly impair keratinocyte glucose utilization thereby altering both proliferation and differentiation (26). Inhibition of nitric oxide production diminishes wound-healing activities of fibroblasts and keratinocytes and causes delay in wound healing (27,28). Deficiencies in wound concentrations of platelet activating factor are associated with impaired healing of chronic venous ulcers (29). Given the variety of causes for retarded wound healing, no "most important" electromagnetic target has been defined. However, because blood supply plays a major role in many of the processes, increases in blood flow and/or oxygen supply are often intrinsic targets.

III. EMF METHODS AND STRATEGIES FOR WOUND HEALING

Therapeutic approaches using ET (direct skin contact using electrodes) and EMFT (non-contact) may be divided into two broad categories: (1) those applied at the wound site and (2) those applied remote from the wound site. Included in category (1) are electric currents and fields, generated in variety of ways, with a range of excitation patterns, in which the wound itself is directly exposed to the currents or fields. In the case of ET, an electrode may be placed directly in the wound bed or the wound may be in the path of electrode pairs that straddle the wound. Included in category (2) is electrostimulation (ET or EMFT) of either nerves or tissue regions that functionally connect with, and potentially alter, wound-site processes, either directly or via reflex effects. Both categories have been reviewed as they relate to different wound conditions (30,31).

Another useful broad distinction between devices that has been used for wound healing is whether they are mainly electric or mainly electromagnetic. In electromagnetic devices, no electrodes are needed and target tissues are exposed to electric and magnetic fields and their associated induced currents. Among electromagnetic devices, all use time-varying or pulsed excitation, some of which modulate a carrier frequency, commonly 27.12 MHz. A further distinction among pulsed radio-frequency devices is made with respect to their potential tissue-heating effects, which is related to the energy they deliver to the tissue. Commercially available EMF devices usually specify device average or peak power, but these do *not* specify the energy or field strengths delivered to target tissues. Pulse width and shape generated by most commercial devices is fixed (65–95 µs), with the power per pulse usually controlled by varying pulse amplitude. Total power is adjusted by varying the pulse repetition frequency, which, for "nonthermal" devices, typically ranges between 80 and 600 pps (Diapulse and Sofpulse). Devices that function in nonthermal and thermal ranges may allow both variable pulse width and rates (Magnatherm, 700–7000 pps), whereas other devices provide no control features (Regenesis). Tissue thermal effects are thought to be minimized by use of low duty cycles, on the assumption that heating due to high power single, short pulses, will be dissipated during a much longer off-time between successive pulses. In general, for ET or EMFT, the parameter variants include generated power, excitation frequency, pulse width, repetition rate and duty cycle, carrier frequency, current magnitude, and magnetic field intensity. In addition there are variants with respect to specific features of the excitation patterns, i.e., whether stimulation is continuous or pulsed, galvanic or frequency modulated, biphasic or monophasic, symmetrical or asymmetrical, sinusoidal or not, and whether high-voltage or low-voltage stimulation is used (30–32).

It is partly because of this wide range of physical excitation parameters that it has been impossible to correlate specific features with wound-healing efficacy. However, it has been argued that the use of pulse radio-frequency EMF (PREMF), with its inductive coupling to tissue, provides for a more uniform and predictable electromagnetic field signal in the target tissue than is currently achieved with surface contact electrodes (33). Thus, the tissue dose is more reliably characterized. It has also been argued that, because of the large spectral range of PREMF, there are more possibilities for coupling of the field to produce effects in a wider range of possible (but as yet unspecified) biological processes. More detailed technical descriptions may be found in several sources (30–34).

IV. CLINICAL FINDINGS OF EMF THERAPY FOR SPECIFIC WOUND TYPES

A. Venous Ulcers

Venous ulcers occur on the lower extremities and are the most common chronic skin wounds in humans. Venous disease increase with age and results in venous ulcers in about 0.3% of the adult population (35). Venous reflux and venous hypertension due to incompetence of deep and communicating vein valves and thrombosis of deep vein segments are linked to the development of venous ulcers. The evolution of skin ulcers from venous hypertension is not fully understood, but contributory factors probably include inflammatory processes, intercellular and vascular adhesion molecule upregulation (36), protein rich edema, leukocyte trapping, oxygen deprivation, and microcirculatory deficits (37–40). Microangiopathy due to venous hypertension may have several manifestations that include abnormally dilated and tortuous capillaries, loss of some functional capillaries, microvascular thrombosis, increased capillary permeability and transcapillary fluid efflux, tissue edema, and altered function of microlymphatics. Compression therapy has been reported to help normalize capillary numbers and size (41) and to tend to normalize the abnormally elevated limb blood flow (42). Healing has been reported to occur only after aspects of the dermal microangiopathy have improved (43). Increased activation of platelets, monocytes, and neutrophils leading to microvascular aggregation (44) and microvascular entrapment of neutrophils (45) has been shown.

In a review of randomized controlled trials (RCT) (46), only three eligible studies were identified (47–49). The reviewers state that there is "currently no reliable evidence of benefit of electromagnetic therapy" in the healing of venous leg ulcers. Although this conclusion may be warranted for one of the reviewed studies, (too few subjects and mixed results), one may question judgments based on the other studies. One was double-blind and compared sham vs. active pulsed EMF therapy (75 Hz, peak field of 2.8 mT) in 37 patients (19 sham) for 90 days (47). At the beginning of the study, ulcers had been present for an average of 30 months in the actively treated group, versus 23 months in the controls. Stimulation was applied with an enclosed coil placed over the wound by patients, at home, for 3–4 h/day. After 90 days, of the actively treated ulcers, 12 were healed, as compared to six in the sham group ($p < 0.02$). Further, granulation tissue, not present prior to active treatment, was present in all patients actively treated by day 15, whereas only seven of the sham group showed new granulation tissue.

The other study (48) was a prospective, randomized, double-blind, placebo controlled multicenter investigation of 27 patients with recalcitrant venous ulcers (mean duration of 39–47 weeks). Patients were treated for 8 weeks at home for 3 h/day with a wearable portable EMF device (22-G, bidirectional pulse of 3.5 msec, 25% duty cycle). All received compression bandaging and daily 3-h leg elevation. At week 8 the active group ($N = 17$) had a 47.7% decrease in wound surface area vs. a 42.3% increase for placebo ($P < 0.0002$). The investigators' global evaluations indicated that 50% of ulcers in the active group had healed or were markedly improved vs. 0% in the placebo group. Other studies have directly indicated a beneficial effect of EMF therapy for venous ulcer healing. In one of these, twin 100-V pulses (0.1 ms, 100 Hz) were applied directly to the ulcers, which resulted in healing rates that were superior to standard therapy alone (50). In another study, EMF patterns were first tailored to interact with human monocytes, as judged by an in vitro assay, and then the EMF pattern was used as the sole treatment for patients with predominantly venous ulcers (51). Results, which were assessed with each patient's long standing and nonresponding ulcer as a control, were suggestive of a beneficial action of the stimulation.

B. Arterial-Ischemic Ulcers

The main predisposing condition for arterial-ischemic ulceration is advanced peripheral artery disease affecting arteries supplying the lower leg and foot. These ulcers, which can be particularly painful and difficult to treat, frequently occur in areas subject to pressure or trauma such as between the toes or at the malleolus or posterior heel regions. Adjunctive therapies for ischemic ulcers for which standard available medical approaches have failed are sorely needed. In this author's opinion they could become one of the most important targets of EMF therapy in the future. Recent pilot work (52) using high voltage-pulsed currents to treat ischemic ulcers in six diabetic patients with very poor initial microcirculation suggests that treatment can raise local oxygen levels sufficiently to save some legs from amputation.

Because the main impediment to wound healing in this condition is inadequate blood flow, effective EMFT would be expected to affect blood flow. There is substantial evidence that this is indeed a realizable goal. Although effects of EMFT on blood circulation are dealt with in detail elsewhere in this book, it is useful here to examine certain aspects that may be tightly linked to wound-healing potential. Early work using PREMF addressed the issue of augmenting blood flow to ischemic regions via reflex effects. PREMF (27.12 MHz) was applied to the epigastric region using low duty cycle excitation in normal persons (53) and in persons with peripheral arterial disease (54). The idea was that the use of short but intense pulses could deliver useful therapeutic excitation without causing significant tissue heating. The physiological strategy of targeting a remote site (epigastric area), rather than the ischemic region itself (foot or ulcer), is to reflexively increase blood flow to the ischemic region without imposing added metabolic demand via local heating on the distant (ischemic) region.

Results on 20 normal subjects showed a dose-dependent increase in foot perfusion as judged by toe-volume plethysmography and toe temperature, which rose an average of $2\,°C$, without a significant core temperature elevation (53). A series of 12 similar PREMF treatments (65 μs, 600 pps) given over a period of 2 weeks to 18 patients with intermittent claudication, also resulted in an increase in toe temperature ($>3.0\,°C$), with no significant increase in core temperature (54). Although the duration of toe temperature elevation was short-lived after each 20-min stimulation was ended, the cumulative effects appeared to be sustained, as measured by increased pain-free walking distance at the end of the 2-week treatment sequence. A toe temperature increase was also noted in normal subjects but to a lesser degree than in patients.

More direct measures of blood flow have used laser-Doppler perfusion monitoring (55–57), which permits skin blood flow to be directly monitored before, during, and after EMF exposures. PREMF (65 μs, 600 pps, 1 G) was applied 1.5 cm above open foot ulcers in diabetic patients. Results showed an EMF-treatment related increase in periulcer blood perfusion. Based on the observed flow patterns, these authors judged that the increase was predominantly caused by an increase in the number of capillaries with active blood flow. This flow feature was consistent with an EMF-field-related capillary recruitment process (57) that may have reflected precapillary vasodilation. Similar microcirculatory flow increases were reported for forearm skin of normal persons (58) and for persons with postmastectomy arm lymphedema (59), but interestingly, no effects of a static magnetic field (500 G) were observed in the hands (60) or forearms of normal subjects (61).

To date there have been no reported clinical trials using PREMF directly for ischemic ulcers, but other forms of electrical stimulation have produced similar changes in blood flow. A particularly promising approach is epidural spinal cord electrical stimulation (ESES), which appears to benefit patients with severe lower extremity ischemia secondary to atherosclerotic disease. This therapeutic approach requires implanted electrodes at the T10–T11 level and usually the use of an implanted pulse generator. This therapy significantly increased microscopically measured blood velocity in capillaries and density of skin capillaries in the foot (62). In patients with rest pain and ischemic ulcers, this technique resulted in immediate pain reduction, and in most patients was accompanied by microscopically verified increases in capillary blood velocity and density, and a significant increase in postocclusive microvascular hyperemia (63). In more than half of these patients, the ulcers subsequently healed, resulting in significant limb salvage. Other studies using ESES have shown similar limb salvage rates and ulcer healing potential (64,65). In patients with and without ulcers, the degree of therapeutic success tends to correspond to an increase in transcutaneous oxygen tension (66–68) (which is itself dependent on blood flow increases in the foot).

C. Diabetes-Related Ulcers

Persons with diabetes are more susceptible to developing skin ulcers due to neuropathy, ischemia, and poor glycemic control. The higher likelihood of peripheral arterial disease and the presence of microvascular deficits increase the chances of ischemia, tissue to breakdown, and ulcer formation. Ulcers in diabetic patients are generally more difficult to heal for reasons that include reduced blood flow and wound oxygenation, deficits in wound cell function, and infection. Recent work has shown that it takes much less local pressure to reduce skin blood flow in regions of bony prominence in persons with diabetes (69). When sensory neuropathy is present, normal pressure and/or pain signals are diminished or absent, thereby removing warning of developing tissue injury. Most of these types of ulcers develop on the foot, with plantar ulcers often associated with neuropathy. Effective therapy should include elimination of elevated foot pressures combined with standard wound care, but this is not always adequate to effect wound healing. Statistics suggest that about 15% of persons with diabetes will get a foot ulcer (70), with an annual incidence rate of 2.2% (71). In this population, nonhealing ulcers account for 54,000 extremity amputations per year (72), and an annual amputation incidence rate between 0.5–0.8% (number of amputations per patient-year) (73).

Pulsed-galvanic electric stimulation (50 V, 100 μs), delivered through a conductive stocking for 8 h every night, was used as an adjunct to standard care for healing diabetic foot ulcers in 40 patients (74). The study was of a randomized, double-blind, placebo controlled pilot trial design, with half of the patients receiving ET and half receiving sham treatment. All received standard wound care including off-loading with removable cast walkers.

Patients were followed for 12 weeks or until healing, whichever occurred first. Considering only patients who were protocol compliant, 71% of those actively treated healed, compared with 29% in the sham treatment group ($p = 0.038$). From these data the authors concluded that the ET improved wound healing. A different ET regime was employed to treat the ulcers of a group of 80 diabetic patients. Daily treatment included a biphasic stimulation pattern consisting of either asymmetric or symmetric square wave pulses at amplitudes set to activate intact peripheral nerves in the skin. Controls consisted of groups that received either very low levels of stimulation current or no electrical stimulation. Average healing rates, measured weekly as changes in ulcer perimeter, were significantly greater than in controls only when the asymmetric treatment was used (75). In a group of 64 diabetic patients with chronic ulcers, electrical nerve stimulation was used therapeutically for 20 minutes twice daily for 12 weeks (76). The excitation parameters in this study consisted of an 80-Hz pulse train with a 1 ms pulse width and an intensity sufficient to evoke strong paresthesias. All patients received standard treatment with half also receiving either sham or active electrical stimulation. At 12 weeks, the active treatment group was reported to have significantly reduced ulcer area and more healed ulcers ($p < 0.05$).

In many ways, plantar ulcers in persons with leprosy resemble diabetic ulcers. In a pilot, randomized, double-blind, controlled clinical trial (77), 40 leprosy patients with plantar ulcers received standard treatment and half of them (EMF group) received exposure to pulsed sinusoidal magnetic fields (0.95 to 1.05 Hz, 2400 nT) for four weeks. Outcome measures were the calculated ulcer volume recorded on the day of admission and at the end of treatment. In the control group, mean ulcer volume at entry was 2843 mm^3 which was reduced to 1478 mm^3 at the end of treatment ($P = 0.03$); corresponding values in the EMF-treated group were 2428 mm^3 and 337 mm^3 ($P < 0.001$). These data indicate that the EMF therapy caused a significantly more rapid healing of plantar ulcers in these leprosy patients.

D. Pressure Ulcers

Pressure (decubitus) ulcers result from sustained or inadequately relieved pressure, most frequently on bony prominences such as the heel and sacral region. These ulcers represent an important clinical, humanitarian and economic problem with an average prevalence in acute care facilities of 10.1% (78) and a reported incidence in persons age 65 and older of 0.18 to 3.36 per 100-person years depending on age (79). Ulcer development depends on many factors including age, nutritional status, mobility, skin irritations, and general health status (80–82), but a final common pathway is associated with blood flow changes within pressure-loaded tissue (83–88). Some experimental evidence suggests that both ischemia and ischemia-reperfusion injuries are involved (89).The clinical stages of pressure ulceration range from nonblanching erythema (stage I) through full-thickness skin loss with extensive destruction and tissue necrosis involving muscle or bone (stage IV).

Examining available literature-based randomized controlled trials led reviewers to the judgment that there is insufficient data from too few clinical trials to conclude that electromagnetic therapy to treat pressure sores is beneficial (90,91). In spite of this conclusion, data from these reviewed studies, and others not included, do provide interesting and strongly suggestive findings of potential benefits of PREMF therapy. One small study (92) used PREMF (27.12 MHz) on patients with long-standing pressure ulcers and found significant improvement over standard treatment alone. Another study (93) was randomized and double-blind and used similar PREMF therapy or sham to treat a total of 30 spinal-cord-injured patients who had either stage II or III pressure ulcers. Wounds were treated for

30 min, twice daily, for 12 weeks, or until healed. The authors indicate that, after controlling for the baseline status of the pressure ulcers, PREMF treatment was independently associated with a significantly shorter median time to complete healing. An additional study (94) using the same PREMF method to treat patients with either stage II or stage III long-standing pressure ulcers, also reported improved healing. PREMF (20 and 110 pps) was also reported to trigger healing progress in five elderly males with trochanteric or sacral pressure ulcers (95). Similar positive results of pulsed ET (300–600 µA) were reported in a double-blind, placebo controlled study of long-standing stage II and III pressure ulcers in which healing rates were significantly improved with active treatment (96). High-voltage pulsed galvanic stimulation (200 V, 100 pps) was used to treat 17 persons with spinal cord injury for 20 days. One electrode was placed on the ulcer and one on the thigh. The reported outcome was a greater reduction in ulcer area as compared to a placebo group (97). In an extensive study of 150 persons with spinal cord injury, the use of pulsed biphasic ET (0.25 ms, 40 Hz, 15–25 ma), with electrodes applied across pressure ulcers, resulted in significantly faster healing (98).

Based on available clinical data, it appears to this author that a strong, if not conclusive, case is made for a beneficial effect of electromagnetic therapy for pressure ulcers. In fact, the National Pressure Ulcer Advisory Committee (NPUAC) has included electrotherapy as an adjunctive therapy for pressure ulcers that have failed to heal by other means. Further, aside from treatment benefits, there is some experimental evidence that ET of the gluteal muscles may have preventative effects related to beneficial buttock shape changes (99) and by increasing muscle thickness and blood flow (100,101). High-voltage pulsed galvanic treatment (75 V, 10 Hz) of 29 persons with spinal cord injuries resulted in a 35% increase in sacral skin oxygen tension (102). Further studies of the role of EMF stimulation as a potential preventative modality would thus appear warranted.

V. POTENTIAL PHYSIOLOGICAL TARGETS OF EMF WOUND THERAPY AND MECHANISMS

The mechanisms by which externally applied EMFs alter cellular properties and biological processes to effect improved wound healing are unknown, although there are many theories that describe how EMF interactions may occur at cellular and subcellular levels. Whatever the specific mechanisms turn out to be, it is this author's opinion that clinical efficacy depends on determining the proper therapeutic parameters and timing to optimally modulate cellular features and their interacting processes within the context of the wound healing cascade. Specific targets for any of the postulated mechanisms could theoretically be any of the cells, or functions, involved in the wound healing process. In the following subsections the focus is only on some of the main relevant experimental cellular targets and findings.

A. Endothelial Cells

A role of EMF stimulation on the growth rate of endothelial cells was suggested by studies in which partially denuded cell layers reacted to an external field in a manner similar to in vivo angiogenisis, but with an accelerated rate as compared to nonexposed cells (103). Other in vitro studies, in which cells derived from human umbilical vein and bovine aorta were subjected to repetitive 5 ms pulse bursts from a Helmholtz device at 15 Hz, produced corresponding results (104). In these studies the calculated electric field at the center of the tissue culture dish containing the cells was 1.3 mV/cm and the measured magnetic field was about 1 G. By examining the rate at which the cells transformed from a monolayer configuration to tubular structures, after cell-layer wounding, the authors determined that vascularization rate was increased in the presence of the EMF stimulation.

Studies on human umbilical vein cells showed that endothelial cell migration to a wounded area is accelerated if cell cultures are exposed to a sawtooth pulse train (2 mT peak, 25 Hz) (105). These results were demonstrated in the presence of growth factor and an induced electric field (0.04–0.11 V/m) perpendicular to the wound edges. Further evidence of an angiogenesis-electrical connection stems from studies on skeletal muscle in which chronic stimulation of rat muscles resulted in an increase in blood vessel density, thought by the authors to involve both angiotensin and vascular endothelial growth factor pathways (106). Various pulsed EMF waveform patterns applied to the rabbit ear chamber (107) also suggested an EMF-affected increase in vessel growth, but results were highly selective and limited to a specific excitation pattern. Evidence that vascular smooth muscle relaxation may be induced by EMF exposure due to endothelial cell mediated processes is provided by studies of rings of bovine aorta (108). The rings, which were initially contracted with phenylephrine, were found to relax when exposed to the effluent from bovine endothelial cells treated with a pulsating electric field (one 5-s pulse train every 30 min, pulse width 0.1 ms, 30 V, 100–500 mA). Threshold levels for relaxation were found to be between 0.5 to 1 Hz with a maximum relaxation at 16 Hz. The authors concluded in part that the EMF-induced endothelium-dependent relaxation was due to nitric oxide released from endothelial cells. Taken together, these findings offer strong evidence for an endothelial cell-electric connection which may affect both angiogenisis within the wound bed and vaso-active changes that mediate blood flow delivery. Whether these are related to enhancement of nitric oxide release, alone or in combination with other factors, represents an important research question.

B. Fibroblasts

Sinusoidal currents (300 Hz) applied for 15 min to rat incision wounds was reported to improve microcirculation and to stimulate proliferation and differentiation of fibroblasts (109). Sinusoidal magnetic fields (0.06–0.7 mT; 50, 60, and 100 Hz) increased chick embryo fibroblast proliferation (26–31%) with excitation frequency or intensity when the other was held constant (110). However, treatment of rat incision wounds with PEMF of the type and intensity used for bone healing failed to produce significant increases in soft tissue fibroblast counts or improvement in wound closure (111). More recent work on normal human fibroblasts exposed to 50 Hz, 20 or 500 mT for 1 or 4 days failed to show any significant effects on measured fibroblast parameters (112).

High-voltage pulsed galvanic stimulation (HVPGS) of cultured human fibroblasts showed that increases in protein and DNA synthesis could be demonstrated, but only for specific combinations of voltage (50–75 V) and pulse rates (100/s) (113). HVPGS also increased the rate of fibroblast formation and wound contraction in a pig burn wound model (114). When human dermal fibroblasts in a type I collagen dermal matrix were exposed to electric fields ranging from 18 to 1000 mV/m at frequencies of 10 and 100 Hz, only a narrow amplitude window between 37 and 50 mV/m at 10 Hz yielded increases in cell proliferation, which, at the reported maximum (41 mV/m), resulted in a 70% increase in total DNA (115,116). Fibroblast proliferation and collagen synthesis were also demonstrated in a tendon explant model when exposed for 4 days to 1-Hz, 1-ms duration pulses (peak 7 A/m^2, average 7 mA/m^2). Exposures to lower (1.8 mA/m^2) or higher (10 mA/m^2) current densities had either no effect or an inhibitory effect on fibroplasia (117). Dermal fibroblast growth into a collagen sponge matrix was found to be increased in the presence of direct currents between 20 and 100 μA, with maximum effects near the cathode at a current of 100 μA (118). Experimental surgical abdominal wounds in rats, when treated with an implanted stimulator (bipolar pulses, 0.87 Hz, 25 μA), showed earlier fibroblast formation and collagen deposition, and more rapid maturation and longitudinal alignment of the collagen fibers, which resulted in stronger scars (119). In rabbits, patellar ligament healing, with increased capillary and fibroblast densities and more mature longitudinally oriented collagen fibers occurred earlier with pulsed (10 Hz, 25 μs) EMF therapy. The most consistent results were obtained at a field strength of 50 G (120). Recent work has indicated that when cultured fibroblasts are exposed to PREMF (27.1 MHz, 32 mW/cm^2, 15 min), there is a significant enhancement in cell proliferation (121,122). Taken together these findings suggest that EMF affects aspects of fibroblast activities that are important to wound healing. However, the forms and patterns of excitation needed to consistently affect the fibroplasia features must to be further elucidated, an aspect that likely depends on a better understanding of the mechanisms involved.

Regarding possible mechanisms, it has been proposed that EMF stimulation of fibroblasts induces transmembrane currents that open voltage-controlled calcium channels causing ATP resynthesis, activation of protein kinase mechanisms to synthesize cell protein, and DNA replication for mitotic cell division (123). Sinusoidal EMF exposure (20 Hz, 8 mT) of human skin fibroblasts (124) has been shown to change cellular calcium oscillation activity within 40 min, with responses (increase or decrease in dynamics) depending on a cell's differentiation state. It has been hypothesized that modulation of proliferation and differentiation phases is triggered by immediate but transient increases in cAMP-dependent protein kinase activity (125).

Based on stimulation experiments (10–100 Hz, 0–130 μA/cm^2) with human dermal fibroblasts in a collagen matrix, an amplitude and frequency windowing process that may predict fibroblast proliferation conditions has been proposed (126). The proposed ion-interference mechanism considers the effects of induced electric gradients on protein-bound substrate ions. Tissue cultures of human foreskin fibroblasts, when exposed to 2 V/cm fields at either 1 or 10 Hz, demonstrated a sixfold increase in internal calcium, but excitation at 100 Hz had no significant effect (127). The fact that the internal calcium increase depended on external calcium concentration, and was blunted by a calcium channel entry blocker, suggested that the stimulation-induced calcium increase was due to increased calcium influx via voltage-gated calcium channels. Since the channel-gating process may be initiated by a membrane depolarization of 30–40 mV (128), it has been argued that the coupling with the applied external oscillatory field may be due to forced vibrational effects on free ions on either side of the plasma membrane, which in turn alter transmembrane potentials sufficiently to open voltage-gated channels (129). However such an oscillatory mechanism would not directly explain the fact that DC fields (10 V/cm) cause an even greater calcium increase (127). The fact that the kinetics of the calcium entry process saturate after about 30 min of continued field exposure may provide initial guidelines for durations of electrotherapy treatments.

In view of the many linkages between EMF stimulation and verified selective modulations of intracellular calcium, it would seem to this author that the search for optimal stimulation parameters to selectively control calcium fluxes is narrowing and represents an exciting and useful research target. However, it is important to bear in mind that although calcium entry into fibroblasts is associated with fibroblast stimulation (130,131), calcium entry effects on vascular caliber, and thus on blood flow, depends on the specific cell type experiencing the field-induced calcium influx effect. Increased calcium entry into vascular smooth muscle promotes vasoconstriction and blood flow reduction, whereas calcium increase in endothelial cells promotes synthesis of nitric oxide (132–134), which normally produces vasodilation and a blood flow increase.

C. Leukocytes and Macrophages

Much of the contribution of leukocytes to wound healing depends upon their activation during the inflammatory phase. This activation is associated with a respiratory burst, the release of cytokines and oxygen radicals, and an upregulation of cell surface receptors that increases adhesion between leukocytes and endothelial cells. Although entry of neutrophils into the wound area is needed for their antibacterial actions, a process perhaps initiated by electric field gradients via galvanotaxis (135), their continued entry, sustained presence, and activation may be associated with diminished local blood flow due to capillary plugging, abnormal vasoconstriction, and tissue damage associated with continued enzyme release. Evidence of such involvement in impaired healing comes from studies on genetically diabetic mice, in which the inflammatory phase is prolonged and dermal wound healing is significantly retarded (136). The sustained inflammatory phase was related to prolonged expressions of inflammatory and chemoattractant proteins that were expressed by keratinocytes and resulted in the persistence of both neutrophils and macrophages within the wound site. Under conditions in which the inflammatory phase is abnormally prolonged, actions of EMF stimulation that affect these and other features of activated leukocytes could influence the wound healing process. Of particular note is the fact that neutrophil activation is accompanied by oscillations in intracellular free calcium concentrations and membrane potentials at frequencies in the range of 0.05 to 0.1 Hz.

In a series of elegant experiments it has been shown that the intensity of these oscillations could be increased in the presence of electric fields (20-ms pulses) that were delivered during the trough of the oscillations at a rate that matched the intrinsic oscillatory frequency (137). The effect, termed *metabolic resonance*, was found to occur with electric fields of 1×10^{-4} through 2×10^3 V/m. An additional finding revealed that reactive oxygen metabolites, normally generated at the 0.05–0.1 Hz rate from migrating neutrophils, could be increased or terminated depending on the phase relationship between applied field and the intrinsic oscillatory process. Electrical stimulation has also been proposed to promote neutrophil, monocyte, and macrophage migration to the wound area (138) by virtue of the interaction between their surface charge and the prevailing electric field. Selection of initial polarity (anode or cathode) placed on the wound in the case of electrode type stimulation may enhance this effect.

D. Keratinocytes

Normal wound healing depends on epithelial cell proliferation and migration to effect wound reepithelialization and closure. Normal early triggering of proliferation is in part related to secretion of granulocyte-macrophage colony stimulating factor from several cell types, including the keratinocytes themselves (139). Deficiencies in adhesion molecules, such as L-selectin and intercellular adhesion molecule-1 (ICAM-1), lead to impaired keratinocyte migration and retarded wound healing (18). Based on the fact that keratinocytes exhibit galvanotaxis (140), it has been proposed that the lateral electric field associated with a wound or injury current is an early stimulus for the initiation of the migration process of epidermal keratinocytes (141). Directed migration of keratinocytes toward a wound is endogenous, associated with wound-associated direct currents corresponding to a field of about 100 mV/mm, a process that depends on growth factors, extracellular calcium (142) and intact keratinocyte β_1-integrins (143). It is significantly reduced if protein kinase activity is inhibited (141). Thus, the field strength required to promote epithelial migration seems to depend on the constituents of the wound environment and on the ambient levels of growth factors, but in a simulated normal wound environment, migration is noted at field strengths close to those generated by the wound (144–146). It has also been observed that exposure of keratinocytes to pulsed electric fields may enhance cellular differentiation at the expense of migratory and proliferative aspects (147).

VI. BLOOD FLOW AND EDEMA AS EMF-RELATED WOUND HEALING TARGETS

A. Blood Flow

Blood flow as a target for EMF-related wound-healing therapy can be conveniently considered in two categories: flow to the wound site and flow within the wound. In the first case, that of flow to the wound, the EMF targets are principally small arteries and arterioles feeding the wound bed site. Changes in vasoactivity of these vessels may be induced either directly, by EMF effects on vascular smooth muscle or endothelial cells, or indirectly, via neural activation, as in transcutaneous electrical nerve stimulation (TENS) (148–150) or by magnetic stimulation (151). Recent histological work indicates that skin blood vessels are innervated by sensory, sympathetic and parasympathetic fibers (152); so any of these may be suitable targets for EMF-effects. In addition, EMF-related reductions in impediments to local flow, such as by release of trapped leukocytes via EMF-related deactivation or by increasing global blood flow to the region, as by spinal cord stimulation, may also be suitable targets. The other flow-related category relates to blood flow *within* the wound bed, which supports granulation and its functions in wound healing. This is a process that depends on angiogenesis and relative flow distribution within the wound. In this case it is unlikely that EMF exposure remote from the wound site would have benefit, unless neural (or other) pathways that selectively innervate (or effect) the wound site can be identified and appropriately stimulated.

Another point that should be considered is that, although blood flow deficits are involved in ischemic and in some diabetic ulcers, it is not necessarily true that greater blood flow means faster wound healing. Nor is it clear that greater tissue oxygenation is always good for the natural wound healing process. It may be argued that effects of blood flow on wound healing depend, at least in part, on the timing of increases or decreases: If blood flow is too high initially, it may affect the trigger for angiogenesis, and if it is sustained at too high a level, it may result in increased edema. On the other hand, if flow becomes too low, it will no longer support wound metabolism and may cause a sustained inflammatory phase that inhibits healing. It is possible that the need to reverse polarity of some forms of ET to effect wound healing may reflect the need for these different requirements for blood flow (153). Of course, polarity also influences the direction of cell migration (154).

Since low oxygen tension triggers angiogenesis, hyperperfusion, occurring at the wrong time, may actually inhibit healing. For example, in patients with venous ulcers, overall limb blood flow is elevated (42,155–157) as is total peri-ulcer skin microvascular blood flow (55,157,158). Yet abnormally dilated precapillary arterioles are present (159), and there is a maldistribution of the total flow between nutritive and nonnutritive pathways (41).

This maldistribution may be related to activated leukocytes that plug nutritional capillaries or other selective flow diminution processes. If leukocytes are involved, then an EMF-related reduction in neutrophil activation and adherence might be beneficial from three perspectives:

Reduction in local ischemia in regions served by obstructed capillaries
Normalization of the effects of enzymes and free radicals released by activated leukocytes
Reduction in the edema associated with their activation.

Further, in patients with venous ulcers, the arteriolar vasoconstriction normally induced by standing is significantly blunted (160). This undoubtedly contributes to the local microvascular hyperperfusion, which exacerbates hypertension within postcapillary venules and capillaries, and causes further tissue edema. Such *high perfusion microangiopathy* may also be involved in neurogenic diabetic ulcers (160). Thus the possibility of global hyperperfusion, with simultaneously reduced wound blood flow and localized tissue edema, is a plausible basis for delayed healing. This scenario suggests that an EMF-related selective *vasoconstriction* of nonnutrient circulation may be of benefit. Alternatively, an EMF-related increase in local nutritional wound blood flow, if it overcomes the relative ischemia without causing substantial edema, might favor wound healing. Normally, edema (such as occurs with venous ulcers) is controlled via compression bandaging, which, among other aspects, is thought to redistribute microcirculation and thereby to normalize the deficient nutritional capillary network (157). Therefore, EMF therapy to increase total blood flow should always be used in conjunction with standard compression bandaging.

Patients with chronic venous insufficiency, and presumably those who go on to develop venous ulcers, appear to have increased vasomotion frequency (161). This vasomotion, which is due to spontaneous changes in blood vessel diameter, manifests itself as measurable rhythmic changes in blood flow at frequencies that range from 0.05 to 0.5 Hz (162). This suggests that EMF-related effects on vasomotion (163) may also have an impact on wound blood flow and wound healing. EMF excitation may alter arteriolar vasomotion through its effect on intracellular calcium ion oscillations and other calcium signaling processes. Although not specifically studied in vascular smooth muscle cells (the effectors for vasomotion), an EMF-related (50 Hz) reduction in total spectral power content of cytosolic calcium ion (Ca^{2+}) oscillations and specific changes in the low-frequency band $(0–10^{-3}$ Hz) have been demonstrated in human leukemia cells (164). Effects were noted only in cells in which such oscillations were already present (165). An argument for the role of spectral power changes as a mode of cellular encoding has been made (166), although both amplitude (167) and frequency (168) may be involved in encoding and decoding. Such a process may be involved in the EMF-related effects that alter the arteriolar vasomotion that is linked to local blood flow changes. Based on these findings and other considerations, it is the author's view that the effectiveness of EMF therapy for altering blood flow to stimulate wound healing may be optimized by linking field–current parameters to rhythms of the healing process using feedback that detects and accommodates naturally occurring physiological and vascular dynamics.

B. Edema

Although the role of the lymphatic system in wound healing has generally received little attention, several aspects of this "orphan" component of the circulatory system may have important consequences with respect to wound healing and the role of EMF therapy.

Interstitial accumulation of fluids as edema or as a protein rich lymphedema retards blood flow by reducing perfusion pressure, reducing oxygen diffusion to tissue, and acts as a breeding area for infection (169,170). In the early phases of a wound, edema is largely due to changes in capillary permeability associated with the inflammatory phase, but damage or dysfunction of the terminal lymphatic system is also probably involved. The presence of edema is obvious under some conditions, but in others its presence is silent, as microedema within the wound environment, and its effects on wound healing are often not considered. Further, the physical features of sustained edema may change over time due to a progressive increase in protein concentration and fibrin cross-linking. These changes further impact the wound healing process.

In view of the well-documented ability of EMF therapy to reduce gross edema, the question arises as to whether EMF-related effects that may reduce microedema, either directly or by its effects on lymphatic pathways, plays a role in the favorable effect of EMFT on wound healing. It has been argued that PREMF affects lymphatic channels as they do blood vessels (59). There is also evidence that lymphatic vessels near ulcers are reduced in number and have partially destroyed endothelium (171), at which site one finds vascular endothelial growth factor receptor-3. In experimental dermal wounds (172), the expected angiogenic derived vessels were observed to evolve into granulation tissue. But, unexpectedly, from day five after wounding and onward, blood vessels that were positive for this growth factor appeared to sprout from periwound lymphatic vessels to become part of the granulation tissue. Although blood vessels remained, the growth factor positive lymphatic vessels regressed (172). This suggests a potentially important role of the lymphatic vessels in processes involved in forming wound granulation tissue. This would be dependent on a transient lymphangiogenesis and, based on data from human wounds, an upregulation of the vascular endothelial growth factor contained therein (172). Preliminary results (59) indicate that PREMF (27.1 MHz) significantly reduces edema in patients with postmastectomy lymphedema. Since in these patients the main deficit is a dearth or absence of normal lymphatic pathways due to surgery and/or radiation, reduction in edema is most likely achieved by the development of alternate lymphatic pathways. This observation suggests the possibility that a new and potentially promising target for EMF therapy is the lymphatic vessels within and surrounding the wound area.

VII. CONCLUSION

The cumulative substantial evidence from cellular and animal experiments and from human studies strongly indicate important positive linkages between forms of electromagnetic therapy and wound healing. The composite findings provide a firm underlying basis for EMF therapy when used in a thoughtful and selective manner in the treatment of certain chronic or recalcitrant wounds. However, the involved mechanisms remain at best speculative, and there remain large gaps in our understanding of the specific cellular and functional targets, therapeutic dose, and regimens to achieve *optimal* treatment of specific wound types. It is suggested that the complexity of the wound healing process in general, and the differential features of specific chronic wound types in particular, demand a selective approach for choosing EMF therapy parameters, timing, and targets. This implies that therapeutic EMF approaches need to be based both on physical and physiological considerations, which ultimately need to be judged on the basis of therapeutic outcomes. The functional concepts and EMF targets described in this chapter in relation to deficits of specific wound types may provide a basis for continued advances in this still evolving adjunctive therapeutic modality.

REFERENCES

1. Becker RO. Augmentation of regenerative healing in man. A possible alternative to prosthetic implantation. Clin Orthop 1972; 83:255–262.
2. Nordenstrom BE. Impact of biologically closed electric circuits (BCEC) on structure and function. Integr Physiol Behav Sci 1992; 27:285–303.
3. Burr HS, Harvey SC, Taffel M. Bio-electric correlates of wound healing. Yale J Biol Med 1938; 11:104–107.
4. Grimes DI, Lennard RF, Swithenby SJ. Macroscopic ionic currents within the human leg. Phys Med Biol 1985; 30:1101–1112.
5. Foulds IS, Barker AT. Human skin battery potentials and their possible role in wound healing. Br J Dermatol 1983; 109:515–522.
6. Barker AT, Jaffe LF, Vanable JW Jr. The glabrous epidermis of cavies contains a powerful battery. Am J Physiol 1982; 242:R358–366.
7. Vanable JW Jr. Integumentary potentials and wound healing. Electric Fields in Vertebrate Repair: Alan R Liss, Inc. 1989:171–224.
8. Lee RC, Canaday DJ, Doong H. A review of the biophysical basis for the clinical application of electric fields in soft-tissue repair. J Burn Care Rehabil 1993; 14:319–335.
9. Carley PJ, Wainapel SF. Electrotherapy for acceleration of wound healing: low-intensity direct current. Arch Phys Med Rehabil 1985; 66:443–446.
10. Gentzkow GD. Electrical stimulation to heal dermal wounds. J Dermatol Surg Oncol 1993; 19:753–758.
11. Bentall RHC. Low-level pulsed radiofrequency fields and the treatment of soft-tissue injuries. Bioelectr Bioenergetics 1986; 16:531–548.
12. Gardner SE, Frantz RA, Schmidt FL. Effect of electrical stimulation on chronic wound healing: a meta-analysis. Wound Repair Regen 1999; 7:495–503.
13. Akai M, Hayashi K. Effect of electrical stimulation on muscoloskeletal systems: A Meta-analysis of controlled clinical trials. Bioelectromagnetics 2002; 23:132–143.
14. Vodovnik L, Karba R. Treatment of chronic wounds by means of electric and electromagnetic fields. Part 1. Literature review. Med Biol Eng Comput 1992; 30:257–266.
15. Yamaguchi Y, Yoshikawa K. Cutaneous wound healing: an update. J Dermatol 2001; 28:521–534.
16. Holzheimer RG, Steinmetz W. Local and systemic concentrations of pro- and anti-inflammatory cytokines in human wounds. Eur J Med Res 2000; 5:347–355.
17. Gillitzer R, Goebeler M. Chemokines in cutaneous wound healing. J Leukoc Biol 2001; 69:513–521.
18. Nagaoka T, Kaburagi Y, Hamaguchi Y, Hasegawa M, Takehara K, Steeber DA, Tedder TF, Sato S. Delayed wound healing in the absence of intercellular adhesion molecule- 1 or L-selectin expression. Am J Pathol 2000; 157:237–247.
19. Efron DT, Most D, Barbul A. Role of nitric oxide in wound healing. Curr Opin Clin Nutr Metab Care 2000; 3:197–204.
20. Tenaud I, Sainte-Marie I, Jumbou O, Litoux P, Dreno B. In vitro modulation of keratinocyte wound healing integrins by zinc, copper and manganese. Br J Dermatol 1999; 140:26–34.
21. Knighton DR, Hunt TK, Scheuenstuhl H, Halliday BJ, Werb Z, Banda MJ. Oxygen tension regulates the expression of angiogenesis factor by macrophages. Science 1983; 221:1283–1285.
22. Lee RH, Efron D, Tantry U, Barbul A. Nitric oxide in the healing wound: a time-course study. J Surg Res 2001; 101:104–108.
23. Frank S, Kampfer H, Wetzler C, Pfeilschifter J. Nitric oxide drives skin repair: novel functions of an established mediator. Kidney Int 2002; 61:882–888.
24. Laplante AF, Germain L, Auger FA, Moulin V. Mechanisms of wound reepithelialization: hints from a tissue-engineered reconstructed skin to long-standing questions. Faseb J 2001; 15:2377–2389.
25. O'Toole EA. Extracellular matrix and keratinocyte migration. Clin Exp Dermatol 2001; 26:525–530.

26. Spravchikov N, Sizyakov G, Gartsbein M, Accili D, Tennenbaum T, Wertheimer E. Glucose effects on skin keratinocytes: implications for diabetes skin complications. Diabetes 2001; 50:1627–1635.

27. Shi HP, Most D, Efron DT, Tantry U, Fischel MH, Barbul A. The role of iNOS in wound healing. Surgery 2001; 130:225–229.

28. Akcay MN, Ozcan O, Gundogdu C, Akcay G, Balik A, Kose K, Oren D. Effect of nitric oxide synthase inhibitor on experimentally induced burn wounds. J Trauma 2000; 49:327–330.

29. Stacey MC, Mata SD. Lower levels of PAI-2 may contribute to impaired healing in venous ulcers - a preliminary study. Cardiovasc Surg 2000; 8:381–385.

30. Markov M. Electric current and electromagnetic field effects on soft tissue: Implications for wound healing. Wounds 1995; 7:94–110.

31. McCulloch JM, Kloth LC, Feedar JA. Wound healing alternatives in management. In: Wolf SE, ed. Contemporay Perspectives in Rehabilitation. Philadelphia: F. A. Davis, 1995:275–310.

32. Sussman C, Bates-Jensen BM. Wound Care: A Collaborative Practice Manual for Physical Therapists and Nurses. Aspen Publishers, 2001.

33. Markov M, Pilla AA. Electromagnetic stimulation of soft tissues: pulsed radio frequency treatment of postoperative pain and edema. Wounds 1995; 7:143–151.

34. Liboff AR, Jenrow KA. Physical mechanisms in neuroelectromagnetic therapies. Neuro-Rehabilitation 2002; 17:9–22.

35. Fowkes FG, Evans CJ, Lee AJ. Prevalence and risk factors of chronic venous insufficiency. Angiology 2001; 52(Suppl 1):S5–S15.

36. Peschen M, Lahaye T, Hennig B, Weyl A, Simon JC, Vanscheidt W. Expression of the adhesion molecules ICAM-1, VCAM-1, LFA-1 and VLA-4 in the skin is modulated in progressing stages of chronic venous insufficiency. Acta Derm Venereol 1999; 79:27–32.

37. Tassiopoulos AK, Golts E, Oh DS, Labropoulos N. Current concepts in chronic venous ulceration. Eur J Vasc Endovasc Surg 2000; 20:227–232.

38. Smith PD. Update on chronic-venous-insufficiency-induced inflammatory processes. Angiology 2001; 52(Suppl 1):S35–42.

39. Valencia IC, Falabella A, Kirsner RS, Eaglstein WH. Chronic venous insufficiency and venous leg ulceration. J Am Acad Dermatol 2001; 44:401–421. quiz 422–404.

40. Gschwandtner ME, Ehringer H. Microcirculation in chronic venous insufficiency. Vasc Med 2001; 6:169–179.

41. Junger M, Steins A, Hahn M, Hafner HM. Microcirculatory dysfunction in chronic venous insufficiency (CVI). Microcirculation 2000; 7:S3–S12.

42. Mayrovitz HN, Larsen PB. Leg blood flow in patients with venous ulcers: relationship to site and ulcer area. Wounds 1994; 6:195–200.

43. Steins A, Hahn M, Junger M. Venous leg ulcers and microcirculation. Clin Hemorheol Microcirc 2001; 24:147–153.

44. Powell CC, Rohrer MJ, Barnard MR, Peyton BD, Furman MI, Michelson AD. Chronic venous insufficiency is associated with increased platelet and monocyte activation and aggregation. J Vasc Surg 1999; 30:844–851.

45. Saharay M, Shields DA, Porter JB, Scurr JH, Coleridge Smith PD. Leukocyte activity in the microcirculation of the leg in patients with chronic venous disease. J Vasc Surg 1997; 26:265–273.

46. Flemming K, Cullum N. Electromagnetic therapy for the treatment of venous leg ulcers. Cochrane Database Syst Rev 2001; 1.

47. Ieran M, Zaffuto S, Bagnacani M, Annovi M, Moratti A, Cadossi R. Effect of low frequency pulsing electromagnetic fields on skin ulcers of venous origin in humans: a double-blind study. J Orthop Res 1990; 8:276–282.

48. Stiller MJ, Pak GH, Shupack JL, Thaler S, Kenny C, Jondreau L. A portable pulsed electromagnetic field (PEMF) device to enhance healing of recalcitrant venous ulcers: a double-blind, placebo controlled clinical trial. Br J Dermatol 1992; 127:147–154.

49. Kenkre JE, Hobbs FD, Carter YH, Holder RL, Holmes EP. A randomized controlled trial of

electromagnetic therapy in the primary care management of venous leg ulceration. Fam Pract 1996; 13:236–241.

50. Franek A, Polak A, Kucharzewski M. Modern application of high voltage stimulation for enhanced healing of venous crural ulceration. Med Eng Phys 2000; 22:647–655.

51. Canedo-Dorantes L, Garcia-Cantu R, Barrera R, Mendez-Ramirez I, Navarro VH, Serrano G. Healing of chronic arterial and venous leg ulcers with systemic electromagnetic fields. Arch Med Res 2002; 33:281–289.

52. Goldman R, Brewley B, Golden M. Electrotherapy reoxygenates inframalleolar ischemic wounds on diabetic patients. Advances in Skin and Wound Care 2002; 15:112–120.

53. Erdman WJ. Peripheral blood flow measurements during application of pulse high-frequency currents. Amer J Orthop 1960; 2:196–197.

54. Hedenius P, Odeblad E, Wahlstrom L. Some prelimnary investigations on the therapeutic effect of pulsed short waves in intermittent claudication. Current Therapeutic Research 1966; 8:317–321.

55. Mayrovitz HN, Larsen PB. Periwound skin microcirculation of venous leg ulcers. Microvasc Res 1994; 48:114–123.

56. Mayrovitz HN, Larsen PB. Standard and near-surface laser-Doppler perfusion in foot dorsum skin of diabetic and nondiabetic subjects with and without coexisting peripheral arterial disease. Microvasc Res 1994; 48:338–348.

57. Mayrovitz HN, Larsen PB. Functional microcirculatory impairment: a possible source of reduced skin oxygen tension in human diabetes mellitus. Microvasc Res 1996; 52:115–126.

58. Mayrovitz HN, Larsen PB. Effects of pulsed electromagnetic fields on skin microvascular blood perfusion. Wounds 1992; 4:197–202.

59. Mayrovitz HN, Macdonald J, Sims N. Effects of pulsed radio frequency diathermy on postmastectomy arm lymphedema and skin blood flow: A pilot investigation. Lymphology, 2002.

60. Mayrovitz HN, Groseclose EE, Markov M, Pilla AA. Effects of permanent magnets on resting skin blood perfusion in healthy persons assessed by laser Doppler flowmetry and imaging. Bioelectromagnetics 2001; 22:494–502.

61. Mayrovitz HN, Groseclose EE, Sims N. Assessment of the short-term effects of a permanent magnet on normal skin blood circulation via laser-Doppler flowmetry. Scientific Rev Altern Med 2002; 6:5–9.

62. Jacobs MJ, Jorning PJ, Joshi SR, Kitslaar PJ, Slaaf DW, Reneman RS. Epidural spinal cord electrical stimulation improves microvascular blood flow in severe limb ischemia. Ann Surg 1988; 207:179–183.

63. Jacobs MJ, Jorning PJ, Beckers RC, Ubbink DT, van Kleef M, Slaaf DW, Reneman RS. Foot salvage and improvement of microvascular blood flow as a result of epidural spinal cord electrical stimulation. J Vasc Surg 1990; 12:354–360.

64. Graber JN, Lifson A. The use of spinal cord stimulation for severe limb-threatening ischemia: a preliminary report. Ann Vasc Surg 1987; 1:578–582.

65. Mingoli A, Sciacca V, Tamorri M, Fiume D, Sapienza P. Clinical results of epidural spinal cord electrical stimulation in patients affected with limb-threatening chronic arterial obstructive disease. Angiology 1993; 44:21–25.

66. Horsch S, Claeys L. Epidural spinal cord stimulation in the treatment of severe peripheral arterial occlusive disease. Ann Vasc Surg 1994; 8:468–474.

67. Claeys LG. Improvement of microcirculatory blood flow under epidural spinal cord stimulation in patients with nonreconstructible peripheral arterial occlusive disease. Artif Organs 1997; 21:201–206.

68. Kumar K, Toth C, Nath RK, Verma AK, Burgess JJ. Improvement of limb circulation in peripheral vascular disease using epidural spinal cord stimulation: a prospective study. J Neurosurg 1997; 86:662–669.

69. Fromy B, Abraham P, Bouvet C, Bouhanick B, Fressinaud P, Saumet JL. Early decrease of skin blood flow in response to locally applied pressure in diabetic subjects. Diabetes 2002; 51:1214–1217.

70. Gonzalez ER, Oley MA. The management of lower-extremity diabetic ulcers. Manag Care Interface 2000; 13:80–87.

71. Abbott CA, Carrington AL, Ashe H, Bath S, Every LC, Griffiths J, Hann AW, Hussein A, Jackson N, Johnson KE, Ryder CH, Torkington R, Van Ross ER, Whalley AM, Widdows P, Williamson S, Boulton AJ. The North-West Diabetes Foot Care Study: incidence of, and risk factors for, new diabetic foot ulceration in a community-based patient cohort. Diabet Med 2002; 19:377–384.

72. Gilcreast DM, Stotts NA, Froelicher ES, Baker LL, Moss KM. Effect of electrical stimulation on foot skin perfusion in persons with or at risk for diabetic foot ulcers. Wound Repair Regen 1998; 6:434–441.

73. Muller IS, de Grauw WJ, van Gerwen WH, Bartelink ML, van Den Hoogen HJ, Rutten GE. Foot ulceration and lower limb amputation in type 2 diabetic patients in dutch primary health care. Diabetes Care 2002; 25:570–574.

74. Peters EJ, Lavery LA, Armstrong DG, Fleischli JG. Electric stimulation as an adjunct to heal diabetic foot ulcers: a randomized clinical trial. Arch Phys Med Rehabil 2001; 82:721–725.

75. Baker LL, Chambers R, DeMuth SK, Villar F. Effects of electrical stimulation on wound healing in patients with diabetic ulcers. Diabetes Care 1997; 20:405–412.

76. Lundeberg TC, Eriksson SV, Malm M. Electrical nerve stimulation improves healing of diabetic ulcers. Ann Plast Surg 1992; 29:328–331.

77. Sarma GR, Subrahmanyam S, Deenabandhu A, Babu CR, Madhivathanan S, Kesavaraj N. Exposure to pulsed magnetic fields in the treatment of plantar ulcers in leprosy patients—a pilot, randomized, double-blind, controlled clinical trial. Indian J Lepr 1997; 69:241–250.

78. Barczak CA, Barnett RI, Childs EJ, Bosley LM. Fourth national pressure ulcer prevalence survey. Adv Wound Care 1997; 10:18–26.

79. Margolis DJ, Bilker W, Knauss J, Baumgarten M, Strom BL. Venous leg ulcer: incidence and prevalence in the elderly. Ann Epidemiol 2002; 12:321–325.

80. Tourtual DM, Riesenberg LA, Korutz CJ, Semo AH, Asef A, Talati K, Gill RD. Predictors of hospital acquired heel pressure ulcers. Ostomy Wound Manage 1997; 43:24–28, 30, 32–24 passim.

81. Byers PH, Carta SG, Mayrovitz HN. Pressure ulcer research issues in surgical patients. Adv Skin Wound Care 2000; 13:115–121.

82. Mayrovitz HN, Sims N. Biophysical effects of water and synthetic urine on skin. Adv Skin Wound Care 2001; 14:302–308.

83. Mayrovitz HN, Smith JR. Adaptive skin blood flow increases during hip-down lying in elderly women. Adv Wound Care 1999; 12:295–301.

84. Mayrovitz HN, Macdonald J, Smith JR. Blood perfusion hyperaemia in response to graded loading of human heels assessed by laser-Doppler imaging. Clin Physiol 1999; 19:351–359.

85. Mayrovitz HN, Smith J. Heel-skin microvascular blood perfusion responses to sustained pressure loading and unloading. Microcirculation 1998; 5:227–233.

86. Mayrovitz HN, Smith J, Delgado M, Regan MB. Heel blood perfusion responses to pressure loading and unloading in women. Ostomy Wound Manage 1997; 43:16–20, 22, 24 passim.

87. Mayrovitz HN. Pressure and blood flow linkages and impacts on pressure ulcer development. Adv Wound Care 1998; 11:4.

88. Mayrovitz HN, Sims N, Taylor MC. Sacral skin blood perfusion: A factor in pressure ulcers? Ostomy Wound Manage 2002; 48:34–42.

89. Peirce SM, Skalak TC, Rodeheaver GT. Ischemia-reperfusion injury in chronic pressure ulcer formation: a skin model in the rat. Wound Repair Regen 2000; 8:68–76.

90. Sheffet A, Cytryn AS, Louria DB. Applying electric and electromagnetic energy as adjuvant treatment for pressure ulcers: a critical review. Ostomy Wound Manage 2000; 46:28–33, 36–40, 42–24.

91. Flemming K, Cullum N. Electromagnetic therapy for the treatment of pressure sores. Cochrane Database Syst Rev, 2001; 1.

92. Comorosan S, Vasilco R, Arghiropol M, Paslaru L, Jieanu V, Stelea S. The effect of diapulse therapy on the healing of decubitus ulcer. Rom J Physiol 1993; 30:41–45.

93. Salzberg CA, Cooper-Vastola SA, Perez F, Viehbeck MG, Byrne DW. The effects of nonthermal pulsed electromagnetic energy on wound healing of pressure ulcers in spinal cord-injured patients: a randomized, double-blind study. Ostomy Wound Manage 1995; 41:42–44, 46, 48 passim.

94. Itoh M, Montemayor JS Jr, Matsumoto E, Eason A, Lee MH, Folk FS. Accelerated wound healing of pressure ulcers by pulsed high peak power electromagnetic energy (Diapulse). Decubitus 1991; 4:24–25, 29–34.

95. Seaborne D, Quirion-DeGirardi C, Rousseau MMRJL. The treatment of pressure sores using pulsed electromagnetic energy (PEME). Physiotherapy Canada 1996; 48:131–137.

96. Wood JM, Evans PE III, Schallreuter KU, Jacobson WE, Sufit R, Newman J, White C, Jacobson M. A multicenter study on the use of pulsed low-intensity direct current for healing chronic stage II and stage III decubitus ulcers. Arch Dermatol 1993; 129:999–1009.

97. Griffin JW, Tooms RE, Mendius RA, Clifft JK, Vander Zwaag R, el-Zeky F. Efficacy of high voltage pulsed current for healing of pressure ulcers in patients with spinal cord injury. Phys Ther 1991; 71:433–442, discussion 442–434.

98. Stefanovska A, Vodovnik L, Benko H, Turk R. Treatment of chronic wounds by means of electric and electromagnetic fields. Part 2. Value of FES parameters for pressure sore treatment. Med Biol Eng Comput 1993; 31:213–220.

99. Levine SP, Kett RL, Cederna PS, Brooks SV. Electric muscle stimulation for pressure sore prevention: tissue shape variation. Arch Phys Med Rehabil 1990; 71:210–215.

100. Bogie KM, Reger SI, Levine SP, Sahgal V. Electrical stimulation for pressure sore prevention and wound healing. Assist Technol 2000; 12:50–66.

101. Levine SP, Kett RL, Gross MD, Wilson BA, Cederna PS, Juni JE. Blood flow in the gluteus maximus of seated individuals during electrical muscle stimulation. Arch Phys Med Rehabil 1990; 71:682–686.

102. Mawson AR, Siddiqui FH, Connolly BJ, Sharp CJ, Stewart GW, Summer WR, Biundo JJ Jr. Effect of high voltage pulsed galvanic stimulation on sacral transcutaneous oxygen tension levels in the spinal cord injured. Paraplegia 1993; 31:311–319.

103. Yen-Patton GP, Patton WF, Beer DM, Jacobson BS. Endothelial cell response to pulsed electromagnetic fields: stimulation of growth rate and angiogenesis in vitro. J Cell Physiol 1988; 134:37–46.

104. Vodovnik L, Miklavcic D, Sersa G. Modified cell proliferation due to electrical currents. Med Biol Eng Comput 1992; 30:CE21–28.

105. Goodman E, Greenebaum B, Frederiksen J. Effect of pulsed magnetic fields on human umbilical endothelial vein cells. Bioelectricity and Bioenergetics 1993; 32:125–132.

106. Amaral SL, Linderman JR, Morse MM, Greene AS. Angiogenesis induced by electrical stimulation is mediated by angiotensin II and VEGF. Microcirculation 2001; 8:57–67.

107. Greenough CG. The effects of pulsed electromagnetic fields on blood vessel growth in the rabbit ear chamber. J Orthop Res 1992; 10:256–262.

108. Geary GG, Maeda G, Gonzalez RR Jr. Endothelium-dependent vascular smooth muscle relaxation activated by electrical field stimulation. Acta Physiol Scand 1997; 160:219–228.

109. Nikolaev AV, Shekhter AB, Mamedov LA, Novikov AP, Manucharov NK. [Use of a sinusoidal current of optimal frequency to stimulate the healing of skin wounds.] Biull Eksp Biol Med 1984; 97:731–734.

110. Katsir G, Baram SC, Parola AH. Effect of sinusoidally varying magnetic fields on cell proliferation and adenosine deaminase specific activity. Bioelectromagnetics 1998; 19:46–52.

111. Glassman LS, McGrath MH, Bassett CA. Effect of external pulsing electromagnetic fields on the healing of soft tissue. Ann Plast Surg 1986; 16:287–295.

112. Supino R, Bottone MG, Pellicciari C, Caserini C, Bottiroli G, Belleri M, Veicsteinas A. Sinusoidal 50 Hz magnetic fields do not affect structural morphology and proliferation of human cells in vitro. Histol Histopathol 2001; 16:719–726.

113. Bourguignon GJ, Bourguignon LY. Electric stimulation of protein and DNA synthesis in human fibroblasts. Faseb J 1987; 1:398–402.

114. Cruz NI, Bayron FE, Suarez AJ. Accelerated healing of full-thickness burns by the use of high-voltage pulsed galvanic stimulation in the pig. Ann Plast Surg 1989; 23:49–55.

115. Goldman R, Pollack S. Electric fields and proliferation in a chronic wound model. Bioelectromagnetics 1996; 17:450–457.

116. Cheng K, Goldman RJ. Electric fields and proliferation in a dermal wound model: cell cycle kinetics. Bioelectromagnetics 1998; 19:68–74.

117. Cleary SF, Liu LM, Graham R, Diegelmann RF. Modulation of tendon fibroplasia by exogenous electric currents. Bioelectromagnetics 1988; 9:183–194.

118. Dunn MG, Doillon CJ, Berg RA, Olson RM, Silver FH. Wound healing using a collagen matrix: effect of DC electrical stimulation. J Biomed Mater Res 1988; 22:191–206.

119. Franke A, Reding R, Tessmann D. Electrostimulation of healing abdominal incisional hernias by low frequency, bipolar, symmetrical rectangular pulses. An experimental study. Acta Chir Scand 1990; 156:701–705.

120. Lin Y, Nishimura R, Nozaki K, Sasaki N, Kadosawa T, Goto N, Date M, Takeuchi A. Effects of pulsing electromagnetic fields on the ligament healing in rabbits. J Vet Med Sci 1992; 54:1017–1022.

121. George FR, Lukas RJ, Moffett J, Ritz MC. In-vitro mechanisms of cell proliferation induction: A novel bioactive treatment for acceleraing wound healing. Wounds 2002; 14:107–115.

122. Gilbert TL, Griffin N, Moffett J, Ritz MC, George FR. The Provant Wound Closure System induces activation of p44/42 MAP kinase in normal cultured human fibroblasts. Ann N Y Acad Sci 2002; 961:168–171.

123. Biedebach MC. Accelerated healing of skin ulcers by electrical stimulation and the intracellular physiological mechanisms involved. Acupunct Electrother Res 1989; 14:43–60.

124. Loschinger M, Thumm S, Hammerle H, Rodemann HP. Induction of intracellular calcium oscillations in human skin fibroblast populations by sinusoidal extremely low-frequency magnetic fields (20 Hz, 8 mT) is dependent on the differentiation state of the single cell. Radiat Res 1999; 151:195–200.

125. Thumm S, Loschinger M, Glock S, Hammerle H, Rodemann HP. Induction of cAMP-dependent protein kinase A activity in human skin fibroblasts and rat osteoblasts by extremely low-frequency electromagnetic fields. Radiat Environ Biophys 1999; 38:195–199.

126. Binhi VN, Goldman RJ. Ion-protein dissociation predicts 'windows' in electric field-induced wound-cell proliferation. Biochim Biophys Acta 2000; 1474:147–156.

127. Cho MR, Marler JP, Thatte HS, Golan DE. Control of calcium entry in human fibroblasts by frequency-dependent electrical stimulation. Front Biosci 2002; 7:a1–a8.

128. Balcavage WX, Alvager T, Swez J, Goff CW, Fox MT, Abdullyava S, King MW. A mechanism for action of extremely low frequency electromagnetic fields on biological systems. Biochem Biophys Res Commun 1996; 222:374–378.

129. Panagopoulos DJ, Messini N, Karabarbounis A, Philippetis AL, Margaritis LH. A mechanism for action of oscillating electric fields on cells. Biochem Biophys Res Commun 2000; 272:634–640.

130. Weimann BI, Hermann D. Studies on wound healing: effects of calcium D-pantothenate on the migration, proliferation and protein synthesis of human dermal fibroblasts in culture. Int J Vitam Nutr Res 1999; 69:113–119.

131. Huang JS, Mukherjee JJ, Chung T, Crilly KS, Kiss Z. Extracellular calcium stimulates DNA synthesis in synergism with zinc, insulin and insulin-like growth factor I in fibroblasts. Eur J Biochem 1999; 266:943–951.

132. Takasugi N. Calcium-induced vasodilation due to increase in nitric oxide formation in the vascular bed of rabbit ear preparation. Jpn J Pharmacol 1993; 61:177–182.

133. Tran QK, Ohashi K, Watanabe H. Calcium signalling in endothelial cells. Cardiovasc Res 2000; 48:13–22.

134. Mizuno O, Kobayashi S, Hirano K, Nishimura J, Kubo C, Kanaide H. Stimulus-specific alteration of the relationship between cytosolic $Ca(2+)$ transients and nitric oxide production in endothelial cells ex vivo. Br J Pharmacol 2000; 130:1140–1146.

135. Rapp B, de Boisfleury-Chevance A, Gruler H. Galvanotaxis of human granulocytes. Dose-response curve. Eur Biophys J 1988; 16:313–319.

136. Wetzler C, Kampfer H, Stallmeyer B, Pfeilschifter J, Frank S. Large and sustained induction of chemokines during impaired wound healing in the genetically diabetic mouse: prolonged persistence of neutrophils and macrophages during the late phase of repair. J Invest Dermatol 2000; 115:245–253.

137. Kindzelskii AL, Petty HR. Extremely low frequency pulsed DC electric fields promote neutrophil extension, metabolic resonance and DNA damage when phase-matched with metabolic oscillators. Biochim Biophys Acta 2000; 1495:90–111.

138. Kloth LC, McCulloch JM. Promotion of wound healing with electrical stimulation. Adv Wound Care 1996; 9:42–45.

139. Mann A, Breuhahn K, Schirmacher P, Blessing M. Keratinocyte-derived granulocyte-macrophage colony stimulating factor accelerates wound healing: Stimulation of keratinocyte proliferation, granulation tissue formation, and vascularization. J Invest Dermatol 2001; 117: 1382–1390.

140. Gruler H, Nuccitelli R. The galvanotaxis response mechanism of keratinocytes can be modeled as a proportional controller. Cell Biochem Biophys 2000; 33:33–51.

141. Pullar CE, Isseroff RR, Nuccitelli R. Cyclic AMP-dependent protein kinase A plays a role in the directed migration of human keratinocytes in a DC electric field. Cell Motil Cytoskeleton 2001; 50:207–217.

142. Fang K. Directional migration of human keratinocytes in direct current electric fields requires growth factors and calcium and is regulated by epidermal growth factor receptor. J Am Acad Dermatol 2000; 43:702–703.

143. Grose R, Hutter C, Bloch W, Thorey I, Watt FM, Fassler R, Brakebusch C, Werner S. A crucial role of beta 1 integrins for keratinocyte migration in vitro and during cutaneous wound repair. Development 2002; 129:2303–2315.

144. Zhao M, Agius-Fernandez A, Forrester JV, McCaig CD. Directed migration of corneal epithelial sheets in physiological electric fields. Invest Ophthalmol Vis Sci 1996; 37:2548–2558.

145. Nishimura KY, Isseroff RR, Nuccitelli R. Human keratinocytes migrate to the negative pole in direct current electric fields comparable to those measured in mammalian wounds. J Cell Sci 1996; 109:199–207.

146. Farboud B, Nuccitelli R, Schwab IR, Isseroff RR. DC electric fields induce rapid directional migration in cultured human corneal epithelial cells. Exp Eye Res 2000; 70:667–673.

147. Hinsenkamp M, Jercinovic A, de Graef C, Wilaert F, Heenen M. Effects of low frequency pulsed electrical current on keratinocytes in vitro. Bioelectromagnetics 1997; 18:250–254.

148. Kaada B, Eielsen O. In search of mediators of skin vasodilation induced by transcutaneous nerve stimulation: I Failure to block the response by antagonists of endogenous vasodilators. Gen Pharmacol 1983; 14:623–633.

149. Kaada B, Emru M. Promoted healing of leprous ulcers by transcutaneous nerve stimulation. Acupunct Electrother Res 1988; 13:165–176.

150. Cramp AF, Noble JG, Lowe AS, Walsh DM. Transcutaneous electrical nerve stimulation (TENS): the effect of electrode placement upon cutaneous blood flow and skin temperature. Acupunct Electrother Res 2001; 26:25–37.

151. Matsuda T. Changes in human peripheral blood flow obtained by magnetic stimulation. IEEE SMC 1999 Conference Proceedings, International Conference on Systems, Man and Cybernetics, 1999, Vol. 6.

152. Ruocco I, Cuello AC, Parent A, Ribeiro-da-Silva A. Skin blood vessels are simultaneously innervated by sensory, sympathetic, and parasympathetic fibers. J Comp Neurol 2002; 448:323–336.

153. Brown M, McDonnell MK, Menton DN. Polarity effects on wound healing using electric stimulation in rabbits. Arch Phys Med Rehabil 1989; 70:624–627.

154. Van Hoek AH, Sprakel VS, Van Alen TA, Theuvenet AP, Vogels GD, Hackstein JH. Voltage-

dependent reversal of anodic galvanotaxis in Nyctotherus ovalis. J Eukaryot Microbiol 1999; 46:427–433.

155. Mayrovitz HN, Larsen PB. Effects of compression bandaging on leg pulsatile blood flow. Clin Physiol 1997; 17:105–117.

156. Mayrovitz HN. Compression-induced pulsatile blood flow changes in human legs. Clin Physiol 1998; 18:117–124.

157. Malanin K, Kolari PJ, Havu VK. The role of low resistance blood flow pathways in the pathogenesis and healing of venous leg ulcers. Acta Derm Venereol 1999; 79:156–160.

158. Sindrup JH, Avnstorp C, Steenfos HH, Kristensen JK. Transcutaneous PO2 and laser Doppler blood flow measurements in 40 patients with venous leg ulcers. Acta Derm Venereol 1987; 67:160–163.

159. Junger M, Klyscz T, Hahn M, Rassner G. Disturbed blood flow regulation in venous leg ulcers. Int J Microcirc Clin Exp 1996; 16:259–265.

160. Belcaro G, Laurora G, Cesarone MR, De Sanctis MT, Incandela L. Microcirculation in high perfusion microangiopathy. J Cardiovasc Surg (Torino) 1995; 36:393–398.

161. Chittenden SJ, Shami SK, Cheatle TR, Scurr JH, Coleridge Smith PD. Vasomotion in the leg skin of patients with chronic venous insufficiency. Vasa 1992; 21:138–142.

162. Mayrovitz HN. Assessment of Human Microvascular Function. In: Drzewiecki G, Li J, eds. Analysis of Cardiovascular Function. New York: Springer, 1998:248–273.

163. Xu S, Okano H, Ohkubo C. Subchronic effects of static magnetic fields on cutaneous microcirculation in rabbits. In Vivo 1998; 12:383–389.

164. Galvanovskis J, Sandblom J, Bergqvist B, Galt S, Hamnerius Y. Cytoplasmic Ca2+ oscillations in human leukemia T-cells are reduced by 50 Hz magnetic fields. Bioelectromagnetics 1999; 20:269–276.

165. Galvanovskis J, Sandblom J, Bergqvist B, Galt S, Hamnerius Y. The influence of 50-Hz magnetic fields on cytoplasmic Ca2+ oscillations in human leukemia T-cells. Sci Total Environ 1996; 180:19–33.

166. Galvanovskis J, JS. Periodic forcing of intracellular calcium oscillators: Theoretical studies of the effects of low frequency fields on the magnitude of oscillations. Bioelectricity and Bioenergetics 1998; 46:161–174.

167. Dolmetsch RE, Lewis RS, Goodnow CC, Healy JI. Differential activation of transcription factors induced by Ca2+ response amplitude and duration. Nature 1997; 386:855–858.

168. De Koninck P, Schulman H. Sensitivity of CaM kinase II to the frequency of Ca^{2+} oscillations. Science 1998; 279:227–230.

169. Hunt TK, Rabkin J, von Smitten K. Effects of edema and anemia on wound healing and infection. Curr Stud Hematol Blood Transfus 1986; 53:101–113.

170. Hunt TK, Hopf H, Hussain Z. Physiology of wound healing. Adv Skin Wound Care 2000; 13:6–11.

171. Eliska O, Eliskova M. Morphology of lymphatics in human venous crural ulcers with lipodermatosclerosis. Lymphology 2001; 34:111–123.

172. Paavonen K, Puolakkainen P, Jussila L, Jahkola T, Alitalo K. Vascular endothelial growth factor receptor-3 in lymphangiogenesis in wound healing. Am J Pathol 2000; 156:1499–1504.

31

Electric Current Wound Healing

David Cukjati

Laboratory of Biocybernetics, Faculty of Electrical Engineering,
Ljubljana, Slovenia

Rajmond Šavrin

Institute of the Republic of Slovenia for Rehabilitation,
Ljubljana, Slovenia

The authors review the existing physical modalities for treatment of chronic wounds and show the advantages of electric current and electromagnetic field stimulation. Direct currents, low frequency pulsed currents, monophasic high voltage pulses and pulsed electromagnetic fields are compared in respect of their efficiency. Wound healing quantification methods, wound healing dynamics and prognostic factors in the prediction of wound healing proposed by the authors represent significant contribution in understanding the mechanisms of electric wound healing.

I. WOUND HEALING

Skin is a vital organ, in the sense that the loss of substantial fraction of its mass immediately threatens the life of the individual. A *cutaneous* wound is any loss of skin integrity. Such a loss can result suddenly, either from fire or mechanical accident, or it can occur in a chronic manner due to illness, as in skin ulcers. Since intact skin is of vital importance to protect the organism against environment, regenerative mechanisms must be activated to resolve a defect. Cutaneous wound healing is a dynamic biological process that begins with tissue injury. It has several goals:

The discontinuation of further injury

The recruitment of injured cells

The formation of new tissue

The remodeling of the new tissue to best approximate the preinjury form and function.

These events have traditionally been divided into three overlapping phases: an inflammatory phase, a proliferative phase, and a maturation phase.

The inflammatory phase refers to immediate vascular and inflammatory response to injury. The immediate response to blood vessel disruption is activation of the coagulation cascade and the production of blood clot. After several minutes, an acute inflammatory response ensues. Subsequently, leukocytes clear the wound of debris and release growth factors to initiate the healing process. Then follows the proliferative phase involving deposition and formation of granulation tissue, which becomes a new and temporary weak tissue, reepitelization, and wound shrinkage. The maturation phase is characterized clinically by gradual shrinking, thinning, and paling of the scar, leading to decreased bulk but increased tensile strength (1). If any of three overlapping phases of cutaneous wound healing is suppressed, wound healing is prolonged or even prevented. Reasons for slower or retarded healing can be local, such as bacterial infection that prolongs the inflammatory phase; lower oxygen tension that prolongs the proliferative phase; or systemic, such as injuries of the nervous system, diabetes mellitus, atherosclerosis and other vascular diseases, metabolic and ageing problems that affect one or more phases of wound healing.

When conservative methods of wound care cannot facilitate wound healing, the wound is considered to be *chronic*. Such chronic wounds can last for weeks, months, or even years despite adequate and appropriate care. They are difficult and frustrating to manage. Typical chronic wounds are pressure ulcers in spinal-cord-injured patients, ischemic ulcers in lower extremities of patients with peripheral vascular disease, ulcers in geriatric patients, and wounds after limb amputations (2). Patients are subjected to discomfort, stress, and high cost of long-term conventional treatment required for such ulceration to heal.

According to statistic reports, 11% of all hospitalized patients and up to 20% of all elderly home residents suffer from decubital wounds (3). The frequency of decubital wounds in spinal-cord-injured (SCI) patients is quite diverse, ranging from 23% to as much as 85%/ year (4). The percentage of SCI patients that will end up with at least one decubital wound in their lifetime is 85% (5–7). Decubital wounds may be directly responsible for death of 7–8% of patients, while frequently an indirect influence upon the mortality rate through different health complications, such as osteomyelitis or sepsis (8). Diabetic foot ulcers are a common problem and result in more than 85,000 lower extremity amputations each year in the United States. Studies were employed to find the most cost effective treatment of nonhealing wounds (9).

Chronic wound healing represent a major social, medical and economic problem. Therefore an extensive effort has been done to find any treatment modality, which may accelerate the wound-healing process.

II. TREATMENT OF CHRONIC WOUNDS

The understanding of the biological and pathologic events in wound healing has led to three areas of treatment that are currently indicated for the treatment of chronic wounds in the clinic practice (10): grow factors, tissue engineered skin, and physical devices. Despite the vast interest in growth factors and cytokine biology and their potential for wound healing (11,12), clinical trials to accelerate chronic wound healing have in most cases been disappointing. Nevertheless several studies have shown that the application of growth factors may induce the acceleration of cutaneous wound healing in animal models (13). Tissue engineered skin offers the possibility of creating physiologically compatible human skin and are successfully used on burn wounds to prevent bacterial infection and allow the wound the chance to heal by normal reparative processes. Unlike in burn patients, the condition in patients with chronic wounds results from underlying diseases therefore closing wound with skin substitutes would not be sufficient to initiate the wound healing (14). A review of the literature revealed that many adjunctive physical devices were employed and reported to facilitate chronic wound healing, including wound dressings (15), low-level laser therapy (16), low-intensity laser therapy–combined phototherapy (17), ultrasound (18), ultrasound/ultraviolet treatment (19), hyperbaric oxygen (20), electric current stimulation (21,22) and magnetic–electromagnetic field stimulation (23).

According to Sheffet et al. (24) only two treatment-related recommendations receive high ratings for reported experimental evidence of validity: use of moist wound dressings and adjunctive electrical stimulation for nonhealing wounds. The recent reviews of literature revealed advances in the knowledge of electrical wound healing.

III. ELECTRIC CURRENT AND ELECTROMAGNETIC FIELD STIMULATION

Electrical interactions are regulators of many basic physiological processes ranging from conformation of molecules within a cell membrane bilayer to the macroscopic mechanical properties of the tissues. However, there is no well-established mechanism that can explain how weak electric currents and electromagnetic field (EMF) applications affect the behavior of living cells and tissues. The use of electric current and EMF stimulation to enhance wound healing is not new. The pioneer clinical studies range in late 1960s (25). In recent years, electric current and EMF stimulation (electrical stimulation) have become increasingly popular treatment modalities of nonhealing wounds. Electrical stimulation was primarily used to accelerate healing of decubitus ulcers and vein insufficiency. Studies revealed that pressure sores react better on electrical stimulation than other types of wounds (26). In the literature following positive effects of electrical stimulation on chronic wound healing can be found:

Accelerated epitelization and healing
Higher percentage of healed wounds in comparing to conservative treatment and activation of healing when conventional treatment failed
Prevention of tissue necrosis and antibacterial effect
Improved blood circulation
Increased wound contraction
Higher scar elasticity
Increased response of fibroblasts
Decrease of neuropath pain
Decreased peripheral neuropathy

There have been many excellent reviews published on electrical wound healing (21,22,24,27). The results of the first meta-analysis showed that electrical wound healing is effective adjective therapy for chronic wound healing, while relative effectiveness of different types of electrical wound healing is inconclusive (28). Nevertheless, more recent meta-analysis on selected pooled trials could not constitute acceptable proof that electrical stimulation has specific effect on health (29). The survey of existing literature indicates a variety of electric and electromagnetic modalities that have been developed to heal wounds (Table 1) (30–35). Only little uniformity can be found in the literature reporting the use of electrical stimulation with respect to electrical signal properties, placement of stimulation electrodes, and treatment regime. Although electrical stimulation produces a substantial improvement in the healing of chronic wounds, further research is needed to identify which

Table 1 Diversity of Electrical Stimulation Modalities for Chronic Wound Healing

Stimulation type	Application time	Electrode polarity and placement	Wounds
Direct current, 0.2–1 mA (25)	2 h of stimulation, 4 h pause, three times a day.	Negative electrode over ulcer, change of polarity as wound progressed.	Ischemic ulcers
High voltage pulses, 100–175 V, frequency of 105 Hz (30)	45 min/day, 5 days a week	Positive electrode over ulcer, switched if wound healing plateau is reached.	Decubitus ulcers
Monophasic pulsed current (frequency of 128 pps, 64 pps as wound progressed, peak amplitude of 29.2 mA) (31)	30 min, twice daily.	Negative electrode over ulcer, polarity was changed every 3 days and daily as wound progressed.	Pressure, vascular ulcers, trauma or surgery wounds
Alternating constant current square wave pulses (80 pps, pulse width 1ms, intensity-evoking paresthesias) (32)	20 min twice daily for 12 weeks	Electrodes placed outside the ulcer surface area, polarity was changed after each treatment.	Diabetic ulcers
Asymmetric biphasic pulses (40 pps, amplitude up to 35 mA) in trains lasting 4 s, followed by 4 s pause. (33)	30, 60, or 120 min/day	Electrodes placed on the intact skin symmetrically on opposite sides of the wound.	Pressure ulcers
Direct current, 0.6 mA (34)	2 h/day	Positive electrode overlaid the ulcer.	Pressure ulcers
Asymmetric and symmetric biphasic square wave pulses, frequency of 50 pps, amplitude below contraction (35)	90 min/day	Electrodes placed on the intact skin symmetrically on opposite sides of the wound.	Ischemic ulcers

electrical properties are most effective and which wounds response to this best. In following subsections electrical waveforms used in electrical wound healing are divided into subsections: direct current, low-frequency pulsed currents, monophasic high-voltage pulses, and pulsed electromagnetic fields.

A. Direct Current Electrical Stimulation

In normal, uninjured human skin, a difference in ionic concentrations is actively maintained between the upper and lower epidermal layer, which can be measured as a difference of electrical potentials, ranging between 10 and 60 mV on different locations on the body surface. The positive terminal of this so-called epidermal battery is located on the inside surface of the living layer of the epidermis (36). After wounding, when the skin layers are interrupted, the epidermal battery at the wound site is short-circuited, producing a conducting pathway, which allows ionic current to flow through the subepidermal region out of the wound and return to the battery by flowing through the region between the dermis and the living layer. The injury current (in µA range) can only flow, as along as wound surface is moist. The active role of endogenous electrical phenomena in wound healing is indirectly confirmed by the fact that the healing of wounds, the surface of which is kept moist, is more successful than in wounds that are left to dry out. Modeling of wound edge has shown relatively steep lateral voltage gradient across the edge, which means that the cells on the wound edge are situated in an electric field (34). Electric fields on order 100–200 mV/mm have been measured lateral to wounds in mammalian epidermis.

Endogenous wound-induced electric fields present in the cornea plays role in the healing process by helping guide the cellular movements that close wounds. It has been shown that externally applied electrical fields of such "physiological" intensities can affect orientation, migration, and proliferation of cells (37), which are of key importance for healing, such as fibroblasts and keratinocytes (38–41). Several studies have confirmed that externally induced electrical fields with endogenous electrical conditions, positive electrode on the wound surface, and negative on the healthy skin around the wound, accelerate wound healing. Electrical currents were in range from 0.2 mA to 1 mA. The application of negative electrode on wound surface was reported to have antimicrobial effect (25,42) and was stipulated to be useful in initial stage of treatment.

B. Low Frequency Pulsed Electric Currents

Low-frequency pulsed electric current applications are quite popular in physical medicine. They are most commonly used for functional electrical stimulation to provoke involuntary muscle contraction for strengthening muscles atrophied by disuse and for eliciting functional movements in patients with motor disfunction (43,44). Such electric current pulses are also known as tetanizing currents. Low-frequency pulsed electric currents were not applied only locally to the wound but also to areas quite distant to the wound. The two major distant locations were the spinal cord and acupuncture points (21). When low-frequency pulsed electric currents are applied locally both electrodes are placed on the healthy skin surrounding the wound. The amplitude of pulses is set to value just below visible tetanic contraction of surrounding muscles. This treatment modality is noninvasive and simple to use. The formation of chronic wounds is principally caused by an insufficient supply of oxygen and nutrients to the tissues due to poor blood flow. Daily use of low-frequency pulsed electric current stimulation was found to significantly increase partial oxygen tension (pO_2) around the chronic wound while no significant changes of pO_2 were found when direct current electrical stimulation was used (45). Increase of pO_2 during low-frequency pulsed electric current stimulation in patients with ischemic ulcers was caused by beneficial effects on the microcirculation. It is assumed that hypoxia or the release of metabolites during electrical stimulation due to insufficient blood flow and lack of oxygen represents stimuli for capillary growth.

C. Monophasic High-Voltage Pulses

Muscle is contracted at application of low pulse amplitudes and longer durations as well as at large amplitudes and shorter pulse durations. For the use of short high-voltage pulses no physiological explanation could be found. The positive electrode is placed over the wound and voltage set just below that capable of producing visible muscle tetanic contraction. The polarity of electrode over the wound was reversed if treatment reached the healing plateau. Reversing electrode polarity was successful when wounds were infected. Negative electrode placed on the wound has disinfection effect. It is reported that high-voltage stimulation improves blood flow and therefore facilitate wound healing (30,46). It is hypothesized that high-voltage pulses stimulation restores sympathetic tone and vascular resistance below the level of the spinal cord lesion, thereby increasing the perfusion pressure gradient in the capillary beds. As such, high-voltage pulses stimulation could be used for preventing pressure ulcers (47).

D. Pulsed Electromagnetic Fields

Since experimental and clinical data suggested that exogenous electromagnetic fields (EMF) at low levels can have a profound effect on a large variety of biological systems, this led to the use of EMF signals in the treatment of large variety of diseases. It is successfully used clinically in all areas of bone fracture management (48,49). The effect of noninvasive EMF on soft tissues is less well defined and it remains unclear though in vivo animal experiments, in vitro cell research and selected clinical studies confirmed accelerated wound healing. Markov and Pilla (27) in their detailed review of EMF stimulation of soft tissues discuss mechanisms of EMF treatment of nonhealing wounds.

IV. WOUND-HEALING QUANTIFICATION METHODS

Despite the fact that different research groups have demonstrated that electrical stimulation can accelerate wound healing, it is still not widely used. Universal efficiency of electrical stimulation, diversity of small studies, unsuitable wound healing quantification methods, and not well established mechanisms that can explain how electrical stimulation affect the behavior of living cells and tissues render optimization of electrical stimulation difficult. Due to different quantification methods used, it is impossible to make a quantitative analysis of the comparative advantages and disadvantages of different treatment modalities. In order to enable quantification and comparison of treatment efficacy, uniform measure of wound healing needs to be generally accepted, which ideally would fulfill the following criteria: simple calculation, suitable for statistical handling, transparency—evident physiological meaning, employability for different wound types, sizes, shapes, and healing and/or non-healing courses. Quantitative measurement of wound healing should enable service providers to assess, improve, and individualize the treatment given to each wound patient. In order to correctly quantify wound healing wound has to be periodically assessed and wound healing process dynamics has to be considered.

A. Wound Status Assessment

Wound assessments provide the foundation of the plan of care and are the only means of determining the effectiveness of the treatment. Regular reassessments are crucial in clinical trials and practice to provide the care provider an insight into the time course of the wound healing by comparing the series of wound data collected over time (50). Documented reassessments can be reanalyzed for treatment optimization. Chronic wound assessment requires quantification of multiple parameters of the wound and surrounding tissue. Lazarus et al. (51) proposed guidelines for wound assessment. They listed attributes that are clues to the cause, pathophysiology, and status of the wound. Clinical assessment should include wound history, anatomic location, stage, size, sinus tracts, undermining, tunneling, exudate or drainage, necrotic tissue, presence or absence of granulation tissue, and epithelization. Intact skin surrounding the wound should be assessed for redness, warmth, induration or hardness, swelling, and any obvious signs of clinical infection (52).

Assessment of wound status should begin with the extent of the wound. Because the extent of the wound changes with time, it requires periodic assessments. There are several techniques that may be employed to assess wound extent. To be clinically acceptable, the assessment of chronic wound healing has to be noninvasive, inexpensive, and practical enough to be regularly used by clinicians. In several past years number of studies to enhance tools for monitoring healing steeply increased. Studies were primarily focused on periodical noncontact wound status assessments and their documenting. Noncontact systems for wound status assessment base on wound size measurements, mostly on wound area. Systems are in various phases of testing on plaster molds and animal wound models:

> Structured lighting pattern captured on a digital photograph of a wound can be used to calculate the area and volume of debrided wound (53,54).
>
> Computer assist planimetric methods using digitalized tracings of the wound (55).
>
> Three-dimensional laser imaging system for wound area and volume assessment (56).
>
> Digital imaging technique and planimetry for wound area assessment (57).
>
> Laser scanner for wound topography measurement and calculation of wound volume and area assessment (58).

The literature reveals that assessment of wound area, wound perimeter, or mutually perpendicular diameters (largest diameter of the wound and diameter taken at right angle to the largest one) are most frequently used. Classical wound volume and depth assessment techniques are invasive because we have to insert our measuring device or material (dental moulds) into the wound (59). Besides the disturbance of the wound, the volume or depth can be underestimated because of invisible edge at the bottom of the wound and degenerative tissue, which fills up the wound. Invasive measurement methods could interfere with healing; therefore, they are generally avoided. Noncontact methods require expensive equipment such as stereoscopy, MRI (60) or above described novel techniques and are rarely used. Since wounds are often irregular in shape and heal asymmetrically, different estimates of wound area are used. Acetate tracings can provide the most accurate description of wound area and perimeter but require manual or computer planimetry. Automatic wound contour detection methods from digitized images of wounds could in future simplify wound area assessment (61). Estimates of wound area can be calculated from the product of two mutually perpendicular perimeters or by calculation of the area of a circle or ellipse from measured diameters. Surface area can also be estimated by simply comparing ulcers to predrawn circles or ellipses of known area. Results of studies suggest that simple and cost-effective wound area measurement techniques such as ellipse estimate may confidently be used to monitor healing in clinical settings (62–64).

Another wound status assessment possibility is scaling systems where scaling of wound status is determined by one or several indicators of wound healing such as wound extent, necrosis, surrounding skin color, peripheral tissue edema and induration, granulation tissue, epithelialization, infection, drainage, eschar and exudates. Shea, in 1975 was one of the first to propose a standard wound classification system (65). It was based mainly on wound depth and did not focus on presence or absence of infection. Additionally, the system did not mention ischemia as a co-morbid factor. Because of these limitations, several classification systems have been proposed since then (66). There are three widely accepted criteria used to classify the stages of ulcers. The most widely used pressure ulcer scaling system is the four stage system developed by the National Pressure Ulcer Advisory Panel (NPUAP), Merck Manual for decubitus ulcers, and Wagner's Classification system for foot ulcers. NPUAP warns that staging should not be used to determine progress toward the wound healing, because stage IV pressure sore is always a stage IV ulcer no matter how it is healing. For this reason several classification systems have been proposed, that are responsive to changes during wound healing. These systems are still in various stages of testing, but two of the most promising appear to be the seven point categorical Sessing scale (67) and Pressure Ulcer Scale for Healing (PUSH) (68). Recently PUSH system was demonstrated on clinical data to be valid and sensitive measure of pressure ulcer healing (69) with the components of length times width, exudates amount, and tissue type, though further testing is needed to confirm these findings. Scaling systems are widely used as a wound assessment alternative, as they are practical for daily monitoring. However it is still not clear if it is appropriate to use them for the follow-up of changes in wound healing. The small number of stages makes them easy to use but at the same time makes them not sensitive enough for wound healing progress description (70). Based on above considerations wound extent should be evaluated for monitoring wound status when progress toward the wound healing has to be determined.

B. Wound-Healing Process Dynamics

If assessment of wound extent is a quantitative value (a scalar) and is periodically assessed, linear or nonlinear regression can reveal wound healing dynamics over time. The majority of researchers use measures of wound extent that incorporate only wound area, while wound volume, depth, and perimeter are rarely used. Gilman (71) defined a measure of wound extent that incorporated wound area and perimeter and was termed the *advance* of the wound margin toward the wound center. Wound extent is mostly defined either as absolute or normalized wound area. Normalized wound area is calculated as wound area divided by the initial wound area and multiplied by 100. Dynamics of the healing processes followed either by measuring absolute or normalized wound area over time are the same.

Researchers generally use either linear or exponential models to present time course of wound-healing process. Both models are distinguished for small number of parameters, however, neither of models has an adequate physiological basis. Most prominent disadvantage of the linear model is that it sets no limit to wound area. Recent research revealed that time course of wound area had in 51% of wounds included in the study decay exponential shape after initial delay longer than 3.5 days. In 40% of wounds the delay was more than 7 days and in 26% of wounds the delay was more then 14 days. Exponential model correctly described only 49% of time courses of wound area during healing. To consider the observed initial delay of healing a delayed exponential model was proposed for the most general mathematical model of chronic wound-healing dynamics (72). An example of such wound-healing dynamics is presented in Fig. 1 and a mathematical description of the delayed exponential model is given by Eq. (1),

$$\hat{S}(t) = \begin{cases} S_{DEX} & 0 \leq t < T_{DEX} \\ \\ S_{DEX}e^{-\theta_{DEX}(t-T_{DEX})} & t \geq T_{DEX} \end{cases} \tag{1}$$

where $\hat{S}(t)$ is the estimated wound area in percent of initial wound area and three parameters S_{DEX}, θ_{DEX} and T_{DEX} describe the wound healing dynamics. Parameter S_{DEX} (%) estimates initial wound area, and parameter θ_{DEX} (day^{-1}) defines the time constant of exponent function and time delay of the healing process is defined by parameter T_{DEX} (day). It has been demonstrated that this model has good predictive capability and in this capacity can be used to predict time needed to complete wound closure after at least 4 weeks of consecutive weekly measurements of wound area. Such model may be very useful in clinical trials, where not all wounds included in the study close within the designated study period.

Incorporating wound shape information (through wound perimeter) in wound extent measure did not improve wound healing dynamics description (73). Since it is easier to measure wound area than wound area and perimeter, estimation of wound healing dynamics from regular wound area measurements is preferred.

C. Wound-Healing Rate Definition

In spite of the evident need for uniform measure of wound healing rate, several measures have been employed in literature to date. The first group of wound healing rate measures base either on wound size assessments the beginning of the observation period and at its end or on periodical wound size assessments in the observation period. Wound healing rate was estimated as percentage reduction of wound area in 4 weeks (74), as percentage reduction of wound area in 12 weeks (32), as percentage reduction of wound area per day in observation

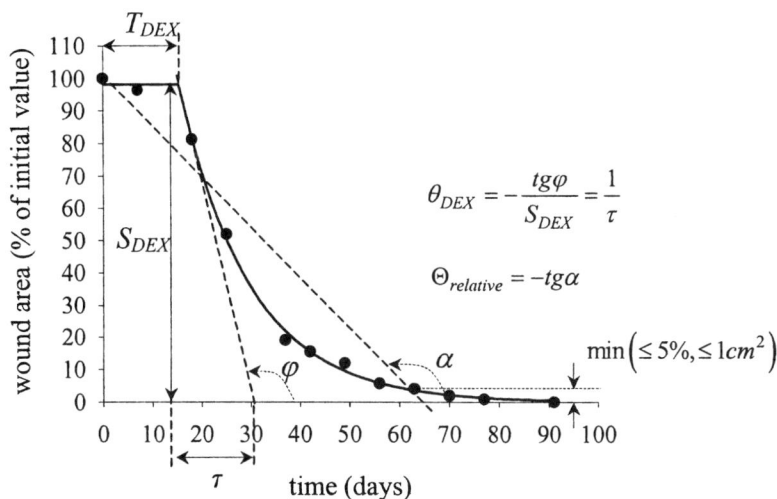

Figure 1 Example of following wound area and application of the delayed exponential model to normalized data. S$_{DEX}$, θ$_{DEX}$, T$_{DEX}$ are calculated parameters of the delayed exponential model, and Θ$_{relative}$ is a measure of wound healing rate. (–) Fitted delayed exponential model; (●) normalized wound area (from Ref. 73).

period (75), as average percentage reduction of wound area per week in 4 weeks (31), as average of the sequentially computed weekly healing rates (normalized difference between two sequential measurements) in percent of initial wound area per week (35), as time needed to complete wound closure (76), as average linear healing of the wound edge toward the center after 2 weeks in distance per day (77), and as time constant of exponential function fit to weekly wound area measurements (33). The second group of wound healing rate measures base on changes in scorings, assessed using classification systems, over time. *Wound-healing rate* was defined as average change in Sessing scale between two consecutive scorings assessed twice per week (67), and as linear regression to PUSH values in the initial, second, fourth, sixth, and eighth week of the observation period (68,78). The majority of authors have used a measure of the wound-healing rate that assumes linear wound extent variation over time. This assumption is misleading since dynamics is nonlinear regardless of how the wound extent is measured.

The goal of wound care is complete wound closure. Therefore, wound healing rate should describe time needed to wound closure and it should be irrespective of wound aetiology, location, and treatment. Wound-healing rate expressed as absolute area healed per day tends to exaggerate the healing rates of larger wounds and healing rate expressed and as percentage of initial area healed per day tends to exaggerate the healing rates of smaller wounds. Wound-healing rate should not be affected by wound size, when wounds of differing sizes are compared. Only wound-healing rate expressed as the advance of the wound margin toward the wound center per day is not influenced by initial wound size (73). The wound-healing rate defined as the advance of wound margin towards the wound center is defined as

$$\Theta = 2\frac{S_0}{p_0}\frac{1}{T} \text{ mm/day} \tag{2}$$

where S_0 is the initial wound area, p_0 is the initial perimeter, and T is the time to complete wound closure. Positive value of wound-healing rate indicates healing wounds and negative value of the wound-healing rate is the estimate of wound growth velocity towards its double initial area. For the wound healing rate Θ to be appropriately calculated, we have to follow the wound-healing process till the complete wound closure. Because clinical trials are financially and time limited, the time to complete wound closure has to be predicted from collected wound extent measurements in observation period, which may be much shorter than time to the complete wound closure. However, prediction of the time to complete wound closure could help clinicians to early detect not efficiently treated wounds. To predict time to complete wound closure wound extent has to be periodically measured and a known model fitted to the collected data. From calculated values of model parameters, the time to complete wound closure can be calculated. Since exponential function reaches its asymptote at infinite time, wound can be defined to be closed when the mathematically predicted wound area is smaller than 5% of initial value and at the same time smaller than 100 mm^2.

V. CLINICAL STUDIES

During more than a decade lasting clinical use of electrical stimulation, data concerning patients, wounds, and their treatment were assessed and documented. The Ethical Committee of the Republic of Slovenia approved the study. The patients were examined by physician for an initial assessment of their wound status and relevant factors. The experimental procedure was explained to them and all patients agreed to participate in the study by signing an informed consent form. Together, 266 patients with 390 wounds were recorded in our computer database up to date. Unfortunately, many patient and wound data are missing, and not all wounds were followed regularly or until the complete wound closure, which is relatively common problem in clinical trials. Wound case inclusion criteria (initial wound area larger than 1 cm^2 and at least four weeks of wound healing process follow-up) were fulfilled in 300 wound cases (214 patients). Our study enrolled wounds of various aetiologies (e.g., vascular ulcerations, amputation wounds, pressure ulcers, neuropathic ulcerations), locations, and different treatments in patients with different primary diagnoses (e.g., spinal cord injury, diabetes mellitus, sclerosis multiplex, vascular diseases).

All patients received conservative treatment of their chronic wounds. The conservative treatment included initial selective debridement, the application of a new standard dressing to the chronic wound two or more times per day, as needed, and broad-spectrum antibiotics in cases of infection, which were rather rare. Fifty-four (18.0%) wounds received only conservative treatment. In addition to the conservative treatment, 23 (7.7%) wounds received sham treatment, where electrodes were applied to the intact skin on both sides of the wound for two hours daily and connected to stimulators, in which, however, the power source was disconnected and they delivered no current. Two different modes of electrical stimulation were used: direct and biphasic current. Forty-two (14.0%) wounds were stimulated with direct current of 0.6mA for 0.5 h, 1 h, or 2 h daily. Positive stimulation electrode overlaid the wound, surface and negative electrode was placed on the intact skin around the wound, or both electrodes were placed on the healthy skin at the wound edge across the wound, one of them being positive and the other negative. We have pooled different electrode placements in direct current stimulation group in spite of the difference in effectiveness of direct current stimulation (34). We did this for two reasons: in literature both electrode placements were shown to accelerate chronic wound healing; and in this way we kept otherwise small direct current stimulation group of wounds at the size that allowed us statistical analysis. One hundred eighty-one (60.3%) wounds were stimulated with biphasic, charge-balanced current pulses (79) for 0.5 h, 1 h, or 2 h daily with electrodes placed on both sides of the wound. The pulse duration was 0.25 ms and at a repetition rate of 40 Hz. The 4-s stimulation trains were rhythmically alternated with pauses of the same duration. The pulsed currents produce tetanic contraction of the stimulated tissue, which is kept at a minimum level (adjusted by the stimulation amplitude, usually at 15 to 25mA) to prevent mechanical damage of the newly formed tissue (Fig. 2).

The currents were applied across the wound by a pair of self-adhesive skin electrodes (Encore TM Plus, Axelgaard Manufacturing Co. Ltd.) attached to the healthy skin at the edge of the wound. In direct stimulation group, where positive stimulation electrode overlaid the wound surface, the wound surface was covered with sterile gauze, soaked in physiological solution, on top of which a conducting rubber electrode was applied. This assured uniform current distribution throughout the entire wound area. Four self-adhesive electrodes were attached to the intact skin around the wound, representing the ring-shaped negative electrode. At the beginning of our study in 1989, wounds were randomly assigned into four treatment groups: conservative treatment, sham treatment, biphasic current stimulation, and direct current stimulation. Since Jerčinović et al. (33) showed that stimulated wounds were healing significantly faster than conservatively or sham treated wounds, it was not ethical to keep including patients in those groups. After Karba et al. (34) reported that electrical stimulation with direct current is effective only if positive electrode is placed on the wound surface, which is an invasive method, only stimulation with biphasic current pulses was used. Therefore, the group of patients stimulated with biphasic current pulses is larger than other groups of patients.

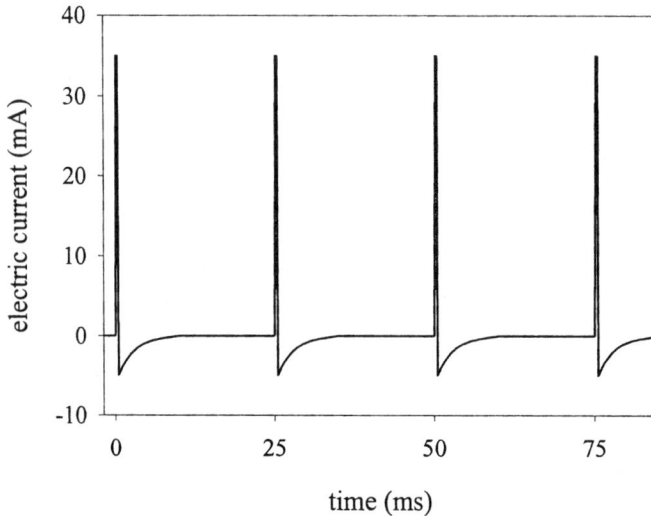

Figure 2   Electrical properties of biphasic electrical current stimulation.

For the evaluation of the efficacy of particular treatment modality or for the evaluation of the influence of wound and patient attributes on wound healing, wound area was periodically followed. Wound shape was approximated with an ellipse and thus it was enough to periodically follow mutually perpendicular diameters of the wound. From wound diameters, the wound area, perimeter, and width-to-length ratio were calculated. As alternative measure of wound extent we used the four-stage Shea grading system (65). Wound depth and grade were collected only at the beginning of treatment. Wounds were treated daily till complete wound closure. If wound did not completely heal within the observation period, the patient continued his treatment at home, but follow-ups were discontinued because the reliability of the home treatment was questionable. Among 300 wound cases, in 174 cases wounds were followed untill complete wound closure, while in 126 cases time to complete wound closure was estimated (72,73). No significant difference between actual time to complete wound closure and estimated one from wound extent measurements in observation period longer than 4 weeks was observed. Because time to complete wound closure was found dependent on initial wound extent, a measure of the wound healing rate an average advance of the wound margin towards the wound centre was used. In Table 2 wound, patient, and treatment data collected in our computer database are listed. These data were selected to be attributes of chronic wound description. All listed attributes except wound extent were collected at the beginning of wound treatment. In addition, wound extent was followed weekly during the observation period or until the complete wound closure.

Plotting percentage of healed wounds against the time elapsed from the beginning of the treatment (Fig. 3) revealed differences between the four treatment groups. Electrically stimulated wounds healed at higher rate and extent than other wounds. Over 90% of electrically stimulated wounds healed within 60 weeks, while only 70% of sham treated wounds and 72% of conservative treated wounds healed within the same period. The wound-healing rate revealed significant differences between four treatment groups. Results of Kolmogorov-Smirnov Two Sample nonparametric test comparing treatment modalities (p values) revealed that wounds treated with biphasic current stimulation healed signifi-

Table 2 Wound, Patient, and
Treatment Data Categories
Collected in a Database
During More Than a Decade
of Using Electrical Stimulation
at the Institute of the Republic
of Slovenia for Rehabilitation

Wound data
  Length of the wound
  Width of the wound
  Depth
  Grade (65)
  Date of wound appearance
  Date of treatment beginning
  Aetiology
  Location
Patient data
  Sex
  Date of birth
  Number of wounds
  Diagnosis
  Date of spinal cord injury
  Degree of spasticity
Treatment data
  Type of treatment
  Daily duration of treatment
  Duration of treatment

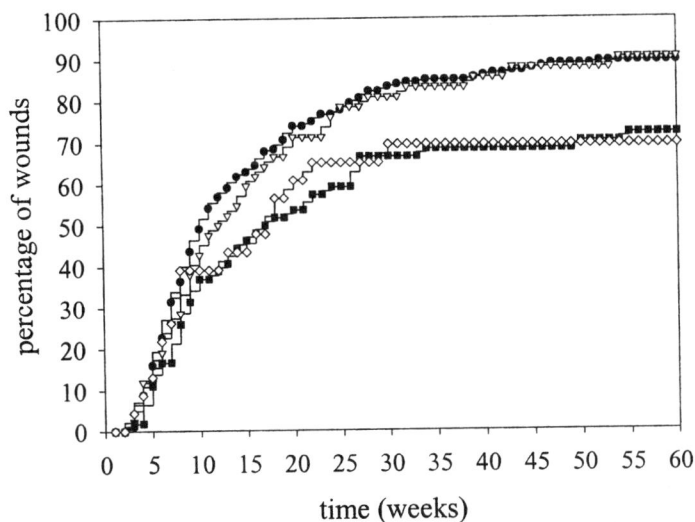

Figure 3 Percentage of healed wounds against time elapsed from beginning treatment for four treatment modalities: (–●–) biphasic current stimulation; (–∇–) direct current stimulation; (–■–) conservative treatment; (–◇–) sham treatment (from Ref. 83).

cantly faster than conservative or sham treated wounds. No significant difference was found in healing rates between wounds treated with direct current and wounds treated with biphasic current pulses. Difference in healing rates between direct current and conservative or sham treatment was considerable, in favor of direct current, although it was not significant. Conservative or sham treated wounds healed at the same rate.

A. Prognostic Factors in the Prediction of Wound Healing

However, dynamics of the wound healing process does not depend only on the type of the treatment, but depends also on wound and patient attributes. The aims of our study were to determine the effects of wound, patient, and treatment attributes on wound-healing process and to propose a system for prediction of the wound healing rate. Only a limited number of groups have investigated wound and patient attributes which affect chronic wound healing (74–76,80,81) and none of them incorporates electrical stimulation as the chronic wound treatment modality. The quantity of available data from our clinical study of electrical wound healing permitted us to employ statistical tools and artificial intelligence methods for analysis of the healing process itself, as well as of the effects of different therapeutic modalities. In the first step of our analysis we determined which wound and patient attributes play a predominant role in the wound-healing process. Then we discussed the possibility to predict wound-healing rate at the beginning of treatment based on initial wound, patient and treatment attributes. Finally we discussed the possibility to enhance the wound healing rate prediction accuracy by predicting it after a few weeks of wound healing follow-up.

1. Wound-Healing Rate Prediction from the Model Wound-Healing Dynamics

We determined that the wound area variation over time has a delayed exponential behavior. Delayed exponential equation is thus the structure of mathematical model of the wound healing process and by fitting this model to a particular chronic wound case; parameters of the model are calculated. At least four measurements of wound area (performed in at least three weeks) are needed before parameters of mathematical model can be estimated. From parameters of mathematical model the time to complete wound closure was estimated.

According to Eq. (2) the estimated wound healing rate was calculated. We found that the estimated wound healing rate after at least 4 weeks of wound follow-up did not differ significantly from the actual one ($p \geq 0.2$). However, if a wound extent was followed less than 4 weeks the difference was found to be significant. In clinical trials 4 weeks is a short period, but in clinical practice a shorter time for treatment outcome prediction may be required.

2. Statistical Analysis

Distribution of the wound healing rate was not normal; non-parametric statistical analysis was therefore employed. To determine differences in distribution of quantitative attributes in groups formed by qualitative attributes we used the Kruskal-Wallis one-way analysis of variance. To test relationship of qualitative attributes, we used a chi-square test. To determine if two quantitative attributes are correlated, we used the Spearman correlation test (rs = Spearman correlation coefficient, p = probability of being wrong in concluding that there is a true association between the variables, and n = number of cases). Statistical analysis revealed that the time to complete wound closure is correlated to wound extent attributes, area ($rs = 0.428$, $p < 0.001$), and grade ($rs = 0.388$, $p < 0.001$). The wound-healing rate is not correlated to initial area, perimeter, or width to length ratio but is moderately correlated to wound grade ($rs = -0.237$, $p < 0.001$, $n = 281$). Wounds of higher grade were healing slower. Wound grade also tends to increase with increasing initial wound area ($rs = 0.292, p < 0.001, n = 281$).

Time elapsed from wound appearance to the beginning of treatment was modestly correlated to wound grade ($rs = 0.181, p = 0.005, n = 243$), which can indicate that wounds should be treated as soon as they appear. Therefore it was also expected that the wound not appropriately treated for a long period would heal slowly (negative correlation coefficient when comparing AppearStart with the wound healing rate) ($rs = -0.215, p < 0.001, n = 243$). A small initial wound area ($rs = -0.261, p < 0.001, n = 178$) of wounds that appeared a long time after spinal cord injury (injuryappear), is probably a result of better patients self care.

Wounds on trochanter healed significantly slower ($p < 0.030$) than wounds on other locations. Locations did not differ with respect to grade ($p = 0.236$) but they differed with respect to area ($p < 0.001$), revealing significantly greater wounds on locations trochanter and sacrum than on gluteus or other locations. Wounds on trochanter, gluteus and sacrum were all pressure ulcers. Patients with wounds on sacrum or trochanter were significantly younger ($p < 0.010$) than patients with wounds on other locations.

Wounds of geriatric (healing rate = 0.271mm/day) and traumatic patients were healing significantly faster ($p = 0.005$) than wounds of patients with other diagnosis: spinal cord injury (0.173 mm/day), vascular insufficiency (0.171 mm/day), diabetes mellitus (0.102 mm/day) and multiple sclerosis (0.138 mm/day). We found diagnosis strongly related to wound aetiology ($p < 0.001$).

Electrically stimulated wounds healed at higher rate and extent than other wounds. Over 90% of electrically stimulated wounds healed within 60 weeks, while only 70% of sham treated wounds and 72% of conservative treated wounds healed within the same period. It was found that wounds treated with biphasic current stimulation healed significantly faster than conservative ($p = 0.031$) or sham ($p = 0.008$) treated wounds. No significant difference ($p = 0.365$) was found in healing rates between wounds treated with direct current and wounds treated with biphasic current pulses. Difference in healing rates between direct current and conservative ($p = 0.085$) or sham treatment ($p = 0.056$) was considerable, in favor of direct current, although it was not significant. Conservative or sham treated wounds healed at the same rate ($p = 0.607$).

Wounds stimulated by biphasic current for 2 h daily healed at the same healing rate as those stimulated for 0.5 h daily, while wounds stimulated for 1h daily healed significantly ($p = 0.017$) faster than wounds stimulated for 2 h or 0.5 h daily. A lack of wound cases stimulated for 1 h daily ($n = 13$) renders this result statistically unreliable. Further study should be performed to optimise daily duration of electrical stimulation.

3. Machine Learning Approach to Wound-Healing Rate Prediction

From results of statistical analysis reported above, it is obvious that the wound healing rate is directly dependent on wound treatment and wound grade, while interactions of other wound and patient attributes on the wound healing rate are not easy to determine. Prognostic factors of wound healing are rarely analyzed in the literature and our study was first attempt to incorporate electrical stimulation as the chronic wound treatment modality. We employed tree learning algorithms to build regression and classification trees to predict the wound healing rate based on initial wound, patient and treatment data. We tested several algorithms for attribute selection among which RReliefF (82) for regression tree generation was found to be the most effective (83). For models in leaves of the tree, the most appropriate were linear equations. A stopping rule of minimal five wound cases in a leaf was used. Since the sample size ($n = 300$) was moderate, the 10-fold cross-validation was used as the error estimation method. The accuracy of regression trees was measured as relative squared error (relative error) (84), which is always nonnegative and usually less than 1. Trees with relative error close to 0 produce good prediction of the wound healing rate, and trees with the relative error around 1 or even greater than 1 produce poor prediction.

Attributes partitioning powers calculated using machine learning algorithm RReliefF revealed that initial wound area, followed by patient's age and time from wound appearance to treatment beginning are the most prognostic attributes, followed by wound shape (width-to-length ratio), location of wound, and type of treatment. Generated regression trees with linear equations in leaves for the wound healing rate prediction at the beginning of treatment had relative squared error greater than one, which means that resulting regression trees are not usable. Adding the model estimate of the wound-healing rate in a set of variables used for regression tree generation reduced relative error of generated regression tree. Wound-healing rate estimated only after 1 week of wound area follow-up reduced the relative error of generated regression tree to 0.64, similarly after 2 weeks to 0.35, after 3 weeks to 0.18 (Fig. 4) and after 4 weeks of follow-up to 0.09. Afterwards relative error was slowly decreasing to 0.06 in 6 weeks of follow-up. After 5 weeks, the wound-healing rate predicted by regression tree was equal to the healing rate estimated by the delayed exponential model. The predicted wound-healing rate in shorter period in addition depends on wound, patient, and treatment attributes. Rough estimation of wound healing rate can be determined only after 2 weeks of wound healing follow-up. Type of treatment is indirectly included in regression trees as daily duration of treatment, which was zero in case of conservative or sham treated wounds. Important prognostic attributes are wound area, grade, shape (width to length ratio), patients age, elapsed time from spinal cord injury to wound appearance, and elapsed time from wound appearance to the beginning of treatment.

Considering also prognostic factors: deep vein involvement, ankle/brachial pressure index, liposclerosis, edema, exudates and granulation, which are reported in the literature (74,80) as prognostic factors, our prediction might be even more accurate. Regression trees in combination with prediction capability of delayed exponential model of wound healing dynamics are basis for the prognostic system for prediction of chronic wound healing rate.

B. Quantitative and Qualitative Changes in the Tissue After Electrical Wound Healing

The proof weather a method of treating wounds is successful is a matter of histological analyses of the affected soft tissue before and after treatment (85,86). Reports of histological

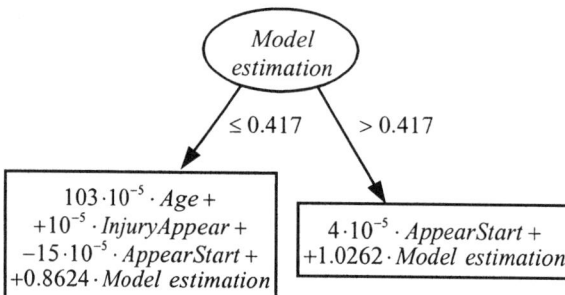

Figure 4 Regression tree with linear equations in leaves for prediction of wound healing rate after 3 weeks of treatment (from Ref. 83).

analyses of electrical wound healing are rare especially in clinical trials. At the Institute of Rehabilitation a histological study of electrical wound healing was done recently. The study enrolled 50 patients with spinal cord injury, suffering from decubital ulcers of III degree according to Shae scale (65) in the sacral area. A half of wounds were treated according to described biphasic electrical stimulation treatment and another half received only conservative treatment. In five patients from each group a qualitative and a quantitative histological analyses of the tissue samples (about 4 mm^3) taken from the wound, on the line between the wound edge and freshly formed scar, were performed before the beginning of treatment and after around 2 months, when the formed scar formed during the electrical stimulation was of considerable size.

Wound healing was followed as described in above clinical study section. Significantly faster healing of wounds in electrically stimulated group was observed. The histological preparations were analyzed by a quantitative stereological method. Content of surface collagen in the preparations stained according to Masson and the surface density of blood vessels was determined in the immunohistochemically stained preparations. The surface percentage of collagen was determined by using test system M-42 and the number of blood vessels per surface unit by a semiautomatic IBAS 1000 image processing and analysis system. Wounds treated by electrical stimulation had lower inflammatory response, higher collagen density as well as more intense process of angiogenesis. In electrically healed group collagen density increased in average 23%, while in the control group decreased by 2% of the initial surface in two months time period. The area density of blood vessels was higher in electrically stimulated wounds, and in poststimulation period the blood vessels were found to be reaching essentially higher towards the wound surface than in the nonstimulated wounds, in fact, almost as far as the crust.

In stimulated wounds endothelial cells were flat, the blood vessels lumina broad with erythrocytes clearly visible within them. In control group endothelial cells were thickened, cubically shaped, with round nuclei, and no erythrocytes were visible within blood vessels lumina. Also previous in vitro studies (37,87) reported flatter endothelial cells exposed to electromagnetic or electric field, which are of cubic shape when not exposed to the field.

The study showed that the intercellular substance is dominated by fibrin whereas more collagen was found in the sample preparations of electrically healed wounds. The conclusion is that electrical stimulation may exert the release of mediators responsible for the increase in collagen synthesis in fibroblasts or the shrinking of myofibroblasts. Furthermore the study showed that electrical healing has a favorable effect on blood circulation in the wound, improves blood circulation in the tissue surrounding the wound and improves the quality of posttreatment scar.

VI. CONCLUSIONS

One of the largest clinical studies of electrical wound healing and its outcomes are presented. Electrically stimulated wounds healed faster and at greater percentage than conservative or sham treated wounds. We noticed slightly slower healing of wounds treated with direct current than wounds treated with biphasic current, but both treatment modalities accelerate wound healing of chronic wounds. Histological analysis confirmed positive effects of biphasic current electrical stimulation, such as improved blood circulation in the wound and surrounding tissue, as well as improved posttreatment scar.

Electrical treatment regime should in future be optimized regarding electrical parameters used and daily duration of treatment. However it should also be determined which treatment regimes apply best for different wound aetiologies. Unified wound-healing quantification and documentation will enable researchers to optimize electrical wound healing and promote it in clinical practice.

It was demonstrated that wound healing process can be weekly followed by simple wound area and perimeter measurements. In future non contact measuring devices will simplify wound extent measurement and documentation. For accurate wound-healing rate estimation, wounds should be followed at least 4 weeks, while using generated regression trees follow-up can be reduced to 3 weeks for wound healing estimation with relative error 0.18. Therefore, the wound-healing rate or the time to complete wound closure can be estimated after 3 weeks of treatment, which can help to formulate appropriate management decisions, reduce the cost, and orient resources to those individuals with poor prognosis.

ACKNOWLEDGEMENTS

The authors are in depth to Prof. Damijan Miklavčič for his valuable help during the chapter preparation. This work was supported by Slovenian Ministry for Education, Science and Sport.

REFERENCES

1. Waldorf H, Fewkes J. Wound healing. Adv Dermatol 1995; 10:77–97.
2. Dagher JF. Cutaneous Wounds. Mount Kisco, NY: Futura Publishing Company, 1985:99–220.
3. Sanders SL. Pressure ulcers, Part 1: Prevention strategies. J Am Acad Nurse Pract 1992; 4(2):63–70.
4. Whiteneck GG, Charlifue SW, Frankel HL, Fraser MH, Gardner BP, Gerhart KA. Mortality, morbidity, and psychosocial outcomes of persons spinal cord injured more than 20 years ago. Paraplegia 1992; 30(9):617–630.
5. Richardson RR, Meyer PR. Prevalence and incidence of pressure sores in acute spinal-cord injuries. Paraplegia 1981; 19(4):235–247.
6. Mawson AR, Biundo JJ, Neville P, Linares HA, Winchester Y, Lopez A. Risk-factors for early occurring pressure ulcers following spinal-cord injury. Am J Phys Med Rehabil 1988; 67(3):123–127.
7. Fuhrer MJ, Garber SL, Rintala DH, Clearman R, Hart KA. Pressure ulcers in community-resident persons with spinal-cord injury—prevalence and risk-factors. Arch Phys Med Rehabil 1993; 74(11):1172–1177.
8. Goodman CM, Cohen V, Armenta A, Thornby J, Netscher DT. Evaluation of results and treatment variables for pressure ulcers in veteran spinal cord-injured patients. Ann Plast Surg 1999; 42(6):665–672.
9. Kantor J, Margolis DJ. Treatment options for diabetic neuropathic foot ulcers: A cost-effectiveness analysis. Dermatol Surg 2001; 27(4):347–351.
10. Braddock M, Campbell CJ, Zuder D. Current therapies for wound healing: electrical stimulation, biological therapeutics, and the potential for gene therapy. Int J Dermatol 1999; 38(11):808–817.
11. Martin P, Hopkinson-Woolley J, McCluskey J. Growth factors and cutaneous wound repair. Prog Growth Factor Res 1992; 4(1):25–44.
12. Kunimoto BT. Growth factors in wound healing: the next great innovation? Ostomy Wound Manage 1999; 45(8):56–64.
13. Limova M. New therapeutic options for chronic wounds. Dermatol Clin 2002; 20(2):357–+.
14. Beele H. Artificial skin: Past, present and future. Int J Artif Organs 2002; 25(3):163–173.
15. Kannon GA, Garett AB. Moist wound healing with occlusive dressings. A clinical review. Dermal Surg 1995; 21:583–590.
16. Lucas C, Coenen CHM, de Haan RJ. The effect of low level laser therapy (LLLT) on stage III

decubitus ulcers (pressure sores); a prospective randomised single blind, multicentre pilot study. Lasers in Medical Science 2000; 15(2):94–100.

17. Lagan KM, McKenna T, Witherow A, Johns J, McDonough SM, Baxter GD. Low-intensity laser therapy/combined phototherapy in the management of chronic venous ulceration: A placebo-controlled study. J Clin Laser Med Surg 2002; 20(3):109–116.

18. Brown M. Ultrasound for wound management. In: Gogia Prem P, ed. Clinical Wound Manage. Thorofare: SLACK, 1995:197–206.

19. Nessbaum EL, Biemann I, Mustard B. Comparison of ultrasound/ultraviolet-C and laser for treatment of pressure ulcers in patients with spinal cord injury. Phys Ther 1994; 74(9):812–825.

20. Kalani M, Jorneskog G, Naderi N, Lind F, Brismar K. Hyperbaric oxygen (HBO) therapy in treatment of diabetic foot ulcers—Long-term follow-up. J Diabetes Complications 2002; 16(2): 153–158.

21. Vodovnik L, Karba R. Treatment of chronic wounds by means of electric and electromagnetic fields, Part 1 Literature review. Med Biol Eng Comput 1992; 30:257–266.

22. Markov MS. Electric-current and electromagnetic-field effects on soft-tissue-implications for wound-healing. Wounds—A Compendium of Clinical Research and Practice 1995; 7(3):94–110.

23. Markov MS, Colbert AP. Magnetic and electromagnetic field therapy. J Back Musculoskel Rehabil 2000; 15(1):17–29.

24. Sheffet A, Cytryn AS, Louria DB. Applying electric and electromagnetic energy as adjuvant treatment for pressure ulcers: a critical review. Ostomy Wound Manage 2000; 46(2):28–33, 36–40, 42–44.

25. Wolcott LE, Wheeler PC, Hardwicke HM, Rowley BA. Accelerated healing of skin ulcers by electrotherapy: preliminary clinical results. South Med J 1969; 62:795–801.

26. Cuddigan J, Frantz RA. Pressure ulcer research: pressure ulcer treatment. A monograph from the National Pressure Ulcer Advisory Panel. Adv Wound Care 1998; 11(6):294–300.

27. Markov MS, Pilla AA. Electromagnetic-field stimulation of soft-tissues-pulsed radio-frequency treatment of postoperative pain and edema. Wounds—A Compendium of Clinical Research and Practice 1995; 7(4):143–151.

28. Gardner SE, Frantz RA, Schmidt FL. Effect of electrical stimulation on chronic wound healing: a meta-analysis. Wound Repair Regen 1999; 7(6):495–503.

29. Akai M, Hayashi K. Effect of electrical stimulation on musculoskeletal systems; A meta-analysis of controlled clinical trials. Bioelectromagnetics 2002; 23(2):132–143.

30. Kloth LC, Feedar JA. Acceleration of wound-healing with high-voltage, monophasic, pulsed current. Phys Ther 1988; 68(4):503–508.

31. Feedar JA, Kloth LC, Gentzkow GD. Chronic dermal ulcer healing enhanced with monophasic pulsed electrical stimulation. Phys Ther 1991; 71(9):639–649.

32. Lundeberg TCM, Eriksson SV, Malm M. Electrical nerve stimulation improves healing of diabetic ulcers. Ann Plast Surg 1992; 29:328–331.

33. Jerčinović A, Karba R, Vodovnik L, Stefanovska A, Krošelj P, Turk R. Low frequency pulsed current and pressure ulcer healing. IEEE Trans Rehabil Eng 1994; 2(4):225–233.

34. Karba R, Šemrov D, Vodovnik L, Benko H, Šavrin R. DC electrical stimulation for chronic wound healing enhancement. Part 1. Clinical study and determination of electrical field distribution in the numerical wound model. Bioelectrochem Bioenerg 1997; 43:265–270.

35. Baker LL, Chambers R, DeMuth SK, Villar F. Effects of electrical stimulation on wound healing in patients with diabetic ulcers. Diabetes Care 1997; 20(3):405–412.

36. Barker AT, Jaffe LF, Vanable JW, Jr. The glabrous epidermis of cavies contains a powerful battery. Am J Physiol 1982; 242(3):358–366.

37. Robinson KR. The responses of cells to electrical fields—a review. J Cell Biol 1985; 101(6):2023–2027.

38. Sheridan DM, Isseroff RR, Nuccitelli R. Imposition of a physiologic DC electric field alters the migratory response of human keratinocytes on extracellular matrix molecules. J Invest Dermatol 1996; 106(4):642–646.

39. Nishimura KY, Isseroff RR, Nuccitelli R. Human keratinocytes migrate to the negative pole in

direct current electric fields comparable to those measured in mammalian wounds. J Cell Sci 1996; 109:199–207.

40. Farboud B, Nuccitelli R, Schwab IR, Isseroff RR. DC electric fields induce rapid directional migration in cultured human corneal epithelial cells. Exp Eye Res 2000; 70(5):667–673.

41. Pullar CE, Isseroff RR, Nuccitelli R. Cyclic AMP-dependent protein kinase a plays a role in the directed migration of human keratinocytes in a DC electric field. Cell Motil Cytoskeleton 2001; 50(4):207–217.

42. Gault WR, Gatens PF. Use of the low intensity direct current in management of ischemic skin ulcers. Phys Ther 1976; 56:265–269.

43. Munih M, Ichie M. Current status and future prospects for upper and lower extremity motor system neuroprostheses. Neuromodulation 2001; 4(4):176–185.

44. Bajd T, Cikajlo I, Šavrin R, Erzin R, Gider F. FES rehabilitative systems for re-education of walking in incomplete spinal cord injured persons. Neuromodulation 2000; 3(3):167–174.

45. Likar B, Poredoš P, Prešern-Štrukelj M, Vodovnik L, Klešnik M. Effects of electric current on partial oxygen tension in skin surrounding wounds. Wounds-A Compendium of Clinical Research and Practice 1993; 5(1):32–36.

46. Feedar JA, Kloth LC. Acceleration of wound healing with high-voltage pulsating direct current. Phys Ther 1985; 65(5):741.

47. Mawson AR, Siddiqui FH, Connolly BJ, Sharp CJ, Stewart GW, Summer WR, et al. Effect of high-voltage pulsed galvanic stimulation on sacral transcutaneous oxygen-tension levels in the spinal-cord injured. Paraplegia 1993; 31(5):311–319.

48. Bassett CAL. Bioelectromagnetics in the service of medicine. Electromagnetic Fields 1995; 250:261–275.

49. Bassett CAL. Beneficial-effects of electromagnetic-fields. J Cell Biochem 1993; 51(4):387–393.

50. vanRijswijk L. Wound assessment and documentation. Wounds—A Compendium of Clinical Research and Practice 1996; 8(2):57–69.

51. Lazarus GS, Cooper DM, Knighton DR, Margolis DJ, Pecoraro RE, Rodeheaver G, et al. Definitions and guidelines for assessment of wounds and evaluation of healing. Arch Dermatol 1994; 130:489–493.

52. Maklebust JA. Pressure ulcer assessment. Clin Geriatr Med 1997; 13(3):455.

53. Plassmann P, Jones TD. MAVIS: a non-invasive instrument to measure area and volume of wounds. Med Eng Phys 1998; 20(5):332–338.

54. Krouskop TA, Baker R, Wilson MS. A noncontact wound measurement system. J Rehabil Res Dev 2002; 39(3):337–345.

55. Richard JL, Daures JP, Parer-Richard C, Vannereau D, Boulot I. Of mice and wounds reproducibility and accuracy of a novel planimetry program for measuring wound area. Wounds-A Compendium of Clinical Research and Practice 2000; 12(6):148–154.

56. Patete PV, Bulgrin JP, Shabani MM, Smith DJ. A non-invasive, three-dimensional, diagnostic laser imaging system for accurate wound analysis. Physiol Meas 1996; 17(2):71–79.

57. Rajbhandari SM, Harris ND, Sutton M, Lockett C, Eaton S, Gadour M, et al. Digital imaging: an accurate and easy method of measuring foot ulcers. Diabet Med 1999; 16(4):339–342.

58. Marjanovic D, Dugdale RE, Vowden P, Vowden KR. Measurement of the volume of a leg ulcer using a laser scanner. Physiol Meas 1998; 19(4):535–543.

59. Covington JS, Griffin JW, Mendius RK, Tooms RE, Clifft JK. Measurement of pressure ulcer volumes using dental impression matherials: suggestions from the field. Phys Ther 1989; 69:690–694.

60. Helbich TH, Roberts TPL, Rollins MD, Shames DM, Turetschek K, Hopf HW, et al. Non-invasive assessment of wound-healing angiogenesis with contrast-enhanced MRI. Acad Radiol 2002; 9:S145–S147.

61. Jones TD, Plassmann P. An active contour model for measuring the area of leg ulcers. IEEE Trans Med Imaging 2000; 19(12):1202–1210.

62. Stefanovska A, Vodovnik L, Benko H, Turk R. Treatment of chronic wounds by means of electric and electromagnetic fields. Part 2. Value of FES parameters for pressure sore treatment. Med Biol Eng Comput 1993; 31:213–220.

63. Mayrovitz HN. Shape and area measurement considerations in the assessment of diabetic plantar ulcers. Wounds—A Compendium of Clinical Research and Practice 1997; 9(1):21–28.

64. Kantor J, Margolis DJ. Efficacy and prognostic value of simple wound measurements. Arch Dermatol 1998; 134(12):1571–1574.

65. Shea JD. Pressure sores-classification and management. Clin Orthop 1975; 112:89–100.

66. Russell L. Pressure ulcer classification: the systems and the pitfalls. Br J Nurs 2002; 11(12):49–59.

67. Ferrell BA, Artinian BM, Sessing D. The sessing scale for assessment of pressure ulcer healing. J Am Geriatr Soc 1995; 43:37–40.

68. Bartolucci AA, Thomas DR. Using principal component analysis to describe wound status. Adv Wound Care 1997; 10(5):93–95.

69. Stotts NA, Rodeheaver GT, Thomas DR, Frantz RA, Bartolucci AA, Sussman C, et al. An instrument to measure healing in pressure ulcers: Development and validation of the Pressure Ulcer Scale for Healing (PUSH). Journals of Gerontology Series A—Biological Sciences and Medical Sciences 2001; 56(12):M795–M799.

70. Johnson M, Miller R. Measuring healing in leg ulcers: Practice considerations. Appl Nurs Res 1996; 9(4):204–208.

71. Gilman TH. Parameter for measurement of wound closure. Wounds 1990; 3:95–101.

72. Cukjati D, Reberšek S, Karba R, Miklavčič D. Modelling of chronic wound healing dynamics. Med Biol Eng Comput 2000; 38(3):339–347.

73. Cukjati D, Reberšek S, Miklavčič D. A reliable method of determining wound healing rate. Med Biol Eng Comput 2001; 39(2):263–271.

74. Johnson M. Using cluster analysis to develop a healing typology in vascular ulcers. J Vasc Nurs 1997; 15:45–49.

75. Lyman IR, Tenery JH, Basson RP. Corelation between decrease in bacterial load and rate of wound healing. Surg Gynecol Obstet 1970; 130(4):616–620.

76. Birke JA, Novick A, Patout CA, Coleman WC. Healing rates of plantar ulcers in leprosy and diabetes. Leprosy Rev 1992; 63:365–374.

77. Gorin DR, Cordts PR, LaMorte WW, Menzoian JO. The influence of wound geometry on the measurement of wound healing rates in clinical trials. J Vasc Surg 1996; 23:524–528.

78. Cuddigan J. Pressure ulcer classification: What do we have? What do we need? Adv Wound Care 1997; 10(5):13–15.

79. Karba R, Vodovnik L, Prešern-Štrukelj M, Klešnik M. Promoted healing of chronic wounds due to electrical stimulation. Wounds 1991; 3(1):16–23.

80. Skene AI, Smith JM, Doré CJ, Charlett A, Lewis JD. Venous leg ulcers: a prognostic index to predict time to healing. BMJ 1992; 305:1119–1121.

81. Kantor J, Margolis DJ. A multicentre study of percentage change in venous leg ulcer area as a prognostic index of healing at 24 weeks. Brit J Dermatol 2000; 142(5):960–964.

82. Robnik-Šikonja M, Kononenko I. An adaption of Relief for attribute estimation in regression. In: Dough F, ed. Machine Learning: Proceedings of the Fourteenth International conference on Machine learning. San Mateo, California: Morgan Kaufman Publ., 1997:296–304.

83. Cukjati D, Robnik-Šikonja M, Reberšek S, Kononenko I, Miklavčič D. Prognostic factors in the prediction of chronic wound healing by electrical stimulation. Med Biol Eng Comput 2001; 39(5):542–550.

84. Breiman L, Friedman JH, Olshen RA, Stone CJ. Classification and regression trees. Belmont, California: Wadsworth International Group, 1984.

85. Herrick SE, Sloan P, Mcgurk M, Freak L, Mccollum CN, Ferguson MWJ. Sequential changes in histologic pattern and extracellular-matrix deposition during the healing of chronic venous ulcers. Am J Pathol 1992; 141(5):1085–1095.

86. Reger SI, Hyodo A, Negami S, Kambic HE, Sahgal V. Experimental wound healing with electrical stimulation. Artif Organs 1999; 23(5):460–462.

87. Yenpatton GPA, Patton WF, Beer DM, Jacobson BS. Endothelial-cell response to pulsed electromagnetic-fields-stimulation of growth rate and angiogenesis in vitro. J Cell Physiol 1988; 134(1):37–46.

32

Pulsed Magnetic Therapy for the Treatment of Incontinence, Disuse Atrophy, Muscle Spasm, and Muscle Reeducation to Increase Mobility

Kent Davey

American Maglev Technology, Edgewater, Florida, U.S.A.

A novel FDA approved device for the treatment of urinary incontinence and muscle atrophy and spasm is described, and the mechanisms of action responsible for its efficacy are explained.

The effects of electrical stimulation on nerve, muscle, and other structures have been studied for over 200 years, starting with Galvani's frog experiments. Faraday allegedly experimented with the use of rapidly changing magnetic fields to induce a flow of current in tissue (1), and in recent years, there has been a particular interest in magnetic field stimulation to evaluate brain dysfunction. Devices generally use aircore simulators to induce cranial stimulation for diagnostic purposes (2). The use of specially fabricated magnetizable cores can significantly improve the efficiency of this procedure because less power is required, there is more flexibility in frequency selection, and a more precise focus can be directed to the targeted area. This proprietary enhanced containment structure allows us to stimulate muscle groups at frequencies up to nearly 50 Hz in a stimulus cycle having a period of 2 to 10 s. By using multiple cores, a smaller section area or muscle group can be specifically stimulated thus reducing effects on adjacent tissues.

It is generally held that magnetic fields cannot have biological effects unless there is motion of or within the field. The static magnetic fields emanating from the poles of permanent magnets are motionless. By contrast, time-varying magnetic fields induce an electrical field whose magnitude is proportional to its rate of change. These induced electrical fields circulate around magnetic field lines. Unlike the fields produced by functional electrical stimulation procedures, they require no electrodes and have no discretely defined input and exit points. Nevertheless, they perform in an identical fashion with respect to transmitting a charge through a neuron boundary, thus increasing the potential inside that boundary. When that increase in potential exceeds the threshold necessary for an action potential, the nerve fires. Unlike heat or x-rays, magnetic fields are unaffected by bone or body tissues, which is one of the advantages of magnetic resonance imaging as a diagnostic aid, particularly with respect to intracranial pathology. Pulsed magnetic field stimulation therapy provides similar advantages because its ability to freely penetrate bone and other structures make it a convenient and safe way to penetrate internal sites.

As shown in Fig. 1, a quiescent nerve has a characteristic resting potential of −90 mV with respect to the extracellular fluid. The time-variable magnetic field is indicated by the circle and X on the figure is commensurate with an electric field depicted by the dotted arrow, and it is the electric field gradient that gives rise to the current that drives the charge into the intercellular space and raises its internal potential. If the rise in internal potential is sufficient to initiate an action potential, the sodium gates in the cell membrane wall open followed subsequently by the opening of the potassium gates. The influx of sodium ions and subsequent efflux of potassium ions gives rise to the characteristic action potential that propagates in both directions away from the stimulus site. The electric field in the cell interior has a spacial gradient that gives rise to a change in the intercellular field potential. It is important to reemphasize that there is *no physiologic difference* between the action potential initiated by an electric field delivered via surface electrodes and the action potential that can be induced by specific electromagnetic fields.

As illustrated in Fig. 2a, an AC line voltage is transformed to higher voltage and then fed to a diode bridge to deliver a high-voltage DC field level. The major function of this DC field is to charge a capacitor to supply the energy that excites the stimulation core. The remaining components of the device merely act as switches and can be more easily appreciated by the simplified equivalent circuit shown in Fig. 2b.

The sequence of events describing a stimulation cycle is summarized above in Fig. 3. Before the cycle begins ($t < 0$) a switch S2 is closed and S1 is open shown in inset Fig. 3a. During this portion of the cycle, the capacitor is charged to match the voltage from the DC power supply. At the initiation of the firing sequence ($t = 0$), switch S1 is closed and S2 is opened as shown in Fig. 2b and the energy from the capacitor begins to discharge into the

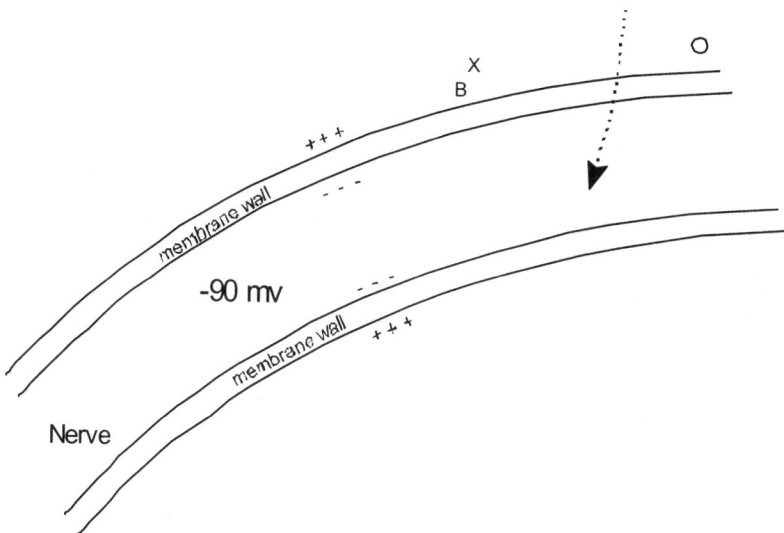

Figure 1 Induced electric field set up by a magnetic field drives charges into the nerve cell.

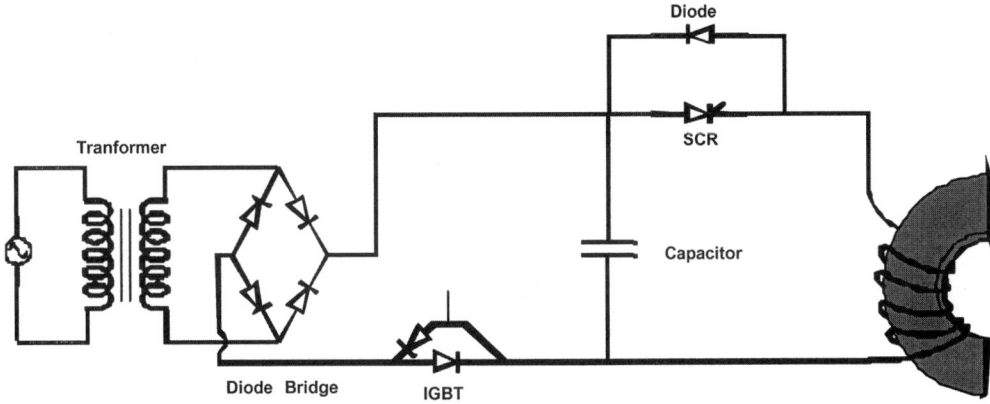

(a) Full Circuit

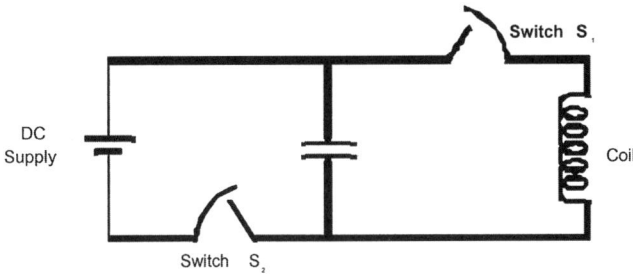

(b) Simplified equivalent

Figure 2 Electrical circuit used to produce electrical stimulation.

coil. It has a characteristic frequency which is given by $1/(2B\sqrt{LC})$. This current I continues to flow until time $t = t_1$, at which time the capacitor becomes reverse charged as in Fig. 3c. At this instant the charge on the capacitor begins to discharge back through the coil in the opposite direction from which it first began as suggested in inset Fig. 3d. It continues to flow until the capacitor becomes charged again with the polarity that it first began as in inset Fig. 3e. At this point in time ($t = t_3$) switch S1 is opened and switch S2 is closed, allowing the capacitor C to charge back to the supply voltage level V as in Fig. 3f.

Figure 4 above shows the representative changes in time of the current through the core, the voltage on the capacitor, the magnetic field experience by the patient, and most importantly the induced electric field within the targeted tissue. The current (Fig. 4a) goes through one complete cycle from time $t = 0$ to $t = t_3$. The magnitude of the current in its upward swing is slightly greater compared to the negative swing due to resistive losses in the wire and the core. Because the diode switch does not shut off completely at time t_3, a very slight over ring is often noticed for $t > t_3$. The voltage (Fig. 4b) on the capacitor starts at a level equal to the supply DC voltage falls to nearly the reverse of that and then rises back again to a level slightly less than the point at which it started. The quantity $C(V_1^2 - V_2^2)$ represents the energy loss in the resistive winding, the core, and the patient tissue. The

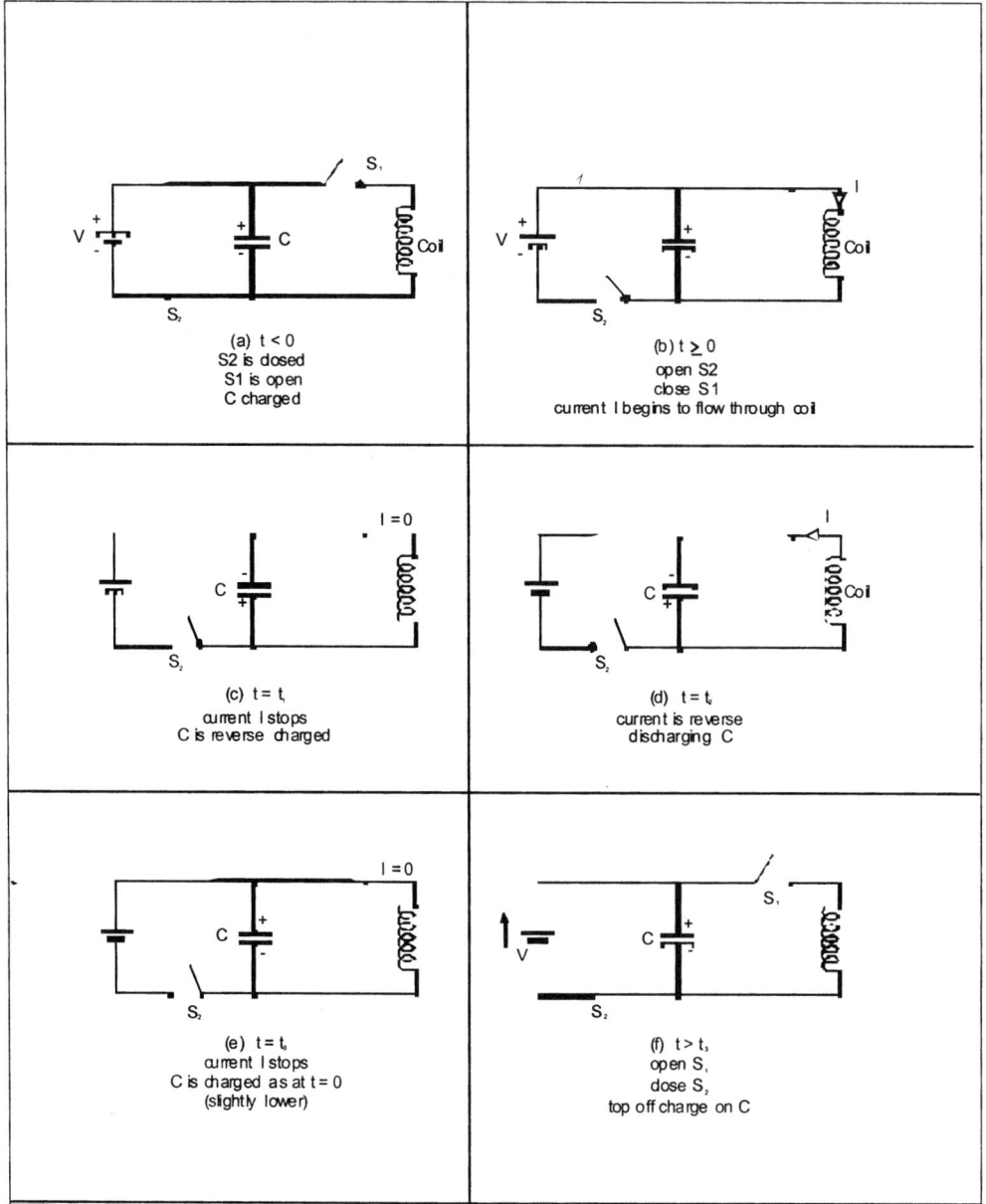

Figure 3   Sequence of circuit events defining a stimulation cycle.

magnetic field B (Fig. 4c) is directly proportional at any point in space to the current, and thus has the same profile in time. The induced current in the tissue is proportional to the rate of change of the magnetic field B with respect to time. Its spatial dependence is dictated by Faraday's law. Figure 4d shows the profile of the induced current in the tissue, which mirrors, incidentally, the voltage on the capacitor.

     How does the changing current in the core induce current in targeted tissue? This secondary induction can be explained by Lenz's law, which states that an electric current induced by a changing magnetic field will flow such that it will attempt to oppose the original

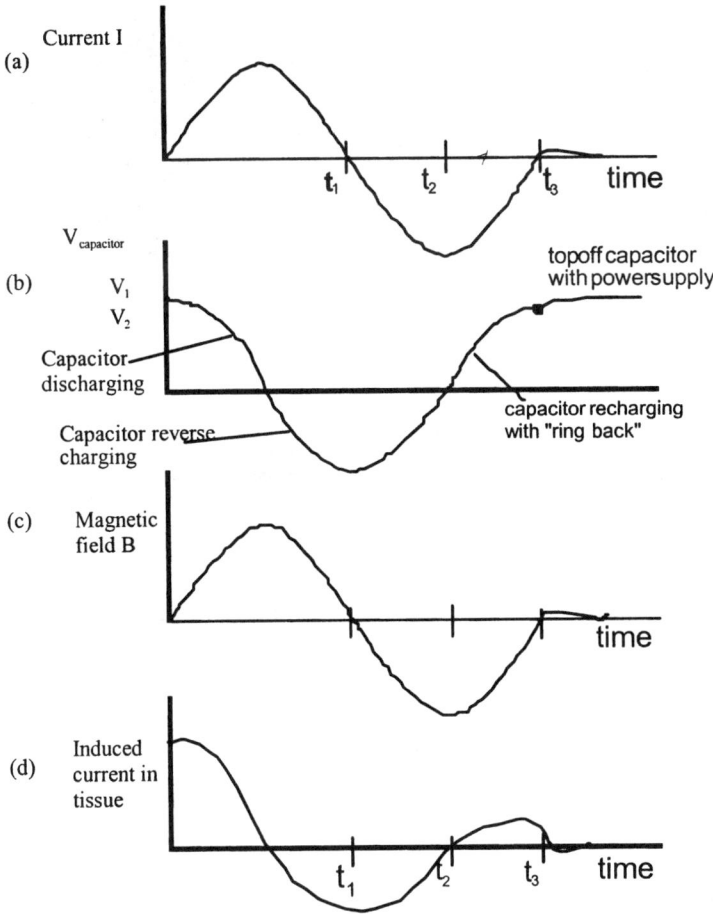

Figure 4   Current, capacitive voltage, magnetic field, and induced electric field in tissue exposed to pulsed magnetic stimulation.

magnetic field. Thus the magnetic field from the secondary induced source opposes the field from the original source; this results in an opposing force analogous to that from two opposing magnetic poles. This can be felt by attempting to push a conductive plate down quickly over a permanent magnet; the action results in a force opposing the movement.

Consider a loop of wire carrying a sinusoidally varying current as suggested above in Fig. 5a. Any loop of wire that carries a current generates a magnetic field B. This magnetic field easily penetrates both conductive and nonconductive media. It is, however, stopped by strong ferromagnetic material such as iron. When this magnetic field is changing with respect to time, it induces a current in any conducting medium that will attempt to resist or oppose the change in that magnetic field. That is, the induced current always flows in such a way as to continue the magnetic field that it experienced in a previous instant in time. When the secondary medium is a good conductor, this induced current will be opposite to the primary current.

However, when the medium is highly resistive as with human tissue, induced secondary current will lag behind the primary current by 90 electrical degrees. In the case of transient stimulus as in Fig. 5b, the induced current is simply proportional to the rate of change of the

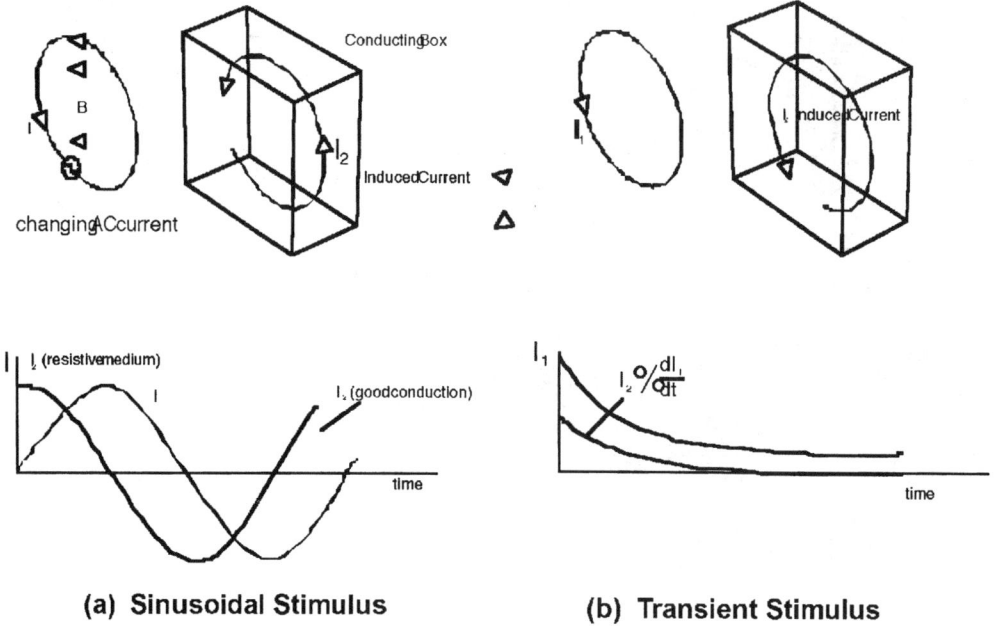

(a) Sinusoidal Stimulus   **(b) Transient Stimulus**

Figure 5   Types of current induced in a secondary medium due to a primary current I_1 changing in a loop of wire.

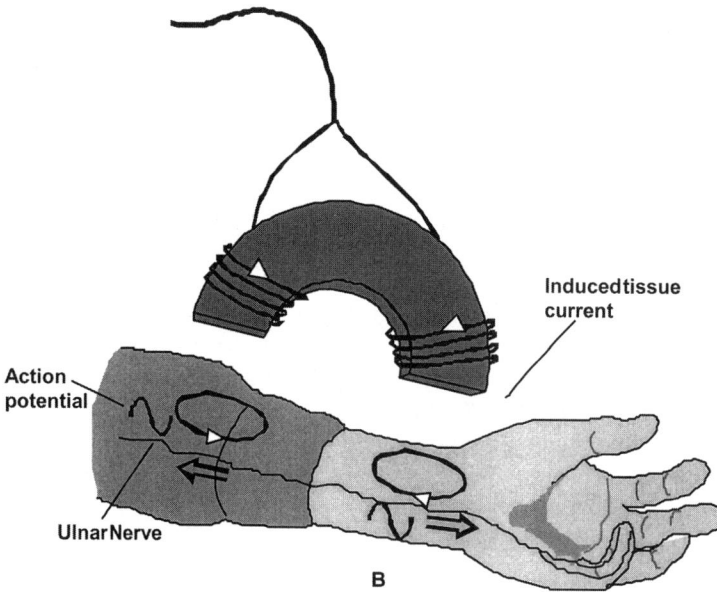

Figure 6   Action potential generation with pulsed magnetic stimulation to prevent disuse atrophy or increase range of motion.

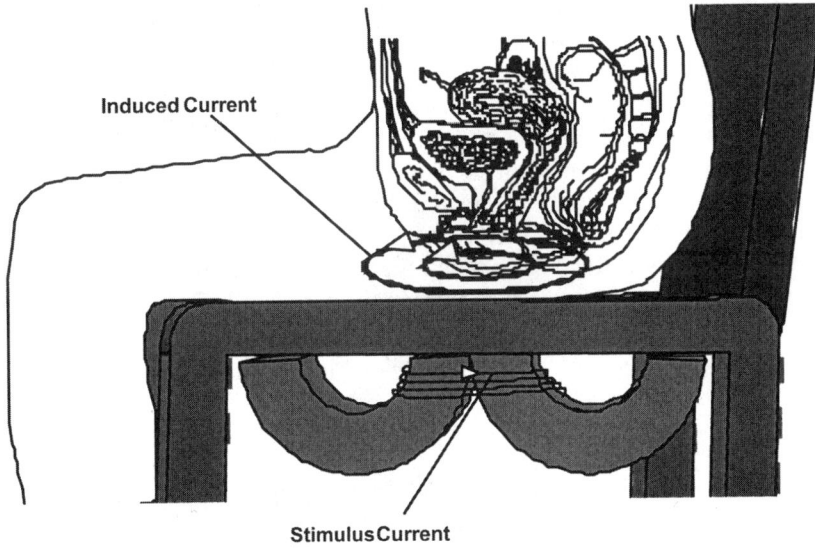

Figure 7 Cross-sectional view of female anatomy.

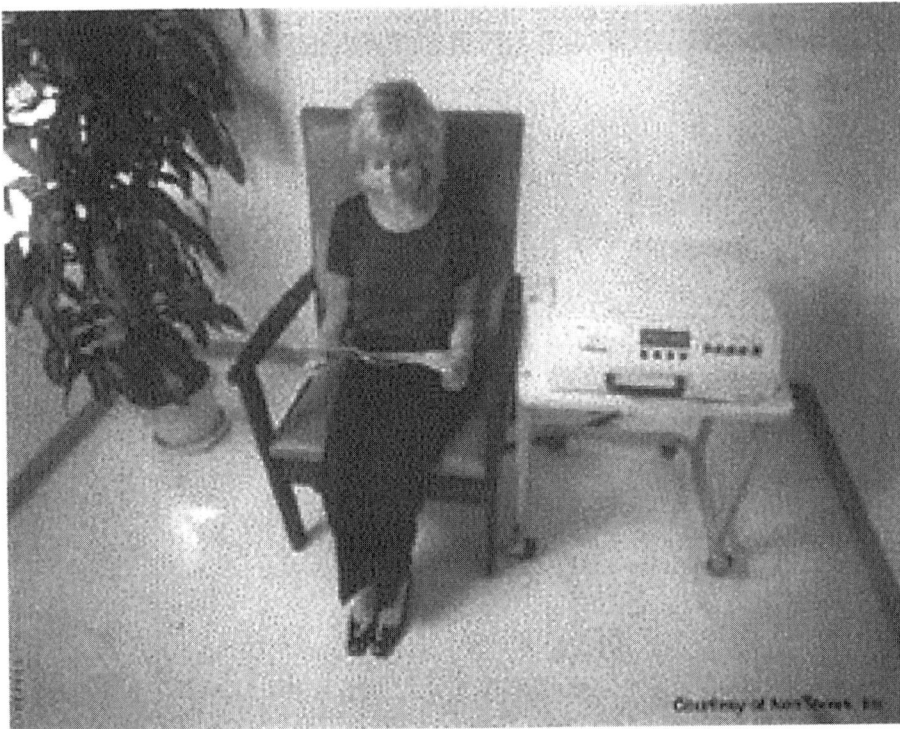

Figure 8 The NeoControl Pelvic Floor Therapy System.

primary current with respect to time. In a nonsuperconducting medium this induced current is always lower in magnitude than the primary source current.

How does this induced current result in the stimulation of nerve and muscle tissue? Consider the placement of a stimulator core over the forearm as suggested in Fig. 6 to treat a local injury. When a changing magnetic field penetrates the forearm, it induces a secondary current similar to that depicted. If this current, or rather the induced electric field that causes the current is localized, it has the ability to move positive charges through a nerve wall, increasing the potential of the intercellular space of the neuron with respect to the surrounding cellular space. This is the requirement necessary for the initiation of an action potential, caused by the sodium and potassium gates in the nerve wall opening. The action potential will move along the nerve away from the site of stimulus in both directions.

It is comparatively difficult to focus a magnetic field to an area of a few inches as would be required for an isolated nerve. Larger muscle nerve groups can be more readily targeted and fired to cause the desired muscles to contract as noted in the sketch in Fig. 7 of the device used to treat female urinary incontinence.

The goal in treating urinary incontinence in females is to strengthen the muscles around the pelvic floor and to specifically target those responsible for contraction of the bladder and urethra. An artificial contraction of these muscles is accomplished using a magnetic field that induces the desired degree of stimulation of these muscle groups. As illustrated in Fig. 7, this is best accomplished with the patient in a seated position and the magnetic stimulator core affixed to the bottoms of the seat so that the magnetic field can be focused to the targeted area directly above. The effective depth of penetration is 5 cm, thus achieving the goal of

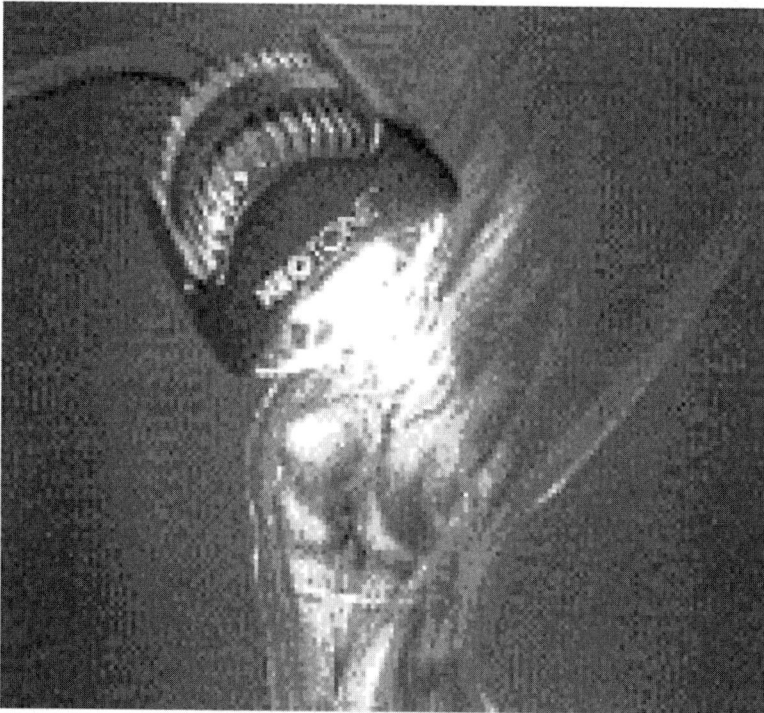

Figure 9 Neotone device.

cyclic contraction of the pelvic floor muscles without significantly affecting neighboring structures.

The NeoControl Pelvic Floor Therapy System shown in Fig. 8 was developed based on the principles noted above. Clinical trials designed to correct loss of pelvic floor muscle strength , the most common cause of urinary incontinence, have confirmed its efficacy and safety with long-term follow-up (3–9). FDA approval for this indication was obtained in June 1998, and it has been used in more than 200 urology and obstetrics and/or gynecology practices throughout the United States and 12 other countries. Pilot studies and clinical trials also suggest that this approach may be useful in treating fecal incontinence and pelvic pain syndrome in males following prostatectomy (10–12).

More recently, FDA approval has also been obtained for using this technology for "use in stimulating neuromuscular tissues for bulk muscle excitation for rehabilitative purposes" based on studies with the Neotone device shown in Fig. 9 (13,14). This includes a broad range of applications including relaxation of muscle spasm, prevention of disuse atrophy, increasing local blood circulation, muscle reeducation to maintain or increase range of motion, and prevention of deep vein thrombosis. Research in how best to design these stimulation devices continues (15–17).

It is likely that other indications will surface as greater experience is obtained with the use of these existing devices and possibly the development of others due to improvements in this exciting new technology. Updated information can be obtained by visiting www. neotonus.com.

REFERENCES

1. Jalinous Reza. A Guide to Magnetic Stimulation. On-line document, Magstim Company, http:// www.magstim.com/Documents.html, 2002:3.
2. Cadwell J. Optimizing magnetic stimulation design. Electroencephalog Clin Neurophysiol 1991; 43(suppl):238–248.
3. Jalinous R. Technical and practical aspects of magnetic stimulation. J Clin Neurophy 1991; 8:10–25.
4. Chokroverty S, Hening W. Magnetic brain stimulation: safety studies. Electroencephalogr Clin Neurophys 1995; 97:36–42.
5. Galloway N, El-Galley S, Appell S, Russell, Carlan. Extracorporeal Magnetic Innervation Therapy for Stress Urinary Incontinence. Urology June 1999.
6. Wilson PD, Bo K, Bourcier A, Hay-Smith J, Staskin D, Nygard I, Wyman J. Conservative management in women. In: Abrams P, Khoury S, Wein A, eds. Incontinence. Plymbridge Ltd, Plymouth, 1998:579–636.
7. Bo K, Hagen RH, Kvarstein B, Jorgensen B, Laarson S. Pelvic floor muscle exercise for treatment of female stress urinary incontinence: III Effects of two different degrees of pelvic floor muscle exercises. Neurourol and Urodyn 1990; 9:489–502.
8. Fall M, Ahlstrom K, Carlsson CA, Ek A, Erlansdson BE. Contelle: pelvic floor stimulator for stress-urge incontinence. A multicenter study. Urol 1986; 27:282–287.
9. Galloway NTM, Appell RA. Extracorporeal magnetic stimulation therapy for urinary incontinence. In: Appell RA, Bourcier AP, LaTorre F, eds. Pelvic Floor Dysfunction: Investigations and Conservative Treatment. Rome: C.E.S.I., 1999:291–294.
10. Carlan SJ, Bhullar A, Followup of patients who underwent extracorporeal magnetic ennervation, therapy for urinary incontinence. American Urological Annual Meeting, Anaheim, CA, June 2–7, 2001.
11. Brodak PP, Bidair M, Joseph A, Szollar S, Saad J. Magnetic stimulation of the sacral roots. Neurol Urodynamics 1993; 12:455–462.

12. McFarlane JP, Foley SJ, DeWinter P, Shah JPR, Craggs MD. Acute suppression of detruser instability by magnetic stimulation of the sacral nerve roots. Brit J Neurol 1997; 80:734–741.

13. Struppler A, Jakob C, Muller-Barna P, Schmid M, Lorenzen HW, Paulig M, Proseigal M. A new method for early rehabilitation in extreme palsy of central origin by magnetic stimulation. EEG-EMG 1996; 27:151–157. German.

14. Mills KR, Thompson CCB. Human muscle fatigue investigation by transcrannial magnetic stimulation. Neuroreport 1995; 6:1966–1968.

15. Davey K, Epstein CM. Magnetic stimulation coil and circuit design. IEEE Trans Biomed Eng 2000; 47(11):1493–1499.

16. Epstein CM, Davey KR. Iron core coils for transcranial magnetic stimulation. J Clin Neurophysiol 2002; 19(4).

17. Barker AT, Janinous R, Freeston IL. Non-invasive magnetic stimulation of human motor cortex. Lancet 1985; 2:1106.

33

Coblation Radio-Frequency Diskal Nucleoplasty: A Novel Approach To The Management of Acute Disk Herniation

Arra S. Reddy and Joshua A. Hirsch

Harvard Medical School, Beth Israel Deaconess Medical Center, Boston, Massachusettes, U.S.A.

Coblation radiofrequency discal nucleoplasty is new procedure that offers advantages over other percutaneous decompression of herniated disk techniques such as chemonucelolysis, laser discectomy and intradiscal electrothermoplasty. It utilizes a radiofrequency probe inserted through a needle rather than a heated wire, to generate a highly focused plasma field that breaks up the molecular bonds of the gel in the nucleus in a safer and more efficient fashion. The procedure is described in detail and illustrative case histories are presented.

The percutaneous decompression of herniated disks is a well-established clinical approach with over 500,000 procedures performed during the past 20 years. Several percutaneous techniques are in practice including chemonucleolysis, percutaneous lumbar discectomy, laser discectomy, and intradiscal electrothermoplasty (IDET) (1–6). These procedures have a reported success rate of approximately 70–75% but are associated with various individual limitations. During the IDET procedure, a needle is inserted into the affected disk under x-ray guidance. A special wire is then threaded through the needle into the disk, and after proper positioning has been achieved, it is heated. This causes partial melting of the annulus or wall of the disk, which, in turn, stimulates the growth of new protein fibers to provide annular reinforcement. In addition, small nerve fibers that have invaded the degenerating disk are also destroyed resulting in pain relief since many episodes of low back pain are due to annular tears.

The coblation radio-frequency diskal nucleoplasty (CRDN) procedure described herein is newer procedure that is similar to IDET but utilizes a special radio-frequency probe (Wand) that is inserted into the disk through a needle rather than a heated wire. This Wand generates a highly focused plasma field with enough energy to break up the molecular bonds

(a)

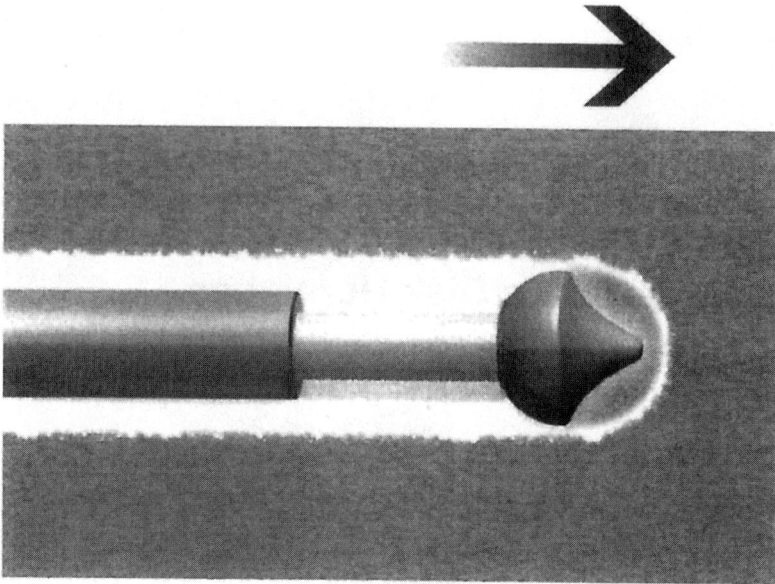

(b)

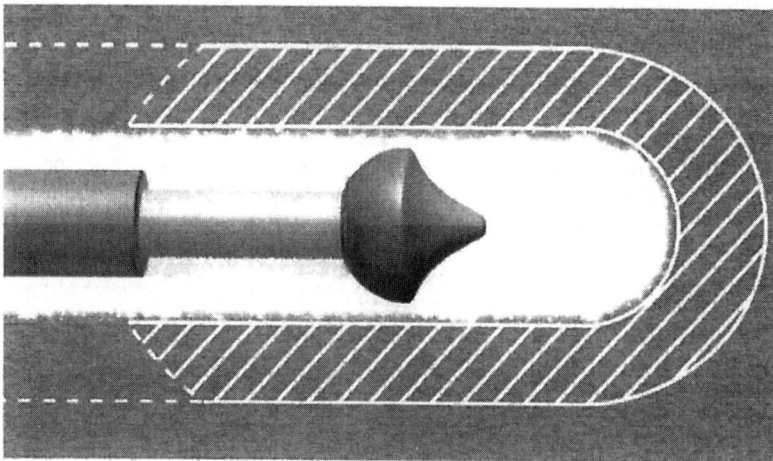

Figure 1 Coblation radio-frequency diskal nucleoplasty. (a) Coblation: advancing the wand creates a small, controlled channel in the disk. (b) Coagulation: withdrawing the wand coagulates tissue adjacent to the channel during decompression of the disk.

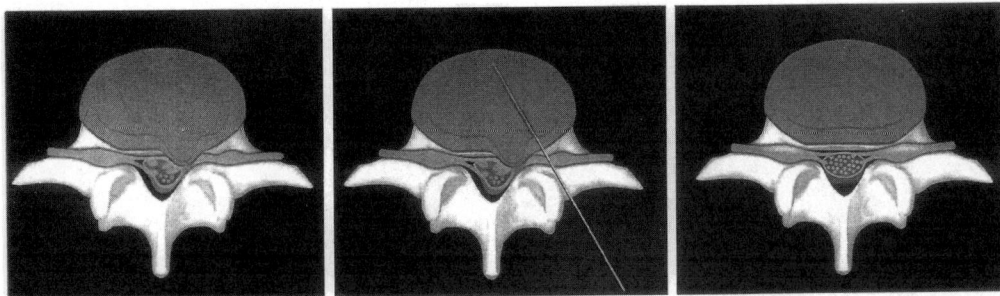

Figure 2   Sequence of events following coblation radio-frequency diskal nucleopasty.

of the gel in the nucleus. As a result, 10–20% of the nucleus is "vaporized," which decompresses the disk and reduces the pressure both on the disk and surrounding nerve roots. Since the high-energy plasma field is generated at relatively low temperatures, damage to surrounding tissues is minimized so that CDRN may be more effective and safer than IDET for relieving sciatic pain. A coagulation mode can subsequently be used to thermally provide further decompression of the intervertebral disk, as illustrated in Fig. 1a and b.The results of this dual action are depicted in Fig. 2.

Coblation radio-frequency diskal nucleoplasty is minimally invasive and appears to be safer and more cost effective than open surgery for selected patients, as illustrated by the following two fairly typical case reports.

Case 1.   A 55-year-old male had recently begun to experience left-sided radiculopathy in an L3 distribution. There was a large far lateral disk herniation at L3 affecting the left exiting L3 nerve root as illustrated in Fig. 3.

The patient had failed conservative medical management and presented for possible pain relief via percutaneous nucleoplasty. The risks, benefits, and alternatives of the procedure were explained in detail to the patient and his wife who understood and signed the consent form. The patient was given premedication including 25 mg of vistaril, 0.5mg of ativan, and 0.5 mg of xanax approximately a half hour before being brought to the neurointerventional suite, where a gram of intravenous ancef was administered. He was positioned prone on the table and the back prepped and draped in the usual sterile fashion.

Using standard techniques, the back was evaluated fluoroscopically and L3-4 opened up on the frontal view by rotating in a craniocaudal direction and also seen on the lateral view. Under fluoroscopic guidance, initially 25-gauge tuberculin needle was inserted followed by a 6-in. 22-gauge spinal needle followed ultimately by a 17-gauge 6-in. Crawford needle to access the disk. When the Crawford needle was placed inside the nucleus pulposus, at the junction of the nucleus and the annulus, intravenous contrast was administered. As illustrated in Fig. 4, diskograms demonstrate the far lateral and posterior left-sided disk herniation. Contrast fills from side-to-side and throughout the disk. It is a normal appearing disk other than this large far lateral disk herniation.

Percutaneous discectomy was performed with the aid of the Arthrocare Wand. While monitoring the patient, a series of channels were created by advancing the wand into the disk while ablating tissue. After stopping at a predetermined depth, the wand was slowly withdrawn, while coagulating, to the starting position. Advancing the wand creates a small, controlled channel in the disk, and withdrawing it coagulates tissue adjacent to the channel during decompression of the disk providing a dual effect. The wand is then rotated

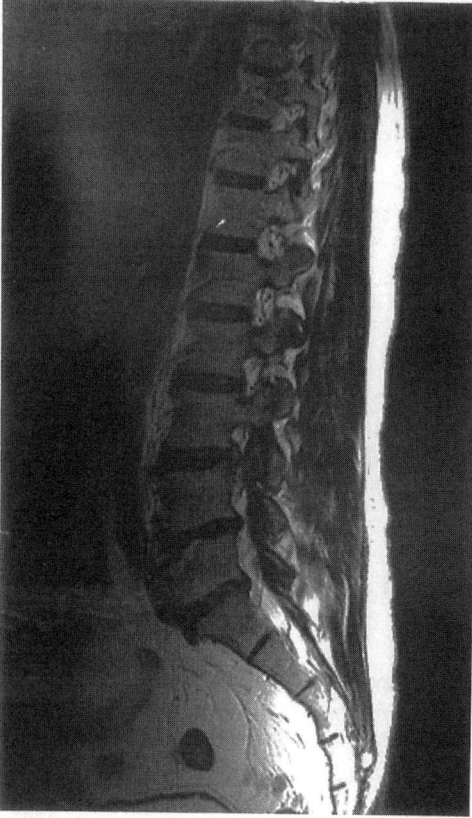

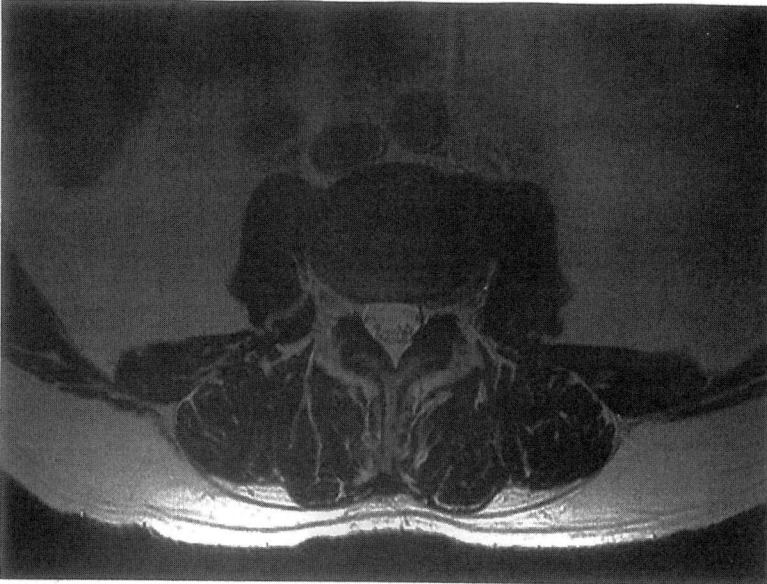

Figure 3 Sagittal and axial T2WI of the lumbar spine demonstrates a left lateral disk herniation at the level of L3/4 and slightly displacing the left L3 nerve root.

(a)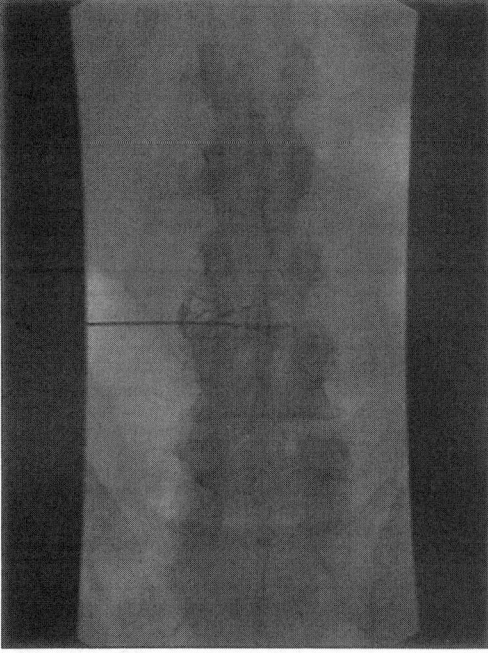

(b)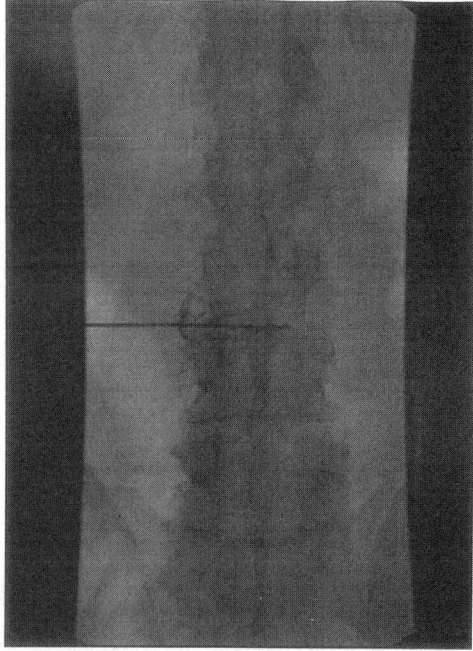

(c)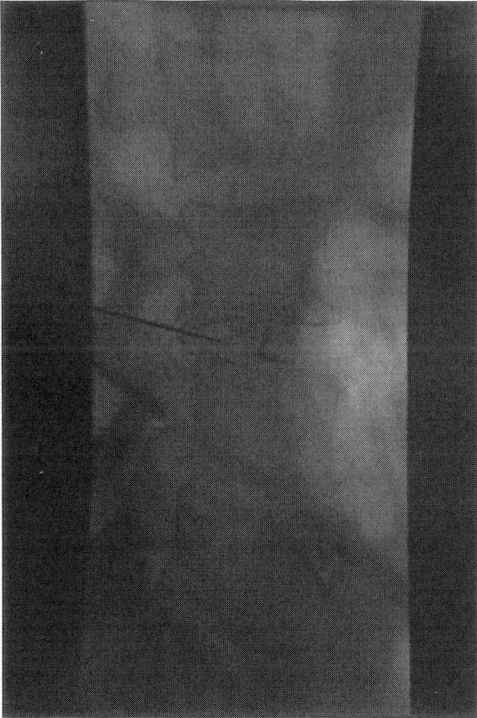

(d)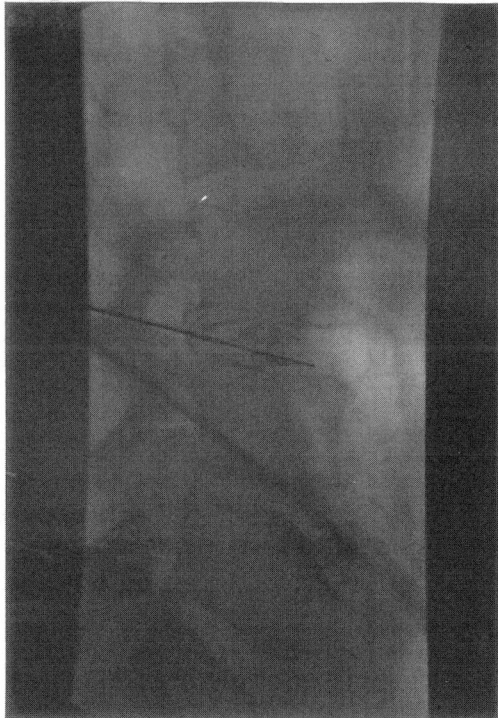

Figure 4 Contrast opacifies the disk indicating the accurate placement of the needle. Also note the contrast opacifying the left lateral disk herniation. (a) and (b) AP spot images showing the proximal and distal position of the Arthrocare Wand. (c) and (d) Lateral spot images showing the proximal and distal position of the Arthrocare Wand.

clockwise, and another channel is created. Approximately six channels were created as per the manufacturer's recommendations, although this can vary depending on the desired amount of tissue reduction.

Following percutaneous discectomy, the trocar was pulled back into the Crawford needle, and selective nerve root block was performed using $2\,cm^3$ of 0.25% preservative free bupivacaine. The needle was removed and a Syvek patch was placed over the wound site. There was no hematoma. The patient tolerated the procedure well and received only some additional sedation.

On 2-week follow up the patient's pain had significantly improved and he had resumed his normal active lifestyle.

Case 2. A 30-year-old male had recently begun to experience left-sided radiculopathy in an L4 distribution from a disk herniation at L3/4 that had not responded to conservative

(a)

(b)

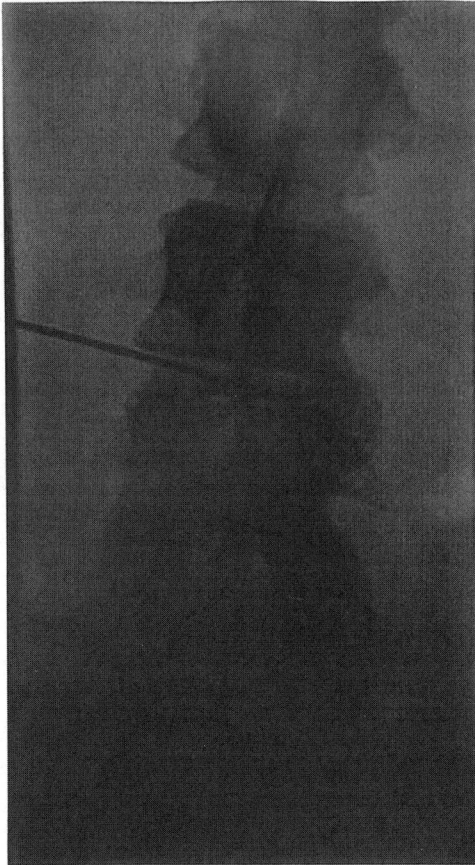
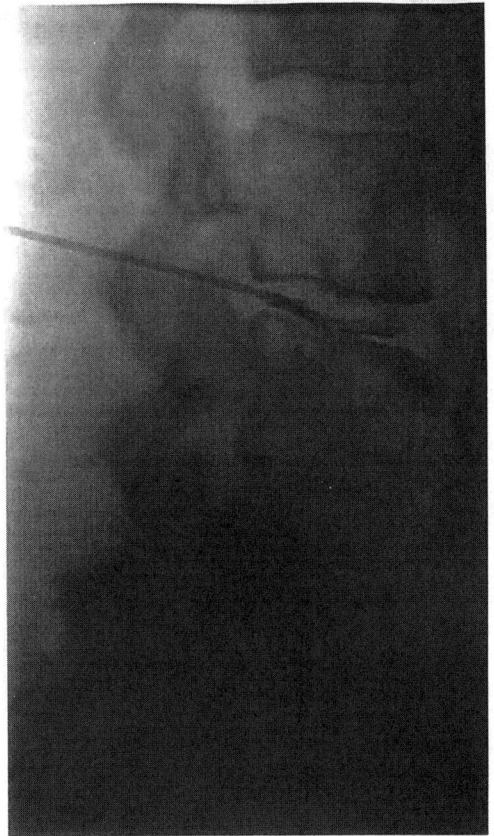

Figure 5 Diskograms demonstrating the proximal and distal positions of the Arthrocare Wand as described in Fig. 4. (a) and (b) AP spot images showing the proximal and distal position of the Arthrocare Wand. (c) and (d) Lateral spot images showing the proximal and distal position of the Arthrocare Wand.

(c) (d)

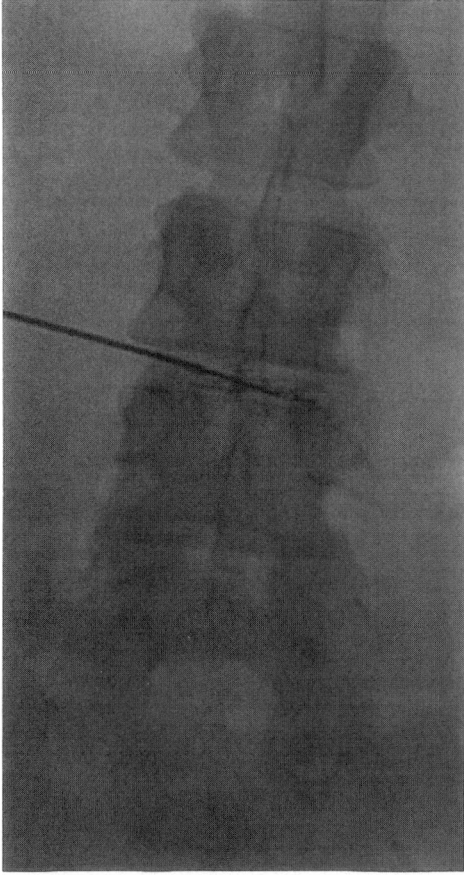 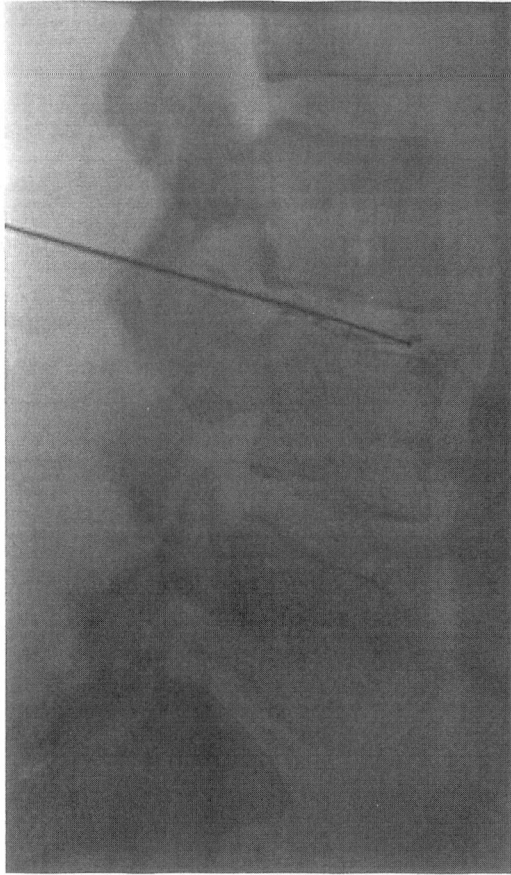

Figure 5 Continued.

medical management. The sequence of events and treatment was similar to that described in case 1. Diskograms demonstrate the far lateral and posterior left-sided disk herniation. Contrast fills from side to side and throughout the disk. It is a normal appearing disk other than this large far lateral disk herniation as illustrated in Fig. 5.

The patient's pain significantly improved and was able to completely resume his active normal lifestyle within a week.

As minimally invasive procedures for treating herniated discs and similar problems become more widely used, it is important to understand and emphasize the safety of various devices and approaches This is particularly true with respect to temperature measurements of vital structures in and around the intervertebral disk tissue (7). We believe that the Coblation procedure described above represents a significant advance in this regard and provides a greater degree of safety without sacrificing efficacy.

The authors would like to express their appreciation to Drs. Darren Crawford and Norman Sanders for supplying artwork and support and to Dr. Paul Rosch for contributing to and editing this chapter.

REFERENCES

1. Brown D. Update on chemonucleolysis. Spine 1996; 21:585–625.
2. Onik G. Percutaneous lumbar diskectomy using a new aspiration probe. Am J Neuroradiol 1985; 6:290–296.
3. Choy DS, et al. Percutaneous laser disk decompression. Spine 1992; 17:949.
4. Choy DS. Percutaneous laser disk decompression (PLDD): Twelve years experience with 752 procedures in 518 patients. J Clin Laser Med Surg 1988; 16(6):325–331.
5. Saal, Saal. Management of chronic discogenic low back pain with a thermal intradiscal catheter. SOAR, pp. 382–389) Physiatry Medical Group, 1999:382–389.
6. Sherk HH. Laser diskectomy. Lasers in Orthopedic Surgery. Medical College of Pennsylvania, 1993; 16:5.
7. Yetkinler DN, Nau WH, Brandt LI, Diederich C. Intervertebral Disc Temparature Measurements During Nucleoplasty and IDET Procedures. European Spine J 2002; 11(4):418.

34

Electricity and the Heart: Innovation and the Evolution of Cardiac Pacing

Kirk Jeffrey

Carleton College, Northfield, Minnesota, U.S.A.

Resuscitation by the administration of electrical shocks was reported in the 1770s. While electrical stimulation of the heart was subsequently attempted with varied degrees of success, it was not until 50 years ago that an effective implantable pacemaker was developed. The evolution of current transistorized devices is reviewed, and new applications are discussed.

The implantation and management of cardiac pacemakers constitute a vast subsystem within cardiology (but not a formal subspecialty) that did not exist half a century ago. The pacemaker, first fully implanted within the body in 1958, delivers pulsed stimuli to the heart so as to speed up an unduly slow heart rate and coordinate the action of the upper and lower chambers.

National policies that encouraged medical research, socialized the cost of implantations through state payment schemes, and insisted that life-sustaining technologies be safe and effective have all affected the ongoing development of the pacemaker. In turn, these policies have embodied the public's changing beliefs about needs and possibilities in medicine (1). A closer examination of the history of cardiac pacing reveals that its dominant theme has been unending innovation encouraged by medical innovators and device manufacturers.

No one had a long-range plan for pacemaker development. The decade-by-decade history of pacing can be traced as a series of improvements addressing critical problems or "needs" as defined by physicians, engineers, and manufacturers. These critical problems represented technological failures or bottlenecks thought to be impeding progress and, equally important, thought to be solvable. Each critical problem arose out of earlier choices that had come to be accepted as given (Table 1).

The recursive process of addressing critical problems and moving on began in the 1950s and is still going on today, but the field of pacing is far larger and includes many more stakeholders than it did 40 years ago. Defining critical problems in cardiac pacing and

525

Table 1 Critical Problems in Cardiac Pacing

Decade	Critical problem
1950s	Defining the basic requirements for chronic pacing
1960s	Making the pacemaker safe and reliable
1970s	Creating smaller and longer-lived pacemakers
1980s	Achieving physiological pacing
1990s	Moving toward automaticity
2000s	Broadening the spectrum of diseases

achieving consensus about the next steps for the field remain vital; what persons or institutions can manage these tasks (2)?

I. CARDIAC ELECTRORESUSCITATION: PREHISTORY

From the discovery of the Leyden jar in 1746, scientific investigators were interested in medical uses of electricity. Resuscitation by administering electric shocks to persons apparently dead from falls or drowning was reported in Britain in the 1770s and later (3). However, the idea of electrotherapeutics soon fell into disfavor among physicians and scientists, partly owing to Aldini's macabre experiments on the corpses of executed criminals in 1803 (work that helped inspire Mary Shelley's novel Frankenstein, 1818) and partly because medical empiricists and quacks to some degree appropriated the field—especially in the United States—by introducing galvanic belts, electro-baths, and other technologies to treat such conditions as impotence, dropsy (renal disease), and heart failure. These treatments almost always understood electricity as a sort of tonic that would pep up the body's processes (4,5).

As far as is known, only one scientist of that era, the Scottish physiologist J. A. MacWilliam (1857–1937), thought of delivering electrical pulses (stimuli) in emulation of the heart's own electrical behavior (6). MacWilliam's suggestion fell on barren ground: physiologists had not yet worked out the basic geography of the heart's conduction system. It was only in the early twentieth century that a modern physiological understanding of the behavior and maladies of the heart, including disorders of heart rhythm, began to take hold among biomedical scientists (7,8).

An interest in so-called Stokes–Adams attacks—chronic severe bradycardia with episodes of syncope, from which the sufferer usually, but not always, revived—contributed to physiologists' invention of the polygraph and the electrocardiograph (ECG), devices that opened the way to analysis of the heartbeat. By the early 1920s, medical scientists who employed the ECG had gained a basic understanding of heart block (the chronic condition that could eventually lead to Stokes–Adams attacks) as well as atrial and ventricular fibrillation and some tachyarrhythmias (9). However, improved understanding of the heartbeat and its disorders did not yield immediate improvements in treatment. Clinicians relied on pharmacological therapy to suppress certain arrhythmias or alter the heart rate, but the mechanisms of these treatments were not well understood (10). Clinical use of electrical stimuli or shocks was still far outside the realm of the acceptable. It took many years for the newer thinking, including a fuller understanding of how ECG tracings revealed the workings of the diseased heart, to affect the outlook of practitioner cardiologists (11).

The developments just set forth had little to do with the isolated invention of two pacemaker like devices between the world wars. In Australia, anesthetist Mark C. Lidwill

(1878–1968) announced (1929) that he had revived a stillborn infant by means of an electrical device featuring a needle electrode that he had inserted in the infant's right ventricle. Lidwill suggested that his invention might be useful in cardiac arrest from anesthesia, drowning, acute illness such as diphtheria, and when underlying heart disease disrupted normal cardiac rhythm. This miscellaneous list perhaps convinced listeners that the device verged on old-fashioned quackery. No photograph or additional documentation of Lidwill's invention has been discovered (12).

A few years later, U.S. practitioner cardiologist Albert S. Hyman (1893–1972) invented a tabletop machine that delivered an interrupted current flow to the heart via a bipolar needle electrode that he believed should be inserted into the right atrium close to the sinus node. This invention is better documented—a patent application and photographs exist—but its efficacy was never demonstrated, even with laboratory animals. Hyman did not distinguish clearly between coronary standstill and ventricular fibrillation; the mechanism of low-amplitude pulsed stimuli was entirely inappropriate for the latter. He made no mention of heart block, the condition for which cardiac pacing was later introduced (13). Both Lidwill and Hyman were technological isolates: their work was inadequately grounded in existing scientific understanding of cardiac arrhythmias, and they proved unable to enlist others in supporting and following up on their work. Aside from Hyman's introduction of the term *artificial pacemaker* and his understanding that such a device ought to deliver pulsed stimuli, the work of the two men had little influence and did not inspire the pacemakers invented after World War II (14).

In 1952, U.S. cardiologist Paul M. Zoll (1911–1999) announced a clinically effective pacemaker consisting of a tabletop pulse generator connected by wires to ECG electrodes strapped to the patient's chest. This machine was able to stimulate the heart to beat and could keep hospitalized patients alive for many hours during episodes of repeated Stokes–Adams attacks. However, capture of the heartbeat required stimuli of 50 to 150 V which could cause involuntary contractions of the chest muscles and considerable pain. Clearly the Zoll pacemaker was of limited utility, but its inventor had conclusively demonstrated that clinical pacing was possible (15). In a promising extension of Zoll's work, cardiologist Aubrey Leatham and technician J.G. Davies in the United Kingdom devised an external pacemaker that would automatically begin to pace the heart if it detected no QRS complexes for 6 s. If the patient's own heartbeat recommenced, the pacer would switch itself off (16).

II. THE 1950s: DEFINING THE BASIC REQUIREMENTS FOR CHRONIC PACING

Two entirely separate streams of innovation came together in the late 1950s to permit the invention of *implantable* cardiac pacemakers suitable for long-term use within the human body.

A. Open-Heart Surgery

Pacing had its real inception in the mid-1950s as a way to manage an unanticipated complication of the new open-heart surgery. Surgical repairs in the septum sometimes damaged the conduction fibers through which the cardiac impulse passed from the atria to the ventricles, creating postsurgical heart block. In 1956 U.S. surgeon C. Walton Lillehei (1918–2000) and associates began to secure the bare end of an insulated wire to the myocardium, bring the wire out through the surgical wound, and connect the other end to a tabletop stimulator that plugged into a wall socket and delivered low-amplitude stimuli to the heart. With this improvised arrangement, postsurgical patients (usually children) could be paced in the hospital for a few days until their hearts had healed sufficiently to beat reliably on their own. Lillehei's myocardial pacing wire was the first electrical device ever to be implanted in the human body and left there for a period of time (14).

B. Transistors: The Revolution in Miniature

Uneasy about the implications of connecting the patient's heart to the hospital AC electrical system, Lillehei in early 1957 discarded the stimulator in favor of a pulse generator powered by a 9-V battery and small enough for the patient to carry on a cord around the neck (17). Invented at Lillehei's request by engineer Earl Bakken, the new device included two transistors. Bakken had in fact adapted a metronome circuit that he had discovered in a hobbyists' magazine. The pulse generator could not sense intrinsic electrical activity within the heart and could not alter its behavior in any way, but as an early and successful application of transistor technology to medical devices it helped launch a new era of innovation in the field then called *medical electronics* (18).

At this stage cardiothoracic surgeons controlled the pacemaker because only they could expose the surface of the beating heart and attach an electrode to it. Surgeons soon began to apply the new technology—the myocardial wire connected to an external, battery-powered pulse generator—not only in cases of postsurgical heart block but for a broader range of patients including many who had developed chronic complete heart block in middle age, not as the result of heart surgery. Between 1959 and the mid-1960s, dozens of men and women lived at home for months and even years with wires emerging from their chests that connected to external pulse generators. Some of the important early work went forward in Sweden, the United States, and the United Kingdom (2,14).

Pacing the heart through a port in the skin invited infections. News of Lillehei's and Bakken's innovations led several groups to investigate pacemaker designs that would permit the implanting of the entire system, an obvious requirement if pacing were to come into general use for chronic complete heart block. In that long-ago era, innovative physicians and engineers were free to introduce new devices into clinical use without first conducting time-consuming studies of their safety and efficacy. Because most patients were at death's door with multiple and severe heart problems, it seemed acceptable to offer an essentially untried therapy; what was the alternative?

In Sweden, surgeon Åke Senning (1915–2000) and engineer Rune Elmqvist (1906–96) devised a fully implantable pacemaker with a nickel-cadmium battery that could be recharged from outside the body. Hurried into clinical use in 1958 to manage the heartbeat of a 43-year-old man suffering several Stokes–Adams attacks daily, the pacer failed within hours; a replacement lasted 7 weeks. The patient, Arne Larsson, survived and beginning in 1961 was given a succession of implanted pacemakers. Paced for nearly half his life, Larsson experienced nearly every major advance in cardiac pacing. He died in 2001 at the age of 86 (2).

The clinical successes and failures of the 1950s focused investigators' attention on three remaining critical problems in the new technology of pacing:

C. Batteries for Implantable Devices

For their power source, most first-generation implantables looked to the mercury-zinc cell invented during World War II to power portable military field telephones. In the United

States, engineer Wilson Greatbatch was designing an implantable pulse generator; he was impressed with the small size and high energy density of the mercury-zinc cells. Though several groups besides Senning's experimented with rechargeable batteries, ultimately Greatbatch and most others chose mercury-zinc. In the original Greatbatch pulse generator, the battery consisted of 10 such cells (19).

D. Encapsulation

The early implantable pacemakers could not be hermetically sealed because the battery chemistry produced hydrogen gas as a by-product. Inventors looked for materials that would permit hydrogen to exit the pulse generator while still shielding the electronic components from both body fluid and the corrosive electrolyte of the battery. Working in 1959–1960, Greatbatch and his partner, surgeon William Chardack, potted the circuitry in epoxy and enclosed the entire assemblage in a silicone shell. Other groups arrived at similar solutions. Greatbatch later recalled that although hydrogen diffused out of the pulse generator, water vapor could readily enter, "raising the interior to an eventual 100% humidity. Thus our electronics were essentially operating under water, but distilled water" (19).

Clinical experience during the 1960s showed that epoxy and silicone would not reliably protect pacemaker electronics. The devices had a disconcerting tendency to fail suddenly. As late as 1973–1975, a leading manufacturer had to issue advisories on thousands of units suspected of susceptibility to short circuits from dendrites that formed in the presence of body fluid, solder flux, and a voltage (14).

E. Myocardial Pacing Lead

At 70 beats per minute, a wire lead attached to the heart flexed some 36.8 million times in a year. Leads sometimes broke within the body; but a more subtle problem puzzled designers for several years: the threshold of stimulation (the minimum stimulus that would reliably induce ventricular contraction), quite low just after implantation of a myocardial lead, would begin to rise within a few days. Eventually it was discovered that fibrosis around the electrode was separating the electrical stimulus from excitable myocardial tissue and effectively reducing the current density. In 1961 Chardack invented a highly flexible coiled-spring lead terminating in an electrode that remained reasonably stable on the heart's surface. Though physicians experimented for a time with numerous alternatives, the Chardack electrode eventually was widely adopted (20).

F. Invention of Implantable Cardiac Pacing: A Summary

Developments in several fields made the implantable pacemaker possible, but they did not make any one design inevitable. In the early 1960s some investigators tested an alternative design in which an external transmitter sent radio-frequency signals through the intact skin to an implanted receiver; others followed up on Elmqvist's earlier work with batteries rechargeable from outside the body; later, still others developed isotopic ("nuclear") pacemakers that boasted extreme longevity. These developmental paths, explored but ultimately not taken, remind us that a new invention can be quite malleable: it can assume a variety of forms depending on the choices of its designers. Each of these alternative designs had drawbacks, but the design that came to be accepted as *the* cardiac pacemaker was not at first clearly superior from a technical standpoint.

The Chardack-Greatbatch Implantable Pacemaker (introduced commercially in 1961) with its mercury-zinc battery gained acceptance for several reasons:

1. Chardack, its coinventor, made an effective case for the device to the medical community.
2. It was commercially available earlier than other models, so that surgeons gained experience with it and a shared body of "know-how" (informal technical knowledge) quickly began to develop around it.
3. Unlike competing designs, the Chardack-Greatbatch pacemaker placed no responsibility on the patient to manage his own implanted device by, for example, remembering to recharge it every few days (14).

III. THE 1960s: MAKING THE PACEMAKER SAFE AND RELIABLE

By the early 1960s, the pacemaker had effectively been redefined as a fully implantable device that provided long-term therapy for a chronic heart rhythm disorder, the ventricular bradycardia caused by complete heart block. To perfect the pacemaker as a long-term treatment, innovators from clinical medicine and private industry introduced several new features:

A. Transvenous Catheter Lead

Until the mid-1960s, most implantable pacemakers used myocardial leads; but this lead required that the patient undergo a thoracotomy. In 1958 (shortly before the Arne Larsson case in Sweden), U.S. surgical trainee Seymour Furman conceived of the idea of passing a catheter lead through the venous system into the right ventricle, then connecting it to an external pulse generator. This arrangement proved able to manage the heartbeat over sustained periods. By 1959 Furman's patients were leaving the hospital and living at home with portable external generators and leads that emerged from the external jugular vein at the base of the neck (21,22). Within a few years surgeons began to introduce the lead via the cephalic vein in the patient's upper chest and to implant the generator close by instead of below, the diaphragm. Numerous clinical cases in Sweden and the United Kingdom established that the procedure was both safe and effective; it spread rapidly in the United States after 1965 (23,24). Chardack's report that transvenous placement of the electrode reduced postoperative mortality contributed to a general switch to the new technique (25). Though this was little noted in the 1960s, transvenous pacing also set the stage for cardiologists (eventually) to dominate the field of pacing (26).

B. Diagnosis of Impending Pacemaker Failure

Before the inception of regulatory oversight of medical devices in North America and Europe, innovative devices and treatments often found their way into general use before their reliability and effectiveness had been fully established. In cardiac pacing, incremental improvements gradually reduced the risk of device failure after 1961 so that by the early 1970s, average pacemaker longevity had reached 3 years and the number of unexpected crises had declined steeply. Physicians who managed pacemaker patients discovered that a slight reduction in the firing rate of the implanted devices heralded impending battery failure. By checking the rate regularly, a doctor could anticipate failure and carry out a pulse generator replacement on a scheduled instead of an emergency basis. With the introduction of transtelephonic monitoring equipment at the end of the 1960s—an innovation that came from the physician community—doctors' offices or commercial follow-up services could obtain basic information about the behavior of the implanted pacemaker from the patient's home or other remote locations (27).

C. The Earliest "Physiologic" Pacing: QRS-Inhibited Pacemakers

Since the 1950s, physicians had been interested in more physiologic pacing, by which they meant devices that would emulate the heart's "natural" behavior to a greater degree. Possibilities were limited until hybrid integrated circuitry (see below) replaced discrete circuitry, but in the late 1960s, manufacturers introduced new pacemaker models capable of withholding their stimulus on sensing a normal QRS complex—thus pacing only "on demand," in the argot of the day (28). Within 5 years they had completely replaced the earlier nonsensing (*asynchronous*) pacers. Because many pacemaker patients experience a mixture of aberrant and normally conducted heartbeats, this ability to "choose" not to fire extended the life of the battery and avoided the risk that the pacemaker, by firing into the vulnerable period of a normal heartbeat, might induce ventricular fibrillation (29).

Improvements in the implantable pacemaker and the introduction of new techniques of implantation led to a broad acceptance of pacing as a standard treatment by the end of the 1960s. As cardiac pacing found its place among the accepted therapies available for maladies of the heart, the number of implanting physicians began to grow rapidly—especially in the United States. Physicians were also beginning to use pacing to treat nonlethal arrhythmias such as lesser degrees of heart block or simple slowing down of the sinus rhythm of the heart. Pacing was being redefined as a way to improve an older person's quality of life even if he or she was not in imminent danger of dying.

IV. THE 1970s: CREATING SMALLER AND LONGER-LIVED PACEMAKERS

With the achievement of reasonable reliability by 1970, pacing technology did not stabilize; instead, the rate of change began to accelerate. On one hand, medical researchers discovered new arrhythmias that could be treated with electrostimulation. On the other, the manufacturers intensified their research and development so as to develop portfolios of patents that would demonstrate their technological prowess, keep them ahead of their competitors, and stave off the stabilization and commodification of the pacemaker (14).

Beginning in the 1970s, the medical device manufacturing companies (often acting on the advice of leading physicians) have guided technological innovation in cardiac pacing. During the second decade of implantable pacing, practitioner implanters made it clear that they desired longer-lived pacemakers that would be smaller and easier to implant. The manufacturers responded effectively to these requests but also went beyond them to introduce noninvasively adjustable (*programmable*) pacemakers.

A. The Discovery of New Rhythm Disorders

Clinical research inspired in part by the dramatic strides in heart surgery and electrostimulation enabled cardiologists to characterize more fully a number of heart rhythm disorders that had never been clearly defined. Especially important for cardiac pacing was the "discovery" of sinus node disease at the end of the 1960s. These names lumped together several known disturbances of the heartbeat involving default of the sinus node, the heart's natural pacemaker (30). By the mid-1970s, pacemaker physicians were implanting pacers in thousands of patients diagnosed with sinus node disease. The surge in pacing for sinus conditions in retrospect raised questions about physicians' uncritical embrace of the treatment: almost all pacers of the 1970s delivered stimuli to the ventricle, but was it not obvious that some forms of sinus disorder called for atrial or dual-chamber pacing (14)?

B. Lengthening the Worklife of the Pacemaker

In 1970 most physicians and manufacturers would have agreed that the principal remaining obstacle to acceptable pacemaker reliability—an obstacle that seriously impeded the further development of cardiac pacing—was the short worklife and general unreliability of the mercury-zinc battery. The manufacturers had made improvements to subsystems of the pacemaker so as to use the battery more efficiently. With QRS-inhibited pacing, the device would fire only when needed and its sensing function required little power. Manufacturers also configured the pulse generator to prolong its escape interval between the last natural R wave and the first pacemaker impulse. This meant that the device would not begin to pace during minor variations in the natural heart rate such as occur during sleep; it would go to work only during a true episode of bradycardia or block (31).

Since the mid-1960s, researchers had investigated a variety of alternatives to the mercury-zinc cell; the most famous of these was an isotopic generator, versions of which came into use in France and the United States during the 1970s. "Nuclear" pacemakers proved an intriguing side path in ongoing pacemaker development (32). In the 1970s, a more acceptable alternative to mercury-zinc at last appeared. Manufacturers' introduction of a new pacemaker battery based on lithium (1973) completed the 15-year process of transforming the implantable pacemaker from an experimental and somewhat refractory technology into a reliable and long-lived device (33). The lithium battery proved able to deliver power for 7 years or more, and its chemical reaction produced no gas by-product—thus the implanted pulse generator could at last be hermetically sealed within a titanium shell. Failure of pulse generators from incursion of body fluid became a thing of the past (19). Greatbatch, the leading advocate of lithium, was correct when he wrote that "the pacemaker battery is no longer a significant clinical problem" (34).

C. Hybrid Circuits and "Programmable" Pacemakers

Despite its popular reputation as a high-tech medical device, the pacemaker has never incorporated the newest advances in microcircuitry but has lagged many military, national security, and civilian applications. In the early 1970s, pacemaker manufacturers began a transition from discrete circuit components to hybrid circuitry. The hybrid circuits used in implantable pacemakers during the 1970s represented partial integration with some circuit elements printed on a ceramic substrate and others individually mounted. These assemblies were certainly more compact and were intended to be more reliable because the manufacturing process was partly automated and the circuit package could be sealed off. A hybrid circuit also drew power from the battery only when performing a function such as opening or closing a switch. Overall, hybrid circuitry enabled manufacturers to meet physicians' request for smaller pulse generators at no sacrifice of reliability or longevity. The generators of the mid-1970s were thinner than the Chardack-Greatbatch device of 1961 and weighed half as much. Smaller generators helped make pacemaker implantation simpler and quicker, thereby reducing complication rates and easing stress on the patient (2,35).

Hybrid circuitry also permitted more flexible pacemaker behavior. In 1973 one U.S. company announced a new pacemaker model that included an integrated sensing amplifier and two integrated digital logic circuits in an overall hybrid design. With this device the physician could noninvasively choose from six pacing rates and four stimulus amplitudes by transmitting a series of magnetic pulses that opened and closed a miniature magnetic reed switch. Despite its new capabilities, the pacemaker made less demand on the battery than a conventional pacer of that era. A follow-on model added a third programmable parameter, stimulus duration (36).

These innovations portended a coming era in which engineers would design complex, fully integrated circuits comprising thousands of elements. The new circuitry promised pulse generators that would be capable of more flexible action than any pacer of the 1960s. Pacing specialists recognized by the mid-1970s that if lithium-powered pacemakers were going to remain in use for 5 or more years, it would be desirable to alter their behavior from time to time as patients aged or their rhythm disorders progressed. By reprogramming the pacemaker, a physician could repeatedly optimize its settings for the individual patient. But this was not yet a vision that the broader community of implanting physicians generally shared. Surveys of physician practice in the United States, indicated that many programmable pacemakers were never reprogrammed but remained on the factory settings (37,38).

The acceleration of innovation in pacing during the 1970s tended to destabilize efforts to contain health-care expenditures by intensifying patients' and physicians' demands for higher levels of health-care consumption (39). With the Medicare program in place (1965) to cover the cost of the pacemaker and the implantation procedure for elderly Americans, the

Table 2 Number of First Implantations and Rates per Million Population, 1981, Selected Countries

	Number of first implantations, 1981	Implantation rate per million population, 1981
Federal Republic of Germany	31,600[a]	519
United States	117,800	518
Austria	1,780	238
France	18,500[a]	236
Canada	5,369	224
Sweden	1,782	215
Netherlands	2,786	198
Norway	776	190
Italy	9,500	167
Argentina	4,500	162
Finland	630	130
United Kingdom	6,400[a]	115
Greece	944	101
Spain	3,550[a]	95
Japan	2,983	26

[a] Estimated.

Source: Feruglio GA, Steinbach K. Pacing in the world today: world survey on cardiac pacing for the years 1979 to 1981. In: Steinbach K, ed. Proceedings of the Seventh World Symposium on Cardiac Pacing, Vienna, May 1 to 5, 1983. Darmstadt: Steinkopff, 1983, Table 5.

number of first-time implantations grew rapidly in the United States. Implantation rates in western Europe generally trailed those in the United States—but the upward trend was unmistakable everywhere (Table 2).

V. THE 1980s: ACHIEVING PHYSIOLOGICAL PACING

During the 1980s, pacemaker manufacturers moved on from lithium and programmability to compete in a new technological arena, dual-chamber pacing. By mid-decade, state-of-the-art pacers boasted both an atrial and a ventricular lead. Manufacturers and leading pacemaker physicians argued that dual-chamber pacing more closely emulated nature and offered important physiological benefits to the patient. Dual-chamber pacing entailed far more complex sensing and pacing behavior; this innovation depended on the enormous flexibility of the newer pulse generators and on new technologies enabling the physician to comprehend and control the behavior of the implanted device.

A. Multiprogrammable Pacemakers with Telemetry

In 1978 a U.S. device manufacturer introduced a pacemaker that could be reprogrammed on four parameters, the highest number yet and an indication that manufacturers would compete with one another by introducing ever more flexible pacemakers (38). The new model also included a novel two-way telemetry system through which the doctor or a technician could download information about the behavior of the implanted device: its stimulation rate, battery voltage and impedance, lead impedance, and the integrity of the encapsulation (40). Soon some implanted pacers had added the capability of storing and yielding up such information as model number, date of implantation, and the patient's diagnosed rhythm disorders. They could transmit intracardiac electrograms that the physician could read in combination with surface ECGs. The new models could be configured to save in memory and later download a record of unusual events in the heart such as episodes of tachycardia (41).

Programmers proved to be an important competitive tool for the device manufacturers, for each programmer would communicate only with pacemakers produced by the same company. Manufacturers offered the programmers *gratis* to hospitals and clinics. Once familiar with a particular programmer and the pacemakers it could manage, the typical physician was likely to remain loyal year after year to the pacing products of that company. Only at large centers did physicians make a continuing effort to implant all the major pacemaker brands.

B. Physiological Pacing: Dual-Chamber Devices

A second pacemaker lead in the atrium was a physicians' concept; it had been attempted repeatedly since the 1950s because sensing in the atrium and pacing in the ventricle would effectively bridge a blocked atrioventricular node and give back to the patient variability in the heart rate. Further, it was understood by the 1980s that simple ventricular pacing was not optimal for many patients who had sinus node disorders (42,43).

The limitations of pacemaker circuitry and problems of stabilizing an electrode in the atrium were finally overcome by 1980. In 1982 the first "AV-universal" dual-chamber pacemaker, capable of sensing and pacing both the atrium and the ventricle, was introduced; the leading manufacturers all followed suit within 3 to 5 years. This new generation of pacemakers behaved in complex ways involving sensing and pacing in both chambers of the heart; they required new programmable features beyond anything required in a single-chamber pacer. Pacemaker engineers could choose a complex custom-designed hybrid circuit or take the more radical course of installing a general-purpose microprocessor to be programmed by software (44).

As pacemakers emulated nature more nearly, they became increasingly difficult for doctors to manage because new programmable functions for dual-chamber pacing now accompanied the more familiar functions for stimulus rate, amplitude, and duration. For example, the physician could set the sensitivity thresholds for both leads so that they reliably sensed spontaneous P and R waves within the heart. It was necessary to choose an appropriate AV interval (the interval between the atrial and ventricular stimuli) and program the postventricular atrial refractory period to avoid pacemaker-mediated tachycardias (PMTs) by rendering the atrial sensing circuit temporarily blind. Physicians could individualize the settings and revise them later as necessary. Even in uncomplicated cases, setting up a dual-chamber pacemaker required that the physician combine information from the patient's ECG and the programmer's telemetered data to form a detailed and insightful picture of how the implanted pacemaker and the heart were interacting. In more complex cases, the heart's own erratic behavior plus the pacemaker's stimuli in both chambers could produce ECGs requiring great skill to interpret (45,46).

As late as 1989 three-fourths of the pacemakers sold in the U.S. market were still single-chamber devices that fired unless inhibited by sensed QRS complexes; this kind of pacing behavior had been around for over 20 years. Physicians could quickly place a ventricular lead in most cases, but adding an atrial lead could be challenging and time-consuming. Many physicians also perceived dual-chamber pacers to be complex, difficult to understand, and likely to require frequent reprogramming. Until the 1990s, many implanters remained unpersuaded that the benefits to the patient of dual-chamber pacing outweighed the troubles it made for both doctor and patient (47,48).

A shift toward dual-chamber pacing occurred rather tardily in the early 1990s. In the United States, this coincided with a growing dominance of cardiologists, including electrophysiologists, in the field of pacing and a corresponding decline in the participation of surgeons. An additional factor may have been that the pacemaker companies' programmers, the auxiliary devices through which doctors communicated with implanted pacemakers, were becoming more user friendly. The newer programmers pointed out unusual patterns in the patient's heartbeat, prompted the doctor with suggested settings, and issued warnings when settings contradicted each other or endangered the patient (49).

C. Rate-Adaptive Pacing

The complexity of dual-chamber pacemakers and the risk of problems such as PMTs led the manufacturers simultaneously down two paths of innovation. The first was to add a biosensor to a single-chamber pacemaker so that the device would vary its firing rate in response to changes in the patient's activity level. In the earliest such system to gain regulatory approval and go into general production (1986), the sensor picked up high-frequency sounds from the movement of muscles. Other researchers and manufacturers varied the stimulus rate based on such indicators of increased metabolic demand as central venous oxygen content, respiratory rate, or changes in the Q-T interval of the heartbeat. Though some found this less elegant than dual-chamber pacing because it continued to ignore the atrium, the *rate-adaptive* pacemaker held out the promise of physiologic pacing with less complexity (50). The second path led toward greater automaticity in pacing devices, an approach to be discussed below.

VI. THE 1990s AND AFTER: BROADENING THE SPECTRUM OF DISEASES

Just as the pacemaker was in effect redefined at the end of the 1950s to treat chronic rhythm disorders, and in the 1970s to manage sinus node disease, beginning in the 1990s specialists and manufacturers redefined it once again. The pacemaker and its close relatives including the implantable defibrillator (ICD) have become instruments that manage a spectrum of chronic heart diseases including atrial and ventricular tachycardia, atrial fibrillation, and congestive heart failure. Modern ICDs are typically able to carry out cardioversion, antitachycardia pacing, and traditional bradycardia pacing as needed. The aging of populations in western Europe and the United States, the greater number of indications for pacemaker implantation, and the growth of markets beyond Western Europe and North America all contributed to continued robust growth in the number of pacemaker implantations (51,14).

A. Complexity and Automaticity

In the 1990s manufacturers introduced new models almost annually and continued to make their pacemakers physically smaller and longer-lived with each iteration, in keeping with physicians' well-known preferences. Each new device also usually included some striking feature that showcased the virtuosity of its manufacturer and permitted the exchange of greater amounts of information between physician and implanted pacemaker. Some models took rate-adaptive pacing to new levels of sophistication by sensing two separate physiologic indicators such as activity and respiration.

More information and more programming choices presented the physician with daunting complexity at a time when physicians typically had less time to make diagnostic and programming decisions. To address this problem, manufacturers introduced pacemakers with automatic functionality based on microprocessors. The implanted devices were increasingly capable of performing on their own the core of the tasks formerly assigned to physicians: diagnosing the patient's arrhythmia and selecting an appropriate pacemaker therapy. A manufacturer's press release stated that one new device could "analyze heart rhythm patterns, much as a physician does when reviewing an electrocardiogram." Physician and support staff would still select, implant, and initially program the pacer, address complications at implantation or later, and periodically check on the condition and performance of the implanted device by transtelephone monitoring or at a pacemaker clinic (52).

The physician's point of connection with the pacemaker came through the programmer. From the earliest models in the 1970s, programmers had evolved into specialized laptop computers able to receive data from the implanted pacemaker, display the data for the physician or technician in a variety of tables and graphs (including stored electrograms), and transmit reprogramming instructions back to the device. The manufacturers emphasized that the programmers would save staff time and that nurse specialists and technicians could program a pacemaker appropriately because the pacer and programmer already contained decades of electrophysiological knowledge and could make or recommend appropriate clinical choices in most situations (53). Newer pacemaker leads also boasted features such as "steerability" that were said to make them faster and easier to use.

B. Beyond Traditional Arrhythmia Therapy

By the end of the 1990s, the pacemaker that met most clinicians' every need had been realized. Yet the manufacturers had come to believe that at least in the American market, failure to "improve the product" continually would ruin a firm's pricing strategy, undermine its reputation, and erode its market share. Seeking new ways to use their technological competence in electrostimulation, five leading manufacturers in Europe and the United States set out in the 1990s to develop cardiac resynchonization systems to treat ventricular dyssynchrony, a condition arising from congestive heart failure. Essentially a cardiac resynchronization system is a dual-chamber pacemaker with a third lead introduced via the coronary sinus and established in a cardiac vein to pace the left ventricle. When the device senses an atrial contraction, it stimulates the ventricles to contract simultaneously. This therapy reduces regurgitation of blood at the mitral valve and improves the filling of the left ventricle (54).

One of the five companies also used its knowledge base in electrostimulation of the heart to develop implantable devices that treated neurological conditions including essential tremor and Parkinsonian tremor, spasticity in cerebral palsy and multiple sclerosis, gastroporesis, sleep apnea, and chronic lower-back pain (55). Few if any of these therapies could have been imagined a generation ago, and some may prove to have limited clinical applicability; but collectively they revealed the enormous flexibility of the basic technology of electrostimulation applied to the body and managed by modern microprocessors.

VII. CONCLUDING REMARKS

We recall the heroic age of cardiac pacing—the 1950s and 1960s—when a handful of physicians and electronic engineers invented the pacemaker and resolved many of its early problems. However, the institutional basis for innovation in pacing has changed fundamentally since those days. In the United States, Europe, and elsewhere, pacing has evolved into a complex subsystem of national health-care systems. Innovation has necessarily become routinized. The parties most intensely involved with the ongoing evolution of pacing include the device manufacturers and cardiologists. Hospitals and large clinics, regulatory agencies, the insurance industry, and national health-care institutions also seek to foster or discourage growth and new directions in cardiac pacing (39).

The circle continues to widen: patients and family members increasingly see themselves as stakeholders in cardiac pacing. Through organized advocacy groups, they will make their hopes and fears known in the political realm. Ongoing innovation in electrostimulation will require not only advances in microelectronics and in understanding of disease but the ability of these numerous interested parties to achieve a degree of consensus (39).

One knowledgeable participant–observer of the device industry argues that "only the (medical device) manufacturers as a group, driven by individual physicians who see the possibility to provide their patients with better therapies, have...been in a position to play a key role in coordinating and influencing activities across different disciplines and organizational spheres to drive the innovation process further" (56). It is not difficult to see why this should be so: the device manufacturers are well positioned to explore the opportunities afforded by the ongoing technological progress in microelectronics and the evolving knowledge of cardiovascular diseases. They are able to organize and manage the elaborate clinical studies needed to persuade physicians, regulators, and funding agencies of the safety and cost effectiveness of a proposed new device. By informing investors and the general public about the promise of a new therapy, they can help create the atmosphere of expectation that is vital for its eventual adoption. More than other stakeholders, the manufacturers possess the institutional skills required to encourage and coordinate innovation (57).

REFERENCES

1. Ott K. The sum of its parts: an introduction to modern histories of prosthetics. In: Ott K, Serlin D, Mihm S, eds. Artificial Parts, Practical Lives: Modern Histories of Prosthetics. New York: New York University Press, 2002:1–42.

2. Hidefjäll P. The Pace of Innovation: Patterns of Innovation in the Cardiac Pacemaker Industry. Linköping, Sweden: Linköping University, 1997.

3. Rowbottom M, Susskind C. Electricity and Medicine: History of Their Interaction. San Francisco: San Francisco Press, 1984.

4. Schechter DC. Exploring the Origins of Electrical Cardiac Stimulation. Minneapolis: Medtronic, 1983.

5. Morus IR. Marketing the machine: the construction of electrotherapeutics as viable medicine in early Victorian England. Med Hist 1992; 36:34–52.

6. MacWilliam JA. Electrical stimulation of the heart in man. Brit Med J 1889; i:348–350.

7. Howell JD. 'Soldier's heart': the redefinition of heart disease and speciality formation in early twentieth-century Great Britain. Med Hist 1985; (suppl 5):34–52.

8. Fleming P. A Short History of Cardiology. Amsterdam: Editions Rodopi, 1997.

9. Howell JD. Early perceptions of the electrocardiogram: from arrhythmia to infarction. Bull Hist Med 1984; 58:83–98.

10. Fye WB. A history of cardiac arrhythmias. In: Kastor JA, ed. Arrhythmias. Philadelphia: W.B. Saunders, 1994:1–24.

11. Howell JD. Cardiac physiology and clinical medicine? Two case studies. In: Geison GL, ed. Physiology in the American Context, 1850–1940. Bethesda: American Physiological Society, 1987:279–292.

12. Mond HG, Sloman JG, Edwards RH. The first pacemaker. Pacing Clin Electrophysiol 1982; 5:278–282.

13. Furman S, Jeffrey K, Szarka G. The mysterious fate of Hyman's pacemaker. Pacing Clin Electrophysiol 2001; 24:1126–1137.

14. Jeffrey K. Machines in Our Hearts: The Cardiac Pacemaker, the Implantable Defibrillator, and American Health Care. Baltimore: The Johns Hopkins University Press, 2001.

15. Zoll PM. Resuscitation of the heart in ventricular standstill by external electric stimulation. N Engl J Med 1952; 247:768–771.

16. Leatham A, Cook P, Davies JG. External electric stimulator for treatment of ventricular standstill. Lancet 1956; ii:1185–1189.

17. Braun E, Macdonald S. Revolution in Miniature: The History and Impact of Semiconductor Electronics. 2d ed. Cambridge: Cambridge University Press, 1983.

18. Rhees DJ, Jeffrey K. Earl Bakken's little white box: the complex meanings of the first transistorized pacemaker. In: Finn B, Bud R, Trischler H, eds. Exposing Electronics. London: Harwood, 2000:75–113.

19. Greatbatch W. The Making of the Pacemaker: Celebrating a Lifesaving Invention. Amherst, N.Y.: Prometheus Books, 2000.

20. Chardack WM. A myocardial electrode for long-term pacemaking. Ann N Y Acad Sci 1964; 111:893–906.

21. Furman S, Schwedel JB. An intracardiac pacemaker for Stokes–Adams seizures. N Engl J Med 1959; 261:943–948.

22. Furman S. Recollections of the beginnings of transvenous cardiac pacing. Pacing Clin Electrophysiol 1994; 17:1697–1705.

23. Lagergren H, Johansson L. Intracardiac stimulation for complete heart block. Acta Chir Scan 1963; 125:562–566.

24. Siddons H, Davies JG. A new technique for internal cardiac pacing. Lancet 1963; ii:1204–1205.

25. Chardack WM. Cardiac pacemakers and heart block. In: Gibbon JH Jr, Sabiston DC, Spencer FC, eds. Surgery of the Chest. 2d ed. Philadelphia: W.B. Saunders, 1969:824–865.

26. Parsonnet V, Bernstein AD. Transvenous pacing: a seminal transition from the research laboratory. Ann Thorac Surg 1989; 48:738–740.
27. Furman S, Parker B, Escher DJW. Transtelephone pacemaker clinic. J Thorac Cardiovasc Surg 1971; 61:827–834.
28. Castellanos A Jr, Lemberg L, Jude JR, et al. Repetitive firing occurring during synchronized electrical stimulation of the heart. J Thorac Cardiovasc Surg 1966; 51:334–340.
29. Bilitch M, Cosby RS, Cafferky EA. Ventricular fibrillation and competitive pacing. N Engl J Med 1967; 276:598–604.
30. Ferrer MI. The sick sinus syndrome in atrial disease. J Am Med Assoc 1968; 206:645–646.
31. Sutton R, Bourgeois I. The Foundations of Cardiac Pacing, Part I. Mount Kisco, N.Y.: Futura, 1991.
32. Parsonnet V, Gilbert L, Zucker R, Werres R, Atherley T, Manhardt M, Cort J. A decade of nuclear pacing. Pacing Clin Electrophysiol 1984; 7:90–95.
33. Greatbatch W, Lee JH, Mathias W, Eldridge M, Moser JR, Schneider AA. The solid-state lithium battery: a new improved chemical power source for implantable cardiac pacemakers. IEEE Trans Biomed Eng 1971; 18:317–324.
34. Greatbatch W. Pacemaker technology: energy sources. Cardiovasc Clin 1983; 14:239–246.
35. Bowers DL. New pacemaker devices from a technical point of view. In: Thalen HJT, Harthorne JW, eds. To Pace or Not to Pace: Controversial Subjects in Cardiac Pacing. The Hague: M. Nijhoff, 1978:126–130.
36. Parsonnet V, Cuddy TE, Escher DJW, Furman S, Morse D, Gilbert L, Zucker IR. A permanent pacemaker capable of external non-invasive programming. Trans Am Soc Artif Intern Org 1973; 19:224–228.
37. MacGregor DC, Furman S, Dreifus LS. The utility of the programmable pacemaker. Pacing Clin Electrophysiol 1978; 1:254–259.
38. Parsonnet V. The proliferation of cardiac pacing: medical, technical, and socioeconomic dilemmas. Circulation 1982; 65:841–845.
39. Moran M. Governing the Health Care State: A Comparative Study of the United Kingdom, the United States and Germany. Manchester and New York: Manchester University Press, 1999.
40. Tyers FO, Brownlee RR. A multiparameter telemetry system for cardiac pacemakers. In: Varriale P, Naclerio EA, eds. Cardiac Pacing: A Concise Guide to Clinical Practice. Philadelphia: Lea & Febiger, 1979:349–368.
41. Sholder J, Levine PA, Mann BM, Mace RC. Bidirectional telemetry and interrogation in cardiac pacing. In: Barold SS, Mugica J, eds. The Third Decade of Cardiac Pacing: Advances in Technology and Clinical Applications. Mount Kisco, N.Y.: Futura, 1982:145–166.
42. Sutton R, Perrins J, Citron P. Physiological cardiac pacing. Pacing Clin Electrophysiol 1980; 3:207–219.
43. Asubel K, Furman S. The pacemaker syndrome. Ann Intern Med 1985; 103:420–429.
44. Hartlaub J. Pacemaker of the future: microprocessor based or custom circuit? In: Barold SS, Mugica J, eds. The Third Decade of Cardiac Pacing: Advances in Technology and Clinical Applications. Mount Kisco, NY: Futura, 1983:417–428.
45. Parsonnet V, Bernstein AD. Cardiac pacing in the 1980s: treatment and techniques in transition. J Am Coll Cardiol 1983; 1:339–354.
46. Sykosch HJ. The new generation of pacemakers. Prog Artif Org 1983; 1:317–323.
47. Bernstein AD, Parsonnet V. Survey of cardiac pacing in the United States in 1989. Am J Cardiol 1992; 69:331–338.
48. Brinker JA. VVI vs. DDD—new twists to the ongoing controversy [editorial]. Intell Reports Cardiac Pacing Electrophysiol 1990; 9:1 (4).
49. Bernstein AD, Parsonnet V. Survey of cardiac pacing and defibrillation in the United States in 1993. Am J Cardiol 1996; 78:187–196.
50. Humen DP, Anderson K, Brumwell D, Huntley S, Klein GJ. A pacemaker which automatically increases its rate with physical activity. In: Steinbach K, ed. Proceedings of the VIIth World

Symposium on Cardiac Pacing, Vienna, May 1st to 5th, 1983. Darmstadt: Steinkopff, 1983:259–264.

51. Bernstein AD, Parsonnet V. Survey of cardiac pacing and implanted defibrillator practice patterns in the United States in 1997. Pacing Clin Electrophysiol 2001; 24:842–855.

52. Ritter P, Cazeau S, Mugica J. Do we really need automatic pacemakers? In: Barold SS, Mugica J, eds. New Perspectives in Cardiac Pacing. Mount Kisco, N.Y.: Futura, 1993:337–346.

53. Increasing efficiency in the pacemaker clinic [panel discussion]. Guidant/CPI Pacing Dynamics 1998; 1 Q:6–7, 12.

54. Abraham WT, Fisher WG, Smith AL, Delurgio DB, Leon AR, Loh E, Kocovic DZ, Packer M, Clavell AL, Hayes DL, Ellestad M, Trupp RJ, Underwood J, Pickering F, Truex C, McAtee P, Messenger J, the MIRACLE Study Group. Cardiac resynchronization in chronic heart failure. N Engl J Med 2002; 346:1845–1853.

55. www.medtronic.com/neuro/, visited July 27, 2002.

56. Hidefjäll P. Can pacemaker innovation go on forever? Unpublished ms, 2001.

57. Gibbons M, Limoges C, Nowotny H, Schwartzman S, Scott P, Trow M. The New Production of Knowledge: The Dynamics of Science and Research in Contemporary Societies. Thousand Oaks, Calif. and London: SAGE Publications, 1994.

35

The Energetic Heart: Bioelectromagnetic Communication Within and Between People

Rollin McCraty

*HeartMath Research Center, Institute of HeartMath,
Boulder Creek, California, U.S.A.*

Evidence is presented demonstrating that internally generated electromagnetic fields from the heart and brain can affect the EEG and ECG wave patterns of individuals who are nearby but not in physical contact. Examples are provided and the nature of physiological coherence is discussed. The importance of coherence in improving synchronization in the internal milieu as well as relationships with others is explained with an emphasis on the implications for promoting emotional and physical health.

Man's perceptions are not bounded by organs of perception; he perceives far more than sense (tho' ever so acute) can discover.—William Blake

This chapter will focus on electromagnetic fields generated by the heart that permeate every cell and may act as a synchronizing signal for the body in a manner analogous to information carried by radio waves. Particular emphasis will be devoted to evidence demonstrating that this energy is not only transmitted internally to the brain but is also detectable by others within its range of communication. The heart generates the largest electromagnetic field in the body. The electrical field as measured in an electrocardiogram (ECG) is about 60 times greater in amplitude than the brain waves recorded in an electroencephalogram (EEG). The magnetic component of the heart's field, which is around 5000 times stronger than that produced by the brain, is not impeded by tissues and can be measured several feet away from the body with superconducting quantum interference device (SQUID)-based magnetometers (1). We have also found that the clear rhythmic patterns in beat-to-beat heart rate variability are distinctly altered when different emotions are experienced. These changes in electromagnetic, sound pressure, and blood pressure waves produced by cardiac rhythmic activity are "felt" by every cell in the body, further supporting the heart's role as a global internal synchronizing signal.

541

I. BIOLOGICAL PATTERNS ENCODE INFORMATION

One of the primary ways that signals and messages are encoded and transmitted in physiological systems is in the language of patterns. In the nervous system, it is well established that information is encoded in the time intervals between action potentials—patterns of electrical activity—and this may also apply to humoral communications. Several recent studies have revealed that biologically relevant information is encoded in the time interval between hormonal pulses (2–4). As the heart secretes a number of different hormones with each contraction, there is a hormonal pulse pattern that correlates with heart rhythms. In addition to the encoding of information in the space between nerve impulses and in the intervals between hormonal pulses, it is likely that information is also encoded in the interbeat intervals of the pressure and electromagnetic waves produced by the heart. Karl Pribram has proposed that the low-frequency oscillations generated by the heart and body in the form of afferent neural, hormonal, and electrical patterns are the carriers of emotional information and that the higher frequency oscillations found in the EEG reflect the conscious perception and labeling of feelings and emotions (5).

A. Detecting Bioelectromagnetic Patterns Using Signal Averaging

A useful technique for detecting patterns in biological systems and investigating a number of bioelectromagnetic phenomena is signal averaging (Fig. 1). This is accomplished by super-imposing any number of equal-length epochs, each of which contains a repeating periodic

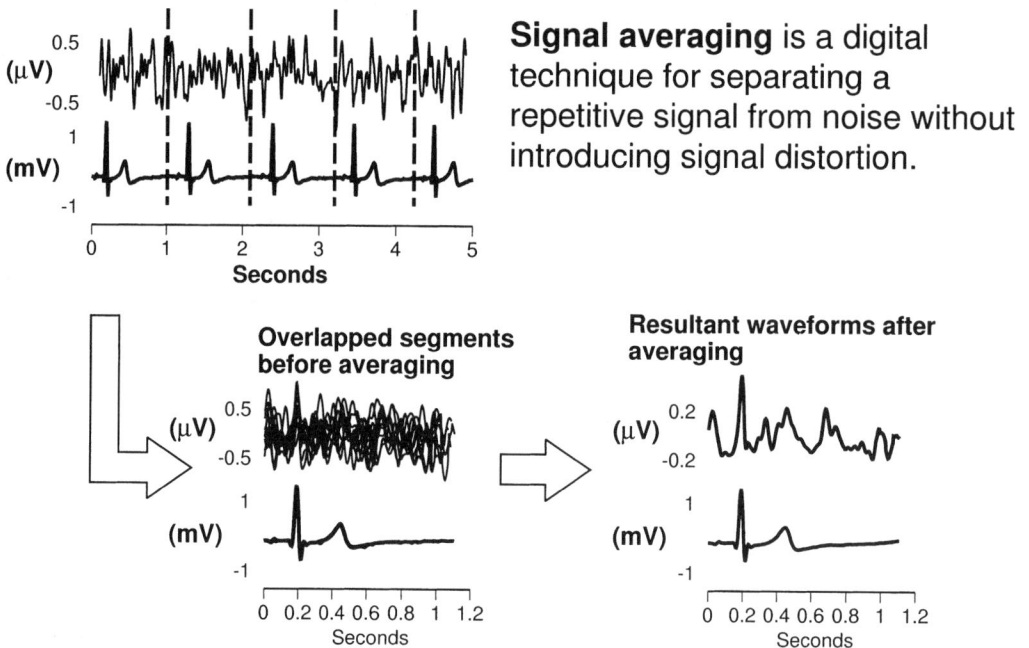

Signal averaging is a digital technique for separating a repetitive signal from noise without introducing signal distortion.

Figure 1 Signal averaging. The sequence of the signal-averaging procedure is shown above. First, the signals recorded from the EEG and ECG are digitized and stored in a computer. The R wave (peak) of the ECG is used as the time reference for cutting the EEG and ECG signals into individual segments. The individual segments are then averaged together to produce the resultant waveforms. Only signals that are repeatedly synchronous with the ECG are present in the resulting waveform. Signals not related to the signal source (ECG) are eliminated through this process.

signal. This emphasizes and distinguishes any signal that is time-locked to the periodic signal while eliminating variations that are not time-locked to the periodic signal. This procedure is commonly used to detect and record cerebral cortical responses to sensory stimulation (6). When signal averaging is used to detect activity in the EEG that is time-locked to the ECG, the resultant waveform is called the *heartbeat evoked potential*.

B. The Heartbeat Evoked Potential

In looking at heartbeat evoked potential data, it can be seen that the electromagnetic signal arrives at the brain instantaneously, while a host of different neural signals reach the brain starting about 8 ms later and continue arriving throughout the cardiac cycle. Although the precise timing varies with each cycle, at around 240 ms the blood pressure wave arrives at the brain and acts to synchronize neural activity, especially the alpha rhythm (Fig. 2). It is also

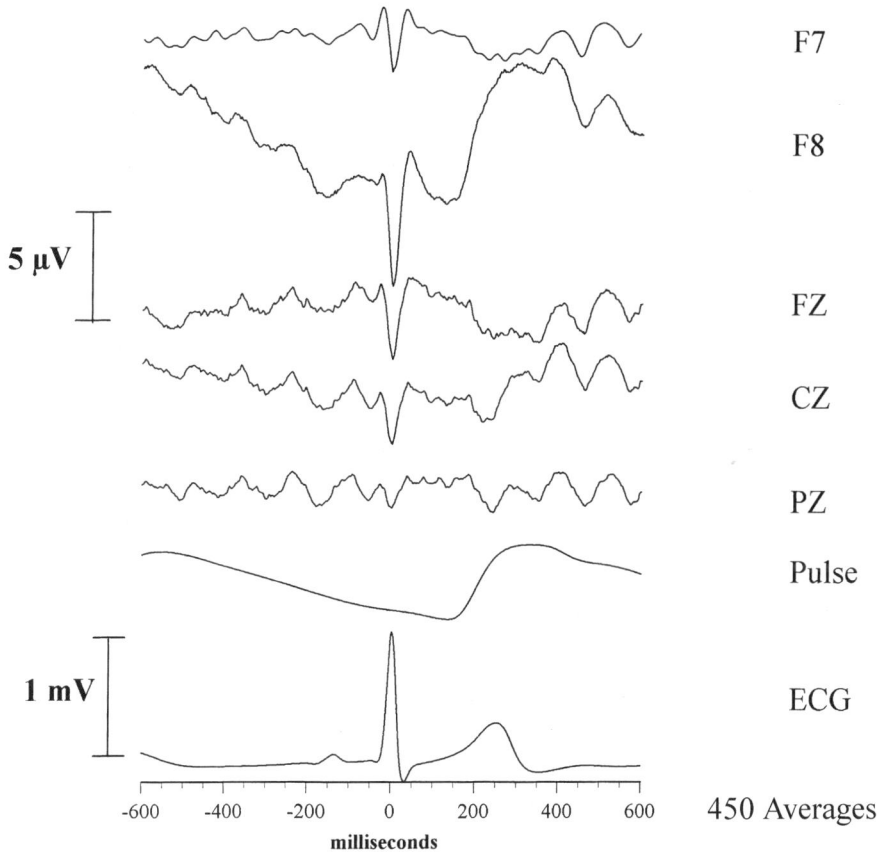

Figure 2   Heartbeat evoked potentials. This figure shows an example of typical heartbeat evoked potentials. In this example, 450 averages were used. The pulse wave is also shown, indicating the timing relationship of the blood pressure wave reaching the brain. In this example, there is less synchronized alpha activity immediately after the R wave. The time range between 10 and 250 ms is when afferent signals from the heart are impinging upon the brain, and the alpha desynchronization indicates the processing of this information. Increased alpha activity can be clearly seen later in the waveforms, starting at around the time the blood pressure wave reaches the brain.

possible that information is encoded in the shape (modulation) of the ECG wave itself. For example, if one examines consecutive ECG cycles, it can be seen that each wave is slightly varied in a complex manner.

As indicated, the heart generates a powerful pressure wave that travels rapidly throughout the arteries much faster than the actual flow of blood that we feel as our pulse. These pressure waves force the blood cells through the capillaries to provide oxygen and nutrients to cells and expand the arteries, causing them to generate a relatively large electrical voltage. These waves also apply pressure to the cells in a rhythmic fashion that can cause some of their proteins to generate an electrical current in response to this "squeeze." Experiments conducted in our laboratory have shown that a change in the brain's electrical activity can be seen when the blood pressure wave reaches the brain around 240 ms after systole.

There is a replicable and complex distribution of heartbeat evoked potentials across the scalp. Changes in these evoked potentials associated with the heart's afferent neurological input to the brain are detectable between 50 to 550 ms after the heartbeat (7). Gary Schwartz and colleagues at the University of Arizona believe the earlier components in this complex distribution cannot be explained by simple physiological mechanisms alone and suggest that an energetic interaction between the heart and brain also occurs (8). They have confirmed our findings that heart-focused attention is associated with increased heart–brain synchrony, providing further support for energetic heart–brain communications. Schwartz and colleagues also demonstrated that when subjects focused their attention on the perception of their heartbeat, the synchrony in the preventricular region of the heartbeat evoked potential increased. From this they concluded that preventricular synchrony may reflect an energetic mechanism of heart–brain communication, while postventricular synchrony most likely reflects direct physiological mechanisms.

II. THE HEART'S ROLE IN EMOTION

Throughout the 1990s, the view that the brain and body work in conjunction in order for perceptions, thoughts, and emotions to emerge gained momentum and is now widely accepted. The brain is an analog processor that relates whole concepts (patterns) to one another and looks for similarities, differences, or relationships between them, in contrast to a digital computer that assembles thoughts and feelings from bits of data. This new understanding of how the brain functions has challenged several long-standing assumptions about the nature of emotions. While it was formerly maintained that emotions originated only in the brain, we now recognize that emotions can be more accurately described as a product of the brain and body acting in concert. Moreover, evidence suggests that of the bodily organs, the heart may play a particularly important role in emotional experience. Research in the relatively new discipline of neurocardiology has confirmed that the heart is a sensory organ and acts as a sophisticated information encoding and processing center that enables it to learn, remember, and make independent functional decisions that do not involve the cerebral cortex (9). Additionally, numerous experiments have demonstrated that patterns of cardiac afferent neurological input to the brain not only affect autonomic regulatory centers, but also influence higher brain centers involved in perception and emotional processing (10–13).

Heart rate variability (HRV), derived from the ECG, is a measure of the naturally occurring beat-to-beat changes in heart rate that has proven to be invaluable in studying the physiology of emotions. The analysis of HRV, or *heart rhythms*, provides a powerful, noninvasive measure of neurocardiac function that reflects heart-brain interactions and autonomic nervous system dynamics, which are particularly sensitive to changes in emotional states (14,15). Our research, along with that of others, suggests that there is an important link between emotions and changes in the patterns of both efferent (descending) and afferent (ascending) autonomic activity (12,14,16–18). These changes in autonomic activity are associated with dramatic changes in the *pattern* of the heart's rhythm that often occur without any change in the *amount* of heart rate variability. Specifically, we have found that during the experience of negative emotions such as anger, frustration, or anxiety, heart rhythms become more erratic and disordered, indicating less synchronization in the reciprocal action that ensues between the parasympathetic and sympathetic branches of the autonomic nervous system (ANS) (16). In contrast, sustained positive emotions, such as appreciation, love, or compassion, are associated with highly ordered or *coherent* patterns in the heart rhythms, reflecting greater synchronization between the two branches of the ANS and a shift in autonomic balance toward increased parasympathetic activity (14,16,17,19) (Fig. 3).

A. Physiological Coherence

Based on these findings, we have introduced the term *physiological coherence* to describe a number of related physiological phenomena associated with more ordered and harmonious interactions among the body's systems (20).

The term *coherence* has several related definitions. A common definition of the term is the quality of being logically integrated, consistent, and intelligible, as in a coherent argument. In this context, thoughts and emotional states can be considered coherent or incoherent. Importantly, however, these associations are not merely metaphorical, as different emotions are in fact associated with different degrees of coherence in the oscillatory rhythms generated by the body's various systems.

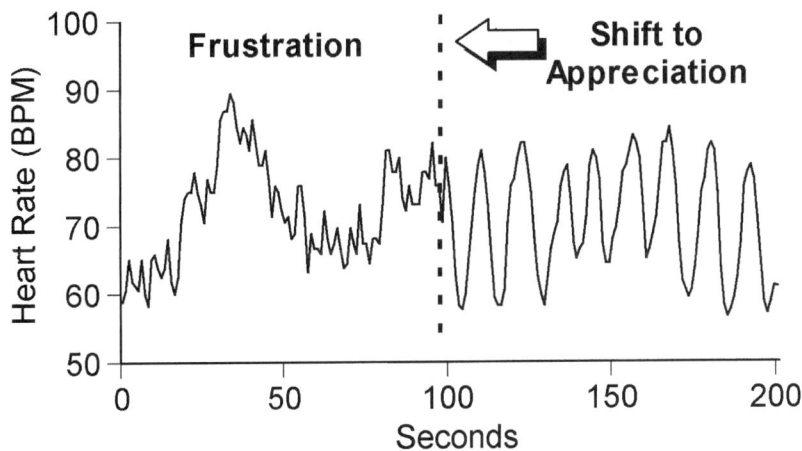

Figure 3 Emotions are reflected in heart rhythm patterns. Real-time heart rate variability (heart rhythm) pattern of an individual making an intentional shift from a self-induced state of frustration to a genuine feeling of appreciation by using a positive emotion refocusing exercise known as the Freeze-Frame technique (at the dotted line). It is of note that when the recording is analyzed statistically, the *amount* of heart rate variability is found to remain virtually the same during the two different emotional states; however, the *pattern* of the heart rhythm changes distinctly. Note the immediate shift from an erratic, disordered heart rhythm pattern associated with frustration to a smooth, harmonious, sine wave-like (coherent) pattern as the individual uses the positive emotion refocusing technique and self-generates a heartfelt feeling of appreciation.

The term *coherence* is used in physics to describe the ordered or constructive distribution of power within a waveform. The more stable the frequency and shape of the waveform, the higher the coherence. An example of a coherent wave is the sine wave. The term *autocoherence* is used to denote this kind of coherence. In physiological systems, this type of coherence describes the degree of order and stability in the rhythmic activity generated by a single oscillatory system. Methodology for computing coherence has been published elsewhere (14).

Coherence also describes two or more waves that are either phase or frequency locked. In physiology, coherence is used to describe a functional mode in which two or more of the body's oscillatory systems, such as respiration and heart rhythms, become *entrained* and oscillate at the same frequency. The term *cross-coherence* is used to specify this type of coherence.

All the above definitions apply to the study of both emotional physiology and bioelectromagnetism. We have found that positive emotions are associated with a higher degree of coherence within the heart's rhythmic activity (autocoherence) as well as increased coherence between different oscillatory systems (cross-coherence or entrainment) (14,20). Typically, entrainment is observed between heart rhythms, respiratory rhythms, and blood pressure oscillations; however, other biological oscillators, including very low frequency brain rhythms, craniosacral rhythms, electrical potentials measured across the skin, and, most likely, rhythms in the digestive system, can also become entrained (20).

We have also demonstrated that physiological coherence is associated with increased synchronization between the heartbeat (ECG) and alpha rhythms in the EEG. In experiments measuring heartbeat evoked potentials, we found that the brain's alpha activity (8–12 Hz frequency range) is naturally synchronized to the cardiac cycle. However, when subjects used a positive emotion refocusing technique to consciously self-generate feelings of appreciation, their heart rhythm coherence significantly increased, as did the ratio of the alpha rhythm that was synchronized to the heart (20,21).

Another related phenomenon associated with physiological coherence is *resonance*. In physics, resonance refers to a phenomenon whereby an unusually large vibration is produced in a system in response to a stimulus whose frequency is identical or nearly identical to the natural vibratory frequency of the system. The frequency of the vibration produced in such a state is said to be the resonant frequency of the system. When the human system is operating in the coherent mode, increased synchronization occurs between the sympathetic and parasympathetic branches of the ANS, and entrainment between the heart rhythms, respiration, and blood pressure oscillations is observed. This occurs because these oscillatory subsystems are all vibrating at the resonant frequency of the system. Most models show that the resonant frequency of the human cardiovascular system is determined by the feedback loops between the heart and brain (22,23). In humans and in many animals, the resonant frequency is approximately 0.1 Hz, which is equivalent to a 10-s rhythm.

In summary, we use coherence as an umbrella term to describe a physiological mode that encompasses entrainment, resonance, and synchronization—distinct but related phenomena, all of which emerge from the harmonious activity and interactions of the body's subsystems. Correlates of physiological coherence include increased synchronization between the two branches of the ANS, a shift in autonomic balance toward increased parasympathetic activity, increased heart–brain synchronization, increased vascular resonance, and entrainment between diverse physiological oscillatory systems. The coherent mode is reflected by a smooth, sine wave-like pattern in the heart rhythms (heart rhythm coherence) and a narrow-band, high-amplitude peak in the low-frequency range of the heart rate variability power spectrum, at a frequency of about 0.1 Hz.

1. Benefits of Coherence

Coherence confers a number of benefits to the system in terms of both physiological and psychological functioning. At the physiological level, there is increased efficiency in fluid exchange, filtration, and absorption between the capillaries and tissues; increased ability of the cardiovascular system to adapt to circulatory demands; and increased temporal synchronization of cells throughout the body (24,25). This results in increased system-wide energy efficiency and conservation of metabolic energy. These observations support the link between positive emotions and increased physiological efficiency that may partially explain the growing number of documented correlations between positive emotions, improved health, and increased longevity (26–28). We have also shown that practicing certain techniques that increase physiological coherence is associated with both short-term and long-term improvement in several objective health-related measures, including enhanced humoral immunity (29,30) and an increased DHEA/cortisol ratio (17).

Increased physiological coherence is similarly associated with psychological benefits, including improvements in cognitive performance and mental clarity as well as increased emotional stability and well-being (20,31). Studies conducted in diverse populations have documented significant reductions in stress and negative affect and increases in positive mood and attitudes in individuals using coherence-building techniques (17,19,29,31,32).

Improvements in clinical status, emotional well being and quality of life have also been demonstrated in various medical patient populations in intervention programs using coherence-building approaches. For example, significant blood pressure reductions have been demonstrated in individuals with hypertension (33), improved functional capacity and reduced depression in congestive heart failure patients (34), improved psychological health and quality of life in patients with diabetes (35), and improvements in asthma (36). Another study reported reductions in pathological symptoms and anxiety and significant improvements in positive affect, physical vitality, and general well-being in individuals with HIV infection and AIDS (37).

Additionally, patient case history data provided by numerous health care professionals report substantial improvements in health and psychological status and frequent reductions in medication requirements in patients with such medical conditions as cardiac arrhythmias, chronic fatigue, environmental sensitivity, fibromyalgia, and chronic pain (38). Finally, techniques that increase physiological coherence have been used effectively by mental health professionals in the treatment of emotional disorders, including anxiety, depression, panic disorder, and posttraumatic stress disorder (38).

2. Drivers of Physiological Coherence

Although physiological coherence is a natural state that can occur spontaneously during sleep and deep relaxation, sustained episodes during normal daily activities are generally rare. While specific rhythmic breathing methods can induce coherence for brief periods, cognitively directed, paced breathing is difficult for many people to maintain. On the other hand, our findings indicate that individuals can produce extended periods of physiological coherence by actively generating and sustaining a feeling of appreciation or other positive emotions. Sincere positive feelings appear to excite the system at its resonant frequency, allowing the coherent mode to emerge naturally. This typically makes it easier for people to sustain a positive emotion for much longer periods, thus facilitating the process of establishing and reinforcing coherent patterns in the neural architecture as the familiar reference. Once a new pattern is established, the brain strives to maintain a match with the new program, thus increasing the probability of maintaining coherence and reducing stress, even during challenging situations (12).

Doc Childre, founder of the Institute of HeartMath, has developed a number of practical positive emotion refocusing and emotional restructuring techniques that allow people to quickly self-generate coherence at will (39,40). Known as the HeartMath system, these techniques utilize the heart as a point of entry into the psychophysiological networks that connect the physiological, mental, and emotional systems. In essence, because the heart is a primary generator of rhythmic neural and energetic patterns in the body—influencing brain processes that control the ANS, cognitive function, and emotion—it provides an access point from which system-wide dynamics can be quickly and profoundly affected. Research studies and the experience of numerous health care professionals indicate that HeartMath coherence-building techniques are easily learned, have a high rate of compliance, and are highly adaptable to a wide range of demographic groups.

3. Promoting Physiological Coherence Through Heart Rhythm Coherence Feedback Training

Used in conjunction with positive emotion-based coherence-building techniques, heart rhythm feedback training can be a powerful tool to assist people in learning how to self-generate increased physiological coherence (41). We have developed a portable heart rhythm monitoring and feedback system that enables physiological coherence to be objectively monitored and quantified. Known as the Freeze-Framer* coherence-building system (Quantum Intech, Inc., Boulder Creek, CA), this interactive hardware and software system monitors and displays individuals' heart rate variability patterns in real time as they practice the positive emotion refocusing and emotional restructuring techniques taught in an on-line tutorial. Using a fingertip sensor to record the pulse wave, the Freeze-Framer plots changes in heart rate on a beat-to-beat basis. As people practice the coherence-building techniques, they can readily see and experience the changes in their heart rhythm patterns, which generally become more ordered, smoother, and more sine wave-like as they experience positive emotions. This process reinforces the natural association between the physiological coherence mode and positive feelings. The software also analyzes the heart rhythm patterns for coherence level, which is fed back to the user as an accumulated numerical score or success in playing one of three on-screen games designed to reinforce the coherence-building skills. The real-time physiological feedback essentially takes the guesswork and randomness out of the process of self-inducing a coherent state, resulting in greater consistency, focus, and effectiveness in shifting to a beneficial psychophysiological mode.

Heart rhythm coherence feedback training has been successfully used in clinical settings by physicians, mental health professionals, and neurofeedback therapists to facilitate health improvements in patients with numerous physical and psychological disorders. It is also increasingly being utilized in corporate, law enforcement, and educational settings to enhance physical and emotional health and improve performance.

B. Heart Rhythms and Bioelectromagnetism

The first biomagnetic signal was demonstrated in 1963 by Gerhard Baule and Richard McFee in a magnetocardiogram (MCG) that used magnetic induction coils to detect fields generated by the human heart (42). A remarkable increase in the sensitivity of biomagnetic

---

* HeartMath, Freeze-Frame, and Heart Lock-In are registered trademarks of the Institute of HeartMath. Freeze-Framer is a registered trademark of Quantum Intech, Inc.

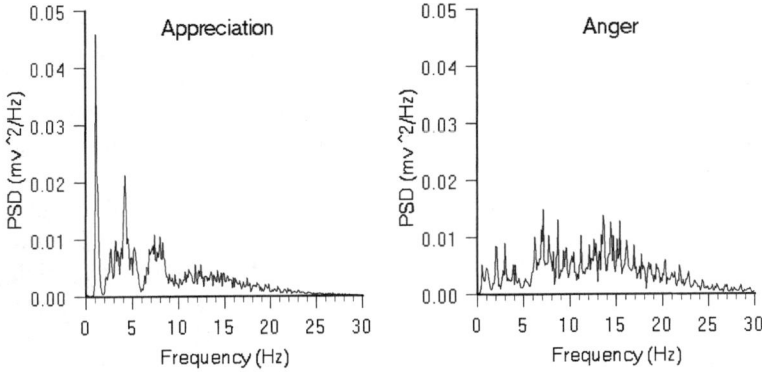

Figure 4 ECG spectra during different emotional states. The above graphs are the average power spectra of 12 individual 10-s epochs of ECG data, which reflect information patterns contained in the electromagnetic field radiated by the heart. The left-hand graph is an example of a spectrum obtained during a period of high heart rhythm coherence generated during a sustained heartfelt experience of appreciation. The graph on the right depicts a spectrum associated with a disordered heart rhythm generated during feelings of anger.

measurements was achieved with the introduction of the superconducting quantum interference device (SQUID) in the early 1970s, and the ECG and MCG have since been shown to closely parallel one another (43).

The heart generates a series of electromagnetic pulses in which the time interval between each beat varies in a complex manner. These pulsing waves of electromagnetic energy create fields within fields and give rise to interference patterns when they interact with magnetically polarizable tissues and substances.

Figure 4 shows two different power spectra derived from an average of 12 individual 10-s epochs of ECG data recorded during differing psychophysiological modes. The plot on the left was produced while the subject was in a state of deep appreciation, whereas the plot on the right was generated while the subject experienced recalled feelings of anger. The difference in the patterns, and thus the information they contain, can be clearly seen. There is a direct correlation between the patterns in the heart rate variability rhythm and the frequency patterns in the spectrum of the ECG or MCG. Experiments such as these indicate that psychophysiological information can be encoded into the electromagnetic fields produced by the heart (14,44).

III. BIOELECTROMAGNETIC COMMUNICATION BETWEEN PEOPLE

The human body is replete with mechanisms for detecting its external environment. Sense organs, the most obvious example, are specifically geared to react to touch, temperature, select ranges of light and sound waves, etc. These organs are acutely sensitive to external stimuli. The nose, for example, can detect one molecule of gas, while a cell in the retina of the eye can detect a single photon of light; and if the ear were any more sensitive, it would pick up the sound of the random vibrations of its own molecules (45).

The interaction between two human beings—for example, the consultation between a patient and her clinician—is a very sophisticated exchange that involves many subtle factors. Most people tend to think of communication solely in terms of overt signals expressed through facial movements, voice qualities, gestures, and body movements. However, evidence now supports the perspective that a subtle yet influential electromagnetic or "energetic" communication system operates just below our conscious level of awareness. The following section will discuss data suggesting that this energetic system contributes to the "magnetic" attractions or repulsions that occur between individuals. It is also quite possible that these energetic interactions can affect the therapeutic process.

The concept of energy or information exchange between individuals is central to many of the Eastern healing arts, but its acceptance in Western medicine has been hampered by the lack of a plausible mechanism to explain the nature of this "energy information" or how it is communicated. However, numerous studies investigating the effects of healers, Therapeutic Touch practitioners, and other individuals have demonstrated a wide range of significant effects including the influence of "energetic" approaches on wound-healing rates (46,47), pain (48,49), hemoglobin levels (50), conformational changes of DNA (51,52), and water structure (52), as well as psychological states (53). Although these reports show beneficial results, they have been largely ignored because of the lack of any scientific rationale to explain how the effects are achieved.

A. Physiological Linkage and Empathy

The ability to sense what other people are feeling is an important factor in allowing us to connect or communicate effectively with others. The smoothness or flow in any social interaction depends to a great extent on the establishment of a spontaneous entrainment or linkage between individuals. When people are engaged in deep conversation, they begin to fall into a subtle dance, synchronizing their movements and postures, vocal pitch, speaking rates, and length of pauses between responses (54), and as we are now discovering, important aspects of their physiology can also become linked and entrained.

Several studies have investigated different types of physiological synchronization or entrainment between individuals during empathetic moments or between clinician and patient during therapeutic sessions. One study by Levenson and Gottman at the University of California at Berkeley looked at physiological synchronization in married couples during empathetic interactions. Researchers examined couples' physiological responses during two discussions: a neutral "How was your day?" conversation, to establish a baseline, and a second conversation containing more emotional content in which the couples were asked to spend 15 min discussing something about which they disagreed. After the disagreement, one partner was asked to leave the room while the other stayed to watch a replay of the talk and identify portions of the dialogue where he or she was actually empathizing but did not express it. Both spouses individually engaged in this procedure. Levenson was then able to identify those segments of the video where empathy occurred and match the empathetic response to physiological responses in both partners. He found that in partners who were adept at empathizing, their physiology mimicked their partner's while they empathized. If the heart rate of one went up, so did the heart rate of the other; if the heart rate slowed, so did that of the empathic spouse (55). Other studies observing the psychophysiology of married couples while interacting were able to predict the probability of divorce (56).

Although studies that have examined physiological linkages between therapists and patients have suffered from methodological challenges, they do support a tendency to autonomic attunement during periods of empathy between the therapist and patient (57). Dana Redington, a psychophysiologist at the University of California, San Francisco, analyzed heart rate variability patterns during therapist-patient interactions using a nonlinear dynamics approach. Redington and colleagues used phase space maps to plot changes in the beat-to-beat heart rate of both the therapist and patient during psychotherapy sessions. They found that the trajectories in the therapist's patterns often coincided with the patient's during moments when the therapist experienced strong feelings of empathy for the patient (58).

Carl Marci at Harvard University found evidence of a more direct linkage between patients and therapists using skin conductance measures. During sessions of psychodynamic psychotherapy, Marci observed a quantifiable fluctuation and entrainment in the pattern of physiological linkage within patient-therapist dyads, which was related to patient perception of the therapist's empathy. In addition, the preliminary results of his studies indicate that during low physiological linkage there are fewer empathetic comments, more incidents of incorrect interpretations, less shared affect, and fewer shared behavioral responses when compared to episodes of high physiological linkage (59).

B. Cardioelectromagnetic Communication

An important step in testing our hypothesis that the heart's electromagnetic field could transmit signals between people was to determine if the field and the information modulated within it could be detected by other individuals.

In conducting these experiments, the question being asked was straightforward. Namely, can the electromagnetic field generated by the heart of one individual be detected in physiologically relevant ways in another person, and if so does it have any discernible biological effects? To investigate these possibilities, we used signal-averaging techniques to detect signals that were synchronous with the peak of the R wave of one subject's ECG in recordings of another subject's electroencephalogram (EEG) or brain waves. My colleagues and I have performed numerous experiments in our laboratory over a period of several years using these techniques (60), and several examples are included below to illustrate some of these findings. In the majority of these experiments, subjects were seated in comfortable, high-back chairs to minimize postural changes with the positive ECG electrode located on the side at the left sixth rib and referenced to the right supraclavicular fossa according to the International 10–20 system. The ECG and EEG were recorded from both subjects simultaneously so that the data (typically sampled at 256 Hz or higher) could be analyzed for simultaneous signal detection in both.

To clarify the direction in which the signal flow was analyzed, the subject whose ECG R wave was used as the time reference for the signal averaging procedure is referred to as the *signal source*, or simply *source*. The subject whose EEG was analyzed for the registration of the source's ECG signal is referred to as the *signal receiver*, or simply *receiver*. The number of averages used in the majority of the experiments was 250 ECG cycles (~4 min). The subjects did not consciously intend to send or receive a signal and, in most cases, were unaware of the true purpose of the experiments. The results of these experiments have led us to conclude that the nervous system acts as an antenna, which is tuned to and responds to the magnetic fields produced by the hearts of other individuals. My colleagues and I call this energetic information exchange *cardioelectromagnetic communication* and believe it to be an innate ability that heightens awareness and mediates important aspects of true empathy and sensitivity to others. Furthermore, we have observed that this energetic communication ability can be enhanced, resulting in a much deeper level of nonverbal communication, understanding, and connection between people. We also propose that this type of energetic communication between individuals may play a role in therapeutic interactions between clinicians and patients that has the potential to promote the healing process.

From an electrophysiological perspective, it appears that sensitivity to this form of energetic communication between individuals is related to the ability to be emotionally and physiologically coherent. The data indicate that when individuals are in the coherent mode, they are more sensitive to receiving information contained in the fields generated by others. In addition, during physiological coherence, internal systems are more stable, function more efficiently, and radiate electromagnetic fields containing a more coherent structure (14).

1. The Electricity of Touch

The first step was to determine if the ECG signal of one person could be detected in another individual's EEG during physical contact. For these experiments we seated pairs of subjects 4 ft apart, during which time they were simultaneously monitored. An initial 10-min baseline period (no physical contact) was followed by a 5-min period in which subjects remained seated but reached out and held the hand of the other person (like shaking hands). Figure 5 shows a typical example of the results.

Prior to holding hands, there was no indication that subject 1's ECG signals were detected in subject 2's EEG. However, upon holding hands, subject 1's ECG could be clearly detected in subject 2's EEG at all monitored locations. While in most pairs a clear signal

The Electricity of Touch
Heartbeat Signal Averaged Waveforms

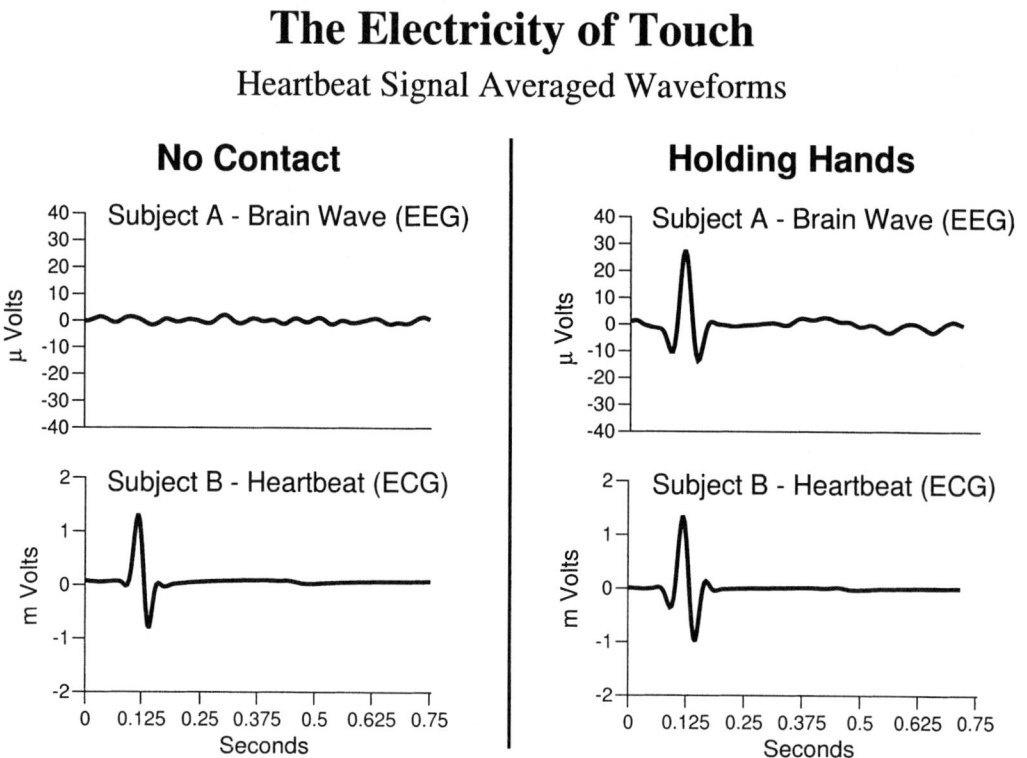

Figure 5 Signal-averaged waveforms showing the detection of electromagnetic energy generated by the source's heart in the receiving subject's EEG. The baseline recording (left side) is from a 10-min period during which time the subjects were seated 4 ft apart without physical contact. The right column shows the recording from the 5-min period during which the subjects held hands. The EEG data shown here were recorded from the C3 site of the EEG.

transfer between the two subjects was measurable in one direction, it was only observed in both directions simultaneously in about 30% of the pairs (i.e., subject 2's ECG could be detected in subject 1's EEG at the same time that subject 1's ECG was detectable in subject 2's EEG). From other experiments we have concluded that this phenomenon is not related to gender or amplitude of the ECG signal. As shown later, an important variable appears to be the degree of physiological coherence maintained.

After demonstrating that the ECG from one individual could be detected in another's EEG during physical contact, we completed a series of experiments to determine if the signal was transferred via electrical conduction through the skin alone or if it was also radiated. In one set of experiments subjects were recorded holding hands under two sets of conditions: barehanded and wearing form-fitting, latex lab gloves. The ECG signal of one subject could be clearly detected in the EEG of the other subject even when they were wearing the gloves; however, the signal amplitude was reduced approximately tenfold. This suggests that while a significant degree of the signal transfer occurs through skin conduction, the signal is also radiated or capacitively coupled between individuals. When conductive gel was used to decrease skin-to-skin contact resistance, the signal amplitude was unaffected. For additional detail, the protocols and data from these and related experiments are described elsewhere (60).

We also conducted several experiments to determine if the transfer of cardiac energy and information is affected by the orientation of the subjects' hand holding (i.e., source's left hand holding receiver's right hand vs. source's right hand holding receiver's left hand, etc.). The subjects were instructed to hold hands in each of the four possible orientations for 5 min. Since we only performed this experiment with three subject pairs, the results should be interpreted with a degree of caution; however, we did find that consistent and measurable differences could be observed. The source's ECG appeared with the largest amplitude in the receiver's EEG when the receiver's right hand was held by either the source's left or right hand. When the receiver's left hand was held by the source's right hand, the signal appeared at a lower amplitude. Finally, when the receiver's left hand was held by the source's left hand, the ECG signal was either very low in amplitude or undetectable (60).

The possibility exists that in some cases the signal appearing in the receiving subject's recordings could be the receiver's own ECG rather than that of the other subject. Given the signal averaging procedure employed, this could only occur if the source's ECG was continually and precisely synchronized with the receiver's ECG. To definitively rule this out, the data in all experiments were checked for this possibility.

Simultaneously and independently, Russek and Schwartz at the University of Arizona conducted similar experiments in which they were also able to demonstrate the detection of an individual's cardiac signal in another's EEG recording in two people sitting quietly, without physical contact (61). In a publication entitled "Energy Cardiology," they discuss the implications of their findings in the context of what they call a "dynamical energy systems approach" describing the heart as a prime generator, organizer, and integrator of energy in the human body (62).

2. Heart-Brain Synchronization During Nonphysical Contact

Since the magnetic component of the field produced by the heartbeat is radiated outside the body and can be detected several feet away with SQUID-based magnetometers (1), we further tested the transference of signals between subjects who were not in physical contact. In these experiments, the subjects were either seated side by side or facing each other at varying distances. In some cases, we were able to detect a clear QRS-shaped signal in the receiver's EEG, but not in others. Although the ability to obtain a clear registration of the

ECG in the other person's EEG declined as the distance between subjects was increased, the phenomenon appears to be nonlinear. For instance, a clear signal could be detected at a distance of 18 in. in one session but was undetectable in the very next trial at a distance of only 6 in. Although transmission of a clear QRS-shaped signal is uncommon at distances over 6 in. in our experience, this does not preclude the possibility that physiologically relevant information can be communicated between people under such conditions.

Figure 6 shows the data from two subjects seated facing one another at a distance of 5 ft, with no physical contact. The subjects were asked to use the Heart Lock-In technique (39), an emotional restructuring exercise that has clearly been shown to produce sustained states of physiological coherence when properly applied (17). There was no intention to "send energy," and participants were not aware of the purpose of the experiment. The top three traces show the signal-averaged waveforms derived from the EEG locations along the medial line of the head.

Note that in this example, the signal-averaged waveforms do not contain any semblance of the QRS complex shape as seen in the physical contact experiments; rather they reveal the occurrence of an alpha wave synchronization in the EEG of one subject that is precisely

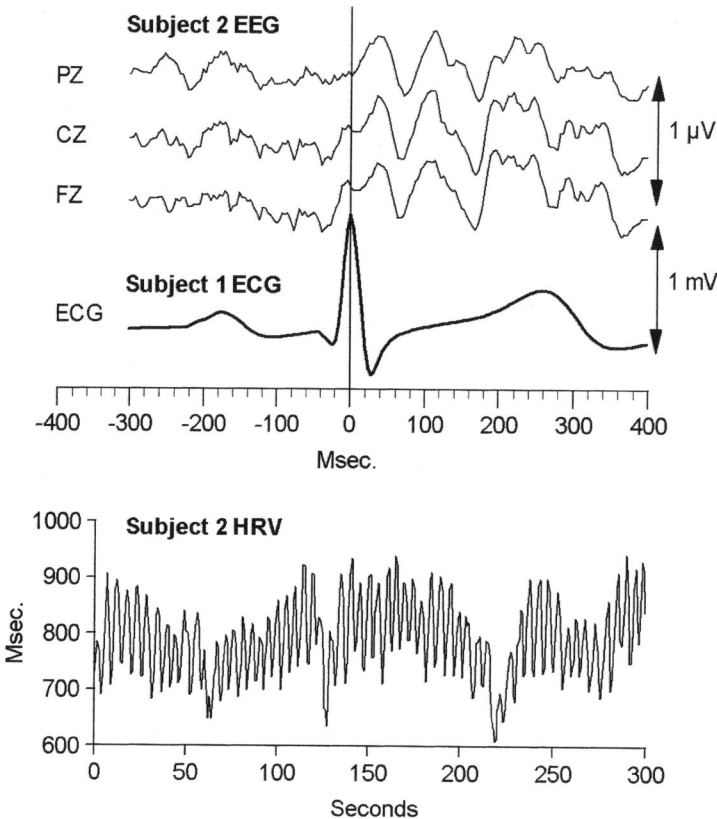

Figure 6 Heart-brain synchronization between two people. The top three traces are subject 2's signal averaged EEG waveforms, which are synchronized to the R wave of subject 1's ECG. The lower plot shows subject 2's heart rate variability pattern, which was coherent throughout the majority of the record. The two subjects were seated at a conversational distance without physical contact.

timed to the R wave of the other subject's ECG. Power spectrum analysis of the signal-averaged EEG waveforms was used to verify that it is the alpha rhythm that is synchronized to the other person's heart. This alpha synchronization does not imply that there is increased alpha activity, but it does show that the existing alpha rhythm is able to synchronize to extremely weak external electromagnetic fields such as those produced by another person's heart. It is well known that the alpha rhythm can synchronize to an external stimulus such as sound or light flashes, but the ability to synchronize to such a subtle electromagnetic signal is surprising. As mentioned, there is also a significant ratio of alpha activity that is synchronized to one's own heartbeat, and the amount of this synchronized alpha activity is significantly increased during periods of physiological coherence (20,21).

Figure 7 shows an overlay plot of one of subject 2's signal-averaged EEG traces and subject 1's signal-averaged ECG. This view shows an amazing degree of synchronization between the EEG of subject 2 and subject 1's heart. These data show that it is possible for the magnetic signals radiated by the heart of one individual to influence the brain rhythms of another. In addition, this phenomenon can occur at conversational distances. As yet, we have not tested this effect at distances greater than 5 ft.

Figure 8 shows the data from the same two subjects during the same time period, only it is analyzed for alpha synchronization in the opposite direction (subject 1's EEG and subject 2's ECG). In this case, we see that there is no observable synchronization between subject 1's EEG and subject 2's ECG. The key difference between the data shown in Fig. 6 and Fig. 8 is the high degree of physiological coherence maintained by subject 2. In other words, the degree of coherence in the *receiver's* heart rhythms appears to determine whether his or her brain waves synchronize to the other person's heart.

This suggests that when one is in a physiologically coherent mode, one exhibits greater sensitivity in registering the electromagnetic signals and information patterns encoded in the fields radiated by the hearts of other people. At first glance these data may be mistakenly interpreted as suggesting that we are more vulnerable to the potential negative influence of

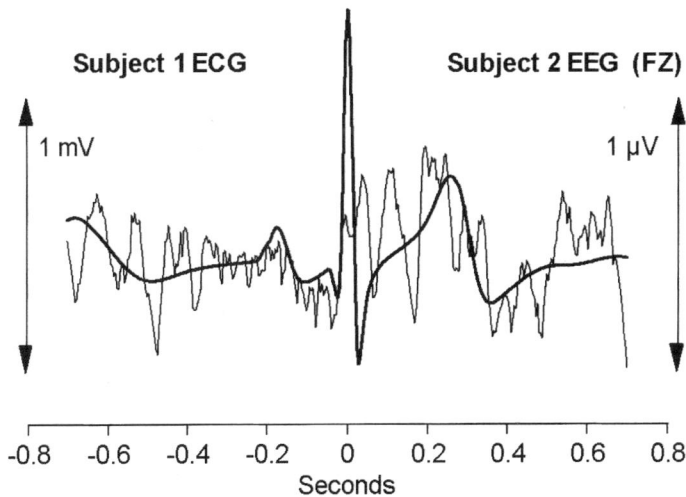

Figure 7 Overlay of signal-averaged EEG and ECG. This graph is an overlay plot of the same EEG and ECG data shown in Fig. 6. Note the similarity of the wave shapes, indicating a high degree of synchronization.

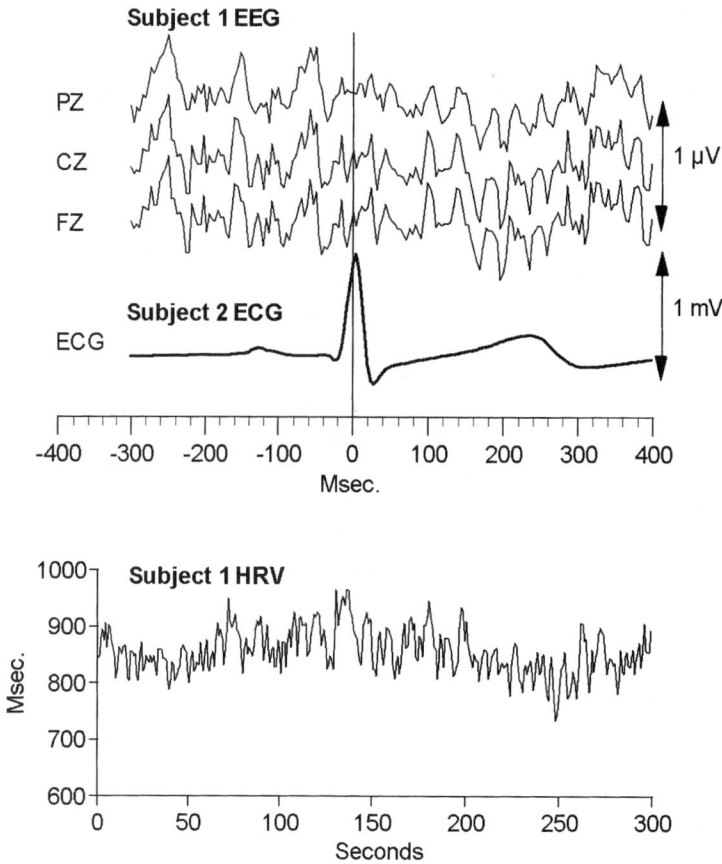

Figure 8 The top three traces are the signal-averaged EEG waveforms for subject 1. There is no apparent synchronization of subject 1's alpha rhythm to subject 2's ECG. The bottom plot is a sample of subject 1's heart rate variability pattern, which was incoherent throughout the majority of the record.

incoherent patterns radiated by those around us. In fact, the opposite is true, because when people are able to maintain the physiological coherence mode, they are more internally stable and thus less vulnerable to being negatively affected by the fields emanating from others. It appears that it is the increased internal stability and coherence that allows for the increased sensitivity to emerge.

This fits quite well with our experience in training thousands of individuals in how to self-generate and maintain coherence while they are listening to others during conversation. Once individuals learn this skill, it is a common experience that they become much more attuned to other people and are able to detect and understand the deeper meaning behind spoken words. They are often able to sense what someone else really wishes to communicate even when the other person may not be clear about that which he is attempting to say. This technique, called *intuitive listening*, helps people to feel fully heard and promotes greater rapport and empathy between people (63).

Our data are also relevant to Russek and Schwartz's findings that people who are more accustomed to experiencing positive emotions such as love and care are better receivers of cardiac signals from others (61). In their follow-up study of 20 college students, those who had rated themselves as having been raised by loving parents exhibited significantly greater registration of an experimenter's ECG in their EEG than others who had perceived their parents as less loving. Our findings, which show that positive emotions such as love, care, and appreciation are associated with increased physiological coherence, suggest the possibility that the subjects in Russek and Schwartz's study had higher ratios of physiological coherence, which could explain the greater registration of cardiac signals.

3. Heart Rhythm Entrainment Between Subjects

When heart rhythms are more coherent, the electromagnetic field that is radiated outside the body correspondingly becomes more organized, as shown in Fig. 4. The data presented thus far indicate that signals and information can be communicated energetically between individuals, but so far have not implied a literal entrainment of two individuals' heart rhythm patterns. We have found that entrainment of heart rhythm patterns between individuals is possible, but usually occurs only under very specific conditions. In our experience, true heart rhythm entrainment between individuals is very rare during normal waking states. We have found that individuals who have a close working or living relationship are the best candidates for exhibiting this type of entrainment. Figure 9 shows an example of heart rhythm entrainment between two women who have a close working relationship and practice coherence-building techniques regularly. For this experiment, they were seated 4 ft apart and, although blind to the data, were consciously focused on generating feelings of appreciation for each other.

A more complex type of entrainment can also occur during sleep. Although we have only looked at couples who are in long-term stable and loving relationships, we have been surprised at the high degree of heart rhythm synchrony observed in these couples while they sleep. Figure 10 shows an example of a small segment of data from one couple. These data were recorded using an ambulatory ECG (Holter) recorder with a modified cable harness

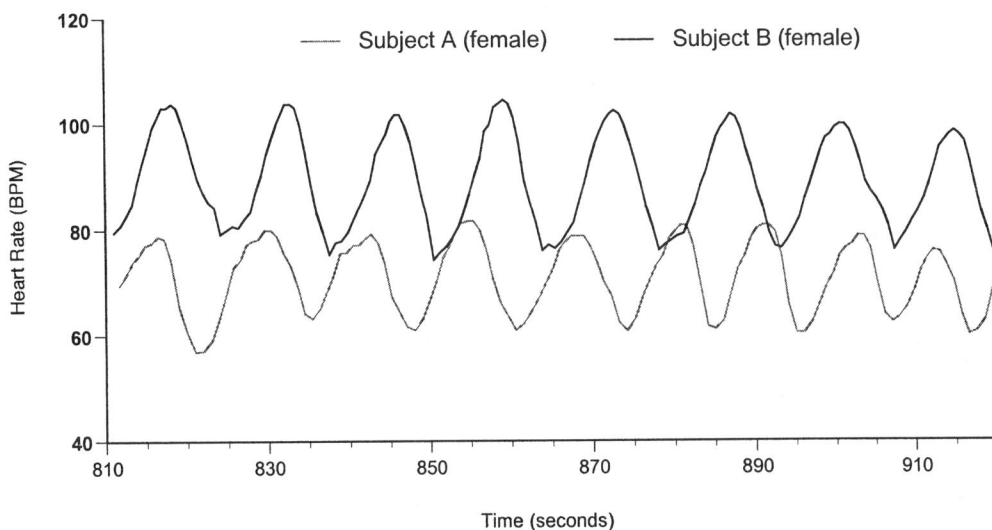

Figure 9 Heart rhythm entrainment between two people. These data were recorded while both subjects were practicing the Heart Lock-In emotional restructuring technique and consciously feeling appreciation for each other. It should be emphasized that in typical waking states, entrainment between people such as in this example is rare.

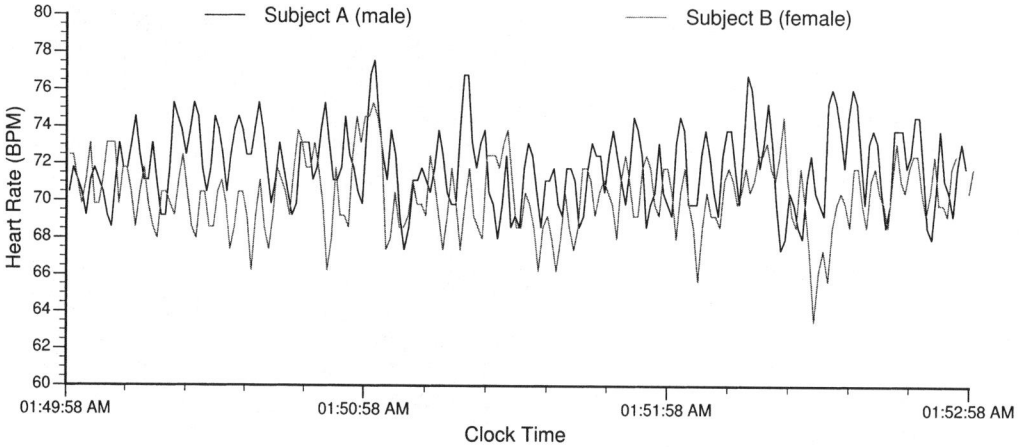

Figure 10 Heart rhythm entrainment between husband and wife during sleep.

A Boy and His Dog
(Heart Rhythms)

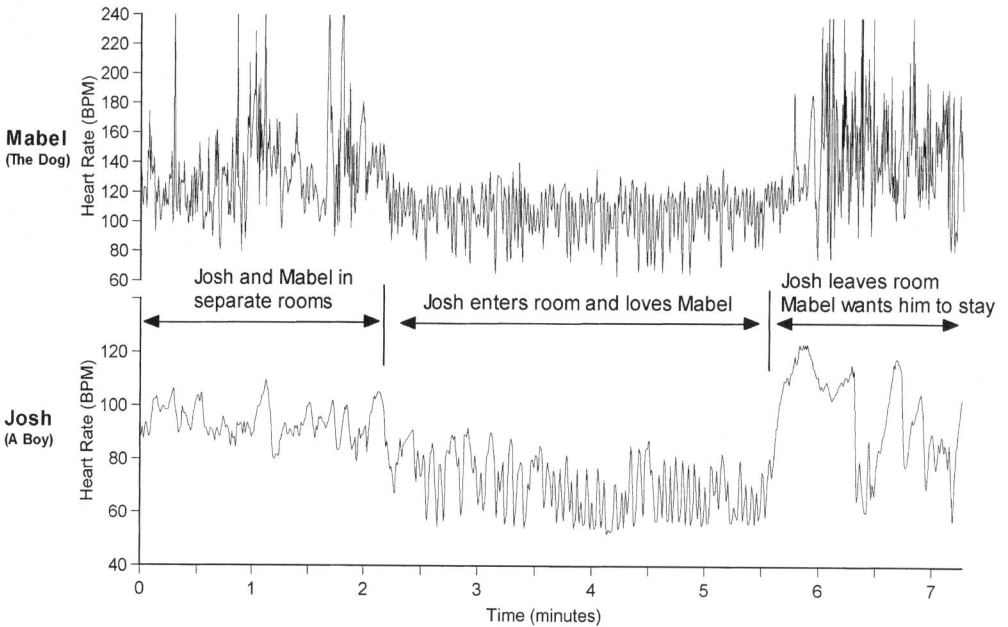

Figure 11 Heart rhythm patterns of a boy and his dog. These data were obtained using ambulatory ECG (Holter) recorders fitted on both Josh, a boy, and Mabel, his pet dog. When Josh entered the room where Mabel was waiting and consciously felt feelings of love and care towards his pet, his heart rhythms became more coherent, and this change appears to have influenced Mabel heart rhythms, which then also became more coherent. When Josh left the room, Mabel's heart rhythms became much more chaotic and incoherent, suggesting separation anxiety!

that allowed the concurrent recording of two individuals on the same tape. Note how the heart rhythms simultaneously change in the same direction and how heart rates converge. Throughout the recording, clear transition periods are evident in which the heart rhythms move into greater synchronicity, maintain the entrainment for some time, and then drift out again. This implies that unlike in most wakeful states, entrainment between the heart rhythms of individuals can and does occur during sleep.

We have also found that a type of heart rhythm entrainment or synchronization can occur in interactions between people and their pets. Figure 11 shows the results of an experiment looking at the heart rhythms of my son Josh (15 years old at the time of the recording) and his dog, Mabel. Here we used two Holter recorders, one fitted on Mabel and the other on Josh. We synchronized the recorders and placed Mabel in one of our labs. Josh then entered the room and sat down and proceeded to consciously experience feelings of love towards Mabel. Note the synchronous shift to increased coherence in the heart rhythms of both Josh and Mabel as Josh consciously feels love for his pet.

IV. CONCLUSIONS AND IMPLICATIONS FOR CLINICAL PRACTICE

Bioelectromagnetic communication is a real phenomenon that has numerous implications for physical, mental, and emotional health. This chapter has focused on the proposition that increasing the coherence within and between the body's endogenous bioelectromagnetic systems can increase physiological and metabolic energy efficiency, promote mental and emotional stability, and provide a variety of health rewards. It is further proposed that many of the benefits of increased physiological coherence will ultimately prove to be mediated by processes and interactions occurring at the electromagnetic or energetic level of the organism.

With the many physiological and psychological benefits that increased coherence appears to offer, helping patients learn to self-generate and sustain this psychophysiological mode with increased consistency in their day-to-day lives provides a new strategy for clinicians to assist their patients on multiple levels. There are several straightforward ways to help patients increase their physiological coherence. Teaching and guiding them in the practice of positive emotion refocusing and emotional restructuring techniques in con-junction with heart rhythm feedback has proved to be a simple and cost-effective approach to improving patient outcomes. These coherence-building methods are not only effective therapeutic tools in and of themselves but by increasing synchronization and harmony among the body's internal systems may also help increase a patient's physiological receptivity to the therapeutic effects of other treatments.

Coherence-building approaches may also help health care practitioners increase their effectiveness in working with patients. In self-generating a state of physiological coherence, the clinician has the potential to facilitate the healing process by establishing a coherent pattern in the subtle electromagnetic environment to which patients are exposed. Since even very weak coherent signals have been found to give rise to significant effects in biological systems (64,65), it is possible that such coherent heart fields may provide unsuspected therapeutic benefits. Furthermore, by increasing coherence, clinicians may not only enhance their own mental acuity and emotional stability but may also develop increased sensitivity to subtle electromagnetic information in their environment. This, in turn, could potentially enable a deeper intuitive connection and communication between practitioner and patient, which can be a crucial component of the healing process.

In conclusion, I believe that the electromagnetic energy generated by the heart acts as a synchronizing force within the body, a key carrier of emotional information, and a mediator of bioelectromagnetic communication between people. As such, the cardiac bioelectromagnetic field is an innate untapped resource that requires further investigation to explore its clinical applications. Such exploration is likely to provide further insight into the dynamics of health and disease that are strongly influenced by emotions and by interactions with others.

REFERENCES

1. Stroink G. Principles of cardiomagnetism. In: Williamson SJ, Hoke M, Stroink G, Kotani M, eds. Advances in Biomagnetism. New York: Plenum Press, 1989:47–57.
2. Prank K, Schofl C, Laer L, Wagner M, von zur Muhlen A, Brabant G, Gabbiani F. Coding of time-varying hormonal signals in intracellular calcium spike trains. Pac Symp Biocomput 1998: 633–644.
3. Schofl C, Prank K, Brabant G. Pulsatile hormone secretion for control of target organs. Wien Med Wochenschr 1995; 145:431–435.
4. Schofl C, Sanchez-Bueno A, Brabant G, Cobbold PH, Cuthbertson KS. Frequency and amplitude enhancement of calcium transients by cyclic AMP in hepatocytes. Biochem J 1991; 273:799–802.
5. Pribram K, Melges F. Psychophysiological basis of emotion. In: Vinken P, Bruyn G, eds. Handbook of Clinical Neurology. Vol. 3. Amsterdam: North-Holland Publishing Company, 1969:316–341.
6. Coles M, Gratton G, Fabini M. Event-related brain potentials. In: Cacioppo J, Tassinary L, eds. Principles of Psychophysiology: Physical, Social and Inferential Elements. New York: Cambridge University Press, 1990.
7. Schandry R, Montoya P. Event-related brain potentials and the processing of cardiac activity. Biol Psychol 1996; 42:75–85.
8. Song L, Schwartz G, Russek L. Heart-focused attention and heart-brain synchronization: energetic and physiological mechanisms. Altern Ther Health Med 1998; 4:44–62.
9. Armour J, Ardell J. Neurocardiology. New York: Oxford University Press, 1994.
10. Sandman CA, Walker BB, Berka C. Influence of afferent cardiovascular feedback on behavior and the cortical evoked potential. In: Cacioppo JT, Petty RE, eds. Perspectives in Cardiovascular Psychophysiology. New York: The Guilford Press, 1982:189–222.
11. Frysinger RC, Harper RM. Cardiac and respiratory correlations with unit discharge in epileptic human temporal lobe. Epilepsia 1990; 31:162–171.
12. McCraty R. Heart-brain neurodynamics: The making of emotions. In: Watkins A, Childre D, eds. Emotional Sovereignty. Amsterdam: Harwood Academic Publishers. In press.
13. van der Molen M, Somsen R, Orlebeke J. The rhythm of the heart beat in information processing. In: Ackles P, Jennings JR, Coles M, eds. Advances in Psychophysiology. Vol. 1. London: JAI Press, 1985:1–88.
14. Tiller W, McCraty R, Atkinson M. Cardiac coherence: a new, noninvasive measure of autonomic nervous system order. Altern Ther Health Med 1996; 2:52–65.
15. McCraty R, Singer D. Heart rate variability: A measure of autonomic balance and physiological coherence. In: Watkins A, Childre D, eds. Emotional Sovereignty. Amsterdam: Harwood Academic Publishers. In press.
16. McCraty R, Atkinson M, Tiller WA, Rein G, Watkins A. The effects of emotions on short term heart rate variability using power spectrum analysis. Am J Cardiol 1995; 76:1089–1093.
17. McCraty R, Barrios-Choplin B, Rozman D, Atkinson M, Watkins A. The impact of a new emotional self-management program on stress, emotions, heart rate variability, DHEA and cortisol. Integr Physiol Behav Sci 1998; 33:151–170.
18. Collet C, Vernet-Maury E, Delhomme G, Dittmar A. Autonomic nervous system response patterns specificity to basic emotions. J Auton Nerv Sys 1997; 62:45–57.
19. McCraty R, Atkinson M, Tomasino D, Goelitz J, Mayrovitz H. The impact of an emotional

self-management skills course on psychosocial functioning and autonomic recovery to stress in middle school children. Integr Physiol Behav Sci 1999; 34:246–268.

20. McCraty R, Atkinson M. Psychophysiological coherence. In: Watkins A, Childre D, eds. Emotional Sovereignty. Amsterdam: Harwood Academic Publishers. In press.

21. McCraty R. Influence of cardiac afferent input on heart-brain synchronization and cognitive performance. Int J Psychophysiol 2002; 45:72–73.

22. Baselli G, Cerutti S, Badilini F, Biancardi L, Porta A, Pagani M, Lombardi F, Rimoldi O, Furlan R, Malliani A. Model for the assessment of heart period variability interactions of respiration influences. Med Biol Eng Comput 1994; 32:143–152.

23. deBoer RW, Karemaker JM, Strackee J. Hemodynamic fluctuations and baroreflex sensitivity in humans: a beat-to-beat model. Am J Physiol 1987; 253:H680–H689.

24. Langhorst P, Schulz G, Lambertz M. Oscillating neuronal network of the "common brainstem system." In: Miyakawa K, Koepchen H, Polosa C, eds. Mechanisms of Blood Pressure Waves. Tokyo: Japan Scientific Societies Press, 1984:257–275.

25. Siegel G, Ebeling BJ, Hofer HW, Nolte J, Roedel H, Klubendorf D. Vascular smooth muscle rhythmicity. In: Miyakawa K, Koepchen H, Polosa C, eds. Mechanisms of Blood Pressure Waves. Tokyo: Japan Scientific Societies Press, 1984:319–338.

26. Danner DD, Snowdon DA, Friesen WV. Positive emotions in early life and longevity: findings from the nun study. J Pers Soc Psychol 2001; 80:804–813.

27. Salovey P, Rothman A, Detweiler J, Steward W. Emotional states and physical health. Am Psychol 2000; 55:110–121.

28. Russek LG, Schwartz GE. Feelings of parental caring predict health status in midlife: a 35-year follow-up of the Harvard Mastery of Stress Study. J Behav Med 1997; 20:1–13.

29. Rein G, Atkinson M, McCraty R. The physiological and psychological effects of compassion and anger. J Adv Med 1995; 8:87–105.

30. McCraty R, Atkinson M, Rein G, Watkins AD. Music enhances the effect of positive emotional states on salivary IgA. Stress Med 1996; 12:167–175.

31. McCraty R, Atkinson M, Tomasino D. Science of the Heart. Boulder Creek, CA: HeartMath Research Center, Institute of HeartMath, Publication No. 01-001, 2001.

32. Barrios-Choplin B, McCraty R, Cryer B. An inner quality approach to reducing stress and improving physical and emotional wellbeing at work. Stress Med 1997; 13:193–201.

33. McCraty R, Atkinson M, Tomasino D, Watkins A. Impact of a workplace stress reduction program on blood pressure and emotional health in hypertensive employees. In preparation.

34. Luskin F, Reitz M, Newell K, Quinn TG, Haskell W. A controlled pilot study of stress management training of elderly patients with congestive heart failure. Prev Cardiol. In press.

35. McCraty R, Atkinson M, Lipsenthal L. Emotional self-regulation program enhances psychological health and quality of life in patients with diabetes. Boulder Creek, CA: HeartMath Research Center, Institute of HeartMath, Publication No. 00-006.

36. Lehrer P, Smetankin A, Potapova T. Respiratory sinus arrhythmia biofeedback therapy for asthma: a report of 20 unmedicated pediatric cases. Appl Psychophysiol Biofeedback 2000; 25:193–200.

37. Rozman D, Whitaker R, Beckman T, Jones D. A pilot intervention program which reduces psychological symptomatology in individuals with human immunodeficiency virus. Complemen Ther Med 1996; 4:226–232.

38. McCraty R, Tomasino D, Atkinson M. Research, clinical perspectives, and case histories. In: Watkins A, Childre D, eds. Emotional Sovereignty. Amsterdam: Harwood Academic Publishers. In press.

39. Childre D, Martin H. The HeartMath Solution. San Francisco: Harper San Francisco, 1999.

40. Childre D, Rozman D. Overcoming Emotional Chaos: Eliminate Anxiety, Lift Depression and Create Security in Your Life. San Diego: Jodere Group, 2002.

41. McCraty R. Heart rhythm coherence—An emerging area of biofeedback. Biofeedback 2002; 30:17–19.

42. Baule G, McFee R. Detection of the magnetic field of the heart. Am Heart J 1963; 55:95–96.

43. Nakaya Y. Magnetocardiography: a comparison with electrocardiography. J Cardiogr Suppl 1984; 3:31–40.

44. McCraty R, Atkinson M, Tiller WA. New electrophysiological correlates associated with intentional heart focus. Subtle Energies 1993; 4:251–268.

45. Russell P. The Brain Book. New York: Penguin Books USA, 1979.

46. Wirth DP. The effect of non-contact therapeutic touch on the healing rate of full thickness dermal wounds. Subtle Energies 1990; 1:1–20.

47. Grad B. Some biological effects of the laying on of hands: review of experiments with animals and plants. J Am Soc Psychical Res 1965; 59:95–171.

48. Keller E. Effects of therapeutic touch on tension headache pain. Nurs Res 1986; 35:101–105.

49. Redner R, Briner B, Snellman L. Effects of a bioenergy healing technique on chronic pain. Subtle Energies 1991; 2:43–68.

50. Krieger D. Healing by the laying on of hands as a facilitator of bioenergetic change: the response of in vivo human hemoglobin. Psychoenergetic Systems 1974; 1:121–129.

51. Rein G, McCraty R. Structural changes in water and DNA associated with new physiologically measurable states. J Sci Explor 1994; 8:438–439.

52. Rein G, McCraty R. Modulation of DNA by coherent heart frequencies. Proceedings of the Third Annual Conference of the International Society for the Study of Subtle Energy and Energy Medicine, Monterey, CA, June 25–29, 1993:58–62.

53. Quinn J. Therapeutic touch as an energy exchange: Testing the theory. ANS Adv Nurs Sci 1984; 6:42–49.

54. Hatfield E. Emotional Contagion. New York: Cambridge University Press, 1994.

55. Levenson RW, Ruef AM. Physiological aspects of emotional knowledge and rapport. In: Ickes W, ed. Empathic Accuracy. New York: Guilford Press, 1997.

56. Levenson R, Gottman J. Physiology and affective predictors of change in relationship satisfaction. J Pers Soc Psychol 1985; 49:85–94.

57. Robinson J, Herman A, Kaplan B. Autonomic responses correlate with counselor-client empathy. J Couns Psychol 1982; 29:195–198.

58. Reidbord SP, Redington DJ. Nonlinear analysis of autonomic responses in a therapist during psychotherapy. J Nerv Ment Dis 1993; 181:428–435.

59. Marci CD. Psychophysiology and psychotherapy: The neurobiology of human relatedness. Practical Reviews of Psychiatry–Audio Tape 2002; 25(3).

60. McCraty R, Atkinson M, Tomasino D, Tiller W. The electricity of touch: Detection and measurement of cardiac energy exchange between people. In: Pribram K, ed. Brain and Values: Is a Biological Science of Values Possible. Mahwah, NJ: Lawrence Erlbaum Associates, 1998: 359–379.

61. Russek L, Schwartz G. Interpersonal heart-brain registration and the perception of parental love: a 42 year follow-up of the Harvard Mastery of Stress Study. Subtle Energies 1994, 5: 195–208.

62. Russek L, Schwartz G. Energy Cardiology: a dynamical energy systems approach for integrating conventional and alternative medicine. Advances 1996;124–24.

63. Childre D, Cryer B. From Chaos to Coherence: The Power to Change Performance. Boulder Creek, CA: Planetary, 2000.

64. Litovitz TA, Krause D, Mullins JM. Effect of coherence time of the applied magnetic field on ornithine decarboxylase activity. Biochem Biophys Res Commun 1991; 178:862–865.

65. Wiesenfeld K, Moss F. Stochastic resonance and the benefits of noise: From ice ages to crayfish and SQUIDs. Nature 1995; 373:33–36.

36

Static Magnetic Fields and Microcirculation

Chiyoji Ohkubo and Hideyuki Okano*

National Institute of Public Health, Tokyo, Japan

The authors review the importance of studying the effects of magnetic field on microcirculation, especially in respect of possibility that vasculature may have direct and indirect role in interaction of magnetic fields with different tissues. Outlining the microcirculation as physiological phenomena, describing relatively new methods of evaluation technique, Dr. Ohkubo and Dr. Okano explained in details the effects of static magnetic field with range of 0.3%–25 mT on microcirculation and blood pressure in experimental animals. Both local and whole body exposure have been investigated. The authors suggested that the results from rabbit experiments could be useful in applying magnetic fields for ischemic diseases and for search of mechanism of action.

I. INTRODUCTION

From the physiological point of view, it is vitally important to study the effects of static magnetic fields (SMFs) on microcirculation and blood pressures (BPs). For the practical application, SMFs ranging from 0.3 to 380 mT for 10 min to 3 months have produced its therapeutic effects on various disorders in patients (Table 1) and experimental mammals (Table 2). The effects by local or whole-body application of SMFs with milliTesla levels could promote healing of various diseases, in particular, inflammation (1–9), wound (10,11), pain (11–16), bone fracture (12–15), and hypertension (16,17). However, the basic physiologicalmechanisms underlying therapeutic effects of SMFs have not been clarified. A few investigations suggest that the therapeutic processes could be explained by enhanced recovery of microcirculation toward normal state during and after exposure to SMFs (2,7). We review the effects of SMFs with milliTesta levels on microcirculation in mammals, which were monitored and analyzed using newly advanced methods: measuring systems for the microcirculation with intravital microscopy and various experimental protocols with application of pharmacological agents.

---

* Pip Tokyo Co., Ltd., Tokyo, Japan.

Table 1 Therapeutic Effects of SMFs on Various Diseases in Patients

Study	Diagnosis	B_{max} (mT)	Duration	Area	Parameters[a]	Reference
Pain	Postpolio pain	30–50	45 min	Pain trigger point	Pain score (D)	3
Pain	Primary dysmenorrhea	80–130	3 h	Suprapubic area	Pain score (D)	1
Pain	Chronic knee pain	180	5–15 days (1–23.5 h/day)	Knee joints	Pain score (D) and physical function (I)	6
Pain	Abdominal and genital pain	190	10 min	Pain trigger point	Pain score (D)	4
Pain	Rheumatoid arthritis	190	1 week	Knee joints	Pain score (D)	5
Wound	Suction lipectomy	15–40	1 day	Operative wound	Pain score (D), edema (D), and discoloration (D)	11
Wound	Spinal cord injury	40–70	2–4 weeks (60–180 min/day)	Injured area	Motor function (I) and sensory function (I)	10
Inflammation	Fibromyalgia	0.3–0.6	6 months	Whole body	Pain score (D) and functional status (I)	9
Hypertension	Essential hypertension	16	10 days (45 min/day)	Chest and neck	Blood pressure (D)	16,17

[a] D and I in parentheses denote decrease and increase as outcomes of parameters.

Table 2 Therapeutic Effects of SMFs on Various Diseases in Experimental Mammals

Study	Animal model	B_{max} (mT)	Duration	Area	Parameters[a]	Reference
Bone healing	Guinea pig with osteotomy	8	9 days (8 h/day)	Whole-body	Rate of bone repair (I)	13
Bone fracture	Rabbit with radial fracture	22–26	4 weeks	Fracture site	Force of bone break (I)	12
Bone formation	Rat with magnet implant in femur	180	12 weeks	Implanted site	Bone mineral density (I)	14
Bone formation	Rat with magnet implant in femur	180	12 weeks	Implanted site	Bone mineral density (I) and bone weight (I)	15
Inflammation	Dog with magnet implant in femoral or cervical artery	6	1 week	Implanted site	Blood coagulation (D) and vascular wall regeneration (I)	7
Inflammation	Dog with femoral artery reconstruction	40	1 week (30 min/day)	Main nervous and vascular area	Blood coagulation (D) and blood flow (I)	7
Inflammation	Rat with inflammatory synovitis	380	3 weeks	Whole body	Inflammatory score (D)	8
Wound	Rat with spinal cord injury	40–70	2–4 weeks (60–180 min/day)	Injured area	Injured area (D) and motor function (I)	10
Pain	Guinea pig with acute ischemic pain	130	10 min	Gastrocnemius muscle	Twitch height of gastrocnemius muscle (I)	2

[a] D and I in parentheses denote decrease and increase as outcomes of parameters.

II. OUTLINE OF MICROCIRCULATION

A. Anatomy and Function

Microcirculation consists of structurally and functionally differentiated small blood vessels: small muscular arteries (vascular diameter range, 50–100 μm), arterioles (20–50 μm), capillaries (5–10 μm), postcapillary venules (20–50 μm), venules (50–100 μm), and lymphatic capillaries (100 μm). In the cutaneous microvascular beds, the connection between the arterioles and the venules is made by some thoroughfare channels or arteriolar-venular shunts (10–15 μm). Smooth muscle cells (SMCs) are found in all of these except the blood capillaries and lymphatic capillaries. The blood capillary wall is composed of a single layer of endothelial cells (ECs). The lymphatic capillaries are composed of endothelium-lined vessels similar to blood capillaries. Fluid and protein that have extravasated from the blood capillaries partially enter the lymphatic capillaries and are transported via the lymphatic system back to the blood vascular system. In most vascular beds, the precapillary resistance vessels are responsible for the largest function of the resistance in a vascular bed (18), and hence are the major components that influence regional hemodynamics and total peripheral resistance (19). Postcapillary venules play an important part in fluid and cellular exchange and are the major site of leukocyte migration into tissues.

The existence of nerves that synthesize, store, and release more than one transmitter is now widely accepted, including acetylcholine (ACh) together with noradrenaline (NA) or 5-hydroxytryptamine (5-HT) with various polypeptides in autonomic and central nervous system (CNS) neurons and ACh or NA with adenosine 5′-triphosphate (ATP) in the neurons of CNS and peripheral nervous system (20). ACh has an inhibitory action in responses to perivascular sympathetic nerve stimulation via prejunctional muscarinic receptors, and NA released from sympathetic nerve terminals reduces the release of ACh from cholinergic nerves. Interactions or cross talk between perivascular adrenergic and cholinergic nerve occur, where the transmitters released from the nerves not only produce antagonistic actions on the vascular smooth muscle (VSM) but also act prejunctionally to reduce the release of each other. Other substances, e.g., adenosine, prostaglandins, 5-HT, and angiotensin, have also been shown to act as prejunctional modulators of perivascular adrenergic nerve transmission (21). Control of VSM by nerves is functionally important in most segments of the microcirculation; however, circulating and locally produced vasoactive substances appear to be more important in controlling the diameter of the terminal arterioles (22).

Rhythmical and spontaneous changes in both the diameter of arterioles and the volume and velocity of blood flow due to constriction and dilation of VSM are known as *vasomotion* (42). Vasomotion is considered to be the results of instability in the interaction of various mechanisms. Tone in VSM is primarily regulated by Ca^{2+} signaling and the intracellular free Ca^{2+} concentration, $[Ca^{2+}]_i$, which plays a key role in the tension-length characteristic of the SMCs: contractile stimuli leading to an increase in $[Ca^{2+}]_i$ trigger vasoconstriction and relaxant signals leading to a reduction in $[Ca^{2+}]_i$ cause vasodilation. As for other possible mechanisms, it has been proposed that the rhythmogenic properties of VSM are closely coupled to a functioning circulation (23). The electrical and mechanical oscillations, which can be traced back to rhythmic activity of the active, electrogenic Na^+/K^+ pump, could originate in the allosteric qualities of a rhythmogenic enzyme, phosphofructokinase (PFK) (23). Extracellular control of the SMCs is exerted through neurogenic, hormonal, local and myogenic mechanisms (24).

The endothelium is an endocrine organ, capable of regulating the function of the microcirculation. The most important compound produced is an endogenous vasodilator, nitric oxide (NO) (25). NO has a physiological antagonist, endothelin-1, a potent vasoconstrictor, and its major effects are to cause local vasodilatation and inhibition of platelet aggregation. NO is produced from L-arginine by the enzyme nitric oxide synthetase (NOS), and its actions are mediated by cGMP. NO is an essential to the normal functioning of the vascular system. It appears that there are two forms of NOS: a constitutive form (cNOS appears to be produced as part of the normal regulatory mechanisms) and an inducible form (iNOS seems to be produced as the pathologic mechanisms). iNOS appears to be produced as an offshoot of the inflammatory response, by TNF and other cytokines. It results in massive production of NO, causing widespread vasodilatation and hypotension.

B. Physiological Significance

The principal function of microcirculation is exchanging physiological substances including O_2, ion, hormones, and nutrients between blood and tissues, and the compensatory adjustments should contribute to the efficacy of the exchange process: lumen dimensions, length, tortuosity, diameter of branch ratios, number of vessels, wall thickness, hemodynamics (vasomotion), blood velocity, blood viscosity, and leukocyte-endothelium interaction. In order to fulfill exchange requirements, changes in the system must allow not only for the delivery of an increased or decreased volumetric flow rate, but also for the distribution of the apportioned volume within the meshwork of capillaries to provide an appropriate surface area for effective exchange.

The quantitative description of spontaneous arteriolar vasomotion requires data on frequency, amplitude, diameter, and branching order of the vessels observed (26). In addition, the ratio of active vessels to total number of arterioles observed should be given (26). Therefore, in situ measurements of microcirculation offer a number of clinical applications: detection of high-risk individuals, index of disease of severity, effectiveness of therapy, and pathogenesis. They can serve as a measure of the effectiveness of a therapeutic regime and for the early detection of disease-related inroads on tissue homeostasis (27). Frequency and amplitude of spontaneous vasomotion could play an important role in disease. In microangiopathies, lymphedema, and essential hypertension, altered patterns of arterioler vasomotion chould constitute an additional pathogenetic factor (26).

C. Evaluation Technique

Various microcirculatory preparations, e.g., rabbit ear chamber (REC) (28–33), dorsal skinfold chamber in mice and hamsters (34,35) and cranial window in mice and rats (35–38), have been used to observe and analyze microcirculation. These preparations allow noninvasive, continuous measurement of hemodynamics, blood velocity, angiogenesis, metabolites, e.g., pH and pO_2, transport of molecules and particles, and cell–cell interactions in vivo (39). The REC offers the advantage of superior optical quality and the use of mice offer the advantage of working with immunodeficient and genetically engineered animals (34). Due to the longer duration of an individual measurement, we have exclusively utilized REC to investigate the effects of SMFs on microcirculation using microphotoelectric plethysmography (MPPG) monitoring system.

1. Rabbit Ear Chamber (REC)

REC is a round-table chamber made of acryl resin for disk with an observing table and three holding pillars, a sustaining ring, and a glass window (Fig. 1a). The methods for installation of REC (28,30,32) and its availability to the bioelectromagnetic research (29–33) have been published in detail. The whole or partial image of a microcirculatory unit at the ocular with a

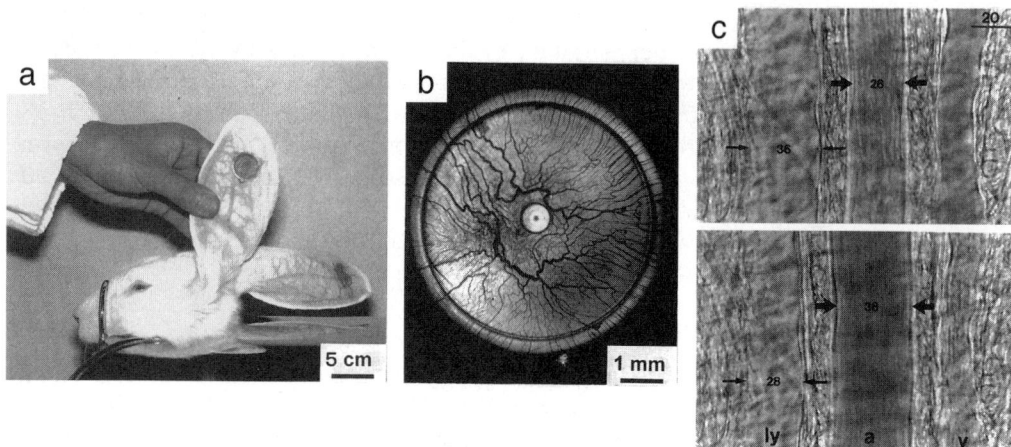

Figure 1 Photographs of general setup for intravital microscopy through rabbit ear chamber (REC). (a) REC was installed to a rabbit ear lobe; (b) a whole view of cutaneous microcircular net within a REC at a low magnification; (c) photomicrographs of the rhythmic change of microcirculatory net within a REC at a high magnification of an arteriole, a venule, and a lymphatic vessel (bar identification in micrometers). Upper panel, phase of full vasoconstriction; Lower panel, phase of full vasodilatation. a = arteriole; v = venule; ly = lymphatic vessel.

suitable microscopic magnification (Fig. 1b,1c). Under optimal conditions, with a well-trained rabbit, rhythmic changes consisting of increase and decrease in both the caliber of vessels and the volume of blood flow are always noticed. Compared to the arterioles, venules and lymphatic vessels have few or no SMCs in their structure and represent for the most part passive vasomotion: the vasoconstriction of an arteriole induced the passive vasodilation of a venules and a lymphatic vessel, and vice versa (Fig. 1c). An arteriole within a REC fixed on an observing stage of the microscope (vascular diameter range, 10–50 μm) was applied to analyzing the temporal changes of microcirculation due to vasomotion using a microphoto-electric plethysmography (MPPG) monitoring system.

2. Microphotoelectric Plethysmography (-gram; MPPG)

A REC or an intact central artery of the rabbit ear lobe fixed on an observing stage of the microscope was applied to analyzing the temporal changes of microcirculation in MPPG monitoring system. MPPG is a modification of a noninvasive technique of photoelectric plethysmography (PPG). The MPPG has been developed to monitor the temporal changes in the microcirculation in various cutaneous tissues by a combination of the intravital microscopic images displayed on a video monitor and the microcirculatory parameters monitored with a data recorder–analyzer (28,30–33,40–42). The MPPG can be adapted repeatedly on the same and different single vessels for the identical microscopic images (42). Two hemodynamic parameters of MPPG profiles, mean DC level (index of the blood flow and contents), and mean amplitude (index of the extent of vasomotion) more accurately and precisely represent the rhythmic fluctuations in microcirculation.

3. Blood Pressures (BPs)

BPs in a central artery contralateral to that of an ear lobe, fixed on the stage of the microscope, were monitored by a BP monitoring system (40,41).

4. Blood Velocity of Microcirculation

For measuring the capillary blood velocity in the muscle tissue, a fluorescence epi-illumination system was used in pentobarbital-anesthetized mice (43). The whole body of each mouse in the prone position, placed on the observing stage of a fluorescence microscope, was exposed to SMFs (0.3, 1.0, and 10.0 mT) for 10 min. Plasma was labeled with fluorescein isothiocyanate (FITC)-dextran, and each FITC-dextran was recognized as a single fluorescent signal between unlabeled blood cells circulating in the capillaries. The peak and mean blood velocity in the capillaries could be calculated from the measured values of several signals.

III. OUTLINE OF RESEARCHING RESULTS REGARDING SMFs AND MICROCIRCULATION

A. Summary of the Methods

The purpose of our study is to examine the effects of SMFs with milliTesla levels (0.3–25 mT) on microcirculation and/or BPs and to demonstrate how SMFs can affect the microcirculation and/or BPs in normal and pharmacologically treated mammals (30,32,40,41,43) or genetically hypertensive mammals (44) (Table 3). The animal husbandry and all the experimental procedures were approved by an institutional animal care and ethic committee.

1. Statistical Analysis

All values were expressed as means $\pm$ SEM. MPPG profiles and BPs were compared between groups by repeated-measures ANOVA followed by post-hoc analysis using Dunnett's multiple comparisons. The differences in the biochemical indices were compared between groups using the two-tailed Wilcoxon rank-sum test. A difference of $P < 0.05$ was considered statistically significant.

B. Results with Regard to Biphasic Action of SMFs on Microcirculation

1. Local Exposure to SMF (1.0 mT, 10–30 min) for Intact Rabbits

This study is attempted to find the effect of 1.0 mT (B_{max}) on the cutaneous microcirculation (30,40) and/or BPs (40) in conscious rabbits.

    a. Experimental Procedures. The SMFs of 1.0 mT were generated by a C-shaped electromagnet device, which was composed of one pair of dipole electromagnets and a DC–AC electric power supply (30,32,40). An animal set on the observing stage of a microscope, laid prone in a holder without anesthesia.

    An intact central artery of the ear lobe fixed on an observing stage of the microscope (vascular diameter range, 500–700 μm) was applied to analyzing the temporal changes of microcirculation in MPPG monitoring system. Two experimental procedures were randomly categorized: (1) sham exposure without pharmacological treatment (CTL) and (2) SMF exposure alone (SMF). MPPG profiles and/or BPs just before exposure (PRE) were compared with those during exposure and postexposure.

    b. Results. SMFs (1.0 mT, 10 min) had a biphasic effect upon the microcirculatory system; when the vascular tone was low, the SMFs induced vasoconstriction, and when it was high, the SMFs induced vasodilation (30). The biphasic effect of SMFs ranging 1.0–50.0 mT was observed in a non-dose-dependent manner.

Table 3 Effects of SMFs with MilliTesla Levels on Microcirculatory Hemodynamics and Blood Pressure

Animal	Description[a]	B_{max} (mT)[b]	Duration	Area[c]	Parameters[d]	Effects	Reference
Rabbit	No treatment	1.0, 5.0, 10.0	10 min	REC	MPPG	Vasodilation/vasoconstriction	30
Rabbit	No treatment	1.0	30 min	Ear lobe	MPPG and BP	Not found	40
Rabbit	No treatment	5.5	30 min	Whole body	MPPG and BP	Not found	41
Rabbit	NA-induced vasoconstriction	1.0	10 min	REC	MPPG, microvascular images, and BP	Suppression of vasoconstriction	32
Rabbit	ACh-induced vasodilation	1.0	10 min	REC	MPPG, microvascular images, and BP	Suppression of vasodilation	32
Rabbit	Ca^{2+}-channel-blocker-induced hypotension	1.0	30 min	Ear lobe	MPPG and BP	Suppression of hypotension	40
Rabbit	NOS-inhibitor-induced hypertension	1.0	30 min	Ear lobe	MPPG and BP	Suppression of hypertension	40
Rabbit	NA-induced hypertension	5.5	30 min	Whole body	MPPG and BP	Suppression of hypertension	41
Rabbit	NOS-inhibitor-induced hypertension	5.5	30 min	Whole body	MPPG and BP	Suppression of hypertension	41
Mouse	Pentobarbital-reduced blood velocity	1.0, 10.0	10 min	Whole body	Blood velocity	Increase of peak blood velocity	43
Rat	Genetically hypertension	10.0, 25.0	3 months	Whole body	BP and hormonal levels	Suppression of elevation of BP and hormones	44

[a] NA, noradrenaline; ACh, acetylcholine; NOS, nitric oxide synthase.
[b] B_{max}, maximum magnetic flux density.
[c] REC, rabbit ear chamber.
[d] MPPG, microphotoelectric plethysmography; BP, blood pressure.

For quantitative analysis, comparing CTL and SMF, there were no statistically significant differences throughout the experiment (Fig. 2). In CTL, the differences of post-PRE values from PRE basal values were within $\pm 10\%$. In SMF, on the other hand, mean DC level and mean amplitude increased by 15–30% during POST 5–10 and during EXP 3–POST 2, respectively. For BPs, comparing SMF with CTL, there were no significant changes throughout the experiment.

2. Whole-Body Exposure to SMF (5.5 mT, 30 min) for Intact Rabbits

This study is attempted to find the effect by whole-body exposure on the cutaneous microcirculation and BPs in conscious rabbits (41).

a. Experimental Procedures. The SMFs of 5.5 mT (B_{max}) were generated by a doughnut-shaped annular electromagnet device (Fig. 3), which was composed of one pair of annular electromagnets and a DC–AC electric power supply (41). A rabbit in a holder was placed into the annular electromagnets (Fig. 3). The measured magnetic flux densities were 5.0–5.5 mT in the trunk, 0.5–4.0 mT in the head, 1.0–4.0 mT in the throat, and <1.0 mT in the ear lobe (Fig. 3).

Two experimental procedures were randomly categorized: (1) sham exposure without pharmacological treatment (CTL) and (2) SMF exposure alone (SMF). These values just before exposure (PRE) were compared with those during exposure and postexposure. Total duration of exposure was 30 min.

b. Results. Comparing SMF with CTL, there were no significant changes throughout the experiment (Fig. 4). In CTL, the differences of post-PRE values from PRE basal values were within $\pm 10\%$. In SMF, on the other hand, mean amplitude increased by 20% during POST 1 and decreased by 10–20% during POST 5–10. For BPs, comparing SMF with CTL, there were no significant changes throughout the experiment.

3. Local Exposure to SMF (1.0 mT, 10 min) for Pharmacologically Treated
Rabbits with Rabbit Ear Chamber

This study is attempted to demonstrate the vasoconstricting effect as well as the vasodilating effect by local exposure on the cutaneous microcirculation within a rabbit ear chamber (REC) under pharmacologically modified vascular tone in the conscious rabbits (32). Based on the hypothesized effects of drugs on hemodynamics, noradrenaline (NA) and acetylcholine (ACh) were chosen to enhance and reduce the vascular tone pharmacologically.

a. Experimental Procedures. Cutaneous microcirculation of REC exposed to SMF (1.0 mT, 10 min) was studied under pharmacological treatment using MPPG method. NA and ACh were used for increase sympathetically (45) and decrease parasympathetically (46) of vascular tone, respectively.

b. Results. The temporal changes of MPPG profiles during and after exposure were quantitatively analyzed. In NA group, the vasoconstriction with reduced vasomotion resulting in decreases of both MPPG profiles were observed throughout the experiment (Fig. 5). In NA + SMF group, the vaconstricting effect with reduced vasomotion following NA infusion were reduced (POST 3) (Fig. 5a). In contrast, in ACh group, the vasodilation with increased vasomotion resulting in increases of both MPPG profiles were observed throughout the experiment (Fig. 5). In ACh + SMF group, however, the vasodilating effect with increased vasomotion following ACh infusion were reduced (EXPOSURE–POST 4) (Fig. 5a). In mean amplitudes of MPPG between ACh + SMF and ACh groups, there were significant differences for up to 60 min after cessation of EXPOSURE (POST 1–6) (Fig. 5b). In CTL group, there were no significant changes throughout the experiment.

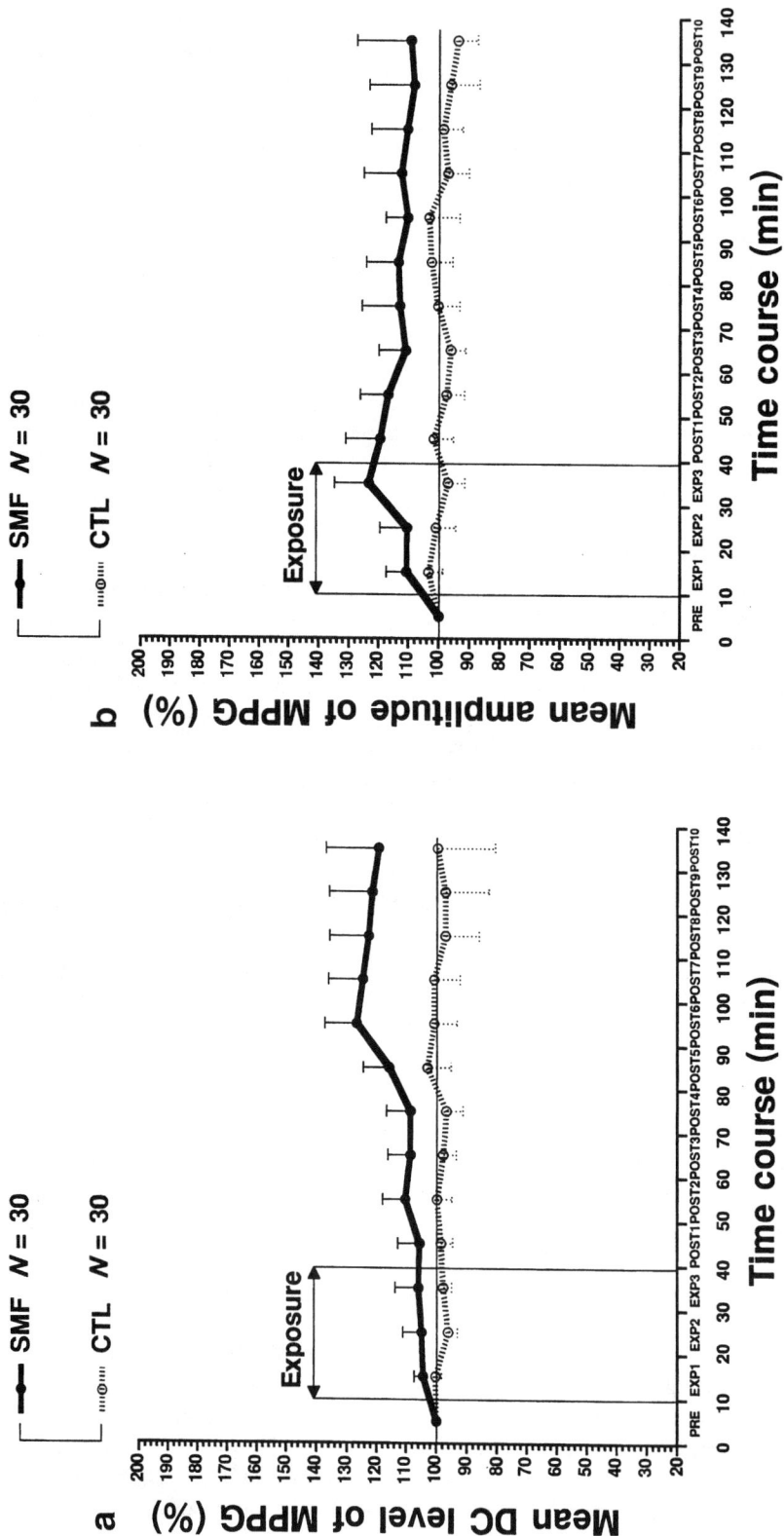

Figure 2 Changes of MPPG profiles in the mean DC level (a) and the mean amplitude (b) in a central artery of an ear lobe, with or without exposure to SMF (1.0 mT, 30 min), in normal (non-drug-treated) rabbits. Each value is calculated as a percentage of each PRE value in the same procedure (mean ± SEM). (Modified from Ref. 40.)

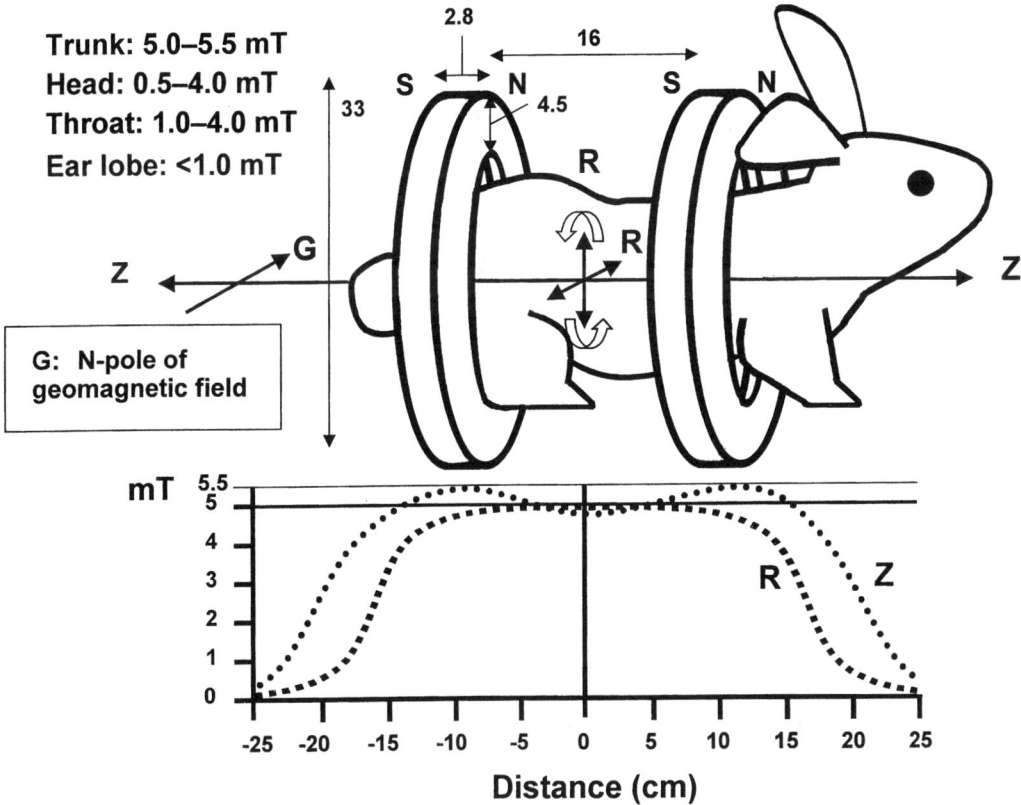

Figure 3 Whole-body exposure to SMF of 5.5 mT (B_{max}) in a rabbit. The applied SMF in the frontal and rear part of the body are generated from an anterior and posterior annular electromagnet (dimensions in centimeters). (Modified from Ref. 41.)

4. Local Exposure to SMF (1.0 mT, 30 min) for Pharmacologically Treated Rabbits Without Rabbit Ear Chamber

The purpose of this study is to elucidate the hypothesized homeostatic effects of SMF on BPs, and to show that it can alter the microcirculation in a cutaneous tissue and hence modify the BPs to minimize its lability. This study was designed to investigate the effects of SMF (1.0 mT, 30 min) on a Ca^{2+} channel blocker, nicardipine-induced hypotension as well as a nitric oxide synthase (NOS) inhibitor, N^{ω}-nitro-L-arginine methyl ester (L-NAME)-induced hypertension in conscious rabbits (40).

a. Experimental Procedures. The effects of SMF on BPs in rabbits were investigated under pharmacological treatment. Hypotensive and vasodilator actions were induced by an L-type voltage-gated Ca^{2+} channel blocker, nicardipine (NIC) (47). Hypertensive and vasoconstrictive actions were induced by a non selective NOS inhibitor, L-NAME (48). The hemodynamic changes in the central artery exposed to SMF were measured continuously and analyzed by penetrating MPPG. Concurrently, BPs in a central artery contralateral to that of the exposed ear lobe were monitored.

b. Results. For quantitative analysis, in NIC alone, the acute and intense vasodilation with increased vasomotion resulting in increases of both MPPG parameters was observed (Fig. 6). In SMF + NIC, by contrast, the vasodilating effect with increased

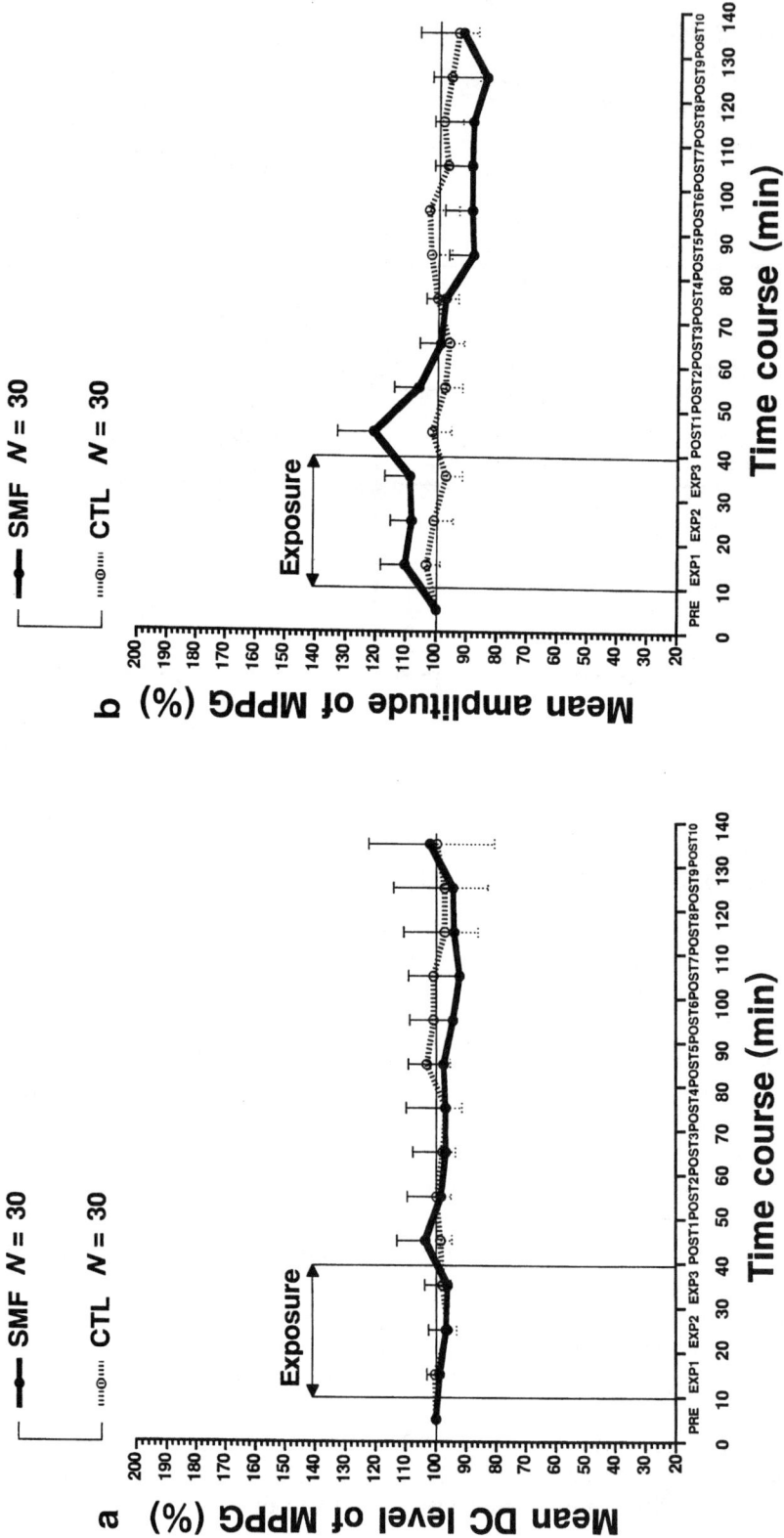

Figure 4 Changes of MPPG profiles in the mean DC level (a) and the mean amplitude (b) in a central artery of an ear lobe, with or without exposure to SMF (5.5 mT, 30 min), in normal (non-drug-treated) rabbits. Each value is calculated as a percentage of each PRE value in the same procedure (mean ± SEM). (Modified from Ref. 41.)

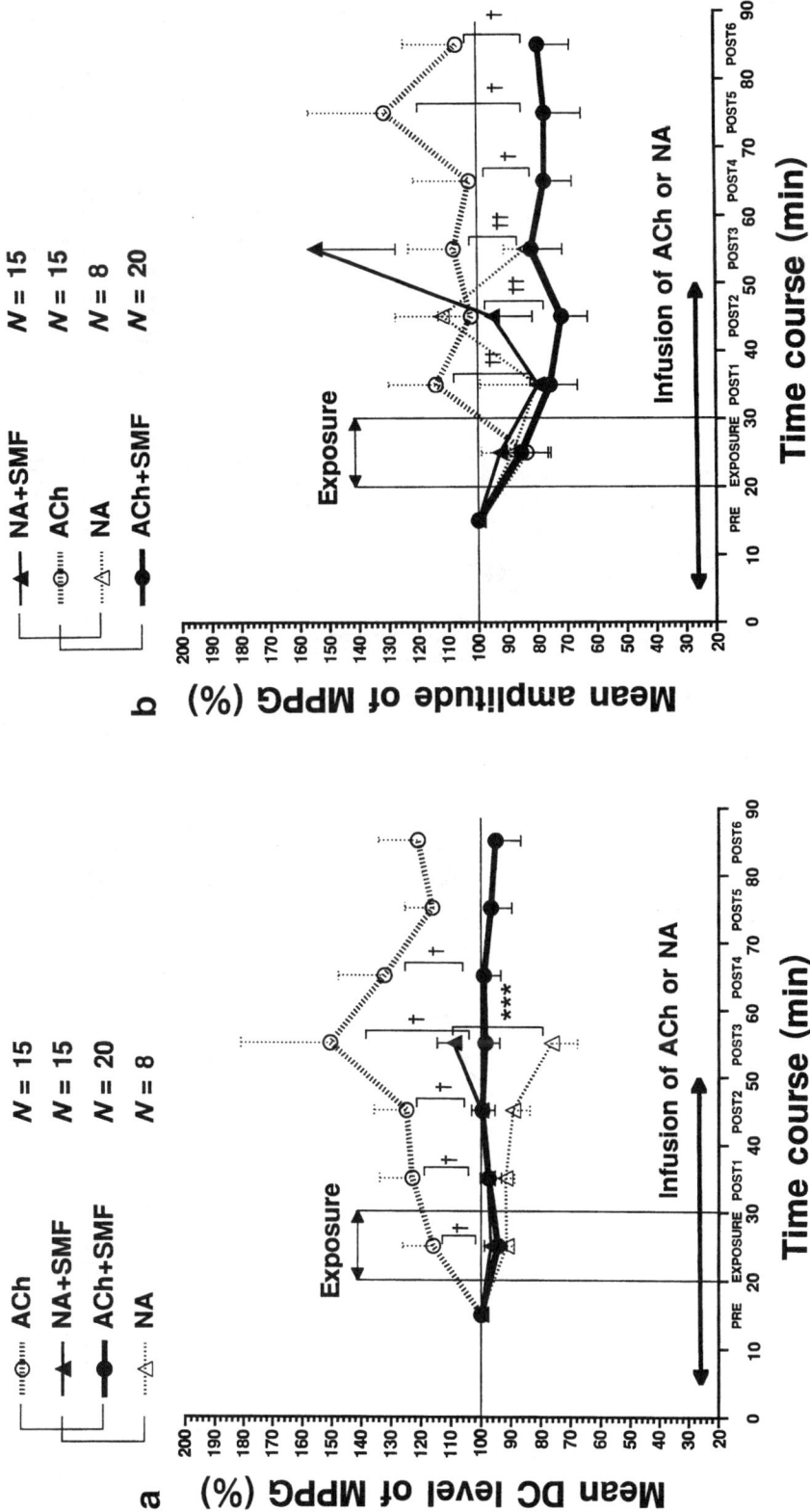

Figure 5 Changes of MPPG profiles in the mean DC level (a) and the mean amplitude (b) in single arteriole-capillary-venule channels following exposure to SMF of 1.0 mT under noradrenaline (NA)-induced high vascular tone and acetylcholine (ACh)-induced low vascular tone. Values are mean ± SEM. ***, $P < 0.001$ for the comparison between NA + SMF and NA. †, $P < 0.05$; ††, $P < 0.01$ for the comparison between ACh + SMF and ACh. (Modified from Ref. 32.)

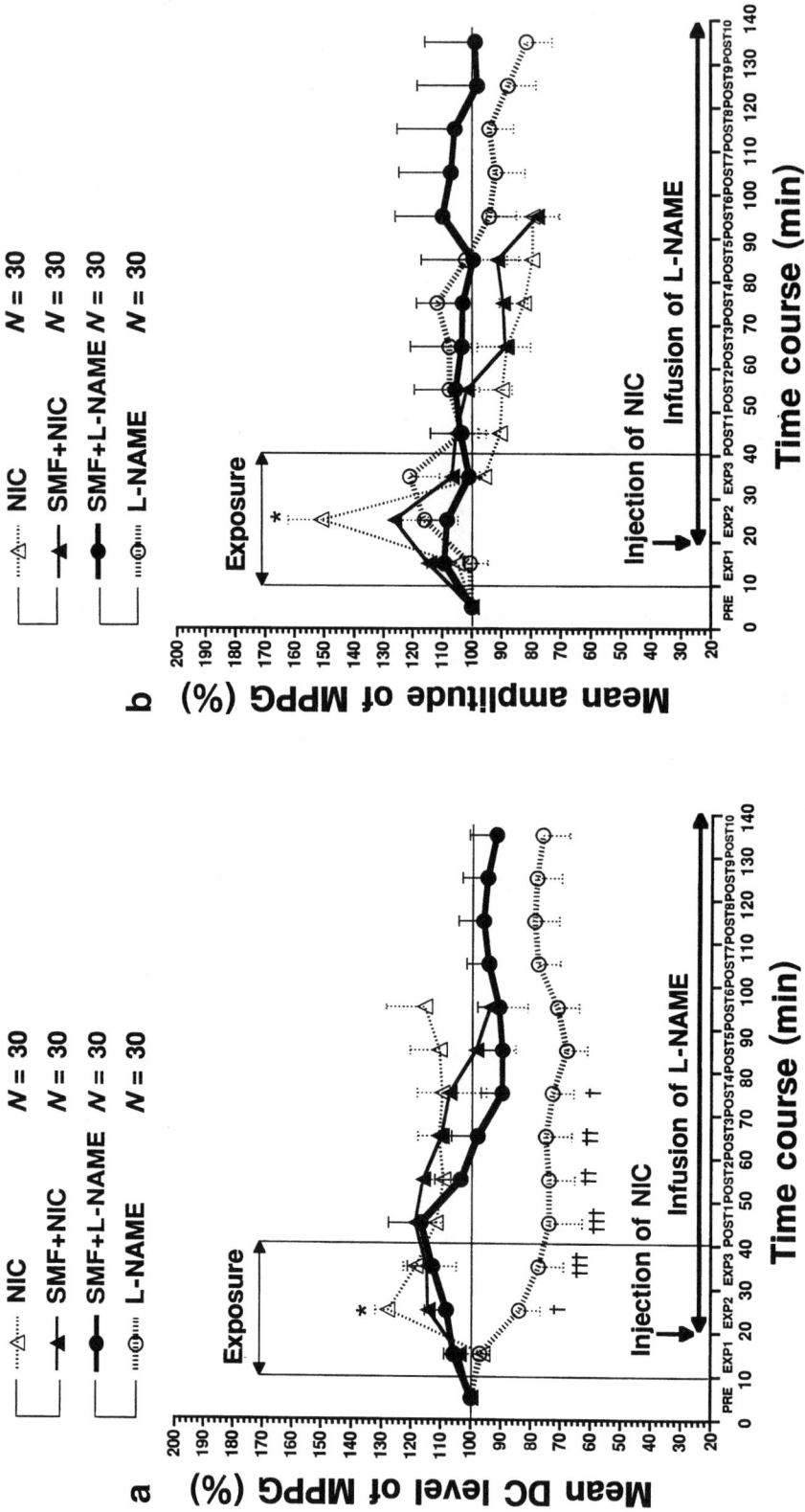

Figure 6 Changes of MPPG profiles in the mean DC level (a) and the mean amplitude (b) in a central artery of an ear lobe, with or without exposure to SMF (1.0 mT, 30 min), under NIC-induced hypotension or L-NAME-induced hypertension. Values are mean ± SEM. *, $P < 0.05$ for the comparison between SMF + NIC and NIC. †, $P < 0.05$; ††, $P < 0.01$; †††, $P < 0.001$ for the comparison between SMF + L-NAME and L-NAME. (Modified from Ref. 40).

vasomotion following NIC injection was reduced (EXP2)(Fig. 6a). In mean amplitude between SMF + NIC and NIC, there was a significant difference during EXP2 (Fig. 6b). In L-NAME alone, 10 min after L-NAME infusion, the vasoconstriction resulting in decreases of mean DC level was observed (Fig. 6a). In SMF + L-NAME, by contrast, the vaso-constricting effect following L-NAME infusion was reduced (EXP2 to POST 4)(Fig. 6a). In mean amplitude between SMF + L-NAME and L-NAME, however, there were no significant differences throughout the experiment (Fig. 6b).

In NIC alone, BPs decreased from baseline immediately after NIC injection (Fig. 7). In contrast, in SMF + NIC, the reduction of BPs was suppressed. In L-NAME alone, BPs gradually increased from baseline after L-NAME infusion (Fig. 7). In contrast, in SMF + L-NAME, the elevation of BPs was suppressed during exposure and post-exposure (Fig. 7).

5. *Whole-Body Exposure to SMFs (0.3, 1.0, and 10.0 mT, 10 min)*
   for Anesthetized Mice

This study was designed to investigate the effects of SMFs for modulating the muscle capillary mirocirculation under pentobarbital-induced hypnosis (43).

a. Experimental Procedures. SMFs were generated by a C-shaped electromagnet device, which was composed of a single dipole electromagnet and a DC-AC electric power supply (43).

Muscle capillary microcirculation of mice exposed to SMFs (0.3, 1.0, and 10.0 mT, 10 min) was studied under pentobarbital anesthesia. FITC-labeled dextran was used for an in vivo fluorescent plasma marker of the muscle capillaries.

b. Results. Significant increases of the peak blood velocities by SMFs of at least 1.0 mT were observed, whereas those of the mean blood velocities were not (Fig. 8). In CTL or SMF exposure at 0.3 mT, on the other hand, there were no significant changes throughout the experiment within either of the peak blood velocities (Fig. 8). In both cases, the differences of post-PRE values from PRE basal values were within ±10%.

6. *Whole-Body Exposure to SMF (5.5 mT, 30 min) for Pharmacologically*
   Induced Hypertensive Rabbits

The purpose of our study is to elucidate the hypothesized hypotensive or antipressor effects of SMFs, and to show that it can alter the microcirculation in a cutaneous tissue and hence normalize the BPs. More particularly, this study was designed to investigate the effects of SMF (5.5 mT, 30 min) on pharmacologically induced hypertension via NA-mediated increases in sympathetic nerve activity, or a NOS inhibitor in vascular ECs and/or neurons (41).

a. Experimental Procedures. Hypertensive and vasoconstrictive actions were induced by NA (45) or a NOS inhibitor, L-NAME (48). As a preliminary intensity-finding experiment using SMFs ranging 1.0–50.0 mT in NA-induced hypertension, whole-body exposure to SMFs under 5.5 mT did not significantly induce antipressor effects. Antipressor effects of SMFs ranging 5.5–50.0 mT were found in a nonintensity dependent manner.

b. Results. In NA alone, just after NA infusion, the acute and intense vasoconstriction resulting in reduction of mean DC level was observed (Fig. 9a). In SMF + NA, by contrast, the vasoconstricting effect following NA infusion was antagonized (EXP 2 to POST 5) (Fig. 9a). Comparing mean amplitude between SMF + NA and NA, there were no significant differences throughout the experiment (Fig. 9b). In L-NAME alone, just after L-NAME infusion, the vasoconstriction resulting in decreases of mean DC level was observed (Fig. 9a). In SMF + L-NAME, the vasoconstricting effect following L-NAME infusion was

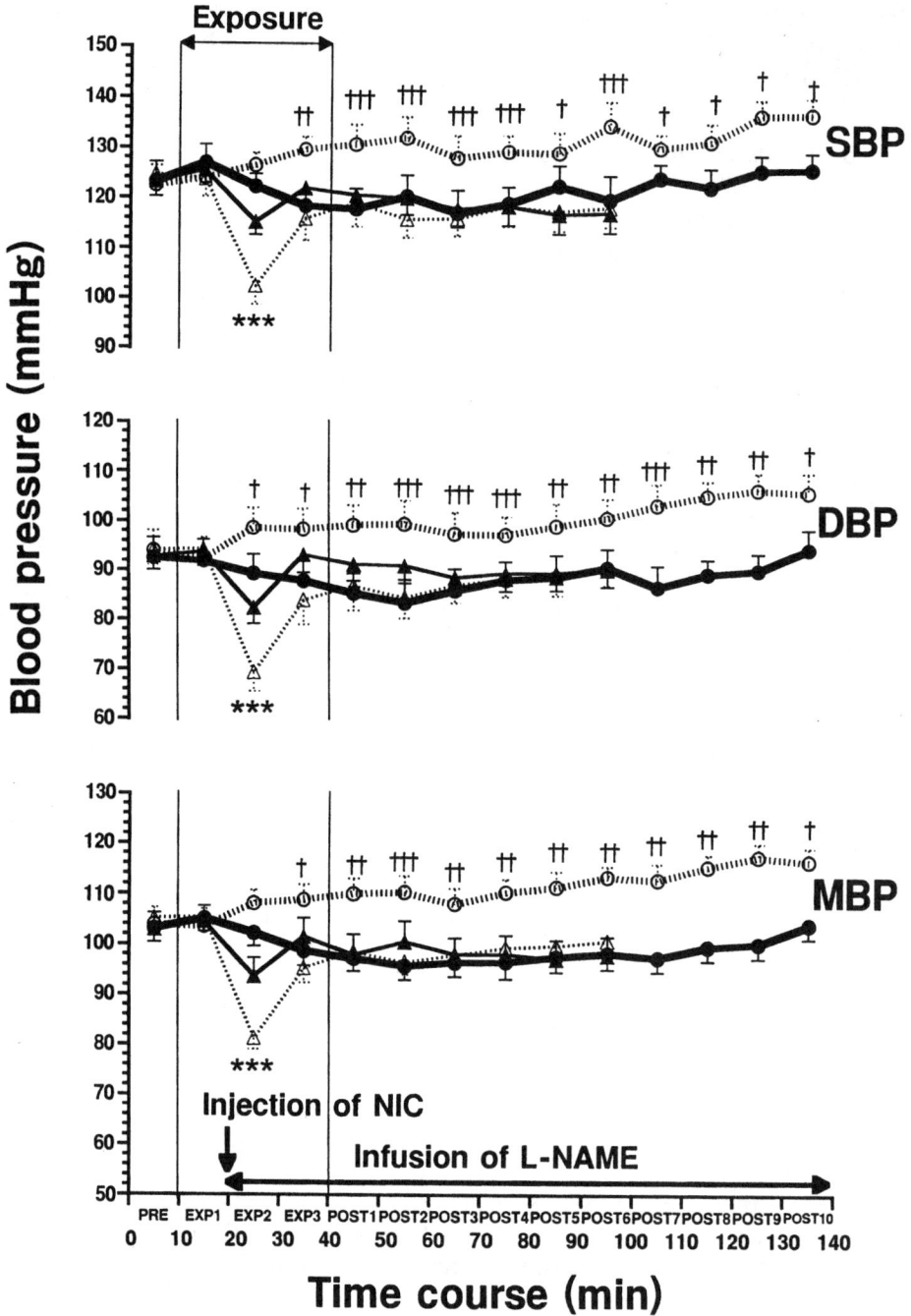

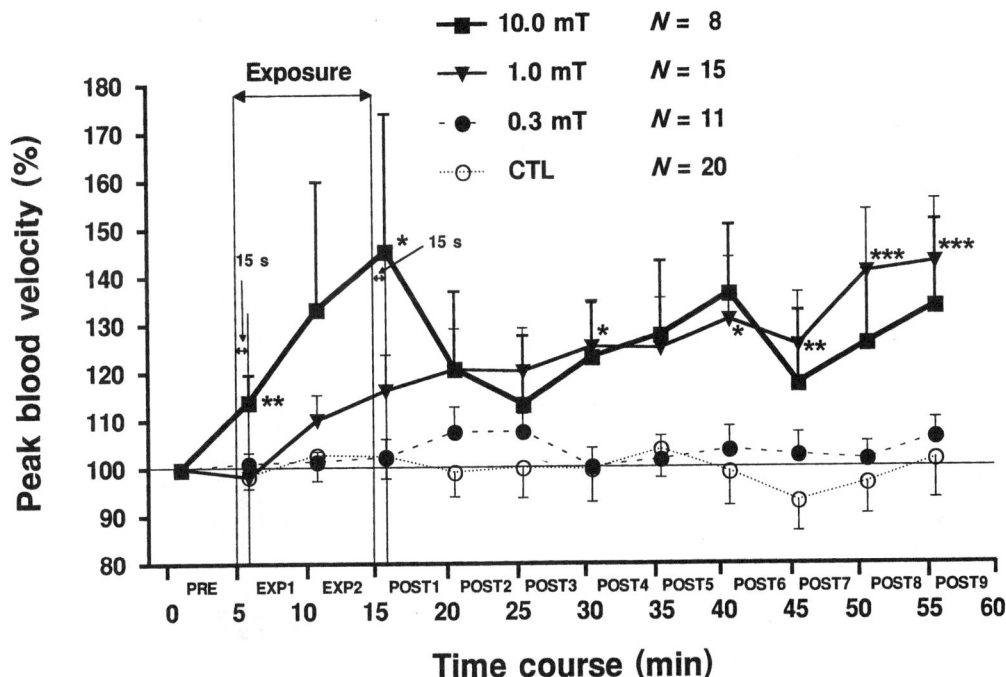

Figure 8 Changes of the peak blood velocity in muscle capillaries, with or without exposure to SMFs (0.3, 1.0, and 10.0 mT), under pentobarbital anesthesia. The capillary plasma velocity was measured for 15 s at each 5-min interval during the observation period. Each value is calculated as a percentage of each PRE value in the same procedure (mean ± SEM). *, $P < 0.05$; **, $P < 0.01$; ***, $P < 0.001$ for the comparison with control. (Modified from Ref. 43.)

reduced (EXP 3 to POST 2 and POST 4) (Fig. 9a). Comparing mean amplitude between SMF + L-NAME and L-NAME; however, there were no significant differences throughout the experiment (Fig. 9b).

In NA alone, BPs increased from baseline after NA infusion (Fig. 10). In contrast, in SMF + NA, the elevation of BPs was antagonized and hypotension was induced. After withdrawal of SMFs, there were significant differences between SMF + NA and NA in BPs. In L-NAME alone, BPs increased from baseline after L-NAME infusion (Fig. 10). In contrast, in SMF + L-NAME, the elevation of BPs was suppressed during exposure and postexposure.

For plasma vasoactive substances, comparing between NA and SMF + NA in PRE and POST 10, there were no significant changes in any vasoactive substances (catecholamines, angiotensin II and aldosterone).

Figure 7 Changes of systolic blood pressure (SBP), diastolic BP (DBP), and mean BP (MBP) in a central artery contralateral to that of an ear lobe, with or without exposure to SMF (1.0 mT, 30 min), under NIC-induced hypotension or L-NAME-induced hypertension. Values are mean ± SEM. ***, $P < 0.001$ for the comparison between SMF + NIC and NIC. †, $P < 0.05$; ††, $P < 0.01$; †††, $P < 0.001$ for the comparison between SMF + L-NAME and L-NAME. (Modified from Ref. 40.)

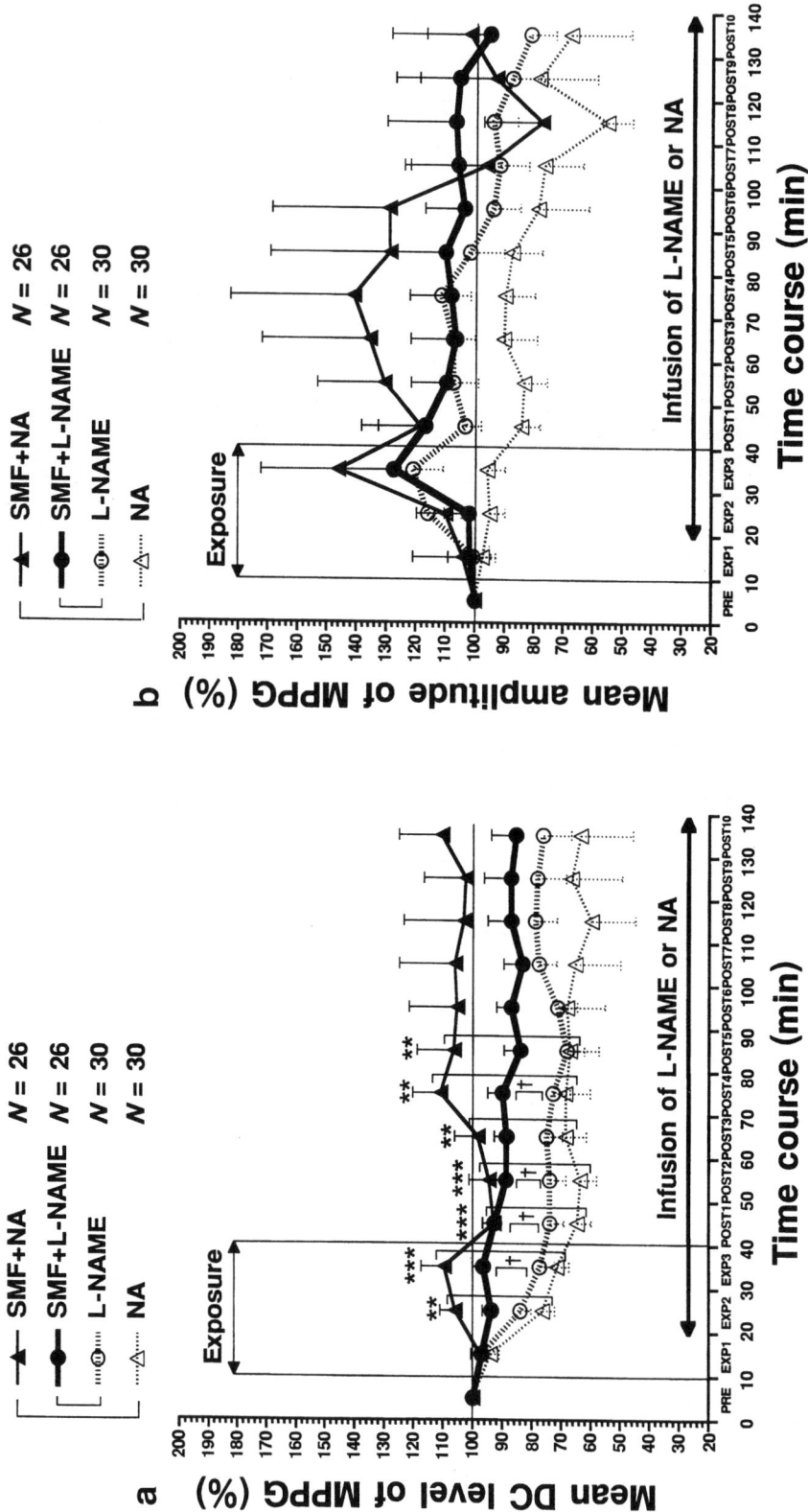

Figure 9 Changes of MPPG profiles in the mean DC level (a) and the mean amplitude (b) in a central artery of an ear lobe, with or without whole-body exposure to SMF (5.5 mT, 30 min), under NA- or L-NAME-induced hypertension. Each value is calculated as a percentage of each PRE value in the same procedure (mean ± SEM). *, $P < 0.05$; **, $P < 0.01$; ***, $P < 0.001$ for the comparison between SMF + NA and NA. †, $P < 0.05$ for the comparison between SMF + L-NAME and L-NAME. (Modified from Ref. 41).

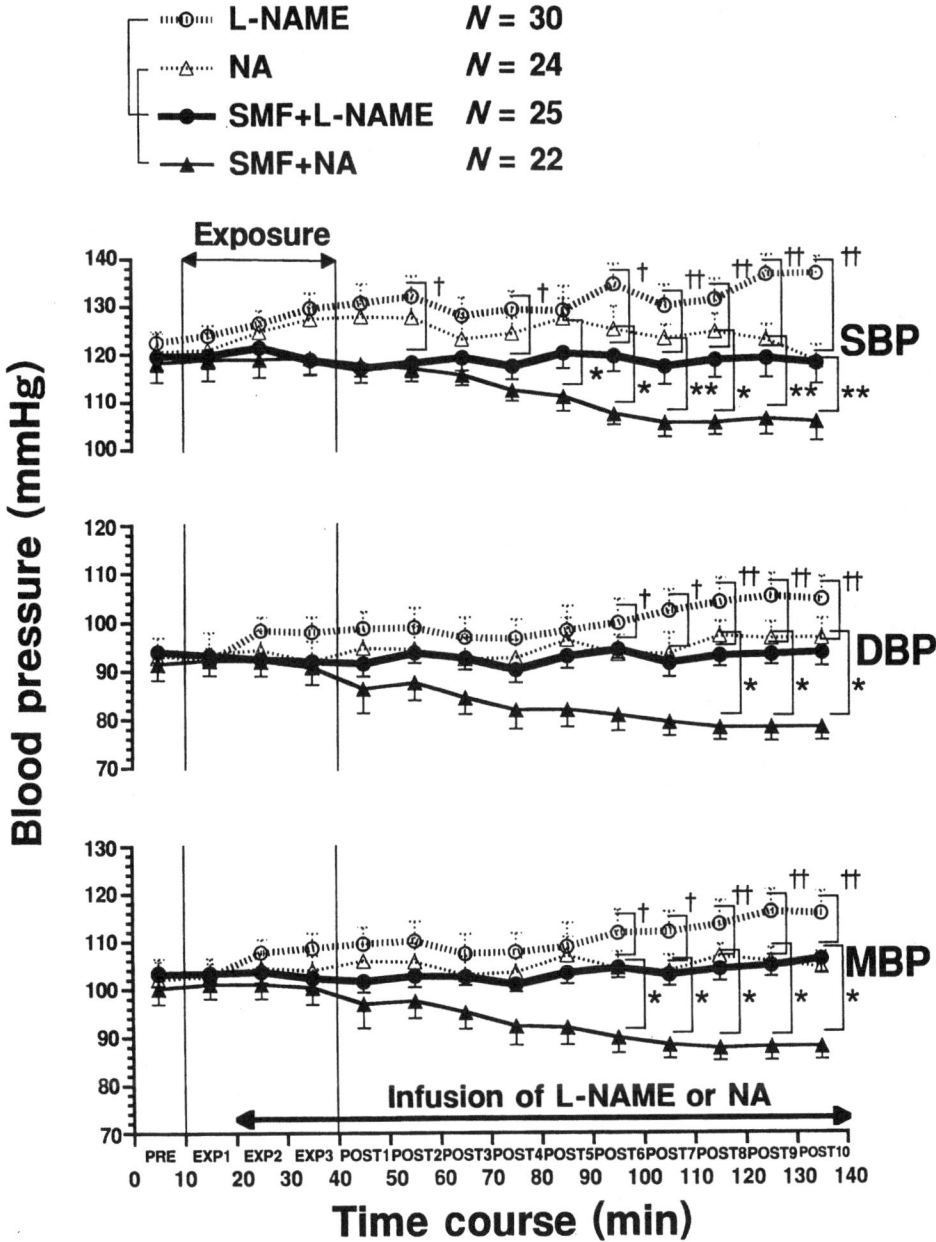

Figure 10 Changes of systolic blood pressure (SBP), diastolic BP (DBP), and mean BP (MBP) in a central artery contralateral to that of an ear lobe, with or without whole-body exposure to SMF (5.5 mT, 30 min), under NA- or L-NAME-induced hypertension. Values are mean ± SEM. *, $P < 0.05$; **, $P < 0.01$ for the comparison between SMF + NA and NA. †, $P < 0.05$; ††, $P < 0.01$ for the comparison between SMF + L-NAME and L-NAME. (Modified from Ref. 41.)

7. Whole-Body Exposure to SMF (10.0 and 25.0 mT, 3 Months) for Genetically Hypertensive Rats

The purpose of our study is to elucidate the hypothesized anti-pressor effects of SMFs with mT levels on a genetically hypertensive animal (44).

a. Experimental Procedures.   A SMF exposure device was composed of a pair of rectangular magnetic plates (strontium-ferrite) externally placed in parallel at a distance of ~1 cm from both sides of an acrylic cage (44). Two types of SMF exposure devices with different magnetic flux densities were prepared (Fig. 11). The mean flux densities in the center of a cage were 5.5 mT ranging from 3.0 to 10.0 mT (B_{max}) here referred to as *SMF 10 mT* (Fig. 11a) and 14.0 mT ranging from 8.0 to 25.0 mT (B_{max}) as *SMF 25 mT* (Fig. 11b). The magnetic gradients of each cage were nearly homogeneous in the center and greater in the peripheral area (Fig. 11).

Effects of SMFs on development of hypertension were investigated using young male stroke-resistant spontaneously hypertensive rats (SHRs) beginning at 7 weeks of age. SHRs were randomly assigned to two different exposure groups or an unexposed group. A rat in a cage with magnetic plates was exposed to either SMF continuously for 12 weeks, except during the short period of measuring BPs and heart rate and blood sampling. The BPs and heart rate in each rat were determined weekly using tail-cuff method.

b. Results.   The changes of SBP with continuous exposure to either SMF for 12 weeks and with crossover exposure to SMF 25 mT for 6 weeks were indicated, as compared with CTL (Fig. 12). The rats exposed to SMFs displayed suppression and retardation in the development of SBP during 2–9 weeks (Fig. 12a). However, at least 1 week after crossover exposure for 6 weeks, significant differences between SBP disappeared (Fig. 12b). Similar suppressions of development of hypertension exposed to SMFs also occurred in DBP during 5–6 weeks in SMF 10 mT and during 3–6 weeks in SMF 25 mT (Fig. 12c). Moreover,

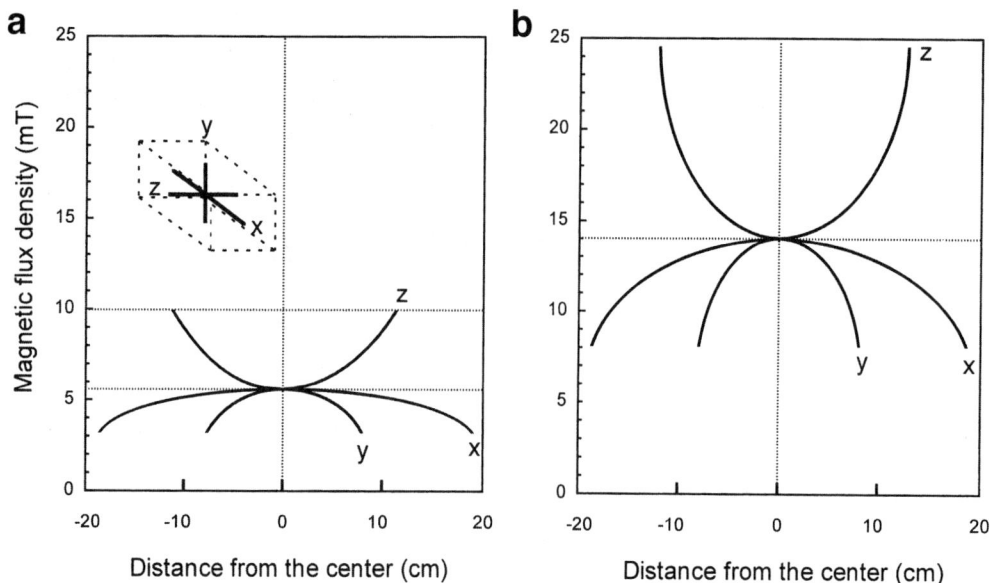

Figure 11   Spatial distribution of SMFs with B_{max} of 10.0 mT (a) and 25.0 mT (b). The mean flux densities in the center of a cage was 5.5 mT ranging 3.0–10.0 mT (a) and 14.0 mT ranging 8.0–25.0 mT (b). (Modified from Ref. 44.)

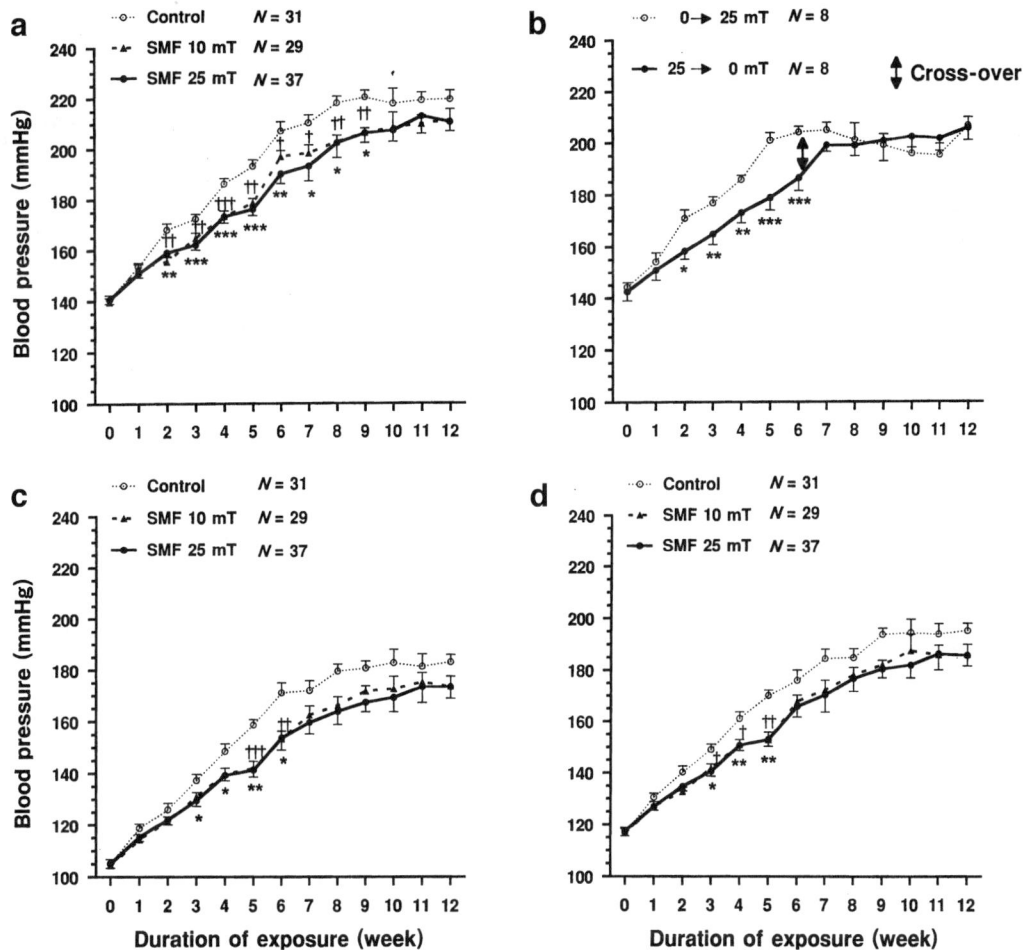

Figure 12 Changes of blood pressures (BPs), with or without exposure to SMF 10 and 25 mT, during the experimental period of up to 12 weeks in groups of SHRs (7– to 19-week-old). (a) Systolic BP (SBP) by continuous exposure for 12 weeks; (b) SBP by crossover exposure for 6 weeks; (c) Diastolic BP (DBP) by continuous exposure for 12 weeks; (d) Mean BP (MBP) by continuous exposure for 12 weeks. Values are mean ± SEM. *, $P < 0.05$; **, $P < 0.01$; ***, $P < 0.001$ for the comparison between SMF 25 mT and control. †, $P < 0.05$; ††, $P < 0.01$; †††, $P < 0.001$ for the comparison between SMF 10 mT and control. (Modified from Ref. 44.)

antipressor effects on MBP were observed during 3–5 weeks in both SMFs (Fig. 12d). Magnetic flux density dependent differences of these BP values between 10 and 25 mT were not significantly noticed throughout the experiment (Fig. 12).

Exposure to SMFs for 5 weeks significantly reduced the concentrations of plasma angiotensin II (Ang II) and plasma aldosterone concentration (Ald), as compared with CTL (Fig. 13). The extent of reduction was 65.3 and 39.6% reduction in Ang II and Ald at 10 mT and 63.8 and 36.6% reduction at 25 mT. The incidences of increased plasma levels of these substances were higher in CTL than in SMFs (Fig. 13). Density-dependent differences of hormones and enzymes between 10 and 25 mT were not noticed at 5 weeks (Fig. 13). There

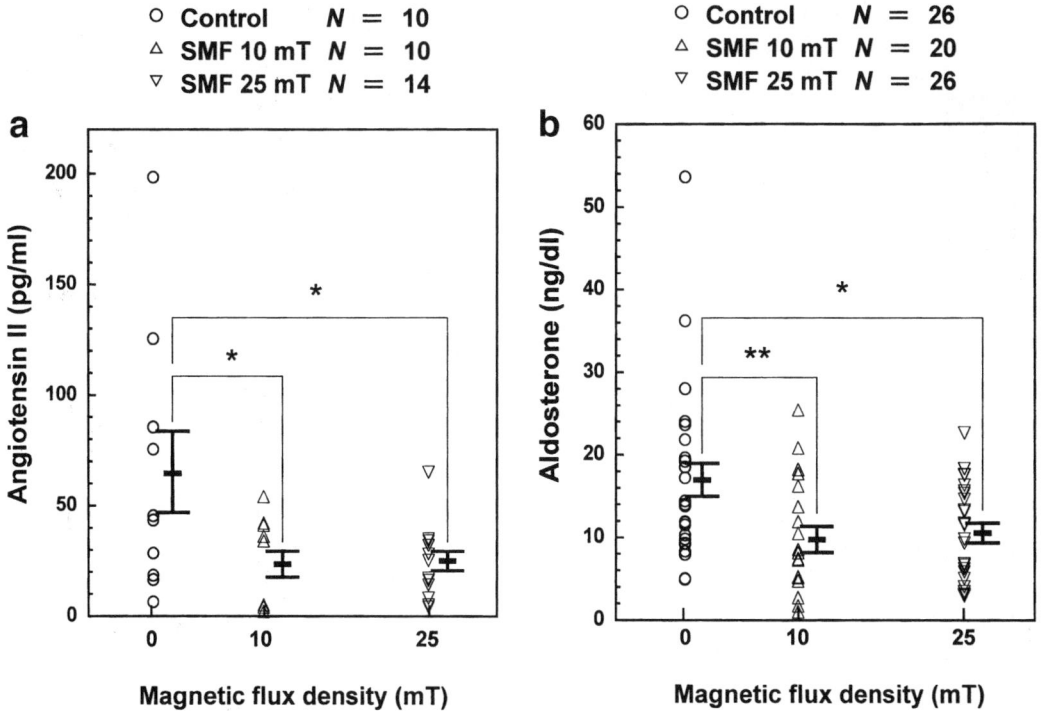

Figure 13 Plasma values of angiotensin II (a) and aldosterone (b), with or without exposure to SMFs (10 and 25 mT), at the experimental period of 5 weeks in groups of SHRs (12 weeks old). O, control; Δ (point up), SMF 10 mT; ∇ (point down), SMF 25 mT. The vertical bars (±) indicate mean ± SEM. *, $P < 0.05$; **, $P < 0.01$ for the comparison with control. (Modified from Ref. 44.)

were no detectable effects of SMFs on the other measured blood substances (renin activity, Ang I, arginine vasopressin and angiotensin I-converting enzyme).

IV. CLINICAL IMPLICATION OF RESEARCHING RESULTS

A. Therapeutic Effects of SMFs on Microcirculation

The acute and subchronic significant effects of SMF with higher densities of 100–500 mT on blood flow (31,49–51), BPs (52–58), heart rate (59), blood oxygen capacity (60), and immune response (61–63) have been reported. Actions of this kind are considered to produce beneficial effects on the systemic circulation as well as microcirculation. Particularly in Japan, SMFs generated by small disk magnets have been more frequently used to provide pain relief from neck and shoulder pain, low back pain, and recovery from muscle fatigue with ischemic conditions of the muscle microcirculation. These magnetic therapies have been found to be effective clinically (49–51). For example, results of a double-blind, randomized, controlled study indicated that a 180 mT SMF for a few days or a few weeks relieved the pain of patients with neck and shoulder stiffness (49), low back pain (50), and osteoarthropathy of the knee joints (51). Coincidentally, the measurable parameters of blood flow, e.g., a thermogram, a deep body thermometer, and a laser Doppler flowmeter, were increased in the ishcemic painful area by exposure to SMFs (49–51).

For a biochemical mechanism of SMF on the promotion of blood flow in the ishcemic conditions, the manners of activation of the cholinergic nerve by 130mT SMF for a few minutes were investigated using an ischemic pain-producing muscle in guinea pigs, and it was suggested that SMF might inhibit cholinesterase (2). The muscle pain relief by SMF is assumed to be induced by recovery of circulation due to the enhanced release of acetylcholine, as a result of activation of the cholinergic vasodilator nerve endings innervated to the muscle artery (2). The recovery of circulation might cause analgesic effects by elimination of a certain accumulated algogenic substance in the ishcemic muscle.

In our studies on the normal conscious rabbits applied SMF alone to the ear lobe (1.0 mT, 30 min) or the whole body (5.5 mT, 30 min), there were no significant changes of the microcirculation in the normal cutaneous tissue up to 100 min after the cessation of exposure. The exact mechanisms of the lack of significant response for SMF exposure alone have not been clarified. Under optimal conditions, regular rhythmic changes were observed irrespective of with or without SMFs. The state of the cells determines their responses to the external fields (64,65). Physiologically significant bioresponses due to therapeutic signals appear to occur only when the state of the target system is far from homeostasis (66). The apparent lack of responses to SMFs might be attributable to biphasic action on the hemodynamics in the physiologically normal cutaneous tissue under optimal conditions (40). The hemodynamics exposed to SMF seemed to reach and maintain the dynamical equilibrium by means of biphasic action.

Moreover, our studies suggested that significant modulatory effects of SMF on hemodynamics provide a mechanism by which SMF could affect a feedback control system on alteration in NOS activity in conjunction with modulation of Ca^{2+} dynamics (40). The delayed and long-lasting effects of SMF would be dependent on not only a magnetic field conduction delay and a lengthened effective refractory period, but also temporal delays on activation, synthesis, transduction, and/or transmission on several vasoactive substances on ECs in conjunction with neurotransmitters on CNS neurons (40).

Accordingly, the transient hemodynamic changes induced by SMFs ranging from 20 μT to 1 T could be in part attributable to some neurogenic factors, especially in the sympathetic nervous system and CNS by modifying neurotransmitter release (2,67), membrane action potentials (64,68–76), ion channel function (77), nerve excitability (78–80), electroencephalogram (EEG) (81–83), and N-methyl-D-aspartate (NMDA) receptor channels (84). There is a possible hypothesis that the responsiveness of hippocampal neurons to SMFs (71,72,81–84) and the ability of hippocampal neurons to generate magnetic signals (85,86) creates the environment where hippocampal neurons can use magnetic signals for interneural communication.

Magnetoreception (87–91) and the presence of biogenic magnetic material (magnetite) (87) in some organs have been reported in animals. Topics on magnetoreception have been reviewed elsewhere (89–91). Some candidate sites for magnetoreception have been identified in several visual centers, e.g., the pineal gland (92), the optic tectum (93), the superior colliculus (94), the nucleus of the basal optic root (95), and the trigeminal nerve system (96). We have not investigated whether the experimental animals are conscious of the acute exposure to SMFs with milliTesla levels exceeding 20 times the earth's magnetic field. If ferrimagnetic deposits, magnetorecepor and/or magnetosensitive ion channels are presented in these experimental animals, the biophysical and/or biochemical mechanisms of SMFs on hemodynamics and BPs could be partially explained using magnetite-based magnetoreception (90) and/or magnetically sensitive chemical reactions (88): this is because small changes in the local SMFs can be coupled chemically to the nervous system and influence the number of ligand–receptor complexes. Further investigations on the effective target region and peak magnetic gradients in living organism are greatly needed for detecting cellular signal transduction pathways concerning vasomotor regulatory mechanisms in situ.

B. Clinical Use of SMF for Hypertension and Future Views

In particular, from a practical point of view, the application of SMFs has been regarded as a feasible method for the treatment of essential hypertensive patients (16,17) (Table 1). In these clinical studies, the local application of SMF to chest and throat together was very effective for inducing hypotension (16). The evaluation of the effects of a SMF on pharmacologically induced hypertensive rabbits indicated that a 10-min exposure of up to 5.5 mT, followed by a 20-min exposure with NA- or L-NAME treatment, suppressed or antagonized the high vascular tone in the NA- or L-NAME-induced hypertensive animals (41) (Fig. 10). One of the most possible actions is that SMF not only can block or antagonize the binding of NA to the receptor but also can up-regulate NOS activity and hence enhance the conversion of L-arginine to NO. These antipressor or hypotensive effects of SMF on pharmacologically elevated BPs were present or enhanced long after the withdrawal of SMF. Further possibility is that the delayed and prolonged effects of SMF would be due to the similar modulatory mechanisms, via neural and humoral regulation systems (40,41). Antipressor effects of SMF might be induced in a tissue-specific manner by other mechanisms than the BP regulation systems concerning the circulating vasoactive substances. Another possible explanation for the antipressor mechanisms is that the increased ACh by SMF lowers BPs via relaxation responses of vascular resistance in hypertensive animals. This is because SMFs could modulate ACh release in vivo (2,32) as well as in vitro (67).

It has been reported that SMFs have antipressor effects on pharmacologically induced hypertensive rabbits under pentobarbital anesthesia (52,56). The intensity levels of locally applied SMFs, which induced reaction to a carotid sinus baroreceptor in the throat, were up to 200–500 mT in rabbits (52–54,56–58). The 30-min exposure of up to 200 mT in the carotid sinus region antagonized the NA-induced pressor action (52). Moreover, the 65-min exposure of up to 350 mT in the carotid sinus region counteracted an α1-adrenoceptor agonist, phenylephrine-induced pressor action (56).

The whole-body exposure of up to 5.5 mT in conscious hypertensive rabbits significantly induced the antipressor effects at much lower intensity (41), as compared with 200–500 mT in anesthetized rabbits (52–54,56–58). The whole-body exposure could exert one of the physiological mechanisms for enhancing baroreceptor sensitivity and improving baroreflex gain in sympathetic nerve activity, thereby inducing antipressor effects.

In genetically hypertensive rats, it became evident that SMFs at 10 and 25 mT might exert regulatory effects on cardiovascular homeostasis via Ang II and Ald levels in BP-controlling renin-angiotensin-aldosterone system (44) (Fig. 13). If these findings are confirmed on a wider scale in long-term clinical trials, then exposure to SMFs might become a valid alternative to current treatments, especially for patients with hypertension who need antihypertensive drugs.

V. SUMMARY

We have brought the tools and techniques of microcirculation to bear on biomagnetic research. The effects of SMFs ranging 0.3–25.0 mT on microcirculation and/or *BPs* in mammals were monitored and analyzed using newly advanced methods. The following conclusions were obtained.

Microcirculation and BPs were modulated by SMFs with milliTesla levels in pharmacologically treated animals and genetically hypertensive animals. By contrast, these physiological parameters were not changed by SMFs in normal animals. Appreciable minimum level for modulating microcirculation and BPs was 1.0 mT in pharmacologically treated animals (Table 3). For the minimum exposure duration of 1.0 mT, it took 10 min to change microcirculation and 30 min to modulate BPs in these animals. To induce antipressor effects of SMFs on pharmacologically induced hypertensive animals, the whole-body exposure to SMF of 5.5 mT for 30 min was needed. To induce antipressor effects of SMFs on genetically hypertensive animals, whole-body exposure to SMFs of 10.0 mT for at least 2 weeks was required.

The effects of SMFs in the mT range were mediated by antagonizing the action of biochemical substances, thereby inducing homeostatic effects biphasically:

1. Suppression of an adrenergic neurotransmitter, NA-induced vasoconstriction, and hypertension
2. Suppression of a cholinergic neurotransmitter, ACh-induced vasodilation
3. Suppression of an anesthetic agent, pentobarbital-induced decrease in the peak blood velocities
4. Suppression of a Ca^{2+} channel blocker, nicardipine-induced vasodilation and hypotension
5. Suppression of a NOS inhibitor, L-NAME-induced vasoconstriction and hypertension
6. Suppression of early BP elevation via inhibition of elevation of vasoconstrictive hormones, Ang II and Ald

The effects of SMFs with milliTesla levels on microcirculation and BPs obtained from different mammals would be used in possible explanation for the therapeutic effects on many ischemic diseases related to dysfunction in circulation and microcirculation. Furthermore, the SMFs might exert regulatory effects on BPs.

REFERENCES

1. Kim KS, Lee YJ. The effect of magnetic application for primary dysmenorrhea. Kanhohak Tamgu 1994; 3:148–179.
2. Takeshige C, Sato M. Comparisons of pain relief mechanisms between needling to the muscle, static magnetic field, external qigong and needling to the acupuncture point. Acupunct Electrother Res 1996; 21:119–131.
3. Vallbona C, Hazlewood CF, Jurida G. Response of pain to static magnetic fields in postpolio patients: a double-blind pilot study. Arch Phys Med Rehabil 1997; 78:1200–1203.
4. Holcomb RR, Worthington WB, McCullough BA, McLean MJ. Static magnetic field therapy for pain in the abdomen and genitals. Pediatr Neurol 2000; 23:261–264.
5. Segal NA, Toda Y, Huston J, Saeki Y, Shimizu M, Fuchs H, Shimaoka Y, Holcomb R, McLean MJ. Two configurations of static magnetic fields for treating rheumatoid arthritis of the knee: a double-blind clinical trial. Arch Phys Med Rehabil 2001; 82:1453–1460.
6. Hinman MR, Ford J, Heyl H. Effects of static magnets on chronic knee pain and physical function: a double-blind study. Altern Ther Health Med 2002; 8:50–55.
7. Lud GV, Demeckiy AM. Use of permanent magnetic field in reconstructive surgery of the main arteries (experimental study). Acta Chir Plast 1990; 32:28–34.
8. Weinberger A, Nyska A, Giler S. Treatment of experimental inflammatory synovitis with continuous magnetic field. Isr J Med Sci 1996; 32:1197–1201.

9. Alfano AP, Taylor AG, Foresman PA, Dunkl PR, McConnell GG, Conaway MR, Gillies GT. Static magnetic fields for treatment of fibromyalgia: a randomized controlled trial. J Altern Complement Med 2001; 7:53–64.

10. Tkach EV, Abilova AN, Gazalieva ShM. Characteristics of the effect of a constant electromagnetic field on reparative processes in spinal cord injuries. Zh Nevropatol Psikhiatr Im S S Korsakova 1989; 89:41–44.

11. Man D, Man B, Plosker H. The influence of permanent magnetic field therapy on wound healing in suction lipectomy patients: a double-blind study. Plast Reconstr Surg 1999; 104:2261–2268.

12. Bruce GK, Howlett CR, Huckstep RL. Effect of a static magnetic field on fracture healing in a rabbit radius. Preliminary results. Clin Orthop 1987; 222:300–306.

13. Darendeliler MA, Darendeliler A, Sinclair PM. Effects of static magnetic and pulsed electromagnetic fields on bone healing. Int J Adult Orthodon Orthognath Surg 1997; 12:43–53.

14. Yan QC, Tomita N, Ikada Y. Effects of static magnetic field on bone formation of rat femurs. Med Eng Phys 1998; 20:397–402.

15. Xu S, Tomita N, Ohata R, Yan Q, Ikada Y. Static magnetic field effects on bone formation of rats with an ischemic bone model. Biomed Mater Eng 2001; 11:257–263.

16. Ivanov SG, Smirnov VV, Solov'eva FV, Liashevskaia SP, Selezneva LI. The magnetotherapy of hypertension patients. Ter Arkh 1990; 62:71–74.

17. Ivanov SG. The comparative efficacy of nondrug and drug methods of treating hypertension. Ter Arkh 1993; 65:44–49.

18. Mellander S, Johansson B. Control of resistance, exchange, and capacitance functions in the peripheral circulation. Pharmacol Rev 1968; 20:117–196.

19. Burnstock G, Griffith SG. Innervation of microvascular smooth muscle. In: Messemer K, Hammersen F, eds. Progress in Applied Microcirculation. Vol. 3. Basel: Karger, 1983:19–39.

20. Osborne NN. Coexistence of neurotransmitter substances in a specifically defined invertebrate neurone. In: Cuello AC, ed. Co-Transmission. London: Macmillan, 1982:207–222.

21. Vizi ES. Presynaptic modulation of neurochemical transmission. Prog Neurobiol 1979; 12:181–290.

22. Furness JB, Marshall JM. Correlation of the directly observed responses of mesenteric vessels of the rat to nerve stimulation and noradrenaline with the distribution of adrenergic nerves. J Physiol 1974; 239:75–88.

23. Siegel G, Malmsten M, Klussendorf D, Hofer HW. Vascular smooth muscle, a multiply feedback-coupled system of high versatility, modulation and cell-signaling variability. Int J Microcirc Clin Exp 1997; 17:360–373.

24. Mulvany MJ. Functional characteristics of vascular smooth muscle. In: Messemer K, Hammersen F, eds. Progress in applied microcirculation. Vol. 3. Basel: Karger, 1983:4–18.

25. Ignarro LJ. Biological actions and properties of endothelium-derived nitric oxide formed and released from artery and vein. Circ Res 1989; 65:1–21.

26. Funk W, Intaglietta M. Spontaneous arteriolar vasomotion. In: Messemer K, Hammersen F, eds. Progress in applied microcirculation. Vol. 3. Basel: Karger, 1983:66–82.

27. Zweifach BW. Microcirculation in health and disease. In: Manabe H, Zweifach BW, Messmer K, eds. Microcirculation in circulatory disorders. Springer-Verlag: Tokyo, 1988:3–9.

28. Asano M, Yoshida K, Tatai K. Microphotoelectric plethysmography using a rabbit ear chamber. J Appl Physiol 1965; 20:1056–1062.

29. Greenough CG. The effects of pulsed electromagnetic fields on blood vessel growth in the rabbit ear chamber. J Orthop Res 1992; 10:256–262.

30. Ohkubo C, Xu S. Acute effects of static magnetic fields on cutaneous microcirculation in rabbits. In Vivo 1997; 11:221–225.

31. Xu S, Okano H, Ohkubo C. Subchronic effects of static magnetic fields on cutaneous microcirculation in rabbits. In Vivo 1998; 12:383–389.

32. Okano H, Gmitrov J, Ohkubo C. Biphasic effects of static magnetic fields on cutaneous microcirculation in rabbits. Bioelectromagnetics 1999; 20:161–171.

33. Gmitrov J, Ohkubo C, Okano H. Effect of 0.25 T static magnetic field on microcirculation in rabbits. Bioelectromagnetics 2002; 23:224–229.

34. Yamada S, Mayadas TN, Yuan F, Wagner DD, Hynes RO, Melder RJ, Jain RK. Rolling in P-selectin-deficient mice is reduced but not eliminated in the dorsal skin. Blood 1995; 86:3487–3492.

35. Pluen A, Boucher Y, Ramanujan S, McKee TD, Gohongi T, di Tomaso E, Brown EB, Izumi Y, Campbell RB, Berk DA, Jain RK. Role of tumor-host interactions in interstitial diffusion of macromolecules: cranial vs. subcutaneous tumors. Proc Natl Acad Sci USA 2001; 98:4628–4633.

36. Yuan F, Salehi HA, Boucher Y, Vasthare US, Tuma RF, Jain RK. Vascular permeability and microcirculation of gliomas and mammary carcinomas transplanted in rat and mouse cranial windows. Cancer Res 1994; 54:4564–4568.

37. Gohongi T, Fukumura D, Boucher Y, Yun CO, Soff GA, Compton C, Todoroki T, Jain RK. Tumor-host interactions in the gallbladder suppress distal angiogenesis and tumor growth: involvement of transforming growth factor beta1. Nat Med 1999; 5:1203–1208.

38. Fukumura D, Gohongi T, Kadambi A, Izumi Y, Ang J, Yun CO, Buerk DG, Huang PL, Jain RK. Predominant role of endothelial nitric oxide synthase in vascular endothelial growth factor-induced angiogenesis and vascular permeability. Proc Natl Acad Sci USA 2001; 98:2604–2609.

39. Jain RK. The Eugene M. Landis Award Lecture 1996. Delivery of molecular and cellular medicine to solid tumors. Microcirculation 1997; 4:1–23.

40. Okano H, Ohkubo C. Modulatory effects of static magnetic fields on blood pressure in rabbits. Bioelectromagnetics 2001; 22:408–418.

41. Okano H, Ohkubo C. Anti-pressor effects of whole-body exposure to static magnetic field on pharmacologically induced hypertension in conscious rabbits. Bioelectromagnetics. In press.

42. Asano M, Brånemark PI. Microphotoelectric plethysmography using a titanium chamber in man. In: Harders H, ed. Advances in Microcirculation. Vol. 4. Basel: S. Karger, 1972:131–160.

43. Xu S, Okano H, Ohkubo C. Acute effects of whole-body exposure to static magnetic fields and 50-Hz electromagnetic fields on muscle microcirculation in anesthetized mice. Bioelectrochemistry 2000; 53:127–135.

44. Okano H, Ohkubo C. Effects of static magnetic fields on plasma levels of angiotensin II and aldosterone associated with arterial blood pressure in genetically hypertensive rats. Bioelectromagnetics. In press.

45. Owen MP, Walmsley JG, Mason MF, Bevan RD, Bevan JA. Adrenergic control in three artery segments of diminishing diameter in rabbit ear. Am J Physiol 1983; 245:H320–H326.

46. Edwards RM. Response of isolated renal arterioles to acetylcholine, dopamine, and bradykinin. Am J Physiol 1985; 248:F183–F189.

47. Matsukawa S, Suzuki H, Itaya Y, Kumagai H, Saruta T. Effects of nicardipine on the systemic and renal hemodynamics in acutely elevated blood pressure induced by vasoactive agents in conscious rabbits. Japan Heart J 1987; 28:435–443.

48. Persson MG, Gustafsson LE, Wiklund NP, Moncada S, Hedqvist P. Endogenous nitric oxide as a probable modulator of pulmonary circulation and hypoxic pressor response in vivo. Acta Physiol Scand 1990; 140:449–457.

49. Kanai S, Okano H, Orita M, Abe H. Clinical study of neck and shoulder pain for therapeutic effectiveness with application of static magnetic field. J Japan Sco Pain Clinicians 1996; 3:11–17.

50. Kanai S, Okano H, Susuki R, Abe H. Therapeutic effectiveness of static magnetic fields for low back pain monitored with thermography and deep body thermometry. J Japan Sco Pain Clinicians 1998; 5:5–10.

51. Kanai S, Taniguchi N, Susuki R. Therapeutic effectiveness of static magnetic fields for osteoarthropathy. J Japan Sco Pain Clinicians 1999; 6:361–366.

52. Gmitrov J, Ivanco I, Gmitrova A. Magnetic field effect on blood pressure regulation. Physiol Bohemoslov 1990; 39:327–334.

53. Gmitrov J, Gmitrova A. Geomagnetic field and artificial 0.2 T static magnetic field combined effect on blood pressure. Electro Magnetobiol 1994; 13:117–122.

54. Gmitrov J, Ohkubo C, Yamada S, Gmitrova A, Xu S. Static magnetic field effects on sino-carotid baroreceptors in rabbits exposed under conscious conditions. Electro Magnetobiol 1995; 14:217–228.

55. Gmitrov J. Static magnetic field effect on sinocarotid baroreceptors in humans. Electro Magnetobiol 1996; 15:183–189.

56. Gmitrov J, Ohkubo C. Static-magnetic-field effect on baroreflex sensitivity in rabbits. Electro Magnetobiol 1998; 17:217–228.

57. Gmitrov J, Ohkubo C. Artificial static and geomagnetic field interrelated impact on cardio-vascular regulation. Bioelectromagnetics 2002a; 23:329–338.

58. Gmitrov J, Ohkubo C. Verapamil protective effect on natural and artificial magnetic field cardiovascular impact. Bioelectromagnetics 2002b; 23:531–541.

59. Bogosav L, Neda PN. Heart rate in rats exposed to constant magnetic fields. Electro Magnetobiol 1993; 12:117–123.

60. Skorik VI, Zhernovoi AI, Sharshina LM, Kulikova NA, Rudakova ZV, Chirukhin VA. Changes in the blood flow oxygen capacity under the action of a permanent magnetic field. Biull Eksp Biol Med 1993; 116:386–388.

61. Jankovic BD, Maric D, Ranin J, Veljic J. Magnetic fields, brain and immunity: effect on humoral and cell-mediated immune responses. Int J Neurosci 1991; 59:25–43.

62. Jankovic BD, Jovanova-Nesic K, Nikolic V. Locus ceruleus and immunity. III. Compromised immune function (antibody production, hypersensitivity skin reactions and experimental allergic encephalomyelitis) in rats with lesioned locus ceruleus is restored by magnetic fields applied to the brain. Int J Neurosci 1993; 69:251–269.

63. Jankovic BD, Jovanova-Nesic K, Nikolic V, Nikolic P. Brain-applied magnetic fields and immune response: role of the pineal gland. Int J Neurosci 1993; 70:127–134.

64. Azanza MJ. Steady magnetic fields mimic the effect of caffeine on neurons. Brain Res 1989; 489:195–198.

65. Eichwald C, Kaiser F. Model for external influences on cellular signal transduction pathways including cytosolic calcium oscillations. Bioelectromagnetics 1995; 16:75–85.

66. Muehsam DJ, Pilla AA. The sensitivity of cells and tissues to exogenous fields: effects of target system initial state. Bioelectrochem Bioenerg 1999; 48:35–42.

67. Rosen AD. Magnetic field influence on acetylcholine release at the neuromuscular junction. Am J Physiol 1992; 262:C1418–C1422.

68. Rosen AD, Lubowsky J. Modification of spontaneous unit discharge in the lateral geniculate body by a magnetic field. Exp Neurol 1990; 108:261–265.

69. Cavopol AV, Wamil AW, Holcomb RR, McLean MJ. Measurement and analysis of static magnetic fields that block action potentials in cultured neurons. Bioelectromagnetics 1995; 16:197–206.

70. McLean MJ, Holcomb RR, Wamil AW, Pickett JD, Cavopol AV. Blockade of sensory neuron action potentials by a static magnetic field in the 10 mT range. Bioelectromagnetics 1995; 16:20–32.

71. Trabulsi R, Pawlowski B, Wieraszko A. The influence of steady magnetic fields on the mouse hippocampal evoked potentials in vitro. Brain Res 1996; 728:135–139.

72. Wieraszko A. Dantrolene modulates the influence of steady magnetic fields on hippocampal evoked potentials in vitro. Bioelectromagnetics 2000; 21:175–182.

73. Rosen AD. Threshold and limits of magnetic field action at the presynaptic membrane. Biochim Biophys Acta 1994; 1193:62–66.

74. Rosen AD. Membrane response to static magnetic fields: effect of exposure duration. Biochim Biophys Acta 1993; 1148:317–320.

75. Balaban PM, Bravarenko NI, Kuznetzov AN. Influence of a stationary magnetic field on bioelectric properties of snail neurons. Bioelectromagnetics 1990; 11:13–25.

76. Ayrapetyan SN, Grigorian KV, Avanesian AS, Stamboltsian KV. Magnetic fields alter

electrical properties of solutions and their physiological effects. Bioelectromagnetics 1994; 15:133–142.

77. Rosen AD. Inhibition of calcium channel activation in GH3 cells by static magnetic fields. Biochim Biophys Acta 1996; 1282:149–155.

78. Rosen AD, Lubowsky J. Magnetic field influence on central nervous system function. Exp Neurol 1987; 95:679–687.

79. Hong CZ, Harmon D, Yu J. Static magnetic field influence on rat tail nerve function. Arch Phys Med Rehabil 1986; 67:746–749.

80. Hong CZ. Static magnetic field influence on human nerve function. Arch Phys Med Rehabil 1987; 68:162–164.

81. Bell GB, Marino AA, Chesson AL. Alterations in brain electrical activity caused by magnetic fields: detecting the detection process. Electroencephalogr Clin Neurophysiol 1992; 83:389–397.

82. Fuller M, Dobson J, Wieser HG, Moser S. On the sensitivity of the human brain to magnetic fields: evocation of epileptiform activity. Brain Res Bull 1995; 36:155–159.

83. Dobson J, St Pierre T, Wieser HG, Fuller M. Changes in paroxysmal brainwave patterns of epileptics by weak-field magnetic stimulation. Bioelectromagnetics 2000; 21:94–99.

84. Hirai T, Nakamichi N, Yoneda Y. Activator protein-1 complex expressed by magnetism in cultured rat hippocampal neurons. Biochem Biophys Res Commun 2002; 292:200–207.

85. Kyuhou S, Okada YC. Detection of magnetic evoked fields associated with synchronous population activities in the transverse CA1 slice of the guinea pig. J Neurophysiol 1993; 70: 2665–2668.

86. Okada YC, Wu J, Kyuhou S. Genesis of MEG signals in a mammalian CNS structure. Electroencephalogr Clin Neurophysiol 1997; 103:474–485.

87. Kirschvink JL, Gould JL. Biogenic magnetite as a basis for magnetic field detection in animals. BioSystems 1981; 13:181–201.

88. Weaver JC, Vaughan TE, Astumian RD. Biological sensing of small field differences by magnetically sensitive chemical reactions. Nature 2000; 405:707–709.

89. Lohmann KJ, Johnsen S. The neurobiology of magnetoreception in vertebrate animals. Trends Neurosci 2000; 23:153–159.

90. Kirschvink JL, Walker MM, Diebel CE. Magnetite-based magnetoreception. Curr Opin Neurobiol 2001; 11:462–467.

91. Ritz T, Dommer DH, Phillips JB. Shedding light on vertebrate magnetoreception. Neuron 2002; 34:503–506.

92. Semm P, Schneider T, Vollrath L. Effects of an earth-strength magnetic field on electrical activity of pineal cells. Nature 1980; 288:607–608.

93. Semm P, Demaine C. Neurophysiological properties of magnetic cells in the pigeon's visual system. J Comp Physiol [A] 1986; 159:619–625.

94. Němec P, Altmann J, Marhold S, Burda H, Oelschlager HH. Neuroanatomy of magnetoreception: the superior colliculus involved in magnetic orientation in a mammal. Science 2001; 294:366–368.

95. Semm P, Nohr D, Demaine C, Wiltschko W. Neural basis of the magnetic compass: Interactions of visual, magnetic and vestibular inputs in the pigeon's brain. J Comp Physiol [A] 1984; 155:283–288.

96. Walker MM, Diebel CE, Haugh CV, Pankhurst PM, Montgomery JC, Green CR. Structure and function of the vertebrate magnetic sense. Nature 1997; 390:371–376.

37

Magneto-Metabolic Therapy for Advanced Malignancy and Cardiomyopathy

Demetrio Sodi Pallares [†]

Mexico City, Mexico

Paul J. Rosch

The American Institute of Stress, Yonkers, and New York Medical College, Valhalla, New York, U.S.A.

The evolution of a novel and highly effective treatment approach for the treatment of metastatic malignancy, pancreatic cancer and terminal cardiomyopathy based on the efficacy of polarizing solution and a low sodium diet in acute myocardial infarction is discussed. Illustrative case histories are provided demonstrating the dramatic benefits derived from the additional administration of electromagnetic fields to this regimen. The mechanisms of action responsible for these rewards are explained as well as implications for future applications.

I. EDITOR'S NOTE:

Demetrio Sodi Pallares passed away on August 12, 2003, at the age of ninety. He was the son of the famous lawyer and Secretary of State of Mexico, Demetrio Sodi Guergue, and grandson of another famous lawyer, Jacinito Pallares, and is survived by five sons, including Mexican Senator Demetrio Sodi. An internationally recognized cardiologist and one of the world's authorities on electrocardiographic interpretation, he was the author of 16 books and more than 300 scientific papers and the recipient of over 100 honorary degrees.

I first became acquainted with Demetrio Sodi Pallares 45 years ago as a result of having been awarded a Fellowship at Hans Selye's Institute of Experimental Medicine and Surgery at the University of Montreal in 1951, shortly after the publication of his magnum opus *Stress*. Selye and I developed a close professional and personal relationship and collabo-

---

[†]Deceased.

rated on several articles and projects over the next three decades. In exploring the role of stress in experimental myocardial infarction, he had demonstrated that the damage was magnified when animals had been previously sensitized by a high salt diet and/or the administration of adrenal cortical hormones like desoxycorticosterone that caused sodium retention. Potassium supplementation had a protective effect and he told me that a Dr. Sodi Pallares was able to subsequently confirm this in such a convincing fashion in humans that Selye replaced all his salt shakers with potassium chloride. It tasted terrible on those occasions when we had dinner at his home but he was confident it would help protect him from a heart attack. Following my internship and residency at Johns Hopkins and postgraduate training at Walter Reed I entered private practice and at Selye's insistence, succeeded Joel Elkes, former Chairman of the Department of Psychiatry at Hopkins, as President of The American Institute of Stress in 1978.

Our First International Montreux Congress on Stress in 1988 included a session entitled "Electromagnetic Energy Effects on Psychophysiologic Function." It was chaired by Björn Nordenström who discussed "The Use of Electrical Energies in the Promotion of Healing and Treatment of Cancer" and included presentations by Norman Shealy and Saul Liss on "The Effect of Electromagnetic Energy on Brain Neurotransmitters" and Boris Pasche on "The Physiological effects of Low Energy Emission Therapy (LEET)." This segment attracted so much interest that we included similar sessions at subsequent events. I had been involved with the development of the Symtonic LEET device and was so impressed with the results of double-blind studies showing its efficacy in insomnia and anxiety that I decided to devote a day to the use of magnetotherapy for the treatment of stress related disorders at our 1997 Ninth International Montreux Congress on Stress. I was anxious to attract leading investigators in this area and particularly any whose research could provide clues about magnetotherapy mechanisms of action. I made some inquiries and two colleagues immediately suggested that I invite a Dr. Sodi Pallares of Mexico City to discuss his remarkable results in patients with advanced metastatic malignancy.

I told them that I was familiar with Demetrio Sodi Pallares, a cardiologist who had now become world renowned for developing a "polarizing solution" to prevent cardiac damage. In the 1960s, I routinely administered this intravenous drip containing potassium chloride and insulin in hypertonic glucose (Fig. 1) as soon as possible to all my acute heart attack patients as did most other cardiologists I knew. There seemed little doubt that it significantly reduced complications of shock, arrhythmia, and congestive failure and shortened duration of hospitalization. However, since this Sodi Pallares would now probably be over 80, it did not seem likely that he was still treating patients much less using magnetotherapy to cure cancer. I assumed that this might be his son or some other relative and wrote to him requesting additional information and related the Selye anecdote.

I was pleased to receive a prompt and very gracious response indicating that he was indeed the same Demetrio Sodi Pallares. His letterhead listed his specialty as "Cardiology and Magnetotherapy," which was like getting a letter from Mike DeBakey indicating "Cardiovascular Surgery and Magnetotherapy." He went on to describe his current research interests and willingness to participate in the congress, where he gave a superb presentation. Demetrio, or Sodi as he is usually referred to, has provided us with updates at subsequent congresses of his astounding achievements not only in patients with seemingly hopeless cancers but also in patients with terminal cardiomyopathy and other disorders. We have become good friends and have cooperated in other presentations, and he has asked me to coauthor this chapter in a narrative fashion based on our conversations and written material that he has provided.

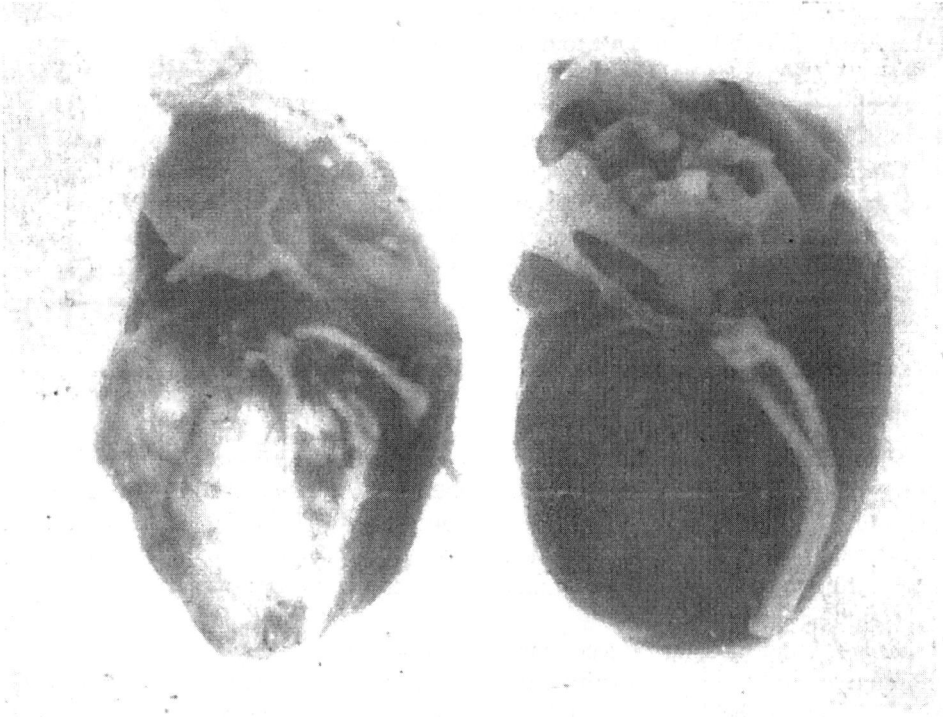

Figure 1 Cadioprotective effect of potassium chloride. Left: Massive necrosis visible as a white patch on the surface of the left ventricle following ligature of the left coronary artery in a control rat. Right: Complete prevention of the necrosis by pretreatment with KCL in a litter made exposed to the same procedure.

He had initially become interested in the antagonistic roles of sodium and potassium in 1944 when his mother developed marked edema of the lower extremities, enlargement of the liver, and tremendous abdominal distention due to ascites. The diagnosis was heart failure due to coronary arteriosclerosis and her electrocardiogram showed a left bundle branch block. In those days, this usually meant a life expectancy of not more than 2 years but it would have been much less for his mother in view of her serious heart failure. She was receiving the standard treatment of mercurial diuretics, digitalis, and a low cholesterol diet but was allowed to have sodium rich foods that were low in fat. The aggressive diuretic therapy required to reduce her fluid retention caused severe cramps and left her feeling exhausted. At the time, Sodi was involved in experimental electrocardiographic investigations at Mexico's National Institute of Cardiology and when he inquired as to why she had to receive so many injections of the mercurial diuretic, his professors explained that it was to eliminate sodium chloride. He asked why they allowed her to eat foods rich in salt and was told that his mother had to be on a low cholesterol diet to delay the atherosclerotic process and that the injections would get rid of the salt.

He was not satisfied with this answer and, although he had little appropriate background, decided to develop a diet for her that would eliminate any food with a sodium content higher than 100 mg/100 g. As it turned out, this was fortuitous, since he ended up with a diet that was not only low in sodium (around 360 mg) but also 10 times higher in potassium, and he did not realize how important this would prove to be. His mother followed the diet faithfully, was able to discontinue her medications, and went on to live a normal life for another 15 years. He began prescribing this dietary regimen for patients with other cardiovascular problems and found that most with congestive failure could be stabilized and usually only required digitalis and/or diuretics if they had acute pulmonary edema. The same was true for many others with essential hypertension, and it was not unusual for angina to disappear in weeks or even days after following the diet. Exhilarated about his results, he tried to convince other physicians to try the diet in their patients to see if they got the same benefits. However, his colleagues not only did not share his enthusiasm but criticized him because his diet was rich in cholesterol like egg yolk, unsalted butter, and other fats that would surely accelerate the progression of atherosclerotic deposits. In addition, he had had relatively little experience in clinical cardiology and was invading other fields not related to the electrocardiographic research he had been assigned, which would not be tolerated by authorities of the National Institute of Cardiology.

In retrospect, we now know that dietary cholesterol and fat have relatively little effect on either serum cholesterol or the development of obstructive atheroslcerotic plaque and that this diet actually proved to have a favorable effect on lipid profiles. Sodi went on to become a superb clinical cardiologist, authored some 20 cardiology texts, including over a dozen on the electrocardiogram alone, and his continued successes with the low salt diet only served to strengthen his belief in its benefits.

In spite of this opposition, he recommended it whenever he could and was encouraged by Hans Selye, who visited the Institute in 1959 during the International Symposium of Arteriosclerosis being held in Mexico City. Selye presented his experiments demonstrating the damaging effects of sodium as well as the cardioprotective effects of potassium in animals subjected to stress. Compared to control animals, more extensive myocardial infarcts were seen in those who had been on a high sodium diet and given adrenal corticoids. Potassium supplementation markedly reduced or prevented myocardial necrosis as seen in Fig. 1.

Since this could be demonstrated in animals with normal coronary arteries, it proved that myocardial infarction was not always due to obstruction of a coronary vessel that deprived the myocardium of oxygen. At the time, *heart attack*, *coronary occlusion,* and *myocardial infarction* were often used interchangeably as if they were synonymous. However, it is now clear that atherosclerotic occlusion of a coronary vessel, which occurs gradually, does not always result in a myocardial infarction and conversely, that myocardial infarction can result from excess catecholamine effects in the absence of coronary occlusion or even ischemia. This is not infrequent in pheochromocytoma and has also been reported as a complication of sympathomimetic drugs (isoproterenol, amphetamines), increased sensitivity to MAO inhibitors, and deaths related to sudden emotional stress, where characteristic "contraction bands" can be seen in the myocardium (1,2).

Selye's presentation also fell on deaf ears since it was contrary to current dogma and many felt that what happened to rats under laboratory conditions had little relevance for people. In commenting on this several years later, Selye wrote (3):

> The very fact that scientists of so many countries have contributed to this monograph on metabolic cardiopathies bears witness to the great change in outlook that has been placed in the interpretation of pathogenesis of heart disease during the last decade. Barely eight years ago, in September 1959, at the International Symposium on Arteriosclerosis and Coronary Disease in Mexico City, I tried to prove that infarcts, like cardiac necroses, can be produced without vascular obstruction, i.e., by combined treatment with electrolytes or corticoids and stress. At that time, with

the notable exception of Dr. Sodi Pallares, few of the participants were prepared to believe that such metabolic factors could play a role in the genesis of true cardiac infarcts in man ..... Although the functional effect of many electrolytes upon the heart has long been known, the finding that sodium increases and potassium and magnesium diminish the susceptibility to cardiac necroses was also received with the greatest reserve.

But what was the mechanism of action that explained the harmful effects of sodium and the benefits of potassium? Why did administering sodium cause fluid retention in patients while potassium did not, since both were monovalent cations? In an acute myocardial infarction, three zones of injury can be distinguished. In the central portion of the damaged area there is a core of necrotic tissue and dead cells due to the absence of oxygen. This is surrounded by an area of severe injury composed of cells that will die unless the metabolic derangement can be stopped or reversed. The damage lessens progressively in the periphery of this section that gradually merges into a larger third zone of cells that are less ischemic. Here, structural damage is not as impressive, and although function is impaired compared to adjacent normal tissue, the abnormalities are reversible.

Sodi demonstrated that in experimental infarction produced by ligature of the left coronary artery in dogs, he could show a clear and consistent correlation between the degree of damage and intracellular concentrations of sodium and potassium as one progressed through these three zones from healthy muscle. The higher the concentration of sodium, the greater the degree of damage, but the reverse was true for potassium. Compared to normal tissue, intracellular sodium in the ischemic area increased around 50%, compared to over 200% in the intermediate area of injury and more than 300% when the central necrotic core was reached. There was a corresponding decrease in potassium of 5% in ischemic tissue, 10% in the intermediate injury zone, and 18% in the necrotic area. Although these figures varied with the location and size of the infarct, they showed the same consistent interrelationships.

Were these abnormalities in sodium and potassium merely a reflection of the degree of damage or could they possibly contribute to it? Was increased intracellular sodium the cause of cellular injury? All atoms have shells orbiting around them filled with electrons to neutralize the positive charge of protons in the nucleus. The first shell contains two electrons and each successive shell contains eight electrons. The sodium atom has 11 electrons, two in the first shell, eight in the second, but only one in the third that it must get rid of to remain stable. The potassium atom has 19 electrons so it has three shells that are filled and a fourth that also has only one electron. In both situations there is a need to remove the extra electron by finding an atom with a shell that needs more electrons to be filled. When this happens, one of the protons in the nucleus is not balanced and these atoms now become monovalent positive ions or cations (Na^+ and K^+). A molecule of water (H_2O) consists of two atoms of hydrogen, each having a positive charge, and 1 atom of oxygen that has a negative charge. Since the radius of the potassium ion, or the distance from the center of the nucleus to the external orbit, is greater than the radius for sodium it is easier for water molecules to cluster around the sodium ion. When the number of intracellular sodium ions increases, they attract more molecules of free water than potassium does and the resultant swelling of the cell interferes with normal function.

The concentration of sodium within the cell is normally much lower than in the extracellular fluid, and the reverse is true for potassium, but what was responsible for this? His further investigations revealed that under healthy conditions, there is a powerful mechanism that constantly pumps excess sodium out of the cell. Because the concentration of sodium ions outside the cell is much higher than inside, a gradient in polarization is produced across the cell membrane known as the *sodium electrochemical potential*. He found that the difference in this gradient decreased progressively as one moved from healthy tissue to zones of increased injury and that this was reflected in the electrocardiogram as illustrated by the typical changes of ST segment depression seen in ischemic tissue noted in Fig. 2.

This progressive decline in the polarization gradient with increased injury mirrored the changes in sodium and potassium alterations noted above were also reflected in the electrocardiogram. As intracellular sodium increased, so did the volume of water in the cell, causing it to swell so that normal function was disrupted. These concomitant changes and correlations are summarized in Fig. 3.

Sodi concluded that increased intracellular sodium caused damage to cardiac muscle fiber cells and that as this became more pronounced, there was a corresponding progressive diminution of the gradient of polarization across the cell membrane and a diminished ability to function optimally. This can be seen more clearly in Fig. 4 taken from his book Deductive and Polyparametric Electrocardiographic Interpretation (4).

He immersed himself in studying physics, biochemistry, bioelectrical phenomena, cybernetics and anything else that might help him understand why his dietary regimen had such cardioprotective effects. This might allow him to convince his colleagues and other physicians of its benefits and more importantly help him learn how to improve his treatment results. The correlation between a healthy cell and its ability to maintain an electrical potential gradient across the cell membrane was consistent and impressive, and by now his mastery of electrocardiographic interpretation made it relatively easy to monitor this. He knew that according to the laws of thermodynamics, energy is neither created nor destroyed. It can only be transformed and that during its conversion from one form to another, some energy is degraded, or "lost" with respect to its availability to do work. This degradation, which is called *entropy*, applies to all chemical, electrical, and mechanical energy transformations, including those in biological systems.

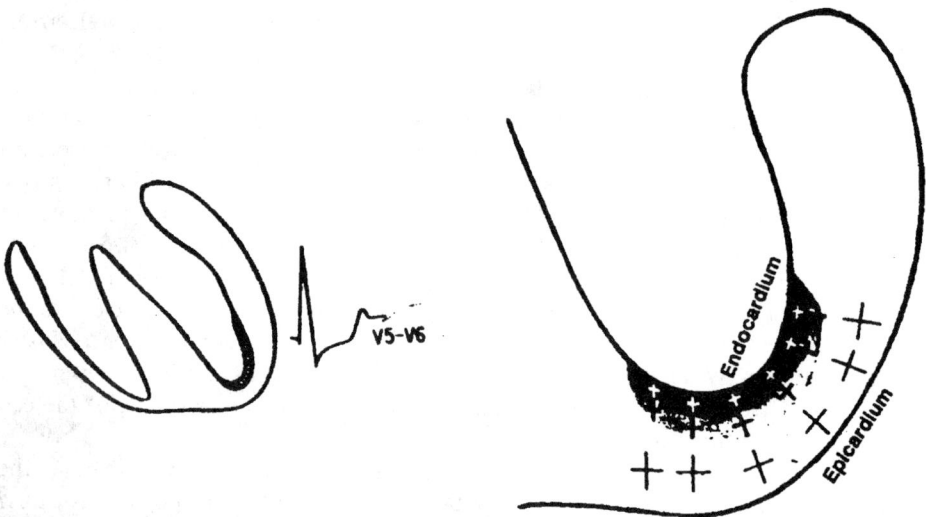

Figure 2 Schematic representation of subendocardial ischemia of the left ventricular wall. The electrocardiogram shows significant S-T segment depression in leads V5-V6.

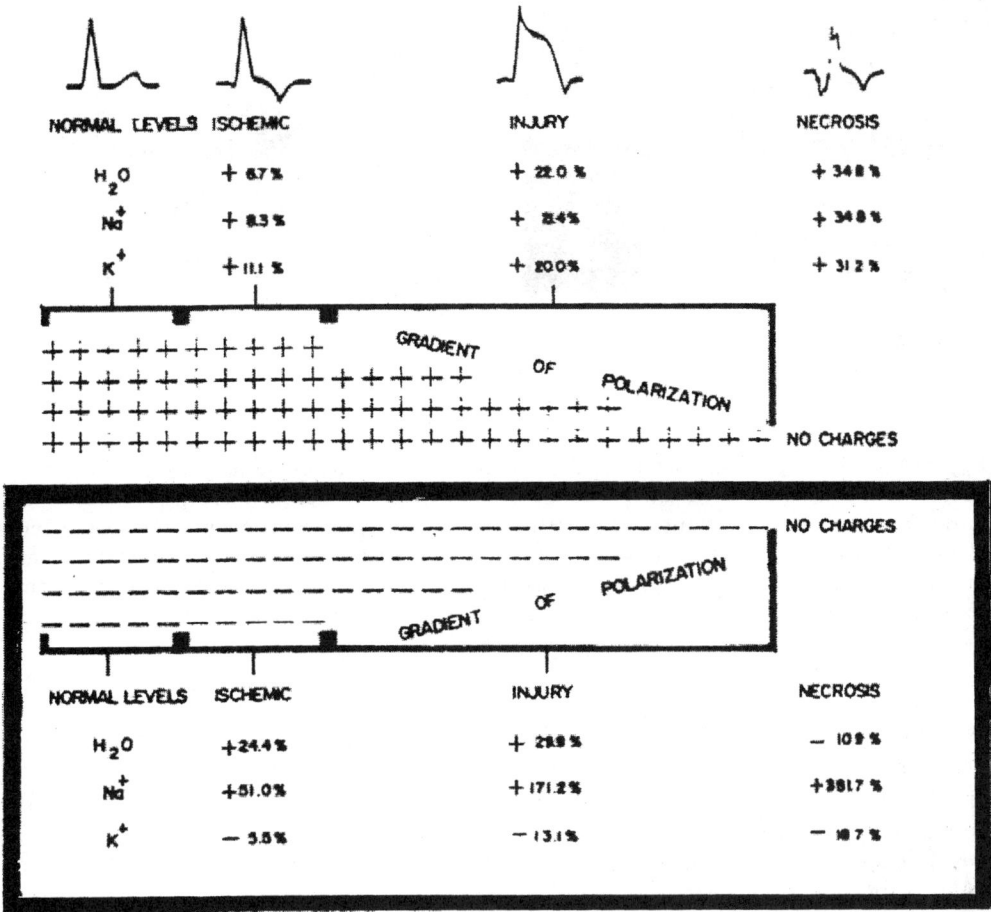

Figure 3 Schematic representation of a recent myocardial infarction showing the progressive change in intracellular and extracelullar concentrations of sodium (Na$^+$), potassium (K$^+$), and water (H$_2$O) as well as the decline in gradient of polarization from normal to ischemic to injured to necrotic tissue with characteristic corresponding ECG changes.

Albert Einstein used the illustration of a roller coaster to explain the different forms of mechanical energy and entropy in a closed system (5). As the car is pushed to the highest point of the track during the first steep rise it acquires potential energy as it progressively resists the force of gravity as shown in Fig. 5a. As it subsequently accelerates down the first bend towards earth, this stored potential energy is steadily converted into kinetic energy, the energy of motion as seen in Fig. 5b When the car ascends the second upward incline, kinetic energy is again progressively transformed into potential energy, and this sequence of energy transformation events is repeated over and over with each successive loop. However, the height reached (potential energy) and the speed of the descent (kinetic energy) progressively diminishes due to entropy, and the car finally stops moving.

If this transfer of energy was absolutely complete without any diminution in its ability to perform work, then the car would always attain the same height on the ascending loop and the same speed during its descent, and we would have perpetual motion. How-

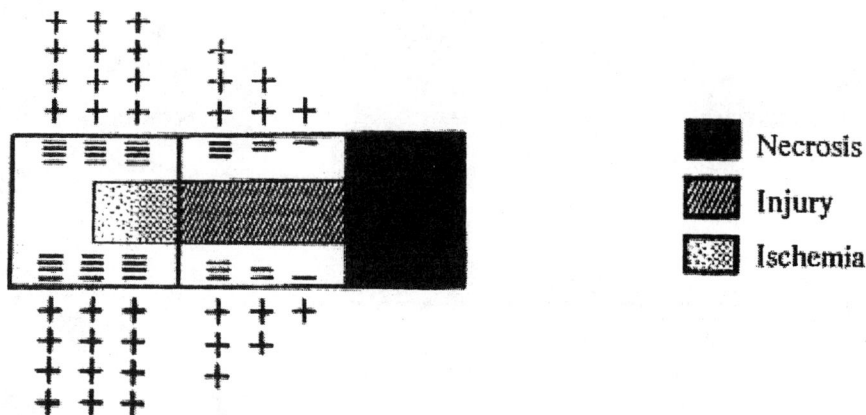

Figure 4 Following an acute myocardial infarction there is a progressive decline in the difference in electrical potential across the cell membrane that is closely related to the degree of injury and intracellular sodium concentration. Much like a battery, heahty tissue maintains a gradient of about 90 mV, whereas no gradient can be detected in necrotic or dead tissue. As this polarization gradient diminishes, so does the ability to do work, and the amplitude of contraction of muscle fibers progressively declines.

ever, we all know that this does not happen because of friction. The friction between the wheels of the car and the rails they ride on create heat. Although this is another form of energy (entropy), it is not available to help the car do its work. Instead, it is conducted to connecting structures, or back into the environment by radiation or convection, during which, some of it is also degraded. The amount of heat, which in this example depends upon the degree of friction or resistance, represents a loss in energy to perform the work of the car. If the surface of either the wheel or the rail becomes damaged so that smooth and continuous contact cannot be maintained, then there will be a corresponding decrease in kinetic and potential energy because of increasing entropy. The total amount of energy remains the same, but the difference between its forms progressively diminishes since entropy keeps increasing over time. Since the laws of thermodynamics also govern biological activities, all three forms of energy in Einstein's roller coaster analogy must be present in the heart. From Sodi's perspective, kinetic energy was the same as what was referred to as

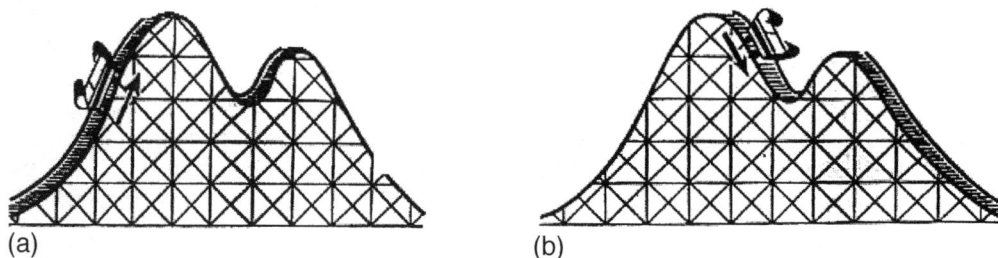

Figure 5 (a) Ascending the track to acquire potential energy; (b) transformation of potential to kinetic energy.

free energy in biological systems, which was supplied by ATP. The free energy concentrated in the phosphate bonds of one molecule of ATP furnishes about 7600–7800 cal. Potential energy was primarily represented by glycogen and triglycerides stored in heart muscle. Under emergency conditions due to fever, trauma, or severe emotional stress, the potential energy in these compounds is converted to ATP free energy similar to the conversion of potential to kinetic energy in the roller coaster. During all cardiac metabolic activities, some energy cannot be converted to do work and these calories (entropy) are dissipated to surrounding tissues.

Sodi reasoned that in heart muscle tissue, entropy is produced when sodium enters the cell, and as this increases, the electrical potential across the cell membrane diminishes and disappears when the cell dies. Under healthy conditions, the power for pumping sodium out of the cell comes from the energy rich phosphate bonds of adenosine triphosphate (ATP). The production of ATP diminishes as intracellular concentrations of sodium rise so that the energy to perform work declines correspondingly. This is what happens when the cell membrane is damaged following a myocardial infarction and sodium enters the cell causing a reduction in the polarization gradient.

When the cell has to do more work, additional energy from ATP is required and the key to this was ATPase, an enzyme that hydrolyzes the ATP molecule to release the free energy in its powerful phosphate bonds. ATP is also the source of energy for normal activities, such as the sodium pump that maintains the difference in concentrations of intracellular and extracellular sodium and potassium. Sodi had shown that his low-sodium high-potassium diet also helped to keep sodium out of the cell and potassium inside by promoting ATP activities. He reported his clinical achievements in cardiovascular disease in 1960 in the Journal of the Canadian Medical Association, possibly because of Selye's encouragement (6). By then, he had become aware of a "polarizing solution" consisting of glucose, insulin, and potassium developed by Henry Laborit, a French researcher (7). It seemed to be even more effective in this regard because insulin facilitates the entry of glucose and potassium into the cell and when this happens, sodium is driven out, thus increasing the polarization gradient across the cell membrane.

Since this was similar to the results he wanted to achieve with his diet, he decided to investigate the effect of different concentrations of the ingredients of this concoction in experimental myocardial infarction produced by ligating a coronary artery in dogs as he had done in previous experiments. He measured extracellular and intracellular sodium (Na^+) and potassium (K^+), and the best results were seen with an intravenous solution of 20% glucose containing 40 units of regular insulin and 40 mEq of potassium chloride given at a rate of 40 drops per minute. Administering polarizing solution significantly reduced the progressive rise in intracellular sodium and decrease in intracellular potassium that correlated with the degree or injury as depicted in Fig. 6.

Polarizing solution also prevented the damage due to experimental myocardial infarction in dogs, as illustrated in Fig. 7.

Encouraged, he studied the effects of administering polarizing solution to patients with acute heart attacks and other cardiovascular disease and was gratified by the clinical numerous benefits it provided as well as significant improvement in electrocardiograms. He reported these results in the early 1960s (8,9) and the rest is history. Cardiologists and researchers all over the world confirmed his results and sent him letters of congratulations. Eugene Braunwald, who would later become one of the most celebrated American cardiologists, Chief of Medicine at the Peter Bent Brigham Hospital with a chair named for him at Harvard, an Award established in his name by the American Heart Association and numerous other honors, received a $100,000 grant to study the effects of polarizing

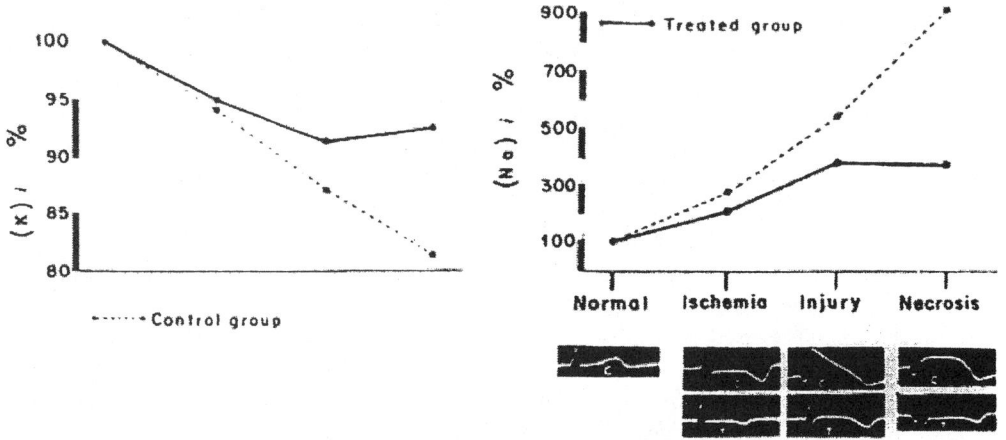

Figure 6 Progressive increase of intracellular sodium and decrease of intracellular potassium (broken lines) from the periphery of the infarct through areas of ischemia and injury to the central core of necrosis. Polarizing solution significantly diminished this trend as shown with the solid lines.

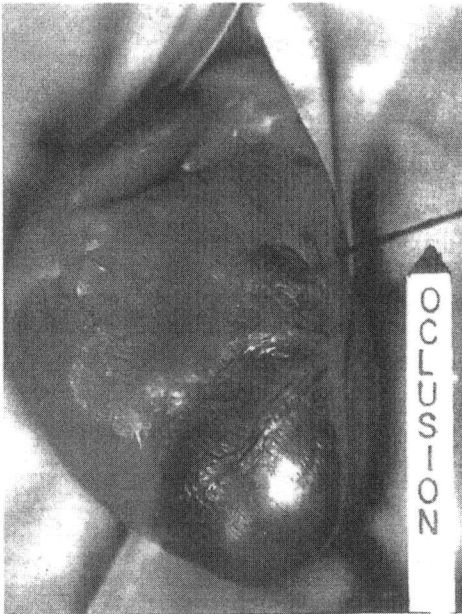
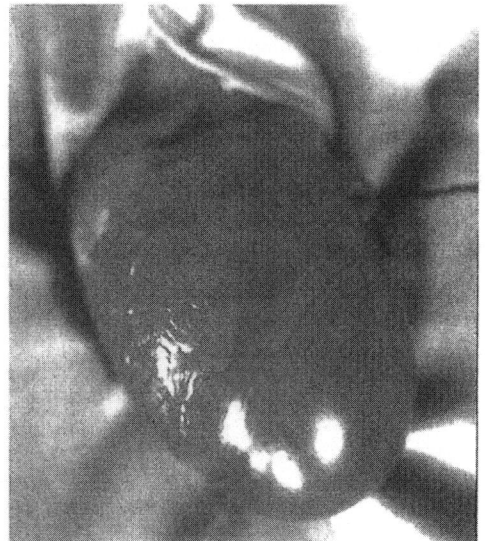

Figure 7 Reduction in necrosis following myocardial infarction in a dog with intravenous infusion of glucose, insulin, and potassium (polarizing solution).

solution in experimental infarction. He and his associates corroborated the results Sodi had reported 10 years previously (10) and subsequently confirmed its clinical benefits (11). Others also reported a decrease in morbidity, mortality, and complications such as arrhythmias (12–14). Studies of polarizing solution effects in experimental infarction in dogs (15), pigs (16), and rats (17), confirmed its ability to boost ATP production and improve free fatty acid metabolism (18) and to protect against hypothermic global ischemia by scavenging free radicals (19).

As Sodi's fame increased, it seemed that the authorities and his colleagues at the Institute became increasingly envious and jealous, rather than praising and supporting his efforts. Instead of improving things, the antagonism to his research increased and became so intense that he was forced to leave the Institute in 1975 and enter private practice to continue his investigations. Over the next decade, Sodi and his associates were able to conclusively show that his polarizing solution speeded up recovery from myocardial infarction, corrected arrhythmias, significantly reduced mortality rates in shock, and boosted ATP and cellular energy mechanisms sufficiently to benefit other conditions including myocarditis, cardiomyopathy, and hepatitis. These results were also confirmed by others in nuclear magnetic resonance studies, patients with diabetes and chronic ischemic cardiomyopathy, as well as clinical trials that acknowledged his seminal contributions (20–23). The use of polarizing solution increased all over the world, but it was often administered in a haphazard or reckless fashion so that optimal or consistent results were not achieved. In other instances, extravagant claims were made suggesting that it was a panacea, and it was prescribed for inappropriate indications. As new drugs were developed to treat shock, congestive failure, hypertension, inflammation, and various arrhythmias they were vigorously promoted to doctors by pharmaceutical companies, and the popularity of polarizing solution declined. However, it continued to be used in heart transplant surgery to maintain the integrity of donor hearts (24) and improve the efficacy of mechanical assist devices (25) and for prophylactic benefits in bypass surgery (26). There has been a recent revival of interest with large clinical trials confirming that it is the most cost-effective treatment for acute myocardial infarction and can reduce mortality by as much as 66 % when damaged cells that are still viable can be restored to normal (27–30).

Polarizing solution was effective because it improved the ability of ATP to provide energy by reducing the entropy produced when sodium enters the cell. As in Einstein's roller coaster illustration, the greater the entropy, the greater the disturbance in the ability to utilize energy to perform work. This principle applies to all forms of energy and all systems but its application to biological processes was first described by the nineteenth century American mathematician-physicist Josiah W. Gibbs. Gibbs conceived the concepts of chemical potential and surface tension and was considered to be one of the world's greatest theoretical physicists by James Clerk Maxwell, who first proposed that electric and magnetic energies travel in transverse waves at the speed of light. One of Gibbs' greatest achievements was devising the equation to express thermodynamic equilibrium in living systems in terms of energy and entropy, and the energy from ATP is often referred to as the *free energy of Gibbs* in his honor. This energy is free for the cell to reproduce itself, manufacture an enzyme or hormone, or use in any way it sees fit. Going back to the roller coaster analogy, it is very much like having a constant source of electricity, that the system can use to control the speed of the cars and provide light, heat, or sound as required. Since the source of energy for all cellular functions comes from ATP, it follows that when ATP synthesis or hydrolysis is impaired by increased intracellular sodium, no cell can function properly and the ability to correct this should resuscitate those with potentially reversible damage.

If this were so, then Sodi's polarizing solution and dietary regimen should prove beneficial for many disorders other than myocardial ischemia, and this has been supported by numerous observations. Ling, a molecular biologist, did not subscribe to the sodium pump theory but also verified the damaging effects of intracellular sodium (31,32) and later confirmed that a high potassium and low sodium environment could partially restore damaged cell proteins to the normal undamaged configuration using nuclear magnetic resonance tecniques (33). Ling had a profound influence on F. W. Cope, who proposed a Tissue Damage Syndrome that could occur anywhere in the body in cells deprived of oxygen and/or nutrients for any reason (34). He regarded the cell as analogous to an ion-exchanger resin granule with structured water in the interstices and potassium and sodium ions associated with fixed negative charges on the protein matrix. In tissues damaged by disease or trauma, there was a configurational change of the protein matrix that resulted in intracellular potassium being replaced by sodium and an abnormal uptake of water by the cell that interfered with ATP production. He advocated diet and medications that could decrease sodium and/or increase potassium concentrations in the body and was later surprised to find that Sodi had already been utilizing this and that Gerson's successful treatment of cancer emphasized this approach (35).

B. F. Trump and colleagues also found that these characteristics of high intracellular sodium and low intracellular potassium in damaged tissue that could be restored to normal could be demonstrated not only in the myocardium but liver cells exposed to carbon tetrachloride, kidney tubules following the mercuric chloride injection, HeLa cells infected with polio virus, ascitic tumor cells treated with cytolytic antibody, and various malignancies. Trump believed that a wide variety of pathological phenomena ranging from acute cell death to chronic processes like neoplasia, hypertension, and aging were all a common series of cellular reactions (36,37).

Sodi's interest in cancer was stimulated by the observation that malignant cells were also depolarized because of failure of the pumping mechanism that keeps sodium out. In some instances, intracellular sodium concentration is 300% higher than normal, and as this progresses, the intracelluar concentrations of protons (H^+) and calcium (Ca^{2+}) increase causing swelling of the cell due to water retention. This seriously disrupts mitochondrial function and the ability to synthesize ATP and lowers membrane potential. Cohen had shown that in very aggressive malignancies like mysoarcoma, the polarization of adjacent healthy tissue was −90 mV in contrast to only −10 mV at the center of the tumor. Furthermore, this decrease in membrane potential could be correlated with increased proliferative activity of malignant cells (38).

Our cells are surrounded by an ocean of salt water very high in sodium and low in potassium that passes through them at a rate of 100 times the cell's volume every second. Since healthy cells contain only 7% of the sodium concentration of extracellular fluid but the concentration of potassium is 342 times greater within the cell, a tremendous amount of energy is required to overcome these very high gradients across the membrane. This energy comes from the hydrolysis of ATP to ADP (Adenosine diphosphate) and phosphorus or to AMP (Adenosine monophosphate) and pyrophosphate with the eventual release of high-energy phosphate bonds. How this was accomplished was not clear until the late 1950s when the Danish biophysicist Jens Christian Skou proposed that an enzyme was responsible (39). Skou was awarded the 1977 Nobel Prize in Chemistry for discovering Na^+-K^- ATPase and showing that when bound to the cell membrane, it was activated by an increase in external potassium and/or internal sodium (40).

Reports that electromagnetic fields could remarkably increase the growth of plants suggested that this was another way to stimulate ATP synthesis, and Sodi investigated this by preparing two small tumblers in which he put five dried beans and a fistfull of soil. One was exposed to a pulsating electromagnetic field for 2 h a day for 5 days, and a highly reputable fertilizer was added to the other according to the prescribed instructions. He was surprised to find that the stem of plant subjected to the electromagnetic field increased as much as 10 cm in a day (Fig. 8a) and was much taller than the fertilized plant (Fig. 8b). Long term studies showed that the fertilizer was effective in promoting increased growth (Fig. 9b) but not to the extent achieved with pulsating electromagnetic fields (Fig. 9a).

Proof that pulsed electromagnetic fields could significantly boost ATP production to provide benefits in other disorders came from a patient with human papilloma virus infection of the cervix that was considered to be a premalignant condition as shown in Fig. 10a. The Schiller test showed an absence of glycogen. She was treated with a low-sodium diet and exposed to a pulsating magnetic field of 70 G for 2 h daily. After 2 months, there was no sign of disease (Fig. 10b) and the Schiller test now confirmed the reappearance of glycogen. This is particularly important since large amounts of ATP are required to form glycogen.

Since then, significantly beneficial results have been found with the use of pulsating magnetic fields in osteoarthritis, rheumatoid disease, discoid lupus, multiple sclerosis cardiomyopathies, severe cardiac insufficiency and other disorders including Kaposi's sarcoma, AIDS, and various malignancies. In most instances the intensity of the magnetic

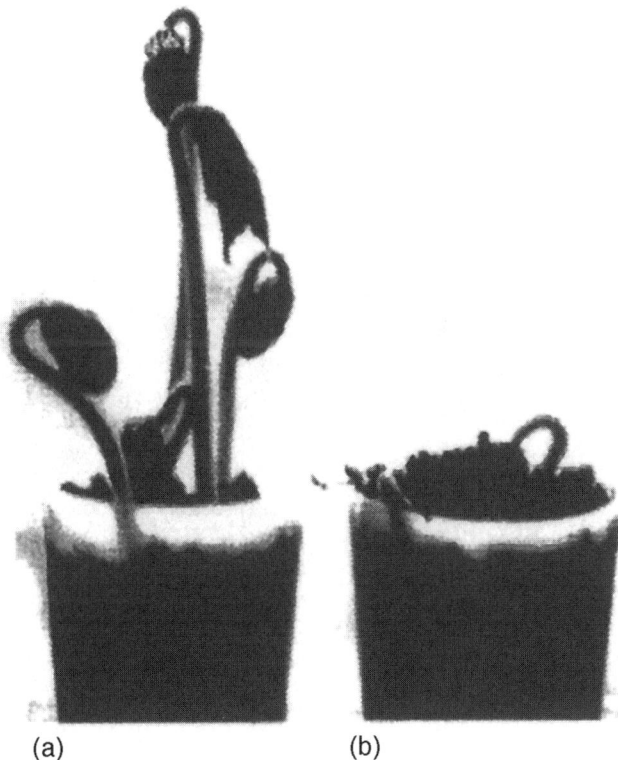

(a)   (b)

Figure 8   After a few weeks, (a) with PEMF and (b) with fertilizer.

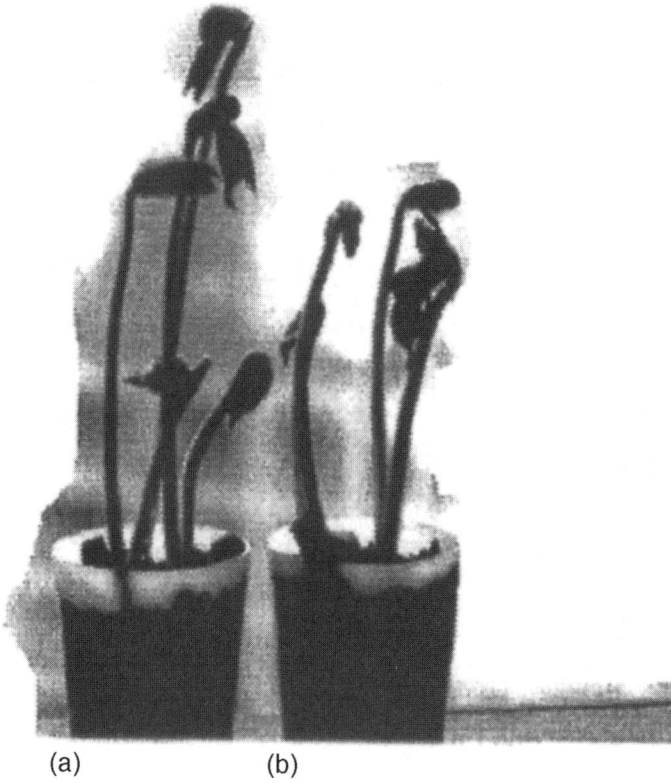

(a)   (b)

Figure 9 After months, (a) with PEMF and (b) with fertilizer.

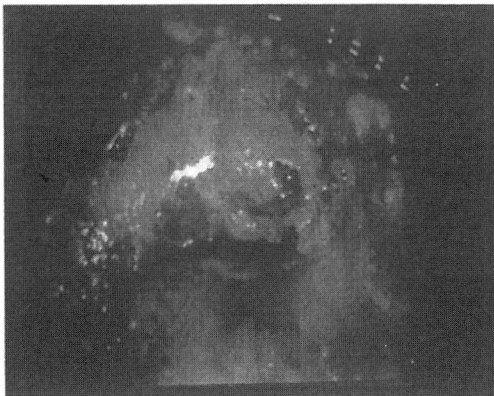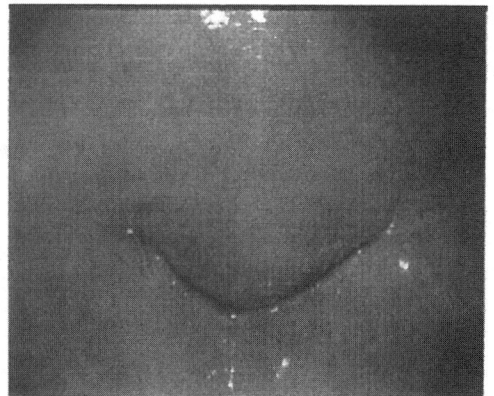

(a)   (b)

Figure 10 (a) Premalignant lesions before treatment and (b) disappearance of lesions after treatment.

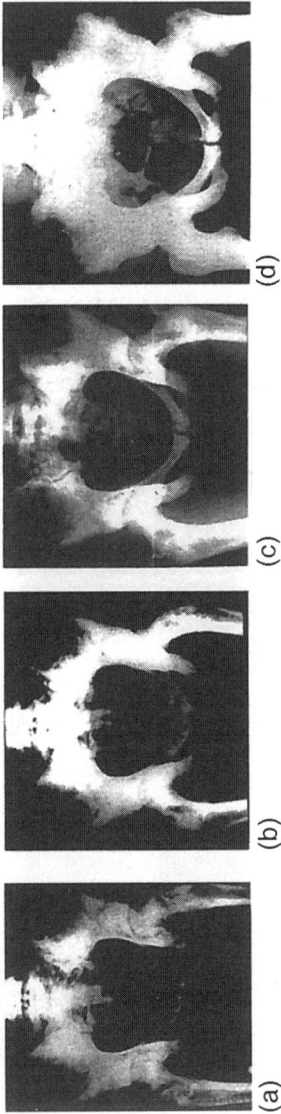

Figure 11 Thirty-nine-year-old female with bilateral breast cancer treated with chemotherapy and radiation with good results for 3 years but subsequently experienced weight loss, shortness of breath, and recurrent breast tumors. X-ray of the pelvis (a) showed an absence of the pubic bones and ischia and numerous metastases. A pleural effusion of 3000 cm^3 was evacuated, but it was generally felt that she would not last a week. Treatment was started with diet, polarizing solution 5 h daily, and application of a pulsating magnetic field of with intensity between 130 and 170 G. She gained 5 lb over the next 3 weeks, continued to improve, and by 6 weeks there was evidence of reappearance of the pubic and ischial structures (b). This continued to improve (c), the breast tumors decreased progressively and she felt so well after 25 weeks she asked if she could continue her treatment at home and appropriate arrangements were made. X-rays at that time (d) showed almost complete remineralization.

field ranges between 40 and 80 G, all patients followed the low-sodium diet, and in resistant cases, polarizing solution was also given. Cancer patients generally require 130–150 G. The pulsating electromagnetic field is delivered by a three-section folding pad containing coils in each section on which the patient can lie or use while sitting in a chair to target specific portions of the body. The wave form is a sinusoidal curve with a frequency of 60 Hz for treating both bone and soft tissue. The reason that cancers respond so well has been clarified by the research of Damadian and Cope, who measured Na^+, K^+, and H_2O in various malignancies and confirmed that the increase in intracellular sodium and water and decrease in potassium were similar to the changes noted in a recent myocardial infarction (41). This had previously been shown by Clarence Cone, who predicted the benefits of restoring intra-cellular potassium but was unaware that Sodi had already demonstrated this (38). Metastatic bone metastases respond especially well to this treatment.

Space constraints preclude an extensive report on clinical successes in various metastatic malignancies as well as brain tumors and primary lung cancer, but these and other triumphs are described in a book published in 1988 (42) that is now being updated and translated into English. It also demostrates how this protocol can prevent cardiac damage due to chemo-therapy and radiation and is effective in a variety of cardiovascular, dermatologic, and other disorders. Figures 11 through 13 are representative of the dramatic results achieved in advanced metastatic breast, prostate, and pancreatic malignancies.

Very positive results have been seen in cardiovascular disorders, including congestive failure, hypertension, and especially end-stage cardiomyopathy requiring heart transplan-tion. In one such 42-year-old male with heart failure resistant to treatment, biopsy at a leading cardiovascular center confirmed coagulative necrosis, and he was told that only a heart transplant would save his life. While waiting for a donor, he developed increasing shortness of breath, abdominal distention angina, and atrial fibrillation and, when seen, had Grade IV enlargement of the heart on x-ray, and ECG showed left ventricular hypertrophy and subendocardial damage. He was started on diet, 5 h of polarizing solution daily and application of 80-G pulsating magnetic field during this period. After only 2 weeks, shortness of breath, angina, and abdominal complaints vanished and heart size was markedly reduced. His electrocardiogram returned to normal following 18 weeks of treat-

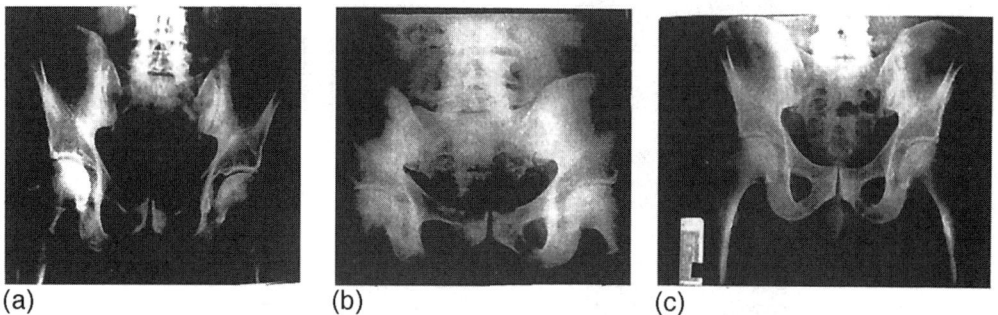

(a)   (b)   (c)

Figure 12 Seventy-two-year-old male with adenocarcinoma of the prostate and metastases to the ribs and pelvis showing destruction of the pubis. (a) Treatment was started on July 7, 1997 with dramatic improvement in general well-being as well as osteolytic lesions in the pelvis after only 4 days. (b) On July 25 the reduction in metastases was even more impressive. (c) The patient had to return to the United States where he intended to find a physician to continue the treatment, but contact was lost because he was apparently unable to accomplish this. Reduction in metastases was even more impressive.

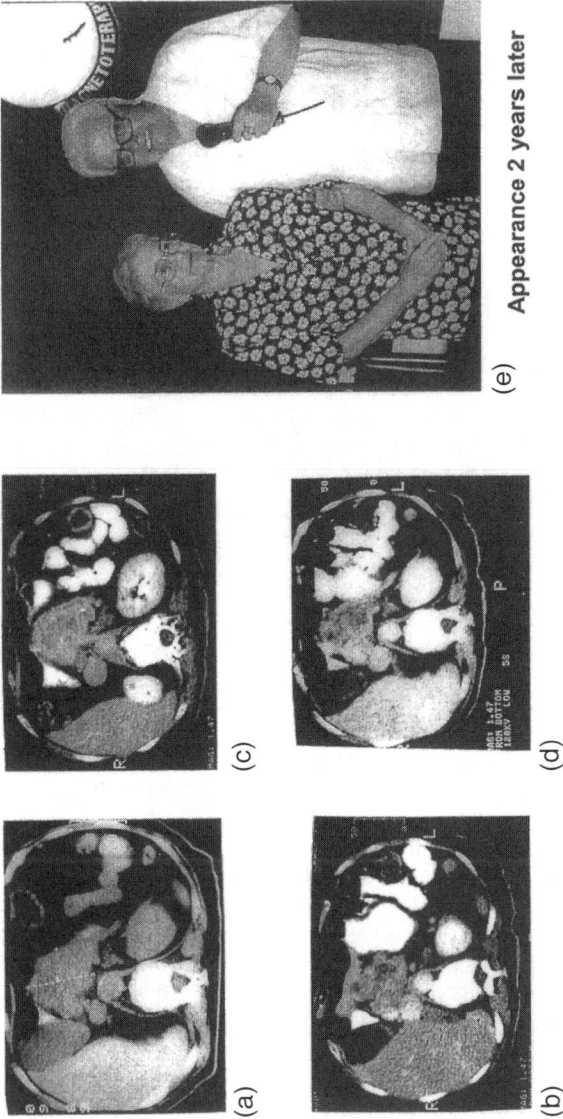

Figure 13 Seventy-five-year-old female seen on March 29, 1998 complaining of progressively severe abdominal pain, weight loss, and fatigue for a month. Tomography revealed a malignancy of the body and head of the pancreas with invasion of regional lymph nodes (a and b). She was started on diet, received polarizing solution twice weekly along with daily application of 150 G to the affected area. She improved rapidly with respect to relief of pain, return of energy, and weight gain, and her general condition was excellent 24 months later. (c) She continued to do well and tomograms at 36 months showed no increase in the tumor size and necrotic areas could be seen (d and e). She was seen by an oncologist who told her that the original diagnosis must have been an error since nobody with this type of pancreatic cancer lives for 3 years, and she could eat as much salt as she wanted and discontinue the treatment. The patient was pleased with this opinion and took his advice but died shortly thereafter.

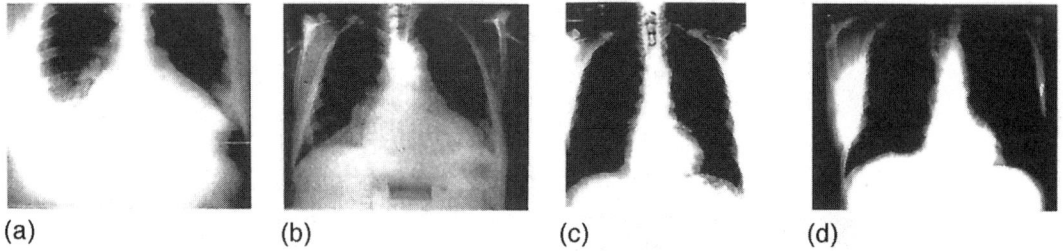

(a)   (b)   (c)   (d)

Figure 14 (a) Before treatment, (b) after 2 months, (c) after 6 months, and (d) after 7 months.

ment, and he continued to improve and was discharged. When contacted 3 1/2 years later, he stated he was in excellent health and living a completely normal life and taking no medication, although he continued to follow the diet. Fig. 14. shows the response of another patient who was treated with the same protocol.

There seems little doubt that this regimen can be improved since it is based on an empiric approach. In some instances, variations in the strength of the polarizing solution and the pulsed electromagnetic field have produced better results, and optimal treatment probably varies with each patient. Unfortunately, we do not have objective parameters to determine this, but advances in measuring biofield characteristics may prove useful. It is also likely that supplementation with ubiquinone (coenzyme Q10) could provide additional benefits since it is a crucial component of the electron transport chain of the Krebs cycle that is required for ATP synthesis and oxidative phosphorylation. Our hope is that others will confirm the benefits of this magnetotherapy-metabolic-thermodynamic approach and find ways to improve it.

REFERENCES

1. Eliot RS. Stress and the Major Cardiovascular Disorders. Mount Kisco: Futura Publishing, 1979:51–52.
2. Rosch PJ. Can stress cause coronary heart disease? Stress Medicine 1994; 10:207–210.
3. Selye H. The pluricausal cardiopathies. Ann N Y Acad Sci 1969; 156(1):195–206.
4. Sodi Pallares D, Medrano G, Bisteni A, Ponce de León JJ. Deductive and Polyparametric Electrocardiography. México D.F.: Inst. Nacional de Cardiol, 1970.
5. Einstein A, Infeld L. The Evolution of Physics. New York: Simon and Schuster, 1961.
6. Sodi-Pallares D, Fisleder B, Cisneros F, Viszcaíno. A low sodium, high water and high potassium regimen in the successful management of some cardiovascular diseases. Can Med Assoc J 1960; 83:243.
7. Laborit H. Stress and Cellular Function. Philadelphia: JB Lippincott, 1959.
8. Sodi Pallares D, Testelli MR, Fishleder BL, Bisteni A. Effect of an intravenous solution of potassium-glucose-insulin solution on the electrocardiographic signs of myocardial infarction. Am J Cardiol 1962; 9:166.
9. Sodi Pallares D, Bisteni A, Medrano GA, Testelli MR, De Micheli A. The polarizing treatment of acute myocardial infarction: possibility of its use in other cardiovascular conditions. Dis Chest 1963; 43:424.
10. Maroko PR, Libby P, Sobel BE, Bloor CM, Sybers HD, Shell WE, Covell JW, Braunwald E. Effect of glucose-insulin-potassium infusion on myocardial infarction following experimental coronary artery occlusion. Circulation 1972; 45(6):1160–1175.
11. Maroko PR, Braunwald E. Effects of metabolic and pharmacologic interventions on myocardial infarct size following coronary occlusion. Circulation 1976; 53(3 suppl):I162–I168.

12. Prasad K, Callaghan JC. Electrophysiologic basis of use of a polarizing solution in the treatment of myocardial infarction. Clin Pharmacol Ther 1971; 12(4):666–675.

13. Thys JP, Cornil A, Smets P, Degaute JP, Rudi N, Bernard R, Denolin H. Significance of the "polarizing" treatment of myocardial infarction. Acta Cardiol 1974; 29(1):19–29.

14. Zukowski SJ. Polarizing solutions in treatment of arrhythmias. J Am Osteopath Assoc 1973; 131–138.

15. Bekheit S, Isber N, Jani H, Butrous G, Boutjdir M, el-Sherif N. Reduction of ischemia-induced electrophysiologic abnormalities by glucose-insulin infusion. J Am Coll Cardiol 1993; 22 (4): 1214–1222.

16. Lazar HL, Zhang X, Rivers S, Bernard S, Shemin R. Limiting ischemic myocardial damage using glucose-insulin-potassium solutions. Ann Thorac Surg 1995; 60(2):411–416.

17. Jonassen AK, Aasum E, Riemersma RA, Mjos OD, Larsen TS. Glucose-insulin-potassium reduces infarct size when administered during reperfusion. Cardiovasc Drugs Ther 2000; 14(6): 615–623.

18. Kobayashi A, Kamiya J, Yamashita T, Ishizaka K, Hayashi H, Kamikawa T, Yamazaki N. Effects of glucose-insulin-potassium solution on free fatty acid metabolism in ischemic myocardium. Jpn Circ J 1984; 48(6):591–595.

19. Hess ML, Okabe E, Poland J, Warner M, Sewart JR, Greenfield LJ. Glucose, insulin, potassium protection during the course of hypothermic global ischemia and reperfusion: a new proposed mechanism by the scavenging of free radicals. J Cardiovasc Pharmacol 1983; 5(1):35–43.

20. Hoekenga DE, Brainard JR, Hutson JY. Rates of glycolysis and glycogenolysis during ischemia in glucose-insulin-potassium-treated perfused hearts: A 13C, 31P nuclear magnetic resonance study. Circ Res 1988; 62(6):1065–1074.

21. Quinones-Galvan A, Ferrannini E. Metabolic effects of glucose-insulin infusions: myocardium and whole body. Curr Opin Clin Nutr Metab Care 2001; 4(2):157–163.

22. Cottin Y, Lhuillier I, Gilson L, Zeller M, Bonnet C, Toulouse C, Louis P, Rochette L, Girard C, Wolf JE. Glucose insulin potassium infusion improves systolic function in patients with chronic ischemic cardiomyopathy. Eur J Heart Fail 2002; 4(2):181–184.

23. Alegria Ezquerra E, Maceria Gonzalez A. Therapy with glucose-insulin-potassium reduces the complications in the acute phase of myocardial infarct. Arguments in favor. Rev Esp Cardiol 1998; 1(9):720–726.

24. Smith A, Grattan A, Harper M, Royston D, Riedel BJ. Coronary revascularization: a procedure in transition from on-pump to off-pump? The role of glucose-insulin-potassium revisited in a randomized, placebo-controlled study. J Cardiothorac Vasc Anesth Aug 2002; 16(4):413–420.

25. Pissarek M, Goos H, Nohring J, Kensicki C, Jonas B, Liebetruth J, Lindenau KF, Krause EG. Beneficial effect of combined glucose-insulin-potassium and mechanical support in acute myocardial ischaemia. Biomed Biochim Acta 1986; 45(5):629–636.

26. Haider W, Hiesmayr M. Glucose-insulin-potassium (GIK) in prevention and therapy of myocardial ischemia. Wien Klin Wochenschr 2000; 112(7):310–321.

27. Apstein CS, Taegtmeyer H. Glucose-insulin-potassium in acute myocardial infarction: the time has come for a large, prospective trial. Circulation 1997; 96(4):1074–1077.

28. Apstein CS. Glucose-insulin-potassium for acute myocardial infarction: Remarkable results form a new prospective, randomized trial. Circulation, 1998, 2223–2226.

29. Diaz R, Paolasso A, Piegas S, Tajer CD, et al. Metabolic modulation of acute myocardial infarction. Circulation. 1998; 2227–2346.

30. Opie LH. Proof that glucose-insulin-potassium provides metabolic protection of ischaemic myocardium? Lancet 1999; 353:768–769.

31. Ling GN. A new model for the living cell: a summary of the theory and recent experimental evidence in its support. Int Rev Cytol 1969; 26:1–61.

32. Ling GN, Ochsenfeld MM. Na^+ and K^+ levels in living cells: do they depend on the rate of outward transport of Na^+? Physiol Chem Phys 1976; 8(5):389–395.

33. Ling GN. A theoretical foundation provided by the Association-induction Hypothesis for

possible beneficial effects of a low Na high K diet and other similar regimens in the treatment of patients suffering from debilitating illnesses. Agressologie 1983; 24(7):293–302.

34. Cope FW. Pathology of structured water and associated cations in cells (ther tissue damage syndrome) and its medical treatment. Physiol Chem Phys 1977; 9(6):547–553.

35. Cope FW. A medical application of the Ling Association-Hypothesis: The high potassium, low sodium diet of the Gerson cancer therapy. Physiol Chem Physics, 1978.

36. Trump BF, Berezesky IK, Chang SH, Pendergrass RE, Mergner WJ. The role of ion shifts in cell injury. Scan Electron Microsc 1979; (3):1–13.

37. Trump BF, Berezesky IK, Phelps PC. Sodium and calcium regulation and the role of the cytoskeleton in the pathogenesis of disease: a review and hypothesis. Scan Electron Microsc 1981; (Pt 2):434–454.

38. Cone CD. Unified theory on the basis of mechanism of normal mitotic control and oncogenesis. J Theor Biol 1971; 30:151–181.

39. Skou JC. Enzymatic basis for active transport of of Na + and K + across the cell membrane. Physiol Rev 1965; 45:596–608.

40. Skou JC, Esmann M. The Na, K-ATPase. Journal of Bioenergetics and Biomembranes 1992; 24:249–261.Trump BF, Berezesky IK, Phelps PC. Sodium and calcium regulation and the role of the cytoskeleton in the pathogenesis of disease: a review and hypothesis. Scan Electron Microsc 1981; (Pt 2):434–454

41. Damadian R, Cope FW. NMR in cancer. V. Electronic diagnosis of cancer by potassium (39K) nuclear magnetic resonance: spin signatures and T1 beat patterns. Physiol Chem Phys 1974; 6(4):309–322.

42. Sodi Pallares D. Lo Que He Descubierto En El Tejido Canceroso. [What I Have Discovered About Cancer Tissue.] Mexico City: D Sodi Pallares, 1998.

38

Electromagnetic Fields as an Adjuvant Therapy to Antineoplastic Chemotherapy

Joseph R. Salvatore

Carl T. Hayden VA Medical Center, Phoenix, Arizona, U.S.A.

Marko S. Markov*

EMF Therapeutics, Inc., Chattanooga, Tennessee, U.S.A.

The treatment of human neoplastic disease incorporates a complex multi-modality approach for maximal benefit. Most malignancies are treated by using combinations of therapies including surgery, radiation therapy, anti-neoplastic chemotherapy, and biologic therapy. However, anti-cancer therapy is usually accompanied by significant adverse effect. This chapter discusses the possibility electromagnetic fields to be applied to human patients through noninvasive means. These fields have been used as an adjuvant to anti-neoplastic chemotherapy in a number of experimental settings including cellular, animal, and human, and applied as time-varying, static, and pulsed fields.

I. INTRODUCTION

The treatment of human neoplastic disease incorporates a complex multimodality approach for maximal benefit. Most malignancies are treated by using combinations of therapies including surgery, radiation therapy, antineoplastic chemotherapy, and biologic therapy. However, anticancer therapy is usually accompanied by significant adverse effects. Advancements have been made in reducing these adverse effects by:

1. Modifying antineoplastic chemotherapy type, timing, or dose of the agents
2. Modifying a surgical procedure or radiation therapy

---

*Current affiliation: Research International, Buffalo, New York, U.S.A.

3. Adding a second or third treatment to the initial designed to reduce overall side effects

4. Incorporation of specific antisymptom treatment.

Primary cancer therapy is usually the single initial therapy that is expected to result in the best outcome; other therapies may be added to that primary therapy. These added or *adjuvant* therapies can be given either prior to the primary therapy (*neoadjuvant*) or after the primary therapy (*adjuvant*).

Two techniques using direct electrical stimulation of tumor tissue have been recently explored. Electrochemical therapy was introduced by Nordenstrom as part of his theory of biologically closed electric circuits (1,2), and used as a technique in the treatment of cancer including lung cancer (3). The core of this method is the use of electric current applied invasively by inserting electrodes into tumor tissue inducing electrochemical reactions. These electrochemical changes (e.g., changes in pH) lead to destruction of the target tumor. (See Chapters 42 and 43.)

Electropermeabilization creates reversible cell membrane pores through the application of short, intensive electrical pulses (4). The presence of these pores allows rapid, direct delivery of antineoplastic chemotherapy into malignant cells. (See Chapter 40.)

These two methods are similar in that they are both invasive and the electrodes used must be introduced into the patient.

Electromagnetic fields, however, can be applied to humans through noninvasive means. These fields have been used as an adjuvant to antineoplastic chemotherapy in a number of experimental settings including cellular, animal, and human, and applied as time-varying, static, and pulsed fields. Electric and magnetic fields have been shown to modify the growth of malignant cells in vitro and malignant tumors in vivo. Early studies on the chemical and biological effects of electromagnetic fields (EMF) measured chemical reactions as well as effects on cell and animal systems (5–9).

More recent studies have used static magnetic fields (SMF), sinusoidal and other waveshapes, and pulsed EMF to affect the growth of malignant cells or tumors. Additional techniques use magnetic fields to draw and retain magnetic treatment particles into malignant cells and tumors (10–12). In some studies EMF has been used to reverse cell resistance to chemotherapy by altering the expression or function of the multidrug resistance (MDR) system (13). Recent publications suggests that EMF can effect angiogenesis in tumors (14,15). (See Chapter 39.) The effects of SMF from very low to very high intensity have been studied for Magnetic Resonance Imaging safety, and as applied to malignant cells with therapeutic intent. EMF has been used to effect the growth of malignant cells in vitro or in vivo, or to improve the efficacy of antineoplastic chemotherapy agents (adjuvant).

II. CELLS SYSTEMS

HL-60 leukemic cells exposed to an SMF of 1 T for 72 h were observed for metabolic activity postexposure. Metabolism of the exposed group was significantly decreased compared to control (Tables 1 and 2) (16). (For continuity, all field strengths in this chapter are reported in Tesla.)

Human colon adenocarcinoma cells exposed to a magnetic field (MF) either 1 Hz or 25 Hz and 1.5 mT peak, for 15 min or 360 min and after 24 h of incubation, were evaluated for cell viability. The group treated for 15 min showed a statistically significant increase in cell growth with both 1 Hz and 25 Hz. In contrast, a significant decrease in cell growth was found

Table 1 Cells and EMF

Cell line	EMF	Strength	Exposure time	Growth rate compared to control[a]	Reference
Human osteosarcoma	75 Hz	2.3 mT	0–18 h	↑	20
A431	Ramp to max 120 μs			↑	24
HT-29	Center of axis: 0.276 mT–0.525 mT. Peak 10.8 mT				
MCF-7	20 Hz	5.3 mT	12 h/day × 14 days	↑	19
				↑	27
Mouse model of LGLL	60 Hz	1.0 mT		↔	29
HTB 63	SMF	7 T	64 h	↓	21
HTB 77 IP3				↓	
CCL 86				↓	
Human adenocarcinoma	1 Hz	1.5 mT	360 min	↓	17
	25 Hz		360 min	↔	
	1/25 Hz		15 min	↑	
HL-60	SMF	1.0 T	72 h	↓	16
MCF-7	15 Hz	0.1 mT	24–96 h	↔	23
HeLa	0.8 Hz	0.18 T	24 h	↓	18
Endometrial ovarian prostate	60 Hz	0.2 mT	Continuous	↑ days 3–7	22

[a] ↑ = increase; ↓ = decrease; ↔ = no change.

with exposure to 1 Hz for 360 min. No significant change was seen for cells exposed to 25 Hz for 360 min (17).

In another study, HeLa cells grown in culture were exposed to a PEMF of 0.8-Hz square wave with a maximum intensity of 0.18 T. Twenty-four hours after exposure there was a 15% decrease in cell proliferation as measured by the methylthiazol tetrazolium (MTT) cell proliferation assay (18).

MCF-7 cells exposed to a sinusoidal EMF of 20 Hz and 5.3 mT for 12 h/day were also tested for cell viability using the MTT assay and showed an increase in mitochondrial activity 14 days after treatment with the EMF (19). Proliferation of human osteosarcoma cells was measured by [³H]thymidine incorporation after culture in a PEMF (75 Hz, 2.3 mT). Exposure times ranged from 0 hours (control) to 18 h; both osteosarcoma cell lines were stimulated to proliferate after 30 min. Minimal time for stimulation of normal human osteoblasts was 6–9 h (20). The cell viability of three human cancer cell lines exposed to a 7-T uniform magnetic field was assessed by the Trypan Blue dye exclusion, and for all three malignant cell lines there was a significant reduction in the number of viable cells compared to controls. This appeared to be due to slower cell growth and not to increased cell death (21).

In another study ovarian, endometrial, and prostate cancer cell lines were exposed continuously to a power frequency magnetic field (60 Hz, 0.2 mT) and the cell proliferation measured by the MTT assay. Assay results showed that the field enhanced the proliferation of all three cell lines (22).

Table 2 Cells Plus EMF Plus Chemotherapy

Cell line	EMF	Chemotherapy	Effect	Reference
U937/CEM	Static	Puromycin etoposide	Decrease in chemotherapy-induced apoptosis with field	28
A431	See Table 1.	Carboplatin Cisplatin Daunorubicin	↑ ed potency — —	24
HT-29		Carboplatin Daunorubicin Cisplatin	↑ ed potency ↑ ed potency —	
Mouse osteosarcoma	10 Hz/0.4 mT/ 25 μs	Doxorubicin	PEMF reverses doxorubicin resistance	25
Human carcinoma	Ref. 24	Daunorubicin	↑ potency when cells pretreated with PEMF	26
Murine osteosarcoma doxorubicin resistant	25 μs/10 Hz/ 0.4–0.8 mT	Doxorubicin	↓ growth rate of resistant cells exposed to PEMF	27
MCF-7 dx	75 Hz	Doxorubicin	↓ cellular thymidine incorporation	13
HL-60	SMF 1T	Cisplatin Doxorubicin Fluorouracil Vincristine In five combinations	↓ cell metabolism in 3/5 combinations compared to no field	16
Endometrial Ovarian Prostate	60 Hz/0.2 mT	Paclitaxel Cisplatin	No effect of field on cytotoxicity of chemotherapy	22
MCF-7	15 Hz/0.1 mT	Cyclophosphamide Doxorubicin Methotrexate	↓ cell viability with all three chemotherapy agents plus field compared to no field	23

Salvatore et al. (23) applied a field of 15 Hz, 0.1 mT to a culture of MCF-7 breast cancer cells. The field alone did not have an effect on the growth of MCF-7 cells compared to controls. A431 and HT-29 cells were exposed to a specifically designed PEMF to assess the effect of the field on cellular growth. Both cell systems showed increase in growth when exposed to the PEMF alone (24).

Improving the efficacy of antineoplastic treatment through combinations of primary and adjuvant therapies may enhance the treatment efficacy, but may also increase side effects. Investigators have added EMF to antineoplastic chemotherapy to modulate the effects of chemotherapy in cell systems. If EMF with chemotherapy can increase cell death and reduce the amount of chemotherapy required, side effects produced by the treatment might be reduced. The mechanisms by which these effects might occur may be mediated through direct cell kill by the field, an enhancement of the cell kill by chemotherapy at the cellular level by changing the characteristics of interaction between the chemotherapy and its cellular or nuclear target, modulation of cell membrane or ion channel function, and changing cell drug resistance.

Cultured A431 and HT-29 cells were exposed to a specifically designed PEMF in addition to multiple chemotherapeutic agents to observe whether cytotoxicity was improved with the combination over chemotherapy alone. The potency of the chemotherapeutic agent carboplatin was enhanced against the A431 cell system after a 1-h exposure to the field. This potentiation was not observed with cisplatin or dauomycin. Against the HT-29 system, the field enhanced the carboplatin and the daunomycin but not the cisplatin (24). Doxorubicin resistance in a mouse osteosarcoma cell line was reversed by the application of a PEMF and appeared to be mediated through inhibition of the P-glycoprotein function (25). Using the PEMF described by Hannan (24), human carcinoma cells were treated with the field and daunorubicin. There was an increase in potency of the daunorubicin against the cell line when the cells were pretreated with the PEMF (26).

A doxorubicin-resistant murine osteosarcoma cell line exposed to doxorubicin with and without a PEMF showed that for all doxorubicin concentrations, the growth rate in resistant cells exposed to PEMF was significantly lower than that in the nonexposed resistant cells, including those in doxorubicin-free culture (27). The multidrug resistant cell line MCF7dx was exposed to a 75 Hz EMF while the cells were cultured in varying concentrations of doxorubicin. [^{3}H]thymidine incorporation was measured in these cells with and without EMF and the results suggest that at the highest concentration used of doxorubicin, 40 μg/ml, there was a significant reduction in [^{3}H]thymidine incorporation by the malignant cells (13).

MCF-7 breast cancer cells were exposed to a 15-Hz, 0.1-mT field with and without the chemotherapy agents cyclophosphamide, doxorubicin, and methotrexate and cell viability was determined by the MTT assay. These three agents were chosen because each has a distinct proposed mechanism of action (Table 3). Cell viability was significantly decreased at 48, 72, and 96 h for cells exposure to the field plus chemotherapy compared to chemotherapy alone (23). Modulation of the influx of calcium ions by a static magnetic field has been suggested as a mechanism for inhibiting apoptosis. U937 and CEM cells were induced to apoptosis by puromycin and etoposide and cells exposed to a SMF by placing a disk-shape magnet under the culture dish. The extent of cell death induced by the chemotherapy agents was reduced by the application of the magnetic field, which the authors felt was due to changes in cellular metabolism of calcium (28). Ovarian, endometrial, and prostate cancer cell lines exposed continuously to a power frequency magnetic field (60 Hz, 0.2 mT) with antineoplastic chemotherapy were assessed for viability by the MTT assay. This field did not enhance the cytotoxicity induced by the antineoplastic agents paclitaxel and cisplatin (22).

III. IN VIVO SYSTEMS

EMF has been applied to animal in vitro systems (Table 4) to observe the effect of EMF alone and EMF plus antineoplastic chemotherapy on the growth of these tumors. The use of these systems increases the difficulty in interpreting field effects by adding complex factors, such as the animal's immune system, which can affect the outcome. Although these studies aim to answer the simple question of whether EMF–SMF can affect the growth of tumor directly or affect the interaction of chemotherapy with malignant tumors in vivo, the com-

Table 3 Chemotherapy Agents Discussed

Chemotherapy drug	Type	Mechanism of action
Carboplatin	Heavy metal complex	Preferential reaction to N7 position of guanine and adenine forming adducts. Leads to intra and inter-strand DNA cross-links.
Cisplatin	Heavy metal complex	Preferential reaction to N7 position of guanine and adenine forming adducts. Leads to intra- and interstrand DNA cross-links.
Cyclophosphamide	Alkylating agent	Converted to active metabolite in liver.
Daunorubicin	Anthracycline antibiotic	DNA strand breaks mediated by inhibition of topoisomerase II, intercalation of DNA, and inhibition of DNA polymerase.
Doxorubicin	Anthracycline antibiotic	DNA strand breaks mediated by inhibition of topoisomerase II, intercalation of DNA, and inhibition of DNA polymerase.
Etoposide	Semisynthetic podophyllotoxin derivative	Single-strand DNA breaks from interaction with topoisomerase II.
Fluorouracil	Antimetabolite	Inhibition of enzyme thymidylate synthetase inhibiting DNA synthesis.
Methotrexate	Antimetabolite	Inhibition of dihydrofolate reductase. Inhibition of the formation of purines and DNA/RNA synthesis.
Mitomycin-C	Aziridine antibiotic	DNA alkylation and strand cross-linking.
Paclitaxel	Antimicrotubule agent	Binds to tubulin polymers (microtubules) with polymerization. Mitosis abnormal
Vincristine	Plant alkaloid	Mitotic spindle microtubule disrupted. Metaphase arrest.

plexity of interaction with the other biologic systems of the model does not provide a simple explanation for positive or negative outcomes.

The effect of a 60-Hz EMF was studied in a rat model of large granular lymphocytic leukemia. There was no significant or consistent differences detected between the EMF exposed group and the ambient control group. The data indicated that exposure to sinusoidal, linearly polarized 60-Hz, 1.0-mT magnetic fields did not significantly alter the clinical progression of this leukemia (29). Exposure to an SMF of ≥600 mT may lengthen the survival of leukemia-prone AKR mice (30).

Female C3H/Bi mice, which develop spontaneous viral mammary carcinoma metastasizing to lungs and other organs, were exposed to 12-, 100-, and 460-Hz fields or were used as nonexposed controls. Exposed mice had lighter spleens and lungs suggesting the possibility

Table 4 In Vivo Systems

Animal System	EMF	Chemotherapy	Effect	Reference
Mouse C3H/Bi	12, 100, 460 Hz/6 mT	—	Tumor weight in 460-Hz exposed animals <12 or 100 Hz	31
Mouse C3H-male	PEMF-average-induced E field = 2.5 mV	Cyclophosphamide	PEMF ↑ cytotoxicity of cyclophosphamide	35
MouseB6C3F1-female	SEF 450,000V/m SMF 110mT	Doxorubicin	↑ tumor regression SEF + doxorubicin, SMF + doxorubicin	36
Nude mouse implanted with A431 HT-29	See Table 1.	Carboplatin Cisplatin Doxorubicin	Smallest tumor volumes: A431:cisplatinum + PEMF HT-29:carboplatinum + PEMF, doxorubicin + PEMF	37
Nude mouse implanted with KB-CH^R-8-5-11 MDR cell line	See Table 1.	Daunorubicin	Tumor volumes smallest in PEMF + daunorubicin	26
WKA rats im planted with fibrosarcoma and hepatocellular carcinoma	200 Hz/4 mT/ 2.0 ms	Mitomycin-C	Best response both cell types: PEMF + Mitomycin	38
Mouse Balb/c; C3H;C57/bl/6 male and female	0.8 Hz/100 mT/ square wave	—	Significant ↓ tumor size and ↑ survival in exposed groups	32
Nude mouse with colon adenocarci-noma cell line	SMF = 3 mT ELF = 50 Hz/ 3 mT	—	Greatest inhibition with+ ELF	33
Mouse C3H, male	75 Hz/1.3 ms	Cyclophosphamide	Peripheral WBC ↓ more rapidly with cyclophosphamide + PEMF	34

that there were fewer metastases. The tumor mass was smaller for 460 Hz, unchanged for 100 Hz, and increased for 12 Hz (31).

Male and female mice were induced to develop tumors by injection of benzo(a)pyrene, and the animals were then exposed to a 100-mT, 0.8-Hz square wave field for 8 h/day. Exposure continued until death or until the tumor reached a predetermined volume. Exposure to this system resulted in a significant decrease in tumor growth and an increase in survival in all treatment groups (32).

A colon adenocarcinoma cell line was established in nude mouse model, and four treatment groups and one control group were created. The four treatment groups were exposed to an SMF of 3 mT and a EMF of 3 mT 50 Hz in varying combinations. The treatment group utilizing the combination of EMF and SMF showed the greatest tumor inhibition of all mouse model groups. The authors speculate that tumor inhibition may be due in part to an increase in cells showing apoptosis (33).

The hematopoietic system of mice provided a system for the study of the effect of a combination of PEMF and chemotherapy. Animals were given either cyclophosphamide or cyclophosphamide plus PEMF; the PEMF was continuous for the treatment time. Peripheral white blood cells, used as a marker of effect, decreased faster in the combined treatment group than in the cyclophosphamide group alone (34).

Another study measured the grafting efficiency of bone marrow cells after mice injected with cyclophosphamide were exposed to PEMF. The work demonstrated that PEMF augments the bone marrow cytotoxicity of cyclophosphamide because of the decrease in grafting efficiency. One mechanism suggested to explain the results is that the PEMF may have moved more cells into the cell cycle, increasing the number of cells affected by the cyclophosphamide (35).

Female B6C3F1 mice were used to study the effect of either an SMF of 110-mT or static electric field (SEF) of 450,000 V/m on the action of antineoplastic chemotherapy against transplanted mammary tumors. On day 7 of the study, four groups of mice were created and injected with doxorubicin; three groups were exposed animals and one was the control group. Statistically significant tumor regression was seen in two groups: one with doxorubicin plus SEF and one with doxorubicin and a nonuniform SMF (36).

Because the immune system is part of the response (or lack of response) to malignant cells, one exposure study used a known PEMF in a system of immune-deficient mice with transplanted A431 and HT-29 cells. The animals were treated with the chemotherapy agents cisplatin, carboplatin, and daunomycin and a 1-h treatment of the PEMF versus control. In measuring the results of the exposure, the tumors with smallest volume were those in the drug-plus-PEMF group. For the A431 tumors, the cisplatin-plus-PEMF group tumor volume was significantly smaller than for the group that received cisplatin alone. In HT-29 tumors, those treated with carboplatin plus PEMF had the smallest tumor volume compared to the carboplatin alone. The doxorubicin-plus-PEMF group showed a smaller volume than the doxorubicin alone (37).

A PEMF, previously described by Sabo et al. (16), was used in the treatment of mice injected with a human carcinoma cell line. Four groups of animals were treated. One of the groups was given daunorubicin plus PEMF while other groups served as controls. Measured tumor volumes in the PEMF-plus-daunorubicin group were smaller than all other groups (26).

Two cell lines, fibrosarcoma and hepatocellular carcinoma, were implanted into WKA rats and exposed to a 200-Hz, 4.0-mT field with and without the antineoplastic agent mitomycin-C. The best responses for both cell types was with the PEMF-plus-mitomycin groups (38).

IV. OTHER STUDIES

Magnetic fields can concentrate chemotherapy modified to be influenced by the magnetic field into a target area. In one study, an external inhomogeneous magnetic field with a magnetic flux density of 1.7 T was used to concentrate chemotherapy within a squamous cell carcinoma implanted into the hind limb of rabbit. Mitoxantrone was attached to ferrofluids and given either as intravenous or intra-arterial injection. Tumors treated with magnetic field plus intra-arterial injection showed a significant remission. Ferrofluids were seen to accumulate within tumors both by histologic examination and by MRI (10).

The stability and positioning of magnetoliposomes for magnetic drug targeting was tested by labeling particles of human serum albumin encapsulated together with phosphatidyl choline/cholesterol liposomes with Technetium-99m. To study in vivo targeting a permanent magnet of approximately 0.35 T was placed near the right kidney. The relative radioactivity of right kidney was $25.92 \pm 5.84\%$ compared to the the left, which was $0.93 \pm 0.05\%$ (11). Doxorubicin has been incorporated into magnetic liposomes and theses particles then injected intravenously into a hamster osteosarcoma model. In this work, the magnetic field was generated by implanting a magnet within the tumor itself as opposed to applying an external field. This resulted in significantly greater antitumor activity in the tumors implanted with a magnet compared to a nonmagnetic control (12).

Alternating magnetic fields have been used to initiate heating in ferromagnetic particles that have been embolized into tumors and exposed to an alternating magnetic field. This then allows the ferromagnetic particles to generate hyperthermic temperatures within the tumor (39).

V. HUMAN STUDY WITH STATIC MAGNETIC FIELD AND CHEMOTHERAPY

One of us (Joseph R. Salvatore) has initiated a Phase I clinical study using a static magnetic field as an adjuvant to antineoplastic chemotherapy used to treat in patients with advanced malignant disease (40,41). Phase I clinical studies are designed to test the safety and establish a toxicity profile of the treatment under study but do not test the efficacy of the treatment. The static magnetic field, averaging 15 mT, was generated by a permanent magnet placed on the patient 15 min prior to and during the time of the chemotherapy infusion. In this pilot study of 10 patients, the data collected was a group of graded toxicity events defined by the Common Toxicity Criteria of the National Cancer Institute, and compared to the graded toxicity events of 10 historical matched treated controls. The event data were for blood tests (hematology and chemistry) and symptoms (gastrointestinal). Results from this work suggest that the static magnetic field plus antineoplastic chemotherapy is safe, and the toxicity profile is acceptable compared to patients receiving chemotherapy without the magnetic field. Further study is needed to definitively establish the safety of this static magnetic field as an adjuvant to chemotherapy in cancer patients, after which studies of efficacy can be conducted.

VI. SUMMARY

The treatment of human malignant disease has evolved from the application of single modality therapy to the complexity of multiple therapies applied simultaneously or sequentially. Researchers using electromagnetic fields have investigated applying these fields for the treatment of malignant disease either alone as an adjuvant therapy to antineoplastic chemotherapy. Possible mechanisms for the effects seen range from a direct interaction with nuclear DNA to interaction with cell membrane structures and receptors. The data from cell and in vivo research on the effects of these fields on malignant cells and tumors as either solo therapy or as an adjuvant therapy to antineoplastic chemotherapy allows us to conclude that these effects are potentially applicable to the treatment of human cancer, although not all data supports a usable effect.

The goal of any cancer therapy should be to obtain the best possible treatment outcome with the least adverse outcome, and electromagnetic fields in the forms reviewed show the potential to augment the effectiveness of chemotherapy against malignancy, but at this point it is not possible to say whether there would be a decrease in the adverse events produced by antineoplastic chemotherapy. Future studies need to address which electromagnetic fields are the most efficacious as an adjuvant to antineoplastic chemotherapy as well as whether these agents, if able to improve neoplastic cell kill, can also help to reduce the adverse events that come with antineoplastic chemotherapy.

REFERENCES

1. Nordenstrom BEW. Biologically Closed Electric Circuits. Stockholm: Nordic Medical Publications, 1983.
2. Nordenstrom BEW. Electrochemical treatment of cancer. I: Variable response to anodic and cathodic fields. Am J Clin Onc 1989; 12:530–536.
3. Xin Y, Xue F, Ge B, Zhao F, Shi B, Zhang W. Electrochemical treatment of lung cancer. BEMS 1997; 18:8–13.
4. Mir L, Orlowski S, Belehradek J, Paoletti C. Electrochemotherapy potentiation of antitumor effect of Bleomycin by local electric pulses. Eur J Can 1991; 27:68–72.
5. Szent-Gyorgi A. Chemical and biological effects of ultra-sonic radiation. Nature 1933; 131:278.
6. Payne-Scott R, Love WH. Tissue cultures exposed to the influence of a magnetic field. Nature 1936; 134:277.
7. Lenzi M. A report of a few recent experiments on the biologic effects of magnetic fields. Radiology 1940; 35:307–314.
8. Levengood W. Cytogenetic variations induced with a magnetic probe. Nature 1966; 209:1009–1013.
9. Weber T, Cerilli J. Inhibition of tumor growth by the use of non-homogeneous magnetic fields. Cancer 1971; 28:340–343.
10. Alexiou C, Arnold W, Klein R, Parak F, Hulin P, Bergemann C, Erhardt W, Wagenpfeil S, Lubbe A. Locoregional cancer treatment with magnetic drug targeting. Can Res 2000; 60:6641–6648.
11. Babincova M, Altanerova V, Lampert M, Altaner C, Machova E, Sramka M, Babinec P. Site-specific in vivo targeting of magnetoliposomes using externally applied magnetic field. Z Naturforsch 2000; 55c:278–281.
12. Kubo T, Sugita T, Shimose S, Nitta Y, Ikuta Y, Murakami T. Targeted systemic chemotherapy using magnetic liposomes with incorporated adriamycin for osteosarcoma in hamsters. Int J Onc 2001; 18:121–125.
13. Petrini M, Matii L, Sabbatini A, Carulli G, Grassi B, Cadossi R, Ronca G, Conte A. Multidrug resistance and electromagnetic fields. J Bioelectric 1990; 9:209–212.
14. Williams C, Markov M. Therapeutic electromagnetic field effects on angiogenesis during tumor growth: A pilot study in mice. Electro Magnetobiol 2001; 20:323–329.
15. Williams C, Markov M, Hardman W, Cameron I. Therapeutic electromagnetic field effects on angiogenesis and tumor growth. Antican Res 2001; 21:3887–3892.
16. Sabo J, Mirossay L, Horovcak L, Sarissky M, Mirossay A, Mojzis J. Effects of static magnetic field on human leukemic cell line HL-60. Bioelectrochemistry 2002; 56:227–231.

17. Ruiz Gomez M, Vega J, de la Pena L, Gil Carmona L, Morillo M. Growth modification of human colon adenocarcinoma cells exposed to a low-frequency electromagnetic field. J Physiol Biochem 1999; 55:79–84.
18. Tuffet S, deSeze R, Moreau J, Veyret B. Effects of a strong pulsed magnetic field on the proliferation of tumour cells in vitro. Bioelectrochem Bioenerget 1993; 30:151–160.
19. Johann S, Lederer, Mikorey S, Kraus W, Blumel G. Influence of electromagnetic fields on morphology and mitochondrial activity of breast cancer cell line MCF-7. Bioelectrochem Bioenerget 1993; 30:127–132.
20. de Mattei M, Caruso A, Traina G, Pezzetti F, Baroni T, Sollazzo V. Correlation between pulsed electromagnetic fields exposure time and cell proliferation increase in human osteosarcoma cell lines and human normal osteoblast cells in vitro. BEMS 1999; 20:177–182.
21. Raylman R, Clavo A, Wahl R. Exposure to strong magnetic field slows the growth of human cancer cells in vitro. BEMS 1996; 17:358–363.
22. Watson J, Parrish E, Rinehart C. Selective potentiation of gynecologic cancer cell growth in vitro by electromagnetic fields. Gyn Oncol 1998; 71:64–71.
23. Salvatore J, Blackinton D, Polk C, Mehta S. Non-ionizing electromagnetic radiation: a study of carcinogenic and cancer treatment potential. Reviews on Env Health 1994; 10:197–207.
24. Hannan C, Liang Y, Allison J, Searle J. In Vitro cytotoxicity against human cancer cell lines during pulsed magnetic field exposure. Antican Res 1994; 14:1517–1520.
25. Hirata M, Kusuzaki K, Takeshita H, Hashiguchi S, Hirasawa Y, Ashihara T. Drug resistance modification using pulsing electromagnetic field stimulation for multidrug resistant mouse osteosarcoma cell line. Antican Res 2001; 21:317–320.
26. Liang Y, Hannan C, Chang B, Schoenlein P. Enhanced potency of Daunorubicin against multidrug resistant subline KB-Ch^R-8-5-11 by a pulsed magnetic field. Antican Res 1997; 17:2083–2088.
27. Miyagi N, Sato K, Rong Y, Yamamura S, Katagiri H, Kobayashi K, Iwata H. Effects of PEMF on a murine osteosarcoma cell line: Drug resistant (P-Glycoprotein-positive) and non-resistant cells. BEMS 2000; 21:112–121.
28. Fanelli C, Coppola S, Barone R, Colussi C, Gualandi G, Volpe P, Ghibelli L. Magnetic fields increase cell survival by inhibiting apoptosis via modulation of Ca^{2+} influx. FASEB J 1999; 13:95–102.
29. Morris J, Sasser L, Miller D, Dagle G, Rafferty C, Ebi K, Anderson L. Clinical progression of transplanted large granular lymphocytic leukemia in Fischer 344 rats exposed to 60 Hz magnetic fields. BEMS 1999; 20:48–56.
30. Bellossi A. Effect of static magnetic field on survival of leukemia-prone AKR mice. Rad Env Biophys 1986; 25:75–80.
31. Bellossi A, Desplaces A, Morin R. Effect of a pulsed magnetic field on tumoral C3H/Bi female mice. Can Biochem Biophys 1988; 10:59–66.
32. de Seze R, Tuffet S, Moreau J, Veyret B. Effects of 100 mT time varying magnetic fields on the growth of tumors in mice. BEMS 2000; 21:107–111.
33. Tofani S, Barone D, Cintorino M, de Santi M, Ferrara A, Orlassino R, Ossola P, Peroglio F, Rolfo K, Ronchetto F. Static and ELF magnetic fields induce tumor growth inhibition and apoptosis. BEMS 2001; 22:419–428.
34. Zucchini P, Cadossi R, Emilia G, Torelli G, Santantonio M, Mandolini G. Effect of pemf on mice injected with cyclophosphamide. In: Brighton C, Pollack S, eds. Electromagnetics in Biology and Medicine. San Francisco: SF Press, 1991:207–209.
35. Cadossi R, Zucchini P, Emilia G, Franceschi C, Cossarizza A, Santantonio M, Mandolini G, Torelli G. Effect of low frequency low energy pulsing electromagnetic fields on mice injected with Cyclophosphamide. Exp Hem 1991; 19:196–201.
36. Gray J, Frith C, Parker J. In vivo enhancement of chemotherapy with static electric or magnetic fields. BEMS 2000; 21:575–583.
37. Hannan C, Liang Y, Allison J, Pantazis C, Searle J. Chemotherapy of human carcinoma xenografts during pulsed magnetic field exposure. Antican Res 1994; 14:1521–1522.

38. Omote Y, Hosokawa M, Komatsumoto M, Namieno T, Nakajima S, Kubo Y, Kobayashi H. Treatment of experimental tumors with a combination of a pulsing magnetic field and an antitumor drug. Japan J Can Res 1990; 81:956–961.
39. Moroz P, Jones SK, Gray BN. The effect of tumor size on ferromagnetic embolization hyperthermia in a rabbit liver tumor model. Int J Hyperthermia 2002; 18:129–140.
40. Salvatore JR. Static magnetic fields in the treatment of human malignancy. Abstract #10-2. Bioelectromagnetics Society Annual Meeting. June 23–27, 2002. Quebec, Canada.
41. Salvatore JR, Harrington J, Kummet T. Phase I clinical study of a static magnetic field combined with anti-neoplastic chemotherapy in the treatment of human malignancy: initial safety and toxicity data. BEMS 2003; 24:524–527.

39

Can Magnetic Fields Inhibit Angiogenesis and Tumor Growth?

Marko S. Markov* and Calvin D. Williams
EMF Therapeutics, Inc., Chattanooga, Tennessee, U.S.A.

Ivan L. Cameron
University of Texas Health Science Center, San Antonio, Texas, U.S.A.

W. Elaine Hardman
Pennington Biomedical Research Center, Louisiana State University, Baton Rouge, Los Angeles, U.S.A.

Joseph R. Salvatore
Carl T. Hayden VA Medical Center, Phoenix, Arizona, U.S.A.

At the time when media and general public raise concern about possible role of EMF in initiation of cancer, this interlaboratory team investigated the possibility of a selected magnetic field to inhibit angiogenesis. Using a proprietary magnetic field signal, authors demonstrate that this modality is capable of preventing formation of new blood vessels from existing tumor vasculature. The potential of magnetic field to not only inhibit angiogenesis, but also reduce tumor growth in animal models should attract interest of main stream medicine since more than 20 different pharmaceutical agents are in clinical trials, but there is not reported success. Moreover, while pharmaceutics may cause adverse effects, magnetic field therapy is free of such hazard.

It is now well established that angiogenesis is an important component in the progression and healing of various diseases, including tumor development. *Angiogenesis* is defined as the process of formation and differentiation of vasculature in which cells induce the growth of new blood vessels from adjacent endothelial cells in order to supply vital

---

**Current affliation*: Research International, Buffalo, New York, U.S.A.

components for cell functioning and to remove toxic products of metabolism. Today this term is widely used to discriminate from *vasculogenesis*, the process of formation of the primordia of blood vessels in the embryo.

Angiogenesis occurs as a normal physiological process during periods of tissue growth, such as embryonic development, any increase in muscle or fat, during the menstrual cycle and during pregnancy. During embryonic life, angiogenesis serves to supplement vasculogenesis, while in postnatal life it is physiological and is related to both normal and pathological conditions.

Angiogenesis is a key factor in the maintenance and progression of several disease states. It may occur either as a natural response to the underlying disease (as in inflammation, wound healing and rheumatoid arthritis) or as a contributing factor to disease progression (as in tumor growth). While angiogenesis is beneficial in wound healing, it is harmful when associated with certain pathologies, particularly cancer, diabetic neuropathy and macular degeneration.

The mechanisms leading to acquisition of the angiogenic phenotype are only partially known and involve complex biochemical, molecular, genetic, and celllular mechanisms. Normally, angiogenesis is a very tightly regulated process which is physiologically controlled through a balance of angio-inhibitory and pro-angiogenic factors.

Some authors consider that angiogenesis requires eight steps (1):

1. Release of proteases from "activated" endothelial cells
2. Degradation of the basement membrane surrounding the existing vessels
3. Migration of endothelial cells into the interstitial space
4. Endothelial cell proliferation
5. Lumen formation
6. Generation of new basement membrane with recruitment of pericytes
7. Fusion of the newly formed vessels
8. Initiation of blood flow

For example, during wound healing these factors allow rapid endothelial cell proliferation, migration, and differentiation (2,3). Imbalance between pro- and antiangiogenic factors has been established for many pathological conditions including diabetic retinopathy (4), rheumatoid arthritis (5), endometriosis (6), and malignant tumors (4).

Growth of the primary tumor, and particularly its metastatic dissemination, is dependent on the tumor's supply of blood vessels. Tumor vasculature usually occurs as extension from the pre-existing network of host vasculature. A neoplastic mass cannot grow beyond a few millimeters in diameter without recruiting new vessels (7–10). In order for tumor to grow, become invasive, and ultimately metastatic, it must firstly induce a blood supply network to support its expansion. The invading blood vessels insinuate into tumor parenchyma, providing nutrition, ions, and oxygen for tumor cell survival. The growing number of capillaries secrete degradative enzymes which digest the extracellular matrix enabling the vascular tubes to "burrow" through the tissues (1).

Additionally, the newly formed blood vessels provide a route for metastatic tumor cells to enter the systemic circulation. The loosening of connective tissue facilitates the movement of tumor cells from the tumor mass into the systemic circulation by infiltrating into immature microvessels (11–15).

The switch to the angiogenic phenotype represents one of the most important tumor progression mechanisms (16) enabling the growth of the primary tumor beyond a critical volume, allowing nutrient supply, and providing metastatic cells with access to the circulatory system. The dependence of tumor growth and metastasis on the growth of new blood vessels has in turn led to the hypothesis that the density of tumor vasculature may reflect its degree of malignancy (17).

Several lines of direct evidence show that angiogenesis is essential for the growth and persistence of solid tumors and their metastases (18–20). In order to determine whether angiogenesis is related to tumor growth, it was first necessary to devise a method to identify and count the microvessels within a tumor. Although some early studies used morphological criteria to identify vessels in histological sections of tumors, only immunochemical methods provide accurate methods for evaluating tissue angiogenesis. Angiogenesis is generally assessed by methods that utilize anti-Factor-VIII antibody, anti-CD-34, anti-CD31, and PAL-E as the primary antibodies (8). An international consensus on the methodology and criteria of evaluation of microvessel density proposed that anti-CD31 monoclonal antibody immunostaining should be the standard for microvessel assessment (9).

Neo-angiogenesis is critical for tumor growth and metastasis and has been proposed as an independent prognostic factor for survival in patients with solid tumors (7). Tumor angiogenesis is characterized by a 30- to 40-fold increase in proliferative activity of endothelial cells (12).

I. ANTIANGIOGENIC THERAPIES

Antiangiogenic therapy is a relatively novel approach to the treatment of solid tumors, macular degeneration, diabetic retinopathy, psoriasis, and other diseases. Since tumor angiogenesis is a fundamental step in tumor growth and metastasis (21), any method that inhibits the formation and development of a blood vessel network in tumor tissue may lead to the reduction or stopping of tumor growth.

Antiangiogenesis was proposed as a cancer therapy more than 30 years ago by Folkman (10) and is currently an exciting target for anticancer drug development. Antiangiogenic compounds have demonstrated success in preclinical models and new agents are rapidly entering preclinical and clinical trials. These compounds are designed to inhibit tumor angiogenesis and thereby to limit blood flow and the delivery of ions, nutrients, and oxygen supply to the tumor.

The effect of antiangiogenic therapy may be seen in decreased tumor growth rate that is associated with a decreased tumor volume. This apparently is due to vascular insufficiency in large tumors or/and insufficient development of the blood-vessel network. Therefore, cells located distal to the vasculature are poorly oxygenated and may find themselves in an acidic environment so that they are not cycling. Results of several studies indicated that growth factors that control tumor growth are different from those involved in endothelial cell growth. Therefore, tumor cell proliferation and microvessel growth and/or density may be regulated by different mechanisms (15). Studies of tumor cell proliferation kinetics have indicated that the growth fraction decreases with increasing distance from the blood vessel (14).

At least 20 antiangiogenic drugs are in various stages of human trials, with many more in early stages of development. Two antiangiogenic proteins, angiostatin and endostatin, have been recently proven to have an important role in reducing angiogenesis and therefore preventing metastasis in a series of animal models (3–5).

Angiostatin, generated by the primary tumor, was shown to potentially inhibit angiogenesis (6,22). Systemic therapy with angiostatin, on the other hand, led to maintenance of metastases in a microscopic dormant state defined by a balance of apoptosis and proliferation of the tumor cells (22,23).

However, despite the promising results in animal studies, the first attempts to use some suggested antiangiogenic drugs in humans appear to be not very successful. One possible reason may be that the human organism is more complex than a rodent.

II. MAGNETIC FIELDS AS POSSIBLE ANTI-ANGIOGENIC THERAPY

There have been some attempts to use various magnetic fields as a adjuvant therapeutic agent in the treatment of various tumors. Because a previous chapter in this book (Salvatore and Markov) discusses the research on use of magnetic fields to treat tumors, we will not review this section of the literature. However, we should note that no studies were found in the available literature on the use of magnetic fields to reduce angiogenesis.

Therefore we designed an approach to investigate the potential of pulsating electromagnetic fields to inhibit angiogenesis in solid tumors.

ANIMALS.   Fifty female mice C3H/HeJ mice, approximately 6 weeks old, were obtained from the Frederick Cancer Research and Development Center of the National Cancer Institute (Frederick, MD). Animal care and handling were performed at Southern Research Institute (Birmingham, AL). Mice were housed in plastic microisolator cages with sterile hardwood bedding and had free access to a standard laboratory diet and filtered tap water. Mice were weighed on the day of tumor implantation, on days 8, 10, 14, and 17 after tumor implantation and at sacrifice. Air temperature and relative humidity in the animal rooms were controlled at $24 \pm 1\,^\circ C$ and $50 \pm 10\%$, respectively. Lights were operated on automatic 12-h light–dark cycles. The ambient magnetic field in the exposure chamber was below 50 μT.

IMPLANTATION OF TUMORS.   The murine 16/C mammary adenocarcinoma cells obtained from the National Cancer Institute collection were implanted subcutaneously in C3H/HeJ mice and the resulting tumor was maintained by routine passages *in vivo* in mice prior to implantation (24). Tumors were implanted via a single subcutaneous injection in the medial left torso (25) of 30 mg of tumor fragments derived from a primitive tumor (26). All implanted tumor fragments were obtained from passage 5 of the adenocarcinoma cell line. The animals were randomized between control (20 animals) and three treatment groups (10 animals per group) after the tumors reached palpable size.

MAGNETIC FIELD DEVICE.   A therapeutic electromagnetic field (TEMF) system having a proprietary signal designed by EMF Therapeutics, Inc. (Chattanooga, TN) was used. The system generates a pulsating half sine wave magnetic field with a frequency of 120 pulses per second (Fig. 1). An ellipsoidal coil with 21-inch large diameter and 14-inch small diameter delivers the signal to the target. In the experiment reported here, three different by magnetic flux density (10 mT, 15 mT, or 20 mT) conditions were created in the exposure chamber. These values of magnetic field flux density were chosen to investigate the dose-response dependence based upon our previous experience and literature data that suggest the existence of a biological window at 15–20 mT magnetic flux density (27,28). A thorough 3-D mapping of the magnetic field was performed for the entire space covered by the coil. The flux density of the magnetic field in the exposure chamber (25 cm long, 10 cm wide and 13 cm high) was consistent within the entire volume of the chamber. The perforation of the walls of the exposure chamber allows air exchange between the exposure chamber and environment. The temperature change inside the exposure chamber during the TEMF treatment did not exceed $1\,^\circ C$, and this change was likely a result of body heat emitted by the mice.

TREATMENT WITH MAGNETIC FIELD.   Treatment of animals started after the tumor volume reached approximately 100 mm^3 (evaluated by caliper and calculated by the

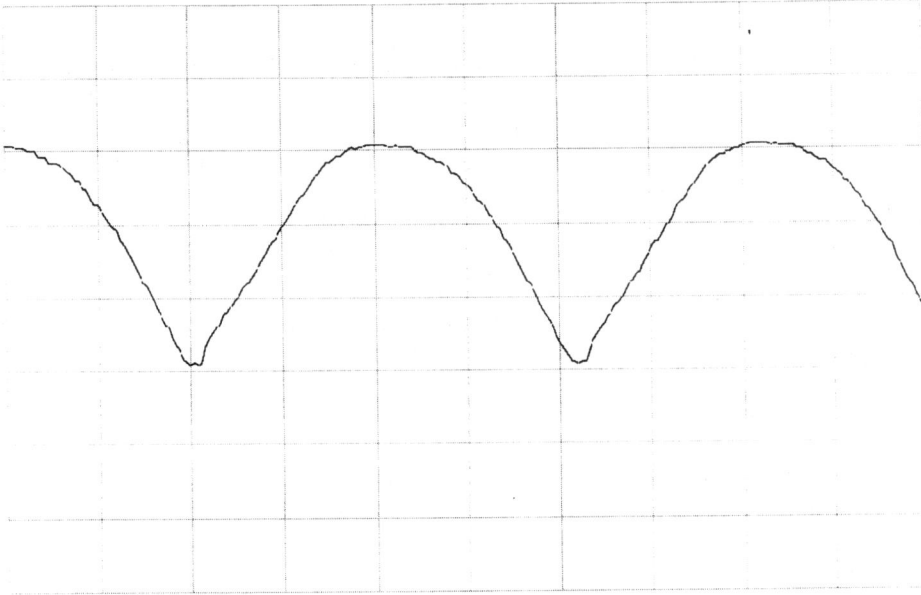

Figure 1 Wave shape of the rectified 60-Hz signal transferred to 120 pulses per second pulsating magnetic field.

standard formula discussed elsewhere) at day 7 after the tumor was implanted. Animals received magnetic field treatment for 10 minutes daily over 12 consecutive days.

TUMOR GROWTH. The tumor volume was calculated by the standard procedure using the formula $V = (AB^2)/2$, where A is the longer diameter and B is the smaller diameter of the tumor. The same formula for tumor volume was used in a recent publication of De Seze et al. (26). The length and width of each tumor was measured with calipers on days 8, 10, 14, 17, and 20 after implantation.

IMMUNOHISTOCHEMISTRY. The effect of TEMF on angiogenesis was evaluated by the expression of CD31. As shown earlier, an international consensus suggest staining with anti-CD31 monoclonal antibody as a standard for evaluation of microvessel density (8). CD31 (platelet endothelial cell adhesion molecule, PECAM-1) is a 130 kDa integral membrane protein that mediates cell-to-cell adhesion and is expressed at the surface of endothelial cells. The tumor sections for CD31 immunohistochemistry were prepared and stained for CD31 at Southern Research Institute, Birmingham, AL (24,25,27). Morphometric analyses for the percent of CD31 viable and necrotic areas were performed on a subset of tumors randomly sampled from the control group and each treatment group. The cryosectioned tumors previously stained for CD31 reactivity were analyzed using phase contrast microscopy to differentiate necrotic, viable, and CD31 stained regions of each tumor. Grid intercept point counting was used to estimate the fraction of an area covered by necrotic, viable, or CD31 positive areas.

STATISTICAL ANALYSES. Differences between groups in mean tumor size at each time point and body weights were evaluated by analyses of variance (ANOVA) followed by a Student-Newman-Kuels (SNK) multiple range test. Fisher's Exact test was used to compare mortality proportions of the groups. Linear regression analysis was used to compare the relationship of vascular (CD31 positive) area to the necrotic fraction in the tumors.

III. RESULTS

The mean body weight of each group before beginning TEMF treatment (day 8) and following TEMF treatment shows that TEMF exposure did not affect the body mass of the mice. All mice in all groups were alive on the 17th day after tumor implantation.

Figure 2 is a graph of the mean tumor size of each group for the first 17 days of the experiment (10 treatment days). The tumor growth curves begin to diverge as early as 2 days after the first TEMF treatment. Following 10 days of TEMF treatment, the control group mice had significantly larger tumors than the TEMF treated mice.

Figure 3 shows that TEMF exposure leads to a significant decrease in the tumor growth estimated by the tumor volume. As is seen on Fig. 4 similar inhibition was found based upon the percent of tumor area stained positive for CD 31. All applied TEMF significantly reduced the percentage of CD31 staining. The percentage of CD31 staining decreased statistically significantly from $7.56 \pm 3.35\%$ in the control group to $4.60 \pm 2.20\%$ in the 10 mT group, to $2.42 \pm 1.13\%$ in the 15-mT group and to $2.86 \pm 1.06\%$ in the 20-mT group. The statistical analysis indicates that the decrease in CD31 staining was statistically significant for all treatment groups when compared to control ($p < 0.001$). Interestingly enough, the difference between the group exposed to 10 mT and the other two experimental groups (15 mT and 20 mT) is also in the range of statistical significance ($p < 0.001$), while there is not a statistically significant difference between the groups exposed to 15 mT and 20 mT ($p < 0.1$). This fact may be considered as an indication that the hypothesis of "biological windows" may be applied to these results (25,32).

The effect of TEMF treatment as measured by changes in CD31 staining expressed as a percent ratio of mean values of CD31 staining in the TEMF treated groups vs. mean values in the control group shows a significant decrease (39% for the group exposed to a 10-mT TEMF, 68 % for the group exposed to 15-mT TEMF and 62% for the group exposed to 20-mT TEMF).

The use of CD31 as a specific marker for blood vessels was confirmed by comparison of bright field with phase contrast microscopy. Phase contrast microscopy of the tumor tissue revealed that viable, necrotic, and CD 31 positive areas could be easily differentiated. We

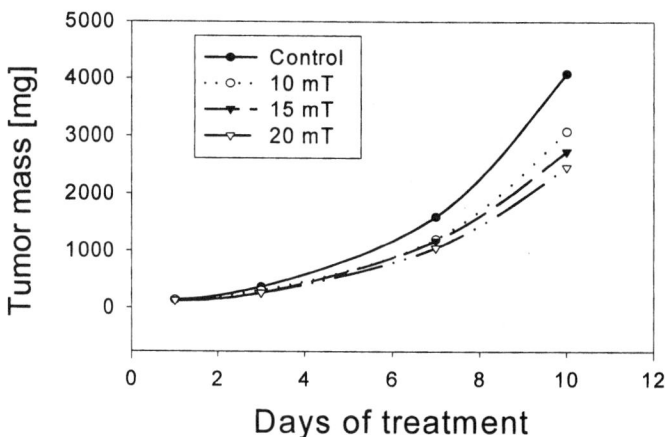

Figure 2 Dynamics of volume changes (Mean $\pm$ SEM) in cubic millimeters of murine 16/C breast adenocarcinoma in control group and in groups of mice exposed for 10 min/day for 10 days to 10 mT, 15 mT, and 20 mT TEMF.

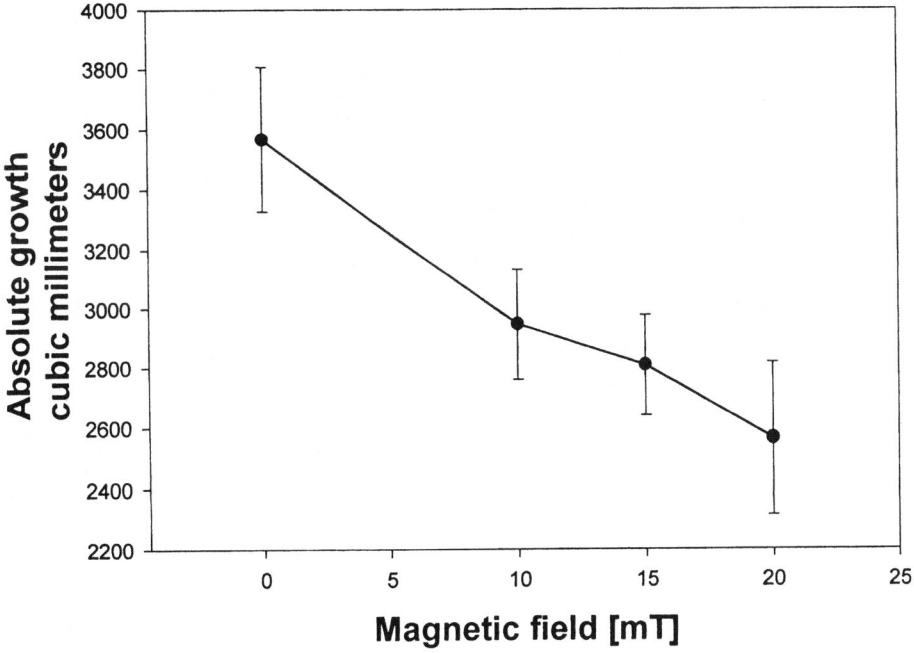

Figure 3 Inhibition of tumor growth as result of 10 days treatment with TEMF. The values represent mean ± standard deviation.

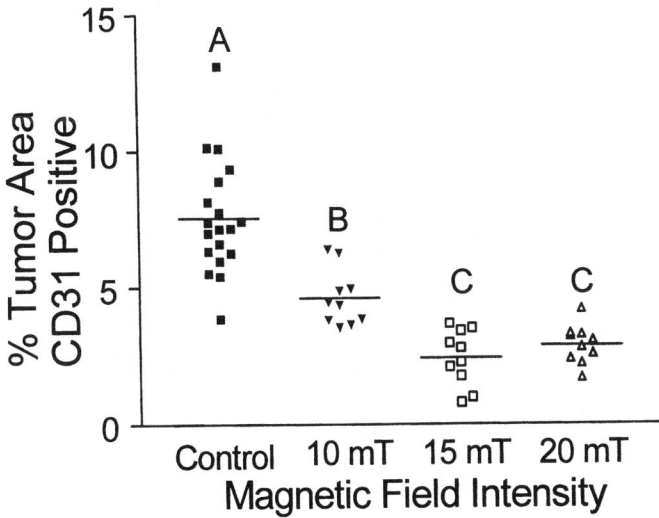

Figure 4 The scattergram of mean CD31-positive area of each tumor for control and EMF-treated groups.

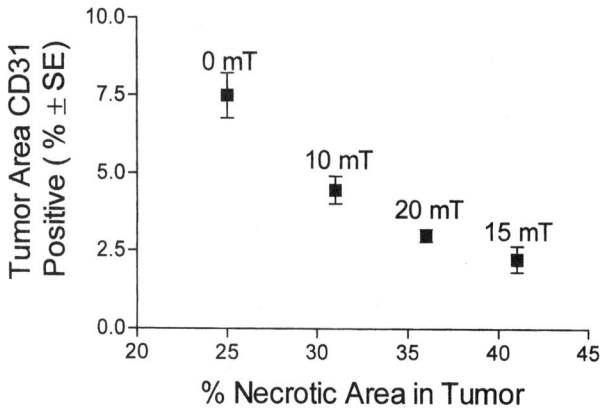

Figure 5 Inverse relationship between the percent of vascular area (CD31 positive) and the percent of necrotic area in mid section of the 16/C murine mammary adenocarcinoma. Linear regression analysis revealed a significant inverse correlation between vascular area and necrosis.

have shown (25) that the TEMF treatments significantly decreased the vascular density of the tumor and increased the volume density of necrotic tissue in the tumors. Figure 5 illustrates the significant inverse correlation between vascular area (CD31 positive) and the necrotic area in the tumors. The largest is the effect for the group of animals that received 15-mT treatment.

In parallel, the data for tumor growth, shown on Figs. 3 and 6 demonstrate a significant reduction in both tumor volume and doublings as a function of the amplitude of the applied magnetic field. Taken together, these results indicate that the TEMF treatment significantly suppressed tumor growth. The significant suppression of tumor growth is likely related to the significant reduction of tumor vasculature and the increase in necrotic tumor tissue.

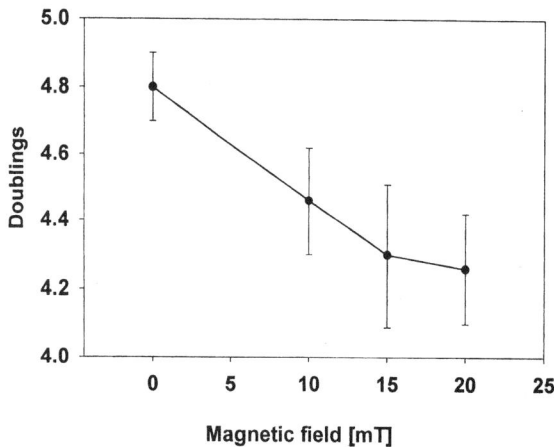

Figure 6 Calculated doublings for 10 days period of treatment of tumors with TEMF. The values represent mean ± standard deviation.

IV. DISCUSSION

It has been shown that the CD31 staining method is based on the densitometric analysis of the percentages of immunostained areas related to total area of interest (28,29). In normal tissues a strong and homogeneous expression of PECAM-1 can be observed exclusively on endothelial cells of glomerular and perturbed capillaries and large vessels (30). Therefore, the diminished percentage of CD31 staining demonstrated in Fig. 4 should be interpreted as a reduction in the number of blood vessels in the tumor area.

The results showing inhibition of angiogenesis and reduction of tumor growth lead to several important observations:

    (i)   TEMFs statistically significantly inhibit both angiogenesis and tumor growth.

   (ii)   The largest changes were observed for the group exposed to 15-mT TEMF(with respect to inhibition of angiogenesis) and for the group exposed to 20-mT TEMF (with respect to tumor growth).

  (iii)   Since the differences between results for both angiogenesis and tumor growth in the 15-mT and 20-mT groups did not show statistical significance, this study supports the hypothesis that a biological window of efficacy exists within the range of 15–20 mT magnetic field amplitude.

It appears that the inhibition of angiogenesis leads to a reduction in tumor growth. One possible reason for this may be found in the suppressed development of the blood-vessel network which in turn leads to a deficiency in supplying tumor cells with oxygen, ions and nutrients. It is known that cells must be located within about 150 μm of a blood vessel for diffusion to adequately meet the oxygen and nutrient requirements for cell viability. Thus, growth and viability of the tumor strongly depends on angiogenesis. This is supported by the observed increase in necrotic tissue in tumors from all animals in the treated groups.

The use of CD31 as a specific marker for blood vessels was confirmed by comparison of bright field with phase contrast microscopy. Observation of the tumor sections by phase contrast microscopy revealed that viable tumor cells were found adjacent to the blood vessels, while tissues at distances greater than 75–150 μm from any blood vessel were necrotic.

The grid intercept method data establishes a relationship between the fraction of CD31 positive area and necrotic fraction. The results were graphed and analyzed by nonlinear regression analysis. A statistically significant ($p < 0.001$) relationship between the fraction of necrotic tissue and the fraction of vascular tissue was found: the area of necrosis decreases logarithmically as the vascular area increases. This negative relationship (i.e., when CD31 was larger, the necrotic area was smaller) was confirmed by the analyses of variance, which revealed a significant difference between the necrotic volume in the control samples and samples from animals exposed to TEMF.

The results suggest that therapeutic effects may be achieved by an appropriate selection of the physical parameters of the applied magnetic fields. It has been shown that it is more appropriate to consider biological response to magnetic fields through the hypothesis of biological windows instead of dose-response dependence. The results shown in this study confirm reports of an amplitude window in the range of 15–20 mT.

The biological response likely depends not only on the amplitude of the applied magnetic field but on some other physical characteristics, such as waveform, frequency, repetition rate, presence or absence of the electric field component, etc. (32).

Even though encouraging, the results of TEMF use for treatment of solid tumors do not suggest a mechanism which could explain the antiangiogenic effect of the TEMF in this tumor model. There are a number of stages and players in the whole machinery of tumor growth that are potential candidates as targets of magnetic field action. Usually, as tumor cells proliferate into the host tissue, tumor angiogenesis leads to the formation of a new tumor vasculature. Tumor microcirculation originates from the normal host vasculature, but the tumor vessels are more dilated, sacular, and tortuous. Furthermore, tumor vasculature has wider intercellular junctions. The extravasion of blood-borne molecules that have reached the tumor vasculature is governed by diffusion and convection (31). The control mechanism underlying the angiogenesis stimulus involves complex interactions between many cell types such as fibroblasts, endothelial cells, growth factors, extracellular matrix enzymes, and cytokines. TEMF may modify the ability of those molecules to move within the tumor tissue.

We discussed elsewhere that the supressed vascularization of the tumor and slowed tumor growth did not lead to regression in TEMF-treated tumors. Folkman et al. (33) make the point that the genome of cancer cells is often too unstable to serve as a fixed therapeutic target. At present there are multiple reports and ongoing studies on the use of antiangiogenic chemotherapy for treatment of cancerous tumors.

The first results on studying the potential of TEMF to treat solid tumors allow us to conclude that a pulsating magnetic field (120 pps) may inhibit the formation of a blood-vessel network in a growing tumor. The suppression of the blood-vessel network is probably the main cause of necrotization of the tumor interior and the reduction of tumor growth rate. Whether this effect is repeatable and valid for all types of tumors and whether the treatment regimen applied to experimental animals will be effective in human tumors remains to be seen.

The findings from TEMF studies add TEMF as a simple, safe and noninvasive physical antiangiogenic method for tumor therapy that warrants further investigation of the combined action of chemotherapy, radiotherapy, and TEMF therapy.

Several studies have indicated a synergistic effect between magnetic fields and commonly used chemotherapeutic agents (34–37). We are pursuing further studies to explore the combined action of TEMF and cytostatic agents. Different tumor models and exposure conditions are under investigation. We are also investigating whether the hypothesis of biological windows is applicable to the observed antiangiogenic effects and tumor growth.

[*Note:* Sects. I, III, and IV were partially published in Anticancer Research v. 21 (2001) (see ref. 25).]

REFERENCES

1. Leek RD. The prognostic role of angiogenesis in breast cancer. Anticancer Res 2001; 21:4325–4332.
2. Mc Namara DA, Harmey JH, Walsh TN, Redmond HP, Bouchier HD. Significance of angiogenesis in cancer therapy. Brit J Surg 1998; 85(8):1044–1055.
3. Folkman J, Shing Y. Angiogenesis. J Biol Chem 1992; 267(16):10931–10934.
4. Murata J, Ishibashi T, Khalil A, Hata Y, Yoshikawa H, Inomata H. Vascular endothelial growth factor play a role in hyperpermeability of diabetic retinal vessels. Ophtalmic Res 1995; 27:48–52.
5. Folkman J. Angiogenesis in cancer, vascular, rheumatoid and other diseases. Nature Med 1995; 1(1):27–31.
6. Mc Laren J, Prentice A, Charnockjones DS, Millican SA, Muller KH, Sharkley AM. Vascular endothelial growth factor is produced by peritoneal-fluid microphages in endometriosis and is regulated by ovarian-steroids. J Clin Invest 1996; 482–489.

7. Sokmen S, Sarioglu S, Fuzun M, Terzi C, Kupelloglu A, Aslan B. Prognostic significance of angiogenesisi in rectal cancer. Anticancer Res 2001; 21:4341–4348.

8. Saito H, Tsujitani S. Angiogenesis, angiogenic factor expression and prognosis of gastric carcinoma. Anticancer Res 2001; 21:4365–4372.

9. Vemeulen PB, Gasparini G, Fox SB, Toi M, Martin L, McCulloch P, Pezzella F, Vilae G, Veidner N, Harris AL, Dirix LY. Quantification of angiogenesis in solid tumors: an international consensus on the methodology and criteria of evaluation. Eur J Cancer 1996; 14:2474–2484.

10. Folkman J. Tumor angiogenesis: therapeutic implications. N Engl J Med 1971; 285:1182–1186.

11. Ribatti D, Vacca A, De Falco G, Roccaro A, Roncali L, Dammacco F. Angiogenesis, angiogenic factors expression and hematological malignances. Anticancer Research 2001; 21:4333–4340.

12. Ausprunk DH, Folkman J. Migration and proliferation of endothelial cells in preformed and newly formed blood vessels during tumor angiogenesis. Microvasc Res 1977; 14:53–65.

13. Sheibani N, Frazier WA. Thrombospondin-1, PECAM-1 and regulation of angiogenesis. Histopathol 1999; 14:285–294.

14. Tannock IF. The relation between cell proliferation and the vascular system in a transplanted mouse mammary tumor. Brit J Cancer 1968; 22:258–273.

15. Vartanian RK, Weidner N. Correlation of intratumoral endothelial cell proliferation with microvessel density (tumor angiogenesis) and tumor cell proliferation in breast carcinoma. Am J Pathol 1994; 144:1188–1194.

16. Hanahan D, Folkman J. Patterns and emerging mechanisms of the angiogenic switch during tumorogenesis. Cell 1996; 86:353–364.

17. Coede V, Fleckenstein G, Dietrich M, Osmers RGW, Kuhn W, Augustin HG. Prognostic value of angiogenesis in mammary tumors. Anticancer Res 1998; 18:2199–2202.

18. Folkman J. Angiogenesis and its inhibitors. In: DeVita VT, Helman S, Rosenberg S, eds. Important Advances in Oncology. Philadelphia: JB Lippincott C, 1985:42–62.

19. Hori A, Sasada R, Matsutani E, Naito K, Sakura Y, Fujita T, Kozai Y. Suppression of solid tumor growth by immuno-neutralizing monoclonal antibody against human basic fibroblast growth factor. Cancer Res 1991; 51:6180–6184.

20. Kim KJ, Li B, Winer J, Armanini M, Gillett N, Phillips HS, Ferrara N. Inhibition of vascular endothelial growth factor-induced angiogenesis supresses tumor growth in vivo. Nature 1993; 362:841–844.

21. Corbett TH, Griswood DP Jr, Roberts BJ, Peckham JC, Schabel FM Jr. Biology and therapeutic response of a mouse mammary adenocarcinoma (16/C) and its potential as a model for surgical adjuvant chemotherapy. Cancer Treatment Rep 1978; 62:1471–1488.

22. Teicher BA, ed. Anticancer Drug Development Guide. Totowa, NJ: Humana Press, 1997.

23. Vanzulli S, Cazzaniga S, Braidot MF, Vecchi A, Montovani A, Weinstok de, Calmanovici R. Detection of endothelial cells by MEC 13.3 monoclonal antibody in mice mammary tumors. Biocell 1997; 21:39–46.

24. Williams CD, Markov MS. Therapeutic electromagnetic field effects of nagiogenesis during tumor growth: a pilot study in mice. Electro Magnetobiol 2001; 20:323–329.

25. Williams CD, Markov MS, Hardman WE, Cameron IL. Therapeutic electromagnetic field effects on angiogenesis and tumor growth. Anticancer Res 2001; 21:3887–3892.

26. De Seze R, Tuffet S, Moreau JM, Veyret B. Effect of 100-mT time-varying magnetic fields on the growth of tumors in mice. Bioelectromagnetics 2000; 21:107–111.

27. Ruifrok AC. Quantification of immunohistochemical staining by color translation and automated thresholding. Analyt Quant Cytol Histol 1997; 19:107–113.

28. De Lisser HM, Christofidou-Solomidou M, Strieter RM, Burdick MD, Robinson CS, Wexler RS, Kerr JS, Garlanda C, Merwin JR, Madri JA, Albelda SM. Involvement of endothelial PECAM-1/CD31 in angiogenesis. Am J Pathol 1997; 151:671–677.

29. Charpin C, Garcia S, Bouvier C, Andras L, Bonnier P, Lavaut M-N, Allasia C. CD31/PECAM Automated and quantitative immunochemical assay in breast carcinomas. Am J Clin Pathol 1997; 107:534–554.

30. Hauser IA, Riess R, Hausknecht B, Thuringer H, Sterzel RB. Expression of cell adhesion molecules in primary renal disease and renal allograft rejection. Neprol Dial Transplant 1997; 12:1122–1131.

31. Jain RK. Delivery of novel therapeutic agents in tumors: physiological barriers and strategies. J Natl Cancer Inst 1989; 81(8):570–576.

32. Markov MS. Influence of radiation on biological systems. In: Allen MJ, ed. Charge and Field Effects in Biosystems II. New York: Plenum Press, 1990:241–250.

33. Folkman J, Hahnfeldt P, Hlatky L. Cancer: looking outside the genome. Nature Reviews. Molecular Cellular Biol 2001; 1:76–79.

34. Hannan CJ, Liang Y, Allison JD, Searle JR. In vitro cytotoxicity against human cancer cell lines during pulsed magnetic field exposure. Anticancer Res 1994; 14(4A):1517–1520.

35. Liang Y, Hannan CJ, Chang BK, Schoenlein PV. Enhanced potency of daunorubicin against multidrug resistant subline KB-ChR-8-5-11 by a pulsed magnetic field. Anticancer Res 1997; 17(3C):2083–2088.

36. Salvatore JR, Blackinton D, Polk C, Mehta S. Nonionizing electromagnetic radiation: a study of carcinogenic and cancer treatment potential. Rev Environmental Health 1994; 10(3–4):197–207.

37. Salvatore JR. Nonionizing electromagnetic fields and cancer: a review. Oncology 1996; 10 (4): 563–570.

40

Electroporation for Electrochemotherapy and Gene Therapy

Damijan Miklavčič and Tadej Kotnik

University of Ljubljana, Ljubljana, Slovenia

The new avenue in treatment of tumors is discussed in this chapter. The possibilities for electroporation of tissues in order to enhance the drug and gene delivery are presented from both basic science and clinical application points of view. In a condensed way, the authors present the journey from first basic experiments with electroporation of single cells through electroporation in cell suspension and in tissue. Discussion of mechanisms of electroporation is followed by discussion of electroporation for electrochemotherapy and electrogenetransfer. A brief review of experimental conditions is linked to electrode requirements and to available commercial devices for electroporation in laboratory and clinical conditions.

I. INTRODUCTION

A. Description of the Phenomenon

When a cell is exposed to an electric field, a transmembrane voltage is induced on the membrane. If this voltage exceeds a certain value, this leads to a significant increase of the electric conductivity and the permeability of the membrane. Typically, each increases by several orders of magnitude. Formation of a state of increased permeability of the membrane caused by an exposure to the electric field is called *electroporation* (also *electropermeabilization*).

As the result of the increased permeability of the membrane, molecules that are otherwise deprived of transport mechanisms can be transported across the membrane. With appropriate duration and amplitude of the electric field, the membrane returns into its normal state after the end of the exposure to the electric field (reversible electroporation). However, if the exposure is too long or the amplitude of the electric field is too high, the membrane does not reseal after the end of the exposure, leading to cell death (irreversible electroporation).

Reversible "electrical breakdown" of the membrane has first been reported by Stämpfli in 1958, but for some time this report has been mostly unnoticed. Nearly a decade later, Sale and Hamilton have reported on nonthermal electrical destruction of microorganisms using strong electric pulses. In 1972, Neumann and Rosenheck have shown that electric pulses induce a large increase of membrane permeability in natural vesicles. This report has motivated a series of further investigations, and from this time on, the data started to accumulate more rapidly and systematically. Most of the early work was done on isolated cells in conditions in vitro, but it is now known that many applications are also successful in situation in vivo. Using electroporation, both small and large molecules can be introduced into cells and extracted from cells, and proteins can be inserted into the membrane and cells can be fused. Due to its efficiency, electroporation has rapidly found its application in gene transfection, preparation of monoclonal antibodies, and electrochemotherapy of tumors. Nowadays, it is finding its way into many fields of biochemistry, molecular biology, and medicine and is becoming an established method used in oncology for treatment of solid tumors. It also holds great promises for gene therapy (1).

B. Schwan's Equation

Although a biological cell is not perfectly spherical, in theoretical treatments, it is usually considered as being such (Fig. 1). Also, the plasma membrane of the cell has a very low conductivity with respect to the intracellular and extracellular environment, and in an approximation it can be considered nonconductive. When a single cell is placed into a homogeneous electric field, the voltage induced on the membrane can be determined by solving Laplace's equation. For a spherical cell with a nonconductive membrane, the solution of Laplace's equation is a formula often referred to as Schwan's equation,

$$\Delta\Phi_m = \frac{3}{2} E R \cos\varphi$$

where $\Delta\Phi_m$ is the induced transmembrane voltage, E is the electric field in the region where the cell is situated, R is the cell radius, and φ is the polar angle measured from the center of the cell with respect to the direction of the field. This formula tells that the maximum voltage

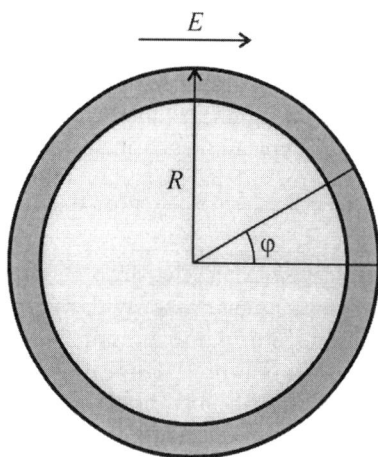

Figure 1 A spherical cell with a nonconductive membrane and the parameters of Schwan's equation: cell radius (R), electric field (E), and the angle measured with respect to the field (φ).

is induced at the points where the electric field is perpendicular to the membrane, i.e., at $\varphi = 0°$ and $\varphi = 180°$, the points we shall refer to as the "poles" of the cell, and varies proportionally to the cosine of the angle in between these poles. Also, the induced voltage is proportional to the applied electric field and to the cell radius.

Schwan's equation as given above describes only the static situation, which is typically established several microseconds after the onset of the electric field. Since durations of exposure to electric field used for electroporation are typically in the range of hundreds of microseconds up to tens of milliseconds, Schwan's equation can safely be applied in electroporation.

C. Electroporation of a Single Cell

Most experimental data suggest that electroporation is a threshold phenomenon—if the induced membrane voltage in a region of the membrane exceeds certain critical value, this leads to electroporation in this region. From Schwan's equation one can deduce that for a single spherical cell (e.g., a cell floating in a medium), electroporation occurs at the caps around the two poles (see Sec. I.A), and it is through these caps that the transport will be established. For stronger fields, the area of these caps gets larger.

A voltage in the range of tens of millivolts is always present on the cell membrane. When a cell is exposed to an electric field, this voltage (the resting transmembrane voltage) combines with the induced voltage. Since the resting voltage is the same all over the membrane, while the induced voltage varies proportionally to the cosine of the angle with respect to the direction of the field, the resultant transmembrane voltage is actually somewhat higher on one pole of the cell than on the other. Since typical transmembrane voltages leading to electroporation are in the range of hundreds of millivolts, this asymmetry is not large. Still, when using bipolar pulses, which compensate for this asymmetry, electroporation is obtained at lower pulse amplitudes than unipolar ones (see Sec. III).

Schwan's equation only describes the transmembrane voltage induced on a spherical cell with a nonconductive membrane. However, more general formulae exist that are valid for spherical cells with a membrane of non zero conductivity (2) and such that apply to spheroidal and ellipsoidal cells (3,4).

D. Electroporation in Cell Suspensions

When cells in suspension are exposed to an electric field, applying Schwan's equation to determine the induced transmembrane voltage is in general not valid. This is due to the fact that the field outside a cell is not homogeneous, as it is distorted by the presence of other cells in the suspension. For suspensions in which the cells represent less than 1% of the total suspension volume, the deviation of the actual induced transmembrane voltage from the one predicted by Schwan's equation is practically negligible. As the volume fraction occupied by the cells gets larger, the prediction obtained from Schwan's equation gets less and less realistic (Fig. 2). For volume fractions over 10% as well as for clusters and lattices of cells, one has to use appropriate numerical or approximate analytical solutions for a reliable analysis of the induced transmembrane voltage (5,6).

In conclusion, the induced transmembrane voltage depends not only on the geometrical and electrical properties of the cell but also on the density of the cells in suspension.

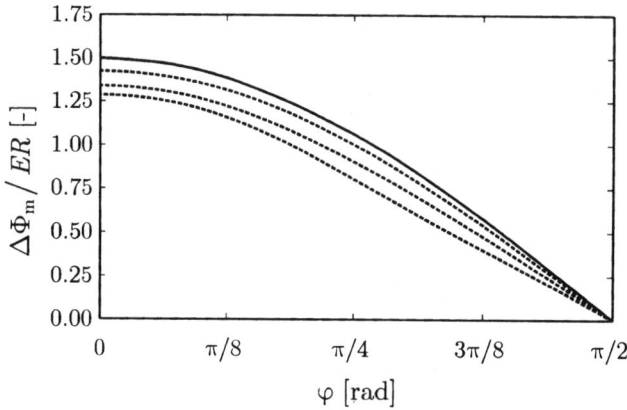

Figure 2 Induced transmembrane voltage normalized to electric field and cell radius. Solid: prediction of Schwan's equation. Dashed: numerical results for cells arranged in a face-centered cubic lattice and occupying (from top to bottom) 10%, 30%, and 50% of the total suspension volume. (Adapted from Ref. 6 with the permission of the authors.)

E. Electroporation in Tissue

In tissues, additional difficulties arise in the analysis of transmembrane voltage induced by an exposure to electric field. First, unlike suspended cells, the cells in tissue are far from spherical. Second, also on a larger scale, most tissues are not homogeneous, e.g., due to the presence of blood vessels. Third, electrical properties of different tissues can differ considerably. Due to these facts, the distribution of electric field in tissues can be quite intricate (7). In addition, after certain regions of tissue are electroporated, this causes a redistribution of electric field, which in general becomes higher around nonporated regions. As a consequence, some of these regions may get electroporated subsequently, and this again leads to a rearrangement of the electric field. Thus, electroporation in a tissue can proceed in a domino-effect manner, with poration of certain regions giving rise to poration of other regions. The actual situation is therefore a dynamical one, and to correctly describe electroporation in a tissue, one must account for ongoing rearrangements of the electric field throughout the exposure. An example is tumor treatment with pulses delivered to the surface electrodes placed on the skin, where the skin gets electroporated first, then the tissue underneath it, and so on (Fig. 3).

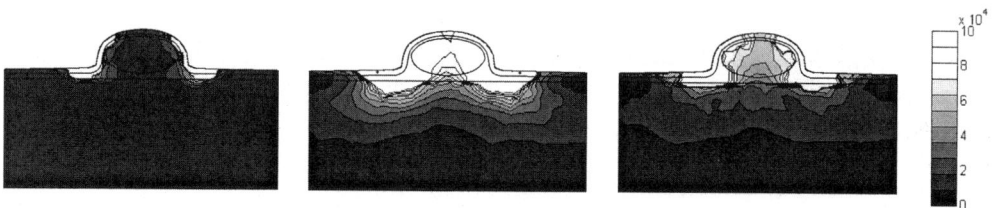

Figure 3 Numerical evaluation of the time course of electric field distribution during electroporation in tissue with a pulse of 1000 V amplitude delivered to plate electrodes placed on the skin at a distance of 8 mm. Units on the scale are in volts per meter (V/m).

F. Mass Transport

There are three general mechanisms of transmembrane transport by which the molecules can pass through an electroporated membrane:

1. Diffusion, driven by the molecular concentration difference across the membrane
2. Electrophoresis, driven by the electric potential difference across the membrane
3. Osmosis, driven by the osmotic pressure difference across the membrane

Most experimental studies imply that diffusion is the main component of transport of small molecules through an electroporated membrane (8–10). On the other hand, it is known that for macromolecules, diffusion itself is often insufficient for adequate uptake into a cell, and the presence of electrophoretic forces can improve such uptake significantly (11,12).

The dependence of the efficiency of transport mechanisms on the size of the transported molecule led to a relatively sharp distinction between the protocols of electroporation used for smaller molecules and those for macromolecules. For smaller molecules, electroporation and a concentration gradient suffice for the transport to occur, and pulses with durations of tens of microseconds up to several milliseconds successfully achieve this aim. On the other hand, electrophoretic transport of macromolecules mostly proceeds during the pulse, and to achieve sufficient uptake of molecules such as DNA, pulses of typical durations of milliseconds to tens of milliseconds are used (11,13). As an alternative, pulses similar to the ones used with smaller molecules are used to obtain electroporation, and a longer pulse with a lower amplitude is applied subsequently to sustain the electrophoretic movement (12,14).

G. Mechanisms of Electroporation

The theory of formation of aqueous pores in the membrane is widely considered as the most convincing theoretical explanation of electroporation (15). According to this theory, a sufficiently long and strong exposure to an electric field leads to a formation of hydrophilic (aqueous) pores, in which the lipids adjacent to the aqueous inside of the pore are reoriented in a manner that their hydrophilic heads are facing the pore, while their hydrophobic tails are hidden inside the membrane. The hydrophilic state of the pore can only be reached through a transition from an initial, hydrophobic state in which the lipids still have their original orientation (Fig. 4). As electric field amplitude increases, the presence of hydrophilic pores becomes energetically ever more favorable, which leads to the formation of pores with an average radius corresponding to the minimum of the free-energy curve (Fig. 5, the upper curve). Further increase of the field amplitude pushes this curve downward, and eventually the energy minimum disappears (Fig. 5, the lower curve), resulting in a complete breakdown of the membrane, which corresponds to irreversible electroporation.

Several studies have recently added to the credibility of the theory of formation of aqueous pores. The measurements of the optical properties of the membrane have shown that during electroporation, the lipid molecules are reoriented, and water penetrates into the bilayer (16). Existence of transient metastable aqueous pores has also been observed in a molecular dynamics simulation of the lipid bilayer formation (17). In a recent experiment, we have also observed that the threshold of irreversible electroporation is lowered if molecules of octaethyleneglycol-dodecylether ($C_{12}E_8$) are incorporated into the membrane (18). These molecules form conical inclusions in the membrane, which makes the reorientation of lipids that is expected to occur in hydrophilic pores more energetically favorable and the pores more stable.

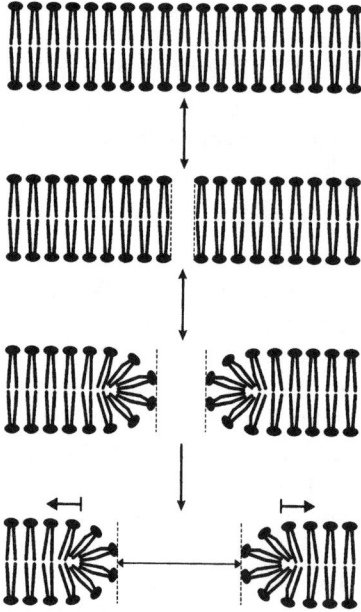

Figure 4 Formation of an aqueous pore. The situation is shown for transmembrane voltage increasing from top to bottom: a nonporated membrane, formation of a hydrophobic pore, transformation into a hydrophilic pore (reversible electroporation), and enlargement beyond the stable size (irreversible electroporation).

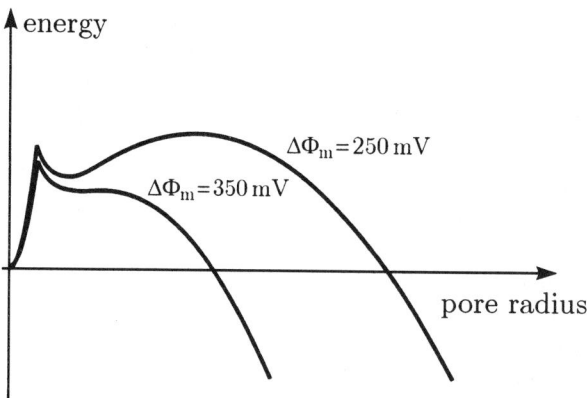

Figure 5 A schematic representation of the amount of energy required for formation of an aqueous pore of a given radius for a transmembrane voltage that yields reversible (the upper curve) and irreversible electroporation (lower curve). The sharp local maximum corresponds to the transition from hydrophobic to hydrophilic state. The local minimum, if it exists, corresponds to the radius at which the pore stabilizes.

II. APPLICATIONS

There are many prospects for application of electroporation in biochemistry, molecular biology, and above all in various fields of medicine. Sections II.A and II.B are devoted to a more detailed description of the two applications that are already finding their way into practice—electrochemotherapy (ECT) and electrogenetransfection (EGT). Here, we outline some other applications.

ELECTROSTERILIZATION. Irreversible electroporation can also be exploited with the aim of sterilization, i.e., killing of bacteria or other microorganisms (19–21). Other techniques of sterilization, such as by antibiotics, detergents, or exposure to radiation, in general lead to some kind of contamination, which is not the case with electrosterilization. However, this approach has proved rather costly with respect to other techniques, and it has not yet found a way into practical applications.

ELECTROINSERTION. Another application of electroporation is insertion of molecules into the cell membrane. As the membrane reseals, it entraps some of the transported molecules, and if these molecules are amphipathic (constituted of both polar and nonpolar regions), they can remain stably incorporated in the membrane. Electroinsertion was observed with several transmembrane proteins, such as CD4 receptors (22) and glycophorin A (23), and could prove valuable in the research of the role of various transmembrane proteins.

ELECTROFUSION. Under appropriate experimental conditions, delivery of electric pulses can lead to the merger (fusion) of membranes of adjacent cells. Electrofusion has been observed between suspended cells (24,25), between suspended cells and cells in tissue (26) and between cells in tissue (27). For successful electrofusion in suspension, the cells must previously be brought into close contact, for example, by dielectrophoresis (24). Electrofusion has proved to be a successful approach in production of vaccines (28,29) and antibodies (30).

TRANSDERMAL DRUG DELIVERY. Application of high-voltage pulses to the skin causes a large increase in ionic and molecular transport across the skin (31). This has been applied for transdermal delivery of drugs, such as metoprolol (32), and also works for larger molecules, for example, DNA oligonucleotides (33).

A. Electrochemotherapy (ECT)

In cancer treatment, some of the drugs aim at damaging DNA. Chemotherapy based on these drugs is only effective for those that readily permeate through the cell membrane and act cytotoxically when reaching their intracellular targets. Unfortunately, some of the very cytotoxic chemotherapeutic drugs permeate the plasma membrane very slowly, or practically not at all. These drugs are good candidates for electrochemotherapy (ECT), which combines chemotherapy and electroporation. The delivery of electric pulses at the time of when a chemotherapeutic drug reaches its highest extracellular concentration considerably increases the transport through the membrane towards the intracellular targets of cytotoxicity.

Two chemotherapeutic drugs, bleomycin and cisplatin, have proven to be much more effective in electrochemotherapy than alone when applied to tumor cell lines in vitro, as well as in vivo on tumors in mice (34–36). Cytotoxicity of bleomycin was shown to be increased for several 100-fold, and of cisplatin up to 70-fold when cells were electroporated. Sarcomas, carcinomas, or melanoma tumors responded with high percentage of complete responses when the drugs were injected intravenously or intratumorally. These experiments provided sufficient data to demonstrate that ECT with either bleomycin or cisplatin is effective in treatment of solid tumors.

Based on these preclinical data, ECT with bleomycin and cisplatin entered clinical trials. Both drugs have proved their value in clinical ECT protocols with cutaneous and subcutaneous tumour nodules of various malignancies in cancer patients (Fig. 6). Most of the treated nodules responded with objective responses in 60–100% (37,38). In the protocols, both intravenous and intratumoral drug administration were used. Current knowledge about antitumor effectiveness of ECT considers this therapy as local treatment being effective on most tumor types tested so far. Since ECT can be performed using surface electrodes, it does not lead to scaring, which is unavoidable with surgical procedures. In addition, the high local concentration of the chemotherapeutic drug in the tumor allows to overcome the developing resistance to the drug (39).

Antitumor effectiveness of ECT is considered to be mainly due to the increased drug uptake into the tumor cells, caused by electroporation. However, other mechanisms, such as prolonged drug entrapment in the tumors due to decrease in tumor blood flow caused by electric pulses and vascular-targeted effects, may also contribute to the effectiveness of ECT (40–42).

The results indicate that electrochemotherapy with bleomycin is equally effective when the drug is given intravenously or intratumorally, while ECT with cisplatin is more efficient when the drug is given intratumorally than when given intravenously. The advantage of electrochemotherapy with cisplatin is that the drug itself, without application of electric pulses, may exert considerable antitumor effect.

It is difficult to foresee all the clinical applications of electrochemotherapy. In the first step, more controlled clinical trials are needed evaluating treatment response of different tumor types. So far, only percutaneously accessible tumor nodules have been treated in the clinical trials, but with development of new electrodes it will become possible to treat tumors in internal organs.

In its concept, electrochemotherapy is a local treatment, and therefore approaches must be exploited to add a systemic component, either by adjuvant immunotherapy or in combination with other systemic treatments. Some chemotherapeutic drugs, including bleomycin and cisplatin, also interact with radiation therapy (43).

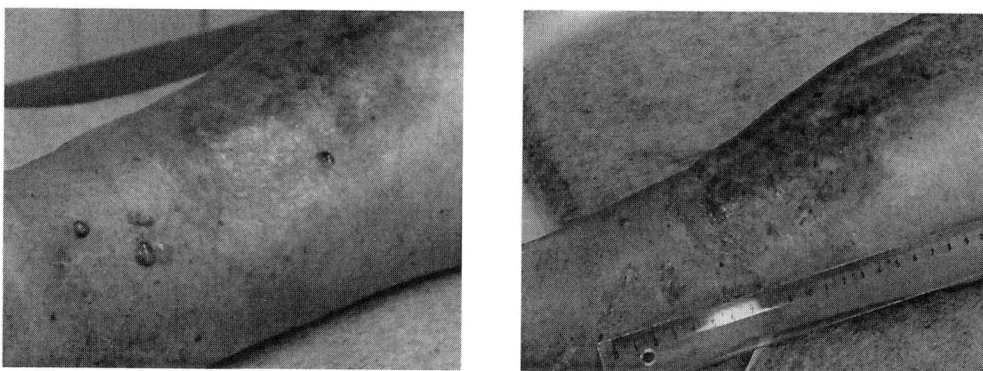

Figure 6 ECT treatment of skin metastases of malignant melanoma with cisplatin: left, before the treatment; right, 1 year after the treatment. The treatment is described in detail in (38). (The photographs were kindly provided by Prof. Zvonimir Rudolf and Prof. Gregor Serša.)

B. Electrogenetransfection (EGT)

Unlike electrochemotherapy, application of electroporation for transfer of DNA molecules into the cell, often referred to as *electrogenetransfection* (EGT), has not yet entered clinical trials. Nevertheless, EGT is devoid of the health risks which are present in viral gene transfection, and it is presently considered to have large potential as a method for gene therapy aimed at correcting genetic diseases.

It has been shown that an injection of naked DNA into a skeletal muscle in itself results in an expression of the injected DNA. The gene expression can last up to several months, which makes the muscle a promising target for gene therapy, but the obtained levels of expression are low and extremely variable, which makes the results of such an approach unpredictable and hence unsuitable for clinical application. However, when DNA injection into the muscle is combined with electroporation, the gene expression is increased by two or three orders of magnitude, and the variability between muscle fibers is significantly reduced (44–46).

Expression of the therapeutic gene coding for erythropoietin has already been reported in animals, and elevated values of erythropoietin have been observed for long periods after the gene transfer (47,48). These results suggest that cell transfection by EGT could be the appropriate method for correction of genetic diseases, vaccination, and cancer treatment. Clinical trials, which can be expected to start in the near future, thus hold great promises for these areas of medicine.

III. PULSE PARAMETERS AND EXPERIMENTAL CONDITIONS

For the large majority of applications in vitro, the efficiency of electroporation is determined by the fraction of reversibly porated cells with respect to the whole treated cell population. In the optimization of electroporation, one thus searches for pulse parameters and other experimental conditions that yield the highest fraction of porated cells that survive the treatment. In addition, for the treatment to serve its purpose, it is often necessary that a certain quantity of exogenous molecules enters into each cell, and in these cases optimal pulse parameters should also ensure a sufficient molecular uptake per cell.

For these reasons, the role of pulse parameters and experimental conditions is usually investigated using a combination of tests, estimating the fraction of porated cells, the fraction of cells surviving the treatment, the average amount of exogenous molecules introduced into the cell, and sometimes also the time of recovery of the cells back into the nonporated state.

A. The Role of the Amplitude, Duration, and Number of Pulses

The role of parameters of rectangular pulses in the efficiency of electroporation was investigated in a number of studies (11,14,49–52). These studies show that poration becomes detectable as the pulse amplitude exceeds a certain critical value. Above this value, with further increase of pulse amplitude, the percentage of porated cells increases, while the percentage of cells surviving the treatment decreases. As a function of pulse amplitude, the percentage of porated cells approximately follows an ascending sigmoidal curve, while the percentage of viable cells resembles a descending sigmoidal curve (Fig. 7). Similar results have been obtained with exponentially decaying pulses (53), where the time constant of pulse decay was used instead of pulse duration.

In a study performed on a number of different cell lines, Čemaar and co-workers have shown that both poration and cell survival as functions of pulse amplitude vary significantly between various types of cells (52). Though some of the observed differences can be

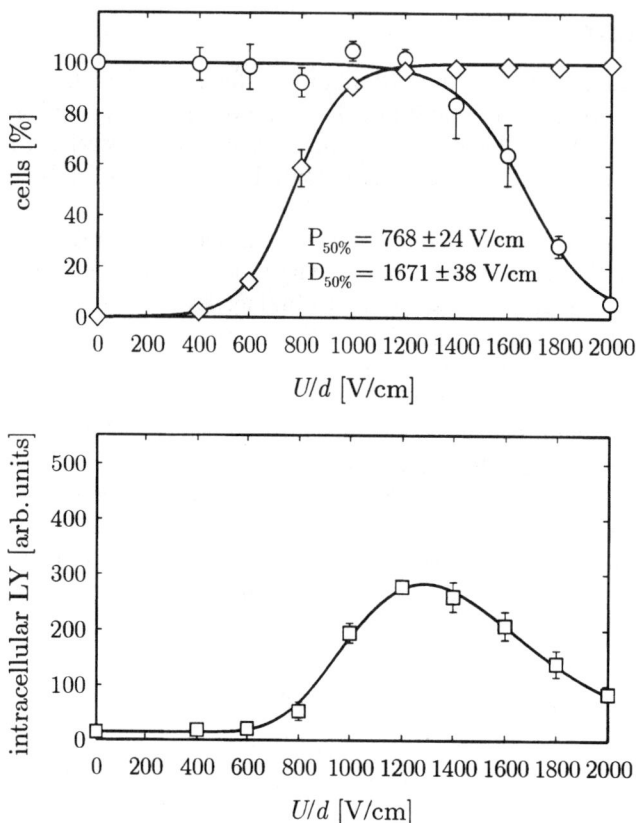

Figure 7 Top: Percentages of porated (diamonds) and viable cells (circles) as functions of pulse amplitude (the ratio between the voltage and the electrode distance). Bottom: uptake of lucifer yellow (LY) into the cells. DC-3F cells (spontaneously transformed Chinese hamster fibroblasts) were porated with eight unipolar rectangular 100-μs pulses delivered in 1-s intervals. $P_{50\%}$ and $D_{50\%}$ denote pulse amplitudes which lead to poration and death, respectively, of 50% of the cells. Extracellular concentration of LY was 1 mM.

attributed to differences in cell size, these results imply that the differences in membrane composition and structure also play an important role.

Experiments show that the critical pulse amplitude of electroporation is lowered if the number and/or duration of the pulses is increased (11,49) (compare Figs. 7 and 8). If the values of these two parameters are not too large, the average amount of molecules introduced into a cell also increases with an increase of the number of pulses. Using four or more pulses, a pronounced peak of molecular uptake is obtained.

Several studies have demonstrated that in the case of macromolecules, electrophoresis plays an important role in the transport of molecules across the membrane, and sufficiently long pulse duration is crucial for adequate uptake (11,14,50). Typically, pulse durations for the uptake of smaller molecules are in the range of hundreds of microseconds, while for macromolecules, durations from several milliseconds to several tens of milliseconds are usually required.

In a study utilizing a broad range of rectangular pulse parameters, Maèek-Lebar and co-workers have shown that the total energy of a train of pulses is not a crucial parameter in

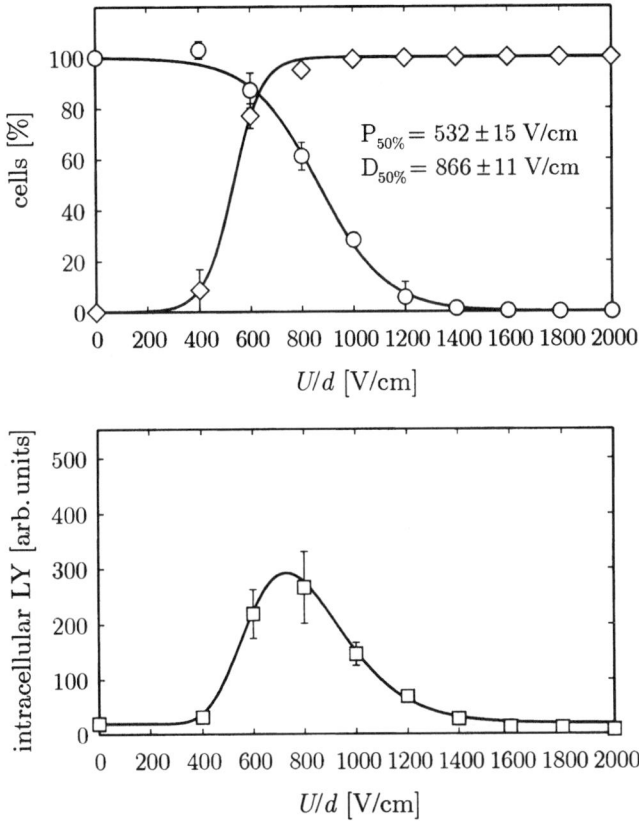

$P_{50\%} = 532 \pm 15$ V/cm
$D_{50\%} = 866 \pm 11$ V/cm

Figure 8 Electroporation and survival of DC-3F cells (top) and uptake of LY (bottom) for eight unipolar rectangular 1-ms pulses delivered in 1-s intervals.

either drug uptake or cell survival. On the contrary, a significant difference was observed in the uptake induced by different trains of the same total energy (51).

B. The Role of Pulse Shape

Because commercially available pulse generators with sufficient voltages for electroporation of cells in suspension are mostly limited to rectangular and exponentially decaying pulses, relatively few studies have dealt with the role of pulse shape in the efficiency of cell electroporation. Chang and co-workers have reported that the efficiency of poration was increased when a sine wave of 30–200 kHz amplitude was superimposed onto a rectangular pulse, though the amplitude of the sine wave was only about 5% of the total pulse amplitude (54,55). Tekle and co-workers found that the efficiency of DNA transfection in vitro was significantly higher with a bipolar 60-kHz square wave of 400-μs duration than with a unipolar wave of the same frequency and duration (56). Schoenbach and co-workers have reported on electropermeabilization with ultrashort (60 ns) pulses (57). In a study comparing unipolar and bipolar rectangular pulses, we have shown that with bipolar pulses, the critical voltage of electroporation is lowered considerably, while cell viability remains practically unaffected (cf. Figs. 8 and 9); at the same time, the peak of the uptake increases with respect to the one obtained by unipolar pulses (58).

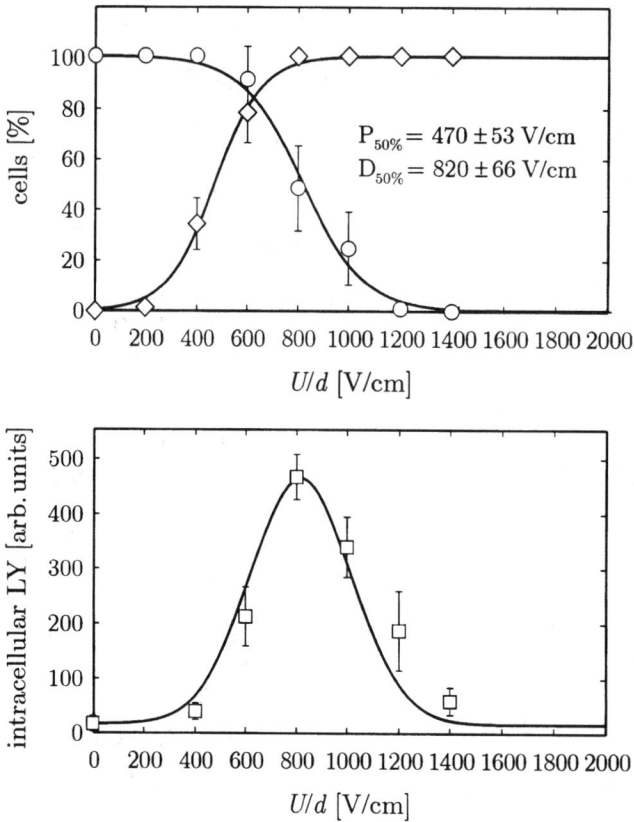

Figure 9 Electroporation and survival of DC-3F cells (top) and uptake of LY (bottom) for eight bipolar rectangular 1-ms (500 μs + 500 μs) pulses delivered in 1-s intervals.

In addition, we have shown that with both aluminum and stainless steel electrodes, the release of metal ions from the electrodes into the cell suspension is reduced significantly if bipolar pulses are used (59). This reduces the electrolytic contamination of the cell suspension and also prolongs the lifetime of the electrodes.

Comparing the results obtained with pulses having 1-ms amplitude duration, but with rise and fall times ranging from 2 μs to 100 μs, we found no detectable differences between the efficiencies of these pulses. Thus, it seems that the rise and fall times of the pulses do not play a significant role in the efficiency of electroporation.

C. Pulse Repetition Frequency

In general, patients find electrochemotherapy tolerable, in spite of unpleasant sensations associated with contraction of muscles located beneath or in the vicinity of the electrodes. These contractions are due to the intensity of the electric pulses required for effective electropermeabilization of tumor cell membranes. Since a train of eight electric pulses with repetition frequency of 1 Hz is usually applied to the tumors, each pulse in the train excites underlying nerves and provokes muscle contractions. The use of pulses with repetition frequency higher than the frequency of tetanic contraction would therefore cause a reduced number of muscle contractions and associated unpleasant sensations. In a recently

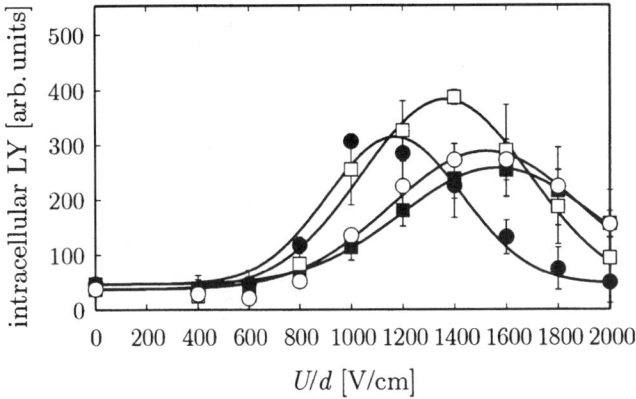

Figure 10 Uptake of LY for eight unipolar rectangular pulses 100-μs pulses delivered with repetition frequencies of 1 Hz (●), 10 Hz (□), 1 kHz (○), and 2.5 kHz (■).

performed study, we have shown that for repetition frequencies ranging from 1 Hz to 8.3 kHz, the uptake of LY into electroporated cells in vitro stays at similar levels (60). Part of these results is shown in Fig. 10. In an ongoing study, similar results are being obtained in vivo. This suggests that there are prospects for efficient use of pulses with high repetition frequency also in clinical electrochemotherapy.

D. Other Experimental Conditions

Besides the pulse parameters, the efficiency of poration also depends on many physical and chemical parameters. An important role is played by the properties of the extracellular medium: its ionic strength and composition (61–63), osmotic pressure (64,65), and its temperature before and after poration (66). In addition, as described in more detail in Sec. IV.B, for successful electroporation in vivo, uniformity of the electric field in the tissue is also important (7,67).

E. Recommendations for the Choice of Pulse Parameters

Based on the studies discussed above, some general advice in the design of experiments involving electroporation can be made. Pulse amplitude (voltage-to-distance ratio) should typically be in the range from 200 V/cm up to 2000 V/cm. Pulse durations should be in the range of hundreds of microseconds for smaller molecules and from several milliseconds up to several tens of milliseconds for macromolecules such as DNA fragments (in the latter case, due to the very long pulse duration, optimal pulse amplitude can even be lower than 100 V/cm). If the equipment allows, bipolar pulses should be used instead of unipolar ones. Bipolar pulses yield a lower poration threshold, higher uptake, and an unaffected viability compared to unipolar pulses of the same amplitude and duration.

These guidelines should provide a starting point for a design of experiments involving electroporation. Still, the optimal values of pulse parameters strongly depend on the cell type used, on the molecule to be introduced, and on specific conditions under which the experiment is performed. Therefore, for best possible results, pulse parameters should be optimized under specific experimental conditions before the actual study is initiated.

IV. ELECTRODES

A. Electrode Designs

The electric field distribution in a cell suspension or in a tissue is to a large extent determined by the geometry of the electrodes. For electroporation of cells in a suspension, typical electrodes consist of two parallel plates at a distance of 1–4 mm. The commercially available electrodes are made of aluminum and usually mounted in a cuvette that also serves as a container for the cell suspension, while several groups also use parallel plate electrodes made of stainless steel or platinum. If the plates are sufficiently large with respect to the distance between them, this design provides a relatively homogeneous field in the suspension. Still, several practical problems arise with electroporation of cells in suspension.

First, it has been reported that with aluminum electrodes, voltage drop at the electrode–solution interface can represent a significant fraction of the total voltage delivered to the electrodes (68). In contrast, this drop is insignificant with stainless steel electrodes (69). Second, electric pulses cause a certain amount of metal ions to be released from the electrodes into the suspension. Aluminum ions released from the electrodes can significantly affect biochemical processes involving inositol phosphates (70). With stainless steel electrodes, which are often used in experimental setups, the release of iron ions is of similar magnitude as that of aluminum ions from aluminum electrodes (59). The problem of electrolytic contamination can be reduced by using bipolar charge-balanced pulses (59), but most commercially available devices for electroporation are unable to generate such pulses. Another option is to use platinum electrodes, but due to the cost of platinum this is not a viable option with experimental setups where the electrodes can only be used once (e.g., for sterile conditions).

A variety of electrode designs have been used for electroporation in vivo. The most widely used are the plate electrodes, either at a fixed or a variable distance between them. In the latter case, the electrode plates can be mounted on a caliper (Fig. 11A). This type of electrode is used for electrochemotherapy of cutaneous and subcutaneous experimental tumors, smaller tumors in patients, and gene delivery in rat mouse and subcutaneous

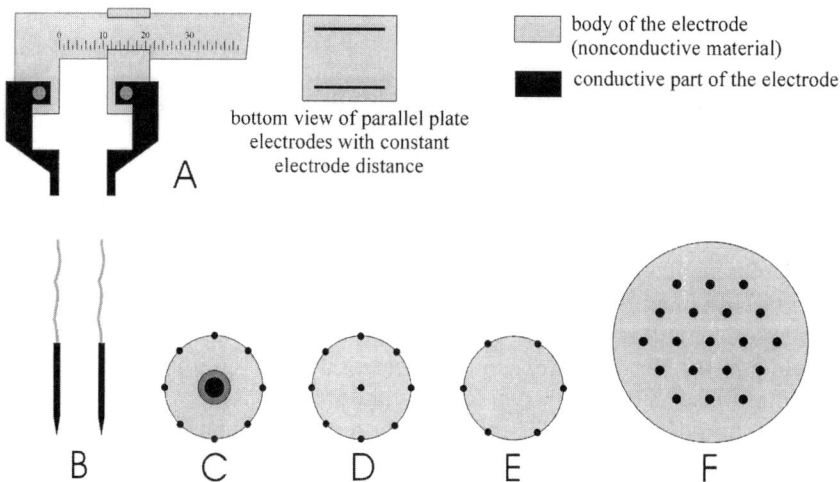

Figure 11 Electrode designs: (A) parallel plate electrodes, (B) simple needle electrodes, (C–F) multiple needles. (Adapted from Ref. 73 with the permission of the authors.)

tumors. Other types of electrodes (Fig. 11 B–E) have been used and compared in electrochemotherapy of experimental subcutaneous mice tumors with variable response (71). Another type of electrode, "honeycomb" (Fig. 11F), has been constructed and used for treatment of larger tumor volumes in rabbits (72). In the latter type, a division of volume to smaller fractions is introduced as pairs of needle electrodes are sequentially fired in a way that eventually the whole (arbitrarily large) volume is being permeabilized. The designs shown in Fig. 11 A and E have also been used in clinical trials (73).

B. Calculations

It is difficult to compare directly the effectiveness of different types of electrodes used in ECT, since they were in many cases used in different experimental setups, with different tumors, and with different voltages. However, it is possible to model numerically the electric field distribution in the tumor obtained with each electrode type. Such modeling clearly shows that the amplitude of electric field in the tumor plays the decisive role in the efficiency of ECT with a given electrode type (7,67). Another important factor to be considered is the homogeneity of the electric field in the tumor. The main reason for this is that in highly nonhomogeneous fields, in the regions with the weakest field, many cells are not electroporated at all, while in the regions where the field is the strongest, for many cells electroporation is irreversible. This is to some extent acceptable for ECT, but not for EGT, where all cells should survive the treatment.

C. Recommendations for the Choice of Electrodes

Mathematical modeling shows that a uniform coverage of a tumor with a sufficiently high electric field is necessary for good effectiveness of electrochemotherapy. This approach can be very useful in further search for electrodes that would make electrochemotherapy and other applications of electroporation in vivo more efficient. The objective of such studies would be to optimize electrode configuration in order to obtain above-threshold electric fields in the whole targeted tissue, e.g., tumor, with the least possible variation of the field amplitude.

V. GENERATORS

In the market, there are a number of pulse generators for electroporation. These devices are usually referred to as *electroporators*. An overview of commercially available electroporators is accessible on the World Wide Web (http://www.the-scientist.com/yr1997/july/shockjok.pdf). Electroporators for clinical use are offered or being developed by Genetronics (http://www.genetronics.com) and IGEA (http://www.igea.it), but the vast majority of electroporators were designed, and are sold, for applications in vitro. Some deliver unipolar rectangular (square wave) pulses, some exponentially decaying pulses, and some are able to deliver more intricate pulse shapes, such as sine-modulated pulses. The main problem, besides the fact that they are designed for in vitro environment, is the fact that the range of pulse parameters is not sufficiently flexible. One of the main reasons for a need of pulse flexibility lies partly in the fact that the exact mechanisms of electroporation are not yet fully known. Therefore, the user has to either rely on protocols and pulse parameters provided by the producers and on protocols from the literature or to develop his own. In the process of developing an efficient protocol and selecting the most effective pulse parameters for a specific need, flexibility is needed.

VI. CONCLUSIONS

Electroporation has been for decades used in cell biology and bioelectrochemistry laboratories for introducing genes into various types of cells. The physical nature of the phenomenon, i.e., increased permeability of plasma membrane, due to exposure to short high-voltage pulses, allows its use in plant, yeast, bacteria, and eukaryotic cells. In addition, electroporation can be used to introduce various sized molecules (from ions up to DNA) that otherwise can not or difficultly pass the membrane into the cells. It has also been demonstrated that proteins can be inserted into the membrane and cells fused, under appropriate experimental conditions.

In the last decade it has been successfully demonstrated by various groups that electroporation can be successfully applied also to cells in tissue in situation in vivo. In preclinical studies on many different tumor models, electropermeabilization has been combined with predominantly two antitumor agents: bleomycin and cisplatin. Both drugs have an intracellular target and the membrane represents a barrier for them. Therefore they are the prime candidates for electrochemotherapy.

In addition to its established role in electrochemotherapy, electroporation might soon become the method of choice for gene transfection in cell biology and bioelectrochemistry, and the existing body of experience and knowledge makes electroporation extremely interesting also as a nonviral method for introduction of therapeutic genes, for immunotherapy and DNA vaccination. As it has been demonstrated for electrochemotherapy, electroporation of cells in tissues in situ can be performed safely and effectively, and electroporation for clinical gene transfection is likely to have a bright future in the era of decoded human genome. It remains, however, extremely important that technology is developed and used with great care. We are just coming into the situation when electroporators and electrodes for clinical use are becoming available.

ACKNOWLEDGMENTS

The research has been supported through various grants from the Ministry of Education, Science and Sports of the Republic of Slovenia. In part, the research was also supported by IGEA, s.r.l. Carpi (MO), Italy. Part of the research was conducted within the frame of the Cliniporator project (Grant QLK3-1999-00484) under the framework of the Fifth Framework PCRD of the European Commission, program Quality of Life and Management of Living Resources, thematic area Cell Factory. In particular, we would like to acknowledge the work done and help offered by our co-workers and students at the Laboratory of Biocybernetics, Faculty of Electrical Engineering at the University of Ljubljana. Special thanks go to Alenka Maèek-Lebar, Dejan Šemrov, Fedja Bobanoviæ, Marko Puc, Maša Kandušer, Mojca Pavlin, Davorka Šel, Nataša Pavšelj, Gorazd Pucihar, Blaš Valiè, Stanislav Reberšek, and Janez Žigon. Early work on cells in vitro and all the work in vivo on animal tumor models and on patients was performed by, or in close collaboration with, colleagues from the Department of Tumor Biology at the Institute of Oncology in Ljubljana, Slovenia headed by prof. Gregor Serša. Prof. Serša and prof. Zvonimir Rudolf also kindly provided the photographs of ECT treatment of tumors in a patient. Many thanks go to our dear friend and colleague dr. Lluis M. Mir from the Institute Gustave-Roussy, Villejuif, France.

We would like to tribute this chapter to the memory of our mentor and friend Prof. Lojze Vodovnik.

REFERENCES

1. Mir LM. Therapeutic perspectives of in vivo cell electropermeabilization. Bioelectrochemistry 2001; 53:1–10.

2. Kotnik T, Bobanović; F, Miklavčič D. Sensitivity of transmembrane voltage induced by applied electric fields—a theoretical analysis. Bioelectrochem Bioenerg 1997; 43:285–291.

3. Kotnik T, Miklavčič D. Analytical description of transmembrane voltage induced by electric fields on spheroidal cells. Biophys J 2000; 79:670–679.

4. Gimsa J, Wachner D. Analytical description of the transmembrane voltage induced on arbitrarily oriented ellipsoidal and cylindrical cells. Biophys J 2001; 81:1888–1896.

5. Susil R, Šemrov D, Miklavčič D. Electric field induced transmembrane potential depends on cell density and organization. Electro Magnetobiol 1998; 17:391–399.

6. Pavlin M, Pavšelj N, Miklavčič D. Dependence of induced transmembrane potential on cell density, arrangement, and cell position inside a cell system. IEEE Trans Biomed Eng 2002; 49:605–612.

7. Miklavčič D, Beravs K, Šemrov D, Čemažar M, Demšar F, Serša G. The importance of electric field distribution for effective in vivo electroporation of tissues. Biophys J 1998; 74:2152–2158.

8. Tekle E, Astumian RD, Chock PB. Selective and asymmetric molecular transport across electroporated cell membranes. Proc Natl Acad Sci USA 1994; 91:11512–11516.

9. Neumann E, Toensing K, Kakorin S, Budde P, Frey J. Mechanism of electroporative dye uptake by mouse B cells. Biophys J 1998; 74:98–108.

10. Gabriel B, Teissié J. Time courses of mammalian cell electropermeabilization observed by millisecond imaging of membrane property changes during the pulse. Biophys J 1999; 76:2158–2165.

11. Rols MP, Teissié J. Electropermeabilization of mammalian cells to macromolecules: control by pulse duration. Biophys J 1998; 75:1415–1423.

12. Satkauskas S, Bureau MF, Puc M, Mahfoudi A, Scherman D, Miklavcic D, Mir LM. Mechanisms of in vivo DNA electrotransfer: respective contributions of cell electropermeabilization and DNA electrophoresis. Mol Ther 2002; 5:133–140.

13. Rols MP, Delteil C, Golzio M, Dumond P, Cros S, Teissie J. In vivo electrically mediated protein and gene transfer in murine melanoma. Nature Biotechnol 1998; 16:168–171.

14. Sukharev SI, Klenchin VA, Serov SM, Chernomordik LV, Chizmadzhev YA. Electroporation and electrophoretic DNA transfer into cells. Biophys J 1992; 63:1320–1327.

15. Weaver JC, Chizmadzhev YA. Theory of electroporation: a review. Bioelectrochem Bioenerg 1996; 41:135–160.

16. Kakorin S, Stoylov SP, Neumann E. Electrooptics of membrane electroporation in diphenylhexatriene-doped lipid bilayer vesicles. Biophys Chem 1996; 58:109–116.

17. Marinkk SJ, Lindahl E, Edholm O, Mark AE. Simulation of the spontaneous aggregation of phospholipids into bilayers. J Am Chem Soc 2001; 123:8638–8639.

18. Kandušer M, Fošnarič M. Šentjurc M. Kralj-Iglič; V, Hägerstrand H. Iglič A, Miklavčič D. Effect of surfactant polyoxyethylene glycol ($C_{12}E_8$) on electroporation of cell line DC3F. Colloid Surf A 2003; 214:205–217.

19. Sale AJH, Hamilton WA. Effects of high electric fields on microorganisms: I. Killing of bacteria and yeasts. Biochim Biophys Acta 1967; 148:781–788.

20. Hamilton WA, Sale AJH. Effects of high electric fields on microorganisms: II. Mechanism and action of the lethal effect. Biochim Biophys Acta 1967; 148:789–800.

21. Vernhes MC, Benichou A, Pernin P, Cabanes PA, Teissié J. Elimination of free-living amoebae in fresh water with pulsed electric fields. Water Res 2002; 36:3429–3438.

22. Mouneimne Y, Tosi PF, Barhoumi R, Nicolau C. Electroinsertion of full length recombinant CD4 into red blood cell membrane. Biochim Biophys Acta 1990; 1027:53–58.

23. Raffy S, Teissie J. Electroinsertion of glycophorin A in interdigitation-fusion giant unilamellar lipid vesicles. J Biol Chem 1997; 272:25524–25530.

24. Abidor IG, Sowers AE. Kinetics and mechanism of cell membrane electrofusion. Biophys J 1992; 61:1557–1569.
25. Sowers AE. Membrane electrofusion: a paradigm for study of membrane fusion mechanisms. Methods Enzymol 1993; 220:196–211.
26. Heller R. Spectrofluorometric assay for cell-tissue electrofusion. Methods Mol Biol 1995; 48:341–353.
27. Mekid H, Mir LM. In vivo cell electrofusion. Biochim Biophys Acta 2000; 1524:118–130.
28. Scott-Taylor TH, Pettengell R, Clarke I, Stuhler G, La Barthe MC, Walden P, Dalgleish AG. Human tumour and dendritic cell hybrids generated by electrofusion: potential for cancer vaccines. Biochim Biophys Acta 2000; 1500:265–267.
29. Orentas RJ, Schauer D, Bin Q, Johnson BD. Electrofusion of a weakly immunogenic neuroblastoma with dendritic cells produces a tumor vaccine. Cell Immunol 2001; 213:4–13.
30. Schmidt E, Leinfelder U, Gessner P, Zillikens D, Bröcker EB, Zimmermann U. CD19+ B lymphocytes are the major source of human antibody-secreting hybridomas generated by electrofusion. J Immunol Methods 2001; 255:93–102.
31. Prausnitz MR, Bose VG, Langer R, Weaver JC. Electroporation of mammalian skin: A mechanism to enhance transdermal drug delivery. Proc Natl Acad Sci USA 1993; 90:10504–10508.
32. Vanbever R, Lecouturier N, Preat V. Transdermal delivery of metoprolol by electroporation. Pharmacol Res 1994; 11:1657–1662.
33. Zewert TE, Pliquett U, Langer R, Weaver JC. Transport of DNA antisense oligonucleotides across human skin by electroporation. Biochim Biophys Res Commun 1995; 212:286–292.
34. Mir LM, Orlowski S, Belehradek J, Paoletti C. Electrochemotherapy potentiation of antitumour effect of bleomycin by local electric pulses. Eur J Cancer 1991; 27:68–72.
35. Mir LM, Orlowski S, Belehradek J Jr, Teissie J, Rols MP, Sersa G, Miklavcic D, Gilbert R, Heller R. Biomedical applications of electric pulses with special emphasis on antitumor electrochemotherapy. Bioelectrochem Bioenerg 1995; 38:203–207.
36. Serša G, Čemažar M, Miklavčič D. Antitumor effectiveness of electrochemotherapy with cis-diamminedichloroplatinum(II) in mice. Cancer Res 1995; 55:3450–3455.
37. Mir LM, Glass LF, Serša G, Teissié J, Domenge C, Miklavčič D, Jaroszeski MJ, Orlowski S, Reintgen DS, Rudolf Z, Belehradek M, Gilbert R, Rols MP, Belehradek J Jr, Bachaud JM, DeConti R, Štabuc B, Čemažar M, Coninx P, Heller R. Effective treatment of cutaneous and subcutaneous malignant tumors by electrochemotherapy. Brit J Cancer 1998; 77:2336–2342.
38. Serša G, Štabuc B, Čemažar M, Milklavčič D, Rudolf Z. Electrochemotherapy with cisplatin: clinical experience in malignant melanoma patients. Clin Cancer Res 2000; 6:863–867.
39. Čemažar M, Serša G, Miklavčič D. Electrochemotherapy with cisplatin in the treatment of tumour cells resistant to cisplatin. Anticancer Res 1998; 18:4463–4466.
40. Serša G, Čemažar M, Miklavčič D, Chaplin DJ. Tumor blood flow modifying effect of electrochemotherapy with bleomycin. Anticancer Res 1999; 19:4017–4022.
41. Serša G, Čemažar M, Parkins CS, Chaplin DJ. Tumour blood flow changes induced by application of electric pulses. Eur J Cancer 1999; 35:672–677.
42. Gehl J, Skovsgaard T, Mir LM. Vascular reactions to in vivo electroporation: characterization and consequences for drug and gene delivery. Biochim Biophys Acta 2002; 1569:51–58.
43. Serša G, Kranjc S, Čemažar M. Improvement of combined modality therapy with cisplatin and radiation using electroporation of tumors. Int J Radiat Oncol Biol Phys 2000; 46:1037–1041.
44. Aihara H, Miyazaki J. Gene transfer into muscle by electroporation in vivo. Nat Biotechnol 1998; 16:867–870.
45. Mir LM, Bureau MF, Gehl J, Rangara R, Rouy D, Caillaud JM, Delaere P, Branellec D, Schwartz B, Scherman D. High efficiency gene transfer into skeletal muscle mediated by electric pulses. Proc Natl Acad Sci USA 1999; 96:4262–4267.
46. Durieux AC, Bonnefoy R, Manissolle C, Freyssenet D. High-efficiency gene electrotransfer into skeletal muscle: description and physiological applicability of a new pulse generator. Biochem Biophys Res Commun 2002; 296:443–450.

47. Rizzuto G, Cappelletti M, Maione D, Savino R, Lazzaro D, Costa P, Mathiesen I, Cortese R, Ciliberto G, Laufer R, La Monica N, Fattori E. Efficient and regulated erythropoietin production by naked DNA injection and muscle electroporation. Proc Natl Acad Sci USA 1999; 96:6417–6422.

48. Bettan M, Emmanuel F, Darteil R, Caillaud JM, Soubrier F, Delaere P, Branelec D, Mahfoudi A, Duverger N, Scherman D. High-level protein secretion into blood circulation after electric pulse-mediated gene transfer into skeletal muscle. Mol Ther 2000; 2:204–210.

49. Rols MP, Teissié J. Electropermeabilization of mammalian cells: quantitative analysis of the phenomenon. Biophys J 1990; 58:1089–1098.

50. Wolf H, Rols MP, Boldt E, Neumann E, Teissié J. Control by pulse parameters of electric field-mediated gene transfer in mammalian cells. Biophys J 1994; 66:524–531.

51. Maček-Lebar A, Kopitar NA, Ihan A, Serša G, Miklavčič D. Significance of treatment energy in cell electropermeabilization. Electro Magnetobiol 1998; 17:253–260.

52. Čemažar M, Jarm T, Miklavčič D, Maček-Lebar A, Ihan A, Kopitar NA, Serša G. Effect of electric-field intensity on electropermeabilization and electrosensitivity of various tumor-cell lines in vitro. Electro Magnetobiol 1998; 17:261–270.

53. Tomov TC. Quantitative dependence of electroporation on the pulse parameters. Bioelectrochem Bioenerg 1995; 37:101–107.

54. Chang DC. Cell poration and cell fusion using an oscillating electric field. Biophys J 1989; 56:641–652.

55. Chang DC, Gao PQ, Maxwell BL. High efficiency gene transfection by electroporation using a radio-frequency electric field. Biochim Biophys Acta 1991; 1092:153–160.

56. Tekle E, Astumian RD, Chock PB. Electroporation by using bipolar oscillating electric field: An improved method for DNA transfection of NIH 3T3 cells. Proc Natl Acad Sci USA 1991; 88:4230–4234.

57. Schoenbach KH, Peterkin FE, Alden RW, Beebe SJ. The effects of pulsed electric fields on biological cells: experiments and applications. IEEE Trans Plasma Sci 1997; 25:284–292.

58. Kotnik T, Mir LM, Flisar K, Puc M, Miklavčič D. Cell membrane electropermeabilization by symmetrical bipolar rectangular pulses. Part I. Increased efficiency of permeabilization. Bioelectrochemistry 2001; 54:83–90.

59. Kotnik T, Miklavčič D, Mir LM. Cell membrane electropermeabilization by symmetrical bipolar rectangular pulses. Part II. Reduced electrolytic contamination. Bioelectrochemistry 2001; 54:91–95.

60. Pucihar G, Mir LM, Miklavčič D. The effect of pulse repetition frequency on the uptake into electropermeabilized cells in vitro with possible applications in electrochemotherapy. Bioelectrochemistry 2002; 57:167–172.

61. Rols MP, Teissié J. Ionic-strength modulation of electrically induced permeabilization and associated fusion of mammalian cells. Eur J Biochem 1989; 179:109–115.

62. Djuzenova CS, Zimmermann U, Frank H, Sukhorukov VL, Richter E, Fuhr G. Effect of medium conductivity and composition on the uptake of propidium iodide into electropermeabilized myeloma cells. Biochim Biophys Acta 1996; 1284:143–152.

63. Pucihar G, Kotnik T, Kanduser M, Miklavčič D. The influence of medium conductivity on electropermeabilization and survival of cells in vitro. Bioelectrochemistry 2001; 54:107–115.

64. Rols MP, Teissié J. Modulation of electrically induced permeabilizaiton and fusion of Chinese hamster ovary cells by osmotic pressure. Biochemistry 1990; 29:4561–4567.

65. Golzio M, Mora MP, Raynaud C, Delteil C, Teissié J, Rols MP. Control by osmotic pressure of voltage-induced permeabilization and gene transfer in mammalian cells. Biophys J 1998; 74:3015–3022.

66. Rols MP, Delteil C, Serin G, Teissié J. Temperature effects on electrotransfection of mammalian cells. Nucleic Acids Res 1994; 22:540.

67. Miklavčič D, Šemrov D, Mekid H, Mir LM. A validated model of in vivo electric field distribution in tissues for electrochemotherapy and for DNA electrotransfer for gene therapy. Biochim Biophys Acta 2000; 1523:73–83.

68. Pliquett U, Gift EA, Weaver JC. Determination of the electric field and anomalous heating caused by exponential pulses with aluminum electrodes in electroporation experiments. Bioelectrochem Bioenerg 1996; 39:39–53.

69. Loste F, Eynard N, Teissié J. Direct monitoring of the field strength during electropulsation. Bioelectrochem Bioenerg 1998; 47:119–127.

70. Loomis-Husselbee JW, Cullen PJ, Irvine RF, Dawson AP. Electroporation can cause artefacts due to solubilizaion of cations from the electrode plates. Biochem J 1991; 277:883–885.

71. Gilbert RA, Jaroszeski MJ, Heller R. Novel electrode designs for electrochemotherapy. Biochim Biophys Acta 1997; 1334:9–14.

72. Ramirez LH, Orlowski S, An D, Bindoula G, Dzodic R, Ardouin P, Bognel C, Belehradek J, Munck JN, Mir LM. Electrochemotherapy on liver tumours in rabbits. Brit J Cancer 1998; 12:2104–2111.

73. Puc M, Reberšek S, Miklavčič D. Requirements for a clinical electrochemotherapy device—electroporator. Radiol Oncol 1997; 31:368–373.

41

Electroporation Therapy: Treatment of Cancer and Other Therapeutic Applications

Dietmar Rabussay and Georg Widera[*]

Genetronics, Inc., San Diego, California, U.S.A.

Martin Burian

University of Vienna Medical School, Vienna, Austria

The principles of electroporation and its advantages of other drug delivery systems for both the prevention and treatment of a wide variety of disorders are discussed. Specific agents and approaches that have been used are reviewed. Experience in the treatment of malignancies is emphasized and other potential clinical applications are presented.

I. INTRODUCTION

Drugs whose effectiveness depends on transmembrane access to the cell interior are often severely limited by their inability to effectively permeate the cell membrane. The methods employed to enhance membrane permeation include chemical modification of the drug (1), appropriate drug formulation (2), and mechanical disturbance or disruption of the membrane (3,4).

A more recent method, known as *electroporation*, or *electropermeabilization* (EP), makes use of short electrical pulses to temporarily increase membrane permeabilization. This method has proven highly effective in increasing transmembrane flux of therapeutically important substances such as anticancer drugs and DNA, by two to four orders of magnitude, without causing significant side effects (5–9). In this chapter we will describe clinical results achieved with EP, as well as selected results from in vitro and animal experiments that open up exciting new clinical approaches.

---

* *Current affiliation*: ALZA Corporation, Mountain View, California, U.S.A.

II. ELECTROPORATION

Early indications of EP were derived 30 to 40 years ago from observations of bacterial cell death and permeabilization of artificial membranes, respectively, after exposure to high electrical fields (10,11). The first application of this phenomenon, the effective delivery of DNA to bacterial cells, was reported in 1982 (12). Ever since, this method has been a valuable tool for in vitro delivery of small and large molecules, particularly DNA, into a large variety of cells (13). Over the last 15 years, EP has also been performed on living plants, animals, and humans (in vivo EP), with an increasing focus on therapeutic uses (7,9,14).

Mechanistic models of EP have been reviewed several times in recent years (15–18). Therefore we will only summarize this subject briefly and direct the reader to these review articles, as well as Chapter 40 in this volume. Electroporation of biological lipid bilayer membranes as evidenced by increased mass transport across the membrane requires electrical pulses of a certain field strength and duration. Both of these parameters must exceed threshold values in order for EP to occur. Depending on the type of cells to be electroporated and the type of molecules to be delivered into the cells, the necessary (nominal) field strengths range from 100 V/cm to several thousand V/cm, and pulse durations vary from approximately 100 μs to tens of milliseconds (ms). Other factors influencing the EP process include size and shape of the cell, the electrical conductivity inside and outside the cell, the thickness and conductivity of the membrane, and mechanical stress on the membrane. Poration of the membrane does not occur uniformly over the surface of the cell. Maximal poration occurs at the "pole caps" (apexes) of the cell in the direction of the external field vector.

Despite extensive experiments and theoretical work the exact mechanism of EP is not well understood, yet interesting medical applications are emerging. The most widely accepted mechanistic model of EP postulates the formation of "primary" hydrophobic and hydrophilic pores of approximately 1 nm diameter. Depending on the pulse conditions and the ionic and molecular environment on either side of the membrane these primary pores may enlarge, reseal, stay open for certain periods of time, or facilitate passive or electromotive transport of ions and molecules through the pores. Permeating molecules encompass low- and high-molecular-weight entities, including DNA. The pore model (pores have not been directly proven) may be too simplistic, at least for electro-permeabilization involving macromolecules such as DNA. This is reflected in significantly different optimal pulse conditions for transmembrane delivery of relatively small molecules (drugs) and large ones (plasmid DNA). Field strengths of approximately 1000 V/cm and pulse lengths of approximately 100 μs are optimal for delivering the drug bleomycin to mammalian cancer cells (5,19), whereas 200 V/cm or less, and tens of milliseconds are optimal for DNA (9). Recently, electropermeabilization of membranes has been achieved with submicrosecond pulses of very high field strengths (tens to hundreds of KV/cm) (20,21) and with alternating current as well (22).

III. ELECTROPORATION THERAPIES

The term *electroporation therapy* (EPT) has been coined to describe the delivery of therapeutic agents across membrane barriers through EP (5,23). The first report foreshadowing the potentially broad use of EP for therapeutic purposes was published by Okino and Mohri in 1987 (24). The authors treated tumor-bearing mice with intramuscular injection of bleomycin and observed retardation of tumor growth only when the tumor was electroporated after drug administration. Four years later, first results of the treatment of cancerous skin lesions in humans, also with bleomycin and EP, were published (25). The authors named the combined treatment with an anticancer drug and EP electrochemotherapy (ECT). Subsequently, several groups treated a variety of cancers in animal models and humans using various drugs and EP conditions (see Sec. IV). In addition, EP was used for imaginative new approaches to treat diseases other than cancer (see Sec. V). Electroporation is distinct from a method called "electrochemical treatment," which has also been used for cancer treatment but employs lower electrical field strengths that don't induce membrane poration (25b). In this chapter, we will use the general term EPT for various electroporation therapies. Specific prefixes will designate specific therapies, e.g., we will use B-EPT for EPT with bleomycin. ECT will be used for the treatment of cancer with drugs delivered by EP.

Electroporation therapy can be performed ex vivo or in vivo. For ex vivo therapies autologous or heterologous cells suspended in aqueous solutions are mixed together with the agent to be transferred into the cells. The suspension is placed between electrodes that can be energized to deliver short, high-voltage EP pulses to permeabilize the cell membranes and allow the therapeutic agent access to the cell interior. After a brief period the cell membrane reseals and the "loaded' cells are either further processed before being administered to the patient, or they can be directly transferred to the patient's body (26). To date, two brief ex vivo Phase I clinical studies have been performed (Sec. V). For in vivo therapy, the therapeutic agent is administered to the patient either systemically or to the site to be treated, followed by EP of the target tissue. Extensive in vivo clinical studies have been conducted on ECT of solid tumors (Sec. IV.F).

IV. ELECTROCHEMOTHERAPY OF CANCER[*]

A. Rationale

It is well known that dosing of chemotherapeutic drugs is limited by their toxic side effects. Administration of limited doses results in corresponding limited systemic drug concentrations, which, in turn, frequently result in insufficient concentrations inside the tumor cells to achieve the desired therapeutic effect. Electroporation of tumor tissue can enhance intracellular drug concentrations to levels that are up to several thousandfold higher than can be obtained in conventional chemotherapy (29,30). Therefore, high intracellular concentrations can be reached in the electroporated tumor cells with relatively low extracellular drug concentrations (8,31).

Since EP enhances cell membrane permeability only transiently, the drug molecules that have entered the cell get trapped when the membrane reseals, thus greatly increasing intracellular drug residence time and efficacy. This results in relatively high local therapeutic efficacy in the absence of systemic toxic side effects. Considering these factors, it follows that drugs with high intrinsic intracellular cytotoxicity and poor cell membrane permeation, such as bleomycin, will show the greatest gain in efficacy when combined with EP.

B. Drugs for ECT

Since the first electrochemotherapy paper appeared over 14 years ago (24), the effect of EP on the activity of different drugs against many specific cancer types has been tested in vitro and in vivo. The effect of EP in vitro can be expressed as the cytotoxicity enhancement ratio

---

* Review articles on this subject include Refs. 5, 6, 8, 19, 27, and 28.

(CER). The CER represents the drug dose necessary to kill 50% of the cells in the absence of EP (LD_{50}) divided by the drug dose required to kill 50% of the cells in the presence of EP ($LD_{50,\ EP}$). For different drugs this ratio varies from 1.0 (no enhancement) to 2500 or more and depends on the cancer cell line tested (5,32). A low CER can either result from a drug that readily passes through the cell membrane without EP [e.g., 5-fluorouracil (5-FU)] or from a drug whose permeation is not enhanced by EP. Suramin may be an example for the latter (5).

In vivo, the effectiveness of EP can be determined by tumor response (growth, shrinkage, or disappearance) or by survival rate. Usually, such tests are performed with human tumors grown subcutaneously in immune-compromised mice. Tumor responses are scored as complete response (CR; no detectable tumor); partial response (PR, tumor volume reduction of 50% or more); objective response (OR, the sum of CR and PR scores); no change (NC, less than 50% tumor volume reduction or less than 25% increase); progressive disease (PD, appearance of new lesions, or increase in tumor volume of more than 25% since beginning of treatment) (33).

Table 1 summarizes the effect of EP on the anticancer activity of different drugs against specific cancer types, tested in vitro and in vivo. Drugs that show enhanced anticancer activity in combination with EP are printed in bold letters; regular type means no enhancement of anticancer activity by EP. Among the drugs tested, bleomycin is exceptional. Bleomycin efficacy is enhanced for every tumor type tested, varying from several hundred to several thousand fold, depending on tumor type. More importantly, the combination of bleomycin and EP yielded the highest antitumor efficacy in essentially all cases. Cisplatin produced CERs between 2 and 10, depending on tumor type, and was the second most effective drug with EP. Out of a total of 22 drugs tested eleven more also yielded enhanced efficacies in combination with EP. Three other drugs showed marginal enhancements.

In vitro results are generally predictive of in vivo results. Exceptions include Carboplatin for melanoma (36), and cisplatin and 5-FU for colorectal cancer (64,66). Also, in most but not all cases, EP enhances the efficacy of a particular drug across all cancer types tested (Table 1). Aside from exceptional cases such as 5-FU, it has not been possible to predict from the physicochemical properties of a drug to what extent its efficacy will be enhanced by EP.

C. Bleomycins

As mentioned, bleomycin is the most effective drug for EPT found so far. Therefore, we will briefly summarize its characteristics. The drug bleomycin marketed in the United States and other countries under different brand names consists of a mixture of eleven molecular species that differ in their terminal amine region. The most prevalent species is A2. All bleomycin components are water-soluble glycopeptide antibiotics of approximately 1500 Da (31). The relatively high hydrophilicity and molecular weight probably account to a large extent for the drug's poor membrane permeation in the absence of EP. However, its high intrinsic cytotoxicity accounts for its exceptional efficacy when ready access to the cell interior is made possible by EP (30). Bleomycins chelate a variety of divalent heavy metal ions and cleave single- and double-stranded DNA and RNA at preferred sequences with high efficiency (31,79,80). The cytotoxicity of bleomycin is considered to be mainly due to DNA double strand breaks induced by free radicals generated by the active bleomycin-Fe^{2+} complex (81,82). In addition to cleaving nucleic acids in the target cells, other effects induced by bleomycin may also contribute to its exceptional efficacy (see Sec. IV.G).

Table 1 Enhancement of Anticancer Activity of Different Drugs by Electroporation Against Various Cancers In Vitro and In Vivo

No.	Cancer type	In vitro[a,b]	In vivo[a,b]
1	Squamous cell carcinoma	(34)**B**; (35)**B**; (36)**B**; Cis, **Carbo**, **Mito**, **Dox**, Vin; (38)and (39)**Borocaptate**	(23)**B**; (37)**B**
2	Tongue (orthotopic)	—	(40)**B**; (41)**B**; (42)**B**
3	Basal cell		
4	Melanoma	(36)**B**, Cis, Carbo, Mito, **Dox**, Vin, (32)**B**, **Cis**	(43)**B**; (44)**B**; (45)**B**; (36)**B**, **Cis**, **Carbo**
5	Pancreas	(46)**Saporin**; (32)**B**, **Cis**, **Carbo**, **Cytarab**, Mito, Vin, Vinbl	(47)**B**, **Cis**, Sur, Neo; (48)**B**, **Mito**, **Carbo**; (49)**B**; (46)**Saporin**
6	Liver	(32)**B**, **Cis**, **Carbo**, Dox, FU*	(24)**B**; (50)**B**; (51)**B**; (52)**B**; (53)and (49)**B**, **Cis**, FU, Dox; (54)**B**; (42)**B**; (55)**Bcl-2**
7	Liver metastases of colorectal cancer	—	(56)**B**
8	Prostate	(57)**B**	(57)**B**
9	Brain (glioma)	(58)**B**, **Carbo**, Nim, Eto, Vin	(59)**B**
10	Breast	(60)**B**; (32)**B**, **Cis**, **Carbo**, **Vin**, Vinbl*, Pac*, Tax	(61)**B**
11	Colorectal	(62)**B**; (63)**B**, Mito, Dox; (64)**B**, Cis, FU, (66)**B**, Cis, FU	(62)**B**; (63)**B**; (65)**B**; (64)**B**, **Cis**, FU*; (67)**B**
12	Bladder	(68)**B**, **Cis**, Adria	(68)**B**, Cis*, Adria; (69)**B**
13	Lung	(46)**Saporin**; (70)**B**, **Cis**, **Carbo**, Dauno, Dox, Eto, Pac; (32)**B**, Cis, Carbo, **Dox***	(71)**B**; (72)**B**; (46)**Saporin** (73)**Pep**, **Cis**, **Cyclo**, **Mito**
14	Cervix	(74)**B**, **Cis**, **Adria**, **Mito**, **Cyclo**	(74)**B**, **Cis**, **Adria**, **Mito**, **Cyclo**
15	Uterus	—	(75)**B**
16	Ovarian	(32)**B**, **Cis**, **Carbo**, **Vin***, Vinbl, **Mito**, **Dox**, Pac, Tax	
17	Soft tissue sarcoma	—	(76)**B**; (G.S. Nanda and D. Rabussay, unpublished)**B**
18	Adeno	(32)**B**, **Cis**	(77)**B**
19	Fibrosarcoma		(78)**TPZ**[c]

[a] Enhancement of the efficacy of 22 different drugs by electroporation against various cancers was tested in vitro and in vivo. Drugs that gained significant anticancer activity are printed in bold letters; drugs whose activity was marginally enhanced are marked with an asterisk*; and drugs printed in normal type showed no efficacy enhancement. Numbers in parentheses correspond to literature references.

[b] Adria, adriamycin; B, bleomycin; Bcl-2, bcl-2 antisense oligonucleotide; Carbo, carboplatin; Cis, cisplatin; Cytarab, Cytarabin; Cyclo, Cyclophosphamide; Dauno, daunorubicin; Dox, doxorubicine; Eto, etoposide; FU, 5-fluorouracil; Mito, mitocycin; Neo, neocarcinostatin; Nim, nimustine; Pac, Paxlitaxel; Pep, Peplomycin; Sur, suramin; Tax, taxotere; TPZ, tirapazamine; Vin, vincristine; Vinbl, vinblastine;

[c] Enhanced antitumor effect is only observed when TPZ is given 20 minutes prior to electroporation. The effect is possibly due to enhanced tumor hypoxia resulting from electroporation-induced diminished tumor blood flow in combination with TPZ's hypoxic bioreductive activity. The effect does not appear to be due to electroporation-enhanced permeation of TPZ across the cell membrane.

Besides the widely marketed heterogeneous bleomycin product isolated from *Streptomyces verticillus* fermentation broth, a largely pure subspecies of bleomycin, A5, has been produced using a subspecies of *S. verticillus*. This compound, marketed as Pingyangmycin, has shown increased efficacy in combination with EP against human prostate tumors in mice (83). The properties of subspecies A2 and deglycosylated A2 in combination with EP have also been investigated (82).

D. Drug Administration and Pharmacokinetics

Intravenous (i.v.), intratumoral (i.t.), intraperitoneal (i.p.), and other parenteral drug administration routes have been used in ECT. Tumors differ from healthy tissue by elevated interstitial pressure, typically in the range of 10–40 mm Hg. The pressure gradient from tumor to normal tissue diminishes the effectiveness of i.v. drug delivery into the tumor (84). Another disadvantage of i.v. injection is the systemic rather than local administration of relatively high doses of drug, which is prone to cause chemotherapeutic side effects. Early animal and human studies successfully used i.v. injection, but later comparative studies resulted in a preference for i.t. delivery (44,71,85–89). When injecting drug intratumorally, it is important to inject the tumor as homogeneously as possible. This can be achieved by employing a "fanning" technique (90), by pushing drug into the tissue while slowly retracting the needle, and by using multiple injection sites for larger tumors.

In some studies 1% lidocaine–epinephrine (1:200,000) was injected into the tissue surrounding the tumor prior to bleomycin injection for the purpose of slowing washout of the drug from the tumor (71,85,88,91). In mouse studies, lidocaine–epinephrine injection had no effect on tissue response and efficacy of EPT (G.S. Nanda and D. Rabussay, unpublished). Drug is injected into the tumor generally several minutes before EP, although injections up to 30 min before or after EP were reported to be effective (44,45,92).

The recommended dose of bleomycin in conventional chemotherapy is 0.25–0.50 U/kg (17.5–35 U for a 70 kg human) once or twice weekly, by one of several parenteral routes (93). However, the approved routes of administration differ from country to country. The maximum recommended cumulative lifetime dose of bleomycin is 400 units. Various doses and modes of drug injection have been used in different ECT clinical studies (summarized in Refs. 5 and 28). Standard conditions used in Genetronics' FDA-authorized Phase II clinical studies for the treatment of recurrent squamous cell carcinomas of the head and neck (SCCHN) included the i.t. injection of 0.25 ml of a 4 U/ml bleomycin solution per cm^3 tumor volume (91). These conditions were based on animal experiments and early clinical studies (44,85,86,94). Later studies with HEp-2 tumors in mice confirmed these conditions as meeting minimal effective dose criteria (see Ref. 91 and G.S. Nanda and D. Rabussay, unpublished).

The pharmocokinetic behavior of bleomycin upon i.v. bolus injection is quite well known. The drug does not bind to serum proteins and the plasma elimination half-life is 2–4 h in patients with normal renal function (4–6 h after continuous infusion). Bleomycin elimination is primarily by renal excretion. In patients with normal renal function 50–70% of the drug appears in the urine within 24 h after administration (93). After injection of [57]Co-labeled bleomycin into SCCs of the oral cavity of patients, 27 % and 95% of the drug, respectively, were detectable in the blood 10 min and 1 h later, respectively. For unknown reasons, the residence time of the drug was significantly prolonged in some of the tumors (95).

Pharmacokinetic data for bleomycin delivery by EP in humans are not available, yet some data derived from animal and in vitro experiments exist. Electroporation increases the accumulation of bleomycin in uterine leiomyosarcoma tissue in mice about 10-fold 1 h after treatment (75) and also in colorectal tumor tissue (64). Ceberg et al. (96) provided evidence for two- and tenfold increases of boronated porphyrin and sulfhydryl boron hydride, respectively, in glial tumors after EP, whereas the corresponding increase in normal brain tissue was much lower. The application of electric pulses was also found to increase and prolong the entrapment of sodium borocaptate in mouse melanoma tumors (97). Engstrom et al. obtained a similar result with [^{111}In]bleomycin in brain tumors (98). Increased drug uptake occurred immediately after EP and the amount of labeled bleomycin remained at a constant ratio between tumor and normal tissue over several days. A similar study with LPB tumors in mice also found elevated bleomycin levels in electroporated tumor tissue compared to nonelectroporated tissue (99). In VX-2 tumors in rabbits, intratumoral injection of [^{111}In]bleomycin resulted in significant levels of drug remaining in the electroporated tumors for three hrs, whereas the drug was almost completely washed out of non-electroporated tumors after only 60 min (100). Cemazar et al. have shown that the amount of both cisplatin in the tumor and bound to DNA is enhanced by EP and that antitumor activity correlates with cisplatin accumulation. Interestingly, tumors resistant to cisplatin in the absence of EP also accumulated the drug intratumorally and intracellularly after EP and were subject to its antitumor effect (101).

Direct measurements of enhanced intracellular drug concentrations in tumor cells in vitro support the above results obtained in various tissues (30,34,39,66,68). Taken together, the in vitro and in vivo results are consistent with the rationale put forward in Sec. IV.A that EP allows increased uptake of the drug during membrane permeabilization and the drug is retained inside the cells after the membrane reseals, while drug present in the interstitial space is washed out relatively quickly.

E. Devices for Electrochemotherapy

A basic electroporation system consists of a pulse generator and an applicator (Fig. 1). The applicator contains the electrodes that are brought in contact with the target tissue and allows the operator to safely deliver the high-voltage, high-current pulses to the treatment site. In addition, accessory instrumentation may be used, such as oscilloscopes, electronic data storage devices and printers to measure and record pulse parameters, treatment times, and other data.

Figure 1 is a schematic representation of the therapy process. The drug is preferentially injected into the tumor, taking care that the drug is distributed as evenly as possible throughout the tumor. In some studies the drug has been delivered intravenously or by other parenteral routes. Subsequently, electroporation is performed using an electroporation therapy system consisting of a pulse generator and an applicator. Shown here is the MedPulser® system. The generator produces the electrical pulse according to specifications programmed into a chip located in the applicator. The applicator contains six needle electrodes, which are inserted into the tumor. The MedPulser system delivers six electrical pulses per treatment cycle, sequentially activating three different double pairs of needles, resulting in the electrical field patterns shown schematically in Fig. 1. Each double pair of needless is pulsed twice, with reversion of electrode polarities after the first pulse (only one polarity is shown here). Electroporation causes permeabilization of the cell membranes (shown as white rings) so that drug molecules (depicted as white dots) can enter the cell efficiently. After the pulses, the cell membrane reseals, trapping the drug molecules inside. The action of the internalized drug molecules results in cell death.

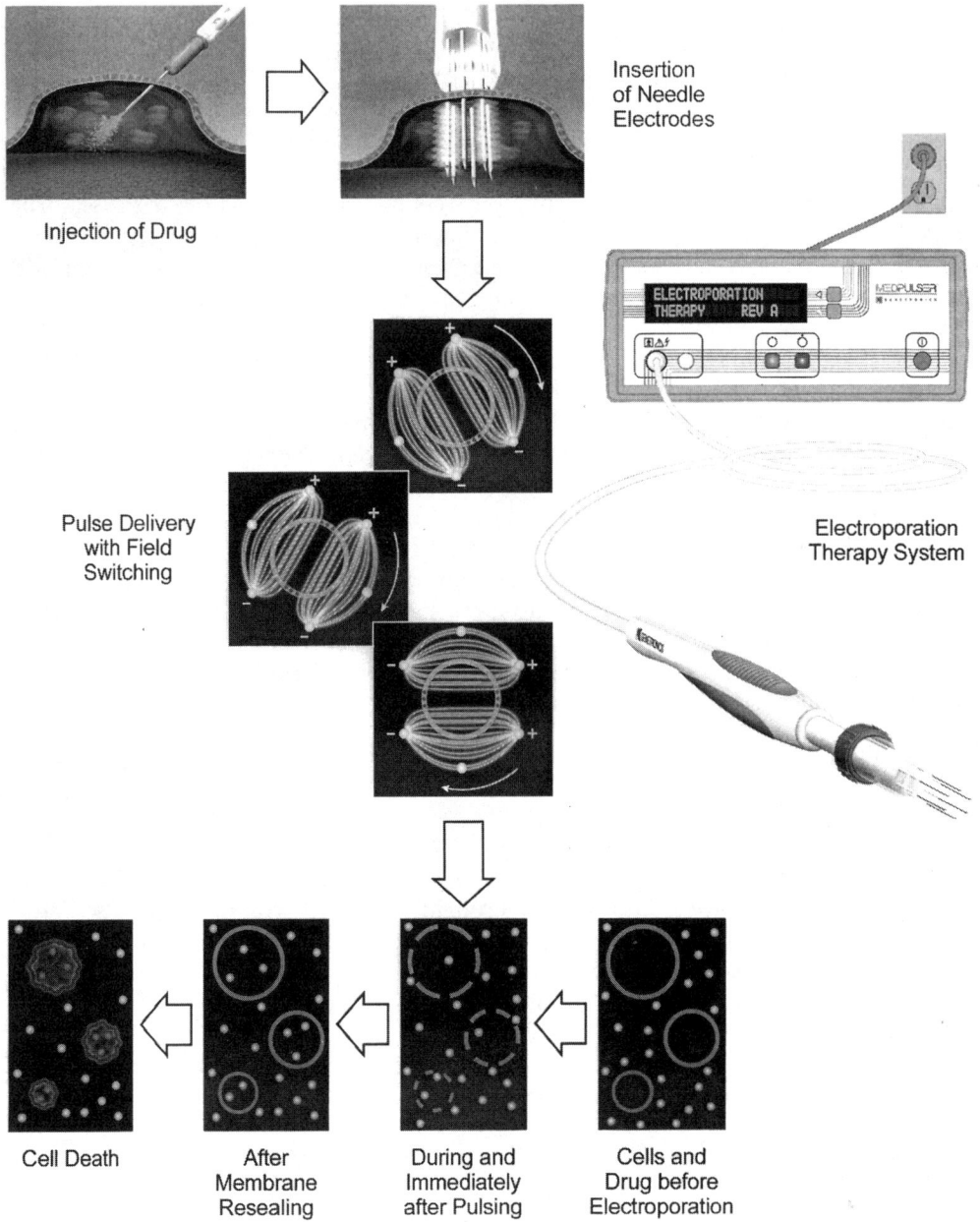

Injection of Drug

Insertion
of Needle
Electrodes

Pulse Delivery
with Field
Switching

Electroporation
Therapy System

Cell Death

After
Membrane
Resealing

During and
Immediately
after Pulsing

Cells and
Drug before
Electroporation

Figure 1 Schematic representation of the electroporation therapy process. (See process description given in text.)

1. Pulse Generators

Early ECT treatments were performed with relatively simple generators designed for research purposes rather than for clinical applications. Some of these instruments delivered exponential pulses generated by discharge capacitors. Such pulses are not very suitable for in vivo applications since the pulse duration and current flow will vary depending on the resistance of the tissue and the surface area and distance of the electrodes. On the other hand, well-designed square-pulse generators allow to preset exact amplitudes and pulse durations independent of variations in tissue resistance and electrode configuration.

The only pulse generator approved to date for therapeutic purposes in Europe and for clinical investigational use in the United States is the MedPulser (Genetronics, Inc., San Diego, CA) (Fig. 1). This instrument delivers square wave pulses of predetermined voltage, duration, and polarity to a six-needle-array applicator; it automatically generates a pulse cycle of six pulses of 100 μs each, delivered at 4 Hz, at a nominal field strength of 1300 V/cm (35). The nominal field strength (V/cm) is the applied voltage (V) divided by the distance of the corresponding electrodes in centimeters. Two parallel needle pairs each are energized simultaneously during each pulse. The polarity and direction of the pulses are varied in such a pattern as to achieve more uniform and effective EP of the tissue within the six-needle array than would be possible with a single pulse or multiple pulses of the same polarity and direction. Directed by a microchip in the applicator, the MedPulser automatically selects the pulse parameters for each type of applicator plugged into this instrument. The same microchip also records data on how and when the applicator was used. Applicators are selected by the surgeon as needed for a particular treatment. The MedPulser also contains hardware and software to assure the safety and accuracy of the treatment and guides the surgeon through the procedure with prompts on the display screen.

2. Applicators

Applicators contain the electrodes that determine the geometry and strength of the electrical field in a particular tissue when a pulse is delivered. In early animal and clinical studies plate (caliper) electrodes were used which consisted of two parallel metal plates of fixed or adjustable distance that can be placed on each side of the tumor. Measuring the distance between the plates allows for easy calculation of the nominal field strength. Plate electrodes have the theoretical advantage of generating a rather homogeneous field. However, the tumor does not fill the space between plates homogeneously. The resulting inhomogeneous field may be insufficient to electroporate the entire tumor. Tumors close to a surface can be treated with this design (25,85,102), although arcing and burns affecting the skin may occur. Efficacy can be improved by rotating the position of the plate electrodes 90 degrees between pulses, thus electroporating cells sequentially in perpendicular fields (103).

The limitations of plate electrodes can be overcome by using needle electrodes that are inserted into the target tissue and allow deeper seated tumors to be effectively electroporated. The invasiveness of needle electrodes is a slight disadvantage, yet it is presently the only feasible approach for generating the critical field strength in larger, subsurface tissue volumes. Single pairs of needles have the disadvantage of generating a relatively inhomogeneous field and electroporating a relatively small tissue volume (71). To overcome this limitation, multineedle arrays have been designed that have proven very effective (71,104,105). Most notably, a six-needle array, energized via a suitable switching pattern (Fig. 1) allows an area of approximately 1 cm² to be covered with fields of acceptable homogeneity and field strength (5,23,48,71,85,86,104,106). As shown by computer generated field plots (5,71) the minimum efficacious field strength of approximately 600 V/cm can easily be achieved with a six-needle array of 1 cm diameter (needles are placed equidistantly around a circle of 1 cm diameter) when pulses of 1130 V are applied in a pattern shown in Fig. 1. An increase in the array diameter is not advisable because the higher voltage necessary to achieve the desired field strength over longer distances between needles would cause unacceptable side effects.

F. Clinical Results

1. Scope

The goal of the clinical studies was to explore the safety, efficacy, clinical feasibility, and merit of this new treatment modality. These studies have now spanned more than a decade and have been performed at over two dozen cancer centers in 11 countries. Studies were either initiated by clinical researchers or by Genetronics Biomedical. The results of 198 treated patients with 635 evaluable lesions have been published (Tables 2 to 5). In addition, we are aware of at least 90 more patients who received ECT, for whom results have not yet been published. Table 6 summarizes the published results of patients and lesions treated per cancer type. The lesions treated included (1) primary tumors (SCCHN, and basal cell carcinoma, BCC), (2) recurrent and/or refractory tumors (SCCHN, adenocarcinomas, BCC), (3) and metastatic lesions (primarily cutaneous) of SCCHN, melanoma, adenocarcinoma, breast, hypernephroma, and transitional cell carcinoma.

ECT has evolved from the treatment of cutaneous permeation nodules with intravenous bleomycin and plate electrodes (e.g., Ref. 102) to the treatment of larger and deeper tumors with intratumoral drug administration and efficient six-needle array electrodes (91,109,112). The development and applications of improved techniques has largely been discussed in Sec. IV.B to IV.E. In addition to surface-accessible tumors, ECT has also been applied to internal tumors that required surgical intervention for drug injection and needle electrode insertions. This was the case for certain head and neck tumors (94,108,109), as well as liver and pancreatic tumors (M. Chazal, personal communication, 1999). The majority of skin lesions, including cutaneous metastases of various cancers, has been treated under local anesthesia or under sedation (19,27). ECT of head and neck carcinomas was usually performed under general anesthesia (91,109).

In the following sections and in Tables 2 to 5 we have attempted to describe every patient who has so far been treated with ECT and for whom results have been published. We have also taken care to count every patient only once even though the same patient may have been included in more than one publication.

2. EPT with Intratumoral Bleomycin

In the context of EPT, intratumoral injection of bleomycin has yielded increased tumor response rates compared to intravenous drug delivery (44,71,85–89). The intratumoral drug dose for most tumors was 1 U/cm^3 tumor volume (slightly different doses were used by Reintgen et al. (88) and Rodriguez-Cuevas et al. (107)), while intravenous doses used for ECT were mostly 18 or 27 U/m^2, respectively (19). Thus, for smaller tumors the intratumoral drug dose is lower than the dose given intravenously. Treatment results for 138 patients with a total of 306 lesions treated with intratumoral bleomycin and EP have been reported in the medical literature (Table 2).

Three patients treated with cutaneous SCC showed partial responses to this treatment modality (Table 2, lines 1 and 2). The largest patient group consisted of 81 SCCHN patients with 96 treated noncutaneous lesions (lines 3–6). Of these lesions 27% responded completely, 35% partially, and 38% did not change significantly. Twelve patients with recurrent

SCCHN who had failed previous therapies were treated at Rush Presbyterian-St. Luke's Medical Center, Chicago, IL, in a study initiated by Genetronics (Table 2, lines 3 and 4). The objective response rate was 83% and a remarkable 50% of the lesions responded completely. The results of a Phase II study designed by Genetronics and performed at about a dozen centers in the United States, Canada, and France are shown on line 5. The initial portion of that study involved treatment of 37 tumors in 25 patients with intratumoral bleomycin, without EP. Only one of the 37 tumors showed a partial response. These tumors and patients are not included on line 5 of Table 2. However, the 17 patients of that group (20 tumors) who crossed over to treatment with bleomycin-EPT (B-EPT) are included on line 5. In addition, another 37 patients who were not candidates for salvage therapy and who suffered from 49 refractory or locoregionally recurring tumors were enrolled.

The standard B-EPT treatment procedure included intratumoral injection of a 4-U/ml bleomycin solution at 0.25 ml/cm^3 tumor tissue. Ten minutes later, a six-needle array electrode was inserted into the tumor and one cycle of EP pulses was delivered (see Sec. IV.E.1). For tumors larger than the volume that fits between the electrodes of a six-needle array, electrode insertion and pulsing were repeated in an overlapping pattern, such that the entire tumor volume was electroporated. Of the 69 lesions treated, 57% yielded an objective response and 25% responded completely. These response rates compare favorably with those obtained with similar patient populations treated with various single and multiple drug regimens (122). Median survival time of the North American patients (42 subjects, 51 treated tumors) was 6.4 months, with 2 years and 11 months as the longest survival time.

The results of 12 patients with primary SCCHN (line 6) are discussed in Sec. IV.F.5. Thirty-six patients with 71 primary BCC were treated at three different centers (Table 2, lines 7–9), the majority of them at the Moffit Cancer Center, in Tampa, FL (line 8). All lesions showed an objective response. The average complete response rate was 91.5% after 1 month. Among the Tampa patients, no recurrences were observed after a mean observation period of 20 months (87). The increase from 17% to 94% in CR rates with intratumoral vs. intravenous drug administration was striking (85,87). After retreatment of three partial responders 53 of the 54 lesions treated at Tampa had responded completely (87). These results, together with the ease of the procedure and the superior cosmetic outcome, make B-EPT a potentially attractive alternative to the present standard therapy of surgical excision. However, additional clinical studies with longer follow-up periods will be required to determine the full potential of this procedure. B-EPT of BCC may also be useful as an adjuvant to surgery for large or multiple tumors or for inoperable tumors (113).

Skin and soft tissue metastases of malignant melanoma were also successfully treated at three different sites (average OR: 97%; average CR: 82%; lines 10–12). The tumors disappeared within 2–3 weeks after therapy. No recurrences at the treated sites were reported during the 20-month mean follow-up period (7–27 months). However, no preventive effect was seen for new metastases at nontreated sites (87). An interesting application of B-ECT is the stopping of bleeding of ulcerating and bleeding metastases. Bleeding stopped immediately and the lesions regressed fully (114).

In addition to SCC, BCC and melanoma metastases, small numbers of other cancer types were treated, with all treatments yielding 100% objective responses (lines 13–16). Thus the clinical results support the conclusion from in vitro and animal studies (Table 1) that B-EPT is potentially an effective treatment for a large variety of solid tumors.

3. EPT with Intravenous Bleomycin

A total of 201 treated nodules of 37 patients were evaluable in the published studies using intravenous bleomycin and parallel plate electrodes (Table 3). Of these nodules 163 shrank

Table 2 Intratumoral Bleomycin ECT Clinical Study Results

No.	Reference[a]	Cancer type[b]	No. of patients	No. of tumors treated	Electrode type[b]	Clinical tumor responses[b] (%)			
						NC	PR	CR	OR
1	Reintgen et al., 1996 (88); Heller et al., 1998 (87)	SCC	1	1	Six-needle array	0	100	0	100
2	Rodriguez-Cuevas et al., 2001 (107)	SCC[c]	2	2	Six-needle array	0	100	0	100
3	Panje et al., 1998, 2000 (94,108)	SCCHN	8	8	Six-needle array	25	25	50	75
4	Allegretti & Panje, 2001 (109)	SCCHN	4[d]	4	Six-needle array	0	50	50	100
5	Rabussay et al., 2003 (91); Goldfarb et al., 1999, 2002 (110,111)	SCCHN	54[e]	69	Six-needle array	43	32	25	57
6	Burian et al., 2002 (112)	SCCHN	12[f]	12	Six-needle array	See Table 5			
7	Greenway (unpublished) (cited in Ref. 5)	BCC	7	8	Six-needle array	0	12.5	87.5	100
8	Reintgen et al., 1996 (88); Glass et al., 1997 (113); Heller et al., 1998 (87); Heller et al., 2000 (27)	BCC	5	13	Parallel plates	0	7.7[g]	92.3	100
			15	41	Six-needle array	0	5[g]	95	100
9	Rodriguez-Cuevas et al., 2001 (107)	BCC	9	9	Six-needle array	0	22	78	100

No.	Reference	Tumor type			Electrode	% NC	% PR	% CR	% OR
10	Glass et al., 1996 (86); Reintgen et al., 1996 (88); Heller et al., 1998 (87); Heller et al., 2000 (27)	Melanoma	2	8	Parallel plates	0	0	100	100
			10	76	Six-needle array	1.3	10.5	88.2	98.7
11	Gehl et al., 2000, (114)	Melanoma	1	9	Needle rows	0	0	100	100
12	Rodriguez-Cuevas et al., 2001 (107)	Melanoma	2	9	Six-needle array	15	61	23	85
13	Panje, 1998 (94)	Adeno[h]	2	2	Six-needle array	0	50	50	100
14	Rodriguez-Cuevas et al., 2001 (107)	Breast cancer	2	14	Six-needle array	0	42	58	100
15	Reintgen et al., 1996 (88); Heller et al., 1998 (87)	Kaposi's sarcoma	1	4	Parallel plates	0	n.s.	n.s.	100
16	Kubota et al., 1998 (115)	Transitional cell carcinoma	1	17	n.s.	0	0	100[i]	100

[a] Where more than one publication per line is given, some or all of the patients described in these publications are the same.

[b] n.s., not stated; BCC, basal cell carcinoma; SCC, squamous cell carcinoma; SCCHN, squamous cell carcinoma of the head and neck; NC, no change; PR, partial response; CR, complete response; OR, objective response.

[c] Cancer of the upper aerodigestive tract metastatic to skin.

[d] In addition to the patients described before in Panje et al., 1998 (94)and 2000 (108), treatment of four new patients is described in this paper.

[e] Phase II multicenter study in the United States, Canada, and France.

[f] Treat-and-resect study of primary tumors (see Table 5).

[g] After retreatment with B-EPT, two of the three partial responders responded completely.

[h] One adenocarcinoma of the ethnoid sinus (PR) and one adenoid cystic carcinoma of the parotid (CR).

[i] Fourteen cutaneous metastases of transitional cell carcinoma disappeared completely. The other three lesions partially regressed, and three months later autopsy specimens revealed complete sterilization with no viable cancer cells detected.

Table 3 Intravenous Bleomycin ECT Clinical Study Results[a]

No.	Reference[b]	Cancer type[c]	No. of patients	No. of tumors treated	Clinical tumor responses[c] (%)			
					NC	PR	CR	OR
1	Mir et al., 1991 (25); Belehradek, 1993 (102)	SCCHN[d]	8	42	31	14	55	69
2	Domenge et al., 1996 (116)	SCCHN[d]	5	19[f,g]	53	26	21	47
3	Mir et al., 1998 (19)	SCCHN[e]	3	10	60[h]	30	10	40
4	Mir et al., 1998 (19); Rols et al., 2000 (92)	SCCHN[e]	1	6	0	17	83	100
5	Heller et al., 1996 (85); Reintgen et al., 1996 (88); Glass et al., 1996 (106); Mir et al., 1998 (19)	BCC	2	6[i]	0	83	17	100
6	Rudolf et al., 1995 (117); Mir et al., 1998[j] (19)	Melanoma	7	30	10	10	80	90
7	Heller et al., 1996 (85); Reintgen et al., 1996 (88); Mir et al., 1998 (19)	Melanoma	3[k]	10[i]	50	20	30	50
8	Rols et al., 2000 (92); Mir et al., 1998 (19); Giraud et al., 1996 (118)	Melanoma	4	55	7	84	9	93

9	Domenge et al., 1996 (116); Mir et al., 1998 (19) (VI 9 and VI 15)	Adeno	2	20[l]	0	0	100	100
10	Heller et al., 1996 (85); Mir et al., 1998 (19)	Adeno[m]	1	2[i]	0	0	100	100
11	Sersa, 2000 (119)	Hypernephroma metastases	1	1	12 month stabilization			0

a All electroporations were performed with parallel plates.

b Where more than one publication per line is given, some or all of the patients described in these publications are the same.

c SCCHN, squamous cell carcinoma of the head and neck; BCC, basal cell carcinoma; NC, no change (includes stable and progressive disease); PR, partial response; CR, complete response; OR, objective response.

d Recurrent or progressive cutaneous permeation nodules.

e Recurrent cutaneous metastatic nodules.

f For 10 out of 29 tumors treated, a response could not be evaluated.

g For different patients, bleomycin (16.5–45 mg) was either administered intravenously or intra-arterially by bolus injection or by infusion.

h Two lesions showed stable disease; four lesions showed progressive disease.

i Bleomycin was administered by i.v. infusion. In all other cases, except as stated in footnote g, bleomycin was injected i.v. as a bolus.

j The two patients in Rudolf et al., 1995 (117) are likely both included in Mir et al., 1998 (19).

k Out of three patients, one did not respond (the number of treated nodules for that patient was not stated [Reintgen et al., 1996 (88)].

l Patient VI 15 had eight breast metastases treated that could not be evaluated because of too short follow-up. Patient VI 9 had 20 metastatic nodules of adenocarcinoma of the salivary gland treated.

m Subclavicular and mid-back metastatic nodules.

Table 4   Cisplatin ECT Clinical Study Results

No.	Reference	Cancer type[a]	No. of patients	No. of tumors treated	Drug administration[a]	Electrode type	Clinical tumor responses[a] (%)				
							PD	NC	PR	CR	OR
1	Sersa et al., 1998 (120)	SCC	1	2	i.t.	Parallel plates	0	0	0	100	100
2	Sersa et al., 1998 (120)	BCC	1	4	i.t.	Parallel plates	0	0	0	100	100
3	Sersa et al., 1998 (120)	Melanoma	2	13	i.t.	Parallel plates	0	0	0	100	100
4	Sersa et al., 2000 (89)	Melanoma	10	82	i.t.	Parallel plates	7[b]	15[b]	10[b]	68[b]	78[b], 77[c]
5	Sersa et al., 2000 (121)	Melanoma[d]	9	27	i.t.	No EP	33[b]	30[b]	19[b]	19[b]	38[b], 19[c]
				27	i.v. infusion	Parallel plates	11[b]	41[b]	37[b]	11[b]	48[b]
				18	i.v. infusion	No EP	39[b]	39[b]	11[b]	11[b]	22[b]

[a] i.t., intratumoral; i.v. intravenous; SCC, squamous cell carcinoma; BCC basal cell carcinoma; PD, progressive disease; NC, no change; PR, partial response; CR complete response; OR, objective response.

[b] Four weeks after treatment.

[c] 124 weeks after treatment.

[d] Skin and lymph node metastases were treated systemically with cisplatin chemo-immunotherapy. Patients were treated with vinblastin (i.v.) and lomustine (orally) on day 1, with cisplatin (i.v. infusion) on days 2–5, and with interferon–α2b on days 4–7. EP was performed on day 4.

Table 5 Treat-and-Resect Study with Primary SCCHN[a]

Patient	DoT[b]	Primary	TNM	Therapy[c]	Histology[d]	pN	Side effects	Add. trtmt.[e]	Outcome[f]
001	02/01	Uvula	T1 N1 Mx	EPT + SND	NECC	pN1	Pain grade I	RT	NED
002	03/01	Lateral tongue	T2 N0 Mx	EPT + END	NECC	pN0	Pain grade II	RT	NED
006	06/01	Retromolar triangle	T2 N0 Mx	EPT + END	NECC	pN0	Pain grade I	0	NED
009	07/01	Base of tongue	T2 N0 Mx	EPT + END	NECC	pN2a	Pain grade II	RT	NED
010	07/01	Lateral tongue	T2 N1 Mx	EPT + SND	NECC	pN2b	Pain grade II	RT	Died due to neck metastases (06/02)
011	08/01	Floor of mouth	T1 N0 Mx	EPT + END	NECC	pN0	Pain grade III	0	NED
012	09/01	Lateral tongue	T2 N2b Mx	EPT + SND	RES	pN2b	Pain grade III	RT	NED
014	10/01	Lateral tongue	T2 N2a Mx	EPT + SND	RES	pN2b	Pain grade I	RT	NED
015	10/01	Floor of mouth	T1 N0 Mx	EPT	NECC	—	Pain grade I	0	NED
016	12/01	Retromolar triangle	T2 N0 Mx	EPT	NECC	—	Pain grade II	0	NED
017	02/02	Soft palate	T2 N1 Mx	EPT + SND	NECC	pN1	Pain grade I	RT	NED
018	03/02	Lateral tongue	T2 N1 Mx	EPT + SND	NECC	pN0	Pain grade II	RT	NED

[a] Twelve patients with primary squamous cell carcinomas of the head and neck (SCCHN) were treated with bleomycin-EPT. Four weeks later, the tumor site was resected and any remaining tumor mass was thoroughly examined histopathologically for viable tumor cells. Observation time ranged between 7 and 20 months (mean: 13.4 months). Depending on the lymphnode status, EPT was performed with or without a neck dissection (122).
[b] DoT: date of treatment.
[c] END: elective neck dissection; SND: selective neck dissection.
[d] NECC: no evidence of cancer cells in histopathological specimen; RES: residual cancer cells in histopathological specimen.
[e] Add. trtmt: additional treatment; RT: radiotherapy.
[f] NED: no evidence of disease.

Table 6 Patients, Cancers, and Lesions Treated with EPT[a]

Treatment[b]	Cancers[c]																	
	SSC		BCC		Melanoma		Adeno		Breast		Kaposi's		TCC		Hyn		Total	
	Patients	Lesions	P	L	P	L	P	L	P	L	P	L	P	L	P	L	P	L
Bleomycin, i.t.	81	96	36	71	15	102	2	2	2	14	1	4	1	17	—	—	138	306
Bleomycin, i.v.	17	77	2	6	14	95	3	22	—	—	—	—	—	—	1	1	36	201
Cisplatin	1	2	1	4	21	122	—	—	—	—	—	—	—	—	—	—	24	128
Total	99	175	39	81	50	319	5	24	2	14	1	4	1	17	1	1	198	635

[a] Summary of patients and evaluable lesions of various cancers treated with EPT as reported in the medical literature. These figures relate directly to those in Tables 2 to 4. Note that the 12 patients with primary head and neck cancer of Table 5 are also included in Table 2 under Burian et al., 2002, (112).
[b] i.t., intratumoral; i.v., intravenous.
[c] SSC, squamous cell carcinoma; BCC, basal cell carcinom; Adeno, adenocarcinoma; TCC, transitional cell carcinoma; Hyn, hypernephroma metastases; P, patients; L, lesions.

by more than half (OR: 81%). Complete responses were observed in 88 lesions (44%). Seventeen patients with cutaneous metastases of SCCHN who had undergone previous radiation, surgery, and/or chemotherapy were treated with B-EPT at three different centers in France (Table 3, lines 1–4). Of the 87 nodules treated, 77 were evaluable. Small lesions were treated under sedation; for larger or more numerous lesions neuroleptanalgesia or general anesthesia were applied. Of the 77 lesions 62% displayed an objective response and 43% responded completely. The complete response rate obtained by Domenge et al. (116) for larger and deeper tumors is somewhat lower than that obtained for smaller and shallower lesions treated by Belehradek et al. (102), probably reflecting the limited effectiveness of the fixed parallel plate electrodes (116). Bleomycin was administered as an i.v. bolus at 18 U/m^2 (102) or 27 U/m^2 (116) (see also Ref. 19). In a few patients bleomycin was injected intra-arterially (116). EP was performed between 8 and 28 min after drug administration.

Melanoma patients enrolled in studies summarized on lines 6–8 of Table 3 had been treated with surgery, chemotherapy, and/or radiation prior to enrollment. Fourteen patients with 95 metastatic lesions were treated and average response rates of 87% OR and 37% CR were obtained. Most lesions responded within 1–2 weeks; no regrowth was observed at the treated sites. Different centers achieved considerably different complete response rates. Comparing the results for metastatic melanomas described in Tables 2 and 3, it appears that the higher efficacies in Table 2 may be primarily due to invasive electrodes, intratumoral drug injection, or both.

Patients tolerated the treatment well, experiencing no or only minor side effects. Each electrical pulse caused localized muscle contraction and, for patients not under general anesthesia, an unpleasant sensation. These side effects lasted only for the duration of the pulse. The sensations differed from individual to individual and were also dependent on the site of treatment. One to two hours after treatment, light erythema and oedema appeared at the treatment site, which usually disappeared within 1 day. In some cases electrode marks on the skin persisted for longer periods of time. EP pulses had no discernible effect on heart function or blood chemistry (19,92,113,117).

4. EPT with Cisplatin

As mentioned, cisplatin shows the second-highest average increase in efficacy (after bleomycin) when delivered by EP (Table 1). The only human treatments with cisplatin-EPT (C-EPT) have been performed at the Institute for Oncology, in Ljubljana, Slovenia (Table 4). Three different studies used essentially the same procedure, namely intratumoral or intravenous cisplatin administration, followed 1–2 min later by eight EP pulses delivered with parallel plate electrodes in two sets of four pulses, in two perpendicular directions. Switching electrical field direction by repositioning the electrodes by 90° enhances EP in a similar way as the field switching in the six-needle array electrodes (103; see also section IV.E).

Four patients were enrolled in the first study (Table 4, lines 1–3). The SSC patient had recurrent nodules after supraglotic laryngectomy and two rounds of radiation therapy. Two treated lesions responded completely, and no recurrence was observed during the 11-month follow-up period. The BCC patient had multiple surgeries and treatments with Interferon-α and vitamin A before being enrolled for ECT. All four lesions treated responded completely without any indication of recurrence after 8 months. Two other tumors treated with cisplatin interestingly showed a partial response lasting 3 months. Three more tumors that were not treated showed no change. The two melanoma patients (line 3) had been treated with surgery, chemotherapy, and/or immunotherapy prior to their enrollment. All 13 metastatic nodules treated responded completely, and no regrowth has been observed in the 7–11 months follow-up periods. Two of three other lesions treated only with i.t. injection of cisplatin also responded completely and one showed no change for seven months. One tumor subjected to EP only (no drug) and untreated tumors continued to grow.

The second study enrolled 10 patients (Table 4, line 4). The objective of this Phase II study was to evaluate the efficacy of ECT with intratumorally administered cisplatin in controlling recurrent or progressive cutaneous tumor nodules in malignant melanoma patients. The ECT effect on 82 tumor nodules was compared to the response of 27 nodules treated with cisplatin only, two nodules treated with electrical pulses only, and 22 nodules that were left untreated. As can be seen in Table 4, C-EPT treatment results in a higher short-term response rate than cisplatin alone; more importantly, the long-term response is even three- to fourfold greater. Nodules that were only electroporated or not treated continued to grow or showed no change. The treatment was well tolerated by all patients and a good cosmetic outcome was achieved, with minimal scarring and depigmentation of the skin.

The objective of the third study was to evaluate the local enhancement of systemic cisplatin treatment of malignant melanoma skin metastases by application of electric pulses to individual tumors. This is an interesting approach since it potentially combines the advantages of easily performed local EP treatment with those of standard systemic treatment. Nine melanoma patients undergoing cisplatin-based chemoimmunotherapy, with skin metastases and metastases in lymph nodes not amenable to surgery, were enrolled in this study (Table 4, line 5). Patients received vinblastine and lomustine intravenously on day 1, cisplatin ($20 \, \text{mg/m}^2$) on days 2–5 and interferon-α2b on days 4–7. Electroporation was performed on day 4 during the daily chemotherapy infusion, at least 3 h after onset of the infusion. Interferon was given no earlier than 6 h after completion of EP. Four weeks post treatment, nodules that had received electrical treatment showed a 48% objective response compared with 22% for nonelectroporated tumors. The complete response rate was the same in both study arms (11%). Median time to progression was significantly longer for electroporated tumors than for nonelectroporated ones (21 weeks vs. 4 weeks). Consistent with preclinical results (123), the response rates achieved in the previous study with intratumoral cisplatin delivery (line 4) were clearly higher than the rates observed with intravenous delivery in this study (line 5). However, this latest study has demonstrated that electrical pulses can be applied advantageously to tumor nodules during ongoing cisplatin-based chemotherapy, which is routinely used in the treatment of metastatic disease in malignant melanoma patients.

5. *Treat-and-Resect Study with Primary Head and Neck Cancers*

The objective of this study was to evaluate the safety and effectiveness of B-EPT in treating primary head and neck cancers. The study design called for treating the tumor with B-EPT and 4 weeks later to excise any remaining tumor mass, including the usual margin. The excised tissue was to be examined histologically for any viable tumor cells. Performing such a treat-and-resect procedure was considered a prudent first step towards the treatment of early stage cancers by B-EPT. This procedure allows to evaluate the degree of tumor eradication by B-EPT without depriving the patient of the benefit of proven conventional surgical treatment. Provided that B-EPT demonstrated equal or greater efficacy as present standard therapy, the next intended step was to solely treat with B-EPT, without subsequent resection. Both patient and care provider could then fully benefit from the inherent potential advantages of B-EPT, which include preservation of patient tissues, organs, and functions and the simplicity and low cost of the procedure.

In a study performed at the Department of Otorhino-laryngology of the University of Vienna Medical School, Vienna, Austria, twelve patients (11 male, 1 female; average age 57 years) with T1 or T2 squamous cell carcinoma of the oral cavity or oropharynx were treated with B-EPT (Table 5). Depending on the lymphnode status, a neck dissection was also performed. Bleomycin (4.0 U/ml, 1.0 U/cm^3 tumor volume) was uniformly injected into the tumor and a 5–10 mm margin. Ten minutes later, the tumor and a safe margin of 5 mm were electroporated using the MedPulser system with appropriate six-needle array applicators. After 4 weeks, resection of the tumor mass was performed exactly as it would have been done without prior ECT. All tissue specimens were systematically and completely evaluated in regard to remaining viable tumor cells.

Table 5 summarizes the medical histories and treatment results. The ECT procedure was tolerated well by all patients. Minor to moderate swelling at the treatment site was observed within 24 h after therapy, lasting three to seven days. Two to 3 days after treatment the tumor surface changed color to yellow-gray to brownish. Step by step the tumors became increasingly necrotic during the 4 weeks after treatment. In two cases (001 and 009), the soft necrotic mass had disintegrated and was completely rejected without surgical intervention at the time of resection. The most significant side effect was pain at the treatment site, which generally increased from a very low level during the first 7 days to a maximum during weeks 3 and 4. Pain grades according to WHO criteria ranged from grade I (41.7%) to grade II (41.7%) and grade III (16.6%).

Histological examination of resected specimens revealed tumor-free tissue in 10 cases. In one case (012) remaining cancer cells were found at the mucosal margin of the specimen. This suggests that the extent of the tumor was underestimated by the surgeon and electroporation or bleomycin injection did not cover the entire cancerous area. In the tumor of patient 014, which extended to the base of the tongue, viable tumor cells were found in the center of the necrotic tumor. This raises the question as to how long it takes for B-EPT to destroy all cancer cells in a bulky tumor and whether the identified malignant cells would have been eliminated if the resection had been performed at a later time.

Follow-up times ranged from 7 to 20 months (mean: 13.4 months). Eleven patients were tumor-free without any sign of local or regional recurrence. One patient (009) died 11 months after treatment due to rapidly growing neck metastases; the primary tumor site showed no evidence of recurrence. The results of this study have been published in Ref. 122.

Two additional patients with primary T1 and T2 oral SCCHN who had received no prior treatment underwent B-EPT at the Benjamin Franklin Center in Berlin, Germany. The residual tumor mass resected 4 weeks after treatment showed no histological evidence of viable tumor cells. Both patients are fully functional with only small scars at the treatment sites and remain tumor-free 14 and 17 months after B-EPT, respectively (T. Plath, personal communication, 2002).

In conclusion, the results indicate that B-EPT is an effective treatment for early stage, primary SCC of the upper aerodigestive tract, and further studies should be conducted to prove its usefulness and to define the criteria for its application.

G. Mechanisms of Electroporation Therapy with Bleomycin

Since bleomycin in combination with EP displays such high and rapid antitumor activity, it is of interest to explore the underlying mechanism. Macroscopically, the typical tumor response to B-EPT in humans involves slight erythema and "oedema" at the treatment site within 24–48 h after treatment. As time progresses, the tumor mass of cutaneous and subcutaneous lesions becomes increasingly necrotic, dries out, and forms an eschar that falls off 2–6 weeks after treatment, revealing healthy tissue underneath (86,89,113–116,120). Tumors in a moist environment such as the upper aerodigestive tract do not form dry eschars; necrotic tissue is either gradually washed away or sometimes separates from healthy tissue in pieces (94,108) (M. Burian, personal communication, 2002). The void left by smaller tumors usually heals well, but necrosis of some large tumors (>100 cm^3) has caused complications (see Sec. IV.I).

Upon histological examination, the "oedema" formed early after treatment of subcutaneous SCCs in mice superficially resembles liquefactive necrosis but differs from the latter by the conspicuous presence of a large number of apoptotic cells and cell fragments (124). Analysis of gene expression patterns shortly after B-EPT supports the histological findings insofar as a number of proapoptotic genes is turned on while antiapoptotic genes are turned off (100,137). Rapid induction of pseudo-apoptosis or apoptosis has also been observed in vitro after B-EPT (34,82,125). Pseudo-apoptosis refers to rapid DNA cleavage by bleomycin rather than apoptotic nucleases, mimicking cell morphological changes and oligo-nucleosomal ladders characteristic of apoptosis (82).

However, it is unknown whether it is solely the induction of pseudo-apoptosis or apoptosis that makes B-EPT so effective against tumors. Most likely, other mechanisms are involved as well:

1. The effect of ECT on tumor blood vessels resulting in reduced or blocked tumor blood flow may play a role in killing tumor cells not killed directly by bleomycin, and in causing necrosis of tumor tissue (52,126–130).
2. Both bleomycin and EP are each capable of raising the level of intracellular reactive oxygen species, leading to membrane lipid peroxidation and other cytotoxic effects (131,132).
3. Bleomycin, even without EP, is known to release cytokines such as IL-2, IL-6, and tumor necrosis factor (133,134) and to upregulate the tumor suppressor protein, p53 (135).

These effects probably contribute to tumor killing and initiate a local and systemic immunostimulatory effect in the patient. The latter point is supported by findings from animal experiments (67,77,136).

The mechanisms involved in producing the remarkable antitumor effect of B-EPT are clearly more complex than the simple model of tumor cell inactivation by DNA cleavage, facilitated by high doses of bleomycin delivered by EP. Some of the puzzling questions that need to be answered to obtain a better understanding of the antitumor effect of B-EPT include:

1. How are tumor cells killed that escape direct destruction by bleomycin? It is unlikely that every single tumor cell receives a sufficient intracellular dose to be killed. Induced immune responses probably play a role (Sec. IV.1).
2. Why do some tumors respond partially or not at all (Tables 2–5)? EP has been shown to essentially permeabilize any cell membrane and bleomycin appears to cleave not only "naked" and replicating DNA but also DNA in stable chromosomal structures (82). How can some tumors be resistant against such an apparently universal, straightforward mechanism?
3. Why are many cancer cells more sensitive to B-EPT than normal cells (see section IV.H)? Will the answer to this question also help to answer the previous one as to why some tumors respond completely and others not at all?

However interesting it might be to speculate about the answers to these questions in the light of existing relevant information, it would exceed the scope of this article.

H. Advantages of ECT

The clinical results shown indicate that ECT is a safe therapeutic approach for primary BCC, for cutaneous and subcutaneous melanoma metastases, and for primary, recurrent and SCCHN tumors, as well as refractory and cutaneous metastases of SCCHN. The same appears to be true for a variety of other solid tumors of which only small numbers have been treated with ECT in humans so far. The treatments performed were tolerated well by all patients enrolled. Tumor response rates achieved with ECT to date match or exceed the values obtained with standard therapies (Tables 2 to 5). Lesions treated with bleomycin or EP alone essentially showed no treatment effect, while intratumoral or intravenous cisplatin produced a small but significant number of objective responses. The main advantage of ECT in treating tumors smaller than approximately 100 cm^3 appears to be its tissue and organ-sparing feature that preserves patient function and appearance to a greater extent than conventional treatments (87,109). The overall low intrusiveness of ECT allows patients to lead more normal, independent, and purposeful lives (87,94,108, 109,114,120). The vast majority of cases required only a one-time treatment, a definite advantage over photodynamic therapy (94,109). However, when performed, retreatment did not cause complications and generally was effective (19,43,109,120). Side effects common for chemotherapy, radiation therapy, or surgery are not observed with ECT. Due to its ease and speed of performance, as well as its efficacy of treating lesions in patients with advanced stages of disease, ECT offers a treatment alternative where no other treatment may be possible or justifiable (19,87,91,94,108,109,120). Drug resistance appears to be overcome with electroporative drug delivery (89,101). In addition, ECT can be performed as an outpatient procedure and is more cost effective than conventional treatments (19,28,89,91,94,108,109,120).

ECT differs from other ablative therapies in one important aspect. The treatment affects tumor cells to a much greater extent than normal cells (91,100,124,137). While radiofrequency, cryo-, and photodynamic therapies destroy any tissue that is treated, ECT preferentially destroys tumor tissue and leaves normal tissue intact, or affects it only temporarily. This is probably the main reason for the observed superior functional and cosmetic outcome achieved with ECT (19,27,87,88,107,109).

Differentiation between malignant and normal tissue by ECT indicated in clinical studies is clearly observable in animal experiments. Normal porcine skin and muscle tissue shows only minor histological changes when subjected to standard ECT treatment and these changes disappear almost completely after about 20 days. Changes induced by EP alone are milder than changes caused by bleomycin and EP. When higher voltages or pulse numbers are applied, histological changes are more pronounced but also largely disappear by day 40 after treatment (91,124). Therefore, it is our recommendation to treat tumor tissue with only one cycle of pulses (Sec. IV.E.1). Multiple cycles generally do not increase efficacy and may impair wound healing, especially in previously irradiated or otherwise compromised tissue (108).

For ECT, as for surgical and radiation therapy, it is important to know how to treat tumors close to vital structures, such as major arteries and nerves, without jeopardizing those structures. When tissue in the immediate vicinity of the carotid sheaths and femoral arteries of dogs was injected with bleomycin, followed by EP of these vital structures and their surrounding tissue, arteries, and nerves did not show significant histological changes and remained fully functional. The only exception was severe loss of smooth muscle cells of arterial walls when bleomycin was injected directly into the vessel walls with subsequent EP, an unlikely, worst-case scenario (91,124). Electrochemotherapy of enlarged dog prostates also resulted in only minor acute changes of prostate tissue (G. S. Nanda and D. Rabussay, unpublished results).

Jaroszeski et al. (54,138) compared the effect of ECT on hepatocellular tumors and healthy liver tissue of rats. Whereas ECT produced a 69% complete response rate of the tumors, comparable ECT conditions barely affected normal liver tissue. At higher than standard field strength and bleomycin concentration, localized liver necrosis was visible on day 14 but not on day 56 after treatment. Other authors have also concluded that ECT preferentially affects tumor tissue as opposed to normal tissue, and that healthy tissue is preserved or restored after B-EPT treatment (41,42).

I. Limitations of ECT

Inherent limitations of ECT include muscle contractions and pain triggered by the electrical pulses, and the limitation of treatment efficacy to local and regional tumors that must be accessible to drug injection and electrode insertion. Pain during pulses can be controlled by local or general anesthesia. Treatment of large SCCHN tumors, although effective in controlling the tumor, has in some cases led to wound-healing complications and to tissue voids after the tumor necrotized and dissipated (T. Plath, personal communication, 2002). Thus, treatment of large tumors, especially if the tumor has invaded adjacent tissue, should be carefully evaluated, and if treatment is performed, the treated site should be closely observed. Prior irradiation of tumors and adjacent tissue seems to exacerbate wound-healing complications. These latter limitations argue for the use of B-EPT as an early treatment where these side effects are not encountered and the greatest efficacy can be obtained. Approaches to increase access to deep-seated tumors and the use of B-EPT for regional and systemic treatments are discussed in Sec. IV.J.

J. Future Directions of ECT

Considering the strengths and weaknesses of ECT discussed in the previous sections, the logical short-term applications of this treatment modality include selected head and neck cancers and various cutaneous lesions. Provided that suitable inclusion and exclusion criteria are applied, the applications make use of the advantages of ECT such as tissue and organ preservation, high efficacy, and ease of use. The lesions are also accessible with presently available applicators. Initially, palliative or salvage treatments may be preferred. However, treatment of primary head and neck and cutaneous tumors could follow soon, as indicated by presently available clinical results. The greatest patient benefit from ECT would clearly be gained by the treatment of primary tumors.

In the medium term, improvement of EP instrumentation could broaden the application of ECT to a wider range of cancer types, including major cancers such as breast and prostate cancer. Preclinical and clinical results support the view that ECT is a promising treatment modality for all or most solid tumors. Novel pulse generators and sophisticated applicators, including endoscopic applicators (22), aim at reducing muscle contraction and pain, and at providing minimally invasive access to deeper-seated tumors.

In the long term, a better understanding of the molecular and cellular mechanisms of ECT may help to increase acceptance of this treatment modality by regulatory agencies and by the medical community. It may also lead to successful regional or systemic cancer treatments in combination with other treatment modalities. For example, Mir's group (139) has shown that mice with established tumors, treated with B-EPT and subsequent peritumoral injection of IL-2 producing cells resulted in cures of almost all directly treated tumors, as well as untreated contralateral tumors. Cured mice were completely protected from developing tumors upon further inoculation with tumor cells. Similarly, Sersa et al. (140) combined intra- or peritumoral injection of TNF-α into SA-1 tumors of mice with the delivery of a suboptimal dose of bleomycin by EP. The results suggested that the effect of adjuvant TNF-α treatment might be immunomodulatory and possibly introduces a systemic component to the localized B-EPT treatment. Another example is the amplification of radiotherapy by C-EPT. The rate of CRs in mice bearing subcutaneous Ehrlich-Lettre ascites tumors increased from 27% after radiation therapy to 92% when radiation was combined with B-EPT. Cisplatin and EP, respectively, enhanced CR rates of radiation therapy to 73% and 54%, respectively. Thus, Cisplatin and EP each enhance the radiation effect, yet the highest efficacy is achieved in combination with C-EPT (141).

Another future approach to regional or systemic cancer treatment may be based on enhancing the immune response triggered by B-EPT. Kuriyama and colleagues (67) obtained a 50% cure rate of mice with established colorectal carcinomas after B-EPT. Tumor-specific cytotoxic lymphocytes were elicited in the spleens of cured animals and were probably responsible for protection against rechallenge with colorectal carcinoma. Similarly, Engstrom et al. (77) observed a 92% cure rate of adenocarcinomas in rat livers after B-EPT. High concentrations of CD 8 lymphocytes were found in the treated tumors, while tumors that received only EP showed mainly macrophage infiltration. These findings and others support the hypothesis that B-EPT stimulates the host's immune system and participates in tumor suppression or eradication by B-EPT.

Last but not least, we would like to emphasize that the excellent DNA delivery results achieved with EP may eventually lead to effective in vivo or ex vivo gene therapies of cancer or to useful DNA cancer vaccines (see Sec. V).

V. OTHER THERAPEUTIC APPLICATIONS OF EP

A. Electroinsertion

During electroinsertion an agent is "inserted" primarily into the membrane rather than delivered into the cytosol. This is achieved by application of an electric field, which is below the critical field strength necessary for electroporation. The most important work in this area, from the clinical point of view, is the electroinsertion of full-length recombinant CD4 molecules into red blood cell (RBC) membranes that can serve as inhibitors of HIV infection (142,143). A limited safety trial involving RBCs from four HIV patients has been published (144). Major observations included

1. The half-life of RBCs (30 days) was not changed by such electroinsertion.
2. The hematological indices or the P50 values of RBCs were not modified.
3. There were neither adverse effects nor an anti-CD4 immune response in patients over the 28 day follow-up period.

Another protein of therapeutic interest is glycophorin A (145,146). Experiments, in vitro, have shown that electroinserted glycophorin A protects target cells from attack by NK cells (147). No clinical application has been published.

B. Electroencapsulation

Electroencapsulation refers to a specific application of EP in which cells are "loaded" with a substance that is carried inside the cell to its therapeutic site of action. One example is the encapsulation of inositol hexaphosphate (IHP), an allosteric effector of hemoglobin, that enhances the oxygen carrying capacity of RBCs. Such loaded RBCs have been shown to improve tissue oxygenation during cardiopulmonary bypass operations (148,149). Max-Cyte, Inc. is developing a closed-loop EP system for clinical use, in which the patient's blood is continuously pumped through an EP chamber where RBCs are loaded with IHP. Another example is the encapsulation of prostacyclin (PGI_2) or iloprost, a prostacyclin analog, into platelets to prevent thrombosis and restenosis of blood vessels. Loaded platelets delivered intravenously were able to reduce or inhibit platelet deposition at the site of blood vessel injury in small and large animal models. Also, when delivered locally by a double-balloon catheter at the site of injury immediately after angioplasty of pig carotid arteries, platelet deposition was reduced over 80% (150,151). Excessive platelet recruitment, along with smooth muscle cell proliferation at the lesion site, is considered to contribute significantly to restenosis of arteries after balloon angioplasty and similar ablative interventions.

C. Ocular Therapy

Interesting applications of EPT in ophthalmology have been pioneered by Japanese researchers. Glaucoma, characterized by an increase of the intraocular pressure (IOP) and atrophy of the optic nerve, is generally caused by occlusion of the filtering system for the aqueous humor of the eye. Glaucoma filtering surgery frequently results in reocclusion of the surgically cleared drain channel, due to fibroblast proliferation. Antiproliferative drugs (5-FU, mitomycin C) are somewhat effective in preventing reocclusion, but produce undesirable long-term side effects. In a rabbit eye model, electroporative delivery of bleomycin to the surgically treated area was performed using specialized miniature electrodes (152, 153). In every case, this B-EPT treatment reduced IOP, whereas EP or drug alone were ineffective.

Cornea (154–156) and retinal ganglion cells (157,158) have been transfected effectively and without side effects by in vivo EP. The advantages of this method over previously used methods might accelerate research in the field of corneal and retinal diseases and lead to useful gene therapies.

D. Vascular Therapy

Areas of vascular therapy which may benefit most from improved local drug and gene delivery technologies include the prevention and treatment of restenosis after angioplasty, stenting, or grafting; revascularization of ischemic tissue; and the prevention or treatment of atherosclerosis and thrombosis. Many potentially effective drugs or genes have been identified which could alleviate or cure the mentioned morbidities if these agents could be efficiently delivered and maintained over a sufficient period of time at the treatment site. Various methods tested have largely been unsuccessful to fill this need in vascular therapy (159). Electroporation has the advantage of acting quickly and therefore impeding blood flow only briefly. Since EP delivers molecules into cells, it enhances drug efficacy and slows or prevents wash out of drugs otherwise located in the interstitium. The method is safe and does not affect heart function, blood chemistry, or the functionality of blood vessels (160,161).

For the delivery of agents into vessel walls EP has been performed intra- and extraluminally. Different types of electroporation catheters were used for intraluminal delivery of marker molecules (159,160) and Heparin (161). The latter resulted in significant (>80%) inhibition of restenosis after angioplasty in all animals when rat carotid arteries were treated with Heparin and EP. Heparin or EP alone had no preventive effect (161). Porous balloon electroporation catheters have also been used successfully for transfecting endothelial and smooth muscle cells of arteries (100).

Extraluminal delivery has been performed with either plate electrodes (162) or a specially designed electrode, which also contained a reservoir for the agent to be delivered (163). In vivo, extraluminal treatment requires surgical access to the vessel. However, for pretreating vascular grafts before splicing (164), or for treating graft junctions to prevent thrombosis or restenosis, this method can be used advantageously to replace viral or other vectors. Ex vivo EP has also greatly improved transfection of entire hearts (165) and may be employed to deliver genes that reduce transplant rejection (166). In addition to therapeutic applications, EP-enhanced transfection is poised to become an attractive method for vascular research, including the functional analysis of genes and gene products involved in the development of vascular diseases (167).

E. Intra- and Transdermal Drug and Gene Delivery

Delivery of drugs or genes into and through the skin has many potential advantages (159). However, only very few drugs (e.g., nicotine, certain steroids) have the ability to penetrate the skin in effective doses without chemical or physical penetration-enhancing measures. Many different approaches have been taken to overcome the effective barrier of the skin, in particular the stratum corneum (SC). The challenge in all these approaches is to achieve maximal penetration while causing minimal skin irritation. Both mechanical and chemical means generally cause significant skin irritation. Similar to permeabilizing cell membranes by EP, the SC, which consists of 20–80 layers of dead cells and is the main entrance barrier, can be permeabilized by EP. Electroporation pulses form new pores or channels across the SC and widen existing weak spots in hair follicles and sweat glands (168). These new pathways allow higher transport rates (flux) through the SC. Several low-molecular-weight drugs have been delivered intra- or transdermally by EP in vitro and in animals, including fentanyl, metropolol, flurbiprofen, and cyclosporin A (reviewed in Refs. 159 and 169). Buprenorphine and vitamin C have also been delivered efficiently (170,171). Recently, anionic lipids have been described to enhance transdermal transport in combination with EP for molecules up to about 4 kDa, but not for larger molecules (172).

The only study involving humans compared the dermal delivery of lidocaine by EP and iontophoresis, respectively. Lidocaine solution was applied topically, followed by EP or iontophoresis, using noninvasive electrodes in contact with the skin surface. Electroporation delivered a higher amount of lidocaine into the skin within 3 min than iontophoresis. Iontophoresis resulted in greater depth of anesthesia (173).

The greatest interest in employing EP for dermal delivery has been for substances which are difficult or impossible to deliver with simpler methods. Such substances include peptides, proteins, oligonucleotides, DNA, and other relatively high molecular weight compounds. The delivery of luteinizing releasing hormone, calcitonin, heparin, and oligonucleotides has been reviewed previously (159,169). Recent progress has been made in transdermal delivery of doses close to therapeutic levels of calcitonin and parathyroid hormone (174). Electroporative delivery of DNA into or across the skin after topical application has not been achieved in biologically relevant quantities. However, noninvasive electroporation has been effective in enhancing plasmid DNA delivery into skin cells after injecting the DNA into skin. This resulted in several hundredfold stimulation of gene expression in a hairless mouse model (175).

F. Erectile Dysfunction

Erectile dysfunction affects an estimated 15 million men in the United States (176). Although oral medication is available, this systemic treatment puts some patients at risk of potentially severe side effects. Local, low-dose drug delivery reduces that risk. Topical application of vasodilators such as prostaglandin E1 to penile skin caused erections in a rabbit model when followed by noninvasive low-voltage EP, but not without EP (177). A clinical study with 20 impotent patients designed to evaluate safety and human tolerance of electrical sensation induced by millisecond EP pulses demonstrated that pulses in the voltage range effective for transdermal delivery were tolerated well by most patients (178). Erectile dysfunction was also corrected by gene therapy in aged rodents when penile neuronal nitric oxide synthase cDNA was delivered by EP (179).

G. Gene Therapy

One of the most persistent technical challenges for gene therapy, whether ex vivo or in vivo, remains the delivery of a sufficient number of DNA molecules to specific target cells to achieve therapeutic expression levels of the encoded gene (180–182). Several modes of DNA transfer into target cells have been pursued. While viral vectors, the most widely used tools for in vivo gene transfer, are efficient in delivering DNA, they also cause side effects and complications, such as immune reactions and insertion mutations (183,184). The DNA "payload" carried by commonly used viral vehicles is limited to about 5 kilobases, too small for many genes of interest. Manufacturing and quality control are very complex and expensive, and regulatory hurdles for approval are high.

Alternatives to viral systems, including liposomes, the "gene gun" and "naked" DNA injection largely eliminate these drawbacks but generally lack transfection efficiency (9,100). The recent finding that EP increases gene expression by two or more orders of magnitude after naked DNA injection has made this combination of methods clinically relevant (9,185–187). One of the most promising tissues for gene transfer in a clinical setting is the muscle. Most studies reporting intramuscular enhancement of gene expression by EP were performed in rodents, but similar increases have been obtained in larger animals, including pigs, dogs, and nonhuman primates (100,188–190). As in vivo EP after intramuscular DNA injection provides long-lasting expression and allows modulation of gene expression levels by DNA dosing, muscle transfection by EP may be most promising for many gene therapy applications. No results of clinical trials involving in vivo electroporation for gene therapy or genetic vaccinations have been published to date. However, results of three ex vivo EP clinical studies are available.

One Phase I clinical study using ex vivo EP has been conducted with the eventual goal of treating hemophilia B. Autologous bone marrow stromal cells were transfected with plasmid DNA coding for blood clotting Factor IX (F.IX), propagated, and returned to the patient. The transfected cells were well tolerated by the patients (191,192). Preclinical trials in hemophilic dogs involving in vivo delivery of F.IX DNA also appear promising. Close to normal clotting times were obtained until an immune response to the newly produced canine F.IX, recognized by the dogs as "foreign," inhibited F.IX activity (100). Several strategies seem feasible to overcome this obstacle.

Another clinical study addresses hemophilia A, caused by a deficiency in Factor VIII (F.VIII). Transkaryotic Therapies, Inc. uses clones of autologous dermal fibroblasts transfected by EP. Cells producing F.VIII are administered to the patient by laparoscopic injection into the omentum. Positive clinical changes in the patient with the highest F.VIII activity (out of six) lasted 10 months. The treatment was well tolerated (193).

In the area of cancer gene therapy, a Phase I clinical trial for the treatment of glioblastoma and a Phase II study for non-small-cell lung cancer have been approved for patients who have undergone conventional therapies (NIH protocol numbers 138 (194) and 331 (195)). H. Fakhrai had shown earlier that all animals implanted intracranially with 9L gliosarcoma cells survived, if immunized with 9L cells transfected by EP with the TGF-β antisense gene (196,197). Initial results from two patients indicated that the treatment did not cause any toxicity and that CD4$^+$ and CD8$^+$ cells were activated, migrated through the blood brain barrier and infiltrated the tumor bed (H. Fakhrai, personal communication, 1999).

H. DNA Vaccines

DNA immunization, a novel method to induce protective immune responses, was recently proven to be very effective in small animal models (198). The method entails the direct in vivo administration of plasmid DNA that encodes defined antigens of a pathogen. De novo production of these antigens in the host's own cells elicits antibody and cellular immune responses that provide protection against live virus challenge and persist for extended periods in the absence of further immunizations. Using a weakly immunogenic hepatitis B surface antigen DNA vaccine as well as a potent HIV gag sequence, we have shown that in vivo EP improves DNA immunization efficacy in three important ways: (1) the immune response is observed earlier than without electroporation, (2) the magnitude of the resulting response is increased, and (3) far less DNA can be used to reproducibly induce an immune response (199). The fast immune response to DNA vaccines can be accelerated even more by using a particle adjuvant (100). In addition to mice, immune responses have been enhanced by EP in both guinea pigs and rabbits (199). Others have confirmed the significant stimulation of both antibody and antigen-specific T cell production by EP (200,201). Recently, it was demonstrated that EP also enables potent humoral and cellular responses in large animals, including pigs and nonhuman primates (189,190), indicating the potential of this approach for human use. With the present emphasis on protection against bioterrorism, fast-acting and potent DNA vaccines appear particularly attractive and may provide a significant advantage over conventional immunizations.

VI. SUMMARY AND OUTLOOK

Electroporation is opening up new avenues to meet therapeutic needs. This new method provides efficient access for drugs, DNA (genes) and gene-regulating molecules to the cell interior by temporarily permeabilizing outer cell membranes. Medical applications of this technology are at various stages of development. Several hundred patients with malignant tumors, particularly cutaneous and head and neck malignancies, have been treated with excellent results. We expect this treatment modality, supported by improved instrumentation, to be expanded to the treatment of other solid tumors and to earlier-stage cancers. A main advantage of EPT is the tissue-sparing aspect of the procedure, which simplifies and shortens local cancer therapy, and reduces cost. The second-most advanced application of EPT concerns the trans-membrane delivery of DNA for gene therapy and DNA vaccination. Clinical studies in cancer gene therapy, cancer DNA vaccines, and vascular therapies are imminent. Intra- and transdermal drug and DNA delivery appears to be an attractive approach but its development has lagged. Promising early developments, e.g., the treatment of erectile dysfunction discussed in Sec. V.F. have been eclipsed by the development of new drugs or drug formulations, obviating the need for device-based delivery. However, EP may play a future role in the dermal delivery of DNA and peptides. Finally, ex vivo EP is poised to have an impact on vascular graft and transplant procedures, cellular and immune therapies, and indications discussed in Sec. V.A. and V.B. In conclusion, we envision increased use of this technology in biomedical and clinical research and eventually in routine therapies, due to the inherent advantages of EP and compelling results achieved so far.

REFERENCES

1. Rose WC, Lee FY, Golik J, Kadow J. Preclinical oral antitumor activity of BMS-185660, a paclitaxel derivative. Cancer Chemother Pharmacol 2000; 46:246–250.
2. Walker RD, Smith EW. The role of percutaneous penetration enhancers. Adv Drug Del Rev 1996; 18:295–301.
3. Inoue N, Kobayaski D, Kimura M, Toyama M, Sugawara I, Itoyama S, Ogihara M, Sugibayashi K, Morimoto Y. Fundamental investigation of a novel drug delivery system, a transdermal delivery system with jet injection. Int J Pharma 1996; 137:75–84.
4. Muddle AG, Longridge DJ, Sweeney PA, Burkoth TL, Bellhouse BJ. Transdermal delivery of testosterone to conscious rabbits using powderject—a supersonic powder delivery system. Proc Int Symp Control Tel Bioact Mater, Controlled Release Society, Inc. 1997; 24:713–714.
5. Hofmann GA, Dev SB, Nanda GS, Rabussay D. Electroporation therapy of solid tumors. Crit Rev Therapeutic Drug Carrier Systems 1999; 16:523–569.
6. Heller R, Gilbert R, Jaroszeski MJ. Clinical applications of electrochemotherapy. Adv Drug Deliv Rev 1999; 4(35):119–129.
7. Dev SB, Rabussay D, Widera G, Hofmann GA. Medical applications of electroporation. IEEE Trans Plasma Sci 2000; 28:206–223.
8. Mir LM. Therapeutic perspectives of in vivo cell electropermeabilization. Bioelectrochemistry 2000; 53:1–10.
9. Smith LC, Nordstrom JL. Advances in plasmid gene delivery and expression in skeletal muscle. Curr Opin Mol Ther 2000; 2:150–154.
10. Sale AJH, Hamilton WA. Effects of high electric fields on microorganisms. I. Killing bacteria and yeasts. Biochim Biophys Acta 1967; 148:781–788.
11. Neumann E, Rosenheck K. Permeability changes induced by electric impulses in vesicular membranes. J Membr Biol 1972; 10:279–290.
12. Neumann E, Schaefer-Ridder M, Wang Y, Hofschneider PH. Gene transfer into mouse lyoma cells by electroporation in high electric fields. EMBO J 1982; 1:841–845.
13. Nikoloff FA. Methods in Molecular Biology. Vol. 47, 48. Totowa, NJ: Humana Press, 1995.
14. Muramatsu T, Nakamura A, Park HM. In vivo electroporation: a powerful and convenient means of nonviral gene transfer to tissues of living animals (Review). Int J Mol Med; 1998; 1:55–62.
15. Weaver JC. Electroporation: a general phenomenon for manipulating cells and tissues. J Cell Biochem 1993; 51:235–426.
16. Weaver JC, Chizmadzhev YA. Theory of electroporation: a review. Bioelectrochemistry and Bioenergetics 1996; 41:135–160.
17. Weaver JC. Electroporation of cells and tissues. IEEE Trans Plasma Sci 2000; 28:24–33.
18. Neumann E, Kakorin S, Toensing K. Principles of membrane electroporation and transport of macromolecules. In: Jaroszeski MJ, Heller R, Gilbert R, eds. Methods in Molecular Medicine. Electrically Mediated Delivery of Molecules to Cells. Vol. 37. Totowa, NJ: Humana Press, 2000:1–35.
19. Mir LM, Glass LF, Serša G, Teissié J, Domenge C, Miklavčič D, Jaroszeski MJ, Orlowski S, Reintgen DS, Rudolf Z, Belehradek M, Gilbert R, Rols M-P, Belehradek J Jr, Bachaud J-M, De Conti R, Štabuc B, Čemažar M, Cininx P, Heller R. Effective treatment of cutaneous and subcutaneous malignant tumours by electrochemotherapy. Br J Cancer 1998; 77:2336–2342.

20. Schoenbach KH, Beebe SJ, Buescher ES. Intracellular effect of ultrashort electrical pulses. Bioelectromagnetics 2001; 22:440–448.

21. Muller KJ, Sukhorukov VL, Zimmermann U. Reversible electropermeabilization of mammalian cells by high-intensity, ultra-short pulses of submicrosecond duration. J Membr Biol 2001; 184:161–170.

22. Kuriyama S, Tsujinoue H, Toyokawa Y, Mitoro A, Nakatani T, Yoshiji H, Tsujimoto T, Fukui H. A potential approach for electrochemotherapy against colorectal carcinoma using a clinically available alternating current system with bipolar snare in a mouse model. Scand J Gastroenterol 2001; 36:297–302.

23. Nanda GS, Sun FX, Hofmann GA, Hoffman RM, Dev SB. Electroporation therapy of human larynx tumors HEp-2 implanted in nude mice. Anticancer Res 1998; 18:999–1004.

24. Okino M, Mohri H. Effects of a high-voltage electrical impulse and an anticancer drug on in vivo growing tumors. Jpn J Cancer Res 1987; 78:1319–1321.

25. Mir LM, Belehradek M, Domenge C, Orlowski S, Poddevin B, Belehradek J Jr, Schwaab G, Luboinski B, Paoletti C. L'électrochimiothérapie, un nouveau traitement antitumoral: premier essai clinique. C R Acad Sci Paris 1991; 313:613–618.

25b. Nordenström B. Survey of mechanisms in electrochemical treatment of cancer. Eur J Surg 1994; 574(suppl.):93–109.

26. Keating A, Nolan E, Filshie R, Dev SB. Ex vivo stromal cell electroporation of factor IX cDNA for treatment of hemophilia B. In: Jaroszeski MJ, Heller R, Gilbert R, eds. Methods in Molecular Medicine. Electrically Mediated Delivery of Molecules to Cells. Vol. 37. Totowa, NJ: Humana Press, 2000:359–368.

27. Heller R, Gilbert R, Jaroszeski MJ. Clinical trials for solid tumors using electrochemotherapy. Jaroszeski MJ, Heller R, Gilbert R, eds. Methods in Molecular Medicine. Electrically Mediated Delivery of Molecules to Cells 2000; Vol. 37. Totowa, NJ: Humana Press, 2000:137–156.

28. In: Jaroszeski MJ, Heller R, Gilbert R, eds. Methods in Molecular Medicine. Electrically Mediated Delivery of Molecules to Cells. Vol. 37. Totowa, NJ: Humana Press, 2000.

29. Orlowski S, Belehradek J Jr, Paoletti C, Mir LM. Transient electropermeabilization of cells in culture. Increase of the cytotoxicity of anticancer drugs. Biochem Pharmacol 1988; 37:4727–4733.

30. Poddevin B, Orlowski S, Belehradek J Jr, Mir LM. Very high cytotoxicity of bleomycin introduced into the cytosol of cells in culture. Biochem Pharmacol 1991; 42(suppl):S67–S75.

31. Mir LM, Tounekti O, Orlowski S. Bleomycin: revival of an old drug. Gen Pharmacol 1996; 27:745–748.

32. Jaroszeski MJ, Dang V, Pottinger C, Hickey J, Gilbert R, Heller R. Toxicity of anticancer agents mediated by electroporation in vitro. Anticancer Drugs 2000; 11:201–208.

33. Miller AB, Hoogstraten B, Staquet M, Winkler A. Reporting results of cancer treatment. Cancer 1981; 47:207–214.

34. Tounekti O, Pron G, Belehradek J Jr, Mir LM. Bleomycin, an apoptosis-mimetic drug that induces two types or cell death depending on the number of molecules internalized. Cancer Res 1993; 53(22):5462–5469.

35. Hofmann GA, Dev SB, Dimmer S, Nanda GS. Electroporation therapy: a new approach for the treatment of head and neck cancer. IEEE Trans Biomed Eng 1999; 46:752–759.

36. Dev SB, Nanda GS, Austin M, Bleecher S, Hofmann GA. Electroporation-mediated drug delivery is highly effective for treatment of solid tumors. Proc Am Assoc Cancer Res 1999; 40:582.

37. Nanda GS, Bleecher S, Dev SB, Rabussay D. Electroporation therapy of head and neck tumors. Oral Oncology 2001; 7:318–322.

38. Ono K, Kinashi Y, Masunaga S, Suzuki M, Takagaki M. Effect of electroporation on cell killing by boron neutron capture therapy using borocaptate sodium (10B-BSH). Jpn J Cancer Res 1998; 89:1352–1357.

39. Ono K, Kinashi Y, Masunaga S, Suzuki M, Takagaki M. Electroporation increases the effect

of borocaptate (10B-BSH) in neutron capture therapy. Int J Radiat Oncol Biol Phys 1998; 42:823–826.

40. Omura S, Tsuyuki Y, Ohta S, Li X, Bukawa H, Fujita K. Rapid tumor necrosis induced by electrochemotherapy with intratumoral injection of bleomycin in a hamster tongue model. Int J Oral Maxillofac Surg 2000; 29:119–125.

41. Omura S, Tsuyuki Y, Ohta S, Bukawa H, Fujita K. In vivo antitumor effects of electrochemotherapy in a tongue cancer model. Int J Oral Maxillofac Surg 1999; 57:965–972.

42. Hasegawa H, Kano M, Hoshi N, Watanabe K, Satoh E, Nakayama B, Suzuki T. An electrochemotherapy model for rat tongue carcinoma. J Oral Pathol Med 1998; 27:249–254.

43. Jaroszeski MJ, Gilbert R, Perrott R, Heller R. Enhanced effects of multiple treatment electrochemotherapy. Melanoma Res Dec. 1996; 6:427–433.

44. Heller R, Jaroszeski M, Perrott R, Messina J, Gilbert R. Effective treatment of B16 melanoma by direct delivery of bleomycin using electrochemotherapy. Melanoma Res 1997; 7:10–18.

45. Serša G, Čemažar M, Miklavčič D. Antitumor effectiveness of electrochemotherapy with cis-diamminedichloroplatinum(II) in mice. Cancer Res 1995; 55:3450–3455.

46. Mashiba H, Ozaki Y, Ikuno S, Matsunaga K. Augmentation of antiproliferative and antitumor effect on human cancer cells in combined use of electroporation with a plant toxin, saporin. Cancer Biother Radiopharm 2001; 16:495–499.

47. Dev SB, Nanda GS, An Z, Wang X, Hoffman RM, Hofmann GA. Effective electroporation therapy of human pancreatic tumors implanted in nude mice. Drug Deliv 1997; 4:293–299.

48. Nanda GS, Sun FX, Hofmann GA, Hoffman RM, Dev SB. Electroporation enhances therapeutic efficacy of anticancer drugs: treatment of human pancreatic tumor in animal model. Anticancer Res 1998; 18:1361–1366.

49. Jaroszeski MJ, Coppola D, Nesmith G, Heller L, Gilbert R, Pottinger C, Dang V, Hickey J, Heller R. Electrically mediated delivery of bleomycin for the treatment of rat hepatomas and hamster pancreatic adenocarcinoma. Proc Am Assoc Cancer Res 1999; 40:582.

50. Okino M, Esato K. The effects of a single high voltage electrical stimulation with an anticancer drug on in vivo growing malignant tumors. Jpn J Surg 1990; 20:197–204.

51. Okino M, Tomie H, Kanesada H, Marumoto M, Esato K, Suzuki H. Optimal electric conditions in electrical impulse chemotherapy. Jpn J Cancer Res 1992; 83:1095–1101.

52. Ramirez LH, Orlowski S, An D, Bindoula G, Dzodic R, Ardouin R, Bognel Cr, Belehradek J Jr, Munck J, Mir LM. Electrochemotherapy on liver tumors in rabbits. Br J Cancer 1998; 77:2104–2111.

53. Jaroszeski MJ, Gilbert RA, Heller R. In vivo antitumor effects of electrochemotherapy in a hepatoma model. Biochim Biophys Acta 1997; 1334:15–18.

54. Jaroszeski MJ, Coppola D, Pottinger C, Benson K, Gilbert RA, Heller R. Treatment of hepatocellular carcinoma in a rat model using electrochemotherapy. Eur J Cancer 2001; 37:422–430.

55. Baba M, Iishi H, Tatsuta M. In vivo electroporetic transfer of bcl-2 antisense oligonucleotide inhibits the development of hepatocellular carcinoma in rats. Int J Cancer 2000; 85:260–266.

56. Chazal M, Benchimol D, Baque P, Pierrefite V, Milano G, Bourgeon A. Treatment of hepatic metastases of colorectal cancer by electrochemotherapy: an experimental study in the rat. Surgery 1998; 124:536–540.

57. Nanda GS, Merlock RA, Hofmann GA, Dev SB. A novel and effective therapy for prostate cancer. Proc Am Assoc Cancer Res 1998; 39:472.

58. Horikoshi T, Naganuma H, Ohashi Y, Ueno T, Nukui H. Enhancing effect of electric stimulation on cytotoxicity of anticancer agents against rat and human glioma cells. Brain Res Bull 2000; 51:371–378.

59. Salford LG, Persson BR, Brun A, Ceberg CP, Kongstad PC, Mir LM. A new brain tumour therapy combining bleomycin with in vivo electropermeabilization. Biochem Biophys Res Commun Jul 1993; 194(30):938–943.

60. Nanda GS, Merlock RA, Hofmann GA, Dev SB. Membrane permeabilizatoin of MCF-7 cells

by electrical pulses enhances cytotoxicity of anticancer drugs. Proc Am Assoc Cancer Res 1997; 38:260.

61. Belehradek JJ, Orlowski S, Poddevin B, Paoletti C, Mir LM. Electrochemotherapy of spontaneous mammary tumors in mice. Eur J Cancer 1991; 27:73–76.

62. Kambe M, Arita D, Kikuchi H, Funato T, Tezuka F, Gamo M, Murakawa Y, Kanamaru R. Enhancing the effect of anticancer drugs against the colorectal cancer cell line with electroporation. Tohoku J Exp Med 1990; 180:161.

63. Kuriyama S, Kikukawa M, Mitoro A, Tsujinoue H, Nakatani T, Yamazaki M, Yoshiji H, Toyokawa Y, Yoshikawa M, Fukui H. Antitumor effect of electrochemotherapy on colorectal carcinoma in an orthotopic mouse model. Int J Oncol 1999; 14:321–326.

64. Kuriyama S, Matsumoto M, Mitoro A, Tsujinoue H, Nakatani T, Fukui H, Tsujii T. Electrochemotherapy for colorectal cancer with commonly used chemotherapeutic agents in a mouse model. Dig Dis Sci 2000; 45:1568–1577.

65. Tada T, Matsumoto K, Suzuki H. Electrochemotherapy significantly inhibits the growth of colon 26 tumors in mice. Surg Today 1997; 27:506–510.

66. Kuriyama S, Matsumoto M, Mitoro A, Tsujinoue H, Toyokawa Y, Nakatani T, Yamazaki M, Okamoto S, Fukui H. Electrochemotherapy against colorectal carcinoma: comparison of in vitro cytotoxicity of 5-fluorouracil, cisplatin and bleomycin. Int J Oncol 1999; 15:89–94.

67. Kuriyama S, Mitoro A, Tsujinoue H, Toyokawa Y, Nakatani T, Yoshiji H, Tsujimoto T, Okuda H, Nagao S, Fukui H. Electrochemotherapy can eradicate established colorectal carcinoma and leaves a systemic protective memory in mice. Int J Oncol 2000; 16:979–985.

68. Ogihara M, Yamaguchi O. Potentiation of effects of anticancer agents by local electric pulses in murine bladder cancer. Urol Res 2000; 28:391–397.

69. Yamaguchi O, Irisawa C, Baba K, Ogihara M, Yokota T, Shiraiwa Y. Potentiation of antitumor effect of bleomycin by local electric pulses in mouse bladder tumor. Tohoku J Exp Med 1994; 172:291–293.

70. Gehl J, Skovsgaard T, Mir LM. Enhancement of cytotoxicity by electropermeabilization: an improved method for screening drugs. Anticancer Drugs 1998; 9:319–325.

71. Hofmann GA, Dev SB, Nanda GS. Electrochemotherapy: transition from laboratory to the clinic. IEEE Eng Med Biol 1996; 15:124–132.

72. Orlowski S, An D, Belehradek J Jr, Mir LM. Antimetastatic effects of electrochemotherapy and of histoincompatible interleukin-2-secreting cells in the murine Lewis lung tumor. Anticancer Drugs 1998; 9:551–556.

73. Kanesada H. Anticancer effect of high voltage pulses combined with concentration dependent anticancer drugs on Lewis lung carcinoma, in vivo. J Jpn Cancer Ther 1990; 25:2640–2648.

74. Yabushita H, Yoshikawa K, Hirata M, Furuya H, Hojyoh T, Fukatsu H, Noguchi M, Nakanishi M. Effects of electrochemotherapy on CaSki cells derived from a cervical squamous cell carcinoma. Gynecol Oncol 1997; 65:297–303.

75. Horiuchi A, Nikaido T, Mitsushita J, Toki T, Konishi I, Fujii S. Enhancement of antitumor effect of bleomycin by low-voltage in vivo electroporation: a study of human uterine leiomyosarcomas in nude mice. Int J Cancer 2000; 88:640–644.

76. Hyacinthe M, Jaroszeski MJ, Dang VV, Coppola D, Karl RC, Gilbert RA, Heller R. Electrically enhanced drug delivery for the treatment of soft tissue sarcoma. Cancer 1999; 85:409–417.

77. Engstrom PE, Ivarsson K, Tranberg KG, Stenram U, Salford LG, Persson BR. Electrically mediated drug delivery for treatment of an adenocarcinoma transplanted into rat liver. Anticancer Res 2001; 21:1817–1822.

78. Čemažar M, Parkins CS, Holder AL, Kranjc S, Chaplin DJ, Serša G. Cytotoxicity of bioreductive drug tirapazamine is increased by application of electric pulses in SA-1 tumours in mice. Anticancer Res 2001; 21:1151–1156.

79. Crooke ST, Bradner WT. Bleomycin, a review. J Med 1976; 7:333–428.

80. Twentyman PR. Bleomycin-mode of action with particular reference to the cell cycle. Pharmacol Ther 1983; 23:417–441.

81. Povirk LF, Austin MJ. Genotoxicity of bleomycin. Mutat Res 1991; 257:127–143.

82. Tounekti O, Kenani A, Foray N, Orlowski S, Mir LM. The ratio of single- to double-strand DNA breaks and their absolute values determine cell death pathway. Br J Cancer 2001; 84:1272–1279.

83. Chang X, Wang J, Shan C. Pingyangmycin (bleomycin A5)-mediated electrochemotherapy for human prostate cancer cell line PC-3M in athymic mice. Chinese J Exp Surgery 1999; 16:510.

84. Jain RK. Barriers to drug delivery in solid tumors. Sci Am 1994; 271:58–65.

85. Heller R, Jaroszeski MJ, Glass LF, Messina JL, Rapaport DP, DeConti RC, Fenske NA, Gilbert RA, Mir LM, Reintgen DS. Phase I/II trial for the treatment of cutaneous and subcutaneous tumors using electrochemotherapy. Cancer 1996; 77:964–971.

86. Glass LF, Pepine ML, Fenske NA, Jaroszeski M, Reintgen DS, Heller R. Beomycin-mediated electrochemotherapy of metastatic melanoma. Arch Dermatol 1996; 132:1353–1357.

87. Heller R, Jaroszeski MJ, Reintgen DS, Puleo CA, DeConti RC, Gilbert RA, Glass LF. Treatment of cutaneous and subcutaneous tumors with electrochemotherapy using intralesional bleomycin. Cancer 1998; 83:148–157.

88. Reintgen DS, Jaroszeski MJ, Heller R. Electrochemotherapy, a novel approach to cancer. Skin Cancer Found J 1996; 14:17–19.

89. Serša G, Štabuc B, Čemažar M, Miklavčič D, Rudolf Z. Electrochemotherapy with cisplatin: clinical experience in malignant melanoma patients. Clin Cancer Res 2000; 6:863–867.

90. Yu NY, Orenberg EK, Luck EE, Brown DM. Antitumor effect of intratumoral administration of fluorouracil/epinephrine injectable gel in C3H mice. Cancer Chemother Pharmacol 1995; 36:27–34.

91. Rabussay DP, Nanda GS, Goldfarb PM. Enhancing the effectiveness of drug-based cancer therapy by electroporation (electropermeabilization). Tech Cancer Res Treat 2002; 1:71–81.

92. Rols M-P, Bachaud J-M, Giraud P, Chevreau C, Roché H, Teissié J. Electrochemotherapy of cutaneous metastases in malignant melanoma. Melanoma Res 2000; 10:468–474.

93. Sikič BI. Beomycin. In: Droz JP, Cvitkovic E, Armand JP, Khoury S, eds. Handbook of Chemotherapy in Clinical Oncology, 1998:143–146.

94. Panje WR, Hier MP, Garman GR, Harrell E, Goldman A, Bloch I. Electroporation therapy of head and neck cancer. Ann Otol Rhinol Laryngol 1998; 779–785.

95. Frölich M, Henke E, Gens J, Seela W, Franke WG. Evaluation of intratumoral bleomycin application in a tumor model and in a clinical pilot study. Deutsche Zeitschrift für Mund. Kiefer und Gesicht-chirurgie 1990; 14:456–462.

96. Ceberg CP, Brun A, Mir LM, Persson BRR, Salford LG. Enhanced boron uptake in RG 2 rat gliomas by electropermeabilization in vivo—a new possibility in boron neutron capture therapy. Anticancer Drugs 1994; 5:463–466.

97. Čemažar M, Skrk J, Mitrovic B, Serša G. Changed delivery of boron to tumours using electroporation for boron neutron capture therapy with BSH. Br J Radiol 2000; 73:195–200.

98. Engstrom PE, Jonsson AC, Persson BRR, Strand S, Salford LG. Enhanced cellular uptake of radiopharmaceuticals with electroporation. Application with ^{111}In-oxine. Tumor Target 1996; 2:251–258.

99. Belehradek M, Orlowski S, Ramirez LH, Pron G, Poddevin B, Mir LM. Electropermeabilization of cells in tissues assessed by the qualitative and quantitative electroloading of bleomycin. Biochim Biophys Acta 1994; 1190:155–163.

100. Rabussay D, Dev ND, Fewell J, Smith LC, Widera G, Zhang L. Enhancement of therapeutic drug and DNA delivery into cells by electroporation. J Phys D 2003; 36:348–363.

101. Čemažar M, Miklavčič D, Mir LM, Belehradek J Jr, Bonnay M, Fourcault D, Serša G. Electrochemotherapy of tumours resistant to cisplatin: a study in a murine tumour model. Eur J Cancer 2001; 37:1166–1172.

102. Belehradek M, Domenge C, Luboinski B, Orlowski S, Belehradek J Jr, Mir LM. Electrochemotherapy, a new antitumor treatment. Cancer 1993; 72:3694–3700.

103. Serša G, Čemažar M, Semrov D, Miklavčič D. Changing electrode orientation improves the efficacy of electrochemotherapy of solid tumors in mice. Bioelectrochem Bioenerget 1996; 39:61–66.

104. Gilbert RA, Jaroszeski MJ, Heller R. Novel electrode designs for electrochemotherapy. Biochim Biophys Acta 1997; 1334:9–14.

105. Gehl J, Skovsgaard T, Nielsen SL, Mir LM. Electroporation of muscle tissue in vivo in mice: sensitivity investigated by uptake of 51chrome-EDTA. Proc Am Assoc Cancer Res 1997; 38:260.

106. Glass LF, Fenske NA, Jaroszeski M, Perrott R, Harvey DT, Reintgen DS, Heller R. Bleomycin-mediated electrochemotherapy of basal cell carcinoma. J Am Acad Dermatol 1996; 34:82–86.

107. Rodríguez-Cuevas S, Barrosco-Bravo S, Almanza-Estrada J, Cristobal-Martínez L, Gonzalez-Rodríguez E. Electrochemotherapy in primary and metastatic skin tumors: phase II trial using intralesional bleomycin. Arch Med Res 2001; 32:273–276.

108. Panje WR, Sadeghi N. Endoscopic and electroporation therapy of paranasal sinus tumors. Am J Rhinol 2000; 14:187–191.

109. Allegretti JP, Panje WR. Electroporation therapy for head and neck cancer including carotid artery involvement. Laryngoscope 2001; 111:52–56.

110. Goldfarb P, Biel M, Hanna E, Houck J, Klotch D, Nathan CO, Panje W, Robbins T, Shaw G, El-Sayed S, Hier M, Jones V, Nasser J, Rice. A phase II study using electroporation (EPT) and intratumoral bleomycin in patient with recurrent head and neck cancer: a safe and active treatment approach. Proceedings of ASCO 1999; 18:39a.

111. Goldfarb P, Biel M, El-Sayed S, Hanna E, Hier M, Houck J, Klotch D, Nathan CO, Panje W, Robbins T, Shaw G, Jones V, Nasser J, Rice D, Vieira F. Treatment of recurrent head and neck cancer utilizing electroporation with intralesional bleomycin: long term results. Proceedings of ASCO 2002; 21:183b.

112. Burian M, Formanek M, Regele H Acta Otolaryngol 2003; 123:264–268.

113. Glass LF, Jaroszeski M, Gilbert R, Reintgen DS, Heller R. Intralesional bleomycin-mediated electrochemotherapy in 20 patients with basal cell carcinoma. J Am Acad Dermatol 1997; 37:596–599.

114. Gehl J, Geertsen PF. Efficient palliation of haemorrhaging malignant melanoma skin metastases by electrochemotherapy. Melanoma Res 2000; 10:585–589.

115. Kubuota Y, Mir LM, Nakada T, Sasagawa I, Suzuki H, Aoyama N. Successful treatment of metastatic skin lesions with electrochemotherapy. J Urol 1998; 160:1426.

116. Domenge C, Orlowski S, Luboinski B, De Baere T, Schwaab G, Belehradek J Jr, Mir LM. Antitumor Electrochemotherapy. Cancer 1996; 77:956–963.

117. Rudolf Z, Štabuc B, Čemažar M, Miklavčič D, Vodovnik L, Serša G. Electrochemotherapy with bleomycin. The first clinical experience in malignant melanoma patients. Radiat Oncol 1995; 29:229–235.

118. Giraud P, Bachaud J-M, Teissié J, Rols M-P. Effects of electrochemotherapy on cutaneous metastases of human malignant melanoma (correspondence). Int J Radiation Oncology Biol Phys 1996; 36:1285.

119. Serša G, Čufer T, Čemažar M, Reberšek M, Rudolf Z. Electrochemotherapy with bleomycin in the treatment of hypernephroma metastasis: case report and literature review. Tumori 2000; 86:163–165.

120. Serša G, Štabuc B, Čemažar M, Jančar B, Miklavčiċ D, Rudolf Z. Electrochemotherapy with cisplatin: potentiation of local cisplatin antitumour effectiveness by application of electric pulses in cancer patients. Eur J Cancer 1998; 34:1213–1218.

121. Serša G, Štabuc B, Čemažar M, Miklavčič D, Rudolf Z. Electrochemotherapy with cisplatin: the systemic antitumour effectiveness of cisplatin can be potentiated locally by the application of electric pulses in the treatment of malignant melanoma skin metastases. Melanoma Res 2000; 10:381–385.

122. Forastiere A, Koch W, Trotti A, Sidransky D. Head and neck cancer. N Engl J Med 2001; 345:1890–1900.

123. Serša G. Electro-chemotherapy. Animal model work review. Methods Mol Med 2000; 37:119–136.

124. Nanda GS, Rabussay D. Safety of head and neck tumor treatment by electroporation therapy: effect on healthy tissues. In: Varma AK, Roodenburg JLN, eds. Oral Oncology. Delhi: Macmillan India Ltd, 2001:326–331.

125. Tounekti O, Belehradek J Jr, Mir LM. Relationships between DNA fragmentation, chromatin condensation, and changes in flow cytometry profiles detected during apoptosis. Exp Cell Res 1995; 217:506–516.

126. Serša G, Čemažar M, Miklavčič D, Chaplin DJ. Tumor blood flow modifying effect of electrochemotherapy with bleomycin. Anticancer Res 1999; 19:4017–4022.

127. Serša G, Čemažar M, Parkins CS, Chaplin DJ. Tumour blood flow changes induced by application of electric pulses. Eur J Cancer 1999; 35:672–677.

128. Gehl J, Skovsgaard T, Mir LM. Vascular reactions to in vivo electroporation: characterization and consequences for drug and gene delivery. Biochim Biophys Acta 2002; 1569:51–58.

129. Čemažar M, Parkins CS, Holder AL, Chaplin DJ, Tozer GM, Serša G. Electroporation of human microvascular endothelial cells: evidence for an anti-vascular mechanism of electrochemotherapy. Br J Cancer 2001; 84:565–570.

130. Engstrom PE, Persson BR, Brun A, Salford LG. A new antitumour treatment combining radiation and electric pulses. Anticancer Res 2001; 21:1809–1815.

131. Voznesenskii AI, Galanova YV, Archakov AI. Covalent binding of bleomycin to concanavalin A and immunoglobulin G enhances the ability of the bleomycin-Fe(II) complex to destroy the erythrocyte membrane. Biomed Sci 1991; 2:147–150.

132. Sauer H, Putz V, Fischer K, Hescheler J, Wartenberg M. Increased doxorubicin uptake and toxicity in multicellular tumour spheroids treated with DC electrical fields. Br J Cancer 1999; 80:1204–1213.

133. Ortiz LA, Lasky J, Hamilton RF Jr, Holian A, Hoyle GW, Banks W, Peschon JJ, Brody AR, Lungarella G, Friedman M. Expression of TNF and the necessity of TNF receptors in bleomycin-induced lung injury in mice. Exp Lung Res 1998; 24:721–743.

134. Micallef M. Immunoregulatory cytokine production by tumor-bearing rat spleen cells and its modulation by bleomycin. Anticancer Drugs 1993; 4:213–222.

135. Nelson WG, Kastan MB. DNA strand breaks: the DNA template alterations that trigger p53-dependent DNA damage response pathways. Mol Cell Biol 1994; 14:1815–1823.

136. Mendiratta SK, Thai G, Eslahi NK, Thull NM, Matar M, Bronte V, Pericle F. Therapeutic tumor immunity induced by polyimmunization with melanoma antigens gp100 and TRP-2. Cancer Res 2001; 61:859–863.

137. Nanda GS, Dev SB, Bleecher S, Rabussay D. A novel treatment modality for head and neck tumors. 8th International Conference on Differentiation Therapy, Montreal, Canada, October 1999, p. 61, Abstract No. 75.

138. Jaroszeski MJ, Coppola D, Nesmith G, Pottinger C, Hyacinthe M, Benson K, Gilbert R, Heller R. Effects of electrochemotherapy with bleomycin on normal liver tissue in a rat model. Eur J Cancer 2001; 37:414–421.

139. Mir LM, Roth C, Orlowski S, Quintin-Colonna F, Fradelizi D, Belehradek J Jr, Kourilsky P. Systemic antitumor effects of electrochemotherapy combined with histoincompatible cells secreting interleukin-2. J Immunother Emphasis Tumor Immunol 1995; 17:30–38.

140. Serša G, Čemažar M, Menart V, Gaberc-Porekar V, Miklavčič D. Anti-tumor effectiveness of electrochemotherapy with bleomycin is increased by TNF-α on SA-1 tumors in mice. Cancer Lett 1997; 116:85–92.

141. Serša G, Kranjc, Čemažar M. Improvement of combined modality therapy with cisplatin and radiation using electroporation of tumors. Int J Radiat Oncol Biol Phys 2000; 46:1037–1041.

142. Mouneimme Y, Tose PF, Barhouni R, Nicolau C. Electroinsertion of full length recombinant CD4 into red blood cell membrane. Biochim Biophys Acta 1990; 272:53–58.

143. Zeira M, Tose PF, Mouneimme Y, Lazarte J, Sneed L, Volsky DJ, Nicolau C. Full-length

CD4 electroinserted in the erythrocyte membrane as a long-lived inhibitor of infection by human immunodeficiency virus. Proc Natl Acad Sci USA 1991; 88:4409–4413.

144. Hollinger FB, Mouneimne Y, Lahart C, Tose PF, Dimitrov D, Nicolau C. Life span of circulating membrane CD4 inserted into the plasma membranes of autologous red blood cells of HIV-infected subjects. Journal of Acquired Immune Deficiency Syndromes and Human Retrovirology 1995; 9:126–132.

145. Raffy S, Teissie J. Surface charge control of electropermeabilization and glycophorin electroinsertion with 1,2-diacyl-sn-glycero-3-phosphocholine (lecithin) liposomes. Eur J Biochem 1997; 250:315–319.

146. Raffy S, Teissie J. Electroinsertion of glycophorin A in interdigitation fusion giant unicellular lipid vesicles. J Biol Chem 1997; 272:25524–25530.

147. El Oaugari K, Teissie J, Benoist H. Glycophorin A protects K562 cells from natural killer cell attack. Role of angiogenesis. J Biol Chem 1995; 270:26970–26975.

148. Mouneimne Y, Barhoumi R, Myers T, Slogoff S, Nicolau C. Stable rightward shifts of the oxyhemoglobin dissociation curve induced by encapsulation of inositol hexaphosphate in red blood cells using electroporation. FEBS Lett 1990; 275:117–120.

149. Ogata Y, Goto H, Sakaguchi K, Suzuki M, Ohsaki K, Suzuki K, Saniabadi AR, Kamitani T, Takahashi A. Characteristics of neo red cells, their function and safety: in vivo studies. Artif Cells Blood Substit Immobil Biotechnol 1994; 22:875–881.

150. Crawford N, Chronos N. Electro-encapsulating drugs within blood platelets: local delivery to injured carotid arteries during angioplasty. Semin Interv Cardiol 1996; 1:91–102.

151. Banning A, Brewer L, Wendt M, Groves PH, Cheadle H, Penny WJ, Crawford N. Local delivery of platelets with encapsulated iloprost to balloon injured pig carotid arteries: effect on platelet deposition and neointima formation. Thromb Haemost 1997; 7:190–196.

152. Sakamoto T, Oshima Y, Sakamoto M, Kawano YI, Ishibashi T, Inomata HH, Ohnishi Y. Electroporation and bleomycin in galucoma-filtering surgery. Invest Ophthalmol Vis Sci 1997; 38:2864–2868.

153. Oshima Y, Sakamoto T, Nakamura T, Tahara Y, Goto Y, Ishibashi T, Inomata H. The comparative benefits of glaucoma filtering surgery with an electric-pulse targeted drug delivery system demonstrated in an animal model. Ophthalmol 1999; 106:1140–1146.

154. Oshima Y, Sakamoto T, Hisatomi T, Tsutsumi C, Sassa Y, Ishibashi T, Inomata H. Targeted gene transfer to corneal stroma in vivo by electric pulses. Exp Eye Res 2002; 74:191–198.

155. Blair-Parks K, Weston BC, Dean DA. High-level gene transfer to the cornea using electroporation. J Gene Med 2002; 4:92–100.

156. Oshima Y, Sakamoto T, Yamanaka I, Nishi T, Ishibashi T, Inomata H. Targeted gene transfer to corneal endothelium in vivo by electric pulse. Gene Ther 1998; 5:1347–1354.

157. Yokoyama A, Oshitari T, Negishi H, Dezawa M, Mizota A, Adachi-Usami E. Protection of retinal ganglion cells from ischemia-reperfusion injury by electrically applied Hsp27. Invest Ophtalmol Vis Sci 2001; 42:3283–3286.

158. Dezawa M, Takano M, Negishi H, Mo X, Oshitari T, Sawada H. Gene transfer into retinal ganglion cells by in vivo electroporation: a new approach. Micron 2002; 33:1–6.

159. Dev SB, Rabussay D, Widera G, Hofmann GA. Medical applications of electroporation. IEEE 2000; 28:206–223.

160. Dev NB, Preminger TJ, Hofmann GA, Dev SB. Sustained local delivery of heparin to the rabbit arterial wall with an electroporation catheter. Cathet Cardiovasc Diagn 1998; 45:337–345.

161. Dev NB, Hofmann GA, Dev SB, Rabussay D. Intravascular electroporation markedly attenuates neointima formation after balloon injury of the carotid artery in the rat. J Interven Cardiol 2000; 13:331–338.

162. Dev SB, Giordano FJ, Brown DL. In vivo delivery of gene to rabbit carotid artery by electroporation. Proceedings of the US Third and Japan Symposium on Drug Delivery Systems, Maui, Hawaii, Dec 17–22, 1995.

163. Martin JB, Young JL, Benoit JN, Dean DA. Gene transfer to intact mesenteric arteries by electroporation. J Vasc Res 2000; 37:372–380.

164. Kupfer JM, Ruan XM, Liu G, Matloff J, Forrester J, Chaux A. High-efficiency gene transfer to autologous rabbit jugular vein grafts using adenovirus-transferrin/polylysine-DNA complexes. Hum Gene Ther 1994; 5:1437–1443.

165. Wang Y, Bai Y, Price C, Boros P, Qin L, Bielinska AU, Kukowska-Latallo JF, Baker JR Jr, Bromberg JS. Combination of electroporation and DNA/dendrimer complexes enhances gene transfer into murine cardiac transplants. Am J Transplant 2001; 1:334–338.

166. Oshima K, Sen L, Cui G, Tung T, Sacks BM, Arellano-Kruse A, Laks H. Localized interleukin-10 gene transfer induces apoptosis of alloreactive T cells via FAS/FASL pathway, improves function, and prolongs survival of cardiac allograft. Transplantation 2002; 73:1019–1026.

167. Mozes G, Mohacsi T, Gloviczki P, Menawat S, Kullo I, Spector D, Taylor J, Crotty TB, O'Brien T. Adenovirus-mediated gene transfer of macrophage colony stimulating factor to the arterial wall in vivo. Arterioscler Thromb Vasc Biol 1998; 18:1157–1163.

168. Prausnitz MR, Bose VG, Langer R, Weaver JC. Electroporation of mammalian skin: a mechanism to enhance transdermal drug delivery. Proc Natl Acad Sci USA 1993; 15:10504–10508.

169. Banga AK. Electrically assisted transdermal and topical drug delivery. Bristol, PA and London, UK: Taylor & Francis, 1998.

170. Bose S, Ravis WR, Lin YJ, Zhang L, Hofmann GA, Banga AK. Electrically-assisted transdermal delivery of buprenorphine. J Control Release 2001; 73:197–203.

171. Zhang L, Lerner S, Rustrum WV, Hofmann GA. Electroporation-mediated topical delivery of vitamin C for cosmetic applications. Bioelectrochem Bioenerg 1999; 48:453–461.

172. Sen A, Zhao Y, Zhang L, Hui SW. Enhanced transdermal transport by electroporation using anionic lipids. J Con Rel 2002; 82:399–405.

173. Walace MS, Ridgeway B, Jun E, Schulteis G, Rabussay D, Zhang L. Topical delivery of lidocaine in healthy volunteers by electroporation, electroincorporation, or iontophoresis: an evaluation of skin anesthesia. Reg Anesth Pain Med 2001; 26:229–238.

174. Chang SL, Hofmann GA, Zhang L, Deftos LJ, Banga AK. The effect of electroporation on iontophoretic transdermal delivery of calcium regulating hormones. J Control Release 2000; 66:127–133.

175. Zhang L, Nolan E, Kreitschitz S, Rabussay DP. Enhanced delivery of naked DNA to the skin by non-invasive in vivo electroporation. Biochim Biophys Acta 2002; 1572:1–9.

176. McKinlay JB. The worldwide prevalence and epidemiology of erectile dysfunction. Int J Impot Res 2000; 12:S6–S11.

177. Zhang L, Azadzoi K, Chang SL, Banga AK, Hofmann GA, Rabussay DP, Goldstein I. Potential noninvasive approach to ameliorate male erectile dysfunction by electroporation: a feasibility evaluation in vitro, in rabbit, in human subjects [abstr]. Int J Impot Res 2000; 13(suppl 1):S17.

178. Zhang L, Rabussay DP. Clinical evaluation of safety and human tolerance of electrical sensation induced by electric fields with noninvasive electrodes. Bioelectrochem 2002; 56:233–236.

179. Magee TR, Ferrini M, Garban HJ, Vernet D, Mitani K, Rajfer J, Gonzales-Cadavid NF. Gene therapy of erectile dysfunction in the rat with penile neuronal nitric oxide synthase. Biol Reprod 2002; 67:20–28.

180. Sokol DL, Gewirtz AM. Gene therapy: basic concepts and recent advances. Crit Rev Eukaryot Gene Expr 1996; 6:29–57.

181. Gottschalk U, Chan S. Somatic gene therapy. Present situation and future perspective. Arzneimittelforschung 1998; 48(11):1111–1120.

182. Knoell DL, Yim IM. Human gene therapy for hereditary diseases: a review of trials. Am J Health Syst Pharm 1998; 55:899–904.

183. DeMatteo RP, Yeh H, Friscia M, Caparrelli D, Burke C, Desai N, Chu G, Markmann JF, Raper SE, Barker CF. Cellular immunity delimits adenoviral gene therapy strategies for the treatment of neoplastic diseases. Ann Surg Oncol 1999; 6:88–94.

184. Muruve DA, Barnes MJ, Stillman IE, Libermann TA. Adenoviral gene therapy leads to rapid

induction of multiple chemokines and acute neutrophil-dependent hepatic injury in vivo. Hum Gene Ther 1999; 10:965–976.

185. Muramatsu T, Nakamura A, Park HM. In vivo elelctroporation: a powerful and convenient means of non viral gene transfer to tissues of living animals. Intl J Mol Med 1998; 1:55–62.

186. Ahira H, Miyazaki J. Gene transfer into muscle by electroporation. Nat Biothechnol 1998; 16:867–870.

187. Mathiesen I. Electropermeabilization of skeletal muscle enhances gene transfer in vivo. Gene Ther 1999; 6:508–514.

188. Mir LM, Bureau MF, Gehl J, Rangara R, Rouy D, Caillaud JM, Delaere P, Branellec D, Schwartz B, Scherman D. High efficiency gene transfer into skeletal muscle by electric pulses. PNAS (USA) 1999; 96:4262–4267.

189. Srivastava I, Kam E, Sun Y, Stamatatos L, Montefiori S, Otten G, O'Hagen D, Sing M, Donelly JJ, Ulmer J, Barnett S. Enhanced neutralizing antibody responses induced in rhesus macaques by 0-gp 140DV2 SF162 in a prime-boost regimen. Abstract 306-W presented at The Ninth Conference on Retroviruses and Opportunistic Infections. Seattle, WA, 2002.

190. Babiuk S, Baca-Estrada ME, Foldvari M, Storms M, Rabussay D, Widera G, Babiuk LA. Electroporation improves the efficacy of DNA vaccines in large animals. Vaccine 2002; 20: 3399–3408.

191. Keating A, Nolan E, Filshie R, Dev SB. In: Jaroszeski MJ, Heller R, Gilbert R, eds. Methods in Molecular Medicine. Totowa, N.J.: Humana, 2000:359–368.

192. Keating A, Berkahn L, Filshie R. A phase I study of the transplantation of genetically marked autologous bone marrow stromal cells. Hum Gene Ther 1998; 9:591–600.

193. Roth DA, Tawa NE Jr, O'Brien JM, Treco DA, Selden RF. Factor VIII transkaryotic therapy study group. Nonviral transfer of the gene encoding coagulation factor VIII in patients with severe A hemophilia. N Engl J Med 2001; 344:1735–1742.

194. Black KL, Fahkrai H. A phase I study of the safety of injecting malignant glioma patients with irradiated TGF-beta-2 antisense gene modified autologous tumor cells. 1995; 138.

195. Fahkrai H, Gutheil JC. A phase II study of antisense TGF-beta +/− IL-2 gene transfected allogeneic tumor cells as a vaccine in patients with stage IIIB and IV non-small cell lung cancer. 1999:331.

196. Fahkrai H, Dorigo O, Shawler DL, Lin H, Mercola D, Black KL, Royston I, Sobol RE. Eradication of established intracranial rat gliomas by transforming growth factor beta antisense gene therapy. Proc Natl Acad Sci USA 1996; 93:2909–2914.

197. Liau LM, Fahkrai H, Black KL. Prolonged survival of rats with tracranial C6 gliomas by treatment with TGF-beta antisense gene. Neurol Res 1998; 20:742–747.

198. Tang DC, DeVit M, Johnston SA. Genetic immunization is a simple method for eliciting an immune response. Nature 1992; 356:152–154.

199. Widera G, Austin M, Rabussay D, Goldbeck C, Barnett SW, Chen M, Leung L, Ottern GR, Thudium K, Selby M, Ulmer JB. Increased DNA vaccine delivery and immunogenicity by electroporation in vivo. J Immunol 2000; 164:4635–4640.

200. Tollefsen S, Tjelle T, Schneider J, Harboe M, Wiker H, Hewinson G, Huygen K, Mathiesen I. Improved cellular and humoral immune responses against Mycobacterium tuberculosis antigens after intramuscular DNA immunisation combined with muscle electroporation. Vaccine 2002; 20:3370–3378.

201. Drabick JJ, Glasspool-Malone J, King A, Malone RW. Cutaneous transfection and immune responses to intradermal nucleic acid vaccination are significantly enhanced by in vivo electropermeabilization. Mol Ther 2001; 3:249–255.

42

The Paradigm of Biologically Closed Electric Circuits and Its Clinical Applications

Björn E. W. Nordenström*

Karolinska Institute and Hospital, Stockholm, Sweden

Jorgen Nordenström

Huddinge University Hospital, Stockholm, Sweden

The origin and evolution of the BCEC concept, early experiments leading to its application for the electrochemical treatment of tumors, mechanisms of action and its relationship to Oriental concepts of Qi and the corona of Kirlian photography are reviewed. This may provide useful background information for additional chapters in this volume that expand on these relationships and present clinical results in a wide variety of malignant and non-malignant tumors.

I. INTRODUCTION

A basis for our physical world is energy (1,2). Energy appears to us in various forms, one of which is electromagnetic energy, (2) also described as a unified electromagnetic field (UEMF), which has a particular relation to matter of our nonbiological (3) and biological (4) world.

Interestingly enough, nonbiological and biological matter consists of identical atoms, the building stones of our world. Furthermore, biological matter has the capacity to transfer and utilize electric energy for function and further structuring. This occurs as field circulation with cotransport of ions in biologically closed electric circuits (BCEC). Therefore, biological matter derived from the EM field is not only structurally modified but also given function by EM energy. Everything in our physical world undergoes "development" from and "regression" back to the EM field, as a circulation of changing forms of energy.

*Recipient of the Linus Pauling Award 1992, and the International Scientific and Technological Cooperation Award of the People's Republic of China, 2001.

The complexity and speed of change vary, but otherwise there is in principle no difference between nonbiological and biological matter.

It is surprising that closed circuit electric flow, with utilization of electrical energy in technology, is a principle largely unrecognized in biology. Structured flow of electricity in biology does, however, exist and is defined to take place in BCEC systems (5,6). These systems are numerous, of varying size and construction, dominated by the flow of ions in circulating fields. The BCEC systems produce structural and functional effects by electric and magnetic influences far beyond what man can produce artificially. This largely depends on the relation between chemistry and physics, here dominated by the EM fields.

II. BIOLOGICALLY CLOSED ELECTRIC CIRCUITS

The first BCEC system identified was the vascular closed circuit (VCC). The walls of blood vessels carry a resistivity 150–200 times that of the conducting plasma of blood (5). Vessels therefore can function as relatively insulated "cables" for transport of ions (5,6). Vessels form multiple loops. An external moving magnetic field can therefore also be shown to induce a flow of ionic current in the loops (7,8).

Across the capillaries an electrical junction exists between the plasma of blood and the extra vascular equally conducting interstitial tissue fluid. The various necessary components for the existence of vascular-interstitial closed circuits (VICC systems) are also identified (5,6). The VICC can be activated by several mechanisms. Firstly, metabolic activities can be considered to be a physiological "disturbance of homeostasis." For example, a working muscle becomes tired. Metabolic activities make the muscle electropositive in relation to blood. Homeostasis is disturbed. The field gradient between muscle and blood will, by ionic exchange via the VICC, restore homeostasis and the muscle can work again. The waste products appearing in the blood will act on the cardiorespiratory centers giving closed circuit "signals" to the heart and respiratory muscles to increase their activity, etc.

Secondly, production of an injury may be looked upon as a pathological disturbance of homeostasis. Traumatic injury, infection, necrosis, and the like produce an injury potential of tissue in relation to blood. Initially, the injured tissue is electropositive but varies its direction of gradient by time under attenuation. This is very purposeful. The injured tissue needs to get rid of both anions and cations and to get new collections of these for the process of healing. The fluctuations of potential are explained as a statistical representation of the varying speed of migration and diffusion of various anions and cations.

Cancers often spontaneously develop necrosis inside a tumour (9). This tissue liberates energy, which is reflected in the developed injury potential in relation to the surrounding tissue. A flow of ionic current in the electric field around the tumour will result in the development of structural modifications (corona structures) (5,9). As many as 12 components of the corona structures have been identified in radiographs. The corona structures are not specific for the lungs. They can also develop around necrotizing cancers, such as breast cancer, or a common injury of any location.

The flow of current in the VICC channels also influences movable cells such as leukocytes, which carry a surplus of fixed negative charge on their surfaces. In spontaneous injury polarization, leukocytes accumulate in the injured electropositive tissue as an in vivo electrophoresis via the VICC channels. This is a biological example of field interferences, leading to cellular cotransport in the VICC system, which allows definition of necessary energy and mechanism of transport in contrast to so-called leukotaxis.

The flow of blood and lymph with their influences of various *charged* and *uncharged* particles will create varying summation of EMFs. Even external EMFs (6–8), gravitation and its "smaller cousins," van der Waals forces, will produce structural and functional, variable electromagnetic effects by interference. It is easy to understand that these field effects by interferences, creating the internal environment of EMF in biology, vary in time, strength, and location both in health and disease.

III. EMF INTERFERENCES INSIDE CELLS

When ionic current is flowing in between cells in tissue, the associated magnetic field will induce eddy currents inside the cells and structural effects may be produced. The flow of current in a tissue may produce entirely new structures of tissue such as fibrous membranes, organ capsules, and various channels. Such channels, produced by the flow of weak current through an excised "dead" tissue sample are possibly representing primitive vessels. It seems that a flow of ionic current in tissue represents an overall structuring principle for the development of biological tissue components such as channels. Depending on from where and to where a *chronical* flow of ionic closed circuit current occurs, blood or lymph vessels or ductal channels or membranes (10), etc., seem to develop (5).

Conductive media other than blood plasma and interstitial tissue fluid, such as the content of urinary or glandular ducts (11,12), and the conductive properties of cerebrospinal liquid and axoplasm of nerves form integrated circuits. An example is the vascular-interstitial-neuromuscular circuit (VINMC) (12–18).

Vessels and interstitial tissue fluid at open membrane channels make contact with the axons of the nerve cell and its muscular connection. In this closed circuit the conductive capacities of the vessels are much larger than those of the axonal channels. Therefore, an electric flow in the nerve should also activate the vascular branch of the closed circuit. This was illustrated by the following experiment.

Partial amputation was made of one hind leg of rats. Only the femoral nerve, the femoral artery and vein were preserved. Through an incision an electrode was positioned in the inferior caval vein or in the abdominal aorta. Via another electrode, 20–50-mV pulses were applied to the femoral nerve in rats in relation to the aorta or the vena cava. Contractions of the leg muscle occurred at each pulse. The femoral vessels were provided with a ligature in the groin. At sudden ligation of the vessels, the leg contractions were immediately suspended. Instead, contractions occurred of abdominal muscles. A shunting of current evidently occurred at the ligation of the leg vessels. In other experiments, without "partial amputation," pinchings of a toe of a rat resulted in spontaneous leg muscle contractions (13), which gave raise to voltage pulses in the vena cava and the aorta.

This example indicate the impact of BCEC systems on structure and functions. The BCEC therefore represents a basic mechanism of an early development of nonbiological matter into biological matter. The electric energy is with this view not only the origin of matter but also a dynamic factor, which provides matter with structural modifications and functions in co-operation with other physical factors.

IV. ELECTROCHEMICAL TREATMENT OF CANCER

The first attempt to utilize the system of biologically closed electric circuits (BCEC) (5) with the aim to treat cancer was performed as an activation of the vascular-interstitial closed circuit (VICC). These treatments are called *electrochemical treatments* (EChT) because they are not exclusively the result of the so-called contact current of Galvani (and Volta), induction current of Faraday, or displacement current of Maxwell. EChT of cancer includes galvanic, faradic, and displacement current, which are all part of electricity, as well as the sequences of electrochemical events and transports that occur at the interactions between the electric and magnetic fields with the biological substrate in the BCEC; the electrochemical system of the body.

EChT represents basically an in vivo electrophoretic treatment, which is entirely different from currently practiced conventional treatments of cancer. EChT consists of two phases, the charging (Phase I) and the discharging (Phase II) of an electrophoretic process. The function of electrochemical cells is presented, partly after Bockris and Drazic (19). It illustrates the technical correspondence with Phases I and II in EChT.

The cell is driven (charged) by an external source of power with the anode ($+$) and cathode ($-$), representing platinum electrodes in contact with the electrolyte (here H_2SO_4 + H_2O). Electrons flow in the metallic parts and ions in the electrolyte. At low voltage, no current flows in the circuit. The reason is that the electrode–electrolyte interphases present resistances together with other resistances of the circuit, which have to be overcome. By gradually increasing the voltage applied to the electrodes, current starts to flow at a certain voltage, which occurs above the so-called equilibrium voltage. The magnitude of voltage difference applied above the equilibrium voltage will drive the circuit and is called the *overpotential*. At the transfer of electrons, which then occurs across the electrode–electrolyte interphases, many effects take place with formation of anodic and cathodic products of reaction. The development of products of reaction and flow of ions when current drives the process corresponds to the charging of an electrophoretic cell (polarization of the system).

When the external source of power has polarized the cell and is replaced by a load or the cables are short-circuited, a self-driving system is created. This means that current will flow in the reverse direction and the cell is discharged. Correspondingly, when current is driven between electrodes in tissue, which is conductive for ions, the electrophoretic EChT system will become polarized (Phase I). When removing the driving source of power, or when, for instance, short-circuiting, the EChT system will also become self-driving with reversal of the current (Phase II). Interestingly enough, biological tissue seems to be capable of reversing current without the presence of metal electrodes or for instance a short-circuiting of their cables. This is possible because of the multiple BCEC systems in tissues, which also contain redox enzymes serving as reversible electrodes (5).

The reactions at the contact of the electrode-electrolyte results in polarization (Phase I). Hydrolysis (decomposition of water) leads to anodic acidity (H^+), pH 2 and cathodic alkalinity (OH^-) pH 12. These compounds and particularly H^+ destroy tissue around the electrodes. The black anodic area in the tissue is formed by acidic haematin, which is derived from extravasation of the blood and its transformation by protons. Similarly, dark base haematin is formed in the cathodic area by OH^- ions. The sectioned tissue also shows a dry anodic and a wet cathodic field area, which correspond to the electro osmotic transport of water. The white center of the acidic black area is due to the bleaching by Cl_2. It represents a small central position, as the relatively large Cl_2 molecules without carrying any excess of charge cannot compete with the destructive effect of H^+ ions. Protons easily diffuse and migrate more rapidly in the anodic field than any other ions. Their effects on tissue is counteracted by the buffering capacity of the tissue fields, which explains the very steep boundary gradient of the protons diffusing and migrating in the tissue.

Besides anodic Cl_2 and O_2 gas, cathodic H_2 gas is also formed. The gaseous materials elevate the pressure in the tissue and produce interference with the tissue circulation and the electrode–electrolyte reactions. They form anodic and cathodic gas bubbles. The electric fields induce a charge displacement in these dielectric materials with secondary gas adsorption onto the electrodes. Small gas bubbles are also "pumped" out into the tissue by gas pressure and in the anodic field, close to the electrode, also into intercellular spaces by dielectrophoresis. Gas bubbles can be seen microscopically in a transparent medium. It is apparent that the gas production at the electrodes will disturb the EChT process by separation of the electrodes from the electrolyte. A decreasing flow of current during Phase I of EChT with oscillations of the voltage is often experienced as pain by the patient and is caused by production of gas bubbles leaving the electrodes. This drawback can be counteracted by flushing the electrode with for instance saline solution.

It is commonly but falsely believed that the H^+ and OH^- ions and other products of the electrode–electrolyte–contact reactions are exclusively responsible for all the effects of the EChT (compare galvanic *contact current*). The situation is considerably more complex, however, due to a multitude of mechanisms connected to BCEC, which lead to the structural and functional effects of the distant field concept.

The circulating electromagnetic field is the basis of induction of all electrically derived interactions in the tissues. The most intensive local reactions occur at the electrode–electrolyte interphases, which we take advantage of for the primary destruction (*killing*) of a diagnosed cancer. The field circulating in the tissues outside the cancer also induces interactions with the biological substrate all the way between the electrodes. But these effects are considerably more complex and superficially less apparent than the primary electrode–electrolyte reactions. In fact, these effects, which are here called *distant field effects*, are of considerable importance and interest but unfortunately as yet only partly understood. Examples of such DF effects will be given below.

One example of transformation of tissue is the development of corona structures by the electric field around an injury-polarized, centrally necrotic cancer (see Ref. 5, pp. 14–44). Edge enhancement, at irregular protrusions of the tumour surfaces produced by dipole induction in dielectric debris from cellular membranes, etc., will result in radiating structures as well as electroosmosis, seen as a dehydrated A zone and a hydrated B zone. Of particular interest are the disappearances of local islands of metastatic cells, which from time to time can be observed in the lung in connection with EChT of a larger primary tumour in the lung.

Small metastases from a previously operated pelvic sarcoma of a 60-year-old woman (5) was present in the lower lobe of the right lung shown. After EChT of two primary tumors in the lower lobe the small metastases in the lung regressed partly or completely. The small metastases were located far away from the electrodes, and no other treatment had been given. It is unlikely that the products of electrode reactions should have caused the regression of the metastases. Therefore another explanation should be sought. It is suggested that there are certain mechanisms related to the DF effects that each or in combination give a plausible explanation.

A. Electroosmosis, Dielectric Transports

Electroosmosis is a particularly important effect of DF. The mechanisms involved depend on the presence of a matrix with narrow interstitial capillaries. These are known to be provided with a surplus of fixed electronegative charges in the walls of closed circuit electrophoretic VICC-channels. Further, the VICC system must be activated by a voltage gradient (see Ref. 5, Chapter IX). The endogenous VICC channels are powered by either metabolic or injury processes or may be powered artificially between implanted electrodes (in EChT). In vivo tissue water always flows electroosmotically from anode to cathode. Even pencil-wide pulmonary arteries in the dog may be narrowed, forming obstructing funnels by an electroosmotic increase of tissue turgor pressure in the cathodic field. This means that also the capillaries in the cathodic field can have a completely suspended circulation (while the micro thromboses block the capillaries in the anodic field). Cancer tissue is often more sensitive than normal tissue to chemotherapeutics, heat, cold, and radiation. A sufficiently long time of vascular obstruction will evidently seriously interfere with the living conditions of the tissues.

These aspects focusing on transport of tissue water are also largely relevant for dielectric particles, e.g., neutral lipids. Such EChT transports can, however, only be predicted on the basis of actual field strengths, of molecular size of particles in relation to capillarity and surface charge of the tissue matrix.

B. Field Activation of the Immunological System

At EChT, the anodic field will attract white blood cells, which are known to be electronegatively charged (20). By making the electrode electronegative, the field will repel the electronegative white blood cells. When they flow in veins directed towards the cathode a field-flow interference will occur, leading to accumulation of white blood cells. The observations show that local accumulation of charged white blood cells is electrophoretically transported in the applied field. This may also indicate that spontaneous so-called leukotaxis might be explained energetically as an in vivo electrophoresis of the VICC system. The in vivo accumulations of leukocytes to the anodic tissue region also seem to indicatate that a field-induced activation of the immunological system, with high probability, is induced at EChT.

Various immunomodulators, activating macrophages with the ability selectively to destroy neoplastic cells are also believed to be put into action by the electrophoretic EChT flow of current. After endocyte formation of liposomes containing immunomodulators, generating cytoaggressive macrophages, the targeting should be provided by the EChT current. Works by Fiedler (21), and others indicate that future treatment of metastases should proceed along these lines.

ELECTRODES.   Platinum as a metal is stable for most anodic and cathodic electrochemical reactions. Its catalytic power, i.e., its ability to permit reactions with the tissue electrolytes is excellent as compared with other metals. It also has the property of enhancing the speed of reactions when increasing the over voltage, also here superior to other metals. However, platinum is expensive and rather brittle. The mechanical properties can be improved by adding 10% iridium. The considerable differences of electrodic material will be described below.

The anode and cathode should have equal surface areas so that the cathode at least will not produce a limiting step for the flow of current. Regression of cancer tissue can take place both around the anode (+) and the cathode (−) in the tumor. It may therefore seem logical to place both anode and cathode in the cancer. Such a positioning of electrodes can, if a sufficient dose of current is given to a T_1 tumor, lead to a treatment result comparable with an initially successful surgical removal of a cancer. Not seldom after surgical removal of the tumor, metastases may, after some time, start growing in the tissue around the former place of the tumor. They may have developed as local metastases in the surrounding tissue of the cancer but have remained undiagnosed at the time of surgery. This kind of peripheral recurrence may also have taken place before local EChT extinction of a cancer with anode and cathode in the tumor. To be able to utilize the DF effect described, the anode and cathode should be positioned far away from each other to create a large field. Thereby a better effect may be expected as compared with local surgical removal or EChT with closely positioned electrodes. These aspects are important and may indicate that EChT of small resectable cancers might be more efficient than conventional surgical resection.

Electrodes positioned very closely to each other will give a relatively small electric field and the risk for a linear breakthrough of current is evident. This also obviates the risk of relatively insufficient diffusion and migration of toxic products caused by local electrode reactions. The latter drawbacks also exist when several anodes and cathodes are used. An uneven distribution of current will occur between pairs of anodes and cathodes, as they will present differences of internal resistances in the conductive fluid of the cancer. In addition, field interferences will occur. By positioning anodic and cathodic electrodes far from each other the dose requirements for treatment will be hampered by a lowering of the flow of current, which has to be compensated for by a longer time of treatment or improvement of the electrodes. The risk of injuring sensitive tissue also requires special attention.

Upon this background it may be evident that a sufficient dose of treatment should be given during Phase I. The electropositive polarity during Phase I will efficiently keep malignant, electronegatively charged cells attached to the anodic tumor. The cells should preferably be devitalised before conclusion of Phase I as the cancer will become cathodic during Phase II. Under no circumstances should a reference electrode be placed on the skin during EChT, similar to what is commonly used in diathermia, when high-frequency alternating current is used. In EChT the applied direct current might choose an unpredictable way to the tumour electrode and damage vital organs such as the heart, spinal cord, and nerve stems.

V. ELECTROSTATIC FIELD INTERFERENCE AND ITS EFFECT ON CELLULAR AND TISSUE FUNCTION

In a colloid, the ions of an electrolyte are attracted to particles with excess charge. Attracted ions form a firm Stern layer and a movable Helmholtz layer around the particle. Instead of a particle, an electrode may be inserted into the electrolyte and charged electrostatically in relation to ground. In an electrolyte with relatively small volume, such as the body electrolytes, ions of opposite polarity, as compared with the electrode, will be attracted. Counterions will give the electrolyte a surplus of charge with the same polarity as the electrode. This can be shown by charging an electrode in 1000 ml of NaCl solution in relation to ground. The voltage in a plastic jar with saline solution was measured at 10 AgCl electrodes in a row in the electrolyte in relation to a distant reference electrode in a 2-m-long rubber tube with saline solution connected to the electrolyte in the jar. By applying plus or minus 300 and 600 V the saline solution reached a voltage of $\pm$ 150–220 mV.

A. Leaking Biological Capacitors

All cells, organs, and the entire body are bidirectional and variably leaking ionic capacitors (7,8). This new principle is one of the integrated important mechanisms of the BCEC systems, the electrical network of the body. Each cell, surrounded by two phospholipid layers, enclose the inside conducting content of the cells. Therefore the cells are ionic microcapacitors, which can leak via open ionic channels of the cellular membranes. These channels can also close, for instance, by the influence of electropositive fields.

Organs such as liver, kidney, brain, lung, muscles, etc., are surrounded by relatively insulating fibrous membranes. Each organ is often also divided into smaller compartments (e.g., lobes of an organ) with the function of capacitors. All capacitors are interconnected via conductive fluids of nerves, blood, and lymph vessels, which are also leaking capacitors. The whole body itself represents a leaking capacitor, leaking as it does by conducting urine, faeces, food, saliva, sweat, etc. The connections are integrated in closed electric circuits of the BCEC system.

By using the principle to charge an electrolyte, an organ, such as the liver, may be electrostatically charged in relation to ground. A field will then be created in relation to the surrounding organs. Via interconnected blood and lymph vessels, for instance, this charging will tend to equilibrate. This takes time in spite of forced convection, etc. Therefore, the time constant can be utilised stepwise to elevate the charging voltage and thereby maintain a voltage gradient of the organ in relation to the surrounding tissue. It is not necessarily so that a high voltage will lead to a high organ surrounding voltage. A relatively low electrode voltage may even result in a locally steeper organ-surrounding tissue gradient than a high one.

The capacitor function of cells is important at an electrostatic charging of the intercellular fluids. A positive charging will counteract the metabolic degradation of ATP to ADP (22), which liberates phosphate and leads to extrusion of Na^+.

B. The Na^+K^+ Membrane Pump: A BCEC Mechanism

A transmembranous cellular gradient of about 70 mV (interior negative, exterior positive) represents an accepted phase of polarization of the cellular membrane. The underlying mechanism is not, however, very well understood but probably related to the function of an anticipated cellular Na^+K^+ *pump*, leading to an outflow of Na^+ and inflow of K^+ across the cellular membrane. Required energy for this process is covered by intracellular ATP, which is degraded by hydrolysis in membrane-bound particles of Na^+K^+-ATPase.

A mechanism of pumping based on this view of energy liberation might exist already at the initial, asymmetrical separation of proton-phosphate ions. By electrostatic electropositive charging the body fluids in relation to ground, it may be possible to create an "uphill" voltage that is too large for the metabolic pumping of Na^+. The cellular function will be depressed or even blocked by such interference. A negative charging should increase the membrane gradient and facilitate the ionic pumping.

This first possibility is shown at an electrostatic charging of the peritoneal fluid in a rat (weight 42 g) with introduction of a platinum electrode with a 6.28 mm^2 area for charging and four nonpolarizable AgCl electrodes in various sites in the abdominal cavity and one electrode in the subcutis of each leg for voltage measurements. These were made in relation to a reference AgCl electrode positioned 2 m away in a plastic tube with saline solution, connected to the peritoneal cavity. Basically the same results as with the experiment in vitro with 1000 ml of saline solution were obtained in the rat. The values of the created field of equal polarity as the electrode is in the rat approximately 1.5–2.5 V at ± 300 to 600 V charging the electrode in relation to ground, which can be explained by the relatively small volume of the body electrolytes in relation to the size of the platinum electrode in the peritoneum positioned in the peritoneal cavity below the liver. Not only the four electrodes in the peritoneal cavity but also the subcutaneous electrodes in the legs reached the same charge of the field of equal polarity as the charged platinum electrode.

C. Application of Electrostatic Treatment (EST)—Initial Experience in Man

The principle of electrostatic treatment (EST) outlined above was tested in three voluntary patients who had received information about the animal experiments in which the body fluids were charged so as to arrest the spread of cancer. Theoretically it was assumed that blocking of the cellular ionic membrane pumps would interfere with the cellular functions, and that this would primarily led to a selective deterioration of metastatic cells. Cancer cells are known to be more sensitive to changes of the microenvironment than normal cells (as in hyperthermia, cryosurgery, chemotherapy, and radiation for instance). Theoretically electrostatic charging is not dangerous and can start at very low voltage differences. Further, charging of the body fluids is a procedure that can be easily controlled and interrupted or reversed instantaneously at any time.

Electrostatic treatment alone has resulted in regression of three cancer metastases in two patients. In a third patient, partial regression of one metastasis also occurred after electrostatic treatment only. Regression of other metastases in the mediastinum, lung, and metastases of the liver was also observed when chemotherapy was supplied. In this patient the possibility remains that the good result was due to (1) a continued but late effect of the electrostatic charging, (2) an unusually good effect of the chemotherapy, or (3) a result of the combined effects of the two modes of treatment.

Selective structural dissolution of small metastases could thus be observed in patients after applying only a fluctuating electrostatic voltage in relation to ground with change of polarity every 12th to 24th hour. Besides anticipated effects on the ionic membrane pumps, a fluctuating voltage of sufficient strength should lead to the separation of loosely attached charged particles of cancerous tissue and thus entail favourable conditions for chemotherapy. The theoretical possibility of displacement of loosely attached cancer cells makes it necessary always to combine this treatment with chemotherapy.

The *leaking body capacitor* has high average conductivity in the conducting fluids (approx. 0.9 Ω-m) but has too complex a mixture of internal leaking capacitors to be defined by one time constant. Various pathways for conductivity between an inserted electrode capacitor and the subcutis are utilized. A flow of current can always be recorded between the electrode and ground. It usually amounts only to about 0.1 μA. Most of the voltage gradient applied between the electrode in the subcutis and ground is present between the patient's outer skin surface and ground. A relatively small fraction of the total field gradient between the body electrode and ground is present between the electrode and the internal body surface representing the applied gradient inside the body. At a sufficiently high voltage difference of electrode to ground and low frequency of fluctuating voltage, the displacement effect should led to partial dissolution of cancer tissue due to the favorable interference by existing forced convection of tissue fluids. Favorable conditions for the effect of applied chemotherapy will then be created.

Electrostatic charging of the body can be performed if certain areas for insertion of electrodes are avoided and if a high voltage is not applied for more than a couple of days at the most. The effect on cellular membrane pumps seems to produce visible regression of small cancer metastases, but not of large tumours. An enhanced effect can, however, be obtained by subsequent chemotherapy. Access to the tumour tissue can be improved by high voltage fluctuation of the applied electrostatic field, which should be given together with the electrostatic treatment. Improved access of chemotherapy agents into the cancer cells is provided by opening of the cellular membrane channels during the electronegative phase of charging.

ACKNOWLEDGMENTS

Due to the author's poor health, this chapter is an abridged version of three articles published in European Journal of Surgery (23–25) which have been compiled by Jörgen

Nordenström, M.D., Ph.D., Professor of Surgery, Department of Surgery, Huddinge University Hospital, Karolinska Institutet, Stockholm, Sweden. Permission to use text has been granted by the editor of the journal. Ms. Kerstin Ersson is acknowledged for her unfailing interest and efforts in preparation of the text.

REFERENCES

1. Curé J. On the identity of Einsteins cosmic ether. Proceeding of the International Congress celebrated in Perugia University, Italy, September 1989.
2. Einstein A. The Meaning of Relativity. Princeton University Press, 1955:82.
3. Erohkin NS. Electromagnetic field as part of matter in problems of charge neutralization. Cambridge: Proceedings PIERS, Mass, 1991:475.
4. Nordenström BEW, Ipavec S, Alfas S. Interferences between electromagnetic field and biological matter—the concept of BCEC. Int J Environ Stud 1992; 42:157–167.
5. Nordenström BEW. Biologically closed electric circuits: clinical, experimental and theoretical evidence for an additional circulatory system. Stockholm: Nordic Medical Publications, 1983.
6. Nordenström BEW. An additional circulatory system: vascular-interstitial closed electric circuits. J Biol Phys 1987; 15:43–55.
7. Nordenström BEW. Link between electromagnetic field and biological matter. Int J Environ Stud 1992; 41:233–250.
8. Nordenström BEW. Hand movements above the unshielded tail of a shielded rat induce differences of voltage inside the animal. Am J Acupuncture 1992; 20:159–163.
9. Nordenström BEW. Fleischner lecture. Biokinetic impact on structure and imaging of the lung: the concept of biologically closed electric circuits. AJR 1985; 145:447–467.
10. Nordenström BEW. Vesicles, basement membranes and the endothelial fibrin film as possible products of biological electrode reactions. In: Eckert GH, Gutmann F, Keyzer H, eds. Electropharmacology. Boca Raton, Boston: CRC Press, 1990:189–203.
11. Nordenström BEW, Kinn A-C, Elbarouni J. Electric modification of kidney function. The excretion of radiographic contrast media and Adriamycin. Invest Radiol 1991; 26:157–161.
12. Nordenström BEW. I. Neurovascular activation requires conduction through vessels. Physiol Chem Phys Med NMR 1989; 21:249–256.
13. Nordenström BEW, Larsson H. II. Slow and rapid electrical pulses in the caval vein at pain-evoked leg contraction in the rat. Physiol Chem Phys Med NMR 1989; 21:257–264.
14. Nordenström BEW. III. The action potential: an effect of fuel cell reactions in the synapse. Physiol Chem Phys Med NMR 1989; 21:265–278.
15. Nordenström BEW. Vascular-interstitial-neurovascular activation: differences in femoral and sciatic nerves in the rat. J Bioelectr 1989; 8:109–117.
16. Nordenström BEW. IV. Electrical pulses appear in the inferior vena cava and abdominal aorta at contraction of leg muscles. Physiol Chem and Phys Med NMR 1992; 24:147–152.
17. Nordenström BEW. V. Potential differences in the inferior vena cava and between cava and extravascular electrode at leg contraction in man. Physiol Chem Phys Med NMR 1992; 24:153–158.
18. Nordenström BEW. VI. Synaptic fuel cell reactions in vascular-interstitial-neuromuscular activation. Electro- Magnetobiol 1992; 11:99–115.
19. Bockris JO'M, Drazic DM. Electro-chemical Science. New York: Barnes and Noble Books, 1972.
20. Weiss L. Studies on cellular adhesion in tissue culture. Exp Cell Res 1968; 53:608.
21. Fidler IJ. Incorporation of immunomodulators in liposomes for systemic activation of macrophages and therapy of cancer metastases. CRS Press 1993; 2:45–63.
22. Skou JC. The relationship of a $(Mn^{2+} + Na^+)$ -activated K^+ stimulated enzyme or enzyme system to the active linked transport of Na^+ and K^+ across the cell membrane. In: Kleinzeller A, Kotyk A, eds. Membrane Transport and Metabolism. New York: Academic Press, 1961.

23. Nordenström B. The paradigm of biologically closed electric circuits (BCEC) and the formation of an international association (IABC) for BCEC systems. Eur J Surg 1994; 574(suppl):7–23.
24. Nordenström B. Survey of mechanisms in electrochemical treatment (ECT) of cancer. Eur J Surg 1994; 574(suppl):93–109.
25. Nordenström B. Electrostatic field interference with cellular and tissue function, leading to dissolution of metastases that enhances the effect of chemotherapy. Eur J Surg 1994; 574(suppl):121–135.

43

Electrochemical Therapy of Tumors

Yuling Xin, Hongchang Zhao, Wei Zhang, Chaoyang Liang, Zaiyong Wang, and Ganzhong Liu

Department of Thoracic Surgery, Electrochemical Therapy Center for Tumors, China-Japan Friendship Hospital, Beijing, P. R. China

The results of EChT (Electrochemical Therapy) based on Björn Nordenström's protocol are presented in 7642 patients with various malignant tumors. Factors influencing selection of patients to treat and long term outcomes are discussed. In addition, our experience with this effective and safe technique in 1369 patients with benign tumors is described.

I. INTRODUCTION

The efficacy of electrochemical therapy (EChT) in mice with implanted Jensen sarcoma tumors was reported in 1953 by Reis and Henniger (1). However, the clinical application of this modality was initiated by the Swedish radiologist, Björn Nordenström. In 1983, he published a book in which he described his theory of biologically closed electrical circuits (BCEC) and the results of two decades of research on EChT treatment of malignancies in animals based on this (2). He also reported the results of EChT in 20 lung cancer patients with 26 tumors in which he used the "skinny needle" he had developed for biopsy purposes as an electrode. Follow-up after 2 to 5 years revealed that 12 tumors had either disappeared or were markedly reduced in size. This study stimulated interest in utilizing EChT for treating lung malignancies, and Japanese researchers subsequently confirmed Nordenström's results in animals and in several patients (3–7).

The advantages of EChT are that it is much safer, easier to administer, and less costly than surgical procedures and can be just as effective in certain instances. In addition, it provides an opportunity to treat tumors in those patients in whom surgery, radiation, and/ or chemotherapy has not been successful or may be contraindicated.

II. EXPERIMENTAL STUDIES ON THE MECHANISM OF ACTION OF EChT

It has been well established that tumor cells are more sensitive to certain changes in their environment than adjacent normal cells. Various treatment approaches, including radiation, chemotherapy, hyperthermia, microwave, laser, and antiangiogenesis strategies, are based on these differences. Nordenström reported that in the catabolic and anabolic phases of tissue growth and degradation, the exchange and transportation of energy may be mediated via unsuspected pathways he referred to as *biologically closed electric circuits* (BCEC). In the BCEC systems, a specific circuit is formed by blood vessels and interstitial fluids called *vascular interstitial closed circuit* (VICC). This VICC system can be activated by direct electric current that causes specific chemical changes in the corresponding environment that have detrimental effects on tumor cells. Multiple pathological changes occur in the tumor tissue during EChT such as pyknosis of nuclei, disruption of cell membranes and mitochondria, as well as coagulation and necrosis of nuclear proteins (2).

The conventional view is that the blood circulation is a nonselective mechanical transportation system for hormones, numerous neuroendocrine secretions and chemicals, oxygen, and other substances that are delivered to tissues at the capillary level by diffusion, filtration, and osmosis. However, Nordenström showed that BCEC systems, including VICC, furnish an energy communication pathway that provides an "electrical circulatory system" in the body as discussed elsewhere in this book. It can be activated by a modification of differences in electrical potential across cell membranes, which results in altered physiological metabolic activities that produce changes in focal structure and function.

On the basis of Nordenström's concepts and research, tumor tissue can be regarded as being deranged and characterized by a difference in electrical potential between tissue damaged by tumor and surrounding normal tissues. The healing process of the damaged tissue is the internal driving process of VICC and also the balancing process of the potential difference. This balancing process could be accelerated by an external activation of the driving process of VICC such as that provided by direct electric current stimulation to promote the healing of injury due to tumor, trauma, and various diseases (8–11).

In animal experiments, histopathological studies have demonstrated that the lethal effect of EChT on tumor tissue in the anode area differs from that around the cathode site. Tumor tissue at the anode shows coagulation necrosis with destroyed cell structures, pyknosis of cells, and denaturation. Tumor tissue around the cathode has a different pattern characterized by necrosis due to liquefaction, complete disruption of cell structures and the accumulation of water molecules due to the presence of positively charged sodium ions and large protein molecules. Although the features of damage are different in anode and cathode areas, the extent of tissue destruction is about the same (2). In the clinical application of EChT, multiple cathodes can be applied in hard and solid types of tumors such as fibroma and osteosarcoma and liquefaction necrosis can be induced by the accumulation of positive ions. On the other hand, when treating softer types of tumors, multiple anodic electrodes could be used to facilitate coagulatory necrosis. These observations stimulated research by Japanese scientists and others to do further experiments to define mechanisms of action that might improve the clinical efficacy of this exciting treatment modality for cancer alone or in combination with conventional approaches (12–15).

On the basis of extensive animal experiments and clinical histopathological studies, we have confirmed that the destruction mechanism of EChT is an electrolytic effect of the direct current. The destruction takes place basically at the surface of electrode. An additional killing effect occurs as a result of the electrolysis of water and electrolytes yielding NaOH and HCl that disseminate a certain distance from the electrode. Na^+ formed after electrolysis will move toward the cathode and combine with OH ions to form NaOH which yields a strong alkaline environment (pH 12–14). Chloride ions accumulate around the anode and combine with H^+ to form HCl, which is strongly acidic (pH 1–2). The strong alkalinity and acidity are the main destructive mechanisms of EChT. During the application of electrochemical therapy, large amount of foam ooze out from the surface of the electrode releasing Cl_2 and H_2O_2 (16). There are, however, additional mechanisms of action which are operative during EChT of tumors. These can be summarized as follows:

1. Electrolysis by direct electric current induces pH changes in the environment that, in turn, results in biological effects.

2. The application of electric current increases the permeability of the cell membrane of tumor cells that allows ions to migrate inside cells and excert antitumor effects.

3. Activity of enzymes in plasma can be released; proteins will be denatured and coagulated and precipitated whereby necrosis may be induced.

4. Electrolysis changes the distribution of ions, which results in coagulation and necrosis around the anode and edema around the cathode.

5. Extensive embolism may occur in blood vessels in the anode area, whereas significant edema in cathode area results in blockage of the microcirculation, and the blood supply to tumor cells is interrupted.

6. White blood cells and T lymphocytes accumulate in the anode area that may also have antineoplastic effects. At the same time, the negatively charged tumor cells are attracted to the anode so that metastasis of tumor cells may be hindered or prevented.

7. Fragments of damaged tumor cells resulting from direct electric current application could serve as antigens and stimulate the body's immune system defences (12–15,17).

III. CLINICAL APPLICATION AND EFFECTIVENESS OF EChT TO TREAT MALIGNANT TUMORS

In 1987, the China–Japan Friendship Hospital took the lead in utilizing EChT, and since then, our group has treated more than 1000 patients with various types of malignant tumors. In order to facilitate the spread of this new technique, 125 EChT training courses have been conducted during the period 1988–2001. More than 2500 doctors from 1200 hospitals have attended these courses and almost 1100 hospitals have used EChT for malignant tumors. This chapter provides a summary of the clinical experience in 9011 tumors (7642 malignant and 1369 benign) from only 28 hospitals (18).

A. Malignant Tumors

Among the 7642 malignant tumors, 4681 were in males and 2961 occurred in females. Among the patients observed, 1284 patients were 20–40 years old, 4084 were 41–60 years old, 1985 were 61–80 years old with 289 older than 81 years old. With respect to types of tumors, 3932 were superficial growths and 3710 were visceral tumors. In regard to tumor staging, there were 749 stage I cases, 2504 with stage II, 2862 with stage III, and 1527 with stage IV. Furthermore, 1723 tumors were 3.0–5.0 cm in diameter, 2758 were 5.1–7.0 cm, 2333 were 7.1–9.0 cm, 628 were 9.1–13.0 cm, and there were 200 cases with a diameter more than 13.0 cm. All tumor typing and staging were confirmed by histopathologic examination.

According to the international standard stipulated by UICC, the short-term effective rates of 7642 cases of malignant tumors were: complete response (CR) 33.2% (2540/7642), partial response (PR) 42.8% (3272/7642), no change (NC) 14.4% (1097/7642), and progressive disease (PD) 9.6% (7330/7642). Taking CR and PR as the effective rate, the total effective rate was 76.0% (Table 1).

The clinical effectiveness varied with the stage, size and location of the tumor as shown in Table 2. The effective rate of stage I and II tumors was 91.0% (2960/3253) and 65.0% (2852/4389) in stage III and IV. The difference in effectiveness between two groups was statistically significant ($P < 0.01$). The effect was closely related to the size of the tumors. The effective rate when treating malignant tumors with a diameter of 7 cm or less was 86.5% (3877/4481), whereas the corresponding figure when treating tumors with diameter greater than 7 cm was 62.5% (1976/3161) ($P < 0.05$). The results showed that the effect in superficial tumors was better than that of visceral tumors. One reason for the better effect observed for superficial tumors could be that needles can be more accurately inserted and better distributed. For this reason we often insert needles under direct vision when treating large visceral tumors.

Long-term effectiveness was as follows: with the follow-up time of 1–5 years, 818 cases (10.7%) died within 1 year after treatment, 6824 (89.3%) survived for more than 1 year, 5883 cases (77.0%) for more than 2 years, 4278 cases (56.0%) for more than 3 years, 3593 cases (47.0) for more than 4 years, and 2752 cases (36.0%) for more than 5 years (Table 3).

The 5-year survival rate of superficial tumors was 49.5% (1946/3932) and that of visceral tumors was 21.7% (806/3710), ($P < 0.01$).

The clinical effectiveness was related to stage. The 5-year survival rate of patients with stage I and II was 61.6% (2004/3253), while the survival rate in patients with stages III and IV was 17.0% (748/4389); $P < 0.01$.

Table 1 Malignant Tumors Treated by EChT According to Localization

Superficial tumors	No. of cases	Visceral tumors	No. of cases
Skin cancer	958	Esophageal cancer	1595
Breast cancer	644	Lung cancer	1113
Head and facial tumor	598	Liver cancer	961
Metastatic cancer of superficial lymph nodes	361	Throat cancer	21
		Prostate cancer	20
Thyroid adenocarcinoma	250		
Vulval tumor	237		
Melanoma	227		
Tumor of abdominal wall	172		
Cancer of oral cavity	138		
Rhabdomyosarcoma	133		
Parotid cancer	84		
Others	130		
Sum	3932	Sum	3710

Table 2 Short-Term Effectiveness of the Treatment of Malignant Tumors

	No. of cases	CR		PR		NC		PD		CR + PR	
		No.	%	No.	%	No.	%	No.	%	No.	%
Esophageal cancer	1595	348	21.8	766	48.0	319	20.0	162	10.2	1114	69.8
Lung cancer	1113	412	37.0	445	40.0	155	13.9	101	9.1	857	77.0
Liver cancer	961	240	25.0	427	44.4	210	21.9	84	8.7	667	69.4
Throat cancer	21	9	42.9	9	42.9	2	9.5	1	4.8	18	85.7
Prostate cancer	20	8	40.0	7	35.0	3	15.0	2	10.0	15	75.0
Skin cancer	958	611	63.8	347	36.2	0		0		958	100
Breast cancer	644	180	28.0	296	46.0	64	9.9	104	16.1	476	73.9
Head and face tumor	598	154	25.8	280	46.8	99	16.6	65	10.9	434	72.6
Metastatic tumor of superficial lymph node	361	135	37.4	145	40.2	57	15.8	24	6.6	280	77.6
Thyroid adenocarcinoma	250	89	35.6	110	44.0	36	14.4	15	6.0	199	79.6
Vulval cancer	237	91	38.4	111	46.8	21	8.9	14	5.9	202	85.2
Melanoma	227	79	34.8	27	11.9	27	11.9	94	41.4	106	46.7
Tumor of abdominal wall	172	44	25.6	81	47.1	29	16.9	18	10.5	125	72.7
Cancer of oral cavity	138	46	33.3	75	54.3	11	8.0	6	4.3	121	87.7
Rhabdomyosarcoma	133	27	20.3	49	36.8	38	28.6	19	14.3	76	57.1
Parotid cancer	84	28	33.3	46	54.8	6	7.1	4	4.8	74	88.1
Others	130	39	30.0	51	39.2	20	15.4	20	15.4	90	69.2
Sum	7642	2540	33.2	3272	42.8	1097	14.4	733	9.6	5812	76.0

Table 3 One to 5 Years Survival Rates in 7642 Patients with Malignant Tumors Treated with EChT

	No. of cases	First year		Second year		Third year		Fourth year		Fifth year	
		No.	%	No.	%	No.	%	No.	%	No.	%
Esophageal cancer	1595	1285	80.6	969	60.8	483	30.3	233	14.6	205	12.9
Lung cancer	1113	1063	95.5	933	83.8	746	67.0	600	53.9	432	38.8
Liver cancer	961	771	80.2	577	60.0	209	21.7	184	19.1	145	15.1
Throat cancer	21	21	100	21	100	19	90.5	17	81.0	14	66.7
Prostate cancer	20	20	100	19	95.0	18	90.0	16	80.0	10	50.0
Skin cancer	958	958	100	958	100	890	92.9	890	92.9	767	80.1
Breast cancer	644	618	96.0	569	88.2	404	62.7	404	62.7	323	50.2
Head and face tumor	598	501	83.8	428	71.6	338	56.5	327	54.7	245	41.0
Metastatic tumor of superficial lymph node	361	336	93.1	295	81.7	258	71.5	184	51.0	139	38.5
Thyroid adenocarcinoma	250	242	96.8	232	92.8	192	76.8	191	76.4	133	53.3
Vulval cancer	237	223	94.1	209	88.2	188	79.3	188	79.3	104	43.9
Melanoma	227	194	85.5	157	69.2	91	40.1	19	8.4	0	
Tumor of abdominal wall	172	140	81.4	130	75.6	115	66.9	102	59.3	74	43.0
Cancer of oral cavity	138	129	93.5	124	89.9	111	80.4	99	71.7	85	61.6
Rhabdomyosarcoma	133	121	91.0	88	66.2	51	38.3	9	6.8	0	
Parotid cancer	84	78	92.9	76	90.5	67	79.8	59	70.2	45	53.6
Others	130	124	95.4	99	76.2	98	75.4	71	56.6	31	23.8
Sum	7642	6824	89.3	5883	77.0	4278	56.0	3593	47.0	2752	36.0

Table 4 Tumor Size (cm) in 1369 Benign Tumors

	No. of cases	3.0–5.0 cm		5.1–7.0 cm		7.1–9.0 cm		9.1–18.0 cm	
		No.	%	No.	%	No.	%	No.	%
Hemangioma	874	223	25.5	384	43.9	175	20.0	92	10.5
Thyroid tumor	116	35	30.2	44	37.9	27	23.3	10	8.6
Thyroid cyst	102	30	29.4	49	48.0	21	20.6	2	2.0
Hypertrophy of prostate gland	191	85	44.5	106	55.5	0		0	
Keloid	86	55	64.0	31	36.0	0		0	
Sum	1369	428	31.3	614	44.9	223	16.3	104	7.6

B. Benign Tumors

In total, 1369 patients (582 M; 787 F) with benign tumors have been treated with EChT. The youngest patient was 6 months old and the oldest was 68 years old. There were 874 cases of cavernous hemangiomas, 116 thyroid tumors, 191 hypertrophy of the prostate gland, 102 thyroid cysts, and 86 keloids. Regarding the size of tumors, 428 cases (31.3%) were 3.0–5.0 cm in diameter, 614 cases (44.9%) were 5.1–7.0 cm, 223 cases (16.3%) were 7.1–9.0 cm, and 104 cases (7.6%) were 9.1–18.0 cm. We consider tumors with a diameter more than 7.0 cm to be exceptionally large tumors, and these constituted 24.0% of all the benign tumors (Table 4).

Short-term effectiveness was as follows: in 874 cases of cavernous hemangioma, 858 cases (98.2%) were cured; in 218 cases of thyroid tumors and cysts, 205 cases (94.0%) were cured; in 191 cases of hypertrophy of prostate gland, 126 cases (66.0%) were cured; and in 86 cases of keloid, 69 cases (80.2%) were cured (Table 5).

The best results were observed in patients with cavernous hemangiomas and thyroid tumors with a clinical effectiveness (CR + PD) of 98.2% (858/874) and 96.6% (112/116), respectively. The effectiveness of treating hypertrophy of the prostate gland was lower (66.0%; 126/191). There was an inverse relationship between tumor diameter and clinical effectiveness. The effective rate when treating tumors with a diameter greater than 7 cm was 83.2% (400/481) The difference was statistically significant ($P < 0.05$).The long-term effectiveness of EChT for benign tumors was assessed by yearly follow-up for 3 years. The survival rate was 99.3% after 1 year, 98.5% after 2 years and 97.8% after 3 years. All of the

Table 5 Short-Term Effectiveness of 1369 Cases of Benign Tumors

	No. of cases	CR		PR		NC		PD		CR + PR	
		No.	%	No.	%	No.	%	No.	%	No.	%
Hemangioma	874	598	68.4	260	29.8	16	1.8	0		858	98.2
Thyroid tumor	116	77	66.4	35	30.2	4	3.4	0		112	96.6
Thyroid cyst	102	62	60.8	31	30.4	9	8.8	0		93	91.2
Hypertrophy of prostate gland	191	68	35.6	58	30.4	48	25.1	17	8.9	126	66.0
Keloid	86	54	62.8	15	17.4	14	16.3	3	3.5	69	80.2
Sum	1369	859	62.7	399	29.1	91	6.6	20	1.5	1358	91.9

Table 6 One to 3 Years Survival Rates of 1369 Patients with Benign Tumors

	No. of cases	First year		Second year		Third year	
		No.	%	No.	%	No.	%
Hemangioma	874	874	100.0	874	100.0	874	100.0
Thyroid tumor	116	116	100.0	116	100.0	116	100.0
Thyroid cyst	102	102	100.0	102	100.0	102	100.0
Hypertrophy of prostate gland	191	181	94.8	170	89.0	161	84.2
Keloid	86	86	100.0	86	100.0	86	100.0
Sum	1369	1359	99.3	1348	98.5	1339	97.8

30 patients who died during the follow-up period had hypertrophy of the prostate gland. Ten patients died within 1 year, 11 patients within 2 years, and 9 patients within 3 years (Table 6). The major causes of death were genitourinary infections and renal failure.

The major factor affecting the long-term effectiveness was recurence after treatment. The highest recurrence rate 31.9% (61/191) was observed in cases with hypertrophy of the prostate gland. Recurrence rates for cavernous hemangioma and keloid were 14.4% (126/874) and 12.8% (11/86), respectively. There were no recurrences of thyroid tumors or thyroid cysts.

IV. INDICATIONS FOR ELECTROCHEMICAL TREATMENT

The choice of treatment for cancer patients needs to be individualized. The first choice is usually a surgical procedure with radiation and/or chemotherapy generally being second

Table 7 Indications for EChT

	Clear indication	Relative indication	Contraindication
Lung cancer	Peripheral type; I, II stages, <6 cm in diameter	III stage or 7–9 cm in diameter	IV stage, >10 cm in diameter or central type
Esophageal cancer	Intraluminal type, length <6 cm or postoperational narrowing of anastomosis	Intraluminal type, length >7 cm	Ulcer type or tumor invaded the outer membrane of the lumen, length >9 cm
Liver cancer	I, II stages, <7 cm in diameter	III stage, 8–10 cm in diameter	IV stage, >12 cm or tumor invaded porta hepatis
Breast cancer	I, II stages, <5 cm or local recurred tumor with 5–7 cm in diameter	III stage, 6–7 cm or 8–15 cm recurred tumor postoperatively	IV stage or >15 cm of recurred tumor postoperatively
Oral cancer	I, II stages, <3 cm	III stage, 4 cm invaded root of tongue	IV stage, >5 cm or tumor
Superficial tumor	I, II stages, 3–6 cm	III stage, 7–10 cm	IV stage, >10 cm, invaded nerves and vessels

options. However, EChT has specific features which makes this method useful in some cases where surgery, radio-, or chemotherapy is not indicated.

Based on clinical experience gained over several years, we have established relative indications for EChT in cancer patients based on the clinical stage as classified in Table 7.

Most patients with a well founded indication for EChT can achieve a complete response (CR); many patients with a relative indication for EChT can get a partial response (PR). If EChT is administered to patients where this method might be contraindicated, only temporary relief of symptoms can be expected with no chance for cure (19–21).

V. COMPLICATIONS OF EChT AND ITS MANAGEMENT

EChT is relatively nontraumatic so that even fragile patients are able to tolerate the procedure without difficulty. A moderate rise in body temperature and in white blood cell (WBC) count may occur but a return to normal generally takes place after 3–5 days. DC is not harmful under 30 V, so EChT can be considered to be quite safe. During EChT a voltage much lower than 30 V is used but if the insulation around the cannula is not properly arranged, surrounding normal tissue and skin may be damaged. Such damage is usually limited and typically restricted to an area of about 0.5–1.0 cm in diameter around the electrode, and no treatment is needed since spontaneous healing takes place. When the cannula is inserted into the liver and the stylet is withdrawn, bleeding may be observed through the cannula. If this happens, the electrode should be inserted rapidly and treatment should be started at once. Since DC has the property of causing coagulation, bleeding usually ceases within a few minutes. On the day after treatment, patients may experience pain; body temperature can reach 38°C and WBC can increase slightly. Local tenderness may occur if a small amount of alkaline (or acidic) liquid from dissolved necrotic cancer tissue reaches the abdominal cavity and causes a chemical reaction or even local peritonitis. Such symptoms will subside after 3–5 days of treatment with anti-inflammatory and analgesic medications (22).

It has been reported that during the treatment of metastatic tumors of the lymph node of neck, the brachial plexus nerves may be injured. Therefore, if severe pain in the upper extremity appears during EChT, the treatment should be stopped at once in order to avoid damage of brachial plexus nerves and the position of electrodes readjusted.

Traumatic pneumothorax may occur while treating lung cancer due to damage of the visceral pleura during the insertion of electrodes. Localized pneumothorax (compression less than 20%) does not affect treatment results and no special management is needed. A small pneumothorax is absorbed spontaneously but a drainage tube should be inserted whenever collapse of lung tissue is extensive. If pneumothorax seems likely, a drainage tube should be inserted prior to the procedure to prevent respiratory distress and discomfort during the treatment as well as electrode dislocation caused by movement of tumor (23–26).

Measures to reduce problems associated with pneumothorax include

1. Injection of codeine before treatment to prevent cough.
2. Inhalation of oxygen to have a calm respiration, especially in patients with chronic bronchitis.
3. Start the treatment immediately after insertion of needles on the X-ray table.

This is important especially in patients with chronic emphysema since these individuals are easily provoked to cough which may cause the electrodes to damage healthy lung tissue. Insuring that the patient is kept calm so that respiration is regular and natural will help prevent pneumothorax.

Atrial fibrillation occurred during the treatment of lung cancer in one patient but disappeared when the procedure was stopped and appropriate medications were given. Another patient went into ventricular fibrillation and cardiac arrest but recovered following defibrillation. The cause of this complication was placement of the electrode too close to the mediastinum (16).

VI. THE PROCEDURE OF ELECTROCHEMICAL THERAPY

The electric current, voltage, and electric quantity should be determined according to histological type, size, and location of the tumor. If the tumor is large or hard, a higher electric quantity should be employed. The general condition of the patient is also important to consider. For EChT we use a computer controlled BK2000 multifunctional instrument that has four outputs with data storage, specialist system, and print function. Electric current, voltage, and electric quantity can be preset.

Electrodes are made of platinum with a 0.7-mm diameter and 160 mm in length with high electrical conductivity and good antierosive properties. Hard needles are usually used to treat superficial tumors, while more elastic needles are often used to treat visceral tumors. Needles are also coated with plastic for insulation to protect normal tissue against electrical injury and strict sterilization is necessary. Various needle shapes are used for different types of tumors and applications, such as catheter-like electrodes for esophageal, prostate and rectal cancer, etc. Proper electrodes should be selected according to the tissue type and location of tumor. Cathodes are usually placed in the center of tumor and anodes in the periphery However, cathodes and anodes can alternatively be placed one beside the other, but both must be inserted into the full diameter of tumor to avoid incomplete treatment.

The manipulation during treatment of superficial tumors is rather easy. The location and the size of the tumor can be determined by palpation and under direct vision. Based on the data obtained from our experiments, the destruction radius of each electrode is about 1.0 cm. Since the distance between two electrodes should be less than 1.5 cm., the number of electrodes can be calculated according to tumor size. For example, if the diameter of a tumor is 5.0–6.0 cm, four to five cathodes should be inserted in its center and seven or eight anodes in the periphery so that the lesion is covered completely by the electric field. For large tumors, it is advisable to use two sets of outputs. In such cases there will be two groups of electrodes in the same tumor and a multioutput instrument provides this advantage.

The treatment of visceral tumors should be monitored using appropriate imaging techniques. For example, when treating esophageal cancers, the pathologic type, length, and condition of obstruction should be determined by x-ray barium meal examination and by esophageal endoscopy. CT scan can determine the thickness of the tumor so that the quantity of DC current can be ascertained. The patient should sit erect and given a local anesthetic before the catheter electrode is inserted in the pharynx through the nostril cavity. The patient is asked to swallow to let the catheter electrode pass into the esophagus, following which a cup of barium solution is given under x-ray fluoroscopy. The location and the length of the tumor is visualized, and the catheter electrode is then inserted to the narrowed portion of the esophagus. Electricity is then given in a quantity of 60–80 C per 1.0 cm length of the lesion. For severe anastomotic stenosis after surgical-procedures or radiotherapy, it may be difficult to insert an electrode, and in such cases, endoscopy is helpful to locate the orifice of stenosis, dilate it, and then insert the electrode (19,20).

For treatment of lung cancers, electrodes can be inserted percutaneously under local anesthesia and continous x-ray monitoring. Closed chest drainage in advance of treatment is helpful in order to avoid pneumothorax. Thoracotomy is necessary when treating central types of lung cancers in order to insert needle electrodes accurately and to avoid injury of the main vessels at the hilus of lung (19,20). When treating liver cancers, there are two ways of inserting needles. If the tumor is located in the left lobe of the liver, needles can be inserted through the skin under ultrasound guidance. If the tumor is located in the right lobe, needles should be inserted under ultrasound guidance in order to avoid the injury of neighboring organs. If the diameter of the tumor is over 10 cm or if there are multiple liver tumors, it is preferable to open the abdomen and insert the needles under direct vision in order to ensure a good distribution of electrodes (21). Advanced stages of prostate cancer are usually complicated by severe urethral narrowing and the urethra should be dilated before inserting the catheter electrode into the isthmus of the prostate.

At the beginning of treatment, the voltage should be increased gradually, e.g., by 0-, 2-, 4-, 6-, 8-, and 10-V intervals for several minutes in order to adjust the patient to the treatment. If the patient's respiratory rate or heart rhythm changes, treatment should be interrupted immediately (27). Generally speaking, a voltage of the order of 6–8 V and electric current in the range of 30–80 mA is recommended. It is important that the electric current is kept at 30–50 mA at the beginning with a gradual increase to 60–80 mA. The electric quantity is determined by tumor size, usually 100 C per 1.0 cm diameter of tumor mass. If the diameter is larger than 8.0 cm, the electric quantity should be increased to 150 C per 1.0 cm diameter. The duration for the treatment is also dependent on tumor size. Our clinical experience is that the duration of therapy needs to be 15 to 20 min for treating a tumor with 1.0 cm diameter and the electric current should be kept below 140 mA. The belief that increasing electric current to high level to shorten treatment time is not correct because the electrolytic action of EChT needs a certain amount of time to be effective.

Patients usually have some sensation of pain during EChT. Local anesthesia usually suffices when treating superficial tumors, but luminal, dilantin, or morphine should be injected intramuscularly if necessary and patients should be in a prone position for longer procedures. When treating tumors in the lower part of the abdomen, extradural anesthesia is recommended. When treating visceral (liver, kidney, etc.) tumors, general anesthesia is preferable.

To improve the effectiveness of EChT when treating malignant tumors, the following measures are recommended (27,28):

1. The indications for EChT should be strict. In patients with advanced tumors who can not be treated with other therapies, EChT could relieve suffering and improve quality of life.

2. Multiple electrodes should be used for large tumors. Under the condition that short circuit does not occur, the distance between electrodes could be reduced to 1.0 cm in order to enhance the destructive effect.

3. EChT should be combined with radiochemotherapy in large tumors, since EChT may render tumor cells more sensitive to radiochemotherapy; 40 Gy radiation could be given either before or after EChT. Positively charged antitumor agents, such as adriamycin and bleomycin, could be injected into the tumor, whereby the electric gradient will move the chemotherapeutic agent toward the cathodic area and destruct tumor cells. Systemic chemotherapy, intervenion therapy, and immunotherapy could also be considered in combination with EChT.

4. Chinese herbs could improve the immune response and inhibit the growth of tumors, and may be a supplementary treatment to be combined with electrochemical therapy.

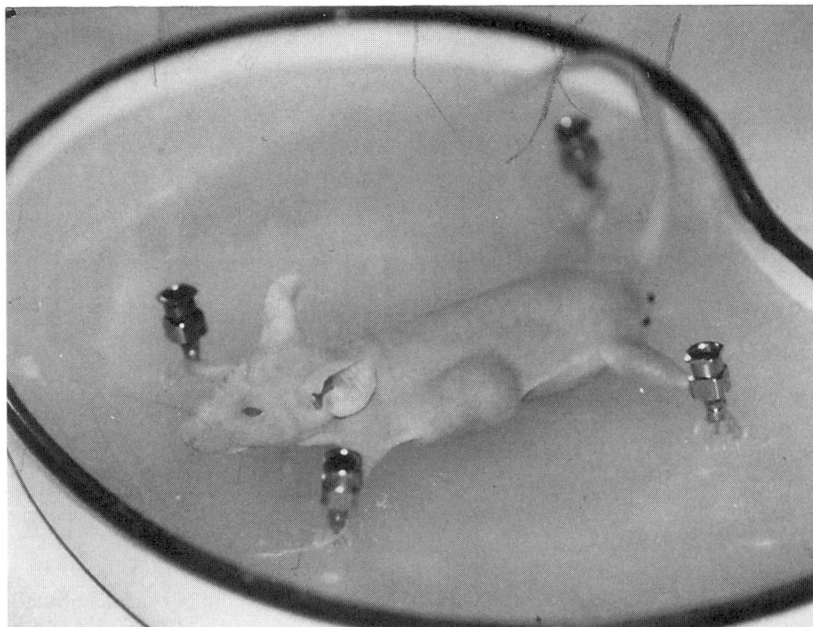

Figure 1   Transplanted carcinoma on nude mouse (tumor size 2.0 × 1.8 cm). Before EChT.

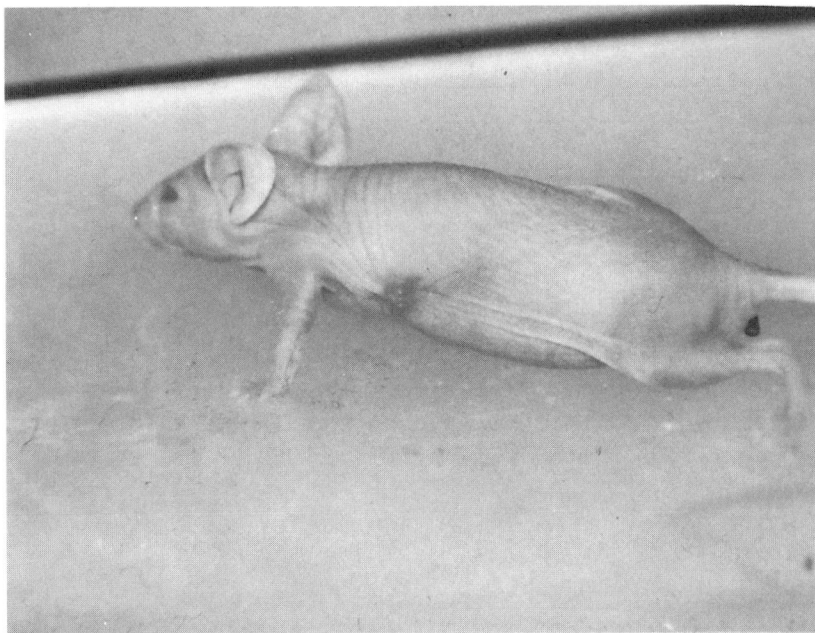

Figure 2   8 weeks later, after EChT, the wound healed.

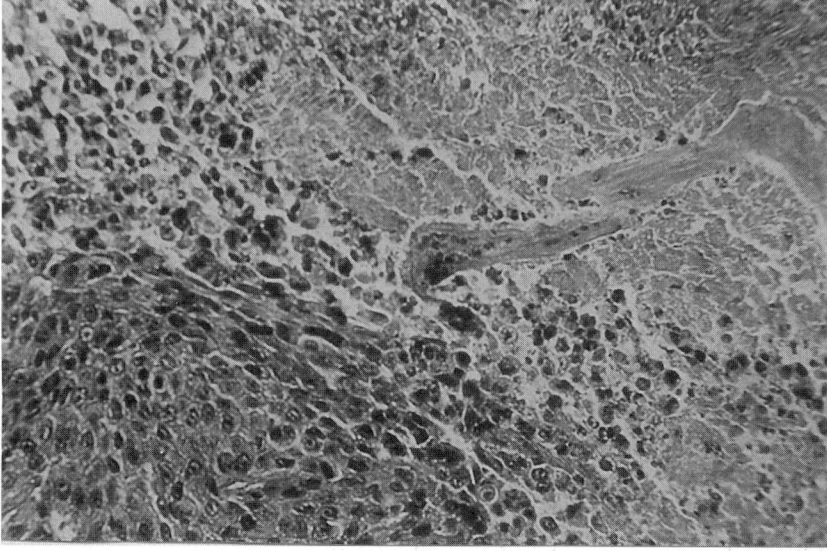

Figure 3 In low electric quantity group (45 C for 1.0 cm diameter), survived tumor cells were found.

VII. THE FUTURE OF EChT

In 1987, Professor Björn Nordenström was invited to come to Beijing to give lectures on his BCEC theory and demonstrate the use of EChT in malignant tumors. After 3 years of animal and clinical practice, good therapeutic efficacy was achieved. EChT was approved by the Ministry of Public Health as a new therapeutic method for the treatment of tumors and quickly spread to many medical centers. There were 9011 cases with various kinds of

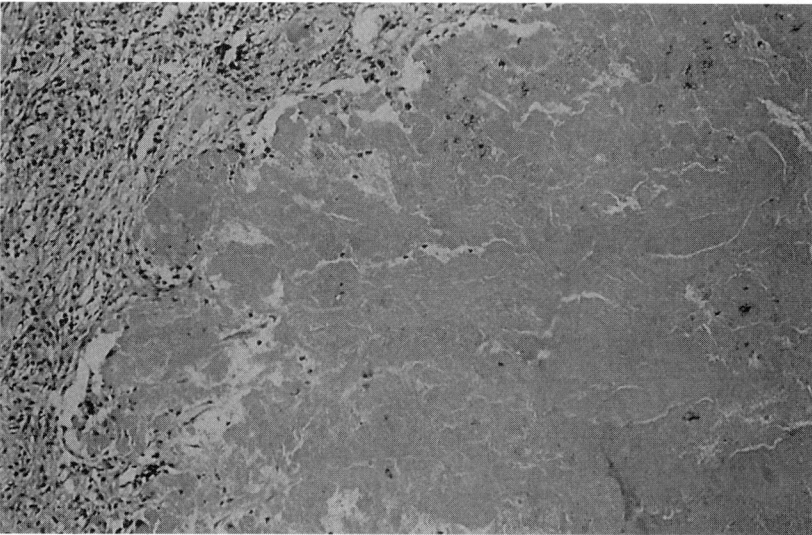

Figure 4 In large electric quantity group (100 C for 1.0 cm diameter), tumor cells were killed completely.

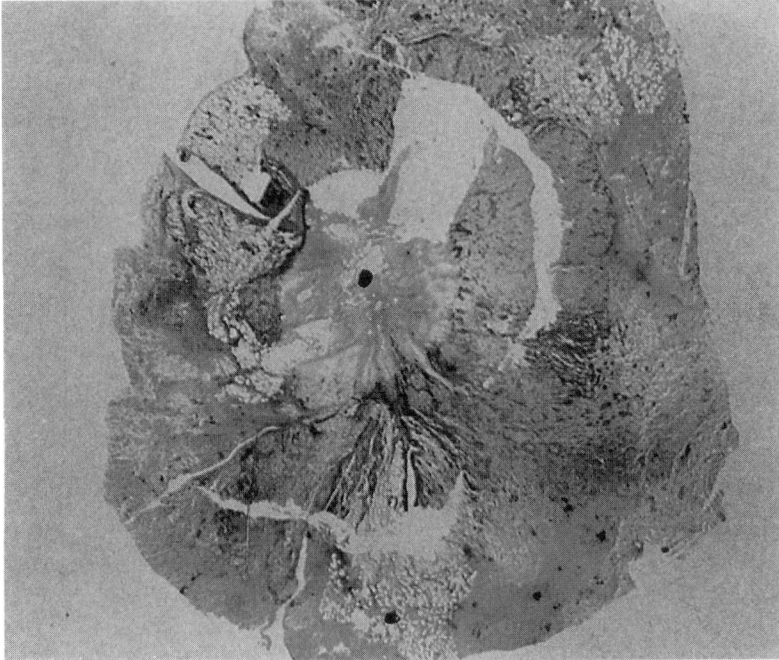

Figure 5 Coagulatory necrosis around anode.

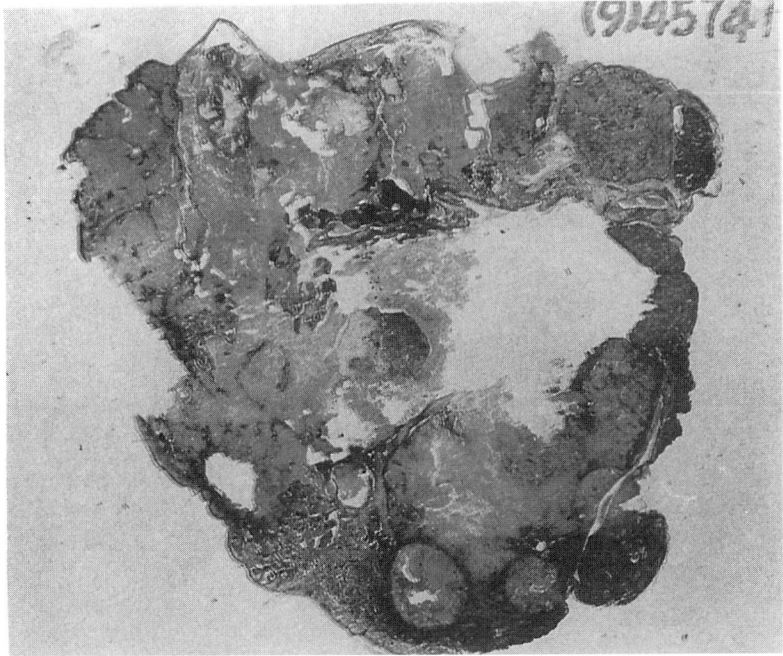

Figure 6 Liquid necrosis around cathode area.

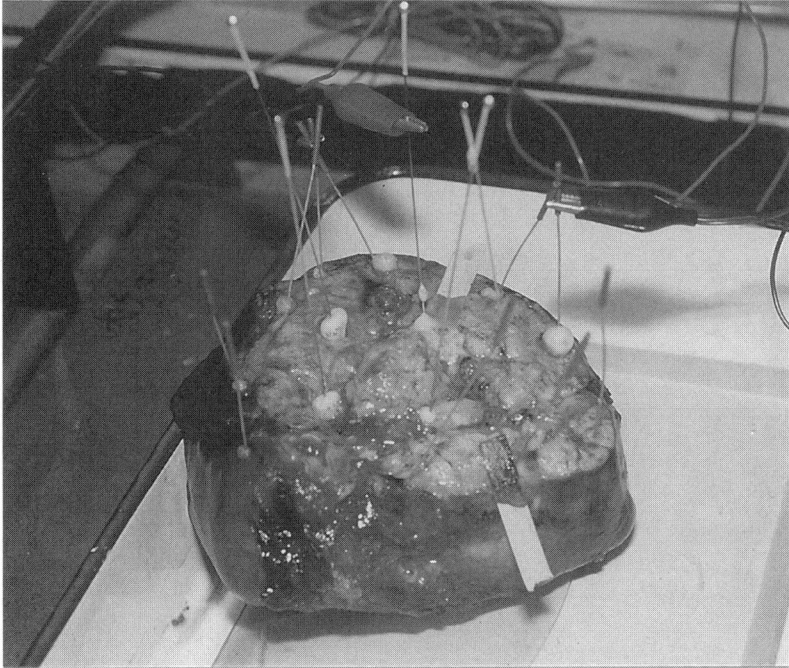

Figure 7 Experiment of ECHT on human lung cancer showed presence of tumor necrosis and much gas.

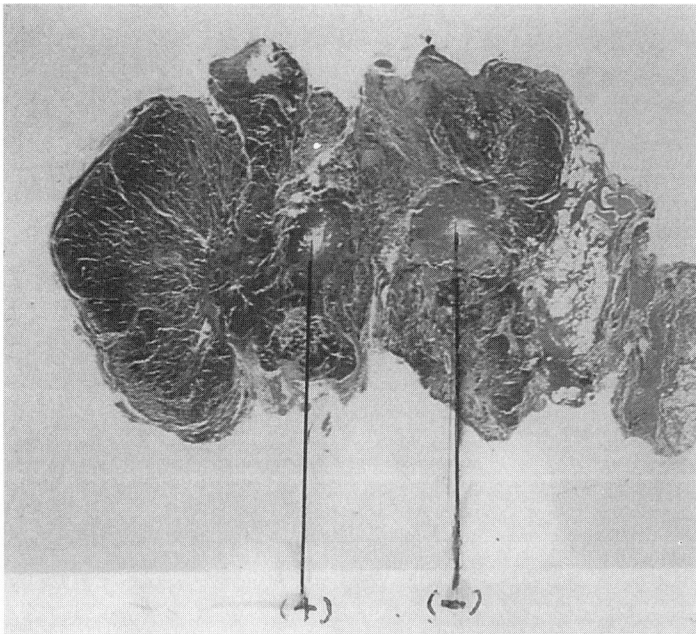

Figure 8 Experiment of ECHT on resected lung cancer to observe different biological effects of anode and cathode. It showed that the killing effect of a cathode is stronger than an anode.

tumors have been treated with EChT in 208 hospitals in China during the past 12 years. It has been shown that EChT can be used not only for treating malignant tumors but also with excellent results in benign tumors, such as cavernous hemangiomas. In fact, EChT has been shown to be a unique therapeutic method for cavernous hemangiomas (29).

In comparing the effectiveness of various methods for treating tumors, EChT proved to be the most effective treatment for cancer. The short-term efficacy of EChT in 7642 malignant tumors has been found to be 76% with a 5-year survival rate of 36%. Next to surgical operation (short-term effectiveness is about 80–90%; 5-year survival rate is 40–50%) ECht is obviously more effective than radio- or chemotherapy (short-term effectiveness is 20–30%; long-term effectiveness is 8–18%). Due to its efficacy in treating malignant tumors, the use of EChT has spread throughout China.

As a result of our accumulated experience and technical improvements, the indications for EChT have broadened. While initially limited to lung, esophageal and breast malig-

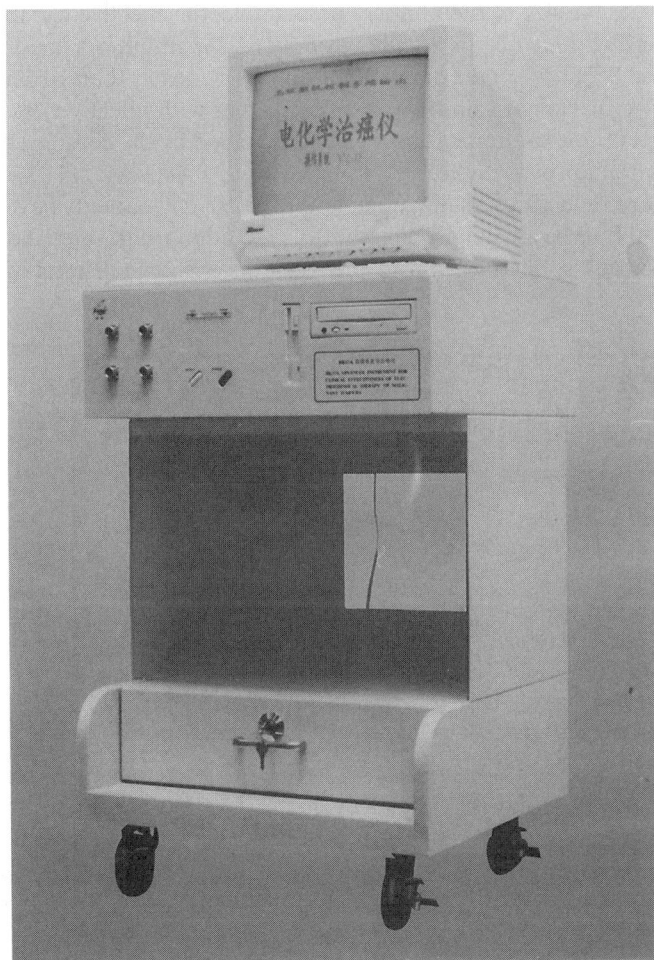

Figure 9 BK 2000 instrument of ECHT. Four outputs controlled by computer. AC 200–240 V, 50–60 Hz, 150 W, voltage: 0–25V + 0.1V, electric current: 0–200mA + 2mA, electric quantity: 0–9999 C. (The instrument is made by Prof. Hongbin Pang.)

nancies, it has subsequently been used for treatment of over 30 kinds of tumors. The effectiveness of treating benign tumors is even more impressive. ECht has been shown to be the best method and far superior to surgery for treating cavernous hemangioma since there is no bleeding and no scar formation so that in addition to a good cosmetic result, function is maintained.

The technical aspects are important. If possible, the needles should be inserted under direct vision, whenever possible and the distribution of and the distance between electrodes should be rational and adjusted when necessary. The electric quantity should be adjusted to the type and the size of the tumor. In general, a quantity of 80–100 C for 1 cm diameter of solid tumors and 30–40 C for hemangiomas should be given. It is important to select the most approprriate cases to achieve the best results. Clinical data for 7642 malignant cases show that the short-term rate (76.0%) and 5-year survival rate (36.0%) are significantly better in stages I and II than in stages III and IV (61.6% and 17.8%, respectively. The main indication of EChT is stages I and II, whereas stages III and IV are relative indications. EChT is contraindicated to cases with general metastases in critical illness.

It is also important to consider the size of the tumor. For example, the effectiveness in malignant tumors with diameter less than 7 cm is 86.5% but only 62.5% in tumors larger than 7 cm. It is not suitable to use EChT when the diameter of tumors is greater than 10 cm (the effective rate 18%). The size of benign tumors is also correlated with effectiveness. EChT is a local treatment and recurrence and metastases can be curtailed by the combined use of radio- and chemotherapy to improve results.

EChT has been used for more than 10 years in China, and over 10, 000 patients have now been treated. We have found it to be amazingly effective, easy to administer, safe, and minimally invasive, and because of this, doctors all over the world have shown interest in

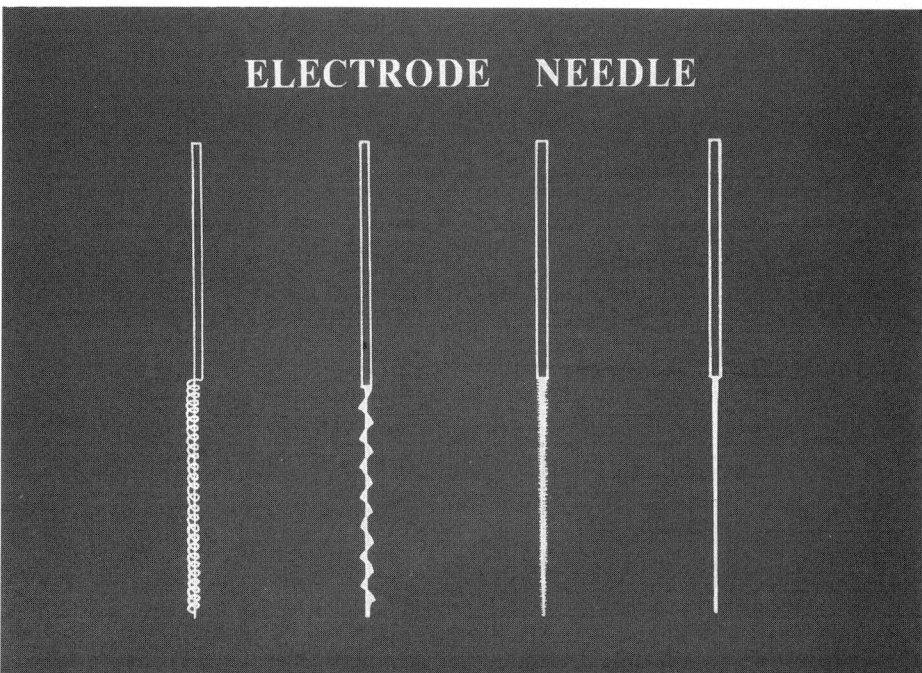

Figure 10   Electrodes made of platinum.

using EChT in their practices. As EChT becomes further refined, it may also be indicated in patients with advanced or recurrent cancers where surgical procedures, radiation, or chemotherapy have not proved effective (Figures 1–10).

REFERENCES

1. Reis A, Henninger T. Experimental study on biological response of ECT in animals. Klin Wochenschrift 1953; 1:39–42.
2. Nordenström B. Biologically Closed Electric Circuits. Stockholm, Sweden: Nordic Medical Publications, 1983.
3. Fu Y. The experimental research of malignant tumors treated by direct current. Mie Med Univ 1985; 19:9.
4. Manabe T. The direct current therapy and experimental research of malignant tumors. J Japan Cancer 1988; 23(3):696–699.
5. Nisiguchi I. The direct current therapy of malignant tumors. J Japan Radiol Assoc 1987; 47(4):621–628.
6. Ito H. The suppression effect of tumor proliferation by direct current. J Japan Cancer Ther 1988; 23:696–702.
7. Nakayama T. The clinical evaluation of radioactive ray sectioning irradiation combined with direct current theapy. J Japan Radiol Assoc 1988; 48:1269–1273.
8. Nordenstrom BEW. Biokinetic impact on structure and imaging of the lung: The concept of biologically closed electric circuits.
9. Nordenstrom BEW. Clinical trials of electrophoretic ionization in the treatment of malignant tumors. IRCS Med Su 1987; 6:537.
10. Nordenstrom BEW. Impact of biologically closed electric circuits (BCEC) on structure and function. Integrative physiological and behavioral science. 1992; 27:285–303.
11. Nordenstrom BEW. Electrochemical treatment of cancer. I. Variable response to anodic and cathodic fields. Am J Clin Oncol (CCT) 1989; 12:530–536; Fu Yu. The experimental research of malignant tumors treated by direct current. Mie Med Univ 1985; 19:9.
12. Manabe T. The direct current therapy and experimental research of malignant tumors. J Japan Cancer 1988; 23(3):696–699.
13. Nisiguchi I. The direct current therapy of malignant tumors. J Japan Radiol Assoc 1987; 47(4):621–628.
14. Ito H. The suppression effect of tumor proliferation by direct current. J Japan Cancer 1988; 23(3):671–696.
15. Nakayama G. The clinical evaluation of radioactive ray sectioning irradiation combined with direct current therapy. J Japan Radiol Assoc 1988; 48(10):1269–1273.
16. Xin Yuling, et al. Experimental Research of Electrochemical Therapy Mechanism. People's Health Publication, 1995.
17. Yokoyama Mi. Local tumor therapy by direct current. J Japan Cancer 1988; 23(9):2040.
18. Xin Yuling. The advancement of electrochemical therapy of tumors in China. Chinese Oncol 1993; 2(11):20–22.
19. Xin Yuling. 334 cases of malignant tumors treated with electrochemical therapy. J Cancer 1995; 10(4):258–261.
20. Xin Yuling. The clinical application of electrochemical therapy of malignant tumors. Gen Clin J 1990; 6(5):25–28.
21. Yuling Xin. Hepatoma therapy with direct current guided by ultrasound. J of China-Japan Friendship Hospital 1989; 3(4):247–251.
22. Xin Yuling. The clinical application of electrochemical therapy of malignant tumors. J Med Theoret Exper Study 1993; 6(3):14–20.
23. Xin Yuling. The clinical effect of lung cancer by electrochemical therapy. J Cancer 1993; 12(4):318–321.

24. Xin Yuling. Advances in the treatment of malignant tumors by electrochemical therapy. Eur J Surg 1994; 574(suppl):31–33.
25. Xin Yuling. The analysis of the clinical effect in 211 cases in middle and later stages lung cancer treated by ECT. Chinese J Integr Trad West Med 1991; 13(3):135–139.
26. Xin Yuling. Electrostatic therapy of lung cancer and pulmonary metastasis. Eur J Surg 1994; 574(suppl):35–37.
27. Xin Yuling. Effects of radiotherapy combined with traditional Chinese medicines of large mass liver cancer. Chinese J Oncol 1992; 14(1):57–61.
28. Xin Yuling. Modern Diagnosis and Treatment of Lung Cancer. People's Health Pub, 1993.
29. Xin Yuling. Verschiedene Tumoren, die mit eletrochemichen methoden in letaten 12, Jahren therapiert wurden. Die Biologische und die Medizinsche Tragodie 2002; 239–260.

44

Cranial Electrotherapy Stimulation for Anxiety, Depression, Insomnia, Cognitive Dysfunction, and Pain

Daniel L. Kirsch and Ray B. Smith

Electromedical Products International, Inc., Mineral Wells, Texas, U.S.A.

The origin and evolution of cranioelectrical stimulation is reviewed, possible mechanism of action are explained as well as problems related to FDA approval because of the extravagant claims made by manufacturers of spurious devices. In contrast, three new meta-analyses of results in depression, insomnia and cognitive dysfunction are presented that are supported by an evidence-based cranioelectrotherapy approach.

I. INTRODUCTION AND HISTORY OF CES

While the use of electric currents in medical practice dates back more than 2000 years, today's interest in cranial electrotherapy stimulation (CES) probably had its beginnings in the research thrusts that began in France in 1903 by Leduc and Rouxeau. Leduc's student, Robinovitch, made the first claim for inducing sleep from electrical treatment in 1914 (1).

Subsequent research interest revolved around electronarcosis and then electroconvulsive shock treatments through the late 1930s. Interest in the smaller amounts of electric current involved in CES did not begin in earnest until work by Anan'ev and his group, in 1957, and in 1958 when Gilyarovski published a book entitled: Electrosleep (2). That work initiated the interest in CES that has lead linearly to the present research and clinical use of CES in America and elsewhere.

The term *cranial electrotherapy stimulation* is used in the United States for what in much of the rest of the world is still called *electrosleep*. The treatment arrived in America as electrosleep, but American researchers soon found that it did not necessarily induce sleep during treatment and that its clinical effects were obtained whether or not sleep occurred (3,4). Today, any small electrical current that is passed across the head for therapeutic purposes is called cranial electrotherapy stimulation, officially, though many related terms such as *transcranial electrical stimulation, cerebral electrostimulation, alpha induction*

727

therapy, neuromodulation, and *neuroelectric therapy* can be found in the titles of many research articles, making it difficult to find and index CES studies in the literature (5,6). A recently revised annotated bibliography of CES research summarized 126 human studies, 29 animal studies, and 31 review articles (7).

Another cause of confusion was the great number of stimulus parameters that fell under the CES rubric. An earlier report found that frequencies used in CES treatment ranged from 1 to 15,000 Hz, the pulse width varied from 0.1 to 20 ms, and the maximum peak pulse amplitude varied from 0 to 20 mA, while the output potential ranged up to 50 V and the supply voltage ranged from a 3.6-V battery source to line voltage of 120 V AC (8).

The United States is the only country in the world that requires a prescription from a licensed health care practitioner to dispense a CES device, and the Food and Drug Administration's (FDA) officially accepted marketing claims for its use are for the treatment of anxiety, depression, and insomnia. Other clinical disorders have been found to be positively affected by CES, however, including several types of cognitive dysfunction, the substance abstinence syndrome, and more recently such widely disparate areas as reflex sympathetic dystrophy, multiple sclerosis, and fibromyalgia.

Possibly underlying the large variety of claims for CES effectiveness were the early findings of Jarzembski and his research group at the University of Wisconsin. When CES was applied to the head of primates in whose brains sensors had been implanted, they found that 42% of the current applied externally actually penetrated through every region of the brain, though it canalized especially along the limbic system (9). More recent research conducted by Ferdjallah at the Biomedical Engineering Department of the University of Texas at Austin has calculated that from 1 mA of current, about 5 $\mu A/cm^2$ of CES reaches the thalamic area at a radius of 13.30 mm, which is sufficient to affect the manufacture and release of neurotransmitters (10).

Accordingly, CES stimulates regions of the brain responsible for pain messages, neurotransmitter genesis, and the hypothalamic-pituitary axis that controls hormone production and control. If one assumes that such stimulation, even at the microampere level, is sufficient over time to generate activity in each of those areas of the brain, then one has cause to suspect symptom reduction in a multiplicity of areas of the body.

This chapter will focus on the scientific clinical studies of CES and will report primarily on the three treatment claims for CES presently permitted by the FDA: anxiety, depression and insomnia. We will then report on promising emerging clinical uses of CES that have been scientifically demonstrated, as published in the peer-reviewed scientific literature.

II. SUMMARY OF SCIENTIFIC STUDY RESULTS

A. Depression

Many studies of depression have appeared in the American literature. While some studies found a remission of depression serendipitously while researching other symptoms (11) others, while researching depression specifically, did so with varying protocols which ranged from open clinical designs with no controls (12) to single blind with sham treated controls (13) to double blind with placebo controls (14).

Measuring strategies have also ranged widely from clinical estimates of no known reliability or validity (15) to measurement with standardized tests of known reliability and validity (16).

While the typical study reported significant changes at the 0.05 or 0.01 level or above, some reported the percent of patients showing clinical improvement of 25% or more as having improved significantly (12). When other studies report results as significant, it may mean that the patients only improved 5% more than the controls if that difference is found to be significant in statistical analysis. Most clinicians find it more helpful for a study to concentrate on finding the actual amount of improvement effected by the treatment. The amount of improvement is known as the *effect size* and can be thought of as an overall percentage of the improvement found. Effect size is the basic unit reported in the increasing number of meta-analytic studies appearing in the literature in which a reviewer statistically combines a large number of studies, the outcomes of which can vary widely. This is done to learn what improvement a new group of patients should experience from a given treatment on average and what the upper and lower limits of the mean (given by the standard error of the mean) of that expected outcome would ordinarily be 95% (when $P < 0.05$) or 99% (when $P < 0.01$) of the time when the treatment is applied. Those numbers are reported in the meta-analyses given here as the r effect size.

What can a practitioner expect for his depressed patients when he recommends CES treatment? Summarizing more than 30 years of CES studies and clinical application in the United States, a recent meta-analytical summary of 25 studies of depression dating from 1972 through 2001 found that the mean r effect size, which is the correlation from 0 to 1.00 of the means of the studies combined for the meta-analysis weighted for the number of subjects in each study, was 0.57 ± 0.06, in which an r effect size of 0.30 is considered moderate and 0.50 is considered high. (The detailed meta-analyses reported in this chapter are available from the authors upon request.)

Another source of information that has not appeared in the literature is that gained by an analysis of self-reported improvement by patients when submitting their warranty card. On the warranty cards supplied with the purchase of Alpha-Stim CES devices (Electro-medical Products International, Inc., Mineral Wells, TX, www.alpha-stim.com), there is a survey form in which the patient can volunteer information regarding the diagnosis, the length of time the device has been used to date, and the treatment results. While most patients do not send in warranty cards, the company has a return for credit policy for patients buying the device and not receiving benefit. Since the cost is not always covered by insurance and fewer than 1% of the units are returned for refund, it is assumed that the vast majority of purchasers feel they are receiving benefit from the treatment, even though they do not remit their warranty card.

When the most recent 300 warranty cards of depressed patients were analyzed, it was found that the average age of the respondent was 47 years, 62% were females, and they reported an average improvement of 58%, which can be translated directly from the binomial effect size distribution as an r effect size of 0.58 ± 0.05. This is very much in line with the overall 0.57 effect size gained from the aforementioned meta-analysis of the research and would seem to add additional confirming value to the CES literature.

As noted above, the study designs have varied widely in terms of the scientific controls employed, and many modern-day reviewers tend to ignore less well controlled studies, scrutinizing more closely the results only of those that employ a double-blinded protocol. After many years of evaluating multiple studies, Glass and his colleagues are reported to have presented convincing evidence that in the typical meta-analysis there is no strong relation between the quality of the study and the average size of the effect obtained. If anything, the effect sizes tend to be higher in both the less well controlled and the most strongly controlled, with other effect sizes falling toward the middle (17).

Another question often arises regarding the type of depression that responds to CES treatment. Most readers will recall the internecine struggles that have gone on regarding the diagnosis of depression in its various forms over the past 30 plus years that CES has been in clinical use in America. The various forms of depression that may be present have often centered diagnostic attention, as has the various levels of depression that may be involved in a given group of patients. Clearly there is some distinction between a patient who "feels blue" and a patient experiencing psychotic depression, though whether that distinction is of a physiological nature or whether the two are only at different points along a continuum is sometimes still debated.

Since no type of deliberate selection factor was reported to be at work in any of the above studies, it may reasonably be assumed that CES was an effective treatment regardless if it was used as a treatment of addicts undergoing the depression of the substance abstinence syndrome, or in those patients who were hospitalized for inpatient treatment of their depression; from the depression that accompanies the difficult stressful studies of graduate students to that accompanying the often times debilitating attention deficit hyperactivity disorder (ADHD) syndrome.

B. Anxiety

This section presents a review and meta-analyzed results of more than 40 published studies of anxiety, plus the results of a survey completed by 47 physicians who evaluated the effectiveness of CES as a treatment for anxiety and stress in 500 of their patients. Also given are self-reported improvement as indicated on the warranty cards submitted by 500 patients who had been prescribed CES for the treatment of their anxiety and/or anxiety related disorders.

The recommended research protocol for the treatment of anxiety with the various CES devices is typically to apply CES for 1 h each day for 2 to 3 weeks, with the patient determining the comfortable stimulation intensity. By the end of the first week or two presenting symptoms have usually subsided significantly or resolved completely in the vast majority. Four studies support the effectiveness of managing some types of situational anxiety during a single treatment session making it an efficient anxiolytic therapy in dentistry and other procedures (5,18–20).

Among the more than 40 CES studies of anxiety published in the United States, few reported the required means and standard error of the means that were required in the early days of meta-analyses for such studies. Meta-analyses were performed, however, at the University of Tulsa by O'Connor and by Klawansky at the Department of Health Policy and Management, Harvard School of Public Health (21,22). Both concluded that CES was unquestionably effective for the treatment of anxiety.

In the very early days of CES treatment in the United States, it began to be used for treating the substance abstinence syndrome in which patients suffering from various addictive substances suffered intensively from anxiety, depression, and sleep disturbance. Because that group has proven susceptible to cross addiction to psychoactive medications, and because they are also more resistant to the effects of such medications than are nonaddicted patients, CES soon became a treatment of choice in both inpatient and outpatient treatment programs for this group of patients (13,14,23–25).

The physicians' poll cited above also reported that of their 500 patients, 349 were previously treatment-resistant anxiety patients. The physicians stated that 94% achieved significant improvement in their anxiety symptoms with the use of CES (7).

Recently, self-reports from the warranty cards of 500 patients suffering from various anxiety states were analyzed to see how they rated the effects of CES treatment on their symptoms. Of the 500 cards, 311 (62%) were submitted by female patients. The ages ranged from 3 years to 89 years of age, so it can be seen that patients were prescribed treatment with CES throughout the life span, with the majority falling between the ages of 40 and 59.

Many of the cards were sent in following 1 or 2 days of treatment, but several were sent in following 12 months of treatment and two were sent in following 156 weeks of treatment. When a correlation was run between the length of treatment and the results of treatment, it was found that while some patients responded at the 100% improvement level within the first week, and at least two patients had received no treatment benefit from 3 months of treatment, there was an overall correlation of 0.63 between the length of CES use and improvement in anxiety, which had strong statistical significance ($p < 0.001$). The mean effect size for all patients reporting was $r = 0.62 \pm 0.04$, with 81% claiming a significant improvement of 25% or greater.

While 473 of the cards analyzed listed anxiety as the primary diagnostic factor, 27 listed stress but did not name anxiety as such. Another 27 listed both stress and anxiety. For purposes of this evaluation, stress and anxiety were combined. Only 175 (35%) listed anxiety alone, while 100 (20%) listed anxiety and depression, 195 (39%) listed anxiety and pain, and 30 (6%) listed anxiety and sleep problems.

In addition, many listed other anxiety related states and those, along with the self-rated treatment results, were panic disorder ($n = 14$, effect size, $r = 0.45$), obsessive compulsive disorder ($n = 5$, effect size, $r = 0.68$), bipolar disorder ($n = 9$, effect size, $r = 0.71$), posttraumatic stress disorder ($n = 8$, effect size, $r = 0.55$), cognitive problems including ADHD ($n = 23$, effect size, $r = 0.62$), and phobias ($n = 9$, effect size, $r = 0.64$). The combined effect size for these sub groups was $r = 0.58 \pm .04$, with 73% claiming significant improvement of 25% or greater.

Also noteworthy is that among the more than 6000 patients who have been involved in CES studies in the English language literature, and among the 500 patients who submitted the warranty cards reported here, there has been no significant negative side effect reported from the use of CES. As the National Research Council reported to the FDA when asked to evaluate the safety of CES, "Review of these reports reveals that significant side effects or complications attributable to the procedure are virtually nonexistent" (26). Rosenthal agreed, stating that, "As a substitute for medication, CES has several advantages. It is possibly more effective. It avoids the common medication side effects as well as problems of medication abuse, incorrect dosage, and suicidal and accidental overdoses" (27).

C. Insomnia

This section presents the results of published insomnia studies, plus data derived from patient self-reports. Twenty-one insomnia studies in which CES was used as the treatment variable were meta-analyzed. While a diversity of research protocols, numbers of patients studied, and measurement strategies employed were found among the studies, an analysis of heterogeneity indicated that those factors did not significantly contaminate the results, which found a mean effect size of $r = 0.62 \pm 0.05$ and a combined probability estimate of significance of the changes in pretreatment to posttreatment mean $= 0.0018$.

Employing electrical stimulation to improve sleep began some years ago when Christian Gottlieb Kratzenstein, a 20-year-old student attending Krueger's medical lectures in Halle, Germany in 1743 was so impressed by Krueger's lectures on electrical therapy that he wrote a report on it (28). He had decided to try this new electrotherapy on himself and was astonished when it permitted him to sleep better.

While electricity has been used off and on to treat insomnia since then, the treatment attracted substantial enthusiasm beginning in 1954 when Russians, then other Europeans began to explore it scientifically. They examined the possibility of turning down the electrical stimulation level from that used in electroanesthesia, which had earlier been reduced from that used in electroconvulsive shock therapy to a level that would induce natural sleep in their patients. Their new technique was named *electrosleep* and was intended to replace sleep medications and their numerous negative side effects, not the least of which was the addictive properties of many of them (29). Electrosleep treatment quickly spread around the world, arriving in the United States in the early 1960s.

The clinical intent was that electrosleep treatment should induce sleep immediately when the current was applied to the patient's head, and that the patient should remain asleep naturally, once the induced sleep was begun. That did not appear to be happening, however, so many of the earliest clinical studies of electrosleep in the United States were concerned with discovering the stimulus parameters that would induce sleep in patients. The pulse rates were varied from less than one per second to thousands per second, while the pulse duration was varied from microseconds to continuous. The stimulus intensity was varied from just a few microamperes to several milliamperes, while the shape of the pulse wave was varied from sinusoidal to modified square to a modified sawtooth wave, and so forth (30–32).

As the treatment arrived in the United States from Europe, the electrodes were placed over each closed eyelid in front of the head and the mastoids in back of the head (29). Later, because of the discomfort from the pressure on the eyelids and the temporarily distorted vision patients typically experienced immediately following their removal, researchers began to place the frontal electrodes just above each eyebrow, while the rear electrodes remained on the mastoids (33). Still later, the electrodes were placed on the mastoid process just behind each ear only, so that the stimulus current now went from side to side across the head instead of from front to back (24). That placement is still used in the United States, but the most recent placement to enhance efficacy and convenience is on each ear lobe via ear clip electrodes (34).

EEG studies soon followed, when no treatment strategy could be found that would reliably induce sleep in the patients. The EEG studies were to see what, if anything, happened when electrosleep current was applied across a patient's head. The first study was designed to see if there were any sleep changes in the EEG. There were none. Some patients slept when in the treatment condition and some slept when in the control condition, while the rest never slept during any phase of the study (3).

Another EEG study found that one 30-min electrosleep treatment per day for 5 days yielded slower EEG frequencies with increase amplitude in the fronto-temporal areas in all of the patients. Most also showed increased quality and quantity of alpha with increased amplitude in the occipital-parietal leads (35).

Itil and his colleagues gave 10 volunteers 2 days of CES and 2 days of sham CES in a crossover design. They found that the patients who exhibited no decrease of vigilance when CES was off also showed no significant changes in vigilance when CES was on. Those who showed a slight to moderate drowsiness during the off recording did show a slight to moderate sleep pattern when the CES was on (36). What the researchers did find was that while they could not induce sleep in the laboratory, with one exception they all found that CES was associated with patient reports of better sleep at night. One EEG study that was deliberately done during evening hours in a sleep laboratory, simply allowed patients who had been diagnosed with insomnia to sleep in their usual way in the university sleep laboratory while having their EEG monitored. Five patients were given actual subsensation CES treatments 30 min a day for 10 days, and five were given sham treatments. On subsequent monitoring of their EEG pattern it was found that patients receiving actual treatment went to sleep faster when "their head hit the pillow," spent more time in stage IV sleep during the night, had fewer awakenings during the night, went back to sleep sooner when they did awaken in the night, and reported a significantly more restful and restoring sleep upon awakening the next morning than did the sham-treated subjects (37). That study and others found that those results still held up and in some areas even improved somewhat following a 2-year follow-up period (38).

Soon a growing number of researchers discovered that electrosleep not only ensured sound, restful sleep for patients suffering from insomnia but effectively treated stress in the process, as measured by various psychological measuring scales of depression and anxiety. Importantly, it was found that the stress measures, including the patients sleep patterns, improved whether or not the patient slept during the treatment (4).

In addition to more than 20 studies, all of which were published in peer reviewed journals, the physicians participating in the survey were also asked to rate the sleep response of their insomnia patients from CES treatment. The physicians rated overall sleep improvement in their 135 insomnia patients as 79% (7).

More recently, as part of a larger study, 140 CES warranty cards that had been sent in by insomnia patients following a minimum of 3 weeks of treatment were analyzed to assess their perception of its effectiveness in the treatment of their sleep disorder (39). As noted above, patients who submit warranty cards can volunteer information regarding their medical diagnosis. Among the persons who listed insomnia as a major diagnosis were those who also included other areas of stress such as anxiety or depression (29%), while still others (48%) also listed pain as a major accompanying symptom. Fewer than a fourth (23%) of the patients listed insomnia as their only symptom.

It is of interest that while the second, more stressed group used their CES device almost 6 weeks before reporting, the pain group used theirs 10 weeks on average before sending in their cards. While one might assume that the longer the patient used the unit, the better the response they would have, that does not appear to be the case. The majority of patients, no matter what category the fell into, claimed 75 to 99% improvement, and this improvement did not appear to be correlated with the length of time used.

The effect size, in this case, is a measure of the percent improvement in their sleeping pattern reported by this group of patients suffering from insomnia. The average effect size from this sample was $r = 0.87 \pm 0.03$. As stated earlier, that compares quite favorably with Cohen's guidelines for small ($r = 0.10$), medium ($r = 0.30$), and large ($r = 0.50$) treatment effect sizes (17).

A meta-analysis was completed of 21 studies that have been published in the peer reviewed scientific literature (one in an edited book) plus the analysis reported just above. The studies were completed over a 30-year period and involve a total of 940 patients. None reported significant negative side effects during or following any study. The number of patients in each study varied widely, as did the amount of scientific control measures applied and the measurement strategies employed. While all studies involved patients suffering from insomnia, several studied the sleep disorder of patients withdrawing from addicting substances, while others looked at the sleep problems accompanying difficult pain syndromes such as fibromyalgia.

That this variety of approaches to studying CES did not have a significant effect in understanding the role of CES in the treatment of insomnia was ascertained from a test of heterogeneity that yielded a probability of $p < 0.30$. This indicated that the studies could be safely combined without prejudice to the understanding of the overall role of CES in the treatment of insomnia. The mean effect size obtained when the results of all the studies were combined was $r = 0.62 \pm 0.05$.

It can be concluded that CES, while remarkably underutilized as compared to pharmaceuticals, is a safe and very effective treatment for insomnia of various etiologies. The fact that no significant negative side effects were reported in any of the studies analyzed is equally important. Also, once a CES device is prescribed for a patient there are no major costs associated with its use except the occasional replacement of batteries, electrodes, and conducting solution. This may turn out to be the deciding factor for CES in an age of rapidly expanding medical costs.

D. Cognitive Dysfunction

Early in the history of CES in the United States, controlled scientific studies began of the substance abstinence syndrome, with its major symptoms of anxiety, depression, and sleeplessness in withdrawing addicts. Those studies involved patients withdrawing from illegal and/or pharmaceutical drugs, alcohol, and nicotine (13,14,23,25,40,41).

Up until that time in the early to mid-1970s it was taught that with each shot of alcohol that one drank, thousands of brain cells were destroyed, and that these would never return. By the time an alcoholic person entered one of the many inpatient treatment centers he or she was assumed to be significantly advanced down the road toward irreversible Korsakoff psychosis. Among the chief signs of the Korsakoff psychosis syndrome were various cognitive problems, including short-term memory loss, cognitive confusion, the inability to store new information reliably, and mental problems such as confabulation (42–44).

It therefore came as an unexpected surprise to practitioners of CES when they discovered that in the process of successfully treating the depression, anxiety and insomnia in withdrawing patients, they also totally reversed the Korsakoff's psychosis syndrome present in the large majority.

In neuropsychology, Korsakoff type degeneration was often measured with the Benton Visual Retention Scale in which patients were shown a drawing with circles, squares, triangles, and the like, then given a clean piece of paper and asked to reproduce it (45). Also used were the Organic Brain Syndrome subscales of the Weschler Adult Intelligence Scale (or the Weschler Intelligence Scale for Children). Those subscales are the Digit Span, the Digit Symbol, and the Object Assembly subscales, and these three subscales were known to fall significantly below the functional level of the other subscales on those tests in Korsakoff patients. Other researchers in the addiction field used the Maize and Form Design subtests on the nonverbal Revised Beta I.Q. examination comparing them with the remaining three subscales on that test in the same way (46–48).

It was serendipitously found that in every case where patients experienced an improvement in stress level from CES, they also experienced a dramatic improvement in cognitive function, with an average gain of 12 to 18 points on standardized I.Q. tests administered previous to and following 3 weeks of daily CES treatment, 1 h of treatment per day (24). It was in this manner that researchers found that so-called permanent brain damage in drug and alcohol addiction was not permanent at all (49).

We now know that while the cognitive abilities of most such patients will approach normal following 2 years of total abstinence (49–51), they will return to normal with just 3 weeks of daily CES treatment (24,49,52).

By the mid-1970s researchers found that the confusion–bewilderment factor on the widely used profile of mood states (POMS) correlated strongly with these other measures of cognitive dysfunction (13) and began to use it as a cognitive function measuring device. According to the test manual, it is thought to measure "bewilderment and muddleheadedness, and may represent a state of cognitive inefficiency, a mood state, or both. It may also be related to the classical organized-disorganized dimension of emotion, possibly a by-product of anxiety or related states" (53). It was not thought to be a measurement of brain damage when that edition of the manual was written.

Following close on the heels of studies of the substance abstinence syndrome, another study looked at the stress-related cognitive problems of graduate students in a business management training program and found CES offered significant improvement as measured by the POMS (16).

Research attention also turned to patients with acquired closed head injuries, resulting from such things as motorcycle accidents, falls from high elevations on construction projects, inoperable brain tumors, and so forth. That group drew special attention because the majority of them were known seizure patients and little was known of the effects of CES on seizure patients. Under the supervision of a research physician, 21 closed head injured patients who were living in a supervised care home were selected for a double-blind study (54).

It was found that along with their anxiety and depression scores, following 1-h treatments daily, 4 days a week for 3 weeks, the cognitive function score improved significantly in the treatment group, as measured on the POMS. During the study one of the subjects who had brain cancer had a seizure and was immediately removed from the study by the study physician. Following the study, the 11 patients in the two control groups were also given CES for 3 weeks. It had been learned that the patient who had the seizure during the double-blind phase of the study was receiving sham CES treatment. Upon the insistence of his parents, he also received actual CES treatment for three weeks following the study. Neither he nor any of the other subjects in the study experienced a seizure while receiving actual treatment, and their seizure experience in the weeks following the study was unremarkable, according to house attendants.

Another report of the effectiveness of CES in posttraumatic amnesia cited two cases, in which the first was a 21-year-old male who was comatose for weeks following a motorcycle accident recovered much of his tested memory recall functions following 3 weeks of 1-h daily CES treatments. The other patient was a 58-year-old orthopedic surgeon who suffered head injury in a motor vehicle accident. He was diagnosed with diencephalic amnesia secondary to trauma. He had difficulty distinguishing between fantasy and reality and experienced overwhelming anxiety during periods of disorientation. His amnesia improved by 28% on immediate recall and 39% on delayed recall after only 1 week of daily CES treatments. These were accompanied by numerous other behavioral improvements (55).

Some researchers have theorized that the present mass epidemic of fibromyalgia patients is due to brain dysfunction following whiplash injury or similar traumas to the brain (56). That concept is still under investigation; meanwhile several recent published studies have shown CES to be a very effective treatment for fibromyalgia (34,39,57–59).

Perhaps due to its hypothesized ability to functionally stabilize a traumatized brain and return it toward a condition of preinjury homeostatic functioning, CES has proven to be an effective treatment for patients with acquired brain injury. It has also proved to be a significantly beneficial adjunct to other forms of physical and psychological therapies.

A meta-analysis of 13 CES studies in which cognitive function was measured, revealed the following: The over all treatment effect size for the combined studies, when corrected for the size of each study, was $r = 0.62 \pm 0.10$.

A check of heterogeneity showed that the studies separated out statistically with the addiction and head injured patients in one group and the otherwise clinically stressed groups of fibromyalgia patients, graduate students, and ADHD subjects in another group. Upon inspection, the two double-blind studies by Schmitt and the one study by Smith that contained the largest N studied had the strongest effect sizes (24,40,52).

The effect size of the group of seven addiction and one brain trauma studies, when separated out and corrected for effect of study sample size was now increased to $r = 0.71 \pm 0.13$, the effect size of the remaining group of studies dropped to only $r = 0.18 \pm 0.01$ and remained at that level when corrected for sample size. This indicated that these two groupings in the overall meta-analysis were not only significantly different but, while still responding well, responded much differently to CES treatment in terms of the amount of treatment effect recorded in effect size.

More recently, there have been an increasing number of CES research protocols in which the impact of high levels of stress on cognitive functioning is being evaluated. Measures of cognitive functioning are now often included in present and ongoing CES studies of fibromyalgia patients (60) and have been added to an upcoming study of pain in spinal cord injured veterans (61).

III. MECHANISMS OF ACTION

Scientists at the University of Tennessee Medical Center completed a series of five different studies in which various drugs were used to deliberately upset the homeostatic balance of the brains in canine subjects and thereby give them Parkinsonlike symptoms. They found that once the homeostasis was thrown into disarray, the application of CES could bring them back into apparent neurochemical homeostasis within 3 to 7 h. Left to their normal care, but without CES, the animals required 4 to 7 days to return to normal behavior once the drugs had been removed (62). The postulated mechanism of action in the neurotransmitter system studied was that CES stimulated the areas of the brain that were responsible for catecholamine and dopamine production, bringing the experimentally imbalanced neurotransmitter homeostasis back to its original homeostatic condition.

Over the years a number of EEG studies have been done pre- and post-CES treatments, as noted above in the sleep sections. In addition, a study of the P300 wave of outpatients who were addicted to various substances found that the P300 wave anomaly earlier found to be diagnostic of this group returned to normal following CES treatment (63).

In another study presynaptic membranes were analyzed before, during, and following CES stimulation of four squirrel monkeys. It was found that the number of vesicles in the presynaptic membrane declined when stimulation first began, that a greater than normal number of vesicles were found in the presynaptic membrane after 5 min of stimulation, and that the number of vesicles in the presynaptic membrane returned toward normal shortly after cessation of stimulation. The authors concluded that CES induces firing of neurotransmitter substances from presynaptic membrane vesicles into the synaptic space, while stimulating the increased manufacture of replacement neurotransmitter substances at the presynaptic membrane (64).

These studies suggest that CES is quite possibly reestablishing neurotransmitter homeostasis by inducing maximal production of each given neurotransmitter, allowing each to reestablish homeostatic balance with others by means of the known ability of neurons to induce inhibitory effects in each other.

There is a growing body of evidence indicating the ability of stress of various kinds to throw the natural neurotransmitter balance out of control. It is also thought that some stressful life experiences may elevate the serum cortisol level to such an extent that neurons are actually debilitated or killed. It is known now that small electrical pulses can stimulate neuron regeneration and repair, and this will likely be the thrust of our next research efforts.

IV. SUMMARY

Cranial electrotherapy stimulation treatments result in a relaxed body with an alert mind. The quality of life of those who use it is substantially improved. When all the research is viewed in aggregate, and without bias against nondrug interventions, CES has already been proven to be the safest and perhaps most effective treatment for a wide range of centrally mediated disorders. There is now enough evidence to establish it as a first line of treatment. Also, CES is so cost effective that it alone could relieve such a substantial burden from limited health care funds that enough money would be freed up to find more effective treatments for the disorders CES does not address. At the very least, the concomitant use of CES reduces the usage of psychoactive pharmaceuticals by at least one-third, and with that alone comes billions of dollars in savings (20,65–73). The day is rapidly approaching when CES will no longer be the best kept secret in American medicine.

REFERENCES

1. Appel CP. Effect of electrosleep: review of research. Goteborg Psychol Rep 1972; 2:1–24.
2. Brown CC. Electroanesthesia and Electrosleep. Am Psychol 1975; 30:402–425.
3. Taaks H, Kugler J. Electrosleep and brain function. Electroenceph Clin Neurophysiology 1968; 24:62–94.
4. Ryan JJ, Souheaver GT. The role of sleep in electrosleep therapy for anxiety. Dis Nerv Syst 1977; 38:515–517.
5. Gibson TH, O'Hair DE. Cranial application of low level transcranial electrotherapy vs. relaxation instruction in anxious patients. Am J Electromed 1987; 4:18–21.
6. England RR. Treatment of migraine headache utilizing cerebral electrostimulation. MS thesis, North Texas State University, Denton, Texas, 1976
7. Kirsch DL. The Science Behind Cranial Electrotherapy Stimulation. 2d ed. Edmonton, Alberta: Medical Scope Publishing, 2002.
8. Smith RB. Cranial electrotherapy stimulation. In: Myklebust JB, Cusick JF, Sances A Jr, Larson SF, eds. Neural Stimulation. Vol II. Boca Raton: CRC Press, 1985:130.
9. Jarzembski WB, Laarson SJ, Sances A Jr. Evaluation of specific cerebral impedance and cerebral current density. Annals of the New York Academy of Sciences 1970; 170:476–490.
10. Ferdjallah M, Bostick FX Jr, Barr RE. Potential and current density distributions of cranial electrotherapy stimulation (CES) in a four-concentric-spheres model. IEEE Transactions on Biomedical Engineering 1996; 43(9):939–943.
11. Smith RB. Cranial electrotherapy stimulation in the treatment of stress related cognitive dysfunction, with an eighteen month follow up. Journal of Cognitive Rehabilitation 1999; 17:14–18.
12. Rosenthal SH, Wulfson NL. Electrosleep: a clinical trial. American Journal of Psychiatry 1970; 127:175–176.
13. Smith RB, O'Neill L. Electrosleep in the management of alcoholism. Biological Psychiatry 1975; 10:675–680.
14. Bianco F Jr. The efficacy of cranial electrotherapy stimulation (CES) for the relief of anxiety and depression among polysubstance abusers in chemical dependency treatment. Ph.D dissertation, The University of Tulsa, Oklahoma, 1994.
15. Tomosovic M, Edwards RV. Cerebral electrotherapy for tension-related symptoms in alcoholics. Quarterly J Studies Alcohol 1973; 34:1352–1355.
16. Matteson MT, Ivancevich JM. An exploratory investigation of CES as an employee stress management technique. J Health Human Res Admin 1986; 9:93–109.
17. Wolf FM. Meta-analysis; quantitative methods for research synthesis. Newbury Park: Sage Publications, 1986:51.
18. Heffernan M. The effect of a single cranial electrotherapy stimulation on multiple stress measures. The Townsend Letter for Doctors and Patients 1995; 147:60–64.
19. Voris MD. An investigation of the effectiveness of cranial electrotherapy stimulation in the treatment of anxiety disorders among outpatient psychiatric patients, impulse control parolees and pedophiles. Delos Mind/Body Institute, Dallas and Corpus Cristi, Texas, 1995.

20. Winick R. Cranial electrotherapy stimulation (CES): a safe and effective low cost means of anxiety control in a dental practice. General Dentistry 1999; 47(1):50–55.

21. O'Connor ME, Bianco F, Nicholson R. Meta-analysis of cranial electrostimulation in relation to the primary and secondary symptoms of substance withdrawal. 12th Annual Meeting of the Bioelectromagnetics Society, June 14, 1991.

22. Klawansky S, Yeung A, Berkey C, Shah N, Chalmers TC. Meta-analysis of randomized controlled trials of cranial electrotherapy stimulation: efficacy in treating selected psychological and physiological conditions. Journal of Nervous and Mental Diseases 1995; 183(7):478–485.

23. Gomez E, Mikhail AR. Treatment of methadone withdrawal with cerebral electrotherapy (electrosleep). Brit J Psychiatry 1978; 134:111–113.

24. Schmitt R, Capo T, Frazier H, Boren D. Cranial electrotherapy stimulation treatment of cognitive brain dysfunction in chemical dependence. J Clin Psychiatry 1984; 45:60–63.

25. Gold M, Pottash ALC, Sternbach H, Barbaban J, Annitto W. Anti-withdrawal effects of alpha methyl dopa and cranial electrotherapy. 12th Annual Meeting of the Society for Neuroscience, 1982.

26. National Research Council, Division of Medical Sciences. An evaluation of electroanesthesia and electrosleep. FDA Contract 70-22, Task Order No. 20 (NTIS PB 241305), 1974; 1–54.

27. Rosenthal SH. Electrosleep therapy. Current Psychiatric Therapies 1972; 12:104–107.

28. Kratzenstein CG. Schreiben von dem Nutzen der Electricitaet in der Arzneiwissenshaft. Halle, 1745

29. Wageneder FM, Iwanovsky A, Dodge CH. Electrosleep (cerebral electrotherapy) and electro-anesthesia- the international effort at evaluation. Foreign Science Bulletin 1969; 5(4):1–104.

30. Forster S, Bernard S, Bendon JG. Preliminary observations on electrosleep. Arch Phys Med Rehabil 1963; 44:481–489.

31. Straus B, Elkind A, Bodian CA. Electrical induction of sleep. Am J Med Sci 1964; 248:514–520.

32. Magora F, Beller A, Assael MI, Askenazi A. Some aspects of electrical sleep and its therapeutic value. In: Wageneder FM, St. Schuy, eds. Electrotherapeutic Sleep and Electroanaesthesia. Excerpta Medica Foundation, International Congress Series No. 136. Amsterdam, 1967:129–1354.

33. Moore JA, Mellor CS, Standage KF, Strong H. A double-blind study of electrosleep for anxiety and insomnia. Biol Psychiatry 1975; 10(1):59–63.

34. Lichtbroun AS, Raicer MC, Smith RB. The treatment of fibromyalgia with cranial electrotherapy stimulation. J Clin Rheumatol 2001; 7:72–78.

35. McKenzie RE, Rosenthal SH, Driessner JS. Some psychophysiologic effects of electrical transcranial stimulation (electrosleep). In: Wulfsohn NL, Sances A, eds. The Nervous System and Electric Currents. New York: Plenum, 1976:163–167.

36. Itil T, Gannon P, Akpinar S, Hsu W. Quantitative EEG analysis of electrosleep using frequency analyzer and digital computer methods. Electroencephalogr Clin Neurophysiol 1971; 31:294.

37. Weiss MF. The treatment of insomnia through use of electrosleep: an EEG study. J Nervous Mental Dis 1973; 157:108–120.

38. Cartwright RD, Weiss MF. The effects of electrosleep on insomnia revisited. J Nerv Ment Dis 1975; 161(2):134–137.

39. Smith RB. Is microcurrent stimulation effective in pain management? An additional perspective. Am J Pain Management 2001; 11(2):64–68.

40. Schmitt R, Capo T, Boyd E. Cranial electrotherapy stimulation as a treatment for anxiety in chemically dependent persons. Alcoholism: Clin Experiment Res 1986; 10:158–160.

41. Patterson MA, Firth J, Gardiner R. Treatment of drug, alcohol and nicotine addiction by neuroelectric therapy: analysis of results over 7 years. J Bioelectricity 1984; 3(1,2):193–221.

42. Mellow NK, Mendelson JH. Alterations in states of consciousness associated with chronic ingestion of alcohol. In: Zubin J, Shagass C, eds. Neurobiological aspects of psychopathology. 58th Annual Meeting of the American Psychopathological Association, 1969.

43. Clarke JG. Some aspects of intellectual deficit and depression in heavy drinkers. J Irish Med Assoc 1976; 69:29–32.

44. Ornstein P. Cognitive deficits in chronic alcoholics. Psychol Rep 1977; 40:719–724.
45. Kapur N, Butters N. Visuoperceptive deficits in long-term alcoholics and alcoholics with Korsakoff's psychosis. J Studies Alcohol 1977; 38:2025–2035.
46. Sivan AB. Benton visual retention test. 5th ed. San Antonio, Texas: Psychological Corporation, 1991.
47. Wechsler D. Statistical properties of the scale. Manual for the Wechsler Adult Intelligence Scale-Revised. New York: Psychological Corporation, 1981.
48. Kellogg CE, Morton NW. Revised beta examination, second edition (beta-II). San Antonio, Texas: The Psychological Corporation, 1978.
49. Smith RB. Confirming evidence of an effective treatment for brain dysfunction in alcoholic patients. J Nervous Mental Dis 1982; 170:275–278.
50. Sharp JR, Rosenbaum G, Goldman MS, Whitman RD. Recoverability of psychological functioning following alcohol abuse; acquisition of meaningful synonyms. J Consult Clin Psychol 1977; 45:1023–1028.
51. O'Leary MR, Radford LM, Chaney EF, Schau EJ. Assessment of cognitive recovery in alcoholics by use of the Trail Making Test. J Clin Psychol 1977; 33:579–582.
52. Smith RB, Day E. The effects of cerebral electrotherapy on short-term memory impairment in alcoholic patients. Int J Addictions 1977; 12:575–582.
53. McNair DM, Lorr M, Droppleman LF. Edits manual for the profile of mood states. San Diego, California: Educational and Industrial Testing Service, 1992.
54. Smith RB, Tiberi A, Marshall J. The use of cranial electrotherapy stimulation in the treatment of closed-head-injured patients. Brain Injury 1994; 8:357–361.
55. Childs A, Crismon ML. The use of cranial electrotherapy stimulation in post-traumatic amnesia: a report of two cases. Brain Injury 1988; 2:243–247.
56. Bennett RM, Cook DM, Clark SR, et al. Hypothalamic-pituitary-insulin-like growth factor-1 axis dysfunction in patients with fibromyalgia. Journal of Rheumatology 1997; 24:384–389.
57. Tyres S, Smith RB. Treatment of fibromyalgia with cranial electrotherapy stimulation. Original Internist 2001; 8(3):15–17.
58. Tyers S, Smith RB. A comparison of cranial electrotherapy stimulation alone or with chiropractic therapies in the treatment of fibromyalgia. The American Chiropractor 2001; 23 (2):39–41.
59. Lichtbroun AS, Raicer MC, Smith RB. The use of Alpha-Stim cranial electrotherapy stimulation in the treatment of fibromyalgia. 15th Annual International Symposium on Acupuncture and Electro-Therapeutics, Columbia University, New York City, October 21–24, 1999.
60. Cork RC. Alpha-Stim CES for fibromyalgia. Study in progress: Louisiana State University Medical Center, Shreveport, 2002.
61. Tan G. Alpha-Stim CES for spinal cord injury pain. Study in progress: Veterans Affairs Hospital, Houston, 2002.
62. Pozos RS, Strack LE, White RK, Richardson AW. Electrosleep versus electroconvulsive therapy. In: Reynolds DV, Sjoberg AE, eds. Neuroelectric Research. Vol. 23. Springfield: Charles Thomas, 1971:221–225.
63. Braverman E, Smith RB, Smayda R, Blum K. Modification of P300 amplitude and other electrophysiological parameters of drug abuse by cranial electrical stimulation. Current Therapeutic Res 1990; 48:586–596.
64. Siegesmund KA, Sances A Jr., Larson SJ. The effects of electrical currents on synaptic vesicles in monkey cortex. In: Wageneder FM, St. Schuy, eds. Electrotherapeutic Sleep and Electroanaesthesia. Internaliton Congress series No. 136. Amsterdam: Excerpta Medica Foundation, 1967:31–33.
65. Alpher EJ, Kirsch DL. A patient with traumatic brain injury and full body reflex sympathetic dystrophy treated with cranial electrotherapy stimulation. Am J Pain Management 1998; 8:124–128.
66. Champagne C, Papiemik E, Thierry JP, Noviant Y. Transcutaneous cerebral electric stimulation by Limoge current during labor. Ann Fr Anesth Reanim 1984; 3:405–413.

67. Childs A. Droperidol and CES in Organic Agitation. Clinical Newsletter of the Austin Rehabilitation Hospital, 1995.

68. Naveau S, Barritault L, Zourabichvili O, Champagne C, Prieur G, Limoge A, Poynard T, Chaput JC. Analgesic effect of transcutaneous cranial electrostimulation in patients treated by Nd:YAG laser for cancer of the rectum. A double-blind randomized trial. Gastroenterol Clin Biol 1992; 16:8–11.

69. Stanley TH, Cazalaa JA, Atinault A, Coeytaux R, Limoge A, Louville Y. Transcutaneous cranial electrical stimulation decreases narcotic requirements during neurolept anesthesia and operation in man. Anesthesia Analgesia 1982; 61(10):863–866.

70. Stanley TH, Cazalaa JA, Limoge A, Louville Y. Transcutaneous cranial electrical stimulation increases the potency of nitrous oxide in humans. Anesthesiology 1982; 57:293–297.

71. Mantz J, Azerad J, Limoge A, Desmonts JM. Transcranial electrical stimulation with Limoge's currents decreases halothane requirements in rats. Evidence for the involvement of endogenous opioids. Anesthesiology 1992; 76:253–260.

72. Stinus L, Auriacombe M, Tignol J, Limoge A, Le Moal M. Transcranial electrical stimulation with high frequency intermittent current (Limoge's) potentiates opiate-induced analgesia: blind studies. Pain 1990; 42(3):351–363.

73. Warner R, Hudson-Howard L, Hojnson C, Skolnick M. Serotonin involvement in analgesia induced by transcranial electrostimulation. Life Sciences 1990; 46:1131–1138.

45

Low-Intensity Millimeter Waves in Biology and Medicine

O. V. Betskii

Institute for Radio Engineering and Electronics of the Russian Academy of Sciences, Moscow, Russia

N. N. Lebedeva

Institute for Higher Nerve Activity and Neurophysiology of the Russian Academy of Sciences, Moscow, Russia

Both authors of this chapter are pioneers of biological research and clinical application of extremely high frequency electromagnetic fields in GHz-region, known as millimeter waves. For a period of less than 15 years a number of well executed basic science studies has been performed, series of papers were published (mainly in Russian language literature), millions of patients received treatment for various diseases and pathologies. The authors gave English-speaking readers a rear chance to obtain information for biological and clinical effects observed so far and some potential mechanisms of action are discussed in the chapter.

I. INTRODUCTION

Electromagnetic millimeter (MM) waves (λ = 1 to 10 mm) correspond to the extremely high frequency (EHF) band: f = 300 to 30 GHz. In the electromagnetic spectrum, this band lies between the super-high-frequency (microwave) band and the optical (infrared) band.

The first wideband oscillator with an electric tuning of oscillation frequency was developed and brought into lot production in the USSR under the leadership of academician N. D. Devyatkov and Professor M. B. Golant in the mid-1960s. The oscillator was called an O-type backward-wave tube. It was employed both to improve radio navigation systems and to create new communications systems (1,2).

In those days, scientists all over the world discussed possible application of electro-magnetic waves in nontraditional fields—such as biology, medicine, and some others. Creators of the MM-wave oscillator suggested an idea of investigating biological effects of

MM-wave radiation. These waves were of special interest for scientists because they were unlikely to take part in phylogenesis of terrestrial beings. The point is that MM-wave radiation is virtually absent in natural conditions. This is due to its strong absorption by the earth's atmosphere: MM waves are absorbed eagerly by water vapor.

It was hypothesized that low-intensity (nonthermal) MM waves might have a nonspecific effect on biological structures and organisms. Foreground investigations, which have been performed in the USSR and then in Russia for 30 years, made it possible to enunciate a hypothesis that vital functions in cells are governed by coherent electromagnetic EHF waves: The alternating electromagnetic field of these waves maintains interaction between adjacent cells to interrelate and control intercellular processes in the entire being. This hypothesis formed the basis for a new scientific lead that was originated at the turn of several branches of sciences: biophysics, radio electronics, medicine, and some others. This lead was thereafter named *millimeter electromagnetobiology* (3,4).

II. EXPERIMENTAL CLINICAL INVESTIGATIONS

L. A. Sevast'yanova was among the first scientists who launched investigations into the biological effects of low-intensity MM waves on mammals (1969–1971) (5–8). She demonstrated that preliminary MM-wave irradiation may counteract x-ray-induced effects in the bone marrow. She also estimated MM-wave penetration into the skin of animals. L. A. Sevast'yanova determined the distribution pattern of MM-wave power for some animals and human beings. The estimated penetration depth showed that MM waves produce a mediate protective effect.

Investigations that lasted for more than 20 years were performed on more than 12,000 laboratory animals (mice and rats). The response of the hematogenous system was evaluated by the count and state of marrow cells (karyocytes) present in the right and left femoral arteries as well as in the spleen. The results obtained are given below:

The biological effect depends on the power flux density.

The biological effect depends on the wavelength.

The biological effect depends on the MM-wave exposure site location.

The biological effect depends on the MM-wave exposure area.

As far back as the 1970s, W. R. Adey advanced a hypothesis that the electromagnetic spectrum should contain "amplitude-frequency windows" in which biological effects are more pronounced (9). The above-described results served as the first experimental verification of this hypothesis. It was inferred that biological effects of electromagnetic radiation, and particularly of MM-wave radiation, are determined by its biotropic parameters, such as the intensity, frequency, signal waveform, location, and exposure.

It is known that cells exposed to x-rays reveal different types of lesions that depend on the x-ray dose. These lesions manifest themselves in the form of chromosome aberrations, decreased mitotic activity, and inhibited reproductive ability. In turn, this leads to reduced karyocyte and blood-cell counts. Most radioprotectors do not exhibit sufficient selectivity. As the radiation dose increases, they themselves may produce toxic effects. Results obtained by L. A. Sevast'yanova were evidence that MM waves have a protective effect and that they influence karyocytes selectively.

When MM-wave irradiation was followed by x-ray exposure, *intact* animals (without grafts) revealed a smaller damage degree of karyocytes as compared to those exposed to x-rays alone: by the fifth day, the karyocyte deficiency was 15% only, whereas it amounted to 38% in animals exposed sequentially to x-rays and MM waves.

Like radiation, antineoplastic compounds isolate the DNA-membrane complex and retard the DNA and RNA synthesis. At the cellular level, the effect of x-ray exposure has much in common with the effect of chemotherapy compounds: a sluggish cellular cycle, delayed mitosis, chromosome aberrations, as well as reproductive and interphase death.

Investigations were made of the combined influence of MM waves and antineoplastic compounds. They demonstrated that MM-wave radiation with some particular parameters can counteract the detrimental effect of antineoplastic compounds on the hematogenous system. Furthermore, MM waves were found to stimulate the functional activity of stem cells.

With respect to effects on hematopiesis, the combined influence always yielded more karyocytes than were found following the administration of x-rays or antineoplastic compounds alone. This held true for all combinations used in the experiments. When combined with antineoplastic compounds, both single and multiple Millimeter-wave exposures produced a decrease in the damage degree of karyocytes. Millimeter-wave irradiation alone produced no changes in the hematogenous system of animals.

Experimental results demonstrate that MM waves do not affect healthy cells and tissues. At the same time, they favor a more rapid recovery of vital functions in affected tissues. When combined with x-rays or antineoplastic compounds, MM waves have a protective action. This arises from an increased proliferative activity of stem cells in the bone marrow. As a result, mitotic activity of karyocytes increases.

In vitro experiments were made to study the effect of low-intensity MM-waves on hemopoietic cells of the bone marrow (10). With this end in view, L. P. Ignasheva and E. I. Soboleva investigated the problem of survival of mice that had received a lethal radiation dose. In their investigation, they transplanted a cryogenically preserved bone marrow. After defrosting, they exposed the bone marrow to MM waves.

Success for myelotransplantation depends on the preservation quality of hemopoietic (hemopoietic is acceptable but hematopoiesis is preferable) stem cells. Usually, bone marrow sanguification recovers later in animals that underwent transplantation using a defrosted bone marrow: it is delayed by 7 to 8 days as compared to animals which underwent transplantation using an *extempore*-produced bone marrow. It is believed that quality of karyocytes is sufficient when animals that had received a lethal radiation dose stay alive for more than 30 days.

Hybrid mice were used as donors and recipients. Cryogenically preserved karyocytes were subjected to MM-wave irradiation at a wavelength of 7.1 mm. Irradiation was carried out according to an optimum program mode. Animals of the control group did not receive transplantation. By the fifteenth day, they all died of acute radiation sickness. The disease revealed typical clinical manifestations: weight loss, adynamic motion, and receding hair.

When a defrosted bone marrow was transplanted without MM-wave irradiation, only 45% of animals survived by the thirtieth day. When the defrosted bone marrow was subjected to MM-wave irradiation before transplantation, 53% of recipients remained alive within the observation time. The animals of both groups exhibited a slight hypodynamia and an insignificant weight loss that showed tendency towards recovery by the end of the observation time.

Hence, nonthermal low-intensity MM-wave irradiation produced a beneficial effect on the stem cells of cryogenically preserved bone marrow and increased the survival rate of postmyelotransplantation recipients that had received a lethal radiation dose. The above-described technique can be used to enhance the repopulation ability of cryogenically preserved bone marrow.

A research team headed by V. I. Govallo at the Central Research Institute for Traumatology and Orthopedy in collaboration with the "Istok" Research and Production

Association conducted investigations into the effect of MM waves on human lymphocytes and fibroblasts (11). It was demonstrated in vitro that human lymphocytes and fibroblasts produce a *factor-phytokine* under MM waves. It enhances the growth and functional activity of similar cells. In high concentrations, phytokine is contained in destroyed irradiated cells (lysates), and it is released in a cultural medium. Millimeter-wave irradiation itself does not stimulate cell growth, does not change the expression of superficial lymphocyte receptors, and does not have an effect on their sensitivity to mitogens or exogenous immunomodulators. However, when added to a culture, phytokine vigorously stimulates the proliferative potential of lymphocytes and fibroblasts.

This factor-phytokine is produced in cytoplasm. It is bound up with the activation of dehydrogenases: the concentration of lactatedehydrogenase increases by a factor of 3 to 5 in irradiated cells. This activation factor is attributed to a class of cell regulators—cytokines. It does not belong to a group of interleukins or interferons. However, it may be attributed to lymphokines or monokines. This is a low-molecular glycosylation factor, secreted locally or distantly. It acts in a paracrine or autocrine way, but not in the endocrine one.

It is apparent that the described mechanism may underlie the immunomodifying effect of MM-wave radiation. This effect was observed while treating inpatients with suppurative diseases and complications at the Central Research Institute for Traumatology and Orthopedy, Moscow. Difficulty in treatment of such diseases is associated with a high severity of injuries, complicated and long-term operations, insufficient immunologic reactivity of patients, as well as with changes in the properties and behavior of suppurative infections, which appear to be resistant to many antibacterial agents.

MM waves were applied to treat severe missile and shotgun injuries of the locomotor system complicated by suppurative and wound infections. The results obtained are as follows (12):

The duration of separate phases of the wound process, including bad infected wounds, decreased by a factor of 1.5 to 2 as compared to the control group.

Millimeter waves produced a pronounced stimulating effect on wound tissue regeneration (the daily fractional decrease in the wound surface area virtually corresponded to that for uncomplicated wounds).

Grafts revealed a 100% retention.

The osteomyelitic process was eliminated: MM waves relieved pain and subsided inflammation in the injured region of a limb; they also stimulated total and local closing of fistulae as well as epithelization of injured soft tissues.

About 92.3% of the patients showed satisfactory outcomes shortly after operations.

Postoperative relapses decreased by 20%.

Microbial semination of wounds was reduced after opening and excision of festerous-necrotic foci.

Microbiological examinations were conducted in vitro to study the effect of MM waves on microbes. It was found that MM waves produce no direct effect on microbial susceptibility to antibiotics as well as on their biochemical and cultural properties.

Investigations carried out demonstrated that MM waves normalize immune-system parameters, which is of value for MM-wave therapy efficiency. Patients who underwent serious reconstructive operations suffer from secondary immunodeficiency, which complicates their recovery. Millimeter waves brought about pronounced shifts in the patients' immunograms. As a result, the patients showed a fractional and absolute increase in T-lymphocyte and T-helper counts (by 30 to 50% and 30 to 80%, respectively). The patients also revealed an increased natural-killer count (by 40 to 60%).

Hence, instead of a direct antimicrobial effect on pathogenic microflora, MM waves produce an indirect effect on it. They enhance an organism's general reactivity and increase wound-tissue viability.

The immunostimulating effect of MM waves was clearly demonstrated by Ryzhkova et al. (13). These researchers investigated how MM-wave radiation protects against and prevents from influenzal infections. To this end, animals received a lethal dose of the influenza A virus. Millimeter waves were applied to healthy animals (preliminary irradiation) and to infected animals (subsequent irradiation). It was found that they produced a protective effect in both cases. The results obtained were as follows:

Millimeter waves produced favorable therapeutic and preventive effects on the survival rate and average life expectancy in all experimental groups.

The protection efficacy depends on the irradiation procedure: the best protective effect (the death rate was zero) was observed for a long-term *preventive* irradiation of healthy animals before they were infected.

The protective preventive effect was potentiated when exposure time was extended to 7 to 17 days.

Millimeter-wave irradiation proved to be a sufficiently effective therapeutic means.

Besides experimental investigations, the researchers retrospectively analyzed the epidemiological situation of influenzal and acute respiratory viral infections in a group of patients who underwent MM-wave therapy with respect to gastric ulcer. The MM-wave course coincided with the epidemiological period of influenza epidemy caused by the influenza A virus. The group of patients receiving MM-wave therapy was compared to the control group (comparable by the age, health state, and conditions of work). It was found that influenzal and acute-respiratory-disease rates in the group of patients receiving MM-wave therapy were smaller by a factor of 1.75 during the *epidemic* as compared to the control group.

Inasmuch as many diseases cause *secondary immunodeficiency*, most scientists pay special attention to the immunomodifying effect of MM waves. *Gastric* and *duodenal ulcers*, as well as many other diseases, are caused by an imbalance between an organism's aggression and its protective factors. Immunity ranks first among protective factors. In order to compare the efficiency of MM-wave therapy and conventional treatment of ulcer, nonspecific immunity (phagocytosis and lysozyme) and specific immunity (T lymphocytes, B lymphocytes, IgA, IgM, and IgG) were examined (14). Although the ulcer healed over, the conventional pharmacotherapy did not enhance protective factors. When MM waves were applied, the ulcer healed over *without a keloid scar*. Furthermore, protective factors exhibited a pronounced normalizing effect. In particular, this concerned nonspecific and specific immunity. A dynamic observation of the patients revealed that their protective factors were at a maximum 3 months after the cure termination. Since MM waves produced a normalizing effect on an organism's protective factors, *preventive* MM-wave therapy was put forward.

When *atopic dermatitis* was treated using MM-wave therapy (15,16), the patients' immune state was monitored using a number of laboratory techniques. They were as follows: an active T-lymphocyte count; total T-lymphocyte count; B-lymphocyte count; agar-gel radial immunodiffusion for the IgA, IgM, and IgG counts of blood serum; circulating-immune-complex (CIC) count of blood serum; as well as immunoenzymic analysis of the total IgE and allergen-specific IgE counts. Note, the allergen-specific IgE includes antibodies against indoor, pollen, and food allergens. The treatment performed favored the positive dynamics and stable improvement of immunologic indices. This concerned both the cellular immunity (such as rosette-forming cells) and the humoral immunity (such as CIC, IgM, IgG, and IgE). Patients receiving conventional therapy exhibited virtually no changes in cellular and humoral immunity indices.

Geymin et al. (17) investigated the effect of MM waves on the immune state of patients with sarcoidosis of lungs. Investigations were made at the Central Research Institute for Tuberculosis of the Russian Academy of Medical Sciences (Moscow). The researchers counted T lymphocytes and determined their functional and phagocytic activity. They also counted B lymphocytes, immunoglobulins, as well as CICs in blood serum (both before and after the treatment). The application of MM waves gave rise to a *universal* stimulation of functional activity of immunocompetent cells. They stimulated the phagocytic activity of macrophages in the granulomatosis-stricken region, in various lung regions, and in blood. Macrophage activation facilitated the elimination of CICs from the body. They were devoured by macrophages, and their content decreased in 87% to 91% of the patients after MM-wave therapy. This restored the blood flow in lungs. As is known, when the CIC count of blood decreases, it prevents microvessels of many organs from being damaged.

In recent years, there has been a widespreade increase in herpes virus infections that have proven difficult to prevent and are relatively resistant to currently available rugs. Furthermore, the number of immunodeficiency states is growing, which is caused by wide application of antibacterial and hormonal compounds. The immune state was examined when conventional treatment was combined with MM-wave therapy. The examination involved counting T lymphocytes, B lymphocytes, CICs, IgA, IgM, IgG, as well as studying the immune-response-modifier tolerance. It was found that MM waves produced an immunostimulating effect, which manifested itself in stimulated phagocytosis and T-lymphocyte activity. This is of great importance for prevention and treatment of diseases complicated by secondary immunodeficiency (18).

At present, *urogenital inflammatory diseases* are also widespread in men and women. Most often, these diseases are caused by chlamydias, mycoplasmas, and ureaplasmas. A distinguishing feature of these microbes is their ability to cause stable immunodeficiency. When antibiotic therapy is combined with immunomodification, the recovery rate increases up to 70% (as compared to 30% to 50% after conventional therapy) (19).

It is known that immunosuppression exacerbates *acne*. Investigations were made of the effect of MM-wave therapy on the cutaneous microbiocenosis in vulgaris-acne patients. All the patients were recorded an immunogram showing cellular and humoral immunity indices before and after the treatment. It was found that conditionally pathogenic microbes did not grow on the skin of patients whose immunologic indices were normalized by MM-wave therapy. In these patients, clinical results were regarded as a recovery or significant improvement. In general, the immunologic indices of most patients exhibited positive dynamics, which was accompanied by an improved state of skin microbiocenosis (20).

The experimental clinical investigations performed thus provided evidence that low-intensity MM-wave radiation has a pronounced *immunomodifying effect*.

The central nervous system (CNS) is the main regulatory system. It governs almost all processes occurring in a living being. Classical investigations into electromagnetic biology revealed that the CNS is the most sensitive system for electromagnetic fields (21). Studies of the CNS role in the realization of biological effects of low-intensity MM waves began at the earliest stage of MM-wave therapy formation.

Professor Yu. A. Kholodov and Professor N. N. Lebedeva have been heading experimental investigations at the Institute for Higher Nerve Activity and Neurophysiology of the then USSR and now Russian Academy of Sciences since 1989. These investigations deal with the sensory and subsensory (EEG) responses of healthy human beings to peripheral stimuli of low-intensity MM-wave radiation. Investigations of *sensory responses*, i. e., *electromagnetic sensitivity of human beings* (22–24), yielded a number of interesting results. They are as follows:

A human being reliably discerns MM-wave signals from sham signals.

Human sensitivity to MM waves depends both on his or her individual features and on the biotropic parameters of the field.

Perception modality (such as pressure, touch, pricking, and burning) is evidence that MM-wave perception involves skin analyzers.

The latent time of a MM-wave response is tens of seconds.

Millimeter-wave perception exhibits sensory asymmetry: it is different for left and right hands.

An analysis of subjective feelings in human beings demonstrated that a MM-wave stimulus "actuates" mechanoreceptors, nociceptors, and free nerve endings—unmyelinated efferent fibers without corpuscular structures at their ends.

An investigation was made of EEG responses of healthy subjects to a long-term (30- to 60-min) peripheral MM-wave irradiation. It was found that such irradiation produced changes in the spatiotemporal organization of cerebral biopotentials. The alpha rhythm exhibited a significant increase in its power in occipital cortical regions. Furthermore, the theta rhythm revealed an average increase in its coherence in central and frontal regions. Note, this increase was more pronounced in the right brain, independent of exposure site location (25,26).

The effect of EHF radiation on the CNS can also be evaluated by studying *behavioral reactions*. For example, S. V. Khromova in her Ph.D. thesis (27) demonstrated that EHF radiation can modify the behavior-reflex activity of rats. This phenomenon manifested itself both in the accelerated alteration of a developed conditioned food reflex and in the delayed impairment of a conditioned defense reflex.

Investigations of a *stress-protective effect* of MM waves were made on animals at the State Research Center for Narcology, the Russian Federation Ministry of Health. Such investigations were carried out by Yu. L. Arzumanov with co-workers (28,29). The effect of MM-wave radiation on the CNS was evaluated by special tests. They were based on studying the inborn behavior that reflected various fields of motivation-emotion activities. In the case of a conflict-defense situation with stress, MM-wave radiation modified the behavior of an experimental group of animals in such a way that it was identical with the behavior of a passive control group.

A research team headed by Prof. N. A. Temur'yants achieved a pronounced antistress effect of MM waves (30,31). In their experiments, they studied the effect of MM-wave radiation on the development of hypokinetic stress in rats. As distinct from control animals, the experimental ones showed no decrease in the protective functions of blood after a 9-day hypokinesia. Furthermore, they revealed an increase in the examined indices (such as the cytochemical state of neutrophiles and lymphocytes in peripheral blood) as compared to the control animals. However, the efficiency of antistress effect of MM waves depended on the individual features of the higher nerve activity of rats. It was at a maximum in rats with a low and medium moving activity.

It was also demonstrated that MM waves produce a modifying effect on the functional CNS state in human beings under simulated stress conditions (32). This was proven by means of EEG spectrum-correlation analysis, psychological test findings, as well as cardiac-rhythm and exertion indices dynamics.

An investigation of the psychophysiological state of patients (33) and development of new methods for inpatient *psychoemotional rehabilitation* (34) revealed that MM-wave therapy relieves situational and personal anxiety, improves memory, raises attention, accelerates sensorimotor responses, as well as restores and stabilizes the psychoemotional state of human beings.

It was also found that MM waves have an *energizing* effect. Millimeter-wave therapy was administered in combination with light therapy to patients having a depressive symptomatology. These patients suffered from maniac-depressive psychosis, cyclothymia, schizophrenia, as well as vascular and involutional psychosis. It was found that the combined treatment produced a favorable clinical effect in 97% of the patients. A distinguishing feature of patients who revealed a virtual recovery was a different degree of the anxiety component in the depression structure, irrespective of its nosological attribute. Furthermore, the vegetative nervous system revealed hypersympathicotonic phenomena. An improvement was observed when the vegetative nervous system had a mixed type and when apathy predominated in the syndrome structure (35).

A more sophisticated problem is to investigate and comprehend the *physiological mechanisms* of biological and therapeutic effects of low-intensity MM-waves at the level of an entire organism. This is owing to the fact that the investigated object—the human being—is a very complex biological system. It possesses myriad positive and negative feedback loops and regulation levels (36). To begin with, one needs to analyze the primary *physiological* targets present in the MM-wave exposure site. As is known, MM waves penetrate into the human skin at a depth of 300 to 500 μm. In other words, they are absorbed almost completely in the epidermis and the top dermis. Hence, MM waves directly influence CNS receptors (such as mechanoreceptors, nociceptors, and free nerve endings), APUD cells (such as the diffuse neuroendocrine cells, mastocytes, and Merkel cells), and immune cells (such as the T-lymphocyte skin pool). In addition, these waves produce a direct effect on the microcapillary bed and biologically active points.

It is apparent that these five primary physiological targets are the five "entry" gates. They determine the involvement of corresponding systems in realization of biological and therapeutic effects of MM-wave radiation. The latter acts on every basic regulation systems of an organism as a peculiar triggering factor. This has been confirmed by many clinical investigations. The direct and simultaneous "triggering" of the aforementioned systems initiates a complex mediate influence on other organs and systems (such as the hematogenous, humoral, vegetative nervous systems). As a result, a MM-wave-induced reaction involves the entire being. The features of this reaction depend both on the *biotropic* parameters of the MM-wave stimulus and on the functional state of the human being. Millimeter-wave radiation produces both nonspecific and specific effects. The latter include wound healing, injury sanitation, tissue regeneration, pain relief, itch mitigation, and hyperemia elimination.

At present, a nonspecific effect is regarded as a reaction of enhanced nonspecific resistivity of an organism. In turn, this initiates adapting and antistress reactions of higher reactivity levels (37).

III. APPLICATION OF LOW-INTENSITY MM-WAVE RADIATION IN MEDICINE

In the early 1970s, Academician N. D. Devyatkov initiated a program of clinical evaluation of MM waves in respect of treating various diseases. This program was approved by the

USSR and R.S.F.S.R. Ministries of Health and was executed in a number of medical establishments. The MM-wave technique was tested in more than 60 clinics, including large medical centers, such as the All-Union Cancer Research Center of the Russian Academy of Medical Sciences, the Central Research Institute for Traumatology and Orthopedy of the Russian Federation Ministry of Health, the P. A. Hertsen Moscow Cancer Research Institute, as well as clinics affiliated with the State Medical University, Moscow Medical Academy, and Moscow State Institute for Dentistry. The results obtained provided evidence for high efficiency of MM-wave therapy for the following diseases: cardiovascular (stable and unstable stenocardia, hypertonia, and myocardial infarction), neurological (pain syndromes, neuritis, radiculitis, and osteochondrosis), urological (pyelonephritis, impotence, and prostatitis), gynecological (adnexitis, endometritis, and uterine neck erosions), dermatological (neurodermite, including psoriasis, streptoderma, and acne), gastroenterological (gastric ulcer, duodenal ulcer, hepatitis, and cholecystopancreatitis), stomatological (periodontosis, periodontitis, some types of stomatitis, and periostitis), as well as oncological (to protect the hematogenous system and to remove side effects of chemotherapy).

The experience of applying MM waves in clinical practice revealed no ultimate side effects. Millimeter-wave therapy went well with other therapeutic techniques (such as pharmacotherapy, physiotherapy, etc.). Furthermore, it exhibited no absolute contraindications. As distinct from drug therapy, MM-wave therapy had no side effects.

Millimeter-wave therapy reveals some features such as noninvasiveness, polytherapeutic effect, monotherapeutic effect, antistress effect, immunomodifying effect, and painkilling effect. Currently, low-intensity MM-wave radiation (MM-wave therapy) finds wide application in medicine. It is employed both to treat and prevent a wide gamut of maladies.

Cardiovascular diseases are among the most urgent problems of present-day medicine. The ischemic disease of the heart is among the most widespread cardiovascular pathologies. The death rate of this illness ranks high worldwide.

The first report on the application of electromagnetic MM waves in treatment of cardiovascular diseases came to light as far back as 1980. Over the years passed by, researchers have acquired broad experience in using MM waves to treat heart ischemia and hypertonia (38–42). It was demonstrated that MM-wave therapy produced a clinical effect, which was verified by laboratory and instrumental findings. Apart from that, researchers developed techniques for individual selection of MM-wave treatment. It was shown that MM-wave therapy can substantially reduce the dose of antianginal compounds. Moreover, a nitrate therapy was stopped completely in patients having exertion stenocardia of the first and second functional classes. In such patients, MM-wave therapy proved to be most effective in treating both painful and painless myocardial ischemia.

The most severe patients had exertion stenocardia of the third and fourth functional classes and rest stenocardia complicated by one or several stenotic coronary arteries. Although these patients received great doses of nitrates, beta adrenoblockers, calcium antagonists, and disaggregants, the treatment appeared ineffective. By the end of a MM-wave therapy course, 80% of the patients revealed a positive clinical effect. The application of MM waves reduced the number of episodes of painful and painless myocardial ischemia. Hence, MM-wave therapy produced both painkilling and antianginal effects.

Unstable stenocardia is classified among acute ischemic diseases of the heart. It is especially dangerous in the case of an abrupt onset (within a few days) or intensifying anginal attacks. Unstable stenocardia may take a bad course, resulting in myocardial infarction, sudden death, or chronic stenocardia. The clinical application of MM-wave therapy was found to be effective in 60% of the cases. The treatment was successful even when MM waves were used as a monotherapy. Being combined with pharmacotherapy, MM-wave therapy increased the rate of positive clinical effects. The conducted therapy produced favorable effects in every patient of the examined group. According to literature findings, myocardial infarction develops in 12% to 20% of patients having unstable stenocardia. However, after MM-wave therapy, myocardial infarction developed in none of the patients with unstable stenocardia. Thus, the involvement of MM-wave therapy in the combined treatment of unstable stenocardia decreased the risk of myocardial infarction.

Myocardial infarction is the most severe ischemic disease of the heart. At the acute stage, it is most dangerous for the patient to develop such complications as a cardiac-rhythm disorder or acute left ventricular failure. Serious postinfarction complications include the development of chronic circulatory deficiency and early postinfarction stenocardia. When MM-wave therapy was administered within the first hours of myocardial infarction and its complications, it decreased the number of episodes of acute left ventricular failure. It also decreased the rate of postinfarction stenocardia and chronic circulatory deficiency. Furthermore, MM-wave therapy substantially increased the Garkavi-Kvakina-Ukolova index (37). It is known that myocardial infarction shocks a person. Shock reactions worsen the disease course. This forms a vicious pathogenic circle. It was shown that patients with an acute stress reaction revealed a greater leukocyte count and a longer pain syndrome. Such patients exhibit the greatest death rate. Before treatment, stress reactions were observed in 55.6% of patients, whereas calm activation reactions were found in 21.0% of patients. After a course of treatment, stress reactions decreased down to 11.1%. Calm activation reactions and training reactions were observed in 50.4% and 34.2%, respectively. Patients retaining stress reactions develop postinfarction stenocardia more often (as compared to those with reactions of other types). It was also found that patients who received MM-wave therapy revealed a raised degree of antioxidant protection. They exhibited a decrease in the malonic dialdehyde content. This substance is among the products of peroxide oxidation of lipids. It was also established that drug treatment caused no decrease in this index (Table 1).

The superoxide-dismutase (SOD) enzyme is an important component of antioxidant protection. According to present-day views, when the SOD activity decreases below 50% of the norm, the concentration of superoxide anion radicals shows an uncontrolled increase. This may cause irreversible changes in cells and tissues. Millimeter-wave therapy enhances the activity of this enzyme, which increases the degree of cell protection. These changes take place in blood plasma and thrombocytes (Table 2).

The deposition of immune complexes on the arterial wall may cause atherosclerosis. The liberation of vasoactive amines under the action of immune complexes increases the vascular wall permeation. This promotes the penetration of immune complexes into tissues, the arterial wall included. The interaction between immune complexes and thrombocytes enhances the activation and adhesion of thrombocytes, which may cause thrombus formation.

Millimeter-wave therapy was found to significantly decrease the CIC count of blood plasma in patients with cardiac ischemia. This phenomenon was not observed in the control group. This means that conventional drug therapy has no effect on the pathogenic aspect of

Table 1 Malonic Dialdehyde Content in the Blood Plasma of Patients with Unstable Stenocardia (nmol/ml)

Group of patients	MM-wave therapy alone	Combined therapy (MM waves + drugs)	Placebo	Drug therapy
Before treatment	18.52 ± 0.85	18.61 ± 1.07	18.94 ± 1.44	18.14 ± 1.08
After treatment	14.61 ± 1.03	13.76 ± 0.97	17.97 ± 1.17	17.90 ± 1.24

Table 2 Superoxide Dismutase Activity in Patients with Unstable Stenocardia

Group of patients	MM-wave therapy alone	Combined therapy (MM waves + drugs)	Placebo	Drug therapy
Before treatment				
In plasma (a.u./ml)	1.87 ± 0.08	1.82 ± 0.12	1.85 ± 0.12	1.91 ± 0.14
In thrombocytes (a.u./protein mg)	6.95 ± 0.28	6.78 ± 0.24	6.92 ± 0.45	6.81 ± 0.63
After treatment				
In plasma (a.u./ml)	4.52 ± 0.50	4.23 ± 0.29	2.96 ± 0.38	2.94 ± 0.46
In thrombocytes (a.u./protein mg)	8.75 ± 0.61	8.81 ± 0.32	6.64 ± 0.7	6.93 ± 0.49

cardiac ischemia. The complimentary activity of serum was found to decrease. This can be associated with a sluggish stimulation of the compliment by immune complexes. Hence, MM-wave therapy makes it possible to correct for immunologic disorders in patients with cardiac ischemia. This can be of value not only for treating this nosology, but also for treating the atherogenic process on the whole.

Microcirculatory disorders are a serious element of cardiovascular pathologies. Tissue perfusion can be impaired not only in the case of atherosclerosis of main vessels but also in the case of microcirculatory blocking. The latter is caused by microscopic thrombi and inelastic erythrocytes.

Investigations were made of microcirculation in the bulbar conjunctiva of patients with cardiac ischemia who received MM-wave therapy. It was found that the MM-wave therapy produced a significant decrease in the total conjunctival index as well as in the index of vascular and intravascular changes. It also enlarged the arteriole caliber, increased the number of functioning limbic ansae, and decreased the content of erythrocyte aggregants in venules. The cerebral blood circulation was estimated in hypertonic patients administered to MM-wave therapy. This was done with the aid of dynamic scintigraphy of cerebral circulation using ^{99m}technetium-labeled compounds. The results obtained revealed blood flow improvement in affected arteries and improved blood circulation in ischemia-stricken regions.

According to the World Health Organization, the death rate of cancer ranks second to the cardiovascular one.

Clinical evaluation of low-intensity MM-wave radiation and development of therapeutic techniques for cancer treatment have been carried out since 1980. These investigations were pursued at the P. A. Gertsen Moscow Cancer Research Institute (43). They were made in patients with mammary cancer. First, this disease is widespread, and, second, this pathology is often treated using radiotherapy and antineoplastic pharmaceuticals. Such treatment causes changes in human vital functions. The studies were made in patients having mammary cancer of the II-b and III-b stages who received chemotherapy and radiotherapy. The structural and functional state of blood cells was examined before treatment, after three MM-wave irradiation sessions, in the middle of the cure, and after its termination. The human general state was assessed by subjective data, symptomatology, and adapting reactions. The type of such reactions was determined from lymphocyte percentage, leukocyte formula, and the ratio of leukocytes to segmented neutrophils.

Chemotherapeutic compounds were introduced before surgical excision according to the following scheme: 3 g of flu-ruracil, 2.8 g of cyclophosphane, and 60 mg of methotrexate.

Before antineoplastic pharmacotherapy, patients were subjected to a 3-day MM-wave irradiation: 60-min daily sessions. During chemotherapy, irradiation was performed 1 h before the introduction of antineoplastic compounds. When a chemotherapy course was finished, MM-wave irradiation was administered for the next 3 days. Usually, a course of MM-wave therapy consisted of 14 to 15 sessions. This cure was administered to 343 patients. A control group embraced 339 patients who received chemotherapy according to the above-described scheme. When the combined treatment was finished completely, 95.1% of the patients exhibited a satisfactory general state (without blood-circulation stimulants). When the chemotherapy course (without MM-wave irradiation) was finished, 74.2% of patients revealed an unsatisfactory general state as well as a reduced leukocyte count of blood. This occurred in spite of the fact that the patients received blood transfusion and blood-circulation stimulants. This regularity persisted during subsequent (adjuvant) chemotherapy courses. In the first year of treatment, adjuvant chemotherapy was administered every 3 months (not more than three courses). In the second year of treatment, it was administered twice at an interval of 5 months.

The ability of MM waves to normalize the leukocyte count was investigated in patients with leukopenia. The investigation was made in 900 patients whose initial leukocyte count of blood was less than 3000 (from 2300 to 2700). A course of treatment lasted for 12 days. The sessions were administered daily. After the cure, the leukocyte count of blood was normalized in 80% of the patients. This allowed the patients to undergo a complete course of chemotherapy.

The bone marrow was examined in patients taking antineoplastic compounds and receiving MM-wave therapy. The results obtained demonstrated that MM-wave therapy initially ejected reserved blood from blood pools. It increased the total volume of circulating blood, which improved oxygen exchange. This might result in a better tolerance to antineoplastic compounds and reduced side toxic effects. The proliferative activity of the bone marrow was found to grow 4 to 5 days after the MM-wave therapy commencement.

Hence, the clinical findings show that MM waves allow cancer patients to undergo a complete course of chemotherapy without a significant decrease in their blood indices and without blood-circulation stimulants.

Melanoma is a highly malignant tumor of the skin. It spreads to other parts of the body via the bloodstream or the lymphatic channels. The rate of this disease has increased over the last several owing to environmental pollution. Surgical excision is common for treating melanomas. When melanoma has metastases, it is regarded incurable: a 5-year survival remains very rare. According to Russian and foreign scientists, the survival rate constitutes 75% at the first clinical stage, 32% at the second one, and 0% at the third one. Skin melanoma metastases occur in 20% to 25% of primarily treated patients within 6 to 18 months. When the process has spread, chemotherapy is used. However, melanoma remains resistant to antineoplastic compounds. Adjuvant chemotherapy courses following surgical excision postpone neither metastasis development nor tumor relapses. Millimeter-wave radiation was employed to prevent relapses and metastases in patients with primary melanoma of the skin after surgical treatment. The clinical experience gained demonstrated a beneficial effect of MM waves. The first course of treatment consisted of 10 daily sessions lasting for 60 min. The MM-wave irradiation sessions were performed immediately after surgical intervention. The second course was administered 1 month after the first one terminated. The third course was performed 3 months after the second, whereas the fourth course was conducted 6 months after the third. Dynamic observation lasted for 9 to 18 months. None of the patients revealed relapses or metastases. Apparently, MM-wave irradiation stimulated the immune system and thus enhanced the individual's natural antineoplastic protection.

Apart from that, scientists of the P. A. Gertsen Moscow Cancer Research Institute studied the effect of MM-wave radiation on the course of wound processes. The investigations were performed in 1302 patients having both sutured and open wounds (after laser tumor excision). The experimental and control group consisted of 651 patients. The wound process was evaluated by the degree of inflammation, necrosis, and granulation, as well as by the terms of granulation, epithelization, and healing. A course of treatment comprised 15 daily sessions lasting for 60 min. In the case of open superficial wounds, the device's horn was positioned on the skin at a distance of 2 to 2.5 cm from the wound. When operations were performed on the abdominal cavity and thorax, the horn was positioned on the sternum. The results obtained revealed that MM-wave radiation produced a favorable effect on wound healing. The patients noted pain and discomfort alleviation in the wound. At the first stage of wound process (when tissue alteration is most pronounced), MM-wave irradiation suppressed necrosis and perifocal inflammation. When vascular reactions (such as edema and hyperemia) predominated, MM-wave irradiation eliminated them 3 to 5 days after the treatment commencement. In the control, these reactions persisted for not less than 8 days. An antiphlogistic effect of MM-wave radiation was most pronounced in patients with sutured wounds. None of the patients subjected to MM-wave irradiation revealed the opening of sutures, whereas 9% of patients of the control group did not hold their sutures. Presumably, MM waves recovered microcirculation and effective receptors, which normalized wound healing autoregulation. It is significant that MM-wave-based wound healing did not result in ugly scars or keloids. This is of special importance for facial treatment.

When MM-wave radiation was used to heal open wounds, the following results were obtained. Granules revealed an early maturation—on the third to fifth day. Wounds revealed overall mature granulation (as distinct from nonlaser wounds that exhibit insular granulation). Overall mature granulation expedited wound closure by 5 to 7 days. Granulation overgrowth was not observed. Millimeter-wave radiation facilitated wound epithelization. It started uniformly at wound edges. This resulted in the concentric contraction of wound edges and skin regeneration. A daily growth of epithelium reached 2 to 3 mm. So, MM-wave radiation gave rise to optimum wound healing, which curtailed the healing by 3 to 5 days.

The clinical studies of MM waves applied in traumatology and orthopedy were launched at the N. N. Priorov Central Research Institute for Traumatology and Orthopedy. Since 1987, this technique has been used there in thousands of patients with various bone-muscular pathologies. The latter include serious shotgun wounds of limbs, which are often encountered in the Russian Federation. Between 1987 and 1990, this technique was used to treat severe war pathologies of the locomotor system under extreme conditions. MM-wave therapy was approved by the Central Military Hospital of the Defense Ministry of the Afghanistan Republic (the N. N. Priorov Central Institute for Traumatology and Orthopedy had direct scientific contacts with this hospital during that time). MM-wave therapy was also applied to the victims of the Armenian earthquake, various natural disasters, and diverse catastrophes. They were also treated at the N. N. Priorov Central Institute for Traumatology and Orthopedy (44–47). Cytological examinations were conducted to demonstrate that the therapeutic effect of MM waves may result from the enhanced proliferative potential of exposed cells. The action of MM waves stimulates the synthesis of cytotoxins in cytoplasm. Cytotoxins produce an effect that is similar to the growth factor. Although cytotoxins are accumulated in cytoplasm, they can be secreted out. As a result, they can produce both contact and distant effects. It seems that the stimulating effect of MM waves on cell growth is not restricted to cutaneous fibroblasts and blood lymphocytes. Evidently, this effect has a universal character and involves cells of various tissue architectures.

When treating orthopedic and traumatic patients, MM waves should produce an effect on cellular growth regulation and cytodifferentiation. This is essential to stimulate reparation processes in the affected region. Millimeter-wave therapy acts as a biological component of the complex therapy. The latter is targeted at the recovery of functional capabilities of tissue structures that are either affected by or involved in the bone-muscular pathology.

Over the last decade, EHF therapy has been firmly established as one of the most effective methods of conservative treatment of orthopedic, traumatic, and surgical patients. The application of EHF therapy at the N. N. Priorov Central Institute for Traumatology and Orthopedy yielded broad experience of using MM waves in the complex treatment of patients with trophic and tissue-viability disorders (typical of shotgun wounds). It can be stated that MM waves provide a new quality of treatment, which overcomes the previous problems of medical rehabilitation of such patients. This is confirmed by an analysis of the results of using EHF therapy for different bone-muscular pathologies complicated by impaired tissue trophics and inhibited reparation processes in the affected region.

An investigation was made of applying EHF therapy to patients with neurodystrophic changes in tissue trophics. These changes were caused by shotgun wounds of limbs. Clinically, these patients revealed persistently aggravating suppurative-necrotic processes in their amputation stumps. The results of MM-wave treatment are listed in Tables 3 and 4.

The normalizing effect of MM-wave therapy on wound healing was also confirmed by the time history of adapting reactions. Before MM-wave treatment, an absolute majority of patients (91.8%) revealed a stress reaction that was prognostically unfavorable. Under the action of MM-wave therapy, they changed their type of adapting reactions. This resulted from a sharp decrease in the number of patients with stress reactions (13.5%) as well as from a simultaneous increase in the number of patients with raised (59.5%) and calm (24.3%) activation. These findings were evidence that MM waves can produce a beneficial effect on neurodystrophic processes. This improves tissue trophics and viability in the affected region.

Millimeter-wave therapy was also found to be highly effective in treating chronic (shotgun and traumatic) osteomyelitis and pressure sores. It was also demonstrated both to decrease the microbial semination of wounds and to facilitate the jointing of bone fractures.

Millimeter-wave therapy efficiency was investigated at the Central Research Institute for Tuberculosis. To this end, patients with various forms of pulmonary tuberculosis received a basic course of chemotherapy using three or four tuberculostatic compounds (such as isoniazid, rifampin, pyrazinamide, and kanamycin). At different stages, basic

Table 3 Results of Using EHF Therapy to Prepare Ample Festering Wounds of Amputation Stumps for Skin Plasty

		Wound stage duration	
Preparation technique	Number of patients	Exudation	Regeneration
With EHF therapy	15	10 ± 0.4	7 ± 0.2
Without EHF therapy	10	14 ± 0.6	10 ± 0.7

Table 4 Wound Planimetry of Amputation Stumps Under EHF Therapy

Groups of patients	Number of patients	Initial wound area (mm^2)	In-a-week wound area (mm^2)	Daily wound-area decrease (mm^2)
With MM-wave therapy	22	741.6 ± 180.7	539.1 ± 134.4	3.9 ± 0.2
Without MM-wave therapy	26	985.1 ± 250.3	981.0 ± 240.4	0.1 ± 0.04

chemotherapy was combined with a course of MM-wave therapy. Experimental and clinical studies revealed that low-intensity MM waves produced a normalizing effect on many clinical parameters, such as the formed elements of blood and blood plasma proteins. In addition, MM waves stimulated lymphocyte proliferation in immunogenic organs. As a result, macrophages present in the bone marrow actively invaded tuberculosis-stricken organs (mainly, the lungs) to normalized external respiration and regional circulation in them. Additionally, macrophages favored the homeostasis recovery during chronic infections, such as tuberculosis (17).

Millimeter-wave therapy was also employed in the complex treatment of sarcoidosis of lungs and intrathoracic lymph nodes. After a course of treatment (20 sessions), the patients were subjected to x-ray examination. It revealed a noticeable resolution of parenchymal-interstitial infiltration, disappearance of granuloma shadows, as well as reduction of alveolitis symptoms, interstitial edema, and pleural reactions. The size of intrathoracic lymph nodes decreased by half. The phagocyte function of macrophages was substantially activated in granuloma-stricken regions, separate lung regions, and blood. In other words, the functional activity of immunocompetent cells was universal. It is significant that MM-wave therapy reduced the dose of corticosteroid compounds: they were taken at a dose of 10 to 15 mg every other day. Moreover, corticosteroid compounds were completely canceled in half of patients with firstly diagnosed carcoidosis.

Gastric and duodenal ulcers are among widespread digestive diseases. Ulcer strikes 7% to 10% of adult population in developed countries. The last several years have shown tendency to increase the number of primarily diagnosed ulcers, especially in young people.

At present, ulcer is widely treated using complex pharmacotherapy. The latter is targeted at different pathogenic mechanisms of the disease. However, pharmacotherapy is not very effective: chronic ulcers heal over for a long time, therapeutic results are unstable, and 30 to 40% of the patients are resistant to the treatment. When patients simultaneously take up to three drugs, 18% of them may exhibit side effects. A simultaneous intake of five to six drugs may cause side effects in 81% of the patients. This is because many drug compounds suffer from various toxic side effects and may cause allergies.

Millimeter-wave therapy efficiency was assessed in more than 3000 patients with ulcer (experimental group). The results obtained were compared to those obtained for drug-treated patients (control group). These patients received a traditional complex of drug compounds (such as antacids, spasmolytics, secretion inhibitors, and reparants).

Ulcers healed over in 98.6% of patients of the experimental group and in 82% of patients of the control group. The healing lasted for 21.1 ± 1.4 days in the experimental group and for 37.5 ± 1.9 days in the control group. Note, duodenal ulcers healed over faster than gastric ulcers in both groups. For example, the healing of duodenal ulcer lasted for 17.6 ± 1.2 days in the experimental group and for 35.8 ± 2.0 days in the control group, whereas the healing of gastric ulcer lasted for 28.1 ± 2.1 days in the experimental group and for 45.1 ± 5.3 days in the control one.

Patients who underwent MM-wave therapy were subjected to a follow-up study. To this end, a dynamic endoscopic examination was made 3 to 4 months after the treatment. Relapses were revealed in 51% of patients of the experimental group and in 82% of patients of the control group. Millimeter-wave therapy increased the level of antioxidant activity and normalized the rheological properties of blood. For example, it decreased blood viscosity, packed cell volume, and erythrocyte deformability index. It is also significant that patients with erythrocyte aggregation exhibited a decreased aggregation rate, and conversely, patients without erythrocyte aggregation revealed a raised aggregation rate. In addition, MM-wave therapy normalized phagocytosis (14).

Unfortunately, the limited space of this publication disallows us to tell the reader about all MM-wave therapy capabilities. Clinical studies have reliably verified the high efficiency of this technique with respect to more than 120 nosologic forms (and this number is becoming larger). Evidently, MM-wave therapy is a method about which ancient physicians used to dream: it "treats a person, not a disease."

IV. CONCLUSIONS

Summarizing the results of the 30-year study of biological effects of low-intensity MM waves, we may ascertain the following. As it often happens, applied research and commercialization have outdistanced fundamental investigations. The wide application of MM waves in medicine, biotechnology, animal husbandry, and plant cultivation has taken a giant step forward. By this time, Russia has manufactured more than 10,000 MM-wave therapy devices, organized more than 2500 MM-wave therapy rooms, and treated over 2,500,000 patients. Since 1992, 27 volumes of the Journal on Millimeter Waves in Biology and Medicine (*Millimetrovye Volny v Biologii i Meditsine*) have been published as well as 12 symposia on *Millimeter Waves in Biology and Medicine* and 11 workshops have been held. During this time, we have issued 13 volumes of symposium and workshop proceedings, four monographs, three popular scientific brochures, and more than 2600 articles. Furthermore, our scientific attainments have been protected by 22 Russian Federation patents. In the year 2000, we were awarded the Russian Federation State Prize in Science and Technology for our research in this field of science.

However, scientists—biophysicists, physiologists, and physicians—carry on their further scientific investigations into the mechanism of biological effects. By now, they have approached a more complete understanding of the role of low-intensity MM-wave radiation in the vital processes of biological systems at different organization levels.

REFERENCES

1. Golant MB, Vilenskaya RL, Zyulina EA. Lot of wideband low-power oscillators in the millimeter and submillimeter bands. PTE 1965; 4:136–139. In Russian.
2. Devyatkov ND, ed. Backward-Wave Tubes of the Millimeter and Submillimeter Bands. Moscow: Radio i Svyaz', 1985. In Russian.
3. Betskii OV, Kislov VV, Devyatkov ND. Low-intensity MM waves in medicine and biology. Biomed Eng 2000; 28-1,2:247–268.
4. Betskii OV, Devyatkov ND. MM-wave therapy conceptual design. Biomeditsinskaya Radioelektronika 2000; 8:53–63. In Russian.
5. Sevast'yanova LA, Potapov SL, Adamenko VG. Combined influence of x-ray and super-high-frequency radiation on the bone marrow. Nauch Dokl Vyssh Shkoly, Ser Biofizika, Biol Nauki 1969; 6:46. In Russian.

6.   Sevast'yanova LA. Biological effects of MM radio waves on normal tissues and malignant tumors. In: Devyatkov ND ed. Effects of Nonthermal MM-Wave Influence on Biological Objects. Moscow: IRE AN SSSR, 1983:48–62. In Russian.

7.   Sevast'yanova LA, Golant MB, Adamenko VG. Effect of microwave radiation on marrow-bone count variations caused by antineoplastic chemotherapeutic compounds. Proceedings of The Second Congress of Oncologists. Omsk 1980:136. In Russian.

8.   Sevast'yanova LA, Golant MB, Zubenkova ES. Effect of MM radio waves on normal tissues and malignant tumors. In: Devyatkov ND, ed. Application of Low-Intensity MM-Wave Radiation in Biology and Medicine. Moscow: IRE AN SSSR, 1985:37–49. In Russian.

9.   Adey WR. Frequency and power window in tissue interactions with weak electromagnetic fields. Proc of IEEE 1980; 68-1:119.

10. Soboleva EI, Ignasheva LP. Survival rate of animals exposed to a lethal dose during trans-plantation of a cryogenically preserved bone marrow subjected to EHF irradiation. International Symposium on Millimeter Waves of Nonthermal Intensity in Medicine, Moscow Oct. 3–6, 1991; 2:354–452.

11. Govallo VI, Barer FS, Volchek IA. Electromagnetic-radiation-induced human lymphocyte and fibroblast production of a cell proliferation activation factor. International Symposium on Millimeter Waves of Nonthermal Intensity in Medicine, Moscow Oct. 3–6, 1991; 2:340–344.

12. Kamenev YuF, Shaposhnikov YuG, Mussa M, Akimov GV. Physical factors in the complex surgical treatment of a missile limb wound. Aktual'nye Voprosy Voennoi Meditsiny Kabul, 1988; 78–80. In Russian.

13. Ryzhkova LB, Starik AM, Volgarev AP, Gal'chenko SV, Sazonov AYu. Protective effect of low-intensity MM-wave radiation at a lethal influenzal infection. International Symposium on Millimeter Waves of Nonthermal Intensity in Medicine, Moscow Oct. 3–6, 1991; 2:373–377.

14. Poslavskii MV. Physical EHF therapy in ulcer treatment and prevention. International Symposium on Millimeter Waves of Nonthermal Intensity in Medicine, Moscow Oct. 3–6, 1991; 2:142–146.

15. Adaskevich VG. Application efficiency of MM-wave radiation in the complex treatment of patients with atopic dermatitis. Millimetrovye Volny v Biologii i Meditsine 1994; 3:78–81. In Russian.

16. Adaskevich VG. Clinical efficiency and immunoregulatory and neurohumoral effects of MM therapy in patiens with atopic dermatitis. Biomed Eng 2000; 28-3:80–88.

17. Gedymin LE, Erokhin VV, Bugrova KM. Electromagnetic waves of the MM-wave band in therapy of sarcoidosis of lungs and intrathoracic lymph nodes. Millimetrovye Volny v Biologii i Meditsine 1994; 4:10–16. In Russian.

18. Pulyaeva EL, Vetokhina SV. Application of EHF therapy in treatment of genital herpes. Millimetrovye Volny v Biologii i Meditsine 1997; 9–10:55–56. In Russian.

19. Elbakidze IL, Ordynskii VF, Sudakova EV. EHF therapy in treatment of inflammatory sexually transmitted diseases. Millimetrovye Volny v Biologii i Meditsine 1998; 1,11:39–41. In Russian.

20. Donetskaya SV, Zaitseva SYu, Viktorov AM. Effect of EHF therapy on skin microbiocenosis in vulgaris acne patients. Millimetrovye Volny v Biologii i Meditsine 1996; 7:57–59.

21. Kholodov YUA, Lebedeva NN. Responses of the Human Nervous System on Electromagnetic Fields. Moscow: Nauka, 1992. In Russian.

22. Lebedeva NN, Sulimov AV. Sensory indication of electromagnetic fields of the millimeter-wave band. Millimeter Waves in Medicine and Biology. Moscow: IRE RAN, 1989:176–182. In Russian.

23. Lebedeva NN, Kotrovskaya TI. Electromagnetic perception and individual features of human being. Crit Rev Biomed Eng 2001; 29-3:440–449.

24. Kotrovskaya TI. Human being's sensory responses to a weak electromagnetic stimulus. Millimetrovye Volny v Meditsine i Biologii 1994; 3:32–38. In Russian.

25. Lebedeva NN. Sensory and subsensory responses of a healthy human being to a peripheral

influence of low-intensity MM waves. Millimetrovye Volny v Biologii i Meditsine 1993; 2:5–23. In Russian.

26. Lebedeva NN. CNS responses to electromagnetic fields with different biotropic parameters. Biomeditsinskaya Radioelektronika 1998; 1:24–36. In Russian.

27. Khromova SV. Millimeter-Wave-Induced Modification of Behavioral Reactions in Rats. Thesis Summary of Doctor of Philosophy in Biological Sciences. Moscow: Institute for Higher Nerve Activity of the Russian Academy of Sciences, 1990. In Russian.

28. Arzumanov YuL, Kolotygina RF, Khonicheva NM. Investigation of the stress-protective effect of EHF electromagnetic waves on animals. Millimetrovye Volny v Meditsine i Biologii 1994; 3:5–10. In Russian.

29. Kolotygina RF, Khonicheva NM, Arzumanov YuL. MM-wave radiation and alcohol narcosis duration in animals with different types of behavior. . Technical Twentieth Russian Symposium with Foreign Participants on Millimeter Waves in Medicine and Biology, Moscow, Apr 24–26, 1997. In Russian.

30. Temur'yants NA, Chuyan EN, Tumanyants EN, Tishkina OO, Viktorov NV. Dependence of the antistress effect of electromagnetic waves of the MM-wave band on exposure location in rats with different typologic features. Millimetrovye Volny v Biologii i Meditsine 1993; 2:51–58. In Russian.

31. Temur'yants NA, Chuyan EN. Effect of microwaves of nonthermal intensity on the development of hypokinetic stress in rats with different individual features. Millimetrovye Volny v Biologii i Meditsine 1992; 1:22–32. In Russian.

32. Lebedeva NN, Sulimova OP. Modifying effect of MM waves on the human CNS functional state under stress simulation. Millimetrovye Volny v Biologii i Meditsine 1994; 3:16–21. In Russian.

33. Temur'yants NA, Khomyakova OV, Tumanyants EN, Derpak MN. Dynamics of some psychophysiologic indices during microwave therapy. Eleventh Russian Symposium with Foreign Participants on Millimeter Waves in Medicine and Biology, Moscow, Apr 24–26, 1997. In Russian.

34. Krainov VE, Sulimova OP, Larionov IYu. Application of EHF influence in the combined method of psychoemotional rehabilitation. Eleventh Russian Symposium with Foreign Participants on Millimetrovye Volny v Meditsine i Biologii, Moscow, Apr 24–26, 1997. In Russian.

35. Tsaritsinskii VI, Taranskaya AD, Derkach VN. Application of electromagnetic waves of the MM-wave band in treatment of depressive states. . International Symposium on Millimeter Waves of Nonthermal Intensity in Medicine, Moscow, Oct 24–26, 1997.

36. Lebedeva NN. Physiological mechanisms of biological effects of low-intensity electromagnetic waves of the MM-wave band. The Eleventh Russian Symposium with Foreign Participants on Millimeter Waves in Medicine and Biology, Moscow Apr 24–26, 1997. In Russian.

37. Garkavi LKh, Kvakina EB, Kuz'menko TS. Antistress Reactions and Activation Therapy. Moscow: Imedis, 1998. In Russian.

38. Lyusov VA, Lebedeva AYu, Shchelkunova IG. MM-wave correction for hemorheologic disorders in patients with unstable stenocardia. Millimetrovye Volny v Biologii i Meditsine 1995; 5:46–49. In Russian.

39. Lyusov VA, Volov NA, Lebedeva AYu. Some mechanisms of MM-wave radiation effect on unstable stenocardia pathogenesis. Tenth Russian Symposium on Millimeter Waves in Biology and Medicine, Moscow, Apr 24–26, 1997. In Russian.

40. Lyusov VA, Lebedeva AYu, Fedulaev YuN. Application of combined infrared laser and MM-wave therapies in outpatients with exertion stenocardia of the second functional class. Tenth All-Russia Congress of Cardiologists, Chelyabinsk, 1996. In Russian.

41. Lebedeva AYu. The use of millimeter wavelength electromagnetic waves in cardiology. Biomedical Engineering 2000; 28-1(2):339–350.

42. Lebedeva AYu. Application of electromagnetic radiation of the MM-wave band in the combined treatment of cardiovascular diseases. Biomeditsinskaya Radioelektronika 1998; 2:49–54. In Russian.

43. Pletnev SD. The use of millimeter band electromagnetic waves in clinical oncology. Biomedical Engineering 2000; 29-2:573–588.

44. Kamenev YuF, Sarkisyan AG, Govallo VI. To the optimization problem of low-intensity MM-wave treatment of limb injuries complicated by wound infections. Seventh All-Union Workshop on Application of Low-intensity MM-wave Radiation in Biology and Medicine, Moscow, 1989. In Russian.

45. Kamenev YuF, Devyatkov ND, Toporov YuA. Activation MM-wave therapy of limb injuries complicated by wound infections. Meditsinskaya Radiologiya 1992; 7–8:43–45. In Russian.

46. Kamenev YuF, Berglezov MA, Nadgeriev VM. EHF therapy of trophic ulcers of amputation limb stumps. Rehabilitation Treatment of Limb Injuries and Diseases, Moscow, 1993:96–97. In Russian.

47. Kamenev YuF, Shitikov VA, Batpenov ND. Requirements for long-term and stable remission of various types of deforming osteoarthrosis. Vestnik Travmatologii i Ortopedii im. N. N. Pirogova 1997; 4:9–13. In Russian.

46

The Use of Electrical Stimulation to Treat Morbid Obesity

Mitchell Roslin and Marina Kurian

Lenox Hill Hospital, New York, New York, U.S.A.

The current epidemic of obesity will soon approach smoking as the leading contributor to premature mortality. The multifactorial etiology of obesity and the relative resistance to current treatment approaches are discussed. The influence of vagal nerve activity on eating behaviors is reviewed and preliminary results demonstrating that vagal nerve stimulation can be an effective and safe treatment for morbid obesity are presented. Refinements in functional imaging techniques promise to improve our understanding of mechanisms of action and optimal stimulation parameters that will increase the efficacy and indications for this novel approach.

I. INTRODUCTION

The prevalence of obesity is increasing in epidemic proportions in westernized societies. Unfortunately treatment options remain limited for this potentially deadly disease. For years, obesity has been treated with behavior modification programs. Recent data demonstrates that less than 5% of adults who are significantly overweight can maintain weight loss. Surgical options, which include both gastric restrictive and malabsorptive procedures, have reduced the number and severity of co-morbidities in this population by providing sustained weight loss. However, with surgery, there is the potential for short-term and long-term complications. New approaches to weight loss are necessary.

Since obesity is the net result of an energy imbalance, where more calories are consumed than necessary, with the surplus stored as fat, treatment strategies directed at key areas of the central nervous system involved in energy regulation are a logical approach. Ablation or stimulation of the hypothalamus has resulted in altered eating behavior in numerous animal species. However, the use of direct brain stimulation is not an attractive strategy for obesity treatment. To begin, most would be reluctant to have a procedure that places an electrode into the brain. Complications such as bleeding and infection would be disastrous.

The vagus nerve is a conduit between the brainstem and the viscera. It is the communication link between key areas of the brain and the organs such as the lungs, heart, and the gastrointestinal tract. The purpose of this chapter is to review obesity and explain some of the science behind the epidemic, explain the limitations of present treatment modalities, and present our early work with vagus nerve stimulation.

II. OBESITY DEFINED

Obesity is actually defined as having excess adiposity or fat tissue. It is the result of caloric intake exceeding energy expenditure. As the body's most energy dense tissue, adipose tissue is the site where this excess energy is stored. Since it is more practical to measure height and weight, rather than amount of fat, determination of level of obesity is generated using these numbers. The most accurate numerical assessment is obtained by determining the body mass index (BMI). This number is derived by dividing weight in kilograms by height in meters squared. A BMI of more than 40 is considered morbidly obese. As an example, an individual who is 5 ft 10 in. tall and weighs 280 lb has a body mass index of 40. A patient with a BMI of 25–30 is considered overweight, 30–35 has stage I obesity, 35–40 stage II obesity, and over 40 stage III or morbid obesity.

In the opinion of many health care experts, obesity is the largest health problem facing westernized societies. From a medical standpoint, obesity is the primary risk factor for type II diabetes and obstructive sleep apnea. It increases the chances for heart disease, pulmonary disease, infertility, osteoarthritis, cholecystitis, and several major cancers, including breast and colon. From an economic standpoint, it is estimated that $100 billion are spent on obesity and treating its major co-morbidities. This does not even consider the psychological and social costs of this epidemic problem.

Despite these alarming facts, treatment options for obesity remain limited. It is estimated that 50 to 60% of the population are obese or overweight. Of these patients, 5 to 6% are considered morbidly obese because they are approximately 100 lb above their ideal body weight. Treatment options include dietary modification, very low calorie liquid diets, pharmaceutical agents, counseling, exercise programs, and surgery. Surgical procedures that restrict the size of the stomach and/or bypass parts of the intestine are the only remedies that provide lasting weight loss for the majority of morbidly obese individuals. Surgical procedures for morbid obesity are becoming more common based on the long-term successful weight loss results (1).

In 1991, the NIH issued a consensus statement on surgery for morbid obesity and outlined the indications for surgery and endorsed two surgical procedures. Patients who meet criteria for surgery have BMI over 40 or over 35 with severe co-morbidities. The two endorsed surgical procedures are gastric bypass and vertical banded gastroplasty (VBG, also known as stapling or banding of the stomach) (2).

All of these weight loss procedures are being done using open and minimally invasive or laparoscopic techniques. It is estimated that 80,000 operative procedures will be performed for obesity this year in the United States. VBG and gastric banding are restrictive procedures and gastric bypass and biliopancreatic diversion (BPD) are restrictive–malabsorptive procedures. However, these procedures are major surgery and have the potential for short-term complications and long-term nutritional problems. In some respects, surgery for obesity is forced behavior modification. Other less drastic options for weight loss have not been as successful as surgery yet do not have the potential complications of surgical weight loss. Additionally, these aggressive procedures are not indicated for those with less severe obesity, who also would substantially benefit from weight reduction. An optimal treatment for morbid obesity is not yet at hand.

The etiology of obesity is multifactorial and beyond the scope of this review. But it is important to note that excess adiposity is the result of energy intake exceeding energy expenditure. Treatment has focused on reducing caloric intake and encouraging exercise to develop muscle and increase energy utilization. Presently, even surgical interventions are targeted at the gastrointestinal tract and limiting intake. Energy regulation is controlled by the central nervous system. Thus, it has been our contention that ideal long-term treatments would need to target the central nervous system and the gut–brain interaction.

The purpose of this article is to explain why stimulation of the vagus nerve may provide an accessible input to the central nervous system and a potential treatment strategy for morbid obesity.

III. THE ROLE OF VAGUS NERVE AFFERENTS IN EATING BEHAVIOR

The termination of a meal or eating in humans is complex and a full understanding of satiety and food consumption has remained elusive. It involves the interaction of cognitive factors from the cerebrum, feedback from the gastrointestinal tract as well as peripheral signals including messages from fat-storing adipocytes. Hormonal influences and peripheral and central monitors of blood glucose content are also involved. While there is feedback from all areas of the gastrointestinal tract to the brain, distension of the stomach is the single greatest factor in satiety. This has been shown by experiments that have placed a cuff around the pylorus. As a result, the stomach distends, activating mechanical receptors and the animal stops eating. Clinically, this accounts for the success of gastric stapling or banding in reducing food intake. What is most interesting as this happens is that there is an increase in vagus nerve activity (3).

The vagus nerve is best known to physicians for of its roles in acid production and motility. However, it is predominately a sensory nerve and approximately 85% of its fibers are sensory or afferent. While there is a large overlap in the areas innervated by the right and left trunks, they are not mirror images. The anterior vagus nerve provides the bulk of innervation to the proximal stomach. In contrast, the posterior trunk provides the majority of the innervation to the pylorus and duodenum.

Evidence of the vagus nerve's role in eating behavior comes from multiple sources. As mentioned, there is an increase in vagus nerve activity with gastric distension and food intake. More convincing are experiments that have been done with peptides known to reduce food intake in animal models. The most extensively studied is cholecystokinin (CCK). CCK is released after meal consumption. It is known to cause contraction of the gallbladder causing the release of bile to aid in fat digestion. Additionally, it helps control the release of chyme from the antrum of the stomach into the duodenum. The administration of CCK, either intravenously or into the peritoneum, has been shown to reduce food intake in animal models ranging from rodent to primate. These studies have been done with gastric fistulas to prevent distension and activation of mechanical receptors. Interestingly, surgical vagotomy attenuates this response. Furthermore, capsaicin (a chemical that damages or destroys vagal afferents) -preserving efferents also significantly reduces the effect of CCK. These data demonstrate that afferent vagus fibers are responsible for the satiating effect of CCK (4,5). Recent research has indicated that the hepatic branch of the vagus is the area of action for CCK and the location of the bulk of CCK receptors.

Several other peptides have also been studied with similar results. In fact, in a recent review, Dr. George Bray, Director of the Pennington Research Laboratories concluded that the vagus nerve is responsible for the transmission of the majority of afferent signals responsible for satiety (6).

In addition to peptides released and mechanical stretch, meal content is an important determinant of food intake. The administration of intravenous alimentation with fat and sugar has been shown to reduce food intake. Experiments have been performed in which a gastric fistula is created with fatty acids, simple sugars, and amino acids being infused into the duodenum. Administration of oleic acid, a fatty acid, reduces food intake. Vagotomy and capsaicin markedly blunt this effect. Sugar infusion with maltose also reduces intake in a fistula model. While vagotomy blunts this effect, it is not nearly as dramatic as with fatty acids (5,7). This has led to the conclusion that lipoprivic feeding is controlled by vagally mediated peripheral signals. In comparison, glucoprivic feeding is controlled by the GI tract and central nervous system and is only partially vagally mediated. A possible explanation is that glucose is the primary fuel of the central nervous system. As a result, it is reasonable that the brain would preserve a role in monitoring that sugar intake is adequate.

IV. PRECLINICAL PROGRAM

The combination of the anatomic relationship of the vagus nerve to the GI tract and the above physiologic experiments provided the rationale for the investigation of electrical stimulation of the vagus nerve for obesity and development of a preclinical animal experimental program. Despite this appealing theory, there was one major factor that needed to be considered prior to beginning investigation. During the clinical years of study with vagus nerve stimulation for epilepsy, besides a few anecdotal reports, no weight loss was reported. Thus, several modifications were necessary. Since we hoped to stimulate the small unmyelinated C fibers of the nerve, we felt it would be best to be in closer proximity to the gastroesophageal junction. Such positioning would avoid stimulation of fibers that join the trunk from the heart and lungs, and we speculated a greater likelihood of stimulating our target fibers. Additionally, positioning away from the neck and the recurrent laryngeal nerve would allow the delivery of higher levels of current that could be necessary to stimulate these unmyelinated fibers. Finally, since the right and left trunks have different distributions in the abdomen and the contribution of both could be essential, we chose to investigate bilateral stimulation of the vagus nerve.

To test whether VNS could alter food intake, a canine study was conducted. Ten mongrel dogs were divided into two different stimulation patterns: (1) acute studies, which were stimulated with duty cycles for 20 min before and during meal consumption, and (2) chronic studies, which were stimulated with duty cycles continuously (Table 1). Animals were fed twice daily and eating behavior, time of food consumption, and amount of food consumption were recorded.

Table 1 Study Results

Studies	Median	P value
Acute		
% Change in average daily consumption time	13.2	0.75
% Change in average daily consumption amount	−3.5	1.0
Chronic		
% Change in average daily consumption time	86.0	0.02
% Change in average daily consumption amount	−26.4	0.00

An NCP bipolar lead was placed on each of the right and left vagal trunks via a left thoracotomy and attached to separate NCP pulse generators. Animals were allowed 20 min to consume their meal. Intake amount and time of consumption was observed and recorded. When the animal returned to baseline eating behavior and seemed sufficiently recovered from the surgical procedure (5–10 days), the NCP systems were activated. All animals were given unlimited access to water. All dogs were weighed on a weekly basis.

Output current (mA), duty cycle (on/off time), signal frequency (Hz), and pulse width (μs) were adjusted by placing the Cyberonics Model 200 NCP Programming Wand over the pulse generator on the skin. A signal frequency of 30 Hz was used, with a pulse width of 500 ms and a 30 s on/2 min off time. Current was variable and started at 2 mA and adjusted in increments of 0.25 mA until maximal effect or current limit was reached.

No significant surgical complications were observed in any animal. One study was terminated on postimplant day 100 due to an erosion of one of the pulse generators through the skin. This was probably due to a combination of rapid loss of subcutaneous fat and placement of the pulse generator within the subcutaneous plane.

The studies were divided into two groups. Group I studies were performed using thoracic placement of the bipolar leads and acute stimulation parameters (stimulation signals delivered 20 min before and during mealtime only). Group II studies consisted of eight animals, which had thoracic placement of the bipolar leads and chronic stimulation parameters (stimulation signals delivered at various duty cycles continuously throughout the day). As shown, during periods when the vagus nerve was stimulated (stimulation on), the average consumption time (time to consume a meal) increased from approximately 3.5 min to 20 min. When the stimulation was turned off, the consumption time decreased from 20 min back down to approximately 3.5 min. The associated weight was also shown during this time (Fig. 1). Analyses were performed on all studies in both groups and included time of food consumption, amount of food consumed, change in weight, hematologic, and biochemical profiles.

Change in weight (weight at or closest to date of NCP System implant minus weight at on a specific time) was evaluated in the group I and group II animals. Weight loss was observed in all chronically stimulated animals, except for one animal that was done early in the series. Percentage of change in weight from start of stimulation periods was calculated and compared in groups of days (Fig. 2). A marked and statistically relevant change (decrease) in weight was observed in the chronically stimulated (group II) animals as compared to the animals undergoing acute stimulation.

In summary, this study suggests that the use of bilateral vagus nerve stimulation is effective in changing eating behavior, with a corresponding weight loss in a canine animal model. The poor response during acute VNS combined with the delayed effect of chronic stimulation suggests that VNS results in changes in the central nervous system and secondarily alters food intake.

V. HUMAN PILOT PROGRAM

The combination of the results of the above study and the known safety of vagus nerve stimulation in humans served as the basis for initiating a Phase I study. A total of six patients underwent implantation of bilateral vagus nerve stimulators in the thoracic cavity at Lenox Hill Hospital in New York and the University of Texas in Houston. There were five females and a single male. All met clinical criteria for morbid obesity surgery. Following implantation, patients were blinded to the timing of activation of their generators. Settings included a pulse width of 500 ms, on time of 30 s, off time of 3 min, a frequency of 20 Hz, and amplitude

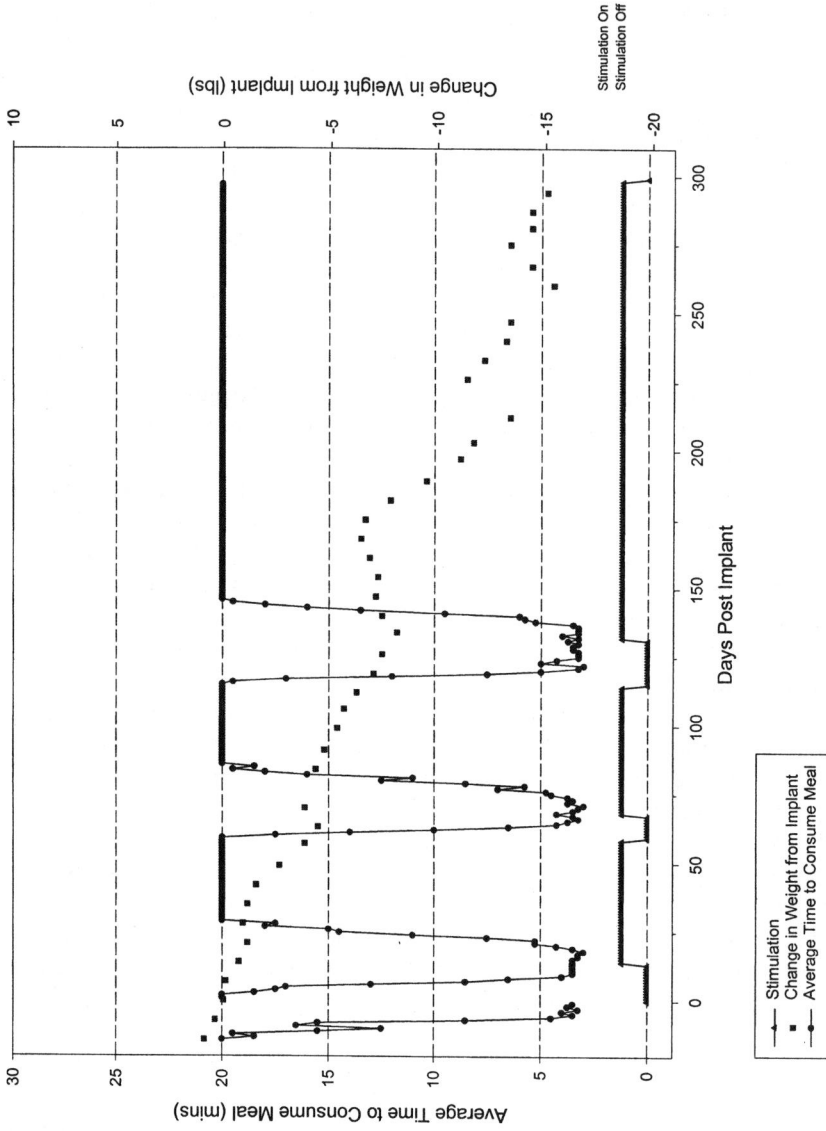

Figure 1 Chronic bilateral VNS for the treatment of obesity. Animal # 1964. Time to consume meal and change in weight.

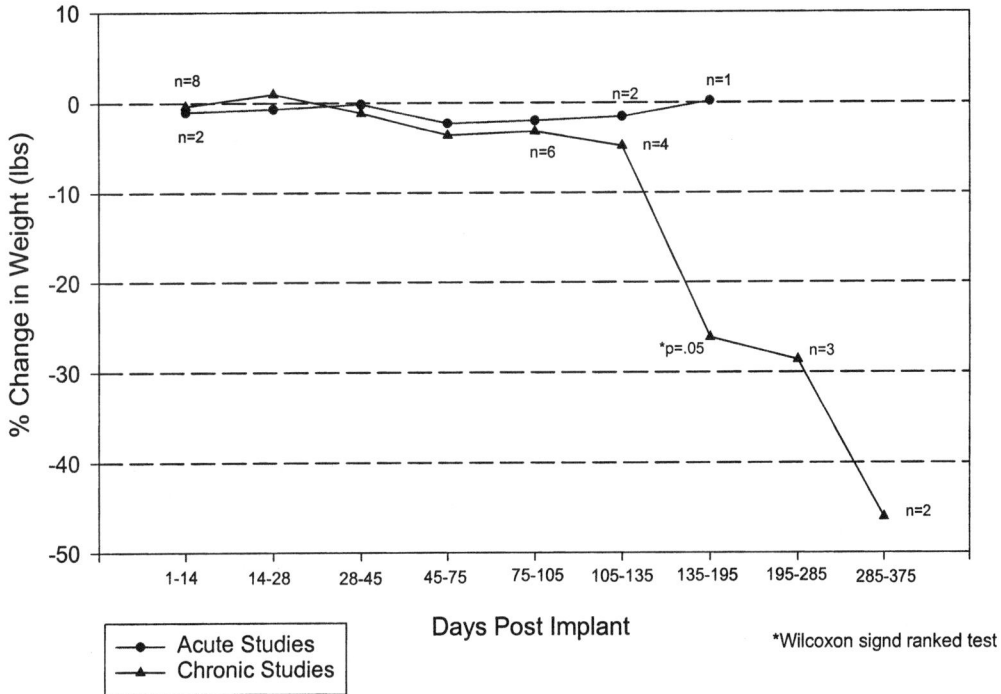

Figure 2 VNS for the treatment of obesity. Percent change in weight from start of simulation. Chronic and acute study animals.

starting at 0.25 mA. Amplitude was raised to maximum allowed by the generators over a several week period of time.

Results of this pilot study were mixed. One female who was over 400 lb, lost over 90 lb and continues to do well. Another lost 40 lb, became pregnant, and had to leave the study. Two others lost approximately 10% of their body weight and then saturated. In the final two, there was no effect.

While these early results compare favorably to current pharmaceutical options, they do not compare to the results that can be accomplished with surgical procedures. There were no device-related complications, and the only source of patient morbidity was a wound infection. Additionally, patients did not complain of significant discomfort from electrical stimulation. No patient needed to deactivate their generators with the magnets.

Another strategy for electrical stimulation for the treatment of obesity has been direct stimulation of the stomach. A multicenter clinical trial (transneuronics) is in progress in the United States and Europe. The original hypothesis was to place electrodes in a position in which they would reduce gastric emptying. As a result electrodes were placed along the greater curvature of the stomach. For a variety of reasons this strategy was abandoned and the electrodes for this trial are now placed along the lesser curvature in proximity to the vagus nerves. Additionally, gastric emptying studies have failed to show any long-term change in motility. As a result, the mechanism of action of this approach is probably similar to what has been discussed above (8,9).

Similar to the results with vagus nerve stimulation, there are responders and non-responders, and it is too early to determine if the results are based on the device or placebo. It is our belief that the two strategies are very similar, and it is not clear whether direct or indirect vagus nerve stimulation is superior.

Thus, our initial clinical experience was not as dramatic as our animal experimentation. What is most striking is the absence of side affects from activation of the small sensory fibers of the vagus nerve, the unmylinated c fibers. In the animal model, we were able to induce retching and emesis, at high currents. Obviously, this would not be desirable for humans, but the absence of any complaints of nausea make us wonder whether we were able to deliver the energy threshold necessary to activate enough c fibers. As a result, we are awaiting a new generation of electrodes that can deliver double the current before continuing the clinical trial.

Additionally, we are actively following the work of Dr. Mark George and his colleagues at the Medical University of South Carolina with functional magnetic resonance imaging. Dr. George has shown that vagus nerve stimulation increases blood flow to areas such as the hypothalamus that are known to control energy regulation (10). The ability to see subtle changes in these area will hopefully provide a rationale framework to determine optimal stimulation parameters. Unfortunately, we still do not know why VNS is only 60% effective for the treatment of epilepsy. Does it not work in certain patients because they have a different disease, or do they have different anatomy, or is there a technical problem with the signal, electrode, or generator. In refractive epilepsy, where there is no other option, this maybe acceptable. However, in other areas with alternatives, higher levels of effectiveness are necessary. Real-time imaging will give us the best chance to answer these difficult questions.

At present, electrical stimulation can not compare to gastric bypass. However, there are numerous reasons to continue to pursue this research. While many predict a magic bullet, this is highly unlikely. It is our belief that the pharmaceutical treatment of obesity will require a cocktail of agents that function in different pathways. Since obesity is a chronic disease these agents will have to be given for a long time period. The combination of lifelong therapy and multiple agents will make undesirable events common. Additionally, while we have focused on morbid obesity, there is an entire group who are overweight and desire help but are not severe enough to justify surgery. Certainly, a device with a good safety profile would be very attractive. Furthermore, it is possible that vagus nerve stimulation can be used with new agents to provide a synergistic effect with some of the over 100 drugs that are in development and lower either the dose or number of medications required for clinical efficacy.

The desire to eat and the body's counter regulatory system when caloric intake is reduced make the treatment of obesity quite a difficult task. While we have taken a cautionary tone with our early data, it is important to point out that our mean weight loss of 14% is double that of pharmaceuticals approved by the Federal Drug Administration for obesity. Thus while this technology is still in the early stages, we are optimistic. The vagus nerve is the link from the abdominal viscera to the brain. The wiring is in place. It is our job to learn the language and find the signal to mimic.

VI. CONCLUSION

There are few options for severe obesity. Despite the success of surgery for obesity, operations that staple the stomach are not an attractive alternative for the majority of morbidly obese adults. Since obesity is the result of an energy imbalance, it seems logical that ideal treatment modalities would be directed at the central nervous system especially areas that control energy intake and expenditure. In this review, we have discussed the rationale for the use of VNS for the treatment of obesity and provided animal data supporting this hypothesis. Recently, Dr. Mark George and his colleagues at Medical University of South Carolina using functional magnetic resonance imaging have demonstrated that activation of vagus nerve stimulation increases blood flow to the hypothalamus (10). These results provide support for our data and demonstrates that the vagus nerve does provide information to the energy control center in the brain.

In addition, vagus nerve stimulation has been shown to be safe and well tolerated. As a result, stimulation of the vagus nerve is a safe portal to the brain and the hypothalamus. In comparison to direct electrical stimulation to the brain, it is our belief that vagus stimulation is safer and a more attractive option to physicians and patients.

At present, we have provided data that suggests that vagus nerve stimulation may represent a treatment option for obesity. Further investigation will be required to determine optimal parameters and timing for stimulation. The development of functional imaging techniques hopefully will provide a method for evaluating parameters and comparing different subjects. As a result, we will be able to determine parameters that maximize input to the eating centers and to titrate patients in this manner.

ACKNOWLEDGMENTS

We would like to thank Cyberonics for their support for providing equipment and supplies. We would like to thank the Maimonides Research and Development Foundation for their support.

REFERENCES

1. Mason EE. Gastric surgery for morbid obesity. Surg Clin N Am 1992; 72:501–513.
2. Gastrointestinal surgery for severe obesity. NIH Consensus Dev Conf Consensus Statement 1991. Am J Clin Nutr 1992; 55:615S–619S.
3. Gonzalez MF, Deutsch JA. Vagotomy abolishes cues of satiety produced by gastric distention. Science 1981; 212:1283–1284.
4. Smith GP, Jerome C, Cushin BJ, Eterno R, Simansky KJ. Abdominal vagotomy blocks the satiety effect of cholecystokinin in the rat. Science 1981; 213:1036–1037.
5. Ritter RC, Ritter S, Ewart WR, Wingate DL. Capsaicin attenuates hindbrain neuron responses to circulating cholecystokinin. Am J Physiol 1989; 257:R1162–R1168.
6. Bray GA. Afferent signals regulating food intake. Proc Nutr Soc 2000; 59:373–384.
7. Houpt TR, Houpt KA, Swan AA. Duodenal osmoconcentration and food intake in pigs after ingestion of hypertonic nutrients. Am J Physiol 1983; 245:R181–R189.
8. Cigaina V, Saggioro A, Rigo V. Long-term effects of gastric pacing to reduce feed intake in swine. Obes Surg 1996; 6:250–253.
9. Cigaina V, Saggioro A. Pacing the stomach: five years experience with an obese patient population [abstr P8]. Obes Surg 2001; 11:171.
10. George MS, Nahas Z, Bohning DE. Vagus Nerve Stimulation therapy: A research update. Neurology 2002; 59(Suppl 4):S56–S561.

47

Biocurrent Therapy for Macular Degeneration

John B. Jarding
Black Hills Regional Eye Institute, Rapid City, South Dakota, U.S.A.

George D. O'Clock
Minnesota State University, Mankato, Minnesota, U.S.A.

Electrotherapy has been used to alleviate various visual disorders for over 200 years but it is only in the past two decades that it has been put on a scientific footing. One of the most promising applications has been for improvement of macular degeneration, an increasingly common problem that is relatively resistant to treatment. A novel safe and effective approach utilized in Europe that has received IRB approval here is described, mechanisms of action are discussed and illustrative case histories are presented.

I. INTRODUCTION

Approximately 15 million Americans, and 100 million people worldwide, are suffering visual acuity loss from the debilitating effects of macular degeneration. Age-related Macular degeneration (AMD or ARMD) is the leading cause of legal blindness for people over the age of 55, affecting more Americans than cataracts and glaucoma combined (1–4). According to the Director of the National Eye Institute, AMD will "soon take on aspects of an epidemic" as baby boomers age and the over 80 age group continues to be the fastest growing segment of the population. Almost 5000 new AMD cases are diagnosed daily. Epidemiologists predict that by the end of this decade, there will be 30 million patients with AMD in the United States.

AMD has an insidious onset. Although it rarely causes total blindness, there is a progressive loss of sharp central vision needed to read, watch TV, identify faces, drive, navigate stairs, and perform other daily tasks that are often taken for granted (5).

Over the past 20 years, there has been a marked increase in research activity to investigate conditions that cause, or have an effect on, the onset and progression of macular degeneration. A significant amount of research activity has been devoted to the improvement of existing therapies and the development of new therapeutic techniques for this, presently, incurable disorder. One of the most promising therapeutic techniques for AMD, electrotherapy, has been revived. Electrotherapy has a 200-year history in the treatment of visual system disease (6,7). If the results that have been achieved up to this point are consistent, electrotherapy will provide health care practitioners with a very effective, patient friendly and relatively low-cost method to mitigate the progress of macular degeneration and other visual system disorders.

From the standpoint of providing the macular degeneration patient with an effective and reliable electrotherapeutic treatment option, the approach taken by Acuity Medical has been to develop a device that is dedicated to the treatment of visual system disease. Some of the electrotherapeutic devices that Acuity Medical health care practitioners previously used to treat macular degeneration patients have been reasonably effective in the office (8). However, many of these electrotherapeutic devices have been designed to address a wide variety of health problems, and the resulting electrical signal or waveform outputs appear to be unusually complex and/or frequency limited. In addition, some of the available devices are a bit difficult to operate for a person who is visually impaired.

Our motivation to provide a dedicated electrotherapeutic system (device and protocol) for the treatment of visual system diseases was highly influenced by size, cost factors, and reliability problems that macular degeneration patients experienced with some of the previously available devices. Some patients complained that their visual acuity became worse as they treated themselves. Upon further investigation, we found that the particular electrotherapeutic device the patients were using was the source of the problem. In some cases, the device output was either very inconsistent, or it was not delivering any current at all.

Macular degeneration patients need a therapeutic device that is portable, affordable, and reliable. In addition, macular degeneration patients need to know the magnitude of the current levels they are receiving during treatment. They need a device that is reasonably simple to operate. They need readout, display, and adjustment control numbers and letters that are large enough in size for a visually impaired person to see.

After recognizing the problems and deficiencies associated with some of the previous electrotherapeutic device models, Acuity Medical developed the TheraMac system. The TheraMac device requires relatively few adjustments on the part of the patient. TheraMac changes frequency automatically, and it provides the types of waveforms and current levels that, for the past 200 years, have proven to be effective in the treatment of visual system health problems.

II. ANATOMY AND PHYSIOLOGY OF A HEALTHY RETINA AND MACULA

The macula, the central and most sensitive part of the retina, is approximately 5.5 mm in diameter and contains between 5 and 6 million photoreceptor cells. This dense collection of light-sensitive cells is, by far, greater in the macular area than anywhere else in the retina. No other retinal area contains a concentration of photoreceptors that is sufficient to prevent the loss of detailed vision that occurs with macular degeneration. The highest concentration of photoreceptors is found in the very center of the macula in an area called the *fovea centralis*, and detailed visual acuity disappears when damage to this site impairs its function.

The lining of the retina is made up of 10 layers of neural tissue, membranes, and photoreceptors. Metabolic support cells, the retinal pigment epithelium (RPE), lie adjacent to the rod and cone photoreceptor cells in the outermost layers of the retina. The RPE is essential for normal metabolic activity and function of rods and cones, which are responsible for visual acuity, detection of image motion and color perception. Below the RPE is a permeable membrane, Bruch's membrane, that separates the neural retinal network from the choroidal circulatory network of blood vessels (9).

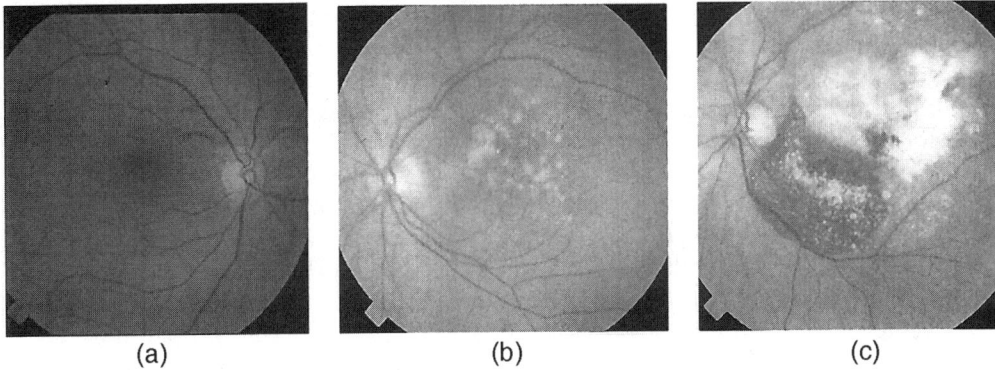

Figure 1 (a) Fundus photo of a healthy retina. (b) Fundus photo for a patient with dry macular degeneration. Notice the mottled appearance of drusen around the macular area. (c) Fundus photo for a patient with wet macular degeneration. Notice the accumulation of blood around the area of the macula.

Since retinal macular metabolic activity is the highest of any tissue in the body, the demand for blood is also the greatest. Nearly two dozen branches of the posterior ciliary arteries create a very dense network of capillaries to supply the increased nutritional and oxygen requirements necessary to support healthy macular function. The complex photo-chemical sequence of events in the visual process and the associated metabolic activity require enormous amounts of nutrients and oxygen from the blood stream. A healthy choroidal vasculature fulfills this requirement as well as the need to continually remove waste products. It has been estimated that 100% of circulating blood passes through our eyes every 80 min. A fundus photograph of a normal retina in the region of the macula is shown in Fig. 1a.

III. MACULAR DEGENERATION PATHOLOGY AND PATHOGENESIS

In the early AMD stage, with dilated pupils, ophthalmoscopy reveals a granular appearance in the macular area, indicating the presence of hard and soft drusen. Drusen can be described as a yellowish clumping of lipids and proteins, representing a macular metabolic exudate (10). Severe disruption of the retinal pigment epithelial cells can produce hyperpigmenta-tion. Hard and soft drusen deposits occur between the retinal pigment epithelium (RPE) and Bruch's membrane. Soft drusen is usually larger in size, with undefined edges, and contributes to the separation of the RPE from Bruch's membrane.

A disruption in normal RPE function triggers the production of vascular endothelial growth factors (VEGF). If a break occurs in the hardened and thickened Bruch's membrane, coroidal neovascularization (11) is stimulated. These abnormalities progress at variable rates over the following months and years. If no retinal blood vessel leakage or bleeding occurs, geographic RPE cell loss occurs. This geographic atrophy is designated as atrophic or "dry" AMD and eventually results in legal blindness due to loss of detailed vision (Figure 1b). For 10 to 15% of AMD patients, neovascularization of the macula and macular bleeding manifests. If this should happen, the course of the disease changes to the exudative or "wet" form (Fig. 1c). If Bruch's Membrane is breached, fragile seeping and bleeding neovascular networks grow into the subretinal space from the choroid. As these thin-walled and weak vessels proliferate and eventually bleed, loss of visual acuity can occur within minutes or hours.

The wet form of AMD causes additional deterioration that results in legal blindness, within 2 years, for almost three out of four patients. It is believed that impaired blood flow to the macula interferes with RPE function and the RPE's ability to provide nourishment and remove metabolic waste products. RPE deterioration affects the recycling or rebuilding process of the rhodopsin/rod-cone cell function.

The cause, or causes, of macular degeneration are not completely clear. The RPE appears to have a reduced activity associated with certain digestive enzymes (12). With aging, ultraviolet (UV) and blue light free radical damage may occur due to the reduction of the UV and blue light blocking macular pigment leutein and zeaxanthin concentrations in the macula. Cross-linking of collagen in Bruch's membrane can promote the accumulation of the retinal debris associated with AMD. There is evidence of a genetic predisposition to AMD in approximately 16% of adult onset AMD and in 100% of the juvenile form of macular degeneration (Stargardt's Disease). Research results have shown that more than one gene may be involved (13–15). Certain environmental and life-style aspects may also contribute to the onset of the disease, including smoking and diet (16,17).

IV. SAMPLE OF MACULAR DEGENERATION TREATMENT OPTIONS

For years, the only approved therapy for wet AMD was Krypton or Argon laser photocoagulation to stop bleeding and destroy neovascular growth (18). However, the heat generated also damaged the overlying retina and underlying choroid, resulting in scar tissue and the formation of a permanent blind spot. As an alternative to laser therapy, proton beam therapy has been used at Loma Linda University Medical Center (CA). Proton beam therapy is painless and avoids retinal burn problems associated with laser therapy (19).

Laser therapy results improved, following FDA approval of photodynamic therapy in April 2000. This procedure utilizes a low-energy laser to activate Verteporphin, a drug that, when activated by a low-energy laser, causes thrombosis to block blood flow and eventual atrophy of neovascular tissue without causing heat damage (20). Other surgical and pharmaceutical advances have also helped to reduce the ravages of wet AMD, but there has been little progress in improving the prognosis for the 85 to 90% of patients with the dry form of the disease.

In 1988, D.A. Newsome published a study (21) showing that a slower progression of AMD occurred over a 2 year period for patients receiving certain vitamin (antioxidant), amino acid, and mineral supplements that were high in zinc compared to unsupplemented patients (controls). Additional research has shown the benefits of leutine, quercetin, rutin, selenium, lycopene, and coenzyme Q10 supplementation.

Early (mid-1800s) drug treatments for diseases of the visual system included strychnine (pills or subcutaneous injections), potassium iodide, bichloride of mercury, and tincture of perchloride of iron. Strychnine, bichloride of mercury, and potassium iodide were often used (with mixed results) because many visual system disease conditions were often complicated by syphilis (7). Recent developments in drug therapy for macular generation patients involve interferon Alfa-2a (minimal or negative results so far) and thalidomide (3), PKC 412, AG 3340, and rhuFab. Many of the drugs used in the treatment of macular degeneration are designed to inhibit angiogenesis.

Other options under consideration or development for the treatment of macular degeneration include submacular surgery, retinal translocation, radiation therapy (strontium 90), and gene therapy.

V. ELECTROTHERAPEUTIC TREATMENT OPTION

Some of the first papers published on the use of electrotherapy in the treatment of various visual diseases appeared in monographs and ophthalmology journals in the mid to late 1800s (7,22,23). The diseases treated included neuropathy, retinitis pigmentosa, diabetic retinopathy, optic atrophy, amaurosis, retinal asthenopia, and other visual problems; some of which may have been due to macular degeneration. According to several sources, electrotherapy to treat eye diseases dates back more than 200 years. The instrumentation used was crude (24).

These treatments (referred to as *galvanotherapy*) often involved relatively high levels of direct current (DC), above 1 mA, using wet-cell batteries as the source (7,22,23). The direct current electrotherapeutic treatment protocol usually required the positive electrode to be placed on the closed lid of the eye to be treated and the negative electrode was placed on the other closed eye lid or temple. Wet cells were added (increasing the levels of applied voltage and current) until the patient started to see flashes of light (phosphenes). Current levels were often in the range of a few milliamperes, which caused considerable discomfort for many patients. Electrodes were held in place for a time frame of 30 s to 5 min. The entire treatment protocol required 5 to 15 min per sitting.

The ability of the patient to self-administer electrotherapeutic treatment was also addressed in the mid- to late 1800s. The relatively low costs associated with an appropriate electrotherapeutic instrument placed a self-administered treatment protocol well within the financial capabilities of most patients with visual disease problems.

Possible mechanisms for the healing effects of electrotherapy in visual disease have been discussed since the mid-1800s. At that time, some of the electrotherapeutic health care practitioners in ophthalmology believed that the direct currents increased the conductivity of the optic nerve and temporarily dilated the retinal blood vessels. Improvements in analytical chemistry, microscopy, spectroscopy, and molecular biology have provided more details concerning the effects of electric currents in living systems. Considering the results of recent research activity in AMD mechanisms, the original assumptions of the 1800s were fairly accurate.

Initially, research results in wound healing mechanisms provided a significant amount of insight into the healing process when an electrotherapeutic device is utilized to treat an injury site or diseased tissue. During the mid-1800s, researchers detected injury currents in the vicinity of fresh wounds. In the 1860s, duBois-Reymond discovered that an injured bleeding finger is electrically positive compared to a neighboring uninjured finger (25). Electrical potentials associated with injury sites were measured and analyzed in the 1940s (26). These results provided valuable insights for improvements in the effective application of electrotherapeutic methods toward the treatment of a variety of disease states. Results, such as these, were useful for the development of Dr. Björn E.W. Nordentström's bioelectric systems theory (27) of Biologically Closed Electric Circuits (BCEC). These results also helped pave the way for Dr. Robert O. Becker's work in the areas of regeneration and cell dedifferentiation and the relationships that these processes have with endogenous and exogenous electrical currents (28).

Recent research results in biochemistry and molecular biology have shown that direct currents in the 10-µA to 1-mA wound-healing range increase ATP concentrations, promote the incorporation of amino acids in tissue, stimulate protein synthesis, and assist in membrane transport of amino acids. Relatively low-level electric field intensities can alter the rate of glycolysis in mammalian astrocytes, or glial cells (29,30). Nordenström discusses the effects of relatively low-level DC electric fields on the porosity of capillaries (27).

Nordenström's descriptions of an electrically induced healing process, and enhancement of capillary porosity, are very important factors for the electrically induced healing process in the eye and reabsorption of protein and lipid exudates that occur when a macular degeneration patient is treated with electrotherapy.

From the late 1880s, alternating current (AC) sources were also used to treat various diseases of the visual system. Electrotherapeutic techniques, using various frequencies, allow the therapeutic device to have an effect on a wide range of healing processes involving metabolism, replication, transcription, translation, transport, and cell proliferation (29–32).

With DC and AC currents, voltages, and electric fields having the kind of influence on the above-mentioned processes involved in healing, regulation, growth, and development, it is obvious that a carefully planned electrotherapeutic protocol can assist and enhance healing, regulation, and growth in the human body.

Over 150 years of research results in wound healing, neurology, cardiology, orthopedics, renal regulation, biochemistry, and molecular biology have proven that the human body regulates and heals itself, using electrical and electrochemical phenomena that involve ion and electron transport mechanisms, under the influence of electric field and magnetic field stimulants. This large body of research has provided enough information, concerning the electrical processes in the human body, to assist in the development of electrotherapeutic devices that are capable of delivering the proper frequencies, voltages, and current levels under the guidance of an appropriate treatment protocol. This will allow an externally applied therapeutic device to supply exogenous voltages and currents to complement the endogenous voltages and currents that naturally occur in the human body and to assist the various processes that are involved in regulation and healing.

VI. BIOCURRENT THERAPY—THERAMAC

The TheraMac device and protocol design incorporates a device12insignificant risk" status for both the patient and the health care practitioner (Fig. 2). The TheraMac device provides electric current and current density levels that are often far below those levels associated with other electrotherapeutic devices, such as pacemakers, TENS units, etc. TheraMac output currents are limited or restricted, and are below the levels that can cause patient discomfort and significant skin irritation problems.

In comparison with other electrotherapeutic devices, if a 170-μA TheraMac treatment current is considered, the resulting TheraMac current densities are more than 1000 times less than the current densities associated with cardiac pacemakers. TheraMac treatment current densities are more than 10 times lower than the localized cellular current density that is required to maintain the basic metabolic rate. In fact, TheraMac current densities, utilized in treatment, are only two to three orders of magnitude higher than the maximum current densities associated with random noise in living systems.

TheraMac automatically varies the output waveform from a very low frequency to approximately 80 Hz. The device output waveform is essentially a frequency-variable square wave that is rich in harmonics. Treatment current levels can vary between 80 μA and 130 μA. Patient comfort is the primary parameter in this case, and the device allows the patient to monitor the output current from the device. Closing the eyelid of the eye to be treated, the patient holds on to one of the TheraMac electrodes while applying the other electrode (a cotton tip electrode covered with gel or a metal electrode covered with gel) to eight specific points located in the orbit of the eye.

Some macular degeneration patients are quite comfortable when treated with current levels of 170 μA (Fig. 3). Others start to feel a slight "sting" at 140 μA. The current levels can

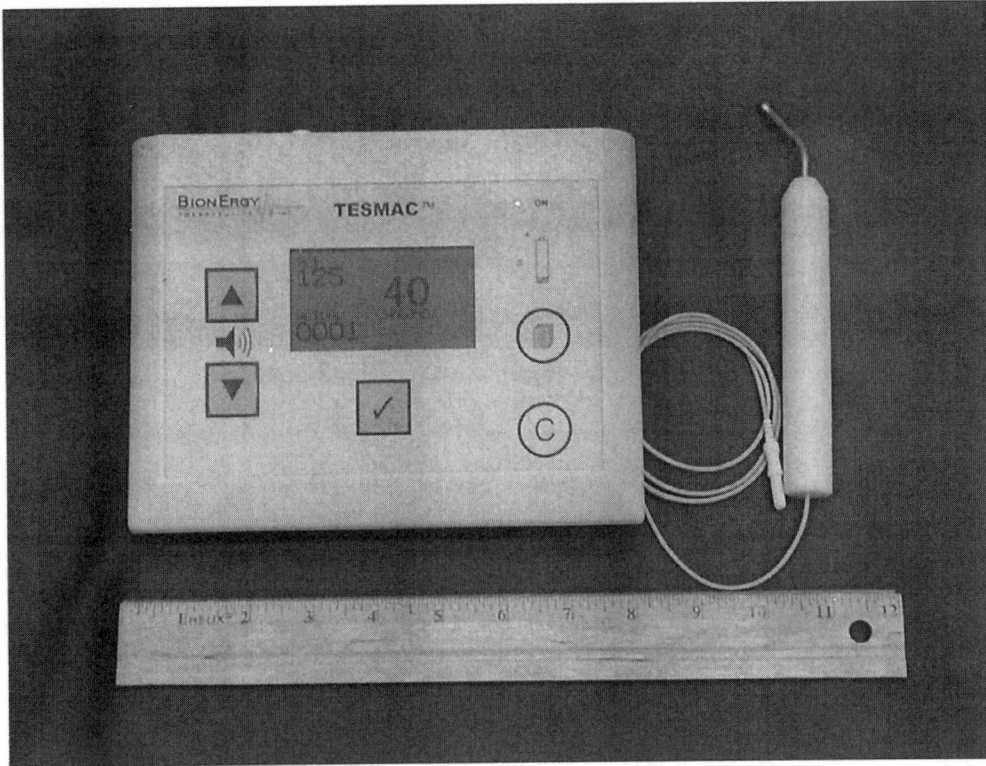

Figure 2 TheraMac device and probe. The above photo depicts the TheraMac device prior to its name change from TESMAC to TheraMac. The BionErgy Therapeutics, Inc. name has now been changed to Acuty Medical, Inc.

be adjusted and reduced to meet the patient's comfort level. In general, when evaluating the therapeutic efficacy of electrotherapeutic devices and their output current levels, more is not necessarily better.

VII. RESULTS

Transcutaneous electrical stimulation of the macula (now designated as *biocurrent therapy*) began with renewed interest and exuberance in 1985. Initial Institutional Review Board (IRB) studies have been completed by Acuity Medical. Phase I FDA trials for TheraMac are now underway in the United States. CE Mark Clearance for TheraMac biocurrent therapy and instrument distribution has been granted in Europe.

The eye color for approximately 50% of the patients treated was blue, 19% had brown eye color, and 18% had hazel eye color. Approximately 50% of the patients treated were in their seventies, 19% were in their sixties and 27% were in their eighties.

The majority of the patients who participated in the initial clinical IRB study noticed positive changes in their vision after treatment. The changes ranged from a decrease in central vision haze to dramatic acuity improvements. Many patients report improvements or recovery of color vision. Of the 808 eyes treated in the first clinical study, 684 (84.7%)

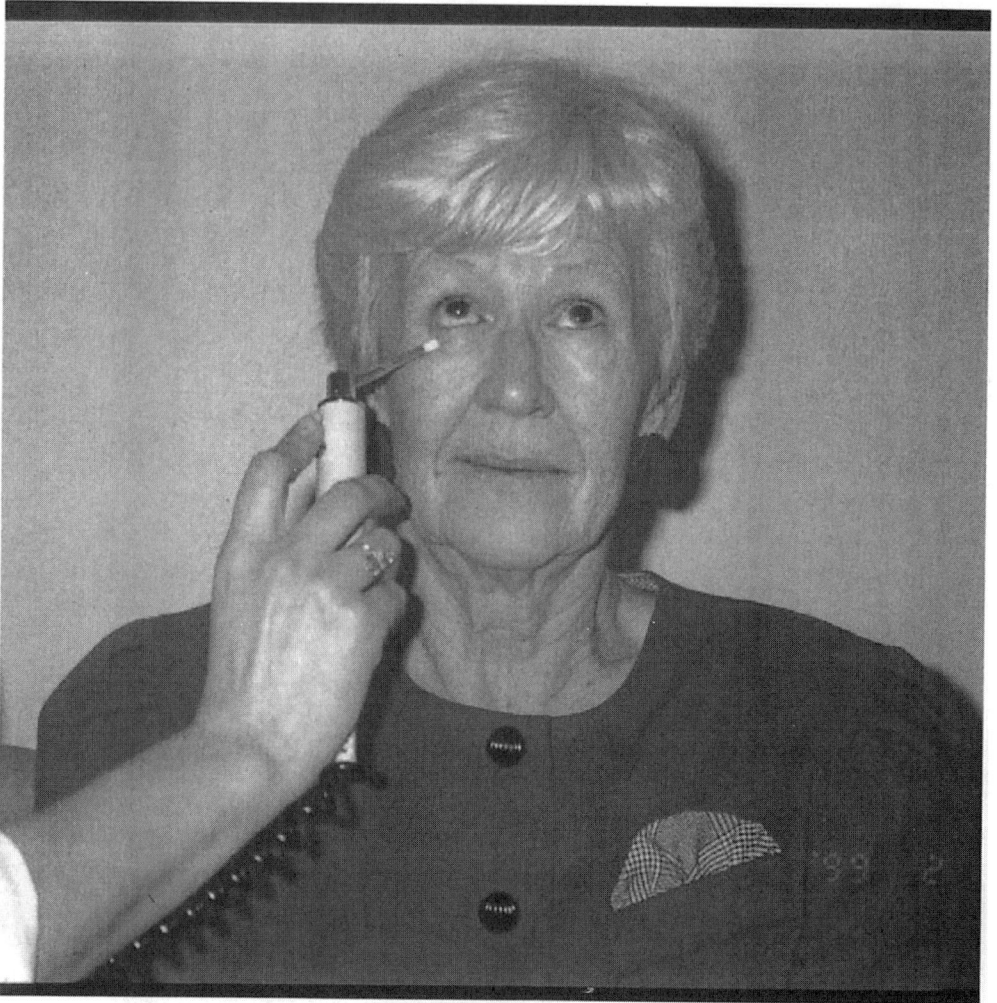

Figure 3 Initiating the TheraMac treatment protocol for a macular degeneration patient. The photo shows the position of the patient's eyes when the probe is placed near the lower orbit of the eye. Normally, during treatment, the eyelids are closed. TheraMac provides a signal to the patient that a particular point has been completed. The probe can then be placed on the next point and the treatment sequence is repeated.

gained one to 19 lines of improvement on the Snellen visual acuity chart. From the standpoint of significant changes in visual acuity, 342 (42.3%) gained 3 to 19 lines of improvement, on the Snellen chart. Approximately 13% of the patients reported no improvement, and only 2% reported further visual deterioration after treatment. Considering the control group (30 patients, 60 eyes, no electrotherapy treatments), 5% exhibited a 1- to 2-line Snellen chart improvement, 20% showed no change in acuity, and 75% exhibited 1- to 10-line Snellen chart losses in visual acuity.

One case report involves a 62-year-old woman who was having difficulty reading small print on the forms that she was required to process at work. She became very distraught and concerned about losing her job because of her vision problems. Her corrected distance visual acuities fluctuated between 20/40 and 20/60, and both maculas were mottled with small to moderate sized drusen. After her first treatment, her corrected distance visual acuities improved to 20/25. With her fourth treatment, her right eye acuity improved to 20/20. However, on the advice of her ophthalmologist, she stopped receiving treatments. Eight months later, her visual acuity had deteriorated to 20/60 in the right eye and 20/80 in the left eye. Alarmed by the dramatic vision loss since her last treatment, she was asked if she would agree to start electrotherapeutic treatment again. She agreed to do this, but she was confused with the negative inputs given by her ophthalmologist. She stated that after taking her ophthalmologists advice, the "visual fog" that used to interfere with her vision returned. After resuming her electrotherapeutic treatments, she reported that the "visual fog" was gone. After five treatments, her corrected acuity improved to 20/25 in her right eye and 20/30 in her left eye. Although she did appear to reacquire most of the visual acuity she lost, it is apparent that her 8-month absence from electrotherapy treatment was not in her best interests.

Some of the most dramatic, and frustrating, electrotherapy treatment results can occur with wet-macular-degeneration patients. After receiving several TheraMac treatments, some wet-macular patients with severe acuity loss improved so much and so fast that they were almost able to read newsprint. Then, after responding so well to electrotherapy, many of them suffer a retinal hemorrhage as the result of a high-blood-pressure event or after taking blood-thinning substances such as the drug coumadin or something as simple as an aspirin. It appears that electrotherapy can be more effective for wet-macular-degeneration patients if they are initially treated with photodynamic therapy (PDT) or transpupilary thermal therapy (TTT). PDT or TTT can help to mitigate the neoplasia problem. Initial treatments with PDT or TTT can control retinal hemorrhaging and reduce the effects that outside substances or cardiovascular problems have in negating the wet-macular-degeneration patient's positive initial responses to electrotherapeutic treatment.

Some of the previously mentioned results were achieved with electrotherapeutic devices that were not designed or optimized for patients with diseases of the visual system. Preliminary results with TheraMac indicate that this device, and the associated protocol, can produce visual improvements for some macular degeneration patients rapidly, sometimes within the first two treatments.

REFERENCES

1. Tielsch JA. Vision problems in the United States: a report on blindness and vision impairment in adults age 40 and older. Prevent Blindness America. Schaumburg, IL: Prevent Blindness America, 1994.
2. Evans J, Wormald R. Is the incidence of registrable age-related macular degeneration Increasing? Br J Ophthalmol 1996; 80:9–14.
3. Fine SL, Berger JW, Maguire MG, Ho AC. Age related macular degeneration. N Engl J Med 2000; 342:483–492.
4. Vingerling JR, Klaver CC, Hofman A, de Jong PT. Epidemiology of age-related Maculopathy. Epidemiol Rev 1995; 17:347–360.
5. Scilley K, Jackson GR, Cideciyan AV, Maguire MG, Jacobson SG, Owsley C. Early Age related maculopathy and self-reported visual difficulty in daily life. Am Acad Ophthalmol 2002; 109:1235–1242.
6. Neftel WB. Galvano-Therapeutics. New York: D. Appleton & Company, 1871.
7. Erb W. Handbook of Electro-Therapeutics. New York: William Wood & Co, 1883.
8. Allen MJ, Jarding JB, Zehner R. Macular degeneration treatment with nutrients and micro current electricity. J Orthomol Med 1998; 13:211–214.

9. Hardy RA. Retina. In: Vaughan D, ed. General Ophthalmology. 15th ed. Stamford, CT: Appleton and Lange, 1999.

10. Holz FG, Wolfensberger TJ, Piguet B. Bilateral macular drusen in age-related macular degeneration: prognosis and risk factors. Ophthalmology 1994; 101:1522–1528.

11. Fine AM, Elman MJ, Ebert JE, Prestia PA, Starr JS, Fine SL. Earliest symptoms caused by neovascular membranes in the macula. Arch Ophthalmol 1986; 104:513–514.

12. Rakoczy PE, Mann K, Cavaney PM, Robertson T, Papadimitreou J, Constable J. Detection and possible functions of a cysteine protease involved in digestion of rod outer segments by retinal pigment epithelial cells. Invest Ophthalmol Vis Sci 1994; 35:4100–4108.

13. Klein ML, Mauldin WM, Stoumbos VD. Heredity and age-related macular degeneration: observations in monozygotic twins. Arch Ophthalmol 1994; 112:932–937.

14. Green WR, Enger C. Age related macular degeneration histopathologic study. Ophthalmology 1993; 100:1519–1535.

15. Allikmets R, Shroyer NF, Singh N, Seddon JM, Lewis RA, Bernstein PS, Peiffer A, Zabriskie NA, Li Y, Hutchinson A, Dean M, Lupski JR, Leppert M. Mutation of the Stargart disease gene (ABCR) in age-related macular degeneration. Science 1997; 277:1805–1807.

16. Hung S, Seddon JM. The relationship between nutritional factors and age-related macular degeneration. In: Bendich A, Deckelbaum RJ, eds. Preventive Nutrition: The Comprehensive Guide for Health Professionals. Totowa, NJ: Humana Press, 1997.

17. Seddon JM, Willett WC, Speizer FE, Hankinson SE. A prospective study of cigarette smoking and age-related macular degeneration in women. JAMA 1996; 276:1141–1146.

18. Macular Photocoagulation Study Group. Laser photocoagulation of subfoveal neovascular lesions in age-related macular degeneration: results of a randomized clinical trial. Arch Ophthalmol 1991; 109:1220–1231.

19. Editor. Eying protons. Scientific American 1999; 275:22.

20. TAP Study Group. Photodynamic therapy of subfoveal choroidal neovascularization in age-related macular degeneration with vertiporfin: two year results of 2 randomized clinical trials. Arch Ophthalmol 1999; 117:1329–1345.

21. Newsome DA, Swartz M, Leone NC, Elston RC, Miller E. Oral zinc in macular degeneration. Arch Ophthalmol 1988; 106:192–198.

22. Gunn RM. On continuous electrical current as a therapeutic agent in atrophy of the optic nerve and in retinitis pigmentosa. Royal London Ophthalmic Hospital Reports 1882; 10:161–192.

23. Derby H. On the possible retardation of retinitis pigmentosa. Am Ophthalmol Soc Trans 1886–1887; 4:217–227.

24. Massey GB. Practical Electrotherapeutics and Diathermy. New York: the Macmillan Company, 1924.

25. Du Bois-Reymond E. Untersuchungen Uber Thierische Elektricitat. Berlin: Reimer, 1860.

26. Barnes TC. Healing rate of human skin determined by the measurement of the electrical potential of experimental abrasions. Am J of Surg 1942; 69:82–88.

27. Nordenström BEW. Biokinetic impacts on structure and imaging of the lung: the concept of biologically closed electric circuits. Am J Roentg 1985; 145:447–467.

28. Becker RO. A method for producing cellular dedifferentiation by means of very small electric currents. Trans NY Acad Sci 1967; 29:606–615.

29. Cheng N, Van Hoof H, Bockn E, Hoogmartens MJ, Mulier J, De Ducker F, Sansen WM, De Loecker W. The effects of electric currents on ATP generation, protein synthesis and membrane transport in rat skin. Clin Ortho and Rel Res 1982; 171:264–271.

30. Huang R, Peng L, Hertz L. Effects of a low-voltage static electric field on energy metabolism in astrocytes. Bioelectromagnetics 1997; 18:77–80.

31. Holian O, Astumian RD, Lee RC, Reyes HM, Attar BM, Walter RJ. Protein Kinase C activity is altered in HL60 cells exposed to 60 Hz AC electric fields. Bioelectromagnetics 1996; 17:504–509.

32. O'Clock GD, Leonard T. In vitro response of retinoblastoma, lymphoma and non-malignant cells to direct current: therapeutic implications. German J Oncol 2001; 33:85–90.

48

Clinical Trials Involving Static Magnetic Field Applications

Agatha P. Colbert

Oregon Center for Complementary and Alternative Medicine, Portland, Oregon, U.S.A.

The chapter reviews the 22 therapeutic trials published in the last two decades in American literature which involve the use of permanent magnets. This chapter shows both positive and negative effects of use of magnetic field generated by permanent magnets. This is very important since the medical community is not very enthusiastic in use of permanent magnets for therapy citing the contradictory discussions around this topic. The author emphasizes on the need of exact evaluation of target location and the parameters of magnetic field this target should receive.

This paper will review 22 therapeutic trials published in the American literature between 1982 and 2002 which evaluated the potential clinical benefits of permanent magnets/static magnetic fields (SMFs). Obstacles encountered when attempting to perform randomized controlled trials in this area of research will be discussed with regard to SMF devices and parameters applied, medical conditions treated, and research designs utilized. Recommendations for more precision in performing and reporting future clinical trials will be made.

I. INTRODUCTION

Widespread public interest in therapy with static magnetic fields (SMF) has advanced more rapidly than the scientific underpinnings needed to validate its mechanism(s) of action. Although magnetic field therapy still lacks a theoretical foundation, empirical evidence substantiating its ability to influence the kinetics of biochemical reactions and tissue growth is accumulating in the basic science as described in previous chapters. The potential therapeutic effects of SMFs on humans are in the early stages of being investigated in controlled clinical trials and reported in pertinent medical and healthcare journals in the United States.

Table 1 Clinical Trials Using Static Magnetic Fields for Chronic Pain Conditions

Author/ year	Number subjects	Diagnosis	Research design	Magnet field strength	Polarity	Exposure time and site application	Results
Hong et al., 1982	52	Neck and shoulder pain	Double-blind, placebo controlled	1300 G	Unspecified	24 h/d × 3 weeks necklace	Both sham and real improved. No statistical difference between groups.
Holcomb et al., 1991	54	Osteoarthritis knee or low back	Randomized double-blind crossover	200 mT (2000 G)	Alternating neg/pos (quadri-polar design)	24 h on back or knee	Statistically significant improvement in pain. No change in sedimentation rate.
Segal et al., 1999	18	Inflammatory arthritis with knee pain	Pilot study no placebo	190 mT (1900 G)	Alternating neg/pos (quadri-polar design)	Continuous × 1 week, 4 points on knee	67% reduction in pain intensity.
Holcomb et al., 2000	2	Chronic abd and genital pain	Case study reports	190 mT (1900 G)	Alternating neg/pos (quadri-polar design)	Low back continuous x > 1 year	Dramatic pain reduction within 10 min of applying.
Segal et al., 2001	64	Knee pain secondary to rheumatoid arthritis	Randomized double-blind	190 mT (1900 G)	Alternating neg/pos (quadri-polar design)	1 week to 4 points around knee	Both reals and controls improve significantly from baseline. No difference between groups.
Collacott et al., 2000	20	LBP × 19 years HNP, radiculopathy DJD, spinal stenosis, spondyl-olisthesis, S/P laminectomy, ankylosing spondylitis fibromyalgia	Randomized double-blind placebo crossover	300 G	Alternating neg/pos	6 h/d, 3 d/week × 1 week to ? low back	Permanent magnet had no effect on low back pain.

Author, Year	N	Condition	Study design	Gauss	Polarity	Application	Results
Valbona et al., 1997	50	Postpolio pain syndrome	Randomized double-blind	300–500 G	Alternating neg/pos	45 min to trigger points	Highly significant improvement 76% of reals vs 19% of shams.
Brown et al., 2000	14	Chronic pelvic pain	Double-blind, placebo controlled	500 G	Unspecified	Abdominal trigger points	No change after 2 weeks. After 4 weeks 60% reals vs. 33% shams improved.
Caselli et al., 1997	34	Plantar heel pain syndrome	Randomized clinical study	500 G	Alternating neg/pos	qd × 4 wks insoles in shoes	Both real and sham improved, but not statistically significant.
Weintraub, 1998	14	Foot pain peripheral neuropathy	Retrospective analysis	475 G	Alternating neg/pos	Insoles worn 24 h/d × 4 months	75% diabetics improved, 50% nondiabetics improved.
Weintraub, 1999	19	Foot pain peripheral neuropathy	Randomized double placebo crossover	475 G	Alternating neg/pos	Insoles worn 24 h/d × 4 months	90% diabetics improved, 33% nondiabetics.
Weintraub et al., 2000		CTS	Single-blind placebo controlled crossover	350 G	Multipolar triangular	carpal tunnel 24 h/d × 1 month	Pain reduction in 57% hands. Progression of electrodiagnostic abnormalities
Carter et al., 2002	30	CTS	Double-blind placebo-controlled	1000 G	Unspecified	Presumed carpal tunnel × 45 min	Significant pain reduction in both groups. No statistical difference between groups.
Colbert et al., 1999	25	Fibromyalgia	Randomized double-blind, placebo controlled	1100 G (surface) (200–600 G to skin)	Negative polarity	Mattress q nightly × 4 months	Statistically significant improvement in pain, ifatigue trigger points, and paindistribution drawings.

Table 1 Continued

Author/ year	Number subjects	Diagnosis	Research design	Magnet field strength	Polarity	Exposure time and site application	Results
Alfano et al., 2001	119	Fibromyalgia	Randomized double-blind, placebo driven	Pad A 3950 G (surface) (6-3 G to target tissue)	Negative polarity	Mattress pad q nightly × 6 months	Statistically significant improvement in pain perception. No significant change in function or trigger point tenderness.
				Pad B 750 G (surface) (33-9 G to target tissue)	Alternating neg/pos	q nightly × 6 months	Reals improved in all measures, but not statistically significant.
Hinman et al., 2002	43	Chronic knee pain	Randomized double-blind, placebo controlled	0.04–0.18 T (400–1800 G)	Negative	0–24 h/d × 2 weeks	Significant improvement in pain physical function and gait.

Table 2 Clinical Trial of Static Magnetic Fields for Wound Healing

Author	Number subjects	Diagnosis	Research design	Magnet field strength	Polarity	Exposure time and site	Results
Man et al., 1999	20	S/P liposuction	Randomized double-blind	150–400 G	Negative polarity	Immediately post-op × 4 days	Statistically significant improvement in pain, edema and ecchymosis.

Table 3 Clinical Trials of Static Magnetic Fields for Sports and Exercise Conditions

Author/year	Number subjects	Diagnosis	Research design	Magnet field strength	Polarity	Exposure time and site application	Results
Borsa et al., 1998	45	Induced muscle microinjury of biceps brachii	Single-blind, placebo controlled	700 G	Alternating neg/pos	Placement at 24 h postinjury for 72 h on biceps	No significant change in pain perception or dysfunction
Chaloupka et al.	35	Strength Improvement	Randomized double-blind crossover	700 G	Unspecified	FDP and FDS then FPB and opponens × 3 min	No increase in muscle strength with either intervention.

Table 4 Clinical Trials of Static Magnetic Fields on Acupuncture Points

Author/year	Number subjects	Diagnosis	Research design	Magnet field strength	Polarity	Exposure time and site application	Results
Colber, 2000	10	Depression	Case series	200 G	Alternating neg/pos connected with ion pumping cords	Sishencong and GV 20 acupoints × 20–40 min, 5–7 times/week × 6–8 weeks or more	Significant improvement in symptoms of depression in 7/10 patients
Liu Shaoxing et al., (1991)	206	Nausea and vomiting postchemotherapy	Clinical observations three-arm trial (magnetic, nonmagnetic diss and point compression)	60 mT (600 G)	Unspecified	6–8 h while receiving IV on acupoint PC 6	Effective in 89% with magnet, in 22% with sham disk, in 0% with point compression
Suen et al.	60	Insomnia	Controlled prospective trial	6.8 mT (68 G)	Negative	3 weeks on ear acupuncture points	Significant improvement in nocturnal sleep time and sleep efficiency

It has been known for some time that a number of phenomena found in living organisms produce subtle but measurable electromagnetic fields (1). These very weak fields emanate from all tissues in the human body and have been quantified by magnetoencephalograms, (2) magnetocardiograms (3), and magnetoretinograms (4).

Although a substantial number of publications have appeared in the European literature documenting the clinical benefits of SMFs, only 22 trials assessing the therapeutic efficacy of static magnetic fields on acupuncture points or other areas of the body have been published in American journals over the last 20 years. Of those identified for scrutiny (5–26) only nine studies were found through the MEDLINE (1960–2002) or CINAHL (1982–2002) databases, using keywords such as *magnet therapy and pain, rehabilitation, permanent magnets, static magnetic fields*, and *magnetism*. It should be noted that this paper will not discuss the numerous clinical trials involving applied electromagnetic fields (EMFs) that have been reviewed by Markov and Colbert in a recent publication (27). The preponderance of studies being examined here were procured from citations in published materials or from presentations at scientific meetings. The novelty of this intervention may account for the fact that many of these clinical trials have been published in somewhat obscure or difficult to find medical or health-related journals. All studies have furnished preliminary findings or pilot data only.

Essential features of the therapeutic trials are summarized in Tables 1 through 4. Clinical improvement in subjects who wore permanent magnets on various parts of their bodies was documented by 15 of the researchers (5,7,11,12,14–16,18,19,21–26). The other seven reported either improvement in both the control and the experimental subjects (8,9,17,20) or no change as a result of SMF application (6,10,13).

The intent of this review, rather than formally critiquing the quality or the methodological strengths and weaknesses of each study, is to provide readers with an overview of current inquiry into magnetic therapy in the United States. It is apparent from this body of literature that

1. Types of magnetic devices and magnetic field dosages being applied vary a great deal.
2. A broad range of medical and healthcare specialists (physicians treating patients with chronic pain syndromes, plastic surgeons, sports medicine experts, physical therapists, podiatrists, and acupuncturists) in the United States are investigating the possible therapeutic benefits of permanent magnets.
3. Patients with diverse, difficult-to-remedy clinical disorders have been effectively treated with SMFs.
4. In many of the studies, the targeted body tissues have not been clearly defined and the actual magnetic fields reaching those tissues have not been precisely documented.
5. Many researchers have reported substantial improvement in patients being treated.
6. No harmful or adverse effects have occurred in any of the clinical trials.

II. ISSUES UNIQUE TO SMF CLINICAL RESEARCH AND PATIENT CARE

A. Polarity, Strength, and Depth of Penetration

Static magnetic fields or permanent magnets for therapeutic use are not at present regulated by the Food and Drug Administration (FDA). Several different types of clinically relevant magnets classified as unipolar, bipolar, multipolar, triangular, and quadipolar are commercially available. All magnets are by nature bipolar, having both a negative and a positive pole usually located on opposite sides. Magnets in therapeutic use should, strictly speaking, be designated *unidirectional* if the configuration of the magnets is such that only one pole is identified on a single surface or *bidirectional* if the magnets are configured in such a way that the magnetic field on a single surface alternates between north and south polarities. A source of misunderstanding comes from the fact that measuring devices indicate a " $+/-$ " magnetic field that does not necessarily correspond to north–south polarity. Gauss meters read $-$ or $+$ depending on the orientation of the measuring probe toward the surface of the magnet. As the probe turns 180° the $-$ reading will become $+$ and vice versa. This has led to some confusion among practitioners who may falsely think that magnetic poles function as electrical charges.

Two opposite nomenclatures are used for identifying south and north poles. The geographic and scientific community names the *south* pole that side of a magnet that rotates toward the geographic south pole when hung freely from a string. Practitioners of bioenergetic medicine on the other hand have designated that same pole *north* and called it *negative* ($-$). These clinicians, particularly acupuncturists, have repeatedly observed different therapeutic effects with the application of north and south magnetic fields, asserting that the side of the magnet that rotates toward the geographic south pole (which they call "north") has a sedating effect and the opposite side of the magnet called *south* a stimulating effect on acupuncture points or areas of the body being treated (28–32). They maintain that their designated "north" pole is more useful in treating painful or "excess" conditions and state that the "south" pole should be applied in conditions of "deficiency," further contending that the south pole is contraindicated for treating infections or cancer. Proponents of the so-called magnetic deficiency syndrome (33) suggest that magnets with alternating polarities best replenish the earth's magnetic field in those people living and working around concrete buildings with heavy steel reinforcements.

Although these claims of north vs. south pole effects have often been repeated in popular books, there are no randomized controlled trials in the peer reviewed scientific literature to authenticate or negate these clinical testimonials. Nor is there any foundation in physics (as of yet) that would support differing biochemical, physiologic, or biologic effects as a result of applying either the north or south poles or both poles of a magnet to the body.

Successful trials have however been reported with the application of unipolar, bipolar, quadipolar, and triangular magnetic arrays (Tables 1–4) Eight of the 13 teams (61%) of researchers applying bidirectional or multidirectional (alternating) magnetic fields found beneficial results in their patients, while all five groups of researchers employing a unidirectional field obtained therapeutic effectiveness in their patient populations. Five researchers (7,9,10,17,21) did not specify the polarity of their magnetic devices. In the two studies involving patients with fibromyalgia, Colbert et al. (11) applied a unidirectional field and found statistically significant improvement in the outcome measures for pain perception and sleep, while Alfano et al. (5) performed a comparison study of a unidirectional and a bidirectional mattress pad. His group found significant improvement only in those subjects sleeping on the unidirectional pad. It is possible that the negative results they observed with the bidirectional pad were due to an insufficient magnetic field reaching the body. A bidirectional magnet with the same manufacturer's gauss rating as a unidirectional magnet has a lower measurable surface field strength.

In addition to ambiguity regarding polarity, the strength of the magnetic field has occasionally been incorrectly measured or inaccurately reported. The strength of a SMF inherent in any particular product is denoted in three ways. The manufacturer's *gauss rating*, a measure of the magnetic field at the core of the magnet is determined by the strength of the electric current used during the manufacturing process. This gauss rating is sometimes quoted by distributors of permanent magnets as the "strength" of a particular magnet, but this description may be misrepresentative and in clinical applications tells us little about the actual dose of magnetic field reaching the target tissue. The *surface field strength*, a more relevant gauge, is the magnetic field measured by a magnetometer probe on the surface of the magnetic device. Of primary importance, however, is the *magnetic field delivered to the target tissue*, which in clinical trials, is usually an estimated value, based on flux density and distance away from the magnet source. To be precise, it is the magnetic field, not the magnet itself, which is the therapeutic agent. Magnetic field intensity declines logarithmically with distance from the source. Misleading information about gauss strength provided by manufacturers and considerable discrepancies between the claimed field flux density of particular commercially available magnets and actual gaussmeter measurements have been reported (34).

The depth of penetration of a SMF, which determines the amount of magnetic flux density reaching the target tissue, depends on the strength, size, volume (bulky or flat), weight, polarity, and configuration of the magnet as well as its distance away from the target tissue. Unlike electric fields, which are stopped at any surface, SMFs are not attenuated or deflected by intervening tissues. All biological tissue including bone, cartilage, muscle, nerve, fat, and other soft tissue are equally transparent to magnetic fields. Unfortunately, very few of the studies have precisely reported either the identity or the depth of the targeted tissue.

B. Types of Magnetic Appliances Used in Clinical Trials

Numerous magnetic appliances are available on the commercial market. In the 22 studies reviewed almost as many different types of magnets varying in size, volume, strength, polarity, and configuration have been tested. In addition to the unidirectional and bidirectional magnets discussed above, researchers have used quadropolar and triangular arrays, concentric circular patterns, and checkerboard alternating poles configurations. Magnetic foil, magnets embedded in $\frac{1}{16}$-in-thick shoe inserts, domino-sized magnets configured in different arrangements in mattress pads, thin magnetic patches that range from 20×30 cm to credit card size, complicated magnetic arrays, and $\frac{1}{6}$-in-thick acumagnets measuring $\frac{1}{8}$ in in diameter have been affixed to various parts of the body. In no studies other than Alfano et al. (5) were products from two different magnet manufacturers compared for greater or lesser efficacy in the same patient population.

C. Health-Related Conditions Treated with SMFs

Medical or health-related conditions for which magnet therapy has been employed also vary widely and will be generally categorized into four major groups. Chronic pain conditions, including neck, shoulder, back, pelvic, abdominal, knee, foot and wrist pain, fibromyalgia, postpolio pain syndrome, carpal tunnel syndrome, and peripheral neuropathy, are the most frequently encountered diagnostic category and include several poorly defined syndromes with unknown etiologies and no clear cut pathological or radiological findings (Table 1).

Wound healing has been successfully managed with EMF application (35) for several years, but the potential benefit of applying a SMF to enhance postoperative wound healing has only recently been evaluated in the United States (Table 2) (18).

A third popular usage for SMFs is in sports or exercise-related activities. Commercially available flexible magnets are being heavily marketed to professional athletes as health and fitness aids. Sports medicine practitioners have a particular interest (both clinical and financial) in determining if magnets are effective in augmenting strength training and reducing the pain perception and recovery time after acute musculoskeletal injuries (Table 3).

Finally, magnets are regularly used in the practice of acupuncture. Permanent magnets are applied to acupuncture points in place of or in addition to needles, especially by practitioners of Japanese style acupuncture. Although several books demonstrate the placement of magnets on acupoints (28–32,36), only three clinical trials have been reported in the American literature. In all three studies therapeutic benefit as a result of applying magnets to acupoints while treating illnesses as diverse as chemotherapy- induced nausea, depression and insomnia has been demonstrated (Table 4).

D. Target Tissues and Site of SMF Application

Although diagnoses were stated in each of the clinical trials, less than half the researchers specified either the nature or the depth of the exact tissue being targeted, i.e., skin, superficial or deep fascia, synovium, tendon, ligament, bone, joint, etc. (5–11,18,20, 23,26)

In almost all disorders of the musculoskeletal system, relevant trigger points contributing to the patient's symptoms can be identified in the muscle or fascial tissue (37,38). The offending trigger points may be some distance from where the patient perceives the pain and not easily identified. If however, these trigger points are detected and successfully deactivated by means of injection, dry needling, massage, ice, or magnet application, the pain is often improved or alleviated entirely. The most statistically significant pain relief ($p <$ 0.0001 for posttreatment pain scores of experimental vs. control groups) evident in these clinical trials was elicited by Valbona et al. (23) who affixed the magnetic patches directly to painful active trigger points. Brown et al.'s patients, (7) also improved when the magnets were applied for 4 weeks to specific abdominal trigger points, related to chronic pelvic pain, with 60% percent of the experimental group and 33% of the control group experiencing a 50% reduction in pain.

Three quarters of Holcomb et al.'s (15) chronic back pain patients' symptoms were attributed to a "musculoskeletal origin" and one quarter were thought to have "neuropathic" pain. With such ill-defined diagnoses, what tissues should be targeted for magnetic field application: nerve, muscle, bone, ligaments, or relevant trigger points? Although these researchers did not explain the rationale for the choice of magnet placement, the site was precisely described and in each case that location corresponded with known trigger and/or acupuncture points. It is likely that the accurate positioning of the magnets contributed considerably to the successful outcomes.

In a case report of two pediatric patients with abdominal and genital pain in whom the correct spinal radicular levels were recognized and site specifically treated both children obtained dramatic relief of symptoms (16). It should also be noted that these two patients required frequent use for up to 2 years before symptoms were completely alleviated. These results suggest that when the correct tissue is targeted with the appropriate strength, SMF subjects derive therapeutic benefit.

Clinicians involved in the care of patients with musculoskeletal disorders are well aware that radiological abnormalities such as degenerative joint disease may be coincidentally present but not the source of the patient's presenting complaints. When the tissue causing the patient's symptoms is not adequately identified, the temptation for practitioners is to either "treat the x-ray findings" or simply place the magnet "where it hurts." The incertitude of this approach is likely to result in less than satisfactory treatment as evidenced in Collacott et al. (13) and Carter et al.'s (9) studies. The former patient population diagnosed with long-standing low back pain had eight different concomitant radiological or clinical diagnoses, any one of which (or none of which) might have contributed to the patients' symptoms. If indeed the source of the patient's complaints was as the author suggested, "degeneration of the 3-joint complex," then the application of a bidirectional 300-G (field strength) magnet was clearly insufficient to reach the depth of those structures. If relevant trigger points (more superficial tissue) had been identified and treated or if a magnet with higher field strength had been applied, the results might have been different.

Attempting to treat the vague medical condition "attributed to carpal tunnel syndrome" (CTS), Carter et al. (9) placed the therapeutic magnet over the wrist at the site of the carpal tunnel despite the absence of any electrodiagnostic or imaging studies confirming compression of the median nerve at that location. Symptoms simulating CTS may be caused by pathology in the forearm, shoulder, or cervical spine, anatomical areas not addressed with this magnetic pad application. Inexplicably both the experimental and control subjects in this study improved.

E. Matching SMFs to a Particular Clinical Disorder

Magnetic field strengths utilized in these studies varied from 68 G to 2000 G. Similar field strengths were used indiscriminately to treat tissues as diverse as the skin and superficial fascia of postoperative wounds, acupoints, intermediate level myofascial tissue such as trigger points and plantar fascia, as well as the deeper tissues involved in degenerative joint disease and carpal tunnel syndrome. Only two research groups (5,11) estimated the field strengths being delivered to their targeted tissues, and these ranged from 7 G to 600 G.

The choice of magnetic field strength is often based on information available from the manufacturer. Basic laboratory science studies have found evidence of an effective biological window between 45 and 50 mT (450–500 G) (39). An obvious question arises as to whether the same in vitro dosimetry applies to clinical situations involving whole human organisms. That query will only be answered as more clinical trials are performed. If 200–600 G turns out to be the correct dosage to be delivered to the target tissues, the identity and exact three-dimensional location of targeted tissues must be more precisely defined in order to apply the appropriate strength magnetic field.

F. Dosing Regimens

Not only where a magnet is positioned but whether the application should be continuous or intermittent, how long it should be left in place, and when in the course of the illness it should be applied are being determined in a trial-and-error fashion based on the personal experience of clinicians and reports of other practitioners. To simulate the typical method in which patients are managed in a clinical setting, Hinman et al. (14) asked their subjects to wear the magnetic device until they noticed pain relief, then remove it and document in a diary the daily frequency and duration of usage. The authors found, however, that when patients achieved a satisfactory level of pain control, they were reluctant to remove the magnet and kept it in place almost continuously for the entire 2-week trial period. Conversely, subjects in the control group finding no relief, removed and replaced their magnets intermittently.

Weintraub (24,25) had successful outcomes in 75% and 90% of his diabetic patients after treating their peripheral neuropathy 24 h/day × 4 months. Less impressive were his results with patients who had a nondiabetic peripheral neuropathy treated for that same period of time (Table 1). Positive results were demonstrated by Colbert et al. (11) and Alfano et al. (5), who treated their fibromyalgia patients nighttime only for 4 and 6 months, respectively, using the unidirectional magnet. Valbona et al. (23) chose 45 min as the trial time for treating active trigger points with excellent results (highly significant improvement in 75% of the experimental subjects and 19% improvement in the control group), while

Carter et al. (9), choosing the same time period to treat presumed CTS found no significant difference in outcome between the experimental group and the control group. In the other carpal tunnel syndrome study (27) patients were required to wear magnetic wrist bands 24 h/day for 1 month, and 57% of the involved hands showed significant pain relief despite the fact that their electrodiagnostic abnormalities continued to worsen. Magnetic therapy practitioners who routinely treat CTS recommend regular nighttime application of magnets for periods of 2–4 weeks before patients notice improvement.

One group of researchers (10) applied magnets for a remarkably short time period planning to refute or substantiate the claims of a sales representative who stated that the 3-min application of a magnet could increase strength in muscles of the hand and forearm. Predictably, the results of this study were negative.

From experience clinicians know that many chronic disorders require prolonged magnetic application (weeks to months) before the beneficial effects become obvious. When performing a controlled trial the time period for wearing the magnet is often necessarily shortened to meet rigorous research methodological requirements with a resultant compromise in the integrity of the therapeutic intervention. In order to conveniently monitor patients with chronic back pain during magnet application, Collacott et al. (13) treated their patients only 3 times/week in 6-h sessions for a total of 18 h. It is quite likely that in this study, not only was the target tissue inappropriate and the magnetic field strength inadequate but the duration of application was a mismatch for the chronicity of the ailment.

During the acupuncture studies patients wore their magnets on selected acupoints for extended periods of time. Patients being treated for nausea and vomiting were requested to wear magnets on PC 6 (a wrist acupoint) for 6–8 h while chemotherapy was being administered (21). Colbert's patients wore scalp acu-magnets for the treatment of depression for periods of 20–40 min daily, 5–7 times/week for a minimum of 6–8 weeks and a maximum of 2 years (12). On that regimen, seven of 10 patients gained significant subjective improvement of their depressive symptoms. The Suen et al. group (22) left magnetic pearls on ear acupoints for a total of 3 weeks (removing and replacing the pearls to alternate ears every 3 days in order to avoid possible skin breakdown) and reported significantly improved sleep in their elderly patient population.

How soon after an injury is it safe and efficacious to apply the magnetic field? Borsa et al. (6) applied magnets 24 h after inducing a microinjury in the biceps brachii and found no difference in outcome between the experimental and control groups. Man et al. (18) in contrast, treated their patients immediately postoperatively and kept the pads in place over the lipectomized area for a total of 4 days. These patients experienced statistically significant decreases in pain, ecchymosis, and edema compared to the control group. Would the Borsa et al. results have been different if the magnet had been applied immediately, rather than 24 h after the injury?

G. Research Design Problems

Randomized double-blind controlled trials comparing outcomes in control and experimental groups are the gold standard required by the National Institutes of Health (NIH) and the FDA when performing clinical research. Unlike the relatively straightforward placebo or so-called sugar pill used in pharmaceutical trials, finding the appropriate control or sham appliance in SMF trials poses some problems. Either a demagnetized or a never magnetized device, similar in every other way to the experimental device has been used in most trials. However, subjects can easily test whether they have the real or sham appliance. Unless observed for the entire duration of wearing their magnets as in the Valbona et al. study (23), it is impossible to assure participant blinding (masking). To circumvent this hurdle, one group of researchers (20) created what they termed a *sham* magnet system with a lower surface field strength than the experimental device (72 mT compared to 190 mT). Both the experimental and the control subjects in this study, however, improved. It is quite likely that this "sham" device with a field strength of 720 G, placed precisely on the four acupuncture points used to treat arthritis of the knee, elicited a positive therapeutic effect.

Debate about placebo effect continues among researchers of complementary and alternative medicine (CAM) as they try to account for the regularly seen 40% or more improvement in the "control" group of subjects who are given special attention by simply being asked to be part of a research protocol. This placebo effect is particularly high among patients treated by alternative medical practitioners (40). One group of researchers (17) told all subjects they were receiving the active device which could have enhanced the placebo effect evidenced by both groups showing similar improvement. During three other clinical trials (8,9,20) subjects in both the control and the experimental groups improved and maintained that status at follow-up. Was this a placebo effect? It is difficult to say, but when the placebo effect and its contrary, the *nocebo effect* (occurring when patients are led to believe they have an inactive device) muddy the waters, it becomes even more problematic to perform and interpret the requisite FDA and NIH randomized controlled, blinded clinical trials.

An additional consideration when researching magnetic fields is the need for complicated and costly long term follow-up studies. Of the studies reviewed only the Colbert et al. report (12) on treating depression and Holcomb et al. (16) case study of two pediatric patients have up to a 2-year follow-up. Both groups of authors were able to demonstrate consistent long-lasting benefit when patients wore their magnetic appliances for extended periods of time.

It is particularly noteworthy when compared with the high incidence of adverse reactions associated with pharmaceuticals (41), that in none of the 22 studies were harmful effects as a result of exposure to magnetic fields detected.

III. CONCLUSION AND RECOMMENDATIONS FOR FUTURE CLINICAL TRIALS

The positive outcomes evident in two thirds of the clinical trials reviewed (Table 4) are encouraging to practitioners, patients, and potential researchers. However, if future trials are to be clinically meaningful and scientifically reproducible certain stringent criteria with regard to research methodology and interventions used must be implemented. Each research protocol should assess only one homogeneous medical or health-related condition with a clearly identified target tissue. The anatomic location of this tissue or organ must be defined and the precise site of external application of the magnetic device described with estimated distance from target tissue.

The SMFs being delivered to the target tissue ought to be documented in terms of magnetic configuration, strength, and polarity. Although more pilot data needs to be gathered to determine when in the course of an illness or after an injury SMFs are best applied, it appears that the closer to the onset of injury or illness is better than 24 h after the fact. Until substantially more evidence is acquired, the choices for duration and frequency of exposure to SMFs should be based on information from knowledgeable practitioners accustomed to treating the selected medical condition.

Lastly, the issue of applying a sham device and masking subjects must be dealt with directly. Research funding agencies such as the NIH and potential publishers of peer reviewed journals must be willing to accept in clinical trials of magnet therapy the same criteria used in randomized surgical trials. When an intervention as obvious as a surgical procedure or an active magnet is used, a suitable sham does not exist, and it is almost impossible to keep the subjects blinded. A far more relevant research design is the outcome study in which a control group of patients are placed on a waiting list while the experimental group receives an active treatment. Although the patients are aware they are receiving a treatment, the examiners and/or evaluators must be blinded as to patient group assignment. After a suitable time period the outcomes between groups are compared and the wait-listed group is then offered treatment. This methodology more closely simulates the everyday practice of magnetic therapy and will certainly provide much more clinically meaningful and therapeutically useful information.

REFERENCES

1. Cohen D, Yoram P, Cuffin BN, Schmid SJ, eds. Magnetic Fields Produced by Steady Currents in the Body. Proc Nat Acad Sci USA 1970; 77:1447–1451.
2. Reite M, Zimmerman JE, Edrich J, Zimmerman J. The human magnetoencephalogram: some EEG and related correlations. Electroencephalogr Clin Neurophysiol 1976; 40:59–66.
3. Saarinen M, Siltanen P, Karp PJ, Katila TE. The normal magnetocardiogram: I Morphology. Ann Clin Res 1978; 10(suppl 21):1–43.
4. Armstrong RA, Janday B. A brief review of magnetic fields from the human visual system. Ophthalmic Physiol Opt 1989; 9:299–301.
5. Alfano AP, Taylor AG, Foresman PA, Dunkl PR, McConnell GG, Conaway MR, Gillies GT. Static magnetic fields for treatment of fibromyalgia: a randomized controlled trial. J Complementary and Alternative Med 2001; 7:53–64.
6. Borsa PA, Liggett MS. Flexible magnets are not effective in decreasing pain perception and recovery time after muscle microinjury. J Athletic Training 1998; 33:150–155.
7. Brown CS, Parker N, Ling F, Wan J. Effects of magnets on chronic pelvic pain. Obstet Gynecol 2000; 95(suppl 1):S29.
8. Caselli MA, Clark N, Lazarus S, Velez Z, Venegas L. Evaluation of magnetic foil and PPT insoles in the treatment of heel pain. J Am Podiatric Med Assoc 1997; 87:11–16.
9. Carter R, Aspy CB, Mold J. The effectiveness of magnet therapy for treatment of wrist pain attributed to carpal tunnel syndrome. J Fam Pract 2002; 51:38–40.
10. Chaloupka EC, Kang J, Mastrangelo MA. The effect of flexible magnets on hand muscle strength: a randomized, double-blind study. J Strength Cond Res 2002; 16:33–37.
11. Colbert AP, Markov MS, Banerji M, Pilla AA. J Back Musculoskeletal Rehabil 1999; 13:19–31.
12. Colbert AP. Magnets on Sishencong and GV 20 to treat depression: Clinical observations in 10 patients. Medical Acupuncture spring/Summer 2000; 12:20–24.
13. Collacott EA, Zimmerman JT, White DW, Rindone JP. Bipolar permanent magnets for the treatment of chronic low back pain: a pilot study. JAMA 2000; 283:1322–1324.
14. Hinman MR, Ford J, Heyl H. Effects of static magnets on chronic knee pain and physical function: a double-blind study. Alternative Therapies 2002; 8:50–55.
15. Holcomb RR, Parker RA, Harrison MS. Biomagnetics in the treatment of human pain-past, present, future. Envir Med 1991; 8:24–60.
16. Holcomb RR, Worthington WB, McCullough BA, McLean MJ. Static magnetic field therapy for pain in the abdomen and genitals. Pediatric Neurol 2000; 23:261–264.
17. Hong CZ, Lin JC, Bender LF, Schaeffer JN, Meltzer RJ, Causin P. Magnetic necklace: its therapeutic effectiveness on neck and shoulder pain. Arch Phys Med Rehabil 1982; 63:462–466.
18. Man D, Man B, Plosker H. The influence of permanent magnetic field therapy on wound healing in suction lipectomy patients: a double-blind study. Plast Reconstr Surg 1999; 104:2261–2266.

19. Segal N, Huston J, Fuchs H, Holcomb R, McLean MJ. Efficacy of a static magnetic device against knee pain associated with inflammatory arthritis. J Clin Rheumatol 1999; 5:302–305.

20. Segal NA, Toda Y, Huston, Saeki Y, Shimizu M, Fuchs H, Shimaoka Y, Holcomb R, McLean MJ. Two configurations of static magnetic fields for treating rheumatoid arthritis of the knee: a double-blind clinical trial. Arch Phys Med Rehabil 2001; 82:1453–1460.

21. Liu S, Chen Z, Hou J, Wang J, Wang J, Zhang X. Magnetic disk applied on Neiguan point for prevention and treatment of cisplatin-induced nausea and vomiting. J Trad Chin Med 1991; 11:81–183.

22. Suen LKP, Wong TKS, Leung AWN. Auricular therapy using magnetic pearls on sleep: a standardized protocol for the elderly with insomnia. Clin Acup Oriental Med 2002; 3:39–50.

23. Vallbona C, Hazlewood CF, Jurida G. Response of pain to static magnetic fields in postpolio patients: a double blind pilot study. Arch Phys Med Rehabil 1997; 78:1200–1203.

24. Weintraub MI. Chronic submaximal magnetic stimulation in peripheral neuropathy: Is there a beneficial therapeutic relationship? Am J Pain Manag 1998; 8:12–16.

25. Weintraub MI. Magnetic bio-stimulation in painful diabetic peripheral neuropathy: a novel intervention–a randomized, double-placebo crossover study. Am J Pain Manag 1999; 9:8–17.

26. Weintraub MI, Cole SP. Neuromagnetic treatment of pain in refractory carpal tunnel syndrome: an electrophysiological and placebo analysis. J Back Musculoskel Rehabil 2002; 15:77–82.

27. Markov MS, Colbert AP. Magnetic and electromagnetic field therapy. J Back Musculoskel Rehabil 2001; 15:17–29.

28. Santwani MT. Magnetotherapy for Common Diseases. Delhi: Hind Pocket Books, 1992.

29. Birla GS, Hemlin C. Magnet Therapy: The Gentle & Effective Way to Balance Body. Rochester, VT: Healing Arts Press, 1999.

30. Schiegl H. Healing Magnetism. London: Century, 1987.

31. Matsumoto K, Birch S. Hara Diagnosis: Reflections on the Sea. Brookline: Paradigm Press, 1988.

32. MA, Manaka Y, Itaya K, Birch S. Chasing the Dragon's Tail. Brookline: Paradigm Press, 1995.

33. Nakagawa K. Magnetic field-deficient syndrome and magnetic treatment. Japan Med J 1976; 2745:24–32.

34. Blechman AM, Oz M, Nair V, Ting W. Discrepancy between claimed field flux density of some commercially available magnets and actual gaussmeter measurements. Alternative Therapies 2001; 7:92–95.

35. Markov MS. Electric Current and Electromagnetic field effects on soft tissue: Implications for wound healing. WOUNDS 1995; 7:94–110.

36. Rose P. The Practical Guide to Magnet Therapy. New York: Sterling, 2001.

37. Travell JG, Simons DG. Myofascial Pain and Dysfunction The Trigger Point Manual Vols 1 & 2. Baltimore: Williams and Wilkins, 1983.

38. Baldry PE. Acupuncture, Trigger Points and Musculoskeletal Pain. 2d ed. Edinburgh: Churchill Livingston, 1993.

39. Markov MS.

40. Kaptchuk TJ. The placebo effect in alternative medicine: can the performance of a healing ritual have clinical significance? Ann Intern Med 2004; 136:817–825.

41. Lazarou J, Pomeranz BH, Corey PN. Incidence of adverse drug reactions in hospitalized patients: a meta-analysis of prospective studies. JAMA 1998; 279:1200–1205.

49

Pain-Free and Mobility-Free Magnetic Force in Orthodontic Therapy

Abraham M. Blechman

Columbia University, New York, New York, U.S.A.

The author reviews the applications of permanent magnets as an alternative to mechanical forces used to move teeth through bone by generating bone remodeling. The original US patent describing the possibility to use magnetic force was awarded to Dr. Blechman in 1967, but the actual application did not start until 1978. At about this time several papers reported successful use of permanent magnets in orthodontics. In this chapter Dr. Blechman reported not only his own experience, but discusses the importance of proper use of magnets mainly in respect to their composition and characterization of such important parameters as magnetization and magnetic flux density. The advantages of using magnetics are described in this chapter.

The relationship between static magnetic and time-varying electromagnetic fields is becoming more clarified as much more importance has been attributed to the magnetic component of the time-varying field. This chapter will amplify the therapeutic similarities between both types of fields.

I. INTRODUCTION

Noninvasive pulsed electromagnetic fields (PEMF) were introduced successfully to orthopedics during the 1970s to stimulate an accelerated osteogenic rate via time-varying inductive coupling to enhance the healing of delayed union or nonunion of long bone fractures. Bassett, Pilla, and Ryaby at Electrobiology, Inc. developed and manufactured this device, which is still available today with considerable improvement (1).

Stark and Sinclair reported in 1987 that their study "suggested that it was possible to increase the rate of orthodontic tooth movement and bone deposition through the application of a noninvasive, pulsed electromagnetic field." Although this was interesting corroborative information, with regard to similar static magnetic field properties, as will be discussed later, this device was extremely clinically impractical because it required lengthy immobilization of the patient's head between the two Helmholtz coils that generated inductive time-varying magnetic fields (2).

Finally, it was demonstrated that static magnetic fields possessed osteogenic properties similar to inductive coupling. In 1995, Darendeliler et al. showed that "both the static magnetic fields produced by (repelling) samarium-cobalt magnets and the pulsed electromagnetic field (PEMF) used in combination with the coil spring were successful in increasing the rate of tooth movement over that produced by the coil spring alone. Both magnetically stimulated groups also showed increases in both the organization and amount of new bone deposited in the area of tension between the orthodontically moved maxillary incisors" (3). This constitutes further confirmation of the bioeffects of the $Sm_2 Co_{17}$ magnets.

Previously further evidence of the osteogenic capability of static magnetic fields was cited in 1987 in two Russian articles; 5–50 mT (50–500 G) were used to accelerate human fracture repair and limb lengthening (4,5).

Golyakhovsky, a Russian orthopedic surgeon on the faculty at the Hospital for Joint Diseases, Orthopedic Institute in New York City, discussed his experiences in 1976 using permanent magnets (static fields) for the treatment of fresh long bone fractures: "Thus permanent magnetic fields of preset parameters promote fragment revascularization earlier with more intensive expansion of vessels into the emergent regenerate and early actuation of the mechanisms of corticogenic osteogenesis" (6). During the treatment of diaphyseal tibial fractures, use of 100–150 oersteds static magnetic fields, Golyakhovsky reported, "Thus the earlier disappearance of the swelling, the higher circulation temperature coefficient, the earlier disappearance of the spastic syndrome, and normalization of the microvascular tension as well as the higher increase in the blood oxygenation rate, all indicates the beneficial effect of magnetotherapy on peripheral circulation." All this "boosted the regenerative capacity of the bone tissue" (7).

In 1991 Holcomb et al. described a four magnet alternating pole device, called a *magna block appliance*, that was reported to reduce low back and knee pain (8). Because of the short-circuiting effect of alternating fields so close to each other, adequate tissue penetration could be challenged. Using the same four-magnet array, in 1995 McLean et al. (9) and Cavopol et al. (10) suggested that a field gradient of 15 G/mm caused an approximate 80% action potential blockade. Field strength alone could not account for this blockade, according to the investigators.

Mainly permanent magnetic fields will be discussed in this chapter, and very little on electrically driven AC fields. Selection of the appropriate permanent magnet and static magnetic field for the desired clinical application, which is usually an open-circuit, nonionizing design, has never been adequately discussed. One choice is over-the-counter commercially available static magnets promoted and marketed vigorously to the public for health maintenance and the treatment of musculoskeletel discomforts and other conditions. Another more sophisticated choice is designing and ordering static permanent magnets from a manufacturer whose main business involves magnets used for industrial applications, such as motors and recording equipment. Unfortunately, the areas delineated by these two choices are riddled with confusion. There is no protocol universally agreed on for testing and characterizing magnets used in medical applications.

To illustrate these problems, five over-the-counter commercially available magnets from different suppliers were tested by Blechman et al. for field flux density, a measurement of magnetic dosage, and it was discovered that these suppliers were not providing reliable information. Measured on the magnet surface, significant discrepancy was demonstrated between field flux density claimed by these suppliers and actual gaussmeter measurements, which were often 10 times lower (11). Therefore, it was necessary for the investigator to confirm the flux density with his own gaussmeter. This problem was intensified when the supplier provided little or no technical information about the magnet.

Another source of confusion were clinical reports in the medical and dental literature that were oversimplified and provided insufficient technical information about the magnet. Absent were parameters such as chemical and physical composition of the magnetic material, the energy product, $(BH)_{max}$, the remanance and coercivity, and any other pertinent information derived from the second quadrant of the hysteresis curve. Almost always the flux density at the target area requiring treatment is not provided, nor is the target area precisely identified.

All this confusion contributes to causing clinical replication of published reports to be impossible. A situation such as that just described would never be tolerated for a pharmaceutical agent. An attempt to correct these deficiencies occurred in the following orthodontic applications of magnetic force.

II. ORTHODONTIC BACKGROUND

In traditional conventional nonmagnetic orthodontic therapy, mechanical forces are used to move teeth through bone, by generating bone remodeling. Biomechanical forces, generated by wires, springs, and elastics, are applied to teeth that then transduce the force that initiates movement and consequently produces localized inflammation in the periodontal ligament. (The periodontal ligament attaches teeth to the surrounding alveolar bone.) This results in stimulation of cellular activity in the periodontal ligament that provokes osteoclastic bone resorption in the direction the teeth are moved and incites osteoblasts, also in the periodontal ligament, that cause bone deposition to occur on the opposite side, the direction from which teeth are moved. This force stimulates the release of various cytokines and incites the deformation of the cytoskeleton of various cells in the periodontal ligament, such as fibroblasts. Force also deforms alveolar bone that surrounds the teeth, generating the transduced piezoelectric effect that is also responsible for bone remodeling.

One very important example of orthodontic movement, derived from the force, that utilizes the information presented above, is maxillary and mandibular molar distalization (upper and lower molar posterior movement). This procedure is the first, most important, and most difficult step in the treatment of common orthodontic malocclusions. Conventional force modalities for this application, such as head gear, Class II elastics or coil springs always cause mobility of the moving teeth, which is attributable to the fact that bone resorption is more rapid than bone deposition. Since the alveolar tooth socket is then temporarily enlarged, tooth mobility ensues. Ultimately normal osteogenesis returns the bony architecture to normal and firm stability results, as part of the remodeling process. Force application is reactivated approximately once a month (usually over a 2 year period) to continue orthodontic treatment. During the mobility phase, pain results since chewing on mobile teeth gives rise to this pain. The localized inflammation in the periodontal ligament that results from force application also contributes to the pain, which is mediated by several factors, including the peptide Substance P.

III. MAGNETIC APPLICATION

The original U.S. patent describing magnetic force in orthodontic therapy was awarded to Blechman in 1967. In 1978 Blechman reported the development of several magnetic devices for orthodontic application (12), which were later modified and miniaturized. These newer designs, described later, form the subject of this chapter (13).

Substituting permanent magnetic force for conventional force modalities has many advantages, attributable to the bioeffect of the magnetic field. However, choosing the correct magnet was critical for its successful use.

One possible material choice was neodymium–iron–boron ($Nd_2Fe_{14}B$), which featured very high saturation polarizations and high magnetic anisotropy, similar to Sm_2Co_{17} but greater magnitudes. Its energy product varied from 28 to 53 MGOe (225–415 kJ/m^3), remanence varied from 10.8 to 14.7 kG or 1.08–1.47 T, and coercivity varied from 10.4 to 11.5 kOe. Similar parameters for Sm_2Co_{17} were energy product varying from 20 to 30 MGOe (160–240 kJm^3), remanence varied from 9.0 to 11.2 kG (0.90–1.12 T) and coercivity varied from 8.3 to 9.2 kOe). However, the preferred magnetic material for this orthodontic application was samarium cobalt (Sm_2Co_{17}—not $SmCo_5$). For this application the chosen energy density or energy product (BH) $_{max}$ equaled 26 MGOe or 210 kJ/m^3, remanence was 10.5 kG or 1.05 T, and coercivity (H_{cB}) is 9.0 kOe—all at room temperature (20°C) (14). Extremely important was the field flux density measured at the target area, not just at the magnet surface. This information should be accurately specified. In this application, 270 G was measured on the magnet surface, but 25 G was measured at the target area, which was the periodontal ligament and alveolar bone on the mesial side of the moving molar. The magnets were positioned close to this target area and maintained a constant distance to the molar as it moved distally.

Sm_2Co_{17} was chosen for several reasons. It provided the ideal orthodontic force level, whereas $Nd_2Fe_{14}B$ was characterized by excessive undesirable force for the intended application. The high Fe content of the latter material also predisposed it to easy corrosion even when adequately protectively coated, and it was particularly vulnerable because it had to function in a wet environment, i.e., the oral cavity. The Co content of Sm_2Co_{17} protected this magnet from excessive corrosion but was coated regardless to be completely biologically safe for the geometric shape used. Parylene C, a biocompatible polymer, was employed as the protective coating.

Full magnetization to saturation by the manufacturer is a precondition for achieving the desired clinical results. Careful attention must be given to the hysteresis curve to ensure that the working point of the magnet is sufficiently above the "knee" of the B(H)-demagnetization curve in the second quadrant.

IV. MAGNETS FOR ORTHODONTIC APPLICATION

Blechman designed the magnetic configuration shown in Figs. 1 and 2 (14). The posttreatment views of repelling magnets shows space generated between the first molar and second premolar resulting from distal movement of the first molar.

Four miniature magnets, two on each side, cylindrical in shape with the following parameters were arranged in repulsion, sliding on a common stainless steel (nonmagnetic) thin-diameter round wire (0.016 in.): SM_2Co_{17} cylinder 3.5 mm in. diameter, 3 mm thick (parallel to the direction of magnetization), 0.5 mm hole in the center of both magnets parallel to the 3 mm thickness, to accommodate the 0.016-in. wire for sliding. The 3 mm thickness dimension was encased by a thin (0.5 mm) stainless steel (316L) sleeve that prevented chipping of the corners since the material was quite brittle. The entire assembly (magnet plus sleeve) was coated by another thin layer (0.25 mm) of a biocompatible polymer-parylene C, to prevent leachout products. Finally, the force generated by the

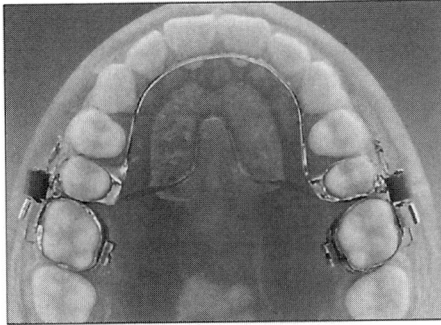

(a)

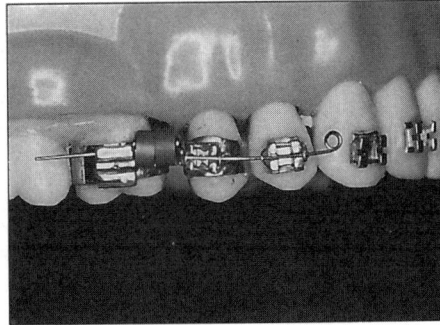

(b)

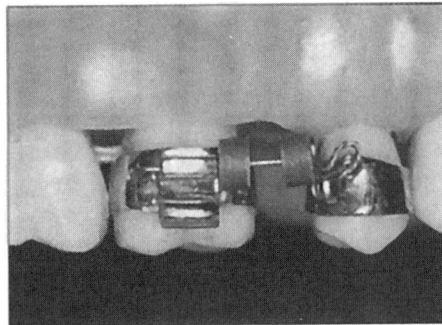

(c)

Figure 1 (a) Shows one pair repelling magnets positioned bilaterally. (b) Shows a buccal view of the initial insertion position. (c) Shows the buccal view of repelling magnets generating space between the first maxillary molar and second premolar. *Source*: Ref. 14.

repelling magnets in contact with each other equaled 160 g. This was sufficient force to distalize maxillary or mandibular first and second molars simultaneously. When conventional force was used, 300–350 g of force was required to accomplish the identical procedure.

Two repelling magnets were temporarily clamped together to prevent loss. Each pair was bilaterally (left and right sides) mounted on the 0.016-in. wire that was inserted distally into buccal steel tubes prewelded to bands cemented on the first maxillary molars. (Maxillary molars were distalized more often than mandibular molars.) The mesial end of the 0.016-in. wire was ligated to the bracket on the first or second premolar bands with steel ligature wires and then simultaneously activated with other steel wires to bring the repelling magnets into total contact. Release of the maximum repelling force was then accomplished by removing the clamp that held the magnets temporarily together on each side.

While the repelling magnets generated a distal or posterior force to move the maxillary molars distally (to provide space into which the maloccluded anterior teeth could be moved), an equal and opposite reactive force from the magnets tended to move the premolars undesirably anteriorly. To control and prevent this a Nance-type palatal acrylic anchorage connected to the premolars was used (14).

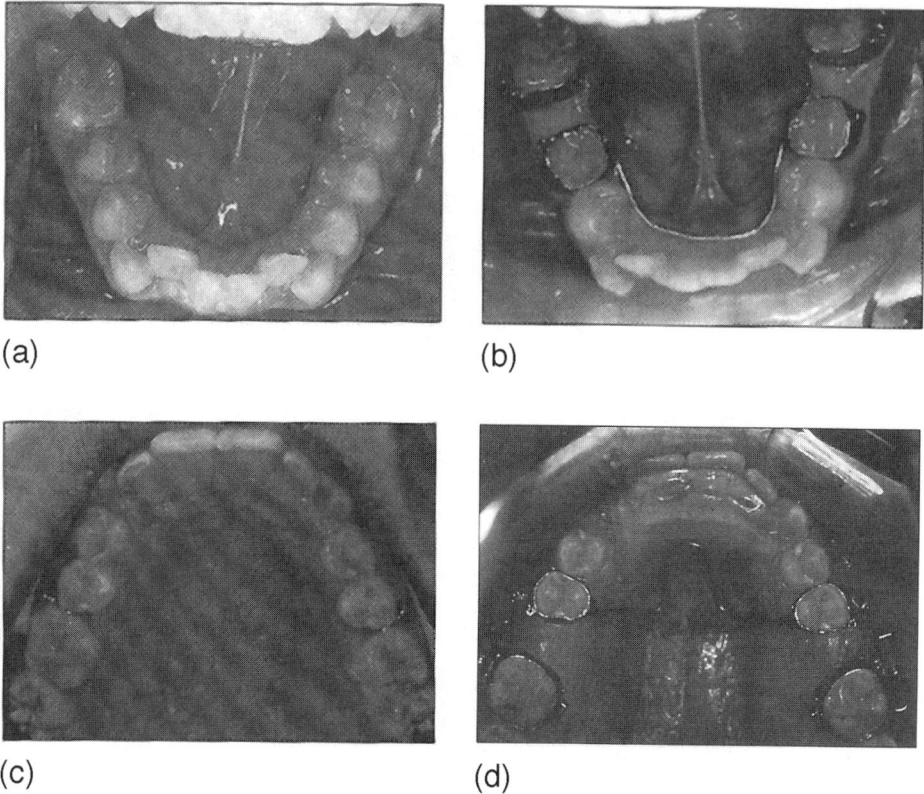

Figure 2 Shows the occlusal view of magnetic pretreatment and posttreatment in the maxilla and mandible. (a) Shows mandibular pretreatment; (b) shows mandibular posttreatment; (c) shows maxillary pretreatment; (d) shows maxillary posttreatment. *Source*: Ref. 14.

V. PARAMETERS RESPONDING TO BIOMAGNETIC FIELD

Alveolar bone remodeling occurred in response to the distally directed magnetic force on the maxillary molars. As the molars moved distally the air gap between the repelling magnets increased, diminishing the force, and required that once a month the steel ligature wires needed to be tightened to bring the repelling magnets into contact again. The magnetic force decayed in accord with the inverse square law. This procedure was repeated until there was sufficient distalization.

One of the advantages of using magnetic force is rapid movement (2 mm/month) without the need for patient cooperation in applying force, thereby shortening treatment. Without the total dependence on patient compliance for applying conventional force, successful treatment fails or lasts for unacceptably long duration with attendant problems. Since magnetic force became available, other designs were developed that do not depend on patient compliance for force application, however, they all continue to use conventional force modalities. Because of this, conventional pain and mobility persist. Rapid movement under conventional force conditions often results in excessive tooth mobility, indicating severe alveolar bone resorption. With magnetic force, mobility is absent, even with rapid movement. A decreased bone resorptive rate cannot account for this lack of mobility because the teeth are moving more rapidly than with conventional force. An increased osteogenic rate that (at least) -matches the bone resorptive rate is the only reasonable explanation.

Interestingly, the magnetic field that generated the force for movement, simultaneously provides the field for an accelerated rate of osetogenisis of the alveloar bone surrounding the moving teeth. Perturbation, altering the local equilibrium, is a necessary activating factor, and accelerated healing are both supplied by the identical magnetic fields simultaneously and bilaterally. Since mobility causes pain, particularly during chewing, magnetic fields also contribute to pain reduction. Magnetic fields also act as anti-inflammatory agents, possibly by increasing vascularity, and this aids in pain reduction because a localized inflammatory reaction in the periodontal ligament always occurs in response to force application. Direct magnetic field effect also seem to occur on the biochemistry of the inflammatory response via the radical pair mechanism—as potential antioxidants. This is the first time in orthodontic therapy that a nonpharmaceutical agent has been able to control both pain and mobility.

This accelerated osteogenic component of the magnetic force hypothesis was then tested in vitro. Employing rabbit calvaria osteoblastlike progenitor cells in tissue culture, Jones and Ryaby used 300-G Sm_2Co_{17} static magnetic fields to demonstrate a twofold increase in alkaline phosphatase compared to controls (15). They found 24-G fields even more effective than the stronger fields, suggesting further evidence of so-called biological windows. These fields decreased mitosis and lysosomal enzyme activity in addition to the increased alkaline phosphatase, as shown in Table 1. The doubling of alkaline phosphatase is consistent with an increase of osteogenesis even with a decrease of mitosis, suggesting a more efficient acceleration of osteogenesis. The lysosomal enzyme activity decrease is usually associated with a decreased rate of bone resorption. This is obviously not consistent with clinical findings, and it can therefore be concluded that the force perturbation cancels the effect of this enzyme.

In an in vivo investigation the following year (1988) DeMarco (16) used orthodontic bihelical springs (for conventional force) to expand the rat's cranial midsagittal sutures in the presence of implanted SM_2Co_{17} magnets over the springs, emitting a static field and dosed similarly to the Jones and Ryaby magnets at the target area (27 G). In the DeMarco investigation, the magnets provided a bioeffect field, but no force. Histomorphometric analysis by the U.S. Army Institute of Dental Research at Walter Reed Medical Center in

Table 1 Effect of Weak Constant Magnetic Fields on Osteoblastlike Cells in Culture

	Metabolic Parameters[a]		
	A	B	C
Control	0.73 ± 0.15	0.79 ± 0.17	0.17 ± 0.06
Magnetic field 1, average field 300 g	0.44 ± 0.13	1.49 ± 0.49	0.05 ± 0.02
Magnetic field 2, average field 24 g	0.39 ± 0.14	1.92 ± 0.7	0.05 ± 0.22

[a] Key: A = mg protein per culture well, B = Alkaline phosphatase activity (arbitary units per mg protein), C = relative activity of N-acetyl-glucosaminidase (NAG). Rabbit calvarial cells were exposed to the magnetic fields of samarium cobalt magnets for 5 days. Cellular protein and alkaline phosphatase were measured at the end of this period. NAG activity was measured in the medium. During this time the controls had increased cell numbers by 3.75 times, and both the magnetic-field-treated cells increased 3 times.
Source: Ref. 15.

Washington, D. C., demonstrated a twofold increase in bone volume in the rat's suture expanded in the presence of magnets, compared to two controls: one with sham magnets and the other with no magnets and both with bihelical springs for force. Expanding the rat's midsagittal sutures was similar to a routine orthodontic–orthopedic clinical procedure in which the midpalatal suture is expanded in patients with deficient transverse maxillary growth. To perform this procedure, a magnetic device exists to expand the maxillary palatal shelves.

Utilizing orthodontic open-circuit static magnetic fields, several different investigator have designed varied application configurations: static magnetic fields for molar distalization, as an aid in the eruption of canines, premolars, and molars, to protract mandibles, expand palatal sutures, apply torque, close extraction spaces, and close diastemas. They have all concluded that pain-free and mobility-free movement was possible. Kawata et al. reported their experience with magnetic force: "Treatment time was shorter, discomfort was eliminated, and orthodontic patients were free from periodontal disturbances, root resorption, and caries" (17). Graber reported that "the magnetic disimpaction of palataly malposed canine teeth with attractive forces resulted in more rapid disimpaction, better directional control, and reduced mobility, together with better control of the gingival margin" (18). Vardimon et al. used 20.3 to 50.9 g force (measured on the magnet surface) of attractive magnetic force to disimpact canines, premolars, and molars and commented, "at no time was there a complaint of pain, nor was there any noticeable mobility. This statement can be made for all teeth that we have erupted magnetically—canines, premolars, molars"(19). In a personal telephone communication, March 1997, Dr. Graber (editor-in-chief emeritus of the American Journal of Orthodontics and Cranio-facial Orthopedics) reported no iatrogenic effects when using magnetic forces. In particular, he noticed an absence of root resorption. Conceivably this desirable clinical finding could be attributable to an accelerated osteogenic rate.

Itoh et al. reporting on their experiences with repelling magnetic force for molar distalization in 1991, indicated that "there were no complaints of pain during tooth movement. It has been found that magnetic forces cause erythrocytes to become one third thinner and longer. Therefore, even if capillaries in the periodontal ligament of the root are compressed by the strong orthodontic forces, the blood flow will still be smooth" (20).

Finally, Blechman and Steger noted that magnetic forces generate "rapid tooth movement without the increased mobility or discomfort normally associated with conventional forces. Magnets also markedly decrease root resorption and alveolar osteopenia, and this was observed within the limits of clinical evidence" (21).

There were no reported cases of adverse side effects in any orthodontic investigations. When static magnetic fields with greater flux density was used to alleviate low back pain, occasionally patients reported warmth and/or erythema at the treatment site, an obvious increase in vascularity or vasodilation.

VI. NEW RESEARCH

New research begins with the relevant introduction of periodontal disease and ends with the pertinence of static magnetic fields to control tooth mobility and potential resultant atheromatous plaque inflammation.

Periodontal disease has been reported to lead to bacterial seeding of atheromatus plaques by periodontal pathogens, resulting from bacteremias. Many different nonperiodontal pathogens (e.g., Chlamydia) have been shown to leave their DNA in the plaques, including periodontal pathogens. As a result, atherosclerotic plaques have been shown to be inflammatory lesions, thereby explaining some of the benefits of aspirin that are used prophylactically, in addition to its antiplatelet activity.

Research has also shown that periodontal pathogens associated with periodontal disease have been found in atherosclerotic plaques. In their experiment, Haraszthy et al. showed that 44% of 50 atheromatous plaques studied were positive for at least one periodontal pathogen, either *Actinobacillus actinomycetemcomitans*, *Bacteroides forsythus*, *Porphyromonas gingivalis*, or *Prevotella intermedia*. Most specimens were found to be positive for more than one species (22). B. Chiu, in his research in 1999, was one of the first to have found two major odontopathogens, bacteria of the teeth and gums, *Porphyromonas gingivalis* and *Streptococcus sanguis*, in atherosclerotic plaques (23). Lastly in a study out of Boston University, Li et al. found that a long-term systemic challenge with *Porphyromonas gingivalis*, as would be seen in periodontal disease, can accelerate atherogenic plaque progression (24).

It is hypothesized that when conventional orthodontic biomechanical force is used for a standard full-term treatment (about 2 years) with the required monthly force reactivation in several different oral areas simultaneously, then a substantial bacteremia is potentially created. Conventional force modalities always cause mobility of the moving teeth that are painful and stimulate (pumping by chewing) the localized inflammation in the periodontal ligament that metastasizes the periodontal pathogens, thereby seeding the atheromatous plaques. The force combined with frequent poor oral hygiene in patients with orthodontic appliances can potentially aggravate the bacterial metastasis.

Literature research reports confirm bacteremias associated with the use of single orthodontic force procedures as well as DNA evidence of periodontal pathogens in atheromatous plaques. In their research, Erverdi et al. (25) found a 7.5% incidence of bacteremias following orthodontic banding and a 6.6% prevalence following band removal (26). In a separate investigation, McLaughlin et al. found a 10% incidence of bacteremias following orthodontic banding (27). Roberts et al. found a significant increase in the intensity of bacteremias following the insertion of an orthodontic separator (28). A study by Glurich et al. compared C-reactive protein (CRP) levels in patients with cardiovascular disease, periodontal disease, both diseases, and neither conditions. He found CRP levels in subjects with either condition alone were elevated twofold above subjects with neither disease, and a threefold increase in CRP in subjects with both diseases (29). Noack et al., in another study, indicated moderate elevation of CRP has been found to be a predictor of increased risk for cardiovascular disease and that elevated CRP levels in patients with periodontal disease has been commonly reported (30). His study supports this by finding statistically significant increases in CRP levels in subjects with periodontal disease as compared to healthy controls.

Finally, in a study by Slade et al., it is indicated that moderate elevation of C-reactive protein is a risk factor for cardiovascular disease among apparently healthy individuals. He also finds that people with extensive periodontal disease had an increase of approximately one third in mean CRP and a doubling in prevalence of elevated CRP compared with periodontally healthy people (31). Since atherosclerosis is now considered to be an inflammatory disease, CRP is now considered to be a more reliable indicator of this disease than cholesterol.

Since many orthodontic patients are adolescents, the question arises whether atherosclerosis is relevant at their age. Autopsies on young soldiers during the Korean War showed a high incidence, already at their age, of established atheromatous plaques.

Current research is focused on the tooth mobility discussed previously. Since this is a constant finding in conventional orthodontic therapy, mobility was hypothesized to be a constant source of bacteremia. If so, conventional force application may be considered a potential cardiovascular risk factor. Because atherosclerosis is now considered to be an inflammatory lesion, correlation with an increase in the mean level of high sensitivity C-reactive protein (over 3 mg/L) (hsCRP), synthesized in the liver, can be considered a significant indicator of periodontial pathogenic invasion of atheromatous plaque. Once this is established, the subsequent step requires magnetic force application, beause elimination of mobility may prevent bacteremias. This can be substantiated by a reduction in hsCRP.

REFERENCES

1. Bassett CAL, Pilla AA, Pawluk RJ. A nonsurgical salvage of surgically resistant pseudoarthroses and nonunions by pulsing electromagnetic fields. Clin Orthop 1977; 124:117–128.
2. Stark TM, Sinclair PM. Effect of pulsed electromagnetic fields on orthodontic tooth movement. Am J Orthod Dentofacial Orthop 1987; 91:91–104.
3. Darendeliler MA, Sinclair PM, Kusey RP. The effects of samarium cobalt magnets and pulsed electromagnetic fields on tooth movement. Am J Orthod Dentofacial Orthop 1995; 107:578–588.
4. Gromak GB, Leis GA. Evaluation of the efficient use of constant magnetic fields in traumatologic patients. Electromagnetic therapy in traumas and diseases of the support motor apparatus. Riga: RMI, 1987:88–95. in Russian.
5. Detlar IE, Blaus AP, Naudinja IJ, Tarauska AV. Magnetic therapy in the treatment of long tubular bone fractures and lengthening of extremities. Electromagnetic therapy in traumas and diseases of the support motor apparatus. Riga: RMA, 1987:110–123. in Russian.
6. Golyakhovsky V. Local and continuous exposure to a permanent magnetic field as a means of boosting repairative osteogenesis. Proceedings of the Kuybyshev Regional Conference on Magnetic Fields in the Clinic, June 1976. Translated from Russian.
7. Golyakhovsky V. Magnetotherapy as part of the treatment strategy for diaphyseal fractures of tubular bones. Proceeding of the Kuybyshev Regional Conference on Magnetic Fields in the Clinic, June 1976. Translated from Russian.
8. Holcomb RR, Parker RA, Harrison MS. Biomagnetics in the treatment of human pain: past, present, future. Environ Med 1991a; 8:24–30.
9. McLean MJ, Holcomb RR, Wamil AW, Pickett JD, Cavapol AV. Blockade of sensory neuron action potentials by a static magnetic field in the 10mT range. Bioelectromagnetics 1995; 16:20–32.
10. Cavapol AV, Wamil AW, Holcomb RR, McLean MJ. Measurement and analysis of static magnetic fields that block action potentials in cultured neurons. Bioelectromagnetics 1995; 16:197–206.
11. Blechman AM, Oz M, Nair V, Ting W. Discrepancy between claimed field flux density of some commercially available magnets and actual gaussmeter measurements. Alternative Therapies 5 Sept/Oct 2001; 7.
12. Blechman AM, Smiley H. Magnetic force in orthodontics. Am J Orthod 1978; 74:435–443.
13. Blechman AM, Alexander C. New miniaturized magnets for molar distalization. Clinical Impressions, Ormco Corp 1995;4(4):14–19.
14. Rare-earth permanent magnets. Vacodym, Vacomax. Edition 2000. Vacuumschmelze GMBH, Hanau, Germany.
15. Jones DB, Ryaby JT. Low energy time—varying electromagnetic field interactions with cellular control mechanisms. In: Blank M, Findl E, eds. Mechanistic approaches to interactions of electric and electromagnetic fields with living systems. London: Plenum Press, 1987:389–397.
16. DeMarco LA. Comparative histologic response of osteogenic capacity of the cranial sagittal suture of Sprague–Dawley rats to tensile orthopedic force applied in a local magnetic field of varying orientations. A research report submitted in partial fulfillment for the requirement for

clinical certification. Dept of Orthodontics, University of Maryland Dental School, Baltimore, MD, June 1988.

17. Kawata T, Hirota K, Sumitomi K, Umehara K, Yano K, Toping HJ. A new orthodontic force system of magnetic brackets. Am J Orthod Dentofacial Orthop 1987; 92:241–248.

18. Graber TM. Magnets and impacted canines. Northcroft Memorial Lecture. British Society for the Study of Orthodontics. Manchester, UK, September 4, 1989.

19. Vardimon AD, Graber TM, Drescher D, Bourauel C. Rare—earth magnets and impaction. Am J Orthod Dentofacial Orthop 1991; 100:494–512.

20. Itoh T, Tokuda T, Kiyosue S, Hirose T, Matsumoto M, Chaconas SJ. Molar distalization with repelling magnets. J Clin Orthod 1991; 25:611–617.

21. Blechman AM, Steger ER. A possible mechanism of action of repelling molar distalizing magnets. Part I. Am J Orthod Dentofacial Orthop 1995; 108:428–431.

22. Haraszthy VI, Zambon JJ, Trevisan M, Zeid M, Genco RJ. Identification of periodontal pathogens in atheromatous plaques. J Periodontol 2000; 71(10):1554–1560.

23. Chiu B. Multiple infections in carotid atherosclerotic plaques. Am Heart J 1999; 138(5):s534–s536.

24. Li L, Messas E, Batista EL Jr, Levine RA, Amar A. Porphymonas gingivalis infection accelerates the progression of atherosclerosis in a heterozygous apolipoprotein E-deficient murine model. Circulation 2002; 105(7):861–867.

25. Ervedi N, Kadir T, Ozkan H, Acar A. Investigation of bacteremia after orthodontic banding. Am J Orthod Dentofacial Orthop 1999; 116(6):687–690.

26. Erverdi N, Biren S, Kadir T, Acar A. Investigation of bacteremias following debanding. Angle Orthod 200; 70(1):11–14. Discussion 15.

27. McLaughlin JO, Coulter WA, Coffey A, Burden DJ. The incidence of bacteremia after orthodontic banding. Am J Orthod Dentfacial Orthop 1996; 109(6):639–644.

28. Roberts GJ, Lucas VS, Omar J. Bacterial endocarditis and orthodontics. J R Coll Surg Edinb 2000; 45(3):141–145.

29. Glurich I, Grossi S, Albini B, Ho A, Shah R, Zeid M, Baumann H, Genco RJ, De Nardin E. Systemic inflammation in cardiovascular and periodontal disease: comparative study. Clin Diagn Lab Immunol 2002; 9(2):425–432.

30. Noack B, Genco RJ, Trevisan M, Grossi S, Zambon JJ, De Nardin E. Periodontal infections contribute to elevated systemic C—reactive protein level. J Periodontol 2001; 72(9):1221–1227.

31. Slade GD, Offenbacher S, Beck JD, Heiss G, Pankow JS. Acute-phase inflammatory response to periodontal disease in the U.S. population. J Dent Res 2000; 79(1):49–57.

50

Concluding Comments: Some Late Breaking Developments and Future Directions

Paul J. Rosch

The American Institute of Stress, Yonkers, and New York Medical College, Valhalla, New York, U.S.A.

Marko S. Markov

Research International, Buffalo, New York, U.S.A.

As indicated in the Preface, the timetable for receipt and review of manuscripts and returning them to authors for suggested revisions was unusually short and had to be rigidly adhered to so that final approval of all chapters could be completed by January 15, 2003. One of the incentives to participate in this work was the promise of exceptionally prompt publication and since a chain is only as strong as its weakest link, it was necessary to strictly enforce this accelerated schedule. This goal was particularly difficult to achieve since our initial outline only provided for up to 30 chapters, and we had received over fifty. As a result, several worthwhile contributions could not be included. In addition, advances were occurring so rapidly in this field that time constraints precluded obtaining chapters on late breaking developments. Nevertheless, we were able to include some, such as radio-frequency nucleoplasty for low back pain due to degenerative disk disease and transcranial magnetic stimulation (rTMS) for tinnitus. It seemed advisable to use this concluding chapter to describe additional approaches that have obtained FDA approval and others that might have merit in an effort to make this presentation as comprehensive and current as possible. In that regard, it should be noted that an interdisciplinary team at NIH has invented a new transcranial magnetic stimulation coil that can stimulate neurons deep within the brain without causing the seizures or tissue damage that limit the use of high intensity TMS fields from conventional coils. Researchers believe this opens up the possibility of numerous applications ranging from Parkinson's disease to energizing the brain's "pleasure center".

I. MAGNETIC GUIDANCE SYSTEMS FOR CARDIAC ARRHYTHMIAS, CEREBRAL ANEURYSMS, AND INOPERABLE BRAIN LESIONS

Magnetic guidance systems have been approved by the FDA to diagnose and treat abnormal cardiac rhythms that are potentially lethal and/or unresponsive to drugs. This requires mapping the heart's electrical system to pinpoint the source of the disturbance by threading a catheter about the size of a piece of spaghetti through a vessel in the groin up to the heart. A wire in the catheter allows the physician to physically twist or turn the catheter using X-rays to determine its precise position and, on occasion, rotating the entire catheter to reorient it before attempting to advance it any further. These manual adjustments are not efficient since twists initiated outside the body near the groin produce much smaller movements at the wire tip several inches away. In addition, after multiple manipulations the wire often becomes kinked and less responsive, and there is always the danger of damaging or puncturing a vessel. These problems have been obviated with a new magnetic guidance system that uses a catheter containing a magnet in its tip. Computer-generated electromagnetic fields are used to direct the catheter to advance in any direction. Commands for each desired direction or movement are "drawn" on a specially designed pen-tablet or by using a three-dimensional computer software interface, with the commands overlaid onto the patient's constantly updated x-rays. A guidewire with a magnetic tip similar to the magnetic catheter, but about the size of a piece of string allows surgeons to position it at any site to localize the focus of irritability so that it can subsequently be destroyed by radiofrequency generated heat, thus avoiding open heart surgery. After a successful radiofrequency ablation procedure, patients are discharged from the hospital the same or the next day and can usually resume normal work and physical activity without any restrictions. Over 200,000 such procedures were performed last year.

A similar approach is being used to treat cerebral artery aneurysms and other brain lesions. Using catheters with guidewires to deliver material to correct an aneurysm is not new but even skilled operators have difficulty because the torque or the ability to turn the guidewire by physical means is limited. In addition to being time consuming, there is always the potential for perforation of an artery. As noted above, a guidewire with a magnetic tip can now snake through tight turns in cranial blood vessels using a computerized road map to allow it to reach an aneurysm. Every second or two, a fluoroscope takes x-rays in two planes of the patient's head. Metal markers show up on the images, which when superimposed, mark the guidewire's position on magnetic resonance images in a computer console. The contours of the magnetic field are determined by the current flow to each of six super-conducting magnets in a helmet-like device that surrounds the head. Altering the contours changes the direction in which the guide wire or magnet tipped catheter moves. Doctors can sit in an x-ray protected control room without wearing a lead apron and steer the magnetized guidewire using a modified joystick. The doctor's commands are interpreted by the computer system, and magnetic fields are applied that enable the operator to move it in any direction, including backward or in a complete circle, until the aneurysm is reached. A catheter is then advanced over the guidewire so that embolizing agents can be deposited in the aneurysm to prevent it from rupturing.

This approach is also being used to treat deep brain lesions that cannot be operated on, as illustrated by the following two cases. A middle-aged roofer who suddenly developed double vision and dizziness whenever he looked down was found to have a fistulous mass of malformed blood vessels that were swelling and putting pressure on crucial sites. Neuro-surgeons were able to snake a catheter with repair glue to the spot but the fistula was too deep and twisted to manually push the catheter to its origin. While there was some initial improvement, the symptoms and swelling returned. The procedure was repeated using a magnet tipped guidewire in accordance with the protocol used for treating aneurysms. This time the wire successfully pulled a catheter to the fistula's core, providing a tunnel through which to squirt healing glue. The three-hour procedure was a success with steady improve-ment being reported over the next weeks and months. A 66-year-old woman who had suffered from seizures for eight years due to blood vessel abnormalities deep in her brain had became severely depressed because she had failed to respond to medications, was unable to drive and was afraid to be alone. A surgical procedure was attempted but it was not possible to reach and repair the abnormal vessels responsible for her seizures. She subsequently underwent a similar magnetic guided procedure with gratifying results. Investigations are under way to see if this approach could also be helpful to treat Parkinson's disease and inoperable brain tumors.

II. RADIOFREQUENCY ABLATION FOR PRIMARY AND METASTATIC MALIGNANCIES, ENDOMETRIOSIS, FIBROIDS, SNORING, AND GASTROESOPHAGEAL REFLUX

Radiofrequency ablation of malignancies is accomplished by inserting a needle under the guidance of computed tomography or ultrasound directly into the tumor. A radiofrequency signal is then sent through the needle that generates heat to destroy malignant tissue. This approach has been used in Europe for decades and has been covered by most insurance companies in the U.S. since its approval by the FDA for primary and metastatic liver malignancies. Radiofrequency ablation of primary and metastatic lung cancers is increasingly being used for tumors that cannot be removed surgically and for metastatic bone disease, where it has proven very effective in reducing pain. The procedure has also been used to treat adrenal and retroperitoneal malignancies such as sarcoma. Some patients can go home the same day and return to normal activities within 48 hours, but most are hospitalized overnight for observation. Doctors recently reported success in treating kidney cancers using radiofrequency ablation. It was initially tried on patients who were not good candidates for surgery but has been so successful that this is no longer a prerequisite. Tumors under 3 cm in diameter located on the surface of the kidney are the most responsive and no recurrences have been reported to date. The procedure does not require general anesthesia, takes about two hours depending on the tumor's size and location and is usually performed on an outpatient basis. Many patients resume normal activities the next day, in contrast to conventional surgery that often necessitates a lengthy hospital stay, weeks of recuperation, and is much more costly. A new variation on this was just reported from Rhode Island Hospital in which a combination therapy was used to treat an inoperable lung malignancy that had recurred despite chemotherapy and radiation. Guided by CT scanning, doctors placed an electrode in the malignancy to deliver radiofrequency heat and then placed a catheter into the tumor to allow high doses of brachtherapy, a form of radiation that uses a very intense local radiation source. This innovative combination of powerful focal radiation and heat was able to successfully destroy the tumor without significantly damaging normal adjacent tissue.

In addition to malignancies, radiofrequency ablation has been approved by the FDA for the treatment of excessive menstrual bleeding, a leading indication for hysterectomy. Precisely measured radiofrequency energy is delivered via a slender, hand-held catheter to remove the endometrial lining of the uterus in women for whom childbearing is complete. The procedure takes approximately 90 seconds, which is significantly shorter than with any other endometrial ablation treatment. Fibroid tumors of the uterus are being treated laparoscopically with two small abdominal incisions that allow the needle electrode to be inserted into the tumor. A recent report on 79 women with symptomatic or enlarging fibroids, most of whom had been advised to have surgery, revealed a 100% success rate, even with tumors as large as 11 cm in diameter. The average patient returned to work in three days.

Radiofrequency ablation of obstructive tissue has been shown to be effective in stopping snoring in most patients with this problem. It has also proved successful in relieving gastroesophageal reflux by creating scar tissue within the muscular layer surrounding the lower esophageal sphincter. Double blind studies with sham treatment that led to FDA approval showed increases in lower esophageal sphincter pressures and improvement in post treatment 24-hour pH monitoring following radiofrequency therapy. Long-term follow-up has confirmed that most patients were able to doscontinue antisecretory drugs, and the remainder reported a marked reduction in their use.

III. PORTABLE DEFIBRILLATORS TO USE AT HOME OR ANYWHERE

More people die from sudden cardiac arrest due to ventricular fibrillation each year than from breast cancer, prostate cancer, AIDS, handguns, house fires, and traffic accidents, combined. It is important to emphasize that most victims have had no previous symptoms or signs of heart disease and are generally in good health. Over 70% of sudden cardiac arrests occur in the home and fewer than 5% of victims survive, largely because they are not defibrillated soon enough. For every minute that goes by without defibrillation, there is a 10% decrease in the likelihood of survival, and the average response time for emergency medical services in a typical community is 6 minutes. The prognosis is good for those who are resuscitated by defibrillation with an 80% one-year survival rate and 57% after five years. Resuscitation is rarely successful after ten minutes have elapsed.

Since the vast majority of sudden cardiac arrests occur at home and places where they are witnessed by others, having a defibrillator readily available that anyone can immediately use would save numerous lives. The American Heart Association has estimated that 50,000 more lives could be saved annually if every community could achieve a 20% cardiac arrest survival rate. New portable defibrillators about the size of a laptop computer have been described as "idiot proof". When placed on the chest, the device automatically analyzes the electrocardiogram and literally talks you through the process of administering shocks to the victim. It is impossible for the operator to increase the voltage sent through the pads on the patient's chest since this is determined by the computerized device and a single shock is usually successful. It may cause the patient to jump a little but not in the exaggerated way portrayed on television. Two studies reported in *The New England Journal of Medicine* confirmed the effectiveness of portable defibrillators in saving lives in airplanes and in a Las Vegas casino. A rule adopted by the Federal Aviation Administration has given airlines three years to train flight attendants and put defibrillators on all planes that carry at least 30 passengers and one attendant. American Airlines already has defibrillators on all its flights, and most other airlines in the United States and abroad have started to include them.

There is also a move on to make these devices available in large office buildings and public places like sports stadiums, train and ferry terminals, airports, amusement parks, health clubs, community and senior citizen centers, and shopping malls. Insuring that qualified personnel know how to use them properly takes an hour or so and when a training course was given to sixth graders, it only took them 20 seconds more to learn what was required compared to adults, so you don't have to be a rocket scientist. Most portable defibrillators weigh four to seven pounds and cost $2,500 to $4,000 and soon may be as common as fire extinguishers in office buildings, schools, and shopping malls. In fact, facilities have already been sued for not having one. The CVS drugstore chain offers defibrillators on its web site by prescription for about $3,000 for people at risk of cardiac arrest, but it is not clear if this will be reimbursed by insurance companies. In contrast, implantable defibrillators for high-risk patients that are approved by Medicare and other fiscal intermediaries are estimated to cost $40,000 to $50,000 per patient.

In one compelling illustration, a 72-year-old man suddenly slumped to the ground at Chicago's O'Hare International Airport on August 20, 1999. A woman who had been making a phone call nearby witnessed the event and ran to help him, finding that he was unconscious but had no detectable pulse. She immediately retrieved an automated defibrillator that was clearly displayed on a nearby wall, followed the instructions, and administered a single shock that resuscitated him. He had suffered a cardiac arrest due to ventricular fibrillation and still talks about that fateful day. Ironically, he was the Chicago Department of Aviation employee in charge of the public access defibrillator program at the city's two airports. Since then, there has been at least one "save" almost weekly using one of the 42 portable defibrillators, spaced approximately one minute apart at O'Hare, which, by coincidence, was the first public place nationwide to make defibrillators readily accessible to the public.

IV. FUNCTIONAL ELECTRICAL STIMULATION FOR CHRONIC HEART FAILURE

Functional electrical stimulation of the legs can enhance the muscle performance and exercise capacity of patients with chronic heart failure. Current guidelines recommend regular exercise for heart failure, but many patients are unable to comply with this because of other problems or limited functional capacity that makes it difficult for them to walk or bicycle for any extended period of time. Functional electrical stimulation can achieve the same benefits as exercise, according to an article in the May 2003 issue of the *European Heart Journal*. Researchers studied 46 patients with stable heart failure who were randomized to participate in a training program that involved stationary bicycling or functional electrical stimulation of the quadriceps and gastrocnemius muscles. Evaluation after six weeks revealed similar significant improvements in 6-minute treadmill walk exercise time as well as maximum leg strength and quadriceps fatigue index testing. Both approaches were also associated with similar improvements in quality-of-life measurements.

V. IMPLANTS TO PREVENT PANIC ATTACKS, SEIZURES, AND HEADACHES?

Most people experience anxiety in certain situations but those suffering from severe anxiety disorders can feel so anxious all the time that they are afraid to leave their house. Others have incapacitating attacks that occur spontaneously that are not prevented by medications that often have debilitating side effects. A novel brain pacemaker approach based on vagal nerve stimulation now promises to provide relief. As noted elsewhere in this book, vagal nerve stimulation has received FDA approval for the treatment of epilepsy and may be effective in certain types of depression and obesity. Pilot clinical trials now suggest that it may be beneficial for certain patients suffering from severe anxiety. Anxiety is associated with a rapid heart rate, and, in some instances, awareness of a rapid heart rate or palpitations can increase anxious feelings. In others, concerns about developing palpitations while driving or during some important presentation can precipitate an anxiety attack. Stimulation of the vagus nerve lowers the heart rate. The procedure involves implanting a pacemaker device in the chest that has wires attached to the vagus nerve in the neck. An electrical signal is sent to the vagus nerve every five minutes to help slow the heart rate and reduce anxiety. One subject who improved remarkably after the procedure said that just knowing the pacemaker was there gave her a sense of control that helped to prevent attacks and reduce her general level of anxiety.

A cardiac pacemaker that also responds to mental demands and emotional stress was recently implanted in an 81-year-old woman who often suffered disabling palpitations when she became excited. Traditional pacemakers are activated only when patients are in motion or there is a change in respiratory rate. The Protos device, recently approved by the FDA, acts more like the sinoatrial node, the heart's natural pacemaker, in that it is also sensitive to autonomic nervous system demands. Signals received directly from the surface of the heart allow it to respond to faster heart rates due to excitement and emotional stress in a manner that mimics the natural rhythm changes of healthy hearts. A built-in microprocessor will allow new features to be installed by upgrading the software.

A brain pacemaker to prevent seizures is also in the works. It was formerly believed that most epileptic seizures come on abruptly with no prior warning signs since standard EEG monitoring of epileptic patients admitted for neurosurgery to remove the focus of irritability has generally failed to demonstrate any antecedent abnormalities. However, when these same EEG recordings were scrutinized using methods derived from chaos theory, certain patterns started to emerge. Most seizures actually start with a tiny spark of activity and can take hours to build up to a surge that is finally discharged. Researchers found that they could predict more than 80 percent of seizures by analyzing them with a computer program and detecting tell tale changes that usually occurred more than an hour before a convulsion. Efforts are now under way to develop a small, implantable computerized device that can predict seizures and abort them with jolts of electricity or tiny squirts of medication directly into the site of increased irritability.

It is estimated that 20 million Americans suffer from severe headaches and 2 million have intractable head or facial pain that does not respond to drugs. Electrodes implanted along the spinal cord have long been used to block pain signals coming from the back or extremities because they could be placed above the site of the problem. Although this is not possible for pain originating in the head, it has been found that stimulating nerves at subcutaneous levels rather than where they enter the spinal cord can provide similar benefits. The procedure has been found to be effective in whiplash-like back of the head pain by targeting the occipital nerve. More recently, it has shown promising if not dramatic results in other types of severe facial pain. One patient had suffered from constant incapacitating headaches for two years. Drugs, including heavy-duty narcotics, failed to prevent the excruciating jolts of pain that could be triggered by the slight touch of wind blowing against her forehead. Resection of the nerve was considered, but in a last-ditch experiment, a tiny electrode was attached to a needle and tunneled under the skin near her left eye to reach the nerve. Her pain disappeared immediately when the electrode was stimulated by a small jolt of electricity. It was then connected to a tiny battery implanted near her collarbone that continually zaps the nerve with weak electric pulses. A magnet can be used to turn the current on and off. Although the pain recurs when the current is turned off, this is necessary in order to pass through certain security devices, such as those in airports. Two implants are needed if pain is on both sides of the head. While still experimental, the procedure has been successful in another patient with intractable headache following brain surgery. A neurosurgeon who has implanted stimulators in the foreheads of four patients is enthusiastic about the results since the first two treated in this fashion have been pain free for over two years.

VI. ELECTROSTATIC FIELDS TO PREVENT HAIR LOSS?

Treating or reducing baldness is a $7 billion-a-year industry, which explains why there are a plethora of products to promote hair growth advertised on TV and in print media. Most are worthless and based on testimonials rather than scientific studies, and there are only two FDA approved products. A Canadian company would like to change this with their electrical stimulation device that they claim is 96% effective in preventing hair loss and/or promoting hair growth and is being administered at 30 treatment centers in 10 countries. Treatment involves sitting in an ergonomically designed chair with a semi-spherical hood containing electrodes positioned over the affected area of the scalp. A low-frequency, low-intensity electrostatic pulse generated in the hood is used to stimulate the scalp without any direct contact, so that tissue penetration is minimal. The 12-minute treatment is administered twice a week, and positive results are usually seen within three to six months. Treatment must be continued on a weekly basis thereafter to prevent shedding the new hair and costs around $50/session. The mechanism of action is not clear, but researchers suspect that dormant hair follicles may be stimulated by the specific current levels and wave characteristics created by the low-level electrostatic field. The electromagnetic fields already approved to promote bone healing and soft tissue repair have very different characteristics. The procedure has been shown to be completely safe in scientific studies, and, although not approved in the U.S., it is available in Canada and Mexico. A New Zealand study published in a peer-reviewed journal recently reported that the treatment was successful in reducing hair loss in women undergoing chemotherapy.

VII. AN "ENERGY" MAT AND VIBRATING PLATFORMS TO PREVENT OSTEOPOROSIS?

A sleeping mat that allegedly creates a "natural energy field" is being tested to determine if it can prevent osteoporosis in postmenopausal women. The mat, which is as thin as a light blanket, is composed of hundreds of interspersed layers of aluminum and polyester and is placed under the bottom sheet. A six-month clinical trial on 70 postmenopausal women is in progress to determine whether sleeping on the mat causes the layers to move against each other to create a "natural energy" field that will stimulate cellular activities to help prevent or treat osteoporosis. Blood samples will be taken periodically to test for biochemical markers of bone formation and breakdown as well as immune system function parameters. The mat was developed based on geophysical research designed to detect new deposits of oil and natural gas that provided coincidental data indicating that such an approach could promote bone growth and stimulate immune system function. It has long been known that bones in casts or in weightless situations like space travel that are not subjected to pressure tend to atrophy. Conversely, physical activity like jogging increases the density of weight bearing bones. However, the predominant skeletal stimulus while awake is not running a 100-yard dash a dozen times a day but weight bearing from standing and sitting that produces high-frequency, low-magnitude energy signals. Weak electromagnetic stimulation is routinely used to heal bone fractures that have failed to unite after years of non-union, and has also been reported to benefit osteoporosis. In both instances the stimulus comes from a piezoelectric signal that is generated when bone is subjected to a load. Because this is diminished in space travel and can pose a significant problem in extended flights, astronauts routinely perform special exercises to in an effort to reduce bone loss. A platform that vibrates at 90 Hz/second with each brief oscillation imparting an acceleration equivalent to one-third of Earth's gravity is now being tested. The vibration is so slight that it cannot be seen, although it can be detected if you touch it with your finger. Nevertheless, these subtle vibrations have had a profound effect on preventing bone loss in turkeys, sheep, and rats. Positive results have also been demonstrated in postmenopausal females with osteoporosis due to estrogen deficiency and children with cerebral palsy who have bone loss due to lack of physical activity. Astronauts might obtain similar benefits by standing on lightly vibrating plates for 10 to 20 minutes a day. The plates are attached to their feet with elastic straps to allow them to work on other tasks while receiving the vibrating stimuli.

It is believed that periodic changes in position when sleeping on the mat causes the layers of aluminum and polyester to rub together and produce a similar weak energy field. In addition, the mat can act like a capacitor that also collects energy that is emitted when stimulated by pressure. Anecdotal evidence obtained in a pilot study of the mat provided support for this hypothesis, and the current trial is designed to confirm these observations by demonstrating changes that are based on more objective and scientific parameters. This product should not be confused with mats containing permanent magnets that make similar claims and are particularly popular in patients complaining of pain due to arthritis and fibromyalgia.

VIII. LIGHT THERAPY FOR SURGERY, ACNE, PSORIASIS, DEPRESSION, DIABETIC AND VENOUS ULCERATIONS, CARPAL TUNNEL SYNDROME, AND MUSCLE PAIN

Although light is part of the electromagnetic spectrum, it would have been almost impossible to thoroughly discuss its numerous therapeutic applications in this volume. Visible and infrared light particularly have been shown to have a variety of effects, including: promoting the formation of new capillaries to increase blood flow and accelerate healing, stimulating collagen production to repair damaged tissue, increasing the production of adenosine triphosphate (ATP—the major source of energy for all cells), enhancing the activities of the lymphatic system to reduce edema, increasing the synthesis of RNA and DNA to rapidly replace damaged cells, stimulating fibroblastic activity to help repair connective tissue injury, increasing phagocytosis to facilitate scavenging and ingesting dead cells, and stimulating acetylcholine release, which lowers heart rate. Exposure to ultraviolet light has been shown to be effective in treating depression due to seasonal affective disorder (SAD syndrome) and is also used to treat psoriasis and other skin disorders.

Lasers have long been used for medical purposes in Europe, and Dr. Markov reviewed these in a book he wrote over two decades ago in Bulgaria (*The Laser's Profession*). Lasers have now become particularly popular here and can be classified as being either "hot" or "cold", depending on the amount of peak power they deliver. "Hot" lasers that emit up to thousands of watts are used in surgical procedures since they make an incision that is very clean with little or no bleeding because the laser cauterizes the incision as it cuts. They are also used in operations that require the removal of diseased tissue without causing damage to surrounding healthy tissue. "Cold" lasers produce a lower average power of 100 milliwatts or less, usually in a pulsating fashion. The light is turned on for only a fraction of a second and then off to deliver a certain number of pulses/second. Laser light is either visible as in red laser pointers or infrared and invisible. Most therapeutic lasers operate at 904 nm, which is in the infrared range. Light emitting diodes (LED) devices are another form of light therapy similar to lasers but differ since most emit a pulse that alternates between being on and off at 0.5-second intervals rather than nanosecond bursts at 1 cycle per second.

They are available in combinations that range from 660 nm (visible red light) to 830 nm to 930 nm (infrared range). L.E.D's are on and off 50% of the time regardless of the frequency setting for pulses/second and are not powerful enough to damage tissue, but they can stimulate the body's innate repair mechanisms. Many consider them safer than lasers since they are less likely to cause accidental eye injury.

Infrared light has been used to treat sun-damaged skin, muscle pain, and acne. Allegedly, a man watching television began pressing his remote control to his sore neck and found that the pain began to disappear. The FDA has now approved such devices for treating carpal tunnel, hand, wrist, and other muscle or tendon pains. Almost a third of all dermatologist visits are for acne-related causes, and about 1.5 billion is spend annually on anti-acne medications and treatment. Some of these are associated with severe side effects, and over 40% of the bacteria that cause acne are resistant to antibiotics. The FDA has now approved a high-intensity narrow band light source (405–420 nm) that triggers the release of chemicals that destroy these bacteria without any side effects. Treatment consists of two fifteen-minute sessions a week for four weeks. An FDA approved 890-nm monochromatic infrared energy device has also been shown to heal venous stasis and diabetic ulcers, and scleroderma related lesions resistant to other therapies. In several cases, the healed wounds have not recurred during 1 to 2 years of follow-up evaluation without the need for additional therapy. Benefits are believed to be due to local increases in nitric oxide concentration, which, if shown to be true, suggests numerous other potential applications.

IX. PERMANENT MAGNETS, BLOOD FLOW, PLANTAR FASCIITIS, DIABETIC NEUROPATHY, AND PELVIC PAIN

Although there are numerous anecdotal reports of the ability of permanent magnets to reduce pain, inflammation, and edema and relieve a variety of other complaints, most scientists remain skeptical. Placebo effects are hard to rule out in double-blind studies because any curious subject can quickly determine whether the product is real or a sham. A magnetic field cannot have biological effects unless there is motion in the field. Unlike electromagnetic fields, which are always fluctuating, permanent magnet fields are static and motionless. In addition, no plausible mechanism of action has been presented and some that have been proposed, such as effects on iron in the hemoglobin of circulating red cells are inane. Other claims that the application of different poles or bipolar applications in a checkerboard or concentric ring configuration produce different or superior biological effects have not been proven. Many believe that permanent magnets increase the flow of blood since they experience a sense of warmth at the site of application but again there are few scientific studies to support this. However, a study presented at an April 11–15, 2003 Experimental Biology meeting sponsored by the American Physiologic Society does suggest that permanent magnet fields can affect microvascular tone in skeletal muscle. Researchers reasoned that local blood flow was directly related to blood vessel diameter based on changes in flow resistance and investigated this in the microvasculature of skeletal muscle. Changes were demonstrated following the application of a static magnetic field but they were not consistent. Microvessels that were initially dilated responded by constricting and those that were constricted became more dilated. The degree of responsivity was related to the initial size or diameter of the vessel. The significance of this biphasic response is not clear but suggests that it may be designed to restore homeostasis. No direct measurements of blood flow were made, and this study hardly proves that permanent magnets increase blood flow. Nevertheless, it does demonstrate that static magnetic fields can affect microvascular tone that could conceivably have such effects under certain circumstances.

Plantar fasciitis is a common condition that is manifested by heel pain, especially in the early morning that increases with standing or exercise. It tends to occur more often in females, people who are overweight, older than 40, or who spend long hours on their feet (especially joggers and runners), and is occasionally associated with heel spurs. Treatment usually consists of arch supports or cushioning devices and nonsteroidal anti-inflammatory drugs, but occasionally cortisone injections or surgery may be required. Magnetic insoles have been reported to provide relief but this is not supported by a Mayo Clinic randomized, placebo-controlled double-blind study reported in the September 17, 2003, issue of *The Journal of the American Medical Association*. Over 100 adults with plantar heel pain either wore magnets embedded in a cushioned shoe insole or the same insole with a sham magnet. At 8 weeks, 33% of the nonmagnetic group and 35% of the magnetic group reported being all or mostly better.

In contrast, the May 2003 issue of *Archives of Physical Medicine and Rehabilitation* reported on a randomized, placebo controlled study headed by Dr. Michael Weintraub conducted at 48 centers of the use of permanent magnet insoles in close to 400 patients suffering from symptomatic diabetic neuropathy. The researchers reported that there was statistically significant and in some instances dramatic reduction in burning, numbness and tingling, and exercise-induced foot pain. This represented a careful follow-up study on the effects of permanent magnetic insoles in diabetic neuropathy, which Weintraub had originally undertaken to prove that there were no benefits. Although the positive results cannot be explained, they are supported by changes in relevant objective parameters that warrant further exploration and confirmation to gain insights into possible mechanisms of action. Well-designed and executed studies such as this are rare, and permanent magnet manufacturers will likely try to capitalize on this by extrapolating the findings to provide a patina of scientific authority for other uses that are not warranted.

For example, a magnetic device was introduced in the U.K. the following month for the relief of menstrual and pelvic pain that apparently became an overnight sensation. According to press releases, "in clinical trials, 94% of the women who tried it experienced some relief from menstrual pain, 47% said it completely relieved pain, and 70% said they felt less irritable. The teardrop-shaped magnet, which is slightly larger than a 50p coin, is designed to be attached to clothing near the womb and lasts forever." The manufacturers claim "it reacts with the ions in the body and works by increasing the oxygen levels in the blood and blood flow to the body's tissues, which eases the contractions that cause the cramps." In most cases the results were immediate and heavy periods were also significantly reduced. As noted in the chapter on permanent magnets, University of Tennessee researchers who investigated the use of permanent magnets for chronic pelvic pain found no change until after three weeks, when 60 percent of the women with active magnets and 33 percent of those with identical placebo products reported less pain. The fact that over half of patients with dummy magnets had the same improvement demonstrates the importance of the placebo effect in pain studies. It is also necessary to reemphasize that true double-blind studies with permanent magnets are almost impossible to conduct in patients who are not under constant observation.

The U.K. device for pelvic pain is now being aggressively promoted in the U.S. The same company states it has "produced a powerful unit that is worn on a main artery. It enables your bloodstream to absorb the correct and balanced amount of natural magnetism. We believe, that in most cases, this enhances the body's own ability to improve its circulation. It will help the body naturally to decrease the level of toxins in the blood and increase oxygen levels, thus reinforcing the bodies own defense mechanism and promoting physical health." Benefits are claimed for a wide variety of disorders ranging from arthritis to circulatory disorders but there is little to back this up other than glowing testimonials. While such devices are generally harmless, they might delay seeking medical attention for disorders that could readily be diagnosed and treated more appropriately. The best advice still seems to be *caveat emptor* (as noted below in Dr. Markov's segment of this chapter, the use of static magnetic fields for the treatment of epilepsy is also being explored).

X. NONTHERMAL EFFECTS OF ELECTROMAGNETIC FIELDS

As noted in the Preface, we have refrained from commenting on the current debate concerning the potential harmful effects of exposure to high power lines and cell phones. However, many believe that important information has been deliberately suppressed by powerful political and financial vested interests. This is especially true for those groups and individuals who continue to deny that ELF and microwave radiation can have significant nonthermal biological consequences. Such interactions have been clearly demonstrated in research ranging from cognitive performance and polysomnography studies to effects on gene expression, enzyme activity, and blood brain barrier permeability. Some feel strongly that the significance of these observations has been consistently rejected or distorted in what is viewed as a well-orchestrated and financed concerted campaign by commercial interests here and abroad who have a lot at stake. If true, this could have significant public health ramifications that might not be detected for decades. In response to this threat, the International Commission For Electromagnetic Safety (ICEMS) was founded and registered in Italy in December 2002 as a not-for-profit organization. Its purpose is to promote research that will protect the public from any adverse effects of electromagnetic fields by developing strategies for the assessment, prevention, management, and communication of risk. These efforts will be guided by what has been referred to as the "precautionary principle". For further information, see www.icems.info.

The above has been an attempt to outline possible future applications of bioelectromagnetic approaches that could not be included elsewhere in this volume for various reasons. Reference has also been made to the current controversy concerning safety with respect to exposure to high power lines, cell phones, and other artificially generated electromagnetic fields from a clinician's viewpoint (PJR). Further discussion of thermal and nonthermal effects and clarification of other relevant issues from the perspective of a physicist (MSM) follows, as well as the latest developments he has gleaned from recent meetings.

XI. THERMAL VS. NONTHERMAL EFFECTS

As Dr. Rosch indicated, the debate over whether nonthermal electromagnetic fields can have biological effects has been discussed and debated by the Bioelectromagnetics community for decades. Scientists, especially physicists and chemists, emphasize that it is really impossible to have any biological effects if one calculates the energy of static magnetic fields and low-frequency magnetic fields. The famous "kT" problem is often a controversial subject. It is correct that from the point of view of equilibrium thermodynamics, the energy of even a 1 T magnetic field is smaller than the energy of a hydrogen bond. Nevertheless, the experimental data show that such effects exist and are manifested at different levels of structural organization of biological systems. Even in the case of static magnetic fields, when cells, tissues, or organisms are exposed to magnetic fields, relative movement is present if one considers dynamic cytoplasmic activities involving ion transport. Therefore, it is difficult to say if the effects are only magnetic field–dependent since induced electric fields should also be considered. On the other hand, one must not forget that most biological effects are nonlinear, and this can apply to their interactions with EMFs. In Chapter 1 of this book, Dr. Ross Adey explains the necessity of application of nonlinear thermodynamics and physics toward these interactions.

One should also consider the fact that most of applied low frequency fields possess one or another modulation and harmonics spectra which additionally complicate the search for and adequate mechanism or mechanisms.

XII. SPECIFIC ABSORPTION RATE (SAR)

SAR is intended to present a physical model and the means to computing the energy delivered to a specific physical or biological body. The guidelines of the International Commission of Non-Ionizing Protection (ICNIRP) emphasize the importance of the energetic characteristics of EMF such as SAR, current density, and power density. This approach is not accepted by experts from a number of countries, especially from Europe, who insist that the standards must be based on biological effects, not upon physical calculation. I have had the privilege of attending several meetings on "harmonization of standards". This program, initiated and funded by the World Health Organization, attempts to help scientists, economists, engineers, and regulatory officers in their efforts to minimize the unfavorable effects of exponentially growing EMF "pollutions", especially from cellular phone communications. It is nearly impossible to get conclusive results for the SAR at the brain level without having information for modulation of the signals during regular conversation. In order to clarify this, experiments with models and real living tissues must be conducted. If the conclusions are based upon biological responses, then thermal vs. nonthermal problems may be avoided.

The public interest—or more precisely the fears about the dangers associated with increasing use of cellular communications—must force scientific and regulatory entities to evaluate and more thoroughly regulate the increasing environmental pollution caused by hundreds and thousands of EMF signals. Mother Nature did not create defense mechanisms against such pollutants. Moreover, the increasing body of evidence that "biological windows" exist should be seriously considered. Such "windows of opportunity" are very successfully used in magnetic and electromagnetic field therapies. This is sometimes based upon systematic research but more often, selected magnetic/electromagnetic fields used for therapy are based upon the intuition of the inventor of the device and the medical staff. Why "selected"? Because these values of the physical characteristics of the MF/EMF correspond to the "windows of opportunities". Living systems are ready to detect, absorb, and utilize signals with specific characteristics, and remain "silent" or unresponsive for the rest of the amplitude and/or frequency spectrum.

While therapeutic applications of the MF/EMF are mostly executed and controlled by medical practitioners for different conditions, EMFs from cellular communications and power lines are uncontrollable. Therefore the "precautionary" principle should be applied in standardization and harmonization of permissible EMF levels from different sources that affect large groups of people who differ in age, gender, and race, as well as educational, socioeconomic, general health, and immune system status.

XIII. IT IS NOT ONLY THE AMPLITUDE BUT THE GRADIENT THAT IS IMPORTANT

Most experiments designed to elucidate biological responses to magnetic fields have traditionally strived for exposures that are as spatially homogeneous as possible. When using permanent magnets to generate fields, it is generally difficult to avoid significant gradients, particularly if the exposure volume is of comparable size to the magnets used and the magnets have to be in close proximity to the sample to counter the sharp drop-off in field strength with distance. The Neuromagnetics group at Vanderbilt University (Holcomb, McLean, and Engstrom) have used permanent magnets for magnetic field exposures, and results from their laboratory indicate that gradients may be a factor in the effects they see on action potentials in cultured neurons, neuronal cell survival, epilepsy, and myosin phosphorylation. Introducing magnetic field gradients generates several new exposure parameters to be controlled in experiments and therapeutic applications. For a macroscopic exposure volume, one must use distributions to describe fields and gradient properties, and independent control of the field variables requires more attention that the spatially uniform case. Novel exposure systems and substantial numerical work have allowed the Vanderbilt group to control field/gradient exposures and the myosin phosphorylation method developed by Markov. This assay has shown remarkable sensitivity to magnetic fields allowing the rate of myosin phosphorylation to be used as sensitive biological dosimeter for complex magnetic fields. This approach is of significant importance for 3-D mapping of the exposure volume to gauge the performance of therapeutic magnetic devices (such as MagnaBloc), which have magnetic fields with gradients perpendicular to the local field vector.

XIV. STATIC MAGNETIC FIELDS FOR THE TREATMENT OF EPILEPSY

Despite the introduction of nine new anti-epileptic drugs during the 1990s, a significant number of patients have chronic seizures that are inadequately treated by currently available modalities. This is a stimulus for the development of novel treatments, including time-varying transcranial magnetic fields to treat seizures in animals and man. Using an alternative field exposure paradigm, a team of scientists from Vanderbilt University, led by Dr. McLean, recently published a study examining the effects of a spatially inhomogeneous static magnetic field, alone and in combination with phenytoin on audiogenic seizures in mice. The origin of this work is an earlier report on how a permanent magnetic field device reversibly blocks action potentials in cultured sensory neurons. In the epilepsy study, the pretreatment with static magnetic fields reduced the incidence of seizure manifestations elicited with auditory stimulation. It was also shown that magnetic field pretreatment potentiates the efficacy of phenytoin, a commonly used anti-epileptic drug.

Three important observations are of clinical importance. First, significant field effects were observed for magnetic fields in the range 5–10 mT, but not at 10-fold lower levels. This suggested that there is a threshold for magnetic field–induced protection. The researchers proposed further experiments to evaluate the field dose-response characteristics in detail and determine the relative contribution of flux density and field gradients. Second, the magnetic field pretreatment shifted the phenytoin dose response curve: three-to four-fold lower concentrations were sufficient in experiments when fields and drugs were given in combination. This may be clinically relevant. Third, the results were strongly dependent on the source mice which were used in the study: later seizure stages (tonic hindlimb extension and death) were similarly affected by pre-exposure to magnetic fields, but the earlier stages (wild running, loss-or-righting, clonus) were only significantly impacted in DBA/2 mice from Charles River Laboratories (Wilmington, MA), while mice obtained from Jackson Laboratories (Bar Harbor, ME) did not respond to magnetic field stimulation. The strain variation could explain, in part, the variable clinical response to treatment with phenytoin.

XV. WATER, CELL CYCLE, INFLAMMATION, AND PAIN

It is said, "The new is well forgotten old". At the XXV Annual Meeting of the Bioelectromagnetic Society which took place in June 2003, Dr. Carlton Hazlewood brought the attention of the audience to the possibility of evaluating the role of water in magnetic fields that appear to provide pain relief. In 1976, it was discovered that the physical properties of the cellular water change depend on the specific phases of the cell cycle. Nuclear magnetic resonance studies showed that in HeLa cells, the relaxation times of water protons were minimum in S-phase and maximum in mitosis. Two decades later, a report was published demonstrating that for patients with various pain syndromes, changes in the cell cycle distribution of circulating T lymphocytes were observed in patients before and after analgesia was achieved.

The link between these two observations was a hypothesis proposing that the changes in the physical properties of water, as well as the changes in T cell distributions, are associated with pain relief. By analyzing different liquids easily obtained from human bodies, one may predict the possibility that a particular pathology can be altered by using magnetic fields. It is remarkable that in a chapter in this book Dr. Nindl and colleagues demonstrate that in order to provoke a response to magnetic field, T-lymphocytes must be "activated", i.e., be in a state out of equilibrium (see Chapter 25). Having in mind that most of diseases and pathologies involve inflammation processes, a possibility emerges that today magnetic resonance technique may be a predictor of the possibility for pain relief when magnetic field is applied and that this MRI data might be connected with the inflammation status of the patient.

XVI. LYMPHEDEMA AS A TARGET FOR ELECTROMAGNETIC THERAPY

EMF's possess promise for providing benefits in the treatment of lymphedema, an accumulation of protein-rich edema in interstitial spaces and tissues. It occurs most frequently as a consequence of lymphatic system dysfunction, but derangements of trans-capillary exchange may also be involved. Effective therapy depends on removal of excess tissue fluid and proteins and kick-starting and maintaining salvageable lymphatic function. Sustained lymphedema often progresses to tissue fibrosis, which makes therapy more difficult and paves the way for other complications.

In view of the numerous examples of EMF-related effects on blood vessels and the flow within them that have been described in this volume, it is tempting to consider that EMF's might be able to restore the ability of lymphatic vessels to promote lymph flow. In part this concept derives from the many similarities between lymphatic and vascular components and controls. The function of each relies on actions of smooth muscle in their walls regulated by both local and sympathetic electrical activities. Lymph circulation, from lymphatic capillaries though its return to the venous system, relies on passive and active changes of lymphatic vessel diameters and pressures. The amount of lymph flow depends on both the frequency and amplitude of these dynamic lymphatic vessel changes. From the point of view of possible EMF connections, the active process is the one of greater interest, since it depends on physiological modulations of lymphatic smooth muscle membrane potentials and ionic currents that result in periodic contraction and relaxation phases. Locally applied electrical stimuli alter calcium, chloride and other ionic currents that affect lymphatic contraction processes. Mechanistically these may be related to release of smooth muscle activating agents from sympathetic nerve terminals that act on lymphatic smooth muscle receptors and by altering interactions between fast sodium currents and L-type calcium currents. Also, applied electrical pulses elicit excitatory junction potentials, which can sum to produce contraction-inducing action potentials. Sympathetic chain stimulation increases the rate of lymphatic contraction which is known to increase lymphatic flow. Other direct actions of imposed local electrical currents are distinctly possible.

In addition to promotion of lymph flow via possible actions on lymphatic vessels, EMF-related effects on the interstitium can be considered, especially with respect to protein clearing, macrophage activation, and adjunctively if fibrosis has developed. Although substantial work has been done using EMF therapies for acute trauma-related edema, little work has been done on the more vexing problem of chronic lymphedema. As a consequence, direct evidence of EMF-related positive (or negative) effects on any aspect of lymphedema therapy is sparse. Preliminary research by Dr. Harvey Meyrovitz suggests that EMF therapy via pulsed radiofrequency signals at 27.12 MHz may be effective in reducing tissue hardness and limb volume in post-mastectomy arm lymphedema. Similar initial findings were found with low-level laser therapy. Application of high-voltage pulses to limbs of experimental animals suggests that excess protein can be cleared via accelerated lymphatic uptake.

Thus, EMF therapy can reduce acute edema, promote blood vessel vasomotion, and alter blood flow in ways that theoretically could benefit lymphedema conditions. It seems reasonable to at least consider that EMF-related effects may positively impact the lymphatic circulation and the lymphedema condition. It is this author's opinion that judicious experimental inquiries need to be now undertaken to investigate this possibility.

XVII. GENE TRANSFECTIONS INTO CELLULAR NUCLEUS

Chapters 40 and 41 in this book have discussed electroporation from the viewpoint of basic science and clinical applications. In June 2003, San Antonio hosted the third ELEC-TROMED conference. This relatively small (by the number of participants) meeting may soon be an historic event. Most of the presentations were oriented toward engineering and studying biological effects of very high amplitude (exceeding 50 kV/cm), very short (in nanosecond range) electric pulses. The fascination over controlling cellular function has reached a new height. It is known that appropriately selected parameters of electric pulses may cause reversible opening of biological membranes. The poration effect is reversible, and the cell survives this "electric shock" if the electric field is neither too high nor too long in duration. In electrochemotherapy, a chemotherapeutic drug is injected into the tumor, and then pulses (within microsecond range and amplitude on the order of 1 kV/cm) are applied to open the pathways and promote drug penetration through the cellular membrane.

Engineers and scientists from several laboratories followed the proposals of the team of Old Dominion University (Norfolk, VA) in improving the technology and applications of electrostimulation of cells. Pulse power technology is capable of delivering high-intensity pulses up to 300 kV/cm and with very short duration of nanoseconds. The original idea was: as the pulse duration decreases, there is a lower incidence of electric field interactions at the level of the cellular membrane and a higher incidence of interactions with intracellular structures. So far, animal studies of mouse fibrosarcoma tumors have shown reduced tumor growth and the possibility of inducing apoptosis. The reasonable question appeared: What is the target for these interactions? The team of Karl Schoenbach and Stephen Beebe suggested the cell nucleus and mitochondria are the most probable targets. Two opportunities exist: direct damaging effect of the pulse expressed on DNA damage (mainly p53 protein), and the possibility to deliver to the nucleus genes which may alter the functioning of the nucleus machinery. In addition, in conjunction with classical electroporation, ultrashort electric pulses could be used to modulate nuclear, mitochondrial, or other intracellular membranes to enhance the delivery of genes or drugs for therapeutic purposes.

XVIII. HYPERSENSITIVITY TO ELECTROMAGNETIC FIELDS

During the last decade, one problem has become discussed more and more frequently, namely: Are there individuals who are hypersensitive to electromagnetic fields? While mainstream medicine in the U.S. simply neglects the problem, governments, scientists, and the general public in Scandinavia and Europe pay serious attention to this possibility. It is not a new problem, and about two decades ago, Dr. Stanislav Szmigelski, one of the most prominent European electromagnetic researchers, wrote: "At about 1–2% of the world population are very sensitive to EMF, but they recall more than 50% of complains against EMF." At that time even the fear of power lines was not popular. Today, exponentially increasing usage of cellular communications, the necessity of building base stations in close proximity to urban areas, and negligence of the regulators who allow building of base stations, even in school yards, makes the problems of hypersensitive individuals even worse.

It is the duty of 21st century health care workers and officials to identify the specific symptoms and criteria which could classify individuals in this category, to search for means of their protection and help, and to press local governments to look for solutions. Yes, we live in an ocean of electromagnetic pollution. Yes, this pollution will increase if society does not react timely to the problem. What may be done for hypersensitive people? Probably nobody knows the exact answer to this question at present. It appears to us that leading scientific societies like Bioelectromagnetics Society (BEMS), the European Bioelectromagnetic Association (EBEA), and the Institute of Electronics and Electrical Engineering (IEEE) should apply more effort in studying the complexity of the problem, to create international programs for this evaluation. And the reasonable question arises: Who will fund this activity? We believe that this should go through W.H.O., the U.N., and the European Community.

XIX. OTHER ITEMS AND TOPICS OF INTEREST THAT COULD NOT BE INCLUDED

Space constraints preclude discussing other approved bioelectromagnetic therapies that are attracting increased attention, such as a report in the August 2003 *Journal of Reproductive Medicine* showing that pelvic pain due to spasm of the levator muscle can be relieved by vaginal electrical stimulation. Painful and unsightly varicose veins seem to respond to the minimally invasive VNUS Closure procedure. Radiofrequency waves are applied directly into the wall of the saphenous vein, which runs from the ankle to the groin. The resultant heat causes the vein to collapse, thus cutting off the blood supply to varicose veins so that they no longer bulge. The procedure has been successfully used in over 30,000 patients around the world but has only been available in the U.S. since 1999. A study reported in the August issue of the *Journal of Vascular Surgery* showed numerous advantages over current surgical vein stripping procedures. A pulsed radiofrequency signal (Diapulse) has been used to successfully treat the pain and swelling of ankle sprains in double-blind studies conducted in the U.S. and Canada.

We have also not been able to adequately address diagnostic techniques that attempt to display or measure "bioenergy fields"; Kirlian photography has long been used to demonstrate energy "auras" around the extremities and other parts of the body that are believed to correlate with health status. Konstantin Korotkoff's gas discharge visualization (GDV) technique now allegedly allows one to capture with a special camera bioenergies emanating to and from people, animals, and plants, and translate this into a computerized model that displays energy intensities and imbalances. The GDV camera may have diagnostic applications and has been approved by the Russian Ministry of Health.

At the VI International Congress of European Bioelectromagnetic Association (EBEA) that took place at November 2003 in Budapest, researchers from the University of Bristol, United Kingdom, presented physical and biophysical background of a new method for early detection of breast tumors: microwave diagnostics. The method is competing with the routine mammogram, ultrasound and MRI. The method is a non-ionizing, potentially low cost and more certain alternative. The main advantage is that it may be repeated frequently without having potential side-effects of existing diagnostics methods.

Bioelectromagnetic resonance therapy, which is popular in Europe, involves identifying unhealthy electromagnetic emanations via electrodes placed on the body. These are then transmitted to a computer where the frequencies are inverted and returned to the patient as a form of healing energy. There are a variety of such devices that are used for diagnostic and therapeutic purposes. Researchers at the Hippocampus Institute in Hungary have developed and patented a new technology for in vivo electro-physiological diagnosis called Functional Electrodynamical Testing. Their "Cerebellum Multifunction Medical Instrument" utilizes sophisticated software and complex ECG and EEG biofeedback monitoring for functional electro-diagnostic testing has apparently been approved by the Ministry of Health Care of the Russian Federation. They have also invented non-invasive bioresonance devices such as the Cell-Com Europe that deliver electromagnetic signals for therapeutic purposes based on this type of information.

Such bioenergy approaches are riding the crest of a tidal wave of interest in "alternative medicine," but their validity has not yet been proven. Some appear to be based on authentic research by qualified investigators, whereas others emanate from well-meaning zealots with no scientific background or entrepreneurs and charlatans who are motivated solely by profit. While it is often difficult to distinguish between all of these, we have tried to provide the tools that will allow readers of this book to separate the wheat from the chaff.

Index

Index was prepared by Publisher.